MAYO
HEALTHQUEST
Guide to Self-Care

Philip T. Hagen, M.D.
Editor-in-Chief

Mayo Clinic
Rochester, Minnesota

Mayo HealthQuest Guide to Self-Care provides reliable, practical, easy-to-understand information on issues relating to good health. Much of its information comes directly from the experience of Mayo's 1,600 physicians and research scientists. This book supplements the advice of your personal physician, whom you should consult for individual medical problems. *Mayo HealthQuest Guide to Self-Care* does not endorse any company or product.

Library of Congress Catalog Card Number 97-73045

ISBN 0-9627865-6-X

Printed in the United States of America

First Edition

1 2 3 4 5 6 7 8 9 10

Preface

Practicing preventive medicine at Mayo Clinic has made me aware of how broad self-care really is. To truly take care of yourself, you must pay attention to all of your needs—spiritual needs and needs for companionship, as well as physical and mental health needs.

In my experience, healthy people develop a collection of resources in their quest for good health. They include friends, professionals and health information materials. In addition, one of the most important resources for good health is learning how to listen to your body.

I hope you use the *Mayo HealthQuest Guide to Self-Care* as one important resource in a complete approach to caring for yourself.

How We Prepared This Book

In preparation for this book, we asked many people around the United States what health topics were important to them. Here's what they told us: Discuss the common problems, and do it simply in easy-to-understand language. Provide tips on prevention as well as self-care. Address important children's health concerns. And, finally, don't forget the workplace. Work is where many of us spend a third of our waking lives.

Those requests were a tall order, which we accepted as our challenge. We reviewed the top 200 reasons why adults and children go to the doctor. We also talked to nurses who respond to telephone calls from people with questions about health and illness. We consulted with health-care professionals, employers and managers of corporate health programs to learn what illnesses and injuries are important in the workplace.

Lastly, but importantly, we looked at health-care costs. We reviewed our experience at Mayo Clinic, which includes providing care annually for more than 400,000 patients and the 20,000 employees of the Mayo Foundation in Rochester, Minnesota; Scottsdale, Arizona; and Jacksonville, Florida.

Using all of this information, we focused our book on how to prevent illness, how to detect illness before it becomes a serious and costly problem and how to avoid an unnecessary trip to the clinic or emergency room.

How to Use This Book

In your quest to become healthy or stay healthy, please put this book to good use. The first time you pick it up, page through it. If you have time, first read the sections titled Staying Healthy and The Healthy Consumer. If you have one of the common conditions such as asthma or diabetes, read the Specific Conditions section. The self-care tips are designed to prevent complications of the condition or to minimize their effect on your life.

If you have questions about health issues and your work, turn to the Your Health and the Workplace section. We believe our approach to topics related to the workplace is unique and instructive.

Finally, when you have a specific symptom or concern, look it up in the Table of Contents or Index. You will almost always find information to guide you in caring for yourself. If you have any questions, suggestions or comments that will make future editions even better, please contact me at the following address:

Philip T. Hagen, M.D.
c/o HealthQuest
Mayo Clinic, Ce9
Rochester, MN 55905

Or send me an E-mail message at
HealthQuest@Mayo.edu.

Introduction

The *Mayo HealthQuest Guide to Self-Care* provides reliable, practical, easy-to-understand information on more than 150 common medical conditions and issues relating to good health.

No book can replace the advice of your physician or other health-care providers. Instead, our intent is to help you manage some common medical problems with techniques that can be performed safely at home or work to relieve your discomfort or resolve your problem. In some cases, this information may help you avoid a trip to the clinic or emergency room; in other cases, we let you know when you need to see a medical professional.

How the Book Is Organized

Each chapter in the *Mayo HealthQuest Guide to Self-Care* begins with a list of symptoms or a summary of the cause and extent of the condition or health topic. The list of symptoms is followed by self-care and prevention suggestions highlighted in yellow shading. Under the heading "Medical Help," you are advised when to see a physician or health-care provider and what kind of treatment you might expect. When there is special information for children, you'll see a "Kids' Care" heading. Finally, articles with bluish gray shading are short pieces with information on related medical topics.

Listed below are summaries of the eight sections that make up the *Mayo HealthQuest Guide to Self-Care.*

Urgent Care

Emergencies are rare and usually require the care of a medical professional. There are some things you can do before medical help arrives, however, to stabilize the person who is in the emergency situation and prepare him or her for treatment. The areas covered in this section include how to perform cardiopulmonary resuscitation (CPR), how to help someone who is choking and how to deal with the following situations: poisoning, bleeding, shock, allergic reactions, bites, burns, cold weather problems, cuts, eye injuries, food-borne illnesses, heat-related problems, poisonous plants, tooth problems and trauma. We encourage you to take a certified first-aid course to learn the lifesaving techniques.

General Symptoms

General symptoms are medical conditions that tend to affect your entire body rather than a specific body part or system. General symptoms might include fatigue, fever, dizziness, pain, sleeplessness, sweating and unexpected weight changes. In this section, we explain the common causes for each of these seven general symptoms. We also provide self-care information on how to treat these symptoms and advice on when to seek medical care.

Common Problems by Body System

This section, which comprises nearly one-half of the book, examines common problems of the body in areas such as the eyes, ears, nose, skin, stomach, throat, back and limbs. There are also chapters on women's and men's health issues. We offer simple remedies for problems such as sore throats, common colds, stomach pains, ingrown toenails and black eyes.

Specific Conditions

In this section, we offer general guidelines on the prevention and management of eight specific conditions: asthma, arthritis, serious respiratory allergies, cancer, diabetes, high blood pressure, heart disease and sexually transmitted diseases. These are common medical conditions for which there is opportunity for self-care. If you have any of these conditions, you need to see a health-care provider for proper diagnosis and treatment.

Mental Health

In this section, we offer helpful information on how to deal with addictive behaviors, such as drug use, compulsive gambling and alcoholism. We discuss other mental health issues, such as anxiety, domestic abuse and memory loss. We also explain the difference between depression and the "blues," how to cope with the loss of a loved one and how to tell whether someone may be contemplating suicide.

Staying Healthy

This section is filled with practical information on how to establish and maintain a healthful lifestyle. You'll find tips on good nutrition, weight control, exercise, stress management and prevention of injury and illness. We also provide suggestions on how to stop smoking.

Your Health and the Workplace

This section focuses on ways to improve your health and well-being at your place of work. We suggest practical tips on reducing stress and job burnout. We also talk about how to avoid strain-related injuries and describe simple exercises for office workers. Other topics include pregnancy and work, workplace safety issues and the potential dangers posed by workers who abuse alcohol and drugs. In the chapter titled "Commonly Asked Questions," we address various topics, ranging from going to work with a cold to returning to work after a back injury.

The Healthy Consumer

In this section, we give you tips on topics such as how to talk with your physician, what you can learn from your family's medical history, home medical testing kits, what you should include in your first-aid kit and potential health risks associated with travel. We also discuss the use of common medications, and we provide easy-to-understand descriptions of cold remedies and over-the-counter pain medications.

Children and Adolescent Health

The *Mayo HealthQuest Guide to Self-Care* is not intended to be a comprehensive resource for all childhood illnesses. We do, however, address the major medical conditions likely to affect your child during his or her preteen years. Many of our chapters include a section on "Kids' Care," which provides information regarding specific concerns in children. We summarize the well-child immunizations in the Staying Healthy section and give many safety tips for children throughout the book. We also discuss how to identify and cope with alcohol and tobacco use in teenagers. Refer to the Index, pages 236 to 245, for a complete list of subjects related to children's health and infant health.

A Few Words About How We Speak

Throughout the *Mayo HealthQuest Guide to Self-Care,* we have used great care in our choice of words and have tried as often as possible to explain medical terms in everyday language. Despite these efforts, there may be occasions when you will find it useful to consult a dictionary for more detailed definitions and explanations of a term.

One term you will see frequently is "health-care provider." We use this phrase because, in addition to "doctor" and "physician," health-care providers include medical personnel such as physician's assistants, nurse-practitioners and certified nurse-midwives.

Table of Contents

Urgent Care

Emergencies don't happen very often, but when they do there's not much time to seek out information. To react effectively, you must know what action to take when a person appears injured, seriously ill or in distress. Your skills may never be required. However, you could someday be the link between life and death for another human being.

We encourage you to take a certified first-aid training course to learn lifesaving skills such as CPR, the Heimlich maneuver and dealing with shock and traumatic injury such as a bone fracture. We offer summary information on rescue techniques as a starting point for learning more. Check with your local Red Cross, county emergency services or public safety office or the state American Heart Association about first-aid courses in your community.

- CPR
- Choking
- Poisoning Emergencies
- Severe Bleeding
- Shock
- Allergic Reactions
- Bites
- Burns
- Cold Weather Problems
- Cuts, Scrapes and Wounds
- Eye Injuries
- Food-Borne Illness
- Heat-Related Problems
- Poisonous Plants
- Tooth Problems
- Trauma

CPR

CPR (cardiopulmonary resuscitation) involves a combination of mouth-to-mouth rescue breathing and chest compression. CPR keeps oxygenated blood flowing to the brain and other vital organs until appropriate medical treatment can restore a normal heart rhythm.

Before starting CPR, you must assess the situation. Is the person conscious or unconscious? If the victim appears unconscious, tap or shake his or her shoulder and ask loudly, "Are you O.K.?" If the person does not respond, think of the ABCs (see below), and get help by calling 911. If you cannot leave the scene, have someone else call.

A: Airway. Your first action is to open the airway, which may be obstructed by the back of the tongue or the epiglottis (the flap of cartilage that covers the windpipe) (see Figures 1 and 2 below).

B: Breathing. Mouth-to-mouth rescue breathing is the quickest way to get oxygen into a person's lungs (see Figures 3 and 4 below).

C: Circulation. Chest compressions replace the heartbeat when it has stopped. Compressions help maintain some blood flow to the brain, lungs and heart (see Figure 7 on page 3). You must perform rescue breathing anytime you perform chest compressions.

The following seven steps and illustrations demonstrate the CPR technique.

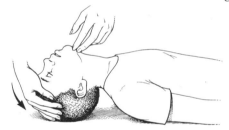

1. *Position the victim so you can check for breathing and a pulse by laying the victim flat on a firm surface and extending the neck.*

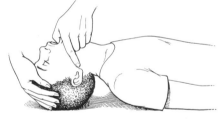

2. *Open the victim's mouth and airway by lifting the chin forward.*

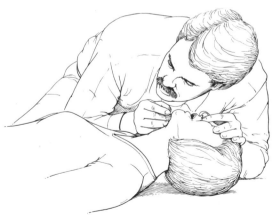

3. *Determine whether the victim is breathing by simultaneously listening for breath sounds, feeling for air motion on your cheek and ear and looking for chest motion.*

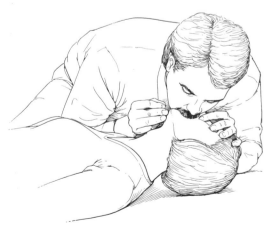

4. *If the victim is not breathing, pinch the person's nostrils closed, make a seal around the mouth and breathe into his or her mouth twice. Give one breath every 5 seconds and completely refill your lungs after each breath.*

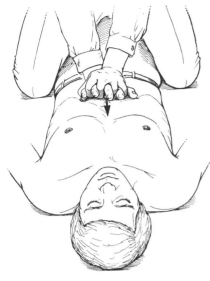

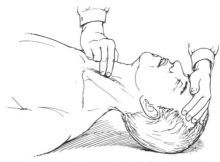

6. *Feel the carotid artery to see whether the victim has a pulse.*

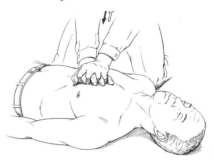

5. *If the victim's chest does not rise when you breathe into his or her mouth, the airway is probably blocked. Try to dislodge the obstruction (such as a piece of food) by performing the Heimlich maneuver. Because the victim will be lying down, place your hands slightly above the navel and press upward, firmly and rapidly. You will need to insert a finger into the victim's mouth to determine whether the obstruction has been expelled and to remove it from the mouth or throat.*

7. *If there is no pulse, begin chest compressions. Your hands should be located over the lower part of the breastbone, your elbows kept straight and your shoulders positioned directly above your hands to make the best use of your weight. Push down 1 1/2 to 2 inches at a rate of 80 to 100 times a minute. The "pushing down" and "letting up" phase of each cycle should be equal in duration. Don't "jab" down and relax. After 15 compressions, breathe into the victim's mouth twice. After every four cycles of 15 compressions and two breaths, recheck for a pulse and breathing. Continue the rescue maneuvers as long as there is no pulse or breathing.*

CPR for Infants

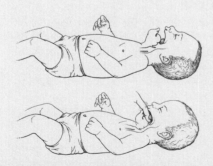

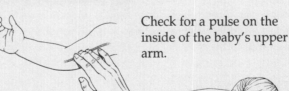

Check for a pulse on the inside of the baby's upper arm.

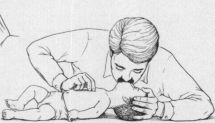

Before giving mouth-to-mouth resuscitation to an infant, tilt the child's head back to open the airway (top). Then, if visual inspection reveals a foreign object in the mouth, remove the object with a sweep of your finger (bottom). Be careful not to push the food or object deeper into the child's airway.

To perform CPR on a baby, cover the mouth and nose with your mouth. Give one breath for every five chest compressions. Compress the chest 1/2 to 1 inch at least 100 times a minute, using only two fingers.

Choking

Choking occurs when the respiratory passage in the throat or windpipe is blocked. This situation requires emergency treatment to prevent unconsciousness or death. Choking, heart disease or other conditions may cause the heart and breathing to stop. To save the life of the person, breathing and blood circulation must be restored immediately (see previous chapter on CPR).

Recognizing and Clearing an Obstructed Airway

Choking is often the result of inadequately chewed food becoming lodged in the throat or windpipe. Most often, solid foods such as meats are the cause.

Commonly, persons who are choking have been talking while simultaneously chewing a chunk of meat. False teeth also may set the stage for this problem by interfering with the way food feels in the mouth while it is being chewed. Food cannot be chewed as thoroughly with false teeth as with natural teeth because less chewing pressure is exerted by false teeth.

Panic is an accompanying sensation. The choking victim's face often assumes an expression of fear or terror. At first, he or she may turn purple, the eyes may bulge and he or she may wheeze or gasp.

If some food "goes down the wrong pipe," the coughing reflex often will resolve the problem. In fact, a person is not choking if he or she is able to cough freely, has normal skin color and is able to speak. If the cough is more like a gasp and the person is turning blue, the individual is probably choking.

If in doubt, ask the choking person whether he or she can talk. If the person is capable of speech, then the windpipe is not completely blocked and oxygen is reaching the lungs. A person who is choking is unable to communicate except by hand motions.

The universal sign for choking is a hand clutched to the throat, with thumb and fingers extended. A person who displays this requires emergency treatment and should never be left unattended.

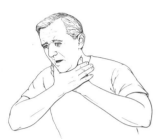

A person who is choking is unable to communicate except by hand motions. Often the hand and arm motions are uncoordinated. It is important to remember that the universal sign for choking is hands clutched to the throat, with thumbs and fingers extended.

The Heimlich Maneuver

The Heimlich maneuver is the best known method of removing an object from the airway of a person who is choking. You can use it on yourself or someone else. These are the steps:

1. Stand behind the choking person and wrap your arms around his or her waist. Bend the person slightly forward.

2. Make a fist with one hand and place it slightly above the person's navel.

3. Grasp your fist with the other hand and press hard into the abdomen with a quick, upward thrust. Repeat this procedure until the object is expelled from the airway.

If you must perform this maneuver on yourself, position your own fist slightly above your navel. Grasp your fist with your other hand and thrust upward into your abdomen until the object is expelled, or lean over the back of a chair to produce this effect.

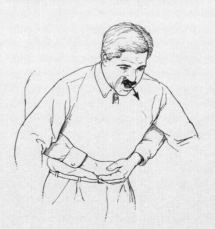

Poisoning Emergencies

A poisoning may or may not be obvious. Sometimes the source of a poisoning can be easily identified—an open bottle of medication or a spilled bottle of household cleaner. Look for these signs if you suspect a poisoning emergency:

- Burns or redness around the mouth and lips. They can result from drinking certain poisons.
- Breath that smells like chemicals (perhaps gasoline or paint thinner).
- Burns, stains and odors on the person, on his or her clothing or on the furniture, floor, rugs or other objects in the surrounding area.
- Vomiting, difficulty breathing, sleepiness, confusion or other unexpected symptoms.

Many conditions mimic the symptoms of poisoning, including seizures, alcohol intoxication, stroke and insulin reaction. If you can find no indication of poisoning, do **not** treat the person for poisoning, but call for emergency help. Meanwhile, make the person as comfortable as possible. Treat the person for shock (see page 7).

Emergency Treatment

If you believe someone has been poisoned, take the following steps:

1. Some products have instructions on the label specifying what to do if a poisoning occurs. Follow the instructions.
2. If the person is alert, give him or her a glass of water or milk to drink. The liquid will slow the rate at which the poison is absorbed by the body. But if the person is weak, lethargic, unconscious or having seizures, do not give anything by mouth.
3. If you cannot identify the poison or there are no instructions on the product label, **call your local poison control center for instructions.** Keep the number near your telephone. Most phone books have the emergency number on the inside cover. If no number is listed, call 911.
4. Certain poisons should be vomited; others should not. If you do not know what substance was swallowed, do not induce vomiting. Overall, you should not induce vomiting unless directed by a poison control authority or your physician.
5. If you are told to induce vomiting in the victim, use syrup of ipecac. An alternative method is touching the back of the throat of the person to initiate gagging. If you have no other alternative, have the person drink a glass of warm water containing 1 teaspoon of dried mustard or 3 teaspoons of salt.
6. After the person has vomited, give a glass of water or milk.
7. If the poison has spilled on the person's clothing, skin or eyes, remove the clothing and flush the skin or eyes with cool or lukewarm water for 20 minutes as you seek medical attention.
8. Get immediate medical attention. If you have identified the poison, take the container with you. If the identity of the poison is unknown, but the person has vomited, take a sample of the vomitus for analysis.

Medications as Poisons

Lifesaving medications also can be killers. Overdoses of seemingly harmless medications such as the common painkillers aspirin and acetaminophen take many lives each year. Numerous other over-the-counter drugs are dangerous if taken in large doses, especially by a child or elderly person. Prominent on the list are sleep medications, antihistamines and vitamin supplements. See page 229 for appropriate use of medications.

Severe Bleeding

To stop a serious bleeding injury, follow these steps:

1. Lay the affected person down. If possible, the person's head should be slightly lower than the trunk, or the legs should be elevated. This position reduces the chances of fainting by increasing blood flow to the brain. If possible, elevate the site of bleeding.
2. Remove any obvious debris or dirt from the wound. Do not remove any objects pierced into the victim. Do not probe the wound or attempt to clean it at this point. Your principal concern is to stop the loss of blood.
3. Apply pressure directly on the wound with a sterile bandage, clean cloth or even a piece of clothing. If nothing else is available, use your hand.
4. Maintain pressure until the bleeding stops. When it does, bind the wound dressing tightly with adhesive tape or a bandage. If none is available, use a piece of clean clothing.
5. If the bleeding continues and seeps through the gauze or other material you are holding on the wound, do not remove it. Rather, add more absorbent material on top of it.
6. If the bleeding does not stop with direct pressure, you may need to apply pressure to the major artery that delivers blood to the area of the wound. In the case of a wound on the hand or lower arm, for example, squeeze the main artery in the upper arm against the bone. Keep your fingers flat; with the other hand, continue to exert pressure on the wound itself.
7. Immobilize the injured body part once the bleeding has been stopped. Leave the bandages in place and get the injured person to the emergency room as soon as possible.

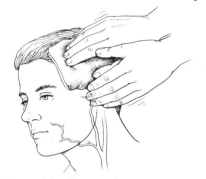

To stop bleeding, apply pressure directly to the wound using gauze or a clean cloth.

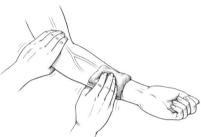

If bleeding continues despite pressure applied directly to the wound, maintain pressure and also apply pressure to the nearest major artery.

Detecting Internal Bleeding

In the event of a traumatic injury, such as an automobile crash or fall, internal bleeding may not be immediately apparent. Look for the following signs:

- Bleeding from the ears, nose, rectum or vagina, or the vomiting or coughing up of blood
- Bruising on the neck, chest or abdomen
- Wounds that have penetrated the skull, chest or abdomen
- Abdominal tenderness, perhaps accompanied by hardness or spasm of the abdominal muscles
- Fracture

Internal bleeding may produce shock. The volume of blood in the body becomes inadequate and the person may feel weak, thirsty and anxious. The skin may feel cool. Other symptoms of shock that may indicate internal bleeding include shallow and slow breathing, a rapid and weak pulse, trembling and restlessness. The person may faint and lose consciousness when standing or seated but recovers when allowed to lie down.

If you suspect internal bleeding, request emergency assistance. Treat the person for shock (see page 7). Keep the person lying quietly and comfortably. Loosen clothing but do not give the person anything to eat or drink.

Internal bleeding, especially in the abdomen, head or chest, is extremely serious and can be life-threatening. Blood loss can be considerable, even if there is no evident external bleeding.

Shock

Shock may result from trauma, heat, allergic reaction, severe infection, poisoning or other causes. Various symptoms appear in a person experiencing shock:

● The skin may appear pale or gray. It is cool and clammy.
● The pulse is weak and rapid, and breathing is slow and shallow. Blood pressure is reduced.
● The eyes lack shine and seem to stare. Sometimes the pupils are dilated.
● The person may be conscious or unconscious. If conscious, the person may faint or be very weak or confused. Shock sometimes causes a person to become overly excited and anxious.

Even if a person seems normal after an injury, take precautions and treat the person for shock by following these steps:

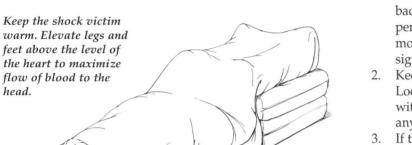

Keep the shock victim warm. Elevate legs and feet above the level of the heart to maximize flow of blood to the head.

1. Get the person to lie down on his or her back and elevate the feet higher than the person's head. Keep the person from moving unnecessarily. Observe for the signs of shock noted above.
2. Keep the person warm and comfortable. Loosen tight clothing and cover the person with a blanket. Do not give the person anything to drink.
3. If the person is vomiting or bleeding from the mouth, place the person on his or her side to prevent choking.
4. Treat any injuries (such as bleeding or broken bones) appropriately.
5. Summon emergency medical assistance immediately. Dial 911.

Anaphylaxis Can Be Life-Threatening

The most severe allergic response is called anaphylaxis. It can produce shock and be life-threatening. Although it is infrequent, each year several hundred Americans die of the reaction.

The anaphylactic response is quick. It can begin within seconds or minutes. Almost any allergen can cause the response, including insect venoms, pollens, latex, certain foods and drugs. Some people have anaphylactic reactions of unknown cause.

If you are extremely sensitive, you may notice severe hives and severe swelling of your eyes or lips or inside your throat which causes difficulty with breathing and shock. Dizziness, mental confusion, abdominal cramping, nausea or vomiting also may accompany a severe reaction.

Many people who know their specific allergies carry medication with them as an antidote to an allergic reaction. Epinephrine is the most common drug used. The effects of the medication are only temporary, however, and you must seek further medical attention immediately.

If you observe an allergic reaction with signs of anaphylaxis, call 911. Check to see whether the person is carrying special medication (to inhale, swallow or inject) to counter the effects of the allergic attack. CPR must be performed as a life-saving measure if there is no breathing or no pulse (see page 2).

Allergic Reactions

An allergy is a reaction to a foreign substance (called an allergen) by the body's immune system. The reaction may take many forms, including rashes, congestion, asthma and, rarely, shock or death. Common allergens include pollen (see Respiratory Allergies, page 154) and insect venoms (see Bites, page 10). This chapter covers food and drug allergies.

■ Food Allergies

Food allergies may be the most misunderstood of all allergies. Two of five Americans believe they are allergic to specific foods. However, fewer than 1 percent have true food allergies.

Ninety percent of food allergies are caused by certain proteins in cow's milk, egg whites, peanuts, wheat or soybeans. Other foods that can cause problems include berries, shellfish, corn, beans and gum arabic (a thickener used in processed foods). Yellow Food Dye no. 5 may produce an allergic response. Chocolate, long thought to cause allergies (particularly among children), is actually seldom a cause of allergy.

Signs and symptoms of food allergies include the following:
- Abdominal pain, diarrhea, nausea or vomiting
- Fainting
- Hives (see page 119), swelling beneath the skin or eczema (see page 117)
- Swelling of the lips, eyes, face, tongue and throat
- Nasal congestion and asthma

Self-Care
- Avoidance is the best way to prevent an allergic reaction.
- When choosing substitute foods, be careful to select foods that provide the necessary replacement nutrients.
- If you have had a severe reaction, wear an alert bracelet or necklace (see page 9); these are available in most drugstores. Ask your doctor about carrying emergency medications.
- Learn rescue techniques, and teach them to family members and friends.

Medical Help

Food allergies can be diagnosed through a careful process that includes the following five steps:

Step 1: History of your symptoms, including when they occur, which foods cause problems, the amount of food needed to trigger symptoms and whether you have a family history of allergies.

Step 2: Food diary to track eating habits, symptoms and medication use.

Step 3: Physical examination.

Step 4: Testing: Skin prick tests using food extracts and a blood test that measures IgE (one of the body's defense proteins) can help. Neither test is 100% accurate. They may be more helpful for determining to what foods you are not allergic.

Step 5: Food elimination-challenge diet is the standard test because it can link symptoms to a specific food. It can't be used, however, if you have severe reactions.

For reactions to foods that are mild, your doctor may prescribe antihistamines or skin creams.

Caution	Severe reactions such as anaphylaxis (see page 7) or acute asthma are very serious because they can be life-threatening. Such reactions are rare. Most reactions are limited to rashes and hives. However, this does not mean they can be ignored. Malnutrition and conditions that suppress your immune system increase the likelihood of developing a food allergy.
Kids' Care	Children are 10 times as likely as adults to have a food allergy. As the digestive system matures, it's less apt to allow absorption of food components that trigger allergies.

Children typically outgrow allergies to milk, wheat and eggs, often by around age 6. Severe allergies and those due to tree nuts and shellfish are more likely to be lifelong. |

■ Drug Allergies

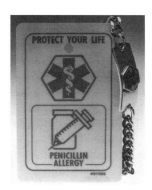

If you have a drug allergy, carry appropriate identification at all times. Drug alert necklaces and bracelets are available at drugstores.

Almost any drug can cause an adverse reaction in some people. Reactions to most drugs are not common, but they can range from merely irritating to life-threatening. Some reactions (such as rashes) are true allergic responses. Most, however, are side effects of a particular drug, typified by dry mouth or fatigue. Some are toxic effects of the drugs, such as liver damage. Still other reactions are poorly understood. Your physician will determine the nature of the reactions and what to do about them.

Penicillin and its relatives are responsible for many drug allergy reactions, ranging from mild rashes to hives to immediate anaphylaxis. Most reactions are minor rashes.

Drugs most likely to cause reactions include sulfas, barbiturates, anticonvulsants, insulin and local anesthetics. These are all common, effective, useful medications. Reactions occur in a minority of people. If you're taking one of them and not having problems, don't stop using it. In addition, contrast dyes that are injected into a person's blood vessels to help outline major organs in some X-ray studies contain iodine and may cause an allergic reaction.

Almost a million Americans, primarily adults, have reactions to a common drug, aspirin. Although not a true allergy, the response mimics one, and it can be serious.

Signs and symptoms of allergic reactions to drugs include the following:
- Wheezing and difficulty breathing
- Rash, hives, generalized itching
- Shock

Self-Care	- Avoid drugs that cause an allergic response.
- If you have a severe reaction, learn the names of related drugs.
- Wear a drug-alert necklace or bracelet to indicate your allergy.
- Alert physicians of your sensitivity before treatment.
- Report possible reactions to your doctor. Reactions can occur days after stopping use of a drug.
Medical Help	The most common drug reactions—rash, itching and hives—are treated with antihistamines or, occasionally, cortisone. Most drug allergies cannot be cured. The allergy to penicillin is an exception. In some cases, this sensitivity can be reduced enough so that the person can tolerate the drug. Small amounts of the drug are given in slowly increasing amounts to desensitize the immune response.

Bites: Animals, Humans, Insects and Spiders

■ Animal Bites

Domestic pets cause most animal bites. Dogs are more likely to bite than cats. However, cat bites are more likely to cause infection. The best treatment is prevention.

Self-Care

- If the bite only breaks the skin, treat it as a minor wound. Wash the wound thoroughly with soap and water. Apply an antibiotic cream to prevent infection, and cover it with a clean bandage.
- Establish whether you have had a tetanus shot within the past 5 years. If not, you should get a booster shot with any bite that breaks the skin.
- Report suspicious bites to local health authorities.
- Follow veterinary guidelines for immunization of your pets.

Medical Help

If the bite creates a deep puncture or the skin is badly torn and bleeding, apply pressure to stop the bleeding and see your doctor. If you have not had a recent tetanus shot, seek medical care. Watch for signs of infection. Swelling, redness around the wound or in a red streak extending from the site, pus draining from the wound or pain should be reported immediately to your doctor.

The Risk of Rabies

Bats, foxes, raccoons and other wild animals may carry rabies, but so can the dog, especially if it runs in the woods. Farm animals, especially cows, may carry rabies, although farm animals rarely transmit rabies to humans.

Rabies is a virus that affects the brain. Transmitted to humans by saliva from the bite of an infected animal, the rabies virus has an incubation period (the time from a bite until symptoms appear) of between 3 and 7 weeks.

Once the incubation period is over, a tingling sensation usually develops at the site of the bite. As the virus spreads, foaming at the mouth may occur because of difficulty with swallowing. Uncontrolled irritability and confusion may follow, alternating with periods of calm.

In the event of an unprovoked bite by a domestic dog, cat or farm animal, the animal should be confined and observed by a veterinarian for 7 to 10 days. Even if the bite is provoked, the animal should be confined for 10 days of observation. Contact a veterinarian if there is any sign of sickness in the animal. If a wild animal has bitten you, the animal should be killed.

■ Human Bites

There are two kinds of human bites. The first is what is usually thought of as a "true" bite—an injury that results from flesh being caught between the teeth. The second kind, called a "fight bite," occurs when a person is cut on the knuckles by an opponent's teeth. Treatment is the same in both cases. Human bites are dangerous because of the risk of infection. The human mouth is a breeding ground for bacteria.

Self-Care

- Apply pressure to stop bleeding, wash the wound thoroughly with soap and water and bandage the wound. Then visit an emergency room. Your health-care provider may prescribe antibiotics to prevent infection or update your tetanus shot if you have not had one for more than 5 years.

■ Snake Bites

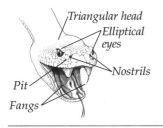

Triangular head
Elliptical eyes
Nostrils
Pit
Fangs

Most snakes are not poisonous. However, because a few are (including rattlesnakes, coral snakes, water moccasins and copperheads), avoid picking up or playing with any snake unless you are properly trained.

If you are bitten by a snake, it is important to determine whether the snake is poisonous. Most poisonous snakes have elliptical, slit-like eyes. Their heads are triangular, with a depression or "pit" midway between the eyes and nostrils on both sides of the head.

Self-Care

- If the snake is not poisonous, wash the bite thoroughly, cover it with an antibiotic cream and bandage it. In general, a snake bite is more scary than dangerous.
- Check on the date of your last tetanus shot. If it has been more than 5 years and the bite broke the skin, get a tetanus booster.

Medical Help

If you suspect that the snake is poisonous, seek emergency medical assistance immediately. Apply ice to the bite if possible, but don't delay.

■ Insect Bites and Stings

Some bites or stings cause little more than an annoying itching or stinging sensation and mild swelling that disappear within a day or so. However, up to 10 to 15 percent of the population is sensitive to insect venom. Bees, wasps, hornets, yellow jackets and fire ants are typically the most troublesome. Mosquitoes, ticks, biting flies and some spiders also can cause problems, but these are generally milder reactions.

Symptoms of an allergic reaction usually appear within a few minutes after the sting or bite occurs. But some take hours or even days to appear. If you are mildly sensitive to the venom, hives, itchy eyes, pain and intense itching around the site of the sting or bite are common. With a delayed reaction, you may experience fever, painful joints, hives and swollen glands. You may experience both the immediate and the delayed reactions from the same bite or sting.

The most severe allergic reactions can be life-threatening. If you are extremely sensitive, you may have severe hives and severe swelling of your eyes, lips or inside your throat; the swelling of the throat can cause breathing difficulty. Dizziness, mental confusion, abdominal cramping, nausea, vomiting or fainting also may accompany a severe reaction.

Self-Care

- Remove the stinger by using tweezers. Grasp the stinger where it enters your skin, or gently scrape the skin with a firm edge such as a credit card. Then swab the site with disinfectant.
- To reduce pain and swelling, apply ice or a cold pack.
- Apply 0.5 or 1 percent hydrocortisone cream, calamine lotion or a baking soda paste to the bite or sting several times daily until your symptoms subside.

If you have experienced a severe reaction in the past:
- Always carry an allergy kit containing epinephrine.
- Obtain a medical alert bracelet.
- Train family members or friends in what to do in an emergency.

Medical Help	If your reaction to an insect bite is severe (shortness of breath, tongue swelling, hives), see your doctor or go to the emergency room immediately.

The most severe allergic reactions to bee stings can be life-threatening. If you experience any breathing problems, swelling of the lips or throat, faintness, confusion, rapid heartbeat or hives after a sting, seek emergency care. Less severe allergic reactions include nausea, intestinal cramps, diarrhea or swelling larger than 2 inches in diameter at the site. See your physician promptly if you experience any of these symptoms.

Your doctor may prescribe shots that can help desensitize your body to insect venom, and an emergency kit containing antihistamine tablets and a syringe filled with epinephrine (adrenaline). Keep the medicine fresh; regularly check the shelf-life.

■ Spider Bites

Only a few spiders are dangerous to humans. Two are the black widow (*Latrodectus mactans*), known for the red hourglass marking on its belly, and the brown recluse (*Loxosceles reclusa*), with its violin-shaped marking on its top.

Both prefer warm climates and dark, dry places where flies are plentiful. They often live in outdoor toilets. You may not notice if you're bitten because bites may feel like a pinprick. But within hours, swelling and breathing problems can occur. Sometimes the black widow bite causes muscle cramping, tingling or weakness.

Seek emergency care immediately. In the meantime, apply a cloth dampened with cold water or filled with ice to the bite. If the bite is on a limb, you can help slow the venom's spread by placing a snug bandage above the bite and applying ice.

■ Tick Bites

By and large, ticks are harmless, but they can be a threat to human health. Some ticks carry infections, and their bite can transmit bacteria that cause illnesses such as Lyme disease (caused by the deer tick, see below) or Rocky Mountain spotted fever. Your risk of contracting one of these diseases depends on what part of the United States you live in, how much time you spend in wooded areas and how well you protect yourself.

Self-Care

 Actual size

Deer tick

Actual size

Wood tick

- When walking in wooded or grassy areas, wear shoes, long pants tucked into socks and long-sleeved shirts. Try to stick to trails, and avoid walking through low bushes and long grass.
- Tick-proof your yard by clearing brush and leaves; keep woodpiles in sunny areas.
- Check yourself and your pets often for ticks after being in wooded or grassy areas. Showering immediately after leaving these areas is a good idea, because ticks often remain on your skin for many hours before biting.
- Insect repellents often repel ticks. Use products containing DEET or permethrin. Be sure to follow label precautions.
- If you find a tick, remove it with tweezers by gently grasping it near its head or mouth. Do not squeeze or crush the tick, but pull carefully and steadily. Once your have the entire tick removed, apply antiseptic to the bite area.
- When you discard a tick, bury, burn or flush it.
- If you've developed a rash or are sick when you find the tick, bring it to your doctor's office.

Burns

Burns can be caused by fire, the sun, chemicals, hot liquids or objects, steam, electricity and other means. They can be minor medical problems or life-threatening emergencies.

Burn Classifications

Distinguishing a minor burn from a more serious burn involves determining the degree of damage to the tissues of the body. The following three classifications and illustrations will help determine your response.

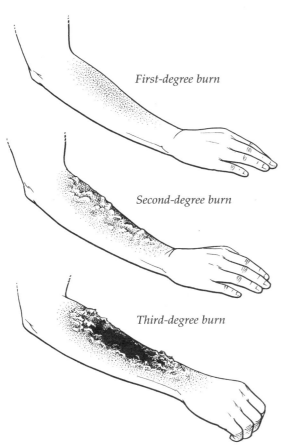

First-degree burn

Second-degree burn

Third-degree burn

First-Degree: Minor

The least serious burns are those in which only the outer layer of skin (epidermis) is burned. The skin is usually reddened, and there may be swelling and pain. However, the outer layer of skin has not been burned through. Unless such a burn involves substantial portions of the hands, feet, face, groin, buttocks or a major joint, it may be treated as a minor burn with the self-care remedies listed on page 14. Chemical burns may require additional follow-up. If the burn was caused by exposure to the sun, see Sunburn, page 15).

Second-Degree

When the first layer of skin has been burned through and the second layer of skin (dermis) also is burned, the injury is termed a second-degree burn. Blisters develop, and the skin takes on an intensely reddened appearance and becomes splotchy. Severe pain and swelling are accompanying symptoms.

If a second-degree burn is limited to an area no larger than 2 to 3 inches in diameter, follow the home remedies listed on page 14. If the burned area of the skin is larger, or if the burn is on the hands, feet, face, groin, buttocks or a major joint, seek urgent care immediately.

Third-Degree: Severe

The most serious burns involve all layers of the skin. Fat, nerves, muscles and even bones also may be affected. There are usually areas that are charred black or appear a dry white. There may be severe pain or, if nerve damage is substantial, no pain at all. You must take immediate action in all cases of third-degree burns.

**Emergency Treatment:
All Major Burns**

Seek emergency treatment immediately for major burns. Dial 911. Until an emergency unit arrives, follow these steps:
- **Do not remove burnt clothing**, but do make sure that the victim is not still in contact with smoldering materials.
- **Make certain that the burn victim is breathing.**
- **Cover the area of the burn** with a cool, moist sterile bandage or with a clean cloth.

Self-Care: Minor Burns Only	For minor burns, including second-degree burns limited to an area no larger than 2 to 3 inches in diameter, take the following action: ● **Cool the burn.** Hold the burned area under cold running water for 15 minutes. If this step is impractical, immerse the burn in cold water or cool it with cold compresses. Cooling the burn reduces swelling by carrying heat away from the skin. ● **Consider a lotion.** Once a burn is completely cooled, a lotion, such as one that contains aloe vera, or moisturizer prevents drying and increases your comfort. For sunburn, try 1 percent hydrocortisone cream or an anesthetic cream. ● **Bandage a burn.** Cover the burn with a sterile gauze bandage. (Fluffy cotton may be irritating.) Wrap it loosely to avoid putting pressure on burned skin. Bandaging keeps air off the area, reduces pain and protects blistered skin. ● **Take over-the-counter pain relievers** (see page 231). ● Minor burns will usually heal in about 1 to 2 weeks without further treatment, but watch for signs of infection.
Caution	**Do not use ice.** Putting ice directly on a burn can cause frostbite and further damage your skin. **Do not break blisters.** Fluid-filled blisters protect against infection. If blisters break, wash the area with mild soap and water, then apply an antibiotic ointment and a gauze bandage. Clean and change dressings daily.

■ Chemical Burns

Self-Care	● **Make sure the cause of the burn has been removed.** Flush the chemicals off the skin surface with cool running water for 20 minutes or more. (If the burning chemical is a powder-like substance such as lime, brush it off your skin before flushing.) ● **Treat the person for shock (see page 7).** Symptoms include fainting, pale complexion or breathing in a notably shallow fashion. ● **Remove clothing or jewelry** that has been contaminated by the chemical. ● **Wrap the burned area** with a dry, sterile dressing (if possible) or a clean cloth. ● **Rewash the burn** for several more minutes if the victim complains of increased burning after the initial washing. **Prevention** ● When using chemicals, always wear protective eyewear and clothing. ● Know about the chemicals you use. ● At work, read appropriate Material Safety Data Sheets, or call your local poison control center listed in your telephone book to learn more about the substance.
Medical Help	Minor chemical burns usually heal without further treatment. However, seek emergency medical assistance (1) if the chemical burned through the first layer of skin and the resulting second-degree burn covers an area more than 2 to 3 inches in diameter or (2) if the chemical burn occurred on the hands, feet, face, groin, buttocks or a major joint. If you are unsure if a given compound is toxic, call a poison control center.
Caution	Common household cleaning products, particularly those that contain ammonia or bleach, and garden chemicals can cause serious harm to the eyes or skin. Read labels. They contain instructions for proper use and treatment recommendations.

■ Sunburn

Although the sun provides a welcome change from gray winter months, it can damage your skin and increase your risk of skin cancer. Symptoms of sunburn usually appear within a few hours after exposure, bringing pain, redness, swelling and occasional blistering. Because a large area is often exposed, a sunburn can cause headache, fever and fatigue.

Self-Care

- Take a cool bath or shower. Adding one-half cup of cornstarch, oatmeal or baking soda to your bath may provide some relief.
- Leave water blisters intact to speed healing and avoid infection. If they burst on their own, apply an antibacterial ointment on the open areas.
- Take over-the-counter pain relievers (see page 231).
- Avoid products containing benzocaine (an anesthetic) because they can cause allergic reactions in many people.

Prevention

- If you plan to be outside, avoid the hours of 10 a.m. to 3 p.m., when the sun's ultraviolet (UV) radiation is at its peak. Cover exposed areas, wear a broad-brimmed hat and use a sunscreen with a sun protection factor (SPF) of at least 15.
- Protect your eyes. Sunglasses that block 95 percent of UV radiation are adequate. But you may need lenses that block 99 percent if you spend long hours in the sun, have had cataract surgery or are taking a prescription medication that increases your sensitivity to UV radiation.

Medical Help

If your sunburn begins to blister or you feel ill, see your physician. Oral cortisone such as prednisone is occasionally helpful.

Caution

Sunburn may not slow you down too much, but a lifetime of overexposure to the sun's UV radiation can damage your skin and increase your risk for skin cancer. If you have severe sunburn or immediate complications (rash, itching or fever), contact your physician.

■ Electrical Burns

Any electrical burn should be examined by a physician. An electrical burn may appear minor, but the damage can extend deep to the tissues beneath the skin. A heart rhythm disturbance, cardiac arrest or other internal damage can occur if the amount of electrical current that passed through the body was large.

Sometimes the jolt associated with the electrical injury can cause a person to be thrown or to fall, and fractures or other associated injuries can result.

Cold Weather Problems

■ Frostbite

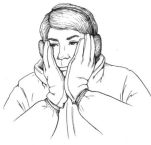

Cover your face if you feel the effects of frostbite.

Frostbite can affect any area of your body. Your hands, feet, nose and ears are most susceptible because they are small and often exposed.

In subfreezing temperatures, the tiny blood vessels in your skin tighten, reducing the flow of blood and oxygen to the tissues. Eventually, cells are destroyed.

The first sign of frostbite may be a slightly painful, tingling sensation. This often is followed by numbness. Your skin may be deathly pale and feel hard, cold and numb.

Frostbite can damage deep layers of tissue. As deeper layers of tissue freeze, blisters often form. Blistering usually occurs over 1 to 2 days.

Persons with atherosclerosis or who are taking medication for a heart condition may be more susceptible to frostbite.

Self-Care

- Carefully and gradually rewarm frostbitten areas. If you are outside, place your hands directly on the skin of warmer areas of your body. Warm your hands by tucking them into your armpits; if your nose, ears or face is frostbitten, warm the area by covering it with your warm hands (but try to keep them protected).
- If possible, immerse your hands or feet in water that is slightly above normal body temperature (100 to 105 F) or that feels warm to someone else.
- Do not rub the affected area. Never rub snow on frostbitten skin.
- Do not smoke cigarettes. Nicotine causes your blood vessels to constrict and may limit circulation.
- If your feet are frostbitten, elevate them after rewarming.
- Don't use direct heat (such as heating pads).
- Do not rewarm an affected area if there is a chance that it will refreeze.

Follow-Up

Frostbitten areas will turn red and throb, or they will burn with pain as they thaw. Even with mild frostbite, normal sensation may not return immediately. When frostbite is severe, the area will probably remain numb until it heals completely. In extreme cases, healing can take months, and the damage to your skin can permanently change your sense of touch. In severe cases, in which infection is present after the affected area has been rewarmed, antibiotics may be necessary. Bed rest and physical therapy may be appropriate. Do not smoke cigarettes during recovery. Once you've had frostbite—no matter how mild—you're more likely to have it again.

Emergency Treatment

If numbness remains during rewarming, seek medical care immediately. A person with frostbite on the extremities also may have hypothermia (see page 17).

Kids' Care

Watch for signs of chilling or cold injury while your child is outside. Watch for wet chinstraps on caps or snowsuits because the skin under the strap can easily freeze. Teach older children the signs of cold injury and have them keep a close watch for changes in skin color on their younger friends.

Teach your child to avoid touching cold metal with bare hands and licking extremely cold metal objects.

How to Prevent Cold Weather Injuries

- **Stay dry.** Your body loses heat faster when your skin is dampened by rain, snow or perspiration.
- **Protect yourself from the wind.** Wind robs more heat from your body than cold air alone. Exposed skin is particularly affected by wind.
- **Wear clothing that insulates,** shields and "breathes." Layers of light, loose-fitting clothing trap air for effective insulation. As an outer layer, wear something that's water-repellent and windproof.

- **Cover your head, neck and face.** Wear two pairs of socks and boots tall enough to cover your ankles. Mittens protect your hands better than gloves.
- If a part of your body becomes so cold that it is starting to feel numb, take the time to rewarm it before continuing your activity.
- Don't touch metal with bare skin—cold metal can absorb heat quickly.
- Plan for trips and outdoor activities. Carry emergency equipment (see page 212).

Hypothermia

Under most conditions, your body maintains a healthy temperature. However, when exposed for prolonged periods to cold temperatures or a cool, damp environment, your body's control mechanisms may fail to keep your body temperature normal. When more heat is lost than your body can generate, hypothermia can result. Wet or damp clothing can increase your chances of hypothermia.

Falling overboard from a boat into cold water is a common cause of hypothermia. An uncovered head or inadequate clothing in winter is another frequent cause.

The key symptom of hypothermia is a body temperature that drops to less than 94 F. Signs include shivering, slurred speech, an abnormally slow rate of breathing, skin that is cold and pale, a loss of coordination and feelings of tiredness, lethargy or apathy. The onset of symptoms is usually slow; there is likely to be a gradual loss of mental acuity and physical ability. The person experiencing hypothermia, in fact, may be unaware that he or she is in a state requiring emergency medical treatment.

The elderly, the very young and very lean people are at particular risk of hypothermia. Other conditions that may predispose you to hypothermia are malnutrition, heart disease, underactive thyroid and excessive consumption of alcohol.

Emergency Treatment

- After getting the person out of the cold, change the victim into warm, dry clothing. If going indoors is not possible, the person needs to be out of the wind, have the head covered and be insulated from the cold ground.
- Seek emergency medical assistance. While waiting for help to arrive, monitor the person's breathing and pulse. If either has stopped or seems dangerously slow or shallow, initiate CPR immediately (see page 2).
- In extreme cases, once the victim has arrived at a medical center, blood rewarming, similar to the procedure in a heart bypass machine, is sometimes used to restore normal body temperature quickly.
- If emergency care is not available, warm the person with a bath at 100 to 105 F (warm to the touch but not hot). Give warm liquids.
- Companions may be able to share body heat.

Caution

Do not give the victim alcohol. Give warm nonalcoholic drinks (unless he or she is vomiting).

Cuts, Scrapes and Wounds

Everyday cuts, scrapes or wounds often don't require a trip to the emergency room. Yet proper care is essential to avoid infection or other complications. The following guidelines can help you in caring for simple wounds. Puncture wounds may require medical attention.

■ Simple Wounds

Self-Care

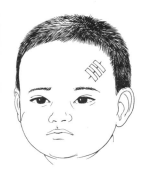

A strip or two of surgical tape (Steri-Strips) may close a minor cut, but if the mouth of the wound is not easily closed, seek a physician's care. Proper closure also will minimize scarring.

- **Stop the bleeding.** Minor cuts and scrapes usually stop bleeding on their own. If not, apply gentle pressure with a clean cloth or bandage.
- **Keep the wound clean.** Rinse with clear water. Clean the area around the wound with soap and a washcloth. Keep soap out of the wound. Soap can cause an irritation. If dirt or debris remains in the wound after washing, use clean tweezers to remove the particles. Apply alcohol to the tweezers before use. If debris remains embedded in the wound after cleaning, contact your health-care provider, and don't attempt to remove it by yourself. Thorough wound cleaning also reduces the risk of contracting tetanus (see page 19).
- Hydrogen peroxide, iodine or an iodine-containing cleanser may be used in the area around the wound. However, these substances are irritating to living cells and should not be used in the wound itself.
- **Consider the source.** Puncture wounds or other deep cuts, animal bites or particularly dirty wounds put you at risk for tetanus infection (see page 19). If the wound is serious, you may require an additional tetanus booster even if you received your last one within the past 10 years. A booster is given for dirty or deep wounds if you have not had one in the previous 5 years.
- **Prevent infection.** After you clean the wound, apply a thin layer of an antibiotic cream or ointment (such as Neosporin or Polysporin) to help keep the surface moist. The products don't make the wound heal faster, but they can discourage infection and allow your body's healing factors to close the wound more efficiently. Be aware that certain ingredients in some ointments can cause a mild rash in some people. If a rash appears, stop using the ointment.
- **Cover the wound.** Exposure to air will speed healing, but bandages can help keep the wound clean and keep harmful bacteria out. Blisters that are draining are vulnerable and should be covered until a scab forms.
- To help prevent infection, **change the dressing** at least once a day or whenever it becomes wet or dirty. If you're allergic to the adhesive used in most bandages, switch to adhesive-free dressings or sterile gauze and paper tape. These supplies generally are available at pharmacies.

Medical Help

If bleeding persists—if the blood spurts or continues to flow after several minutes of pressure—emergency care is necessary.

Are stitches needed? A deep (all the way through the skin), gaping or jagged-edged wound may require stitches to hold it together for proper healing. A strip or two of surgical tape may close a minor cut, but if the mouth of the wound is not easily closed, seek medical care. Proper closure also minimizes scarring (see page 19).

Caution   **Watch for signs of infection.** Every day that a wound remains unhealed, the risk of infection increases. See your health-care provider if your wound isn't healing steadily or if you notice any redness, drainage, warmth or swelling.

A Shot in the Arm: Tetanus Vaccine

A cut, laceration, bite or other wound, even if minor, can lead to a tetanus infection. The result can be lockjaw that occurs days or even weeks later. Lockjaw, or tetanus, is a stiffness of jaw muscles and other muscles. It may be followed by a range of other symptoms and could lead to convulsions, breathing problems and even death.

Tetanus bacteria usually are found in the soil but can occur virtually anywhere. If their spores enter a wound beyond the reach of oxygen, they germinate and produce a toxin that interferes with the nerves controlling your muscles.

Active immunization is vital for everyone in advance of an injury. The tetanus vaccine usually is given to children as a DTP shot. Adults generally need a tetanus booster every 10 years. If the wound is serious, your physician may recommend an additional booster even if your last one was within 10 years. A booster is given if you have a deep or dirty wound and your most recent booster was more than 5 years ago. Boosters should be given within 2 days of the injury.

■ Puncture Wounds

A puncture wound does not usually result in excessive bleeding. Often, in fact, little blood flows and the wound seems to close almost instantly. These features, however, do not mean that treatment is unnecessary.

A puncture wound—such as stepping on a nail or being stuck with a tack—can be dangerous because of the risk of infection. The object that caused the wound may carry spores of the tetanus or other bacteria, especially if the object has been exposed to soil. Follow the same self-care steps and advice on seeking medical help listed on page 18, but a deep, contaminated puncture wound may need to be cleaned by a physician.

What About Scarring?

No matter how you treat them, most deep wounds that penetrate beyond the first layer of skin form a scar when healed. Even superficial wounds can form a scar if infection or re-injury occurs. Following the guidelines on page 18 may help avoid these complications.

When a healing wound is exposed to sunlight, it can darken permanently. This darkening can be prevented by covering the area with clothing or sunblock (sunscreen protection factor more than 15) whenever you are outside during the first 6 months after the wound occurs.

A scar usually thickens about 2 months into the healing process. Within 6 months to a year, it should become thinner and be even with your skin surface.

A large, jagged scar that continues to enlarge is called a keloid, an abnormal growth of scar tissue. Surgical incisions, vaccinations, burns or even a scratch can cause keloids. The tendency to develop keloids is often inherited, and they're more common on deeply pigmented skin than on white skin.

Keloids are harmless. But if they itch or look unattractive, doctors can remove small keloids by freezing them with liquid nitrogen, then injecting with cortisone. Sometimes they stop growing, but they rarely disappear by themselves.

Ask a dermatologist or plastic surgeon to evaluate your scar and advise treatment.

Eye Injuries

Consider some common objects in your home—paper clips, pencils, tools and toys. Used without care, they pose a threat to your windows on the world—your eyes.

The topic of eye injuries offers a "bad news-good news" scenario. Eye injuries are common, and some are serious. Fortunately, you can prevent the vast majority of these injuries by taking simple steps (see page 72 for common eye problems).

■ Corneal Abrasion (Scratch)

The most common types of eye injury involve the cornea—the clear, protective "window" at the front of the eye. The cornea can be scratched or cut by contact with dust, dirt, sand, wood shavings, metal particles or even an edge of a piece of paper. Usually the scratch is superficial, and this is called a corneal abrasion. Some corneal abrasions become infected and result in a corneal ulcer, which is a serious problem.

Everyday activities can lead to corneal abrasions. Examples are playing sports, doing home repairs or being scratched by children who accidentally brush your cornea with a fingernail. Other common injuries to the cornea include "splash accidents"—contact with chemicals ranging from antifreeze to household cleaners.

Because the cornea is extremely sensitive, abrasions can be painful. If your cornea is scratched, you might feel like you have sand in your eye. Tears, blurred vision, sensitivity or redness around the eye can suggest a corneal abrasion.

Self-Care

In case of injury, seek prompt medical attention. Other immediate steps you can take are to:

- Run lukewarm tap water over the eye, or splash the eye with clean water. Many work sites have eye-rinse stations for this purpose. Rinsing the eye may wash out the offending foreign body. The technique is described on page 21.
- Blink several times. This movement may remove small particles of dust or sand.
- Pull the upper eyelid over the lower eyelid. The lashes of the lower eyelid can "brush" the foreign body from the undersurface of the upper eyelid.

Caution

- If abrasion was caused by an object in the eye, refer to page 21.
- Don't apply patches or ice packs to the eye. If on the outside chance you do get an object within the eye itself—typically when hammering metal on metal—the last thing you want to do is press on the eyeball.
- Don't rub your eye after an injury. This action can worsen a corneal abrasion.

■ Chemical Splash

If a chemical splashes into your eye, flush it with water immediately. Any source of clean drinking water will do. It is more important to begin flushing than it is to find sterile water. Flushing water may dilute the chemical. Continue to flush the eye for at least 20 minutes, particularly if your eye is exposed to household cleaners that contain ammonia. After washing the eye thoroughly, close the eyelid and cover it with a loose, moist dressing. Then seek emergency medical assistance.

■ Object in the Eye

Children and adults alike occasionally get foreign objects in their eyes. You can take appropriate steps in some cases to remove the object. In other situations, you need to see a health-care provider.

Clearing the Eye

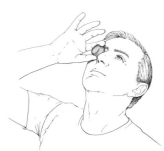

To remove a small object from your eye, flush the eye with a small amount of clean water using a small cup.

Your Own Eye

If no one is nearby to help you, try to flush the eye clear. Using an eyecup or small juice glass, wash your eye with clean water. Position the glass with its rim resting on the bone at the base of your eye socket and pour the water in, keeping the eye open. If you do not succeed in clearing the eye, seek emergency medical help.

Someone Else's Eye

- Do not rub the eye. Wash your hands before examining the eye. Seat the person in a well-lighted area.
- Locate the object in the eye visually. Examine the eye by gently pulling the lower lid downward and instructing the person to look upward. Reverse the procedure for the upper lid. Hold the upper lid and examine the eye while the person looks downward. If you find that the foreign object is embedded in the eyeball, cover the person's eye with a sterile pad or a clean cloth. Do not try to remove the object.
- If the object is large and makes closing the eye difficult, cover it with a paper cup taped to the face and forehead. Seek emergency medical assistance immediately.
- If the object is floating in the tear film or on the surface of the eye, you may be able to flush it out or remove it manually. While holding the upper or lower lid open, use a moistened cotton swab or the corner of a clean cloth to remove the object by lightly touching it. If you are unable to remove the object easily, cover both eyes with a soft cloth and seek emergency medical assistance.
- If you do succeed in removing the object, flush the eye with an eye irrigating solution or with water.
- If pain, vision problems or redness persists, seek emergency medical care.

Common Sense Can Save Your Sight

- **Wear goggles** while working with industrial chemicals, power tools and even hand tools. Some of the most serious eye injuries occur while people are using hammers. Also wear a safety helmet when appropriate.
- **Wear safety glasses** for sports such as racquetball, basketball, squash or tennis. Also wear appropriate headgear, such as batter's helmets for baseball and face masks for hockey.
- **Carefully follow the instructions for using detergents,** ammonia and cleaning fluids. When using fluids that come in spray containers, point nozzles away from your eyes at all times. Store household chemicals safely and out of children's reach.

- **Supervise children at play.** Remove toys that could lead to an eye injury. Examples are BB guns, plastic swords or spring-loaded toys that shoot darts. Don't allow children to have fireworks.
- **Don't lean over a car battery** when attaching jumper cables.
- **Pick up rocks and sticks** before mowing your lawn. While mowing, watch for trees with low-hanging branches.
- **Carefully follow your physician's instructions** for removing and applying contact lenses. Also, investigate any pain or red eye that occurs while you're wearing contact lenses.

Food-Borne Illness

Food-borne illness is a growing problem in the United States. The major reasons for this problem are an increase in restaurant dining and more centralized food processing.

All foods naturally contain small amounts of bacteria. But when food is poorly handled, improperly cooked or inadequately stored, bacteria can multiply in great enough numbers to cause illness. Parasites, viruses and chemicals also can contaminate food, but food-borne illness from these sources is less common.

If you eat contaminated food, whether you'll become ill or not depends on the organism, the amount of exposure, your age and your health. As you get older, immune cells may not respond as quickly and effectively to infectious organisms. Young children are at increased risk of illness because their immune systems haven't developed fully. Conditions such as diabetes and AIDS and cancer treatment also reduce your immune response, making you more susceptible to food-borne illness.

Food poisoning can cause various ailments. If you become ill within 1 to 6 hours after consuming contaminated food or water, you probably have a common type of food poisoning. Symptoms include nausea, vomiting, diarrhea or stomach pain.

Self-Care

- Rest and drink plenty of liquids.
- Don't use antidiarrheal medications because they may slow elimination of the bacteria and toxins from your system.
- Mild to moderate illness often resolves on its own within 12 hours.

Medical Help

If the symptoms last more than 12 hours, or if you have severe symptoms or belong to one of the high-risk groups noted above, see your physician.

Caution

Botulism is a potentially fatal food poisoning. It results from eating foods containing a toxin formed by certain spores in food. Botulism toxin is most often found in home-canned foods, especially green beans and tomatoes. Symptoms usually begin 12 to 36 hours after eating the contaminated food. Symptoms include headache, blurred or double vision, muscle weakness and eventually paralysis. Some people report nausea, vomiting, constipation, urinary retention and reduced salivation. These symptoms require immediate medical attention.

Handling Food Safely

- **Plan ahead.** Thaw meats and other frozen foods in the refrigerator, not on the countertop.
- **When shopping,** don't buy food in cans or jars with dented or bulging lids.
- **When preparing food,** wash your hands with soap and water. Rinse produce thoroughly or peel off the skin or outer leaves. Wash knives and cutting surfaces frequently, especially after handling raw meat and before preparing other foods to be eaten raw. Launder dishcloths and kitchen towels frequently.
- **When cooking,** use a meat thermometer. Cook red meat to an internal temperature of 160 F, poultry to 180 F. Cook fish until it flakes easily with a fork. Cook eggs until the yolks are firm and no longer runny.
- **When storing food,** always check expiration dates. Use or freeze fresh red meats within 3 to 5 days after purchase. Use or freeze fresh poultry, fish and ground meat within 1 to 2 days. Refrigerate or freeze leftovers within 2 hours of serving.

Troublesome Bacteria and How You Can Stop Them

Keep hot food hot. Keep cold food cold. Keep everything—especially your hands—clean. Follow these three basic rules and you're less likely to become ill from the troublesome bacteria listed here.

Bacteria	How Spread	Symptoms	To Prevent
Campylobacter jejuni	Contaminates meat and poultry during processing if feces contact meat surfaces. Other sources: unpasteurized milk, untreated water	Severe diarrhea (sometimes bloody), abdominal cramps, chills, headache. May cause nerve damage. Onset within 2 to 11 days. Lasts 1 to 2 weeks	Cook meat and poultry thoroughly. Wash knives and cutting surfaces after contact with raw meat. Don't drink unpasteurized milk or untreated water
Clostridium perfringens	Meats, stews, gravies. Commonly spread when serving dishes don't keep food hot enough or food is chilled too slowly	Watery diarrhea, nausea, abdominal cramps. Fever is rare. Onset within 1 to 16 hours. Lasts 1 to 2 days	Keep foods hot. Hold cooked meats above 140 F. Reheat to at least 165 F. Chill foods quickly. Store in small containers
Escherichia coli 0157:H7	Contaminates beef during slaughter. Spread mainly by undercooked ground beef. Other sources: unpasteurized milk, unpasteurized apple cider, human stools, contaminated water	Watery diarrhea may turn bloody within 24 hours. Severe abdominal cramps, nausea, occasional vomiting. Usually no fever. Onset within 1 to 8 days. Lasts 5 to 8 days	Cook beef to internal temperature of 160 F. Don't drink unpasteurized milk or unpasteurized apple cider. Wash hands after bathroom use
Salmonella	Raw or contaminated meat, poultry, milk; contaminated egg yolks. Survives inadequate cooking. Spread by knives, cutting surfaces or an infected person who practices poor hygiene	Severe diarrhea, watery stools, nausea, vomiting, temperature 101 F or more. Onset within 6 to 72 hours. Lasts 1 to 14 days	Cook meat and poultry thoroughly. Don't drink unpasteurized milk. Don't eat raw or undercooked eggs. Keep cutting surfaces clean. Wash hands after bathroom use
Staphylococcus aureus	Spread by hand contact, coughing and sneezing. Grows on meats and prepared salads, cream sauces, cream-filled pastries	Explosive, watery diarrhea, nausea, vomiting, abdominal cramps, light-headedness. Onset within 1 to 6 hours. Lasts 1 to 2 days	Don't leave high-risk foods at room temperature for more than 2 hours. Wash hands and utensils before preparing food
Vibrio vulnificus	Raw oysters and raw or undercooked mussels, clams, whole scallops	Chills, fever, skin lesions. Onset 1 hr to 1 wk. Fatal in 50 percent of cases	Don't eat raw oysters. Make sure all shellfish is thoroughly cooked

Heat-Related Problems

Under normal conditions, your body's natural control mechanisms—skin and perspiration—adjust to the heat. However, those systems may fail when you are exposed to high temperatures for prolonged periods.

Heat Cramps

Heat cramps are painful muscle spasms. They usually occur after vigorous exercises and profuse perspiration. Your abdominal muscles and ones you use during exercise are most frequently affected.

Heat Exhaustion

Signs of heat exhaustion include an increased temperature, faintness, rapid heartbeat, low blood pressure, an ashen appearance, cold, clammy skin and nausea. Symptoms often begin suddenly, sometimes after excessive perspiration and inadequate fluid intake.

Heatstroke

Elderly and obese people are particularly at risk of heatstroke. Other risk factors include dehydration, alcohol use, heart disease, certain medications and vigorous exercise. People born with an impaired ability to sweat are particularly at risk. Signs of heatstroke include rapid heartbeat, rapid and shallow breathing, confusion and either increased or lowered blood pressure. Fainting can be the first sign in the elderly. A victim may stop sweating, but this is not a reliable sign.

Self-Care

For Heat Cramps
- Rest briefly; cool down.
- Eat salty foods.
- Drink water with a teaspoon of salt per quart.

For Heat Exhaustion
- If you suspect heat exhaustion, get the person out of the sun and into a shady spot or air-conditioned location. Then, lay the person down and elevate his or her feet slightly. Loosen or remove the clothing.
- Give cold (not ice) water to drink, or give an electrolyte-containing drink such as one of the popular sports drinks.

Medical Help

If you suspect heatstroke, get emergency help immediately, move the victim out of the sun and into a shady spot or air-conditioned space and give the victim a sponge bath.

Monitor victims of heat exhaustion carefully. Although less dangerous than heatstroke, heat exhaustion can quickly become heatstroke.

Tips to Beat the Heat

- **Stay out of the sun.** Avoid going outside during the hottest part of the day, noon to 4 p.m.
- **Limit activity.** Reserve vigorous exercise or activities for early morning or evening.
- **Dress properly.** Wear light-colored, lightweight, loose-fitting clothing that breathes.
- **Drink lots of liquids. (**Avoid alcohol and caffeine.)
- **Avoid hot and heavy meals.**

Poisonous Plants

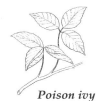

Poison ivy

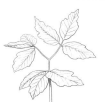

Poison oak

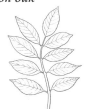

Poison sumac

When it comes to poison oak and ivy, it's wise to heed these words of advice: "Leaves of three, let them be."

With their leaves usually grouped three to a stem, poison ivy and poison oak are two of the most common causes of an allergic skin reaction called contact dermatitis.

Contact with poison ivy and poison oak usually causes red, swollen skin, blisters and severe itching. This reaction typically develops within 2 days after exposure, but it can develop as soon as a few hours. The rash usually reaches its peak after about 5 days, and it is usually gone within 1 to 2 weeks.

The rash is caused by exposure to resin, a colorless, oily substance contained in all parts of these plants. Resin transfers easily from clothing or from pet hair to your skin. Burning the plants is also hazardous because inhaling the smoke can cause internal and external reactions.

It takes only a tiny amount of resin to cause a reaction. Poison ivy and other rashes do not develop as a result of merely being near the plant, nor does the rash spread as a result of washing or scratching open rash blisters. The resin is not present in blister fluid. However, it can be spread by accidentally rubbing the resin on other areas of the skin before all the resin is washed off.

Besides poison ivy and oak, other plants also can cause the reaction. They include sumac, heliotrope (found in the deserts of the Southwest), ragweed (both the leaves and pollen), daisies, chrysanthemums, sagebrush, wormwood, celery, oranges, limes and potatoes.

Self-Care

- Washing the harmful resin off the skin with soap within 5 or 10 minutes after exposure may avert a skin reaction.
- Do not try to remove the resin by taking a bath. Bathing can spread the resin to other areas of your body.
- Wash any clothing or jewelry that may have been in contact with the plant. Note: Footwear and shoelaces also should be washed.
- Try not to scratch. Take cool showers.
- Over-the-counter preparations (calamine lotion or hydrocortisone cream) can ease itching. Or, apply a paste of baking soda or Epsom salts and water.
- Creams and lotions do not help much when the blisters open, but they can be used again when the blisters close.
- Do not apply alcohol because this tends to make the itching worse. Cover open blisters with a sterile gauze to prevent infection.
- To avoid exposure, learn to recognize poisonous plants and wear protective clothing when appropriate. Poison ivy leaves are oval or spoon-shaped. Poison oak leaves resemble oak leaves. The colors of the leaves of these plants change with the seasons, from green in the summer to orange and red in the fall.

Medical Help

If you have a severe reaction, or when your eyes, face or genital area is involved, contact your health-care provider, who may prescribe cortisone or an antihistamine, either orally or topically.

Tooth Problems

◼ Toothache

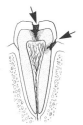

Dental cavities can lead to toothaches.

In most children and adults, tooth decay (cavities, also called caries) is the primary cause of toothaches. Tooth decay mainly is caused by bacteria and carbohydrates. Bacteria are present in a thin, almost invisible film on your teeth called plaque.

Tooth decay takes time to develop, often a year or two in permanent teeth but less in primary teeth. Acid formation occurs within the first 20 minutes after you eat.

The decay-producing acid that forms in plaque attacks the tooth's outer surface. The erosion caused by the plaque leads to the formation of tiny cavities (or openings) in the tooth surface. The first sign of decay may be a sensation of pain when you eat something sweet, very cold or very hot.

Self-Care

Until you are able to get to the dentist, try these self-care tips:
- Try flossing to remove any food particles wedged between the teeth.
- Suck on an ice cube placed in the area of irritation.
- Use an over-the-counter pain reliever.
- Over-the-counter antiseptics containing benzocaine will offer temporary relief. Oil of cloves (eugenol) can relieve pain. It is available at most pharmacies.
- Prevention is the best way to avoid tooth decay and cavities.

Caution

Swelling, pain when you bite, a foul-tasting discharge and redness indicate infection. See your dentist as soon as possible. If you have fever with the pain, seek emergency care.

◼ Tooth Loss

Whenever a tooth is accidentally knocked out, appropriate emergency medical care is required immediately. Today, permanent teeth that are knocked out sometimes can be reimplanted if you act quickly. A broken tooth, however, cannot be reimplanted.

Emergency Treatment

If a permanent tooth is knocked out, save the tooth and consult your dentist immediately. If it is after office hours, call your dentist at home. If he or she is unavailable, go to the nearest emergency room.

Successful reimplantation depends on several factors: prompt insertion (within 30 minutes if possible; no longer than 2 hours after loss) and proper storage and transportation of the tooth. Keeping it moist is essential.

Self-Care

To preserve the tooth until you get to the dentist:
- Handle the tooth by the top (crown) only.
- Do not rub it or scrape it to remove dirt.
- Gently rinse the tooth in a glass of tap water, but not under the faucet.
- Try to replace the tooth in the socket and bite down gently on gauze or a moistened tea bag to help keep it in place.
- If the tooth cannot be replaced in the socket, immediately place it in milk, your own saliva or a warm, mild saltwater solution.

Trauma

Trauma is any injury sustained as a result of external force or violence. A broken bone, a severe blow to the head and a knocked-out tooth are all considered trauma.

Fractures, severe sprains, dislocations and other serious bone and joint injuries also are trauma emergencies and usually require professional medical care.

■ Dislocations

A dislocation is an injury in which the ends of bones in a joint are forced from their normal positions. In most cases, a blow, fall or other trauma causes the dislocation.

The indications of a dislocation include the following:
- An injured joint that is visibly out of position, misshapen and difficult to move
- Swelling and intense pain at a joint

The dislocation should be treated as quickly as possible, but do not try to return the joint to its proper place. Splint the affected joint in the position it is in. Treat it as you would a fracture. Seek immediate medical attention.

For more information on dislocations, see page 89.

■ Fractures

A fracture is, simply, a broken bone. It requires immediate medical attention.

If you suspect a fracture, the proper approach is to protect the affected area from further damage. Do not try to set the broken bone. Instead, immobilize the area with a splint. Also keep joints above and below the fracture immobilized.

If bleeding occurs along with the broken bone, apply pressure to stop the bleeding. If possible, elevate the site of bleeding to lessen the blood flow. Maintain pressure until the bleeding stops.

If the person is faint, pale or breathing in a notably shallow, rapid fashion, use the treatment steps for shock: lay the person down, elevate the legs and cover with a blanket or something for warmth.

Signs of a fracture are as follows:
- Swelling or bruising over a bone
- Deformity of the affected limb
- Localized pain that is intensified when the affected area is moved or pressure is put on it
- Loss of function in the area of the injury
- A broken bone that has poked through adjacent soft tissues and is sticking out of the skin

For more information on fractures, see page 85.

Sprains

A sprain occurs when a violent twist or stretch causes a joint to move outside its normal range. A sprain is the result of overstretched ligaments. Tearing of the ligaments may occur. The usual indications of a sprain are the following:

- Pain and tenderness in the affected area
- Rapid swelling and possible discoloration of the skin
- Impaired joint function

Most minor sprains can be treated at home. However, if a popping sound and immediate difficulty in using the joint accompany the injury, seek emergency medical care.

For more information on sprains, see page 84.

Head Injuries

Most head injuries are minor. The skull provides the brain with considerable protection from injury. Only 10 percent of all head injuries require hospitalization. Simple cuts and bruises can be treated with basic first aid techniques.

The serious types of head injuries that require emergency medical care are listed below. In all cases of worrisome head injury, do not move the neck because it may have been injured.

Concussion: When the head sustains a hard blow as the result of being struck or from a fall, a concussion may result. The impact creates a sudden movement of the brain within the skull. A concussion involves a loss of consciousness. Victims are often described as dazed. Loss of memory, dizziness and vomiting also may occur. Partial paralysis and shock are other possible symptoms.

Blood clot on the brain: This occurs when a blood vessel ruptures between the skull and the brain. Blood then leaks between the brain and skull and forms a blood clot (hematoma), which presses on the brain tissue. Symptoms occur from a few hours to several weeks after a blow to the head. There may be no open wound, bruise or other outward sign. Symptoms include headache, nausea, vomiting, alteration of consciousness and pupils of unequal size. There may be progressive lethargy, unconsciousness and death if the condition is not treated.

Skull fracture: This type of injury is not always apparent. Look for the following:

- Bruising or discoloring behind the ear or around the eyes
- Blood or clear, watery fluids leaking from the ears or nose
- Pupils of unequal size
- Deformity of the skull, including swelling or depressions

Emergency Treatment

Seek emergency medical care if any of the following symptoms are apparent:

- Severe head or facial bleeding
- Change in level of consciousness, even if only briefly
- Irregular or labored breathing
- Vomiting

Caution

- Until emergency help arrives, keep the person lying down and quiet in a dimmed room. Observe the person for vital signs: breathing, heartbeat and alertness. Stop any bleeding by applying firm pressure.

General Symptoms

- **Dizziness and Fainting**
- **Fatigue**
- **Fever**
- **Pain**
- **Sleep Disorders**
- **Sweating and Body Odor**
- **Unexpected Weight Changes**

Fatigue...fever...dizziness...pain...
sleep disorders...sweating...unex-
pected weight changes. In medicine, these conditions are called
"general symptoms" because
they tend to affect your whole
body rather than a particular
body part or system. In this section, we explain the common
causes for each of seven general
symptoms and provide self-care
information and advice on when
to seek medical care.

Dizziness and Fainting

Dizziness has many causes. Fortunately, most dizziness is mild, brief and harmless. It can be caused by many things, including medications, infections and stress. The word "dizziness" actually describes various sensations.

Vertigo and Imbalance

Vertigo is the sensation that you or your surroundings are rotating. You may feel that the room is spinning, or you may sense the rotation within your own head or body. Vertigo usually is associated with problems in your inner ear. The inner ear has an ultrasensitive device for sensing movement. Viral illness, trauma or other disturbance can result in the device sending a false message to your brain.

Imbalance is the sensation that you must touch or hold onto something to maintain your balance. Severe imbalance may make it difficult to stand without falling.

Light-Headedness and Fainting

Light-headedness includes feelings of being woozy, floating or near fainting. Fainting is a sudden, brief loss of consciousness. It occurs when your brain doesn't receive enough blood and the oxygen it carries. Although frightening, fainting generally isn't a reason for alarm. Once you are lying flat, blood flows to your brain and you regain consciousness within about a minute. Fainting may be caused by medical disorders, including heart disease, severe coughing spells and circulatory problems. In other cases, fainting may be related to the following:

- Standing too quickly
- Medications for high blood pressure and erratic heartbeats
- Excessive sweating that results in loss of sodium and dehydration
- Extreme fatigue
- Upsetting news or an unexpected or unusual stress such as the sight of blood

A rapid drop in blood pressure, called *postural hypotension,* occurs when you get up quickly from a sitting or reclining position. Everyone experiences this reaction to a mild degree. You feel light-headed or slightly faint, and it usually passes within seconds. When it leads to fainting or blackouts, it's more serious. It often occurs after a hot bath or in people taking medications to control blood pressure.

Self-Care

- If your vision darkens or you feel faint, lower your head. Lie down and elevate your legs slightly to return blood to the heart. If you can't lie down, lean forward and put your head between your knees.

Prevention

- Stand and change positions slowly—particularly when turning from side to side or when changing from lying down to standing. Before standing up in the morning, sit on the edge of the bed for a few minutes.
- Pace yourself. Take breaks when you are active in heat and humidity. Dress appropriate to the conditions to avoid overheating.
- Drink enough fluids to avoid dehydration and assure good circulation.
- Avoid caffeine, smoking, alcohol and illegal drugs.
- Don't drive a car or operate dangerous equipment if you feel dizzy.
- Don't climb or descend staircases.
- Check medications. You may need to ask your doctor about adjustments.

Medical Help

Mild symptoms that persist for weeks or months may be due to serious nervous system diseases. Because problems of dizziness and balance can have many different causes, making a diagnosis usually requires a complete medical history and several tests.

Treatments for sudden onset of vertigo include avoiding positions or movements that cause dizziness, sedatives, antinausea drugs and a positioning treatment your doctor may suggest.

Contact your health-care provider:
- When the condition is severe, prolonged (more than a few days or a week) or recurrent
- You are taking drugs for high blood pressure
- You have black stools or blood in your stools or other signs of blood loss
  Seek emergency medical care if:
- You faint when you turn your head or extend your neck, or if fainting is accompanied by symptoms such as pain in the chest or head, trouble with breathing, numbness or continuing weakness, irregular heartbeat, blurred vision, confusion or trouble with talking
- The symptoms listed above are present on awakening
- Someone faints without warning
- This was the person's first fainting spell and there were no obvious reasons for it
- The person was injured during the faint
  Until medical help arrives, do the following: If the person is lying down, position him or her on the back. Watch the airway—people often vomit after fainting. If you believe the person is about to vomit, roll him or her onto the side. Listen for breathing sounds and check for a pulse. (If they are absent, the problem is more serious than fainting, and CPR, see page 2, must be started.) Raise the legs above the level of the head. If a person faints and remains seated, quickly lay him or her flat. Loosen tight clothing.

How Your Body Maintains Balance

Maintaining balance requires a complex networking of several different parts of your body. To maintain balance, your brain must coordinate a constant flow of information from your eyes, muscles and tendons, and inner ear. All of these parts of the body work together to help keep you upright and provide you with a sense of stability when you are moving.

Many problems with dizziness are caused by problems within your inner ear. However, problems in any part of the system that controls your balance can cause dizziness and imbalance.

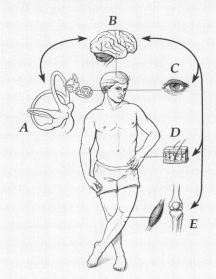

A. The inner ear contains our primary balance structure.

B. The brain relays and interprets information to and from the body.

C. The eyes record the body's position and surroundings.

D. When we touch things, sensors in our skin give us information about our environment.

E. Muscles and joints report bodily movement to the brain.

Fatigue

Almost everyone experiences fatigue at some time. After putting in a long weekend of yard chores or a hectic day with the children or at the office, it's natural to feel tired. This kind of physical and emotional fatigue is normal, and you can usually restore your energy with rest or exercise.

If you feel tired all the time, or if the exhaustion is overwhelming, you might start to worry that your condition is more serious than just fatigue. However, when fatigue is not accompanied by other symptoms, a specific cause often can't be determined. A common cause of chronic fatigue is lack of regular exercise (deconditioning). This problem can be remedied easily by gradually increasing your activity and beginning an exercise program.

Fatigue can be the result of physical or emotional problems. Physical fatigue is usually more pronounced later in the day, and it often resolves with a good night's sleep. Emotional fatigue often peaks first thing in the morning and gets better as the day progresses.

Common Causes

Common causes of physical fatigue include the following:
- Poor eating habits
- Lack of sleep
- Being out of shape
- Warm working or living quarters
- Carbon monoxide poisoning
- Over-the-counter medications, including pain relievers, cough and cold medicines, antihistamines and allergy remedies, sleeping pills and motion sickness pills
- Prescription drugs such as tranquilizers, muscle relaxants, sedatives, birth control pills and blood pressure medications
- Dehydration

Fatigue also can be an early symptom of these conditions:
- A low red blood cell count (anemia)
- Low thyroid activity (hypothyroidism)
- Various acute or chronic infections
- Heart disease
- Sleep disorder
- Electrolyte imbalance (when the levels of salts in your blood such as sodium, potassium and other minerals are too high or too low)
- Cancer
- Diabetes
- Alcoholism
- Rheumatoid arthritis

Most of these illnesses are accompanied by other symptoms such as muscle aches, pain, nausea, fever, weight loss, cold sensitivity or shortness of breath.

Common causes of emotional fatigue include:
- Overextending yourself, especially if you can't say "no"
- Boredom or lack of stimulation from family, friends or coworkers
- A major crisis (losing a spouse or a job), a move or a family difficulty
- Depression
- Loneliness
- Unresolved past emotional issues
- Repressing anger instead of expressing it

Self-Care	Before you talk to a health-care provider, consider the possibility that your fatigue is related to an explainable cause that can be remedied with some of the following lifestyle changes:

- Get an adequate night's sleep—6 to 8 hours of uninterrupted sleep.
- Give yourself a break. Ask others to pitch in.
- Organize your schedule, and prioritize activities.
- Rest and relax—unwind. Do something fun.
- Exercise more, starting gradually. Walk instead of watching television. If you are older than 40, consult your doctor before beginning a vigorous exercise program.
- Increase your exposure to fresh air at home and at work.
- Eat a balanced diet. Steer clear of high-fat foods.
- Lose weight if you are overweight.
- Drink plenty of water (2 or more quarts per day to avoid dehydration).
- Review your medications (over-the-counter and prescription) to determine if fatigue is a side effect.
- Quit smoking.
- Reduce or eliminate your use of alcohol and caffeine.
- If you have problems at your job, find ways to resolve them. (See Keeping Stress Under Control, page 210, and Avoiding Stress in the Workplace, page 216.)

Medical Help

If fatigue persists even when you rest enough, and it lasts for 2 weeks or longer, you may have a problem that requires medical care. See your health-care provider.

Kids' Care

Children and young adults rarely complain of fatigue. If they do, it's usually a sign that they have an acute infection, or that one is developing. Consult your physician.

What Is Chronic Fatigue Syndrome?

Chronic fatigue syndrome is a poorly understood, flu-like condition that can completely drain your energy and may last for years. People who were previously healthy and full of energy experience intense fatigue, pain in joints and muscles, painful lymph glands and headaches.

Experts haven't yet determined the causes of chronic fatigue syndrome, although there are likely to be many. Theories include infections, hormonal imbalances and psychological, immunologic or neurologic abnormalities. In one study, researchers found that some people with the syndrome had a low blood pressure disorder triggering the fainting reflex.

Treatment for chronic fatigue syndrome is aimed at relieving your symptoms. Anti-inflammatory pain relievers, such as ibuprofen, often are prescribed, but they rarely help. Low doses of certain antidepressants may help relieve pain and the depression that often is present with a chronic illness. Because people with chronic fatigue syndrome may become deconditioned, perpetuating the fatigue, physical therapy is crucial. It can help prevent or decrease the muscle weakness that is caused by prolonged inactivity. You may benefit from counseling to help you deal with the illness and the limitations it creates.

Fever

Even when you're well, your temperature varies, and that variation is normal. We consider 98.6 F (37 C) a healthy body temperature. But, your "normal" temperature may differ by a degree or more.

In the morning your temperature is generally lower, and in the afternoon it's somewhat higher. Check your family members' temperatures when they're healthy. Discover their "normal" range.

What Is the Cause?

Fever itself is not an illness, but it is often a sign of one. A fever tells you that something is happening inside your body.

Most likely, your body is fighting an infection caused by either bacteria or a virus. The fever may even be helpful in fighting the infection. Rarely, it's a sign of a reaction to a medicine, an inflammatory condition or too much heat. Sometimes you don't know why you have a fever. But don't automatically try to lower your temperature. Decreasing it may mask symptoms, prolong an illness and delay identifying the cause.

You usually will know what caused a fever in a day or two. If you think it's something other than a viral illness, consult your health-care professional. Other common causes of fever include the following:

- An infection, such as urinary tract infection (frequent or painful urination), strep throat or tonsillitis (often with a sore throat), sinus infection (pain above or beneath the eyes) or dental abscess (tender area in the mouth)
- Infectious mononucleosis, accompanied by fatigue
- An illness you picked up in a foreign country
- Heat exhaustion or severe sunburn

Caution

Never give a child or young adult aspirin for a fever unless directed by your doctor. Rarely, aspirin causes a serious or even fatal disease called Reye's syndrome if given during a viral infection.

Self-Care

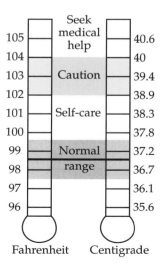

Drink plenty of water to avoid dehydration (because the body loses more water with a fever) and get enough rest.

- **For children and adults with temperatures less than 102 F (38.9 C):**
  - Normally, avoid using medicine for a new fever in this range.
  - Wear comfortable, light clothing and cover yourself with only a sheet or light blanket
- **For children and adults with temperatures between 102 F (38.9 C) and 104 F (40 C):**
  - Give adults or children acetaminophen (Tylenol or generic brand) or ibuprofen (Advil, Motrin or generic), according to the label instructions. Adults may use aspirin instead. Do not give children aspirin.
- **For children and adults with temperatures more than 104 F (40 C):**
  - Give adults or children acetaminophen (Tylenol or generic) or ibuprofen (Advil, Motrin or generic), following the manufacturer's instructions. Adults may use aspirin instead.
  - A sponge bath of lukewarm water may bring the temperature down.
  - Recheck the temperature every half hour.

| **Medical Help** | Call your health-care provider about a fever in any of the following situations: |

- Your temperature is more than 104 F (40 C)
- A baby younger than 3 months whose temperature is 100.5 F (38 C) or higher
- Your temperature has been more than 101 F (38.3 C) for more than 3 days

A fever is only one sign of the illness. Tell the physician what contagious diseases people around you have, including flu, colds, measles or mumps.

Call your health-care provider **immediately** if any of these symptoms accompany a fever:

- A severe headache
- Severe swelling of the throat
- Unusual eye sensitivity to bright light
- Significant stiff neck and pain when you bend your head forward
- Mental confusion
- Persistent vomiting
- Difficulty breathing
- Extreme listlessness or irritability
- A bulging soft spot on a baby's head

Kids' Care

An unexplained fever is a greater cause for concern in children than in adults. A rapid rise or fall in temperature causes a seizure in about 1 in 20 children younger than 4. It generally lasts less than 10 minutes. It usually causes no permanent damage. If a seizure occurs, lay your child on his or her side and hold the child to prevent trauma. Don't place anything in the mouth or try to stop the seizure.

Sometimes a fever accompanies teething. Fever with ear pulling often indicates a middle ear infection. Ask your doctor about fevers associated with shots.

It's usually easier to give medications in liquid form. For a small child, use a syringe with measurements on the side and a bulb on the tip. Gently squirt the medicine in the back corners of the child's mouth.

Encourage children to drink ample water, juice and sugared pop or to eat frozen ice pops.

Taking Temperatures

Several types of thermometers are available: glass-type mercury thermometers, electronic thermometers and tympanic (ear) thermometers. Use disposable temperature strips cautiously; they are often inaccurate.

The most accurate thermometers are the old-fashioned glass type. Learn to read your thermometer, following these steps:

- Clean it with soapy, cool water or alcohol.
- Hold it firmly between two fingers. Flick your wrist to shake the mercury indicator to less than 98.6 F (37 C), ideally down to 92 F.
- **Oral thermometer:** Place the bulb under your tongue. Close your mouth for 3 minutes.

Remove the thermometer and rotate it slowly until you can read the temperature.

- You also can use an oral thermometer for an armpit reading (hold the arms across the chest). Wait 5 minutes. Add 1° to the temperature to convert to an approximate oral temperature.
- **Rectal thermometer** (for infants): Place a dab of petroleum jelly on the bulb. Lay your child on his or her stomach. Carefully insert the bulb 1/2 to 1 inch into the rectum. Hold the bulb and child still for 3 minutes. Subtract 1° from the temperature to convert to an approximate oral temperature.

Pain

Physical pain is a part of life. Perhaps you've slammed your finger in a door, burnt your hand touching the hot handle of a pan on the stove or twisted your ankle while playing your favorite sport. The result is a sensation of pain.

A great deal of the pain you experience in life may be intense, but it is usually short-lived. It may last only moments or might continue for days or weeks, depending on the severity of the injury and how long it takes to heal. Most of the time, however, the pain eventually does go away. This type of temporary pain is known as **acute pain**.

When pain lasts long after the normal healing process, or when there does not seem to be any past injury or bodily damage causing ongoing pain, it is known as **chronic pain.** Generally, chronic pain is considered to be pain that lasts more than 3 months. A 1996 survey of employees in the United States indicated that more than two-thirds of workers have chronic or repeated episodes of pain—more than 80 million people. This type of pain resulted in employees taking nearly 50 million sick days during 1995.

Chronic pain can be overwhelming. But you can learn ways to manage your pain so that your life can be more fulfilling and enjoyable, and you can still carry out your daily activities. Your attitude about your pain, along with medications and therapies, can help you to control it. An important part of managing your pain is understanding it.

Why Doesn't the Pain Stop?

When your body is injured or infected, special nerve endings in your skin, joints, muscles or internal organs send messages to your brain telling it that there has been damage or unpleasant stimulus to your body. Certain nerve fibers instantaneously tell your brain where the pain is, how badly it hurts and how it feels (such as, it is sharp, burning or throbbing). Your brain then "reads" these pain signals and sends back a message to stop you from doing whatever is causing the pain. If you are touching something hot, for example, your brain will send a message to your muscles to contract so that you will pull back your hand.

Your brain also sends a message to your nerve cells to stop sending pain signals once the cause of the pain goes away (for example, when your injury starts to heal). But sometimes this mechanism fails, like a gate that is blocked open. For some reason, your nervous system continues to fire pain signals to your brain for months or even years after the injury heals, or even when there has been no bodily damage. The result is chronic pain.

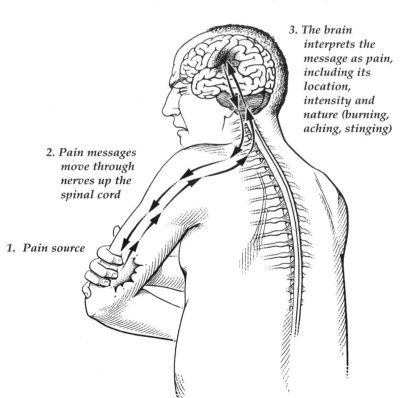

3. The brain interprets the message as pain, including its location, intensity and nature (burning, aching, stinging)

2. Pain messages move through nerves up the spinal cord

1. Pain source

The Role of Emotions in Pain

There is no exact definition for pain. Everybody perceives it differently. Pain is not only a physical experience but also an emotional one. Part of how you interpret and react to your pain is the result of your personal experience and upbringing.

If you learned to ignore or work through pain, for example, it may have less of an effect on you than if you grew up in a family where people talked a lot about the pain they were in and how much they were suffering.

When you experience pain for a long time, it can also increase your level of frustration and irritability and can lead to feelings of depression. You might also fall into a "sick role." This feeling of being a victim of your pain might bring you more attention and relieve you of some responsibilities, but eventually it also can cause you to become more inactive and isolated and even increase your perception of pain. This pain behavior can become a habit. Stress and unhappiness also tend to amplify pain and lessen your tolerance to pain. Finding positive ways to cope with your pain can have physical and emotional benefits.

Common Forms of Chronic Pain

Chronic pain is often debilitating, but still treatable. Many techniques exist. The key to pain control is a careful review of causes and a coordinated approach to management. Early and effective treatment of acute pain, such as after an operation or after a bout of shingles, often can prevent chronic pain. But, if you have chronic pain, there's still hope. Some of the common forms of chronic pain are listed below.

Low back pain: More people have low back pain than any other form of chronic pain. It is caused most frequently by muscular stress or wear due to overuse, injury or poor body mechanics. (See Back and Neck Pain, page 46.)

Cancer pain: Most of the pain you experience with cancer results from the pressure of a growing tumor or the spreading of tumor cells into bones, tissues or other organs. As a result, the pain can increase as the illness progresses. Although they often relieve pain, radiation treatment or chemotherapy also can generate pain. In addition, pain can become worse if you are anxious or depressed. (See Cancer, page 164.)

Headache pain: The most common type of head pain is the so-called tension headache. However, doctors are not certain this is caused by actual muscle tension. The start or worsening of tension headaches is not always related to stressful events. The throbbing pain of migraine headaches may be related to changes in the blood vessels in your head. Genetics, medications, alcohol, certain foods, exertion and anxiety or depression may provoke this kind of headache. (See Headache, page 78.)

Arthritis pain: Arthritis is the general name for affliction of the joints. Osteoarthritis, which usually affects the joints in the knees, hands, hips and spine has no known cause. Rheumatoid arthritis involves inflammation of the tissue around and in the joints and typically affects the hands and feet. (See Arthritis, page 157.)

Rheumatism: Although the term is no longer used, rheumatism refers to generalized aching in most parts of the body. Rheumatism, when confined to the joints, is classified as arthritis.

Neuropathic pain: This pain is caused by damage to your nervous system and can be one of the most difficult types of pain to treat. Some people experience severe, stabbing pain in the cheek, lips, gums or chin on one side of the face. Another form of pain related to nerve damage follows an attack of shingles, which usually affects older adults. It causes burning, searing pain.

Stimulating Your Natural Pain Killers

Studies show that aerobic exercise can stimulate the release of endorphins, your body's own natural pain killers. Endorphins are morphine-like pain relievers that send "stop pain" messages to your nerve cells. Duration of exercise seems to be more important than intensity. Doing low-intensity aerobic exercises for 30 to 45 minutes at a time 5 or 6 days a week may produce an effect. Be sure to build up slowly. Even 3 or 4 days of exercise a week may have some effect.

If you begin an exercise program more vigorous than walking, you should have a medical evaluation if:
- You are older than 40
- You have been sedentary
- You have risk factors for coronary artery disease (see page 172)
- You have chronic health problems

Self-Care

Once serious diseases have been excluded or treated, ask your doctor about the following options:
- **Stay active.** Focus on the things you can do. Try new hobbies and activities. Exercise daily. An activity that initially causes some pain doesn't necessarily cause further damage or worsen chronic pain. If you have arthritis, exercise can improve the range of motion in your joints. Exercises for your back and abdominal muscles may help relieve or even prevent back pain. Begin slowly. Work up to 20 to 30 minutes three or four times a week.
- **Focus on others.** When you pay more attention to the needs of others, you focus less on your own difficulties. Get involved in community, church or other volunteer activities.
- **Accept your pain.** Don't deny or exaggerate how you feel, but be clear and honest with others about your current capabilities. Be practical about what you can accomplish, and let people know when you are overcommitted.
- **Stay healthy.** Eat and sleep on a regular schedule. Reduce the use of stimulants, such as caffeine and nicotine, that may intensify some kinds of pain.
- **Relax.** Muscle tension increases your awareness of pain. Traditional techniques such as massage or enjoying a whirlpool bath can promote muscle relaxation and general comfort. Learn relaxation skills, such as controlled-breathing exercises and visualization. (See Keeping Stress Under Control, page 210.)
- **Keep a pain diary.** A pain diary can be helpful when you are communicating with your doctor about pain.
  - Write a detailed description of your pain while you are having it.
  - Describe the location, intensity and frequency of your pain and what makes your pain better or worse.
  - Use words such as stinging, penetrating, dull, throbbing, achy, nagging or gnawing to describe the quality of your pain.
  - Note what days or time of day the pain is better or worse.

Medical Help

You should see a physician again if pain does not lessen in 4 to 6 weeks, if the pain changes in character or if you have new symptoms.

Using Pain-Relieving Medications Safely

Some over-the-counter medications can be effective for relieving chronic pain. Drugs such as aspirin, ibuprofen and acetaminophen can provide pain relief by stopping the production of certain hormones in your nervous system which carry pain signals to your brain.

Follow these recommendations for using pain medications safely at home:

- Read the label and follow all instructions, cautions and warnings. Never use more than the maximal recommended dose.
- Unless a doctor recommends it, adults should not use pain medication for more than 10 days in a row. The limit for children and teenagers is 5 days.
- Don't take aspirin during the last 3 months of pregnancy unless your doctor recommends it. Aspirin can cause bleeding in both the mother and the child. Children should not take aspirin unless directed to do so by a physician.
- If you are allergic to aspirin, check with your doctor or pharmacist about which pain relievers you can use safely.
- For more on pain medications, see page 230.

■ Chronic Pain Programs

When standard treatments for chronic pain have failed, you may benefit from a pain clinic or pain management center. Before entering a program, you should undergo a thorough physical examination to exclude an unrecognized problem (such as diabetes or cancer) that may be responsible for your pain. Chronic pain programs may use one or a combination of the following treatment approaches:

Comprehensive: Physical and occupational therapy, behavior modification, group interaction, educational experiences, biofeedback and counseling are the mainstays of this type of program. This treatment approach emphasizes the elimination of medications and the initiation of physical activity to gain independence from chronic pain.

Symptom-oriented: This approach focuses on a single form of pain, such as headaches or backache. Clinics that use this approach typically offer an array of treatments that address a specific type of pain.

Treatment-oriented: This type of program emphasizes specific forms of therapy, such as neurosurgery or nerve blocks, which may be appropriate courses of treatment for several types of pain.

Chronic pain programs may offer both inpatient and outpatient services. They usually have a multidisciplinary approach, which means many specialists are involved with the patient's care. When inquiring about a program, ask about its success rate, insurance coverage and follow-up services.

FOR MORE INFORMATION

- American Pain Society, 4700 W. Lake Avenue, Glenview, IL 60025-1485; (847) 375-4715, fax (847) 375-4777, or E-mail aps@dial.cic.net.
- American Chronic Pain Association, P.O. Box 850, Rocklin, CA 95677; (916) 632-0922, fax (916) 632-3208, or E-mail ACPA@pacbell.net.

Sleep Disorders

◼ Insomnia

The most common of 60 or more sleep disorders is insomnia. Insomnia includes difficulty going to sleep, staying asleep or going back to sleep when you awaken early. It may be temporary or chronic. Insomnia is a symptom, not a disease.

Common causes include the following:

- Stress related to work, school, health or family concerns
- Depression
- Use of stimulants (caffeine or nicotine), herbal supplements and over-the-counter and prescription medications
- Alcohol
- Change in environment or work schedule
- Long-term use of sleep medications
- Chronic medical problems, including fibromyalgia or complex diseases of the nerves and muscles
- Behavioral insomnia, which may occur when you worry excessively about not being able to sleep well and try too hard to fall asleep. Most people with this condition sleep better when they're away from their usual sleep environment.

Sleep Cycle

Light Sleep
Body movement decreases. Spontaneous awakening may occur.

REM (Rapid Eye Movement)
Dreaming occurs. Heart rate increases. Lasts about 10 minutes in first cycle, 20-30 minutes in later cycles.

Typically , you have four to six sleep cycles, lasting 70-90 minutes each per night. At the end of each cycle, you are nearly awake.

Intermediate Sleep
Most of the night is spent in this stage. Helps refresh body.

Deep Sleep
Difficult to arouse. Most restorative stage, lasting 30-40 minutes in first few cycles, less in later cycles.

Self-Care

- Establish and follow a ritual for going to bed.
- Avoid afternoon or evening naps.
- Avoid strenuous exercise right before bedtime. However, moderate exercise 4 to 6 hours before bedtime is helpful.
- Limit activities in bed to sex and sleep. Don't read or watch TV.
- Set aside a "worry time" during the day.
- Don't take work materials to bed.
- Take a warm bath 1 to 2 hours before bedtime.
- Drink a glass of milk, warm or cold. A light snack is fine, but don't eat a large snack or meal or consume alcohol close to bedtime.
- Keep your sleeping environment dark, quiet and comfortably cool. If necessary, use eye covers.
- Try relaxation exercises (see page 211).
- Lower or eliminate use of stimulants. Check medication labels for caffeine.
- Do not smoke before bedtime.
- If you still can't sleep, get up. Stay up until you feel tired, and then return to bed. But, as a result, do not shift your rising time.
- Keep a sleep diary. If, after a week or two, you still can't sleep, see your physician. Tests may uncover the cause of your insomnia.

Kids' Care

Bedwetting (enuresis) is the most common reason children ages 3 to 15 wake up at night. Contact the National Enuresis Society (1-800-NES-8080) for helpful suggestions.

Nightmares may be a response to stress or trauma that occurs during waking hours. Calmly reassure your child after an incident.

Night terrors generally occur between ages 3 and 5, and they tend to run in families. Sleepers may awaken screaming, with no recollection of a dream. Emotional tension increases night terrors.

Sleepwalking may include opening doors, going to the bathroom, dressing or undressing. This runs in families and is most common in children ages 6 to 12.

Should You Nap, or Not?

The urge for a mid-day snooze is built into your body's biologic clock. This typically occurs between 1 p.m. and 4 p.m., as indicated by a slight dip in your body temperature.

Napping is not a substitute for a full night's sleep. Don't nap if sleeping at night is a problem. If you find a nap refreshes you and doesn't interfere with nighttime sleep, try these ideas:

- **Keep it short.** A half-hour nap is ideal. Naps longer than an hour or two are more likely to interfere with your nighttime sleep.
- **Take a mid-afternoon nap.** Naps at this time produce a physically invigorating slumber.
- **If you can't nap, just rest.** Lie down and keep your mind on something else.

■ Other Sleep Disorders

Recurrent episodes of breathing stoppage during sleep (sleep apnea): People with this problem snore and stop breathing for short periods, from which they emerge with a jerk or gasp. Sleep apnea may occur when an upper airway is blocked by enlarged adenoids or nasal polyps or as a result of previous nose fractures. If you have these symptoms, see your doctor. It may help to lose weight, sleep on your stomach or side, avoid consuming alcohol before bedtime and use nasal decongestants, but only under the guidance of a physician.

Grinding or clenching your teeth during sleep (bruxism) may be associated with stress. Your dentist can check whether your bite needs adjustment and provide you with a plastic guard to prevent further damage. Attempt to deal with the source of your tension. Learn relaxation skills (see page 211).

Excessive sleepiness may be controlled by getting plenty of sleep at night, taking a daytime nap and eating light or vegetarian meals, especially before important activities. Use caffeinated drinks (coffee, tea and colas) to keep you awake. If you still need help, your physician may prescribe a stimulant after appropriate testing.

Restless legs is the irresistible urge to move your legs and can occur shortly after you go to bed or throughout the night, interfering with your ability to get to sleep or stay asleep. Stress often makes the condition worse. Get up and walk around. Try muscle relaxation techniques and a warm bath before bedtime. If your condition is severe, see your physician.

FOR MORE INFORMATION

- National Sleep Foundation, 1367 Connecticut Ave. N.W., Suite 200, Washington, DC 20036; (202) 785-2300.

Sweating and Body Odor

Sweating is the body's normal response to the buildup of body heat. Sweating varies widely from person to person. Many women perspire more heavily during menopause. Drinking hot beverages, or those containing alcohol or caffeine, can cause temporary increases in sweating.

For most of us, sweating is only a minor nuisance. But for some people, sweaty armpits, feet and hands are a major dilemma. Sweat is basically odorless, but it may take on an unpleasant or offensive odor when bacteria multiply and break down the body's secretions into odor-causing by-products. Odor may be influenced by mood, activity, hormones and food, such as caffeine.

A "cold sweat" is usually the body's response to a serious illness, anxiety or severe pain. A cold sweat should receive immediate medical attention if there are signs of light-headedness or chest and stomach pains.

Self-Care	• **Wear clothing made of natural materials,** especially cotton, next to the skin.
	• **Bathe daily.** Antibacterial soaps may help, but they can be irritating.
	• **Try over-the-counter products,** such as antiperspirant sprays and lotions, that contain aluminum chlorhydrate or buffered aluminum sulfate.
	• **For sweaty feet,** choose shoes made of natural materials that breathe, such as leather. Wear the right socks. Cotton and wool socks can help keep your feet dry because they absorb moisture. Socks made of acrylic, a synthetic material, keep moisture away from your feet. Change your socks or hosiery once or twice a day, drying your feet thoroughly each time. Dry your feet thoroughly after a bath. Microorganisms thrive in the damp spaces between your toes. Use over-the-counter foot powders to help absorb sweat. Air out your feet. Go without shoes when it's sensible. But when you can't, slip out of them from time to time. Women should try pantyhose with cotton soles.
	• **For sweaty armpits,** use antiperspirants. If irritation remains a problem, a 0.5 percent hydrocortisone cream (available without prescription) can help.
	• **Apply antiperspirants nightly** at bedtime to sweaty palms or soles of feet. Try perfume-free antiperspirants.
	• **Try iontophoresis.** This procedure, in which a low current of electricity is delivered to the affected body part with a battery-powered device, may help. However, it may be no more effective than a topical antiperspirant.
	• **Eliminate caffeine and other stimulants** from your diet, as well as foods with strong odors such as garlic and onions.

Medical Help

Your doctor may recommend a prescription antiperspirant. For a few people, surgery may help. The operation removes the troublesome sweat glands. However, this is appropriate for only a few people who have persistent soreness and irritation caused by antiperspirants or excessive sweating.

Consult your doctor if there's an increase in sweating or nighttime sweating without an obvious cause. Infections, thyroid gland dysfunction and certain forms of cancer may produce unusual sweating patterns.

Excessive sweating associated with shortness of breath requires immediate action. This could be a sign of a heart attack.

Occasionally, a change in odor signals a disease. A fruity smell may be a sign of diabetes, or an ammonia-like smell could be a sign of liver disease.

Unexpected Weight Changes

In most cases, the reasons for change in weight are obvious. Changes in diet or activity are the usual explanations. However, physical illness also can affect your weight. An unexpected weight change of 5 to 10 percent of your body weight (7 1/2 to 15 pounds for a 150-pound person) in 6 or fewer months is significant. If you lose or gain weight and can't point to a reason, or if you are losing or gaining weight very rapidly, talk to your health-care provider.

■ Weight Gain

Are you overweight? Refer to the discussion of normal weight and body mass indicator on page 196.

Weight gain is the most common scenario in adulthood. It's usually a gradual creep—a few pounds a year. Careful diet and regular exercise can stop this trend. If you've experienced a rapid gain, consider these possible causes:

1. Diet changes—increased intake of alcohol or soda, a new favorite high-fat food such as ice cream, sweet rolls or fried foods, increased snacking, a switch to fast foods or prepared foods.
2. Decrease in activity—an injury restricting movement, a switch from an active to a sedentary job or a change in a routine such as using stairs or walking to work.
3. New medication—some medicines may contribute to weight gain. Some antidepressants and some hormones, including estrogen, progesterone and cortisone, may produce weight gain.
4. Changes in mood—excessive anxiety, stress or depression can affect activity and food intake. (See Depression and the "Blues," page 188.)
5. Fluid retention—medical conditions such as heart or kidney failure or thyroid conditions cause fluid buildup. Have you noted puffiness of the tissues—tight rings or shoes, progressive swelling of the ankles as the day progresses, unusual shortness of breath or new, frequent trips to the bathroom at night?

Self-Care

If item 1 or 2 listed above applies to you, change your diet and increase your activity. (See Weight: What's Right for You, page 194.) Wait 4 to 6 weeks to see if the changes work. If they don't affect your weight, or if item 3, 4 or 5 applies to you, then see your doctor.

■ Weight Loss

Unexplained weight loss of 5 to 10 percent of your body weight over 6 or fewer months is usually cause for concern, but occasionally it's not. Consider the following causes:

1. Change in diet—skipping meals, eating on the run, a significant reduction in fat intake, a change in meal preparation methods, a change in routines around mealtime, eating alone.
2. Change in activity—job change, from sedentary to active, new exercise program, busy or hectic schedule, seasonal variation.
3. New medication—some antidepressants, stimulants—prescription or over-the-counter (caffeine, herbals).

4. Mood changes—anxiety, stress and depression also can cause weight loss (see page 188).
5. Other medical conditions—dental problems; diabetes with thirst or increased urination; digestive disorders such as malabsorption or ulcer with abdominal pain; inflammatory bowel diseases, such as Crohn's or colitis, causing diarrhea and bloody stools; infections such as HIV, AIDS or tuberculosis; cancer of many types.

Self-Care

If item 1 or 2 listed above applies to you, but none of the other items seem to fit, modify your diet. Eat three balanced meals. For snacks, or when you can't eat a good meal, try a nutritional supplement drink. Instant breakfasts are simple, fairly balanced and less expensive than prepared supplements. If you haven't reversed the weight loss trend in 2 weeks, or if item 3, 4 or 5 seems to fit, see your doctor without delay.

Kids' Care

Weight loss or failure to grow in children may be caused by a digestive problem that prevents important nutrients from being digested or absorbed. Loss of these nutrients can lead to bony changes and other problems. Your child also may have an eating disorder. If your child has unexplained weight loss, consult your child's health-care provider.

Eating Disorders: Anorexia Nervosa and Bulimia Nervosa

Anorexia nervosa is an eating disorder that can lead to drastic weight loss as a result of self-imposed semistarvation. A person with bulimia nervosa is often at normal weight but uses binge-eating and purging as a means of weight control. Both disorders are most common in adolescent girls and young women, but they also can occur in males and older individuals.

The number of people affected by anorexia and bulimia has increased as society has placed more emphasis on being thin and attractive. Decreasing this emphasis and not placing unrealistic expectations on adolescents may be steps in curbing this trend. If you suspect an eating disorder in yourself or others, contact your health-care provider.

Anorexia Nervosa

Symptoms and signs:
● Misperception of body image—the person sees herself as being fatter than she is
● Unrealistic fear of becoming fat
● Excessive dieting and exercise
● Significant weight loss or failure to gain weight during a period of growth
● Refusal to maintain a normal body weight
● Absence of menstrual periods
● Preoccupation with food, calories and food preparation

The cause of anorexia nervosa is unclear, but biologic and psychological factors may be involved. Total recovery is possible if the disorder is diagnosed early. Left untreated, anorexia can lead to death. Treatment involves psychotherapy, diet counseling and family counseling in most cases. Hospitalization may be needed in severe cases.

Bulimia Nervosa

Symptoms and signs:
● Recurrent episodes of binge eating
● Self-induced vomiting or laxative abuse
● Weight usually within fairly normal range
● Fear of becoming fat

Bulimia involves eating large amounts of food and then purging by vomiting or abusing laxatives. It is also a form of semistarvation. Purging depletes water and potassium from the body and can lead to death. People with bulimia often become depressed because they realize that their eating is abnormal. Treatment usually includes behavior modification, psychotherapy and, in some cases, antidepressant medication. Hospitalization may be needed if the disorder is out of control and there are physical complications.

Common Problems by Body System

- **Back and Neck**

- **Digestive System**

- **Ears and Hearing**

- **Eyes and Vision**

- **Headache**

- **Limbs, Muscles, Bones and Joints**

- **Lungs, Chest and Breathing**

- **Nose and Sinuses**

- **Skin, Hair and Nails**

- **Throat and Mouth**

- **Men's Health**

- **Women's Health**

In medicine, there is a saying, "Common things are common." In other words, most pains and ailments are not serious. Often, simple remedies in combination with time can help resolve the problem and save you a trip to the doctor. Of course, if the problem persists or if simple remedies don't help, you need to seek medical care.

This section is organized by body system. Each chapter includes several illnesses or symptoms with appropriate self-care advice and directives on when to see your doctor. Sidebar articles (with light gray shading in the background) address related topics or offer insight into medical issues. We pay special attention to children's health where appropriate throughout the section.

Back and Neck

Almost everyone has a back problem at some time. Back pain sends many people to health-care providers each year. Fortunately, you can do things to prevent back problems. And you can do them most effectively if you know a little bit about your back.

Your back supports your body. It holds and protects your spinal cord and nerves that send signals back and forth from your brain to the rest of your body. And it serves as a place of attachment for muscles and ligaments of the back.

A Bit of Anatomy

Your spine, or so-called backbone, is not one bone, but many. If you look at a healthy spine from the side, it curves inward at your neck and lower back and outward at your upper back and pelvis.

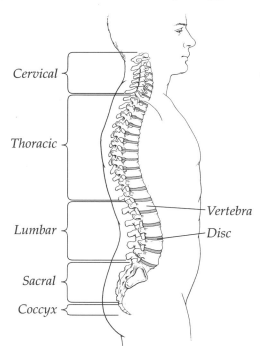

Cervical

Thoracic

Lumbar

Sacral

Coccyx

Vertebra

Disc

Vertebrae: The backbone, or vertebral column, is composed of bones called vertebrae, which are held together by tough, fibrous bands called ligaments. The normal adult vertebral column consists of 7 cervical (neck) vertebrae, 12 thoracic (middle back) vertebrae, and 5 large lumbar (lower back) vertebrae. The lumbar vertebrae are the largest because they bear most of the body weight. The sacrum, made from five vertebrae that are fused together, is below the lumbar vertebrae. The last three vertebrae, also fused together, are called the coccyx or tailbone.

Spinal cord: The spinal cord, part of the central nervous system, extends from the base of the skull to the lower back. Two nerves (called spinal nerves) are sent out at each vertebral level. In the upper lumbar part of the back where the spinal cord ends, a group of nerves (called the cauda equina) continue down the spinal canal. The spinal nerves exit from openings (foramina) on either side of the vertebrae, one leading to the right side of the body and the other to the left. In all, there are 31 pairs of these spinal nerves in the back and neck.

Discs: Between the vertebrae, and close to the point of exit of each pair of spinal nerves, are intervertebral discs. These disks serve as cushions or "shock absorbers" between the vertebrae, preventing the hard and bony vertebrae from hitting one another when we walk, run or jump. A disc is made up of a ring of tough, fibrous tissue that has a jelly-like substance in the center. Damaged outer disc rings may result in a protruded, herniated or ruptured disc (see page 49). This produces pressure on nerves or surrounding tissues, causing pain. (A disc does not actually "slip" because it is firmly attached between the vertebrae.)

Muscles: Muscles are elastic bands up and down your back which support your spine. They contract or relax to help you stand, twist, bend or stretch. Tendons connect muscles to bones. The muscles of your abdomen and trunk support, protect and move your spine.

With age your spine may become stiff and lose its flexibility. Discs become worn, and the spaces between your vertebrae narrow. These changes are part of the aging process, but they are not necessarily painful. Vertebrae sometimes develop jutting bone spurs, which also may or may not produce pain. As the cartilage that cushions joints wears out, bones rub together and you experience the pain of arthritis. But often it's hard to pinpoint the cause of back pain because of the back's complexity.

■ Common Back Problems

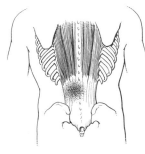

Your lower back, a pivot point for turning at your waist, is vulnerable to muscle strains.

Your lower back carries most of your weight. It's the site of most back pain for people between the ages of 20 and 50. But strains and sprains can injure any part of your neck or back. The most common sources of back pain are one or more strained (overstretched) muscles or sprained (overstretched) ligaments. The cause may be:

- Improper lifting (see Lifting Properly, page 50)
- A sudden, strenuous physical effort; an accident, sports injury or fall
- Lack of muscle tone
- Excess weight, especially around your middle
- Your sleeping position, especially if you sleep on your stomach
- A pillow that forces your neck into an awkward angle
- Sitting in one position a long time; poor sitting and standing postures
- Holding the telephone with your shoulder
- Carrying a heavy briefcase, purse or shoulder bag
- Sitting with a thick wallet in your back pocket
- Holding a forward-bending position for a long time
- Daily stress and tension
- Normal or excessive weight gain during pregnancy

"No Pain, No Gain" —Not True!

You may become sore immediately after you've injured a muscle, or it may take several hours before it feels sore. An injured muscle may uncontrollably tighten or "knot up" (a muscle spasm). Your body is telling you to slow down and prevent further injury. A severe muscle spasm may last 48 to 72 hours, followed by days or weeks of less severe pain. Strenuous use of an injured muscle during the next 3 to 6 weeks may bring back the pain. However, most back pain is gone in 6 weeks.

As you age, muscle tone tends to decrease, and your back is more prone to aches or injury. Maintaining your flexibility and strength and keeping your abdominal muscles strong are your best bets to avoid back problems. Spending 10 to 15 minutes a day doing gentle stretching and strengthening exercises can help a lot.

Self-Care

Healing will occur most quickly if you can continue your usual activities in a gentle manner while avoiding what may have caused the pain in the first place. Avoid long periods of bed rest, which can worsen your pain and make you weaker.

With proper care of a strain or sprain, you should notice steady improvement within the first 2 weeks. Most back pain is much better in 6 weeks. Sprained ligaments or severe muscle strains may take up to 12 weeks to heal. Once you have back pain, you're more prone to experience repeated painful episodes.

Follow these home care steps:
- Use cold packs initially to relieve pain. Wrap an ice pack or a bag of frozen vegetables in a piece of cloth. Hold it on the sore area for 15 minutes four times a day. To avoid frostbite, never place ice directly on your skin.
- You may be most comfortable lying with your back on the floor, hips and knees bent and legs elevated. Get plenty of rest, but avoid prolonged bed rest—more than a day or two may slow recovery. Moderate movement keeps your muscles strong and flexible. Avoid the activity that caused the sprain or strain. Avoid heavy lifting, pushing or pulling, repetitive bending and twisting.

Common Problems

Self-Care *(continued)*

- After 48 hours, you may use heat to relax sore or knotted muscles. Use a warm bath, warm packs, a heating pad or a heat lamp. Be careful not to burn your skin with extreme heat. But if you find that cold provides more relief than heat, you can continue using cold, or try a combination of the two methods.
- Gradually begin gentle stretching exercises. Avoid jerking, bouncing or any movements that increase pain or require straining.
- Use over-the-counter pain medications (see page 231).
- Massage may be helpful, especially for muscle spasms, but avoid placing any pressure directly on your spine.
- If you must stand or sit much of the day, you may consider using a support brace or corset. Worn properly, they may relieve your pain and provide warmth, comfort and support. However, relying on this type of support for a long time, rather than using your muscles, may actually weaken your muscles.

Medical Help

If your back or neck pain hasn't improved noticeably after 72 hours of self-care, contact your health-care provider.

Seek medical care *immediately* if your pain:
- Is severe or tearing in quality.
- Results from a fall or blow to your back. Do not try to move someone who has severe neck pain or can't move his or her legs after an accident. Moving the person can cause further injury.
- Produces weakness or numbness in one or both legs.
- Is new and is accompanied by an unexplained fever.
- Results from an injury that causes pain from your neck to shoot down your arms and legs.
- You also need to seek medical care *immediately* if you have one of the following conditions: poorly controlled blood pressure, cancer, an abdominal aortic aneurysm or a new loss of bowel or bladder control.

The nerves to most of your body travel through your back. Sometimes, back or neck pain may be caused by a problem somewhere else in your body. Your physician may do testing to determine the cause of your pain.

Kids' Care

Low back pain is unusual in children before their teen years. Common causes for back pain are sports injuries or falls. Be sure that your children's athletic programs:
- Use the proper protective equipment
- Have competent coaches
- Use sufficient warmup and conditioning activities

If your injured child has not been unconscious, can move freely and has no numbness or weakness, use the self-care tips listed on page 47. Be careful to avoid excessive heat or cold. Check proper children's doses for over-the-counter medicines. Do not give children aspirin.

If the pain is unrelated to an injury or other known cause, your health-care provider may want to check for an infection (especially if your child has a fever) or for factors in your child's development which may cause the pain. Girls often experience lower back pain with their menstrual period.

Warning signs of serious back problems in children younger than 11 include constant pain that lasts for several weeks or occurs spontaneously at night; pain that interferes with school, play or sports; and pain that occurs with stiffness and fever.

Less Common Back Problems

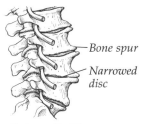

Osteoarthritis

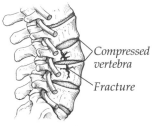

Compressed vertebra

Fracture

Osteoporosis

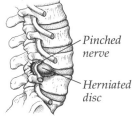

Pinched nerve

Herniated disc

Herniated disc

Back and neck problems often don't result from a single incident. They may be the product of a lifetime of stress and strain for your back and neck. If you have chronic back pain, your health-care provider may look for the following conditions:

Osteoarthritis affects nearly everyone older than 60. Excessive use, injury or aging slowly deteriorates cartilage, the protective tissue that covers the surface of vertebral joints. Discs between vertebrae become worn and the spaces between the bones narrow. Bony outgrowths called spurs also develop. Gradually, your spine stiffens and loses flexibility.

Osteoporosis is the weakening of your bone structure as the amount of calcium in your bones decreases. Weakened vertebrae become compressed and fracture easily. Modern drugs and hormone replacement therapy may slow or halt this process, once considered inevitable for women older than 50.

Herniated or so-called slipped disc occurs when normal wear and tear or exceptional strain causes a disc to rupture. Bulging of discs is common and often painless. It becomes painful when excessive bulging or fragments of the disc herniate or break off and place pressure on nearby nerves. This condition may lead to leg pain (sciatica, named for the sciatic nerve that extends down the back of each leg from your buttock to your heel). Symptoms from herniated discs may resolve over weeks.

Fibromyalgia is a chronic syndrome that produces achy pain, tenderness and stiffness in the muscles and joints where tendons attach to your bones. Pain is usually worse after inactivity and improves with movement.

Some back and neck problems are complex. Rarely is surgery the answer. Surgery is usually reserved for times when a nerve is pinched severely and threatens to cause permanent weakness or is affecting bowel or bladder control. Back pain without nerve injury is rarely a reason for surgery.

Back Injuries in the Workplace

You can avoid many back problems by following these guidelines (see Ergonomics, page 221, and Exercises for "Office Potatoes," page 222, for other ideas):

- Change positions often.
- Avoid high heels. If you stand for long periods, rest one foot on a small box or stool from time to time.
- Use adjustable equipment. Find comfortable (rather than extreme) positions.
- Don't bend continuously over your work. Hold reading materials at eye level.
- Avoid excessive repetition. Take frequent, short breaks to stretch or relax— even 30 seconds every 10 to 15 minutes helps.
- Avoid unnecessary bending, twisting and reaching.
- Stand to answer your phone. If you are on the phone a lot, get a headset.
- Adjust your chair so your feet are flat on the floor. Change leg positions often.
- Use a chair that supports your lower back's curve or place a rolled towel or pillow behind your lower back. The seat of your chair should not press on the back of your thighs or knees.
- Lift objects properly (see page 50).
- Carry objects close to the body at about waist level.

Preventing Common Backaches and Neck Pains

Regular exercise is your most powerful weapon against back and neck problems. Proper exercise can help you:

- Maintain or increase flexibility of muscles, tendons and ligaments
- Strengthen the muscles that support your back
- Increase muscle strength in your arms, legs and lower body to reduce the risk of falls and other injuries and allow optimal posture for lifting and carrying
- Improve your posture
- Increase bone density
- Shed excess pounds that stress your back

If you're over 40 or have an illness or injury, check with your health-care professional before you begin an exercise program. If you're out of condition, start slowly and increase gradually. Exercises that are good for your back include the following:

- Abdominal and leg strengthening exercises.
- Nonjarring exercise on a stationary bike, treadmill or cross-country skiing machine. Bicycling is good, but be sure your bike seat and handlebars are properly adjusted to keep you in a comfortable position.
- If you have back problems or are out of shape, avoid activities that involve quick stops and starts and a lot of twisting. High-impact activities on hard surfaces—like jogging, tennis, racquetball or basketball—may add wear and tear to your back. Avoid contact sports.

Lifting Properly

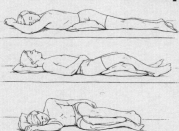

1   2   3

Follow these steps:
1. Position your feet firmly, toes pointed slightly outward, one foot slightly ahead of the other. Stand as close to the load as possible.
2. Bend from your knees, and use your powerful leg muscles to lift the load. Keep your back as upright as possible. As you lift, tighten the abdominal muscles that support your spine.
3. Hold the load close to your body. Avoid turning or twisting while holding the load. Avoid lifting heavy loads above your waist.

Proper Sleeping Positions

To avoid aggravating your backache when you sleep or lie down, sleep on your stomach only if your abdomen is cushioned by a pillow (top). If you sleep on your back, support your knees and neck with pillows (middle). Best option: sleep on your side with your legs drawn up slightly toward your chest with a pillow between your legs (bottom).

■ Your Daily Back Routine

Here are basic exercises to stretch and strengthen your back and supporting muscles. Try to work 15 minutes of exercise into your daily routine. (If you've hurt your back before, or if you have other health problems such as osteoporosis, get medical advice before exercising.)

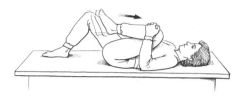

Knee to shoulder stretch: *Lie on your back on a firm surface with your knees bent and feet flat. Pull your left knee toward your chest with both hands. Hold for 15 to 30 seconds. Return to starting position. Repeat with opposite leg. Repeat with each leg three or four times.*

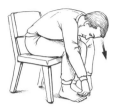

Chair stretch: *Sit in a chair. Slowly bend forward toward the floor until you feel a mild stretch in your back. Hold for 15 to 30 seconds. Repeat three or four times.*

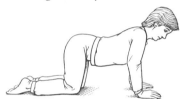

"Cat" stretch: *Step 1. Get down on your hands and knees. Slowly let your back and abdomen sag toward the floor.*

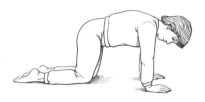

"Cat" stretch: *Step 2. Slowly arch your back away from the floor. Repeat several times.*

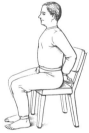

Shoulder blade squeeze: *Sit upright in a chair. Keep your chin tucked in and your shoulders down. Pull your shoulder blades together and straighten your upper back. Hold a few seconds. Return to starting position. Repeat several times.*

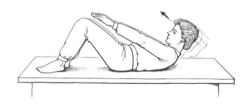

Half sit-up: *Lie on your back on a firm surface with your knees bent and feet flat. With your arms outstretched, reach toward your knees with your hands until your shoulder blades no longer touch the ground. Do not grasp your knees. Hold for a few seconds and slowly return to the starting position. Repeat several times.*

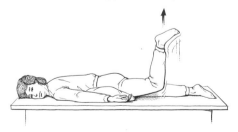

Leg lifts: *Step 1. Lie face down on a firm surface with a large pillow under your hips and lower abdomen. Keeping your knee bent, raise your leg slightly off the surface and hold for about 5 seconds. Repeat several times.*

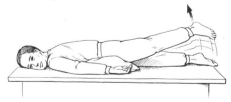

Leg lifts: *Step 2. With your leg straight, repeat the exercise. Raise one leg slightly off the surface and hold for about 5 seconds. Repeat several times.*

Digestive System

Your digestive tract is an extremely complex system. Problems can occur anywhere along this tract, upsetting its delicate balance. Because of the complexity of this system, you should not attempt to diagnose new problems, such as unexplained pain or bleeding, on your own.

Digestion begins when you chew your food. The food is broken into smaller pieces by your teeth and, at the same time, is mixed with saliva secreted by your salivary glands. Your saliva contains an enzyme that begins to change starches (carbohydrates) into sugars.

Food is propelled down your esophagus to the stomach and then on through the intestines by muscular contractions. This process, called digestion, is aided by digestive juices (acid, bile and enzymes) from the stomach, pancreas and gallbladder. They break down food and allow the nutrients to be absorbed. Undigestible food and bacteria are eliminated as feces from the rectum.

Gastrointestinal tract

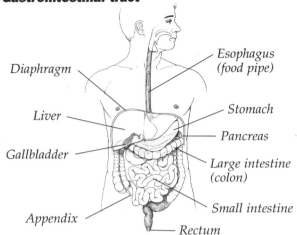

Diaphragm

Liver

Gallbladder

Appendix

Esophagus
(food pipe)

Stomach

Pancreas

Large intestine
(colon)

Small intestine

Rectum

■ Abdominal Pain

Pain in your abdomen can occur anywhere along your digestive tract, from your mouth or throat to your pelvis and rectum. In some cases, pain can signal a mild problem such as overeating. In others, it can be an early warning sign of a more serious disorder that may require medical treatment.

Fortunately, many forms of discomfort respond well to a combination of self-care and supervised medical treatment. See the following pages if your pain accompanies any of these conditions: constipation, page 54; diarrhea, page 55; excessive gas, page 56; gastritis, page 57; or hemorrhoids, page 58.

Caution

Although most abdominal pains are not serious, you should not attempt to diagnose the source of new or unexplained pain. Seek medical attention if you experience any of the following: intense pain lasting longer than a minute or pain that seems to be worsening; pain accompanied by shortness of breath or dizziness; pain accompanied by a temperature of 101 F or more.

What Is Appendicitis?

Your appendix is a worm-shaped structure that projects out from the large intestine. Although it has no known function or importance in humans, this tiny structure can become inflamed, swollen and filled with pus. This condition is called appendicitis.

Appendicitis typically causes acute pain that starts around your navel and settles in the lower right side of your abdomen. These symptoms generally progress over 12 to 24 hours. You also may experience a loss of appetite, nausea, vomiting and the urge to have a bowel movement or pass gas.

Although appendicitis can affect people of all ages, it usually occurs between the ages of 10 and 30.

An infected appendix may burst and cause a serious infection. Seek immediate medical attention if you suspect you have appendicitis.

■ Colic

Generations of families have dealt with colic. This frustrating and largely unexplainable condition affects babies who otherwise seem healthy. Colic usually peaks at 6 weeks of age and disappears in the baby's third or fourth month.

Colic is a difficult experience for everyone. One doctor describes colic as "when the baby's crying—and so is Mom."

Although the term "colic" is used widely for any fussy baby, true colic is determined by the following:

- **Predictable crying episodes:** A colicky baby cries at about the same time each day, usually in the evening. Colic episodes may last minutes or 2 or more hours.
- **Activity:** Many colicky babies pull their legs to their chests or thrash around during crying episodes as if they are in pain.
- **Intense or inconsolable crying:** Colicky babies cry more than usual and are extremely difficult—if not impossible—to comfort.

Doctors call colic a "diagnosis of exclusion," which means other possible problems are ruled out before determining the baby has colic. The parent of a colicky infant, therefore, can be assured that the crying is probably not a sign of a serious medical problem.

Studies of colic have focused on several possible causes: allergies, an immature digestive system, gas, hormones, mother's anxieties and handling. Still, it is unclear why some babies have colic and others don't.

Self-Care

If your health-care provider determines that your baby has colic, these measures may help you and your child find some relief:

- Lay your baby tummy-down on your knees or arms and sway your baby gently and slowly.
- Rock, cuddle or walk your baby. Avoid fast, jiggling movements.
- Play a steady, uninterrupted "white noise" near your baby. Motors with soft noise, such as a clothes dryer, may work.
- Put your baby in an infant swing.
- Give your baby a warm bath or lay him or her tummy-down on a warm water bottle.
- Try singing or humming while walking with or rocking the baby. A soothing song can have a quieting effect on both parent and baby.
- Take your baby for a car ride.
- Leave your baby with someone else for 10 minutes and walk alone.

Medical Help

At this time, there are no medications to relieve colic safely and effectively. In general, consult with your health-care provider before giving your baby any medication.

If you are worried that your baby is sick or if you or others caring for the baby are becoming frustrated or angry because of the crying, call your doctor or bring the baby to the office or emergency department.

Common Problems

■ Constipation

This common problem is often misunderstood and improperly treated. Technically speaking, constipation is the passage of hard stools fewer than three times a week. You also may experience a bloated sensation and occasional crampy discomfort. The normal frequency for bowel movements varies widely—from three bowel movements a day to three a week.

Constipation is a symptom, not a disease. Like a fever, this problem can occur when one of many factors slows the passage of food through your large bowel. These factors include inadequate fluid intake, poor diet, irregular bowel habits, age, lack of activity, pregnancy and illness. Various medications also can cause constipation.

Although constipation may be extremely bothersome, the condition itself usually is not serious. If it persists, however, constipation can lead to complications such as hemorrhoids and cracks or tears in the anus called fissures.

Self-Care

To lessen your chances of constipation:
- Try to eat on a regular schedule, and eat plenty of high-fiber foods, including fresh fruits, vegetables and whole-grain cereals and breads.
- Drink 8 to 10 glasses of water or other liquids daily.
- Increase your physical activity.
- Don't ignore the urge to have a bowel movement.
- Try fiber supplements such as Metamucil, Konsyl, Fiberall or Citrucel.
- Do not rely on laxatives (see below).

Medical Help

Contact your doctor if your constipation is severe or if it lasts longer than 3 weeks. In rare cases, constipation also may signal more serious medical conditions such as cancer, hormonal disturbances, heart disease or kidney failure.

Kids' Care

Constipation is not usually a problem among infants, especially if they are breast-feeding. A healthy breast-fed infant may have as few as one bowel movement a week.

Young children sometimes experience constipation because they neglect to take time to use the bathroom. Toddlers also may become constipated during toilet training because of a fear or unwillingness to use the toilet. However, as few as one bowel movement a week may be normal for your child.

If constipation is a problem, have your child drink plenty of fluids to soften stools. Warm baths also may help relax your child and encourage bowel movements.

Avoid use of laxatives in children unless advised by your doctor.

Excessive Use of Laxatives Can Be Harmful

Habitual or excessive use of laxatives can actually be harmful and make your constipation worse. Overusing these medications can:
- Cause your body to flush out necessary vitamins and other nutrients before they are absorbed. This process disrupts your body's normal balance of salts and nutrients.

- Interfere with other medications you are taking.
- Induce lazy bowel syndrome, a condition in which your bowels fail to function properly because they have begun to rely on the laxative to stimulate elimination. As a result, when you stop using laxatives, your constipation may worsen.

■ Diarrhea

This unpleasant disorder affects adults an average of four times a year. Symptoms include loose, watery stools, often accompanied by abdominal cramps.

There are many causes, most of which are not serious. The most common is a viral infection of your digestive tract. Bacteria and parasites also can cause diarrhea. These organisms cause your bowel to lose excess water and salts as diarrhea.

Nausea and vomiting may precede diarrhea that is caused by an infection. In addition, you also may notice cramping, abdominal pain and other flu-like symptoms, such as low-grade fever, achy or cramping muscles and headache. Bacterial or parasitic infestations sometimes cause bloody stools or a high fever.

Infection-induced diarrhea can be extremely contagious. You can catch a viral infection by direct contact with an infected person. Food and water contaminated with bacteria or parasites also spread diarrheal infections.

Diarrhea can be a side effect of many medications, particularly antibiotics. In addition, the artificial sweeteners sorbitol and mannitol found in chewing gum and other sugar-free products can cause diarrhea. About 40 to 50 percent of healthy people may have difficulty digesting these sweeteners. Chronic or recurrent diarrhea may signal a more serious underlying medical problem such as chronic infection or inflammatory bowel disease.

Self-Care

Although uncomfortable, diarrhea caused by infections typically clears on its own without antibiotics. Over-the-counter medications such as Imodium and Kaopectate may slow diarrhea, but they won't speed your recovery. Take these measures to prevent dehydration and reduce symptoms while you recover:
- Drink at least 8 to 16 glasses (2 to 4 quarts) of clear liquids, including water, clear sodas and broths, gelatin, juices and weak tea.
- Add semisolid and low-fiber foods gradually as your bowel movements return to normal. Try soda crackers, toast, eggs, rice or chicken.
- Avoid dairy products, fatty foods or highly seasoned foods for a few days.
- Avoid caffeine and nicotine.

Medical Help

Contact your health-care provider if diarrhea persists beyond 1 week or if you become dehydrated (excessive thirst, dry mouth, little or no urination, severe weakness, dizziness or light-headedness). You also should seek medical attention if you have severe abdominal or rectal pain, bloody stools, a temperature of more than 101 F or signs of dehydration despite drinking fluids.

Your physician may prescribe antibiotics to shorten the duration of diarrhea caused by some bacteria and parasites. However, not all diarrhea caused by bacteria requires treatment with antibiotics, and antibiotics don't help viral diarrhea, which is the most common kind of infectious diarrhea.

Kids' Care

Diarrhea can cause infants to become dehydrated. Contact your health-care provider if diarrhea persists for more than 12 hours or if your baby:
- Hasn't had a wet diaper in 8 hours
- Has a temperature of more than 102 F
- Has bloody stools
- Has a dry mouth or cries without tears
- Is unusually sleepy or drowsy or unresponsive

Common Problems

■ Excessive Gas and Gas Pains

Belching

Belching and burping are normal ways to get rid of the air you swallow every time you eat or drink. Belching removes gas from your stomach by forcing it into your esophagus and then out your mouth. Swallowing too much air can cause bloating or frequent belching. If you belch repeatedly when not eating, you may be swallowing air as a nervous habit.

Passing Gas

Most intestinal gas (flatus) is produced in the colon. Usually the gas is expelled during a bowel movement. All people pass gas (called flatulence), but some people produce an excessive amount of gas that bothers them throughout the day. Intestinal gas is composed primarily of five substances: oxygen, nitrogen, hydrogen, carbon dioxide and methane. The foul odor usually is the result of small traces of other gases such as hydrogen sulfide and ammonia and other substances. Swallowed air makes up a small fraction of intestinal gas. Carbonated drinks may release carbon dioxide in the stomach and may be a source of gas.

Gas Pains

Sharp, jabbing or crampy pains in your abdomen may be caused by the buildup of gas. They are often intense, but brief (less than 1 minute). They often occur in the right lower and left upper abdomen and change locations quickly. You may notice a "knotted" feeling in your abdomen. Passing gas sometimes relieves these pains.

Any of the sources of intestinal gas or diarrhea can lead to gas pains. Gas pains can occur when your intestines have difficulty breaking down certain foods or when you have a gastrointestinal infection or diarrhea.

Self-Care

To reduce belching and bloating, try the following tips:
- Eat slowly and avoid gulping. Eat fewer rich, fatty foods.
- Avoid chewing gum or sucking on hard candy.
- Limit sipping through straws or drinking from narrow-mouthed bottles.
- Don't smoke cigarettes, pipes or cigars. Cut down on carbonated drinks and beer.
- Try to control stress, which may aggravate the nervous habit of swallowing air.
- Don't force yourself to belch.
- Avoid lying down immediately after you eat.

To reduce flatulence, try the following tips:
- Identify the foods that affect you the most. Try eliminating one of these foods for a few weeks to see if your flatulence subsides: beans, peas, lentils, cabbage, radishes, onions, brussels sprouts, sauerkraut, apricots, bananas, prunes and prune juice, raisins, whole-wheat bread, bran cereals or muffins, pretzels, wheat germ, milk, cream, ice cream and ice milk.
- Temporarily cut back on high-fiber foods. Add them back gradually over weeks.
- Reduce dairy products. Try Lactaid or Dairy Ease for lactose intolerance.
- Try adding Beano to high-fiber foods to reduce the amount of gas they make.
- Occasional use of over-the-counter anti-gas products containing simethicone (Mylanta, Riopan Plus, Mylicon) can help. Activated charcoal pills or capsules may help absorb gas.

◾ Gallstones

About 1 in 10 Americans has or will have gallstones. Most gallstones produce no symptoms. Stones that block the ducts linking your gallbladder with your liver and small intestine can be extremely painful and potentially dangerous.

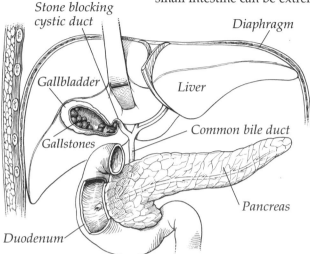

Stone blocking cystic duct

Diaphragm

Gallbladder

Liver

Gallstones

Common bile duct

Pancreas

Duodenum

Gallstones may form in your gallbladder. If a stone obstructs your cystic duct, you may experience a gallbladder attack.

Your gallbladder stores bile, a digestive fluid produced in the liver. The bile passes through ducts from the gallbladder into the small intestine and helps digest fats. A healthy gallbladder has balanced amounts of bile acids and cholesterol. When the concentration of cholesterol becomes too high, gallstones may form. They can be as small as a grain of sand or as large as a golf ball.

Gallstones can cause intense and sudden pain that may last for hours. The pain usually begins shortly after eating. It begins in your upper right abdomen and may shift to your back or right shoulder blade. Fever and nausea also may accompany the pain. After your pain subsides, you may notice a mild aching sensation or soreness in your upper right abdomen. If a gallstone blocks your bile duct, your skin and the whites of your eyes may turn yellow (jaundice). You also may develop a fever or pass pale, clay-colored stools.

The elderly and women tend to be at higher risk, especially women who are pregnant or taking estrogen or birth control pills. Your risk may also be higher if:

- You are overweight or have recently lost weight
- You have a family history of this problem or a disorder of the small intestine

Self-Care	Avoiding rich, fatty foods may help reduce your episodes of gallbladder pain.
Medical Help	Contact your health-care provider if you have recurrent or intense pain. Seek prompt medical attention if you develop yellowing skin or a fever during an attack.

◾ Gastritis (Burning or Sour Stomach)

Gastritis is inflammation of your stomach lining. Upper abdominal discomfort, nausea and vomiting are the more common symptoms. Gastritis may cause bleeding that appears in vomit or turns your stools black. Most often, gastritis is mild and poses no danger. Gastritis may occur when acid damages your stomach lining. Excessive smoking, alcohol and medications such as aspirin also can cause gastritis.

Self-Care	<ul><li>Avoid smoking, alcohol and foods and drinks that irritate your stomach.</li><li>Try taking over-the-counter antacids or medicines such as Pepcid, Tagamet and Zantac. (**Caution:** Excessive use of antacids containing magnesium can cause diarrhea. Calcium- or aluminum-based antacids can lead to constipation.)</li><li>Use pain relievers that contain acetaminophen (see page 231). Avoid aspirin, ibuprofen, ketoprofen and naproxen sodium. They can cause or worsen gastritis.</li></ul>
Medical Help	If your discomfort lasts longer than 1 week, contact your health-care provider.

Common Problems

■ Hemorrhoids and Rectal Bleeding

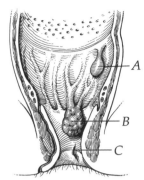

Cross-section view of anus and rectum shows the location of three common causes of rectal bleeding: (A) polyp, (B) hemorrhoids and (C) anal fissure.

More than 75 percent of Americans have problems with hemorrhoids at some time in their lives. Itching, burning and pain around the anus often signal their presence. You also may notice small amounts of bright red blood on your toilet tissue or in the toilet bowl.

Hemorrhoids occur when veins in your rectum become enlarged. They usually form over time as you strain to pass hard stools. Hemorrhoids may develop inside the anal canal or protrude outside the anal opening. Lifting heavy objects, obesity, pregnancy, childbirth, stress and diarrhea also can increase the pressure on these veins and lead to hemorrhoids. This condition seems to run in families.

In addition to hemorrhoids, bleeding from the rectum can occur for other reasons, some of which can be serious. Passing hard, dry stools may scrape the anal lining. An infection of the lining of the rectum or tiny cracks or tears in the lining of your anus called anal fissures also can cause rectal bleeding. With these types of problems, you may notice small drops of bright red blood on your stool, on your toilet tissue or in the toilet bowl.

Black, tarry stools, maroon stools or bright red blood in your stools also may signal more extensive bleeding elsewhere in your digestive tract. Small sacs that protrude from your large intestines (called diverticuli), ulcers, small growths called polyps, cancer and some chronic bowel disorders can all cause bleeding.

Self-Care

Although uncomfortable, hemorrhoids are not a serious medical condition. Most hemorrhoids respond well to the following self-care measures:
- Drink at least 8 to 10 glasses of water each day and eat plenty of high-fiber foods such as wheat bran cereal, whole wheat bread, fresh fruit and vegetables.
- Bathe or shower daily to cleanse the skin around your anus gently with warm water. Soap is not necessary and may aggravate the problem.
- Stay active. Exercise. If at work or home you must sit or stand for long periods, take quick walks or breaks from work.
- Try not to strain during bowel movements or sit on the toilet too long.
- Take warm baths.
- Apply ice packs.
- For flares of pain or irritation, apply over-the-counter creams, ointments or pads containing witch hazel or a topical numbing agent. Keep in mind that these products can only help relieve mild itching and irritation.
- Try fiber supplements (Metamucil, Citrucel) to keep stools soft and regular.

Medical Help

Hemorrhoids become most painful when a clot forms in the enlarged vein. If your hemorrhoids are extremely painful, your health-care provider may prescribe a cream or suppository containing hydrocortisone to reduce inflammation. Some troublesome internal hemorrhoids may require operation or other procedures to shrink or eliminate them.

Diagnosing the cause of rectal bleeding can be difficult. You should see your health-care provider for evaluation. Seek immediate emergency care if you notice large amounts of rectal bleeding, light-headedness, weakness or rapid heart rate (more than 100 beats per minute).

■ Hernias

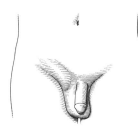

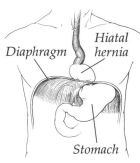

An inguinal hernia can cause a bulge at the junction of your thigh and groin. Bulges can be round or oval.

In hiatal hernia diagram: **Diaphragm**, **Hiatal hernia**, **Stomach**

In hiatal hernia, a portion of the stomach protrudes through the diaphragm into the chest cavity.

A hernia occurs when one body part protrudes through a gap into another body area. Some hernias cause no pain or visible symptoms.

Types of Hernias

Inguinal hernia is the medical name for a hernia in the groin area. It's far more frequent in men than women and accounts for 80 percent of all hernias in men. It occurs along the inguinal canal—an opening in abdominal muscles. In men, the canal is the spermatic cord's passageway between the abdominal cavity and the scrotum. In women, it's the passageway for a ligament that helps hold the uterus in place. With an inguinal hernia, you may be able to see and feel the bulge created by the protruding tissue or intestine. It's often located at the junction of your thigh and groin. Sometimes in men the protruding intestine enters the scrotum. This can be painful and cause the scrotum to swell. The first sign of an inguinal hernia may be a bulge or lump in your groin. You may notice discomfort while bending over, coughing or lifting and a "heavy" or "dragging" sensation.

A *strangulated hernia* occurs when the tissue bulging through the abdominal wall becomes pinched and the blood supply is cut off. The affected tissue dies and then swells, causing extreme pain and a potentially life-threatening situation. Seek immediate medical attention if you think you have a strangulated hernia.

A *hiatal hernia* occurs at the spot called the *hiatus*, which is an opening in your diaphragm through which your esophagus (food pipe) passes into your stomach. If this opening is too large, your stomach may protrude (herniate) through it into your chest, creating a hiatal hernia. Symptoms include heartburn, belching, chest pain and regurgitation. Hiatal hernias are common, occurring in about 25 percent of all people older than 50 years. Most hiatal hernias are minor and show no symptoms. A hiatal hernia is not painful in and of itself, but the condition allows food and acid to back up into your esophagus, causing heartburn, indigestion and chest pain in some people. Obesity aggravates these symptoms.

Self-Care	**For Inguinal Hernia** You can neither prevent nor cure a hernia through self-care. Once you've had the lump evaluated and know it's a hernia and your hernia does not cause you discomfort, you need not take any special precautions. Wearing a corset or truss may give slight relief but will not reduce a hernia or fix it. **For Hiatal Hernia** ● Lose weight if you are overweight. ● Follow self-care precautions for heartburn on page 60.
Medical Help	If your hernia is painful or bothersome, contact your health-care provider to discuss whether an operation is necessary.
Caution	If you cannot reduce the hernia by pushing on the lump, the blood supply to this segment of bowel may be cut off. Symptoms of this complication include nausea, vomiting and severe pain. Left untreated, intestinal blockage or, in rare cases, a life-threatening infection may result. If you have any of these symptoms, contact your health-care provider.

Common Problems

■ Indigestion and Heartburn

Indigestion is a nonspecific term used to describe discomfort in your abdomen which often occurs after eating. Indigestion is not a disease. It is a collection of symptoms, including discomfort or burning in your upper abdomen, nausea and a bloated or full feeling that belching may relieve.

The cause of indigestion is sometimes difficult to pinpoint. In some people, eating certain foods or drinking alcohol may trigger it. In others, your discomfort may be a daily occurrence.

A common form of indigestion is heartburn. Each day, as many as 10 percent of adults experience the burning sensation commonly called heartburn. Technically called gastroesophageal reflux, heartburn occurs when stomach acids back up into your esophagus (food pipe). A sour taste and the sensation of food coming back into your mouth may accompany the burning sensation behind your breastbone.

Why do these acids back up? Normally, a circular band of muscle at the bottom of your esophagus, called a sphincter, closes off the stomach but allows food to enter your stomach when you swallow. If the sphincter relaxes abnormally or becomes weakened, stomach acid can wash back up (reflux) into your esophagus and cause irritation.

Various factors can cause reflux. Being overweight puts too much pressure on your abdomen. Rich, fatty or spicy meals, alcohol, caffeine, peppermint, chocolate, citrus and tomato juices and nicotine relax the sphincter muscle or irritate the esophagus. Overeating or lying down after a meal also can encourage reflux.

Self-Care

Changing what and how you eat is the first step to prevent heartburn.
- Manage your weight. Slim down if you are overweight.
- Eat small meals.
- Avoid foods and drinks that relax the sphincter or irritate the esophagus (such as rich, fatty or spicy meals, alcohol, caffeine, peppermint, chocolate, citrus and tomato juices and nicotine).
- Stop eating 2 to 3 hours before you lie down or go to bed.
- Quit smoking.
- Do not wear tight clothing and tight belts.
- Avoid excessive stooping or bending or heavy exertion for 1 hour after eating.
- Over-the-counter antacids can relieve mild heartburn by neutralizing stomach acids temporarily. However, prolonged or excessive use of antacids containing magnesium can cause diarrhea. Calcium- or aluminum-based products can lead to constipation.

    Another type of medication such as Pepcid, Tagamet and Zantac may relieve or prevent heartburn symptoms by reducing the production of stomach acid. These medicines are available in over-the-counter and prescription strengths.

Medical Help

Most problems with indigestion and heartburn are occasional and mild. But if you have severe or daily discomfort, don't ignore your symptoms. Left untreated, chronic heartburn can cause scarring that can make swallowing difficult. In rare cases, severe heartburn can lead to a condition called Barrett's esophagus, which may increase your risk for cancer.

Heartburn and indigestion symptoms may signal the presence of a more serious underlying disease. Contact your health-care provider if your symptoms are persistent or severe, or if you have difficulty swallowing.

■ Irritable Bowel Syndrome

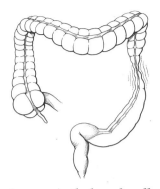

A spasm in the bowel wall may cause abdominal pain and other unpleasant symptoms commonly associated with IBS.

Irritable bowel syndrome (IBS), sometimes known as "spastic bowel" or "spastic colon," is a common medical problem that is not completely understood. IBS is annoying, painful and sometimes embarrassing, but it is not life-threatening. Some physicians rank the disorder with the common cold as the major cause of time lost from work.

Adolescents, young children and women experience this problem more than men. About one in five adult Americans has symptoms of IBS, but less than half of these people seek help.

Although experts cannot pinpoint its exact cause, IBS may be related to abnormal muscle spasms in your stomach or intestines. Stress and depression are often blamed as causes of IBS. But these emotions only aggravate the condition.

Symptoms may include abdominal pain, diarrhea, constipation, bloating, indigestion and gas. Although a bowel movement temporarily relieves the pain, you may feel as if you can't empty your bowels completely. Your stools can be ribbonlike and laced with mucus, or they can be hard, dry pellets. Often, diarrhea alternates with constipation.

Self-Care

Although no single treatment can eliminate IBS, simple diet and lifestyle measures can relieve your symptoms:

- Pay attention to what you eat. Avoid or eat smaller portions of foods that consistently aggravate your symptoms. Common irritants include tobacco, alcohol, caffeine, spicy foods, concentrated fruit juices, raw fruits and vegetables, fatty foods and sugar-free sweeteners such as sorbitol or mannitol.
- Eat high-fiber foods such as fresh fruits, vegetables and whole-grain foods. Add fiber gradually to minimize problems with gas and bloating.
- Drink plenty of fluids—at least 2 quarts per day.
- Try using fiber supplements containing psyllium, such as Metamucil or Konsyl, to help relieve your constipation and diarrhea.
- Reduce your stress through regular exercise, sports or hobbies that help you relax.
- Try over-the-counter medications such as Imodium or Kaopectate to relieve diarrhea.

Medical Help

If self-care doesn't help, your health-care provider may recommend prescription medications designed to relieve muscle spasms. If depression plays a role in your symptoms, treating this problem may be helpful.

Because the symptoms of IBS mimic those of more serious medical disorders such as cancer, gallbladder disease and ulcers, you should contact your health-care provider for evaluation if simple self-care measures don't help within a couple of weeks.

Common Problems

■ Nausea and Vomiting

Nausea and vomiting are common and uncomfortable symptoms of a wide variety of disorders, most of which are not serious.

Feeling queasy and throwing up usually signal a viral infection called gastroenteritis. Diarrhea, abdominal cramps, bloating and fever also may accompany this condition. Other causes include food poisoning, pregnancy, some medications and gastritis (see page 57).

Self-Care

If gastroenteritis is the culprit, nausea and vomiting may last from a few hours to 2 or 3 days. It is also common to have diarrhea and mild abdominal cramping. To keep yourself comfortable and prevent dehydration while you recover, try the following:
- Stop eating and drinking for a few hours until your stomach has settled.
- Try ice chips or small sips of weak tea, clear soda (Seven-Up or Sprite) and broths or noncaffeinated clear sports drinks to prevent dehydration. Consume 2 to 4 quarts (8 to 16 glasses) of liquid per day, taking frequent, small sips.
- Add semisolid and low-fiber foods gradually and stop eating if the vomiting returns. Try soda crackers, gelatin, toast, eggs, rice or chicken.
- Avoid dairy products, caffeine, alcohol, nicotine or fatty or highly seasoned foods for a few days.

Medical Help

Vomiting can lead to complications such as dehydration (if the condition is persistent), aspiration (food in the windpipe) or, in rare instances, a tear in the food pipe. Infants, the elderly and people with suppressed immune systems are particularly vulnerable to complications. Contact your health-care provider if you are unable to drink anything for 24 hours, if vomiting persists beyond 2 or 3 days, if you become dehydrated or if you vomit blood. Signs of dehydration include excessive thirst, dry mouth, little or no urination, severe weakness, dizziness or light-headedness. Vomiting also can be a warning of more serious underlying problems such as gallbladder disease, ulcers or bowel obstruction.

Kids' Care

Spitting up is an everyday occurrence for babies and usually causes no discomfort. Vomiting, however, is more forceful and disturbing to your baby and can lead to dehydration and weight loss.

To prevent dehydration, let the baby's stomach rest for 30 to 60 minutes and then offer small amounts of liquid. If you are breast-feeding, let your baby nurse on one side. Offer bottle-fed babies a small amount of formula or an oral electrolyte solution such as Pedialyte or Infalyte.

If the vomiting does not recur, continue to offer small sips of liquid or the breast every 15 to 30 minutes. Contact your health-care provider if vomiting persists for more than 12 hours or if your child:
- Hasn't had a wet diaper in 8 hours
- Has diarrhea or bloody stools
- Has a dry mouth or cries without tears
- Is unusually sleepy or drowsy or unresponsive

A few newborn babies have a disorder called pyloric stenosis, which can cause repeated and forceful vomiting. This condition usually appears during the second or third week of life. It requires medical care.

■ Ulcers

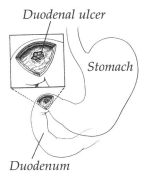

Duodenal ulcer

Stomach

Duodenum

The most common form of ulcer occurs in the duodenum and is called a duodenal ulcer.

Ulcers are holes or breaks in the inner lining of your esophagus or stomach or the uppermost section of your small intestine called the duodenum.

The cause of ulcers is not fully known. Recent research suggests that bacteria called *Helicobacter pylori (H. pylori)* play an important role. This condition also appears to run in families. Contrary to popular belief, there is no clear evidence that emotional stress causes ulcers.

Ulcers can cause considerable distress. Symptoms may include a burning feeling beneath your breastbone in your upper abdomen, gnawing "hunger pangs" or "boring" pain and nausea. At times, ulcers also can cause belching or bloating. These symptoms typically occur when your stomach is empty. Although eating may relieve the symptoms, they often resume 1 to 2 hours later.

In severe cases, ulcers may bleed and cause you to vomit blood or pass black, tarry stools. In rare cases, an ulcer may perforate the wall of your stomach, causing severe abdominal pain.

Self-Care

Diet, lifestyle and medication choices may help prevent or control ulcers.

- If you're using pain relievers, use acetaminophen. Aspirin, ibuprofen, ketoprofen and naproxen sodium can cause ulcer.
- Avoid alcohol, coffee, tea and other caffeinated drinks. Stop smoking.
- Eat small meals and avoid letting your stomach remain empty for long periods.
- Avoid spicy or fatty foods if they seem to make your symptoms worse.
- Take nonprescription antacids to neutralize stomach acids or medicines such as Pepcid, Tagamet or Zantac to stop the production of stomach acid.

Medical Help

Some ulcers disappear with self-care or with over-the-counter medication. If your symptoms do not improve after 1 week or if you have troublesome, recurrent ulcers, see your health-care provider for further evaluation and treatment.

The diagnosis requires visualizing the ulcer with an X-ray or scope, although your doctor may treat you on the basis of your symptoms alone.

Bleeding ulcers can cause serious blood loss. Seek help immediately if you vomit blood, pass black, tarry stools or if you have severe pain.

Ulcers: Are Antibiotics the Answer?

Antibiotics are gaining acceptance among physicians to help treat ulcers, although many doctors reserve their use for recurrent ulcers.

Your physician may order a special test to identify the bacteria *H. pylori*. Antibiotics are used in combination with standard ulcer medications.

There are drawbacks to using antibiotics. Large doses of medication are required. You may take 12 to 15 pills daily for 10 to 12 days. About 20 percent of people who take them in these doses experience nausea and diarrhea. Bacteria may become resistant to antibiotics.

I WANT TO KNOW MORE

- National Digestive Diseases Information Clearinghouse, Box NDDIC, 9000 Rockville Pike, Bethesda, MD 20892; (301) 486-6344.

Common Problems

Ears and Hearing

There's more to the ear than meets the eye. The part of your ear that's visible—your outer ear—is connected inside your head to your middle ear and inner ear, which work together to allow you to hear and help you maintain balance.

How the Ear Works

Your ear is a finely tuned organ that's specially designed to send sound impulses to your brain. When sound waves travel through the ear canal, your eardrum and the three small bones to which it is attached vibrate. This vibration moves through the middle ear to your inner ear, triggering nerve impulses to your brain, where you perceive them as sound.

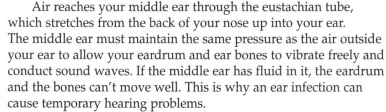

Air reaches your middle ear through the eustachian tube, which stretches from the back of your nose up into your ear. The middle ear must maintain the same pressure as the air outside your ear to allow your eardrum and ear bones to vibrate freely and conduct sound waves. If the middle ear has fluid in it, the eardrum and the bones can't move well. This is why an ear infection can cause temporary hearing problems.

Some common causes of ear pain and ear problems are described in this chapter.

◾ Airplane Ear

The medical name for this condition is "barotrauma." Simply stated, it means an injury caused by changes in pressure. It often occurs if you fly or scuba dive with a congested nose, allergy, cold or throat infection. You may have pain in one ear, a slight hearing loss or a stuffy feeling in your ears. It is caused by your eardrum bulging as a result of change in air pressure. Having a cold or ear infection is not necessarily a reason to change or delay a flight, however.

Self-Care

- Try taking a decongestant an hour before takeoff and an hour before landing. This may prevent blockage of your eustachian tube.
- During flight, suck candy or chew gum to encourage swallowing, which helps open your eustachian tube.
- If your ears plug as the plane descends, inhale and then gently exhale while holding your nostrils closed and keeping your mouth closed. If you can swallow at the same time, it is more helpful.
- Remember, it is better to prevent this type of pain by following the listed suggestions rather than beginning treatment once the pain has occurred.

Medical Help

If your symptoms do not disappear within a few hours, see your physician.

Kids' Care

For babies and young children, make sure they are drinking fluids (swallowing) during ascent and descent. Give the child a bottle or pacifier to encourage swallowing. Give acetaminophen 30 minutes before takeoff to help control discomfort that may occur. Decongestants in young children are not generally recommended.

■ Foreign Objects in the Ear

Objects stuck in your ear can cause pain and hearing loss. Usually you know if something is stuck in your ear, but small children may not be aware of it.

Self-Care

If an object becomes lodged in the ear, follow these steps:
- Do not attempt to remove the foreign object by probing with a cotton swab, matchstick or any other tool. To do so is to risk pushing the object farther into the ear and damaging the fragile structures of the middle ear.
- If the object is clearly visible, is pliable and can be grasped easily with tweezers, gently remove it.
- Try using the pull of gravity: tilt the head to the affected side. Do not strike the victim's head, but shake it gently in the direction of the ground to try to dislodge the object.
- If the foreign object is an insect, tilt the person's head so that the ear with the offending insect is upward. Try to float the insect out by pouring mineral oil, olive oil or baby oil into the ear. It should be warm but not hot. As you pour the oil, you can ease the entry of the oil by straightening the ear canal. Pull the ear lobe gently backward and upward. The insect should suffocate and may float out in the oil bath.
- Do not use oil to remove any object other than an insect. Do not use this method if there is any suspicion of a perforation in the eardrum (pain, bleeding or discharge from the ear).

Medical Help

If these methods fail or the person continues to experience pain in the ear, reduced hearing or a sensation of something lodged in the ear, seek medical assistance.

■ Ruptured Eardrum

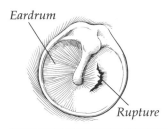

Eardrum

Rupture

An eardrum may rupture after an infection or from trauma. Signs of a ruptured, or perforated, eardrum are earache, partial hearing loss and slight bleeding or discharge from your ear. With an infection, the pain often resolves once the drum ruptures, releasing infected fluid or pus. Usually, the rupture heals by itself without complications and with little or no permanent hearing loss. Large ruptures may cause recurring infections. If you suspect that you have ruptured an eardrum, see your physician as soon as possible. Meanwhile, try the self-care tips listed here.

Self-Care

- Relieve pain with aspirin or another pain medication that is safe for you.
- Place a warm (not hot) heating pad over your ear.
- Do not flush your ear.

Medical Help

Your physician may prescribe an antibiotic to make sure that no infection develops in your middle ear. Sometimes a plastic or paper patch is placed over your eardrum to seal the opening while it heals. Your eardrum will often heal within 2 months. If it has not healed in that time, you may require a minor surgical procedure to repair the tear.

■ Ear Infections

To many parents of young children, coping with ear infections is almost as routine as changing wet diapers. Seven of 10 children will have at least one middle ear infection (otitis media) by age 3. One-third of these youngsters will have repeated bouts of ear infections.

A 1996 Mayo Clinic study pointed out that ear infections are increasing. According to the report, the number of office visits for ear infections in American children younger than age 2 tripled between 1975 and 1990. For children ages 2 to 5, the rate doubled.

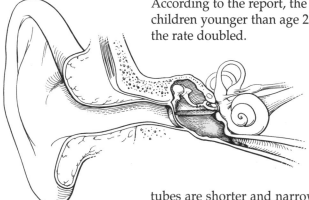

Fluid-filled middle ear creates environment for growth of bacteria.

Most ear infections don't lead to permanent hearing loss. Some infections that aren't treated, however, can spread to other parts of the ear, including the inner ear. Infections of the middle ear can damage the eardrum, ear bones and inner ear structure, causing permanent hearing loss. An ear infection often begins with a respiratory infection such as a cold. Colds cause swelling and inflammation in the sinuses and eustachian tubes. Children's eustachian tubes are shorter and narrower than adults. This size makes it more likely that inflammation will block the tube completely, trapping fluid in the middle ear. This trapped fluid causes discomfort and creates an ideal environment for bacteria to grow. The result is a middle ear infection.

Self-Care

- Consider an over-the-counter pain reliever such as ibuprofen or acetaminophen. (If your child is younger than 2, consult your health-care provider.)
- Eardrops with a local anesthetic may help reduce pain. They won't prevent or stop an infection. They should **not** be used if there is drainage from the ear.
- To administer the eardrops, warm the bottle slightly in water and place the child on a flat surface (not in your arms or on your lap), ear up, to insert the eardrops.
- Place a warm (not hot), moist cloth or heating pad (on lowest setting) over the ear.

Medical Help

Contact your doctor if pain lasts more than a day or is associated with fever. Ear infections usually are treated with antibiotics. Even if your child feels better after a few days, continue giving the medicine for the full length of time recommended (usually 10 days).

The Pros and Cons of Ear Tubes

Recurrent ear infections are sometimes treated by surgically inserting a small plastic tube through your eardrum, which allows pus to drain out of your middle ear.

For the Procedure
- It usually results in fewer infections.
- Hearing is restored.
- The operation allows ventilation of the middle ear, which decreases the risk of permanent

changes in the lining of the middle ear—changes that might occur with prolonged infection.

Against the Procedure
- It requires brief general anesthesia.
- You must avoid getting water in your ear while the tube is in place.
- In rare cases, severe scarring or a permanent hole in the eardrum may result.

Common Questions About Ear Infections in Kids

What are the risk factors for infections?

Although all children are susceptible to ear infections, those at higher risk are children who:

- Are male
- Have siblings with a history of recurrent ear infection
- Have their first ear infection before they are 4 months old
- Are in group child care
- Are exposed to tobacco smoke
- Are of Native American, Alaskan or Canadian Eskimo descent
- Have frequent upper respiratory tract infections
- Were bottle-fed instead of breast-fed

What are the symptoms?

In addition to an earache or a feeling of pressure and blockage in the ear, some children may experience temporary hearing loss. Be aware of other signs of an ear infection such as irritability, a sudden loss of appetite, the development of a fever a few days after onset of a cold, nausea, vomiting or a preference for sleeping in an upright position. Your child also may have discharge in the ear or may tug at the ear.

Does your child need an antibiotic?

Because most ear infections clear on their own, your health-care provider may first recommend a "wait-and-see" approach, especially if your child has few symptoms. In other cases, your doctor may opt to prescribe an antibiotic to treat the infection. Within 2 to 3 days of beginning the medication, symptoms usually improve.

Be sure to follow instructions carefully for giving the antibiotic. Continue to give the medication to your child for the entire recommended time. If you stop giving your child the antibiotic when symptoms improve, you may allow stronger remaining bacteria to multiply and cause another infection. Surviving bacteria may carry genes that make them drug-resistant.

If symptoms don't go away or if your child is younger than 15 months, schedule a follow-up visit as recommended by your health-care provider. If your child is older and symptoms have resolved, a recheck may not be necessary, especially if infections have not been recurrent.

What can you do?

Although an ear infection is not an emergency, the first 24 hours are often when your child's pain and irritability are the worst. Follow the self-care tips on page 66. To make your child more comfortable, don't underestimate the benefits of extra cuddling.

What about recurrent infections?

Time and the use of antibiotics usually resolve ear infections. But sometimes ear infections can become a chronic problem. If so, ask your health-care provider about preventive antibiotic therapy. Persistent fluid buildup may cause temporary or even permanent hearing loss. This can lead to delayed speech development.

Can you prevent infections?

Preventing ear infections is difficult, but consider these approaches to help reduce your child's risk:

- Breast-feed rather than bottle-feed your baby for as long as possible.
- When bottle-feeding, hold your baby in an upright position.
- Avoid exposing your child to tobacco smoke.

Do children outgrow ear infections?

As your child matures, the eustachian tubes become wider and more angled, providing a better means of draining secretions and fluid out of the ear. Although ear infections still may occur, they probably won't develop as often as during the first few years of life.

What are medical researchers working on to help treat ear infections?

In addition to antibiotics, some approaches under investigation include the use of cortisone-like medication, such as prednisone, that would reduce inflammation (more research is needed to determine when this treatment is most effective); a "one-shot" approach using an injection of a particular antibiotic when oral drug therapy is impractical; and vaccines against the influenza virus.

Common Problems

■ Ringing in Your Ear

A ringing or buzzing in your ear when no other sounds are present can have many causes, including ear wax, a foreign object, infection or exposure to loud noise. It also can be caused by high doses of aspirin or large amounts of caffeine. This condition, called tinnitus, uncommonly is a symptom of more serious ear disorders, particularly if it is accompanied by other symptoms such as hearing loss or dizziness.

Self-Care

- If aspirin was recommended to you in high doses (more than 12 per day), ask your doctor for an alternative. If you are taking aspirin on your own, try lower doses or another over-the-counter pain medication.
- Avoid nicotine, caffeine and alcohol, which may aggravate the condition.
- Try to determine a cause, such as exposure to loud noise, and avoid or block it if possible.
- Wear earplugs or some other form of hearing protection if you have excess noise exposure, such as when you are working with yard equipment (leaf blowers or lawn mowers).
- Some people benefit by covering up the ringing sound with another, more acceptable sound (such as music or listening to a radio as you fall asleep).
- Other people may benefit by wearing a "masker," a device that fits in your ear and produces "white" noise.

Medical Help

If tinnitus worsens, persists or is accompanied by hearing loss or dizziness, consider evaluation by your health-care provider. He or she may choose to pursue further evaluation. Although most causes of tinnitus are benign, it can be a difficult and frustrating condition to treat.

■ Swimmer's Ear

This is an infection of your outer ear canal. In addition to pain or itching, you may see a clear drainage or yellow-green pus and experience temporary hearing loss. Swimmer's ear is the result of having persistent moisture in the ear or, sometimes, from swimming in polluted water. Other similar inflammations or infections may occur from scraping your ear canal when you clean your ear or from hair sprays or hair dyes. Some people are prone to bacterial or fungal infections.

Self-Care

If the aching is mild and there is no drainage from the ear, do the following:
- Place a warm (not hot) heating pad over your ear.
- Take aspirin or another pain medication (be sure to follow the label instructions).
- To prevent swimmer's ear, try to keep ear canals dry, avoid substances that might irritate your ear and don't clean inside the ear canal unless you are instructed to do so by your health-care provider.

Medical Help

Seek medical care if you have severe pain or swelling of the ear, a fever, drainage from the ear or an underlying disease. Your doctor may clean your ear canal with a suction device or a cotton-tipped probe. Your doctor also may prescribe eardrops or medications to control infection and reduce pain. Keep your ear dry while it is healing.

■ Wax Blockage

Ear wax is part of the body's normal defenses. It traps dust and foreign objects, protects the ear canal and inhibits growth of bacteria. At times, you may produce too much ear wax, blocking your ear canal, giving you an earache or causing a rattling in your ears. You also may notice a gradual hearing loss as the wax accumulates.

Self-Care

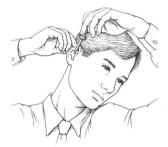

- Soften ear wax by applying a few drops of baby oil, mineral oil or glycerin with an eyedropper twice a day for several days.
- When the wax is softened, fill a bowl with water heated to body temperature (if it is colder or hotter, it may make you feel dizzy during the procedure).
- With your head upright, grasp the top of your ear and pull upward. With your other hand, squirt the water gently into your ear canal with a 3-ounce rubber bulb syringe. Then, turn your head and drain the water into the bowl or sink.
- You may need to repeat this several times before the extra wax falls out.
- Dry your outer ear with a towel or a handheld hair dryer.
- Ear wax removers sold in stores are also effective.
- Other home wax removal methods may also be effective if wax buildup is a recurrent problem. But ask your doctor about these self-care remedies. For example, 5 to 10 drops of Colace, an over-the-counter medication (used for constipation in infants), can be very helpful but needs flushing (leave drops in for 30 minutes). Another "flusher" is a Water-Pik. A few drops of diluted vinegar (half-strength) after flushing returns the ear canal to an acid state, which suppresses bacteria growth after ears are wet. A commercial alcohol-boric acid preparation is available for the same purpose.

Caution

Your ear canal and eardrum are very delicate and can be damaged easily. Do not poke them with objects such as cotton swabs, paper clips or bobby pins.

Flushing wax out of the ears should be avoided if there has been a prior eardrum perforation or prior ear surgery, unless your doctor approves. If infection is a concern, don't flush your ears.

Medical Help

Even if the tips given above are followed, many people have difficulty washing wax out of their ears. It may be best to have this done by your health-care provider. Excessive wax can be removed in a procedure similar to the one described above. A special instrument is used to either scoop the wax out of the ear or suction it out. If this is a recurring problem, your doctor may recommend using a wax-removal medication every 4 to 8 weeks.

■ Noise-Related Hearing Loss

Sound is measured in decibels. An average conversation is about 60 decibels. A loud conversation in a crowded building is about 70 decibels. Your ears can be damaged by prolonged exposure to noise at 90 decibels or louder.

Self-Care

If you are exposed to loud power tools or engines, loud music, firearms or other equipment that produces loud noises, you should take the following precautions:

- Wear protective earplugs or earmuffs. Use commercially made protection devices that meet federal standards (cotton balls will not work, and they could get stuck in your ears). These bring most loud sounds down to acceptable levels. You can obtain custom-molded earplugs made of plastic or rubber to effectively protect against excessive noise.
- Have your hearing tested. Early detection of hearing loss can prevent future, irreversible damage.
- Use ear protection off the job. Protect your ears from any loud recreational activities, such as loud music or concerts, trapshooting or driving snowmobiles.
- Beware of recreational risks. Sensorineural hearing loss related to recreation is becoming more common. Activities with the greatest risk are trapshooting, driving snowmobiles and some other recreational vehicles and, particularly, listening to extremely loud music. If your son or daughter listens to loud music on a headset, use this simple test to determine whether the sound is too loud: if you can identify the music being played while your child is wearing the headset, it is too loud. Tell your child to save his or her ears for a lifetime of music enjoyment.

Maximal Job Noise Exposure Allowed by Law

Duration, Hours Daily	Sound Level, Decibels
8	90
6	92
4	95
3	97
2	100
1 1/2	102
1	105
30 minutes	110
15 minutes	115

Sound Levels of Common Noises

Decibels	Noise
	Safe range
20	Watch ticking; leaves rustling
40	Quiet street noise
60	Normal conversation; bird song
80	Heavy traffic
	Risk range
85-90	Motorcycle; snowmobile
80-100	Rock concert
	Injury range
120	Jackhammer 3 feet away
130	Jet engine 100 feet away
140	Shotgun blast

Age-Related Hearing Loss

A decrease in hearing is common with age. This condition is called presbycusis. If you or a family member suspect you have more serious hearing loss, see a physician. You may be referred to a doctor who is an ear specialist or to an audiologist (a person trained in hearing evaluation). Hearing loss can sometimes be restored with medical treatment or surgery, especially if the problem is in the outer ear or middle ear. If the problem is in the inner ear, however, it is usually not treatable. A hearing aid can improve your hearing. The advice given below may help you select a hearing aid.

Before You Buy a Hearing Aid, Here's Sound Advice

Of the 25 million Americans who have some degree of hearing loss, about 5.8 million use hearing aids. A hearing aid costs from $500 to $2,000. But if it helps you hear better and improves your quality of life, it's worth the money. Yet the Food and Drug Administration (FDA) reports that too often people aren't fully satisfied with their hearing aids. Consumer complaints range from improper fit to poor repair service to lack of hearing improvement.

Here are some tips for selecting a hearing aid:
- **Have a medical and hearing examination.** Before you buy a hearing aid, be examined by a physician, preferably an ear, nose and throat doctor (otolaryngologist). An FDA regulation says it's best to have this examination within 6 months before you buy a hearing aid. An examination can determine whether a medical condition will prevent you from using a hearing aid.
- **Buy from a reputable dispenser.** If you don't get a hearing test (audiogram) from a medical facility, a dispenser will give you one. This person then takes an impression of your ear, chooses the most appropriate aid and adjusts the device to fit well. These are complex tasks, and skills of dispensers vary. Also, contact the Better Business Bureau about a dispenser's complaint record. Be cautious of "free" consultations and dispensers who sell only one brand of hearing aid.
- **Be alert to misleading claims.** For years, a few manufacturers and distributors claimed their hearing aids allowed you to hear speech and eliminate background noise. But this technology doesn't exist. Some newer hearing aids subdue loud sounds and so make wearing a hearing aid

in noisy places more comfortable. But no hearing aid can filter out the voice you want to hear from other voices in a crowded room.
- **Ask about a trial period.** Have the dispenser put in writing the cost of a trial and whether this amount is credited toward the final cost of the hearing aid.
- **Obtain a second hearing test.** To determine if a hearing aid really helps you hear better, have another hearing test while wearing the aid.
- **Understand the warranty**. A warranty should extend for 1 to 2 years and cover both parts and labor.

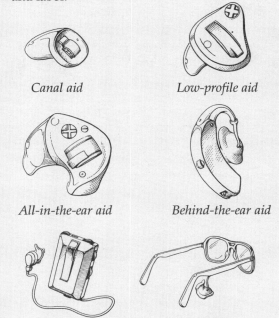

Canal aid

Low-profile aid

All-in-the-ear aid

Behind-the-ear aid

Body aid

Eyeglasses aid

From Hearing Aids for Hearing Problems (patient education brochure). By permission of Mayo Foundation.

Eyes and Vision

Because your eyes are crucial in so many activities, eye problems usually demand attention. Luckily, many eye problems are more bothersome than serious.

Almost everyone has vision changes with age. Age also increases your risk of developing more serious eye problems. Some eye problems can't be prevented, but medications or surgery can slow or stop progression. This section covers the more common eye problems and discusses some of the issues related to declining vision.

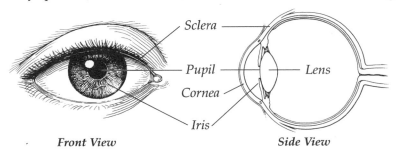

Front View   *Side View*

■ Black Eye

The so-called black eye is caused by bleeding beneath the skin around the eyes. Sometimes a black eye indicates a more extensive injury, even a skull fracture, particularly if the area around both eyes is bruised or there has been head trauma. Although the injury may not be serious, bleeding within the eye (which may turn the white of the eye red) can reduce vision and damage the cornea. In some cases, glaucoma (see page 76) also can result.

Self-Care
- Using gentle pressure, apply ice or a cold pack to the area around the eye for 10 to 15 minutes. Take care not to press on the eye itself. Apply cold as soon as possible after the injury to reduce swelling.
- Be sure there is no blood in the white and colored parts of the eye.

Medical Help
Seek medical care immediately if you experience vision problems (double vision, blurring), severe pain or bleeding in the eye or from the nose.

Taking Care of Your Eyes

- Have your vision checked regularly.
- Control chronic health conditions such as diabetes and high blood pressure.
- Recognize symptoms. Sudden loss of vision in one eye, sudden hazy or blurred vision, flashes of light or black spots or halos or rainbows around lights may signal a serious medical problem such as acute glaucoma or a stroke.

- Protect your eyes against sun damage. Buy sunglasses with UV blocking lenses.
- Eat foods containing vitamin A and beta carotene, such as carrots, yams and cantaloupe.
- Optimize your vision with the right glasses.
- Use good lighting.
- If your vision is impaired, use low-vision aids (such as magnifiers and large-type books).

▍Dry Eyes

Dry eyes feel hot, irritated and gritty when you blink. They may become slightly red. Tear production decreases as you age. Dry eyes usually affect both eyes, especially in women after menopause. Some medicines (such as sleeping medications, antihistamines and some drugs for high blood pressure) can cause or worsen dry eyes. Some rare medical conditions may be associated with dry eyes.

Self-Care
- Use a preservative-free artificial tear preparation such as Cellufresh.
- Because some over-the-counter eyedrops can cause drying, use them for no more than 3 to 5 days.
- Don't direct hair dryers (or other sources of air such as car heaters or fans) toward your eyes.
- Wear glasses on windy days and goggles when swimming.
- Keep your home humidity between 30 and 50 percent.
- Seek medical care if the condition persists despite the self-care efforts.

▍Excessive Watering

Your eyes may actually water in response to dryness and irritation. Watery eyes also commonly occur with infections such as so-called pinkeye (see page 74). They can result from an allergic reaction to preservatives in eyedrops or contact lens solutions. Watery eyes also can result from a blockage in the ducts that drain tears to the inside of your nose. Overflowing tears can cause even more eye irritation and tearing.

Self-Care
- Apply a warm compress over closed eyelids two to four times a day for 10 minutes.
- Don't rub your eyes.
- Replace mascara every 6 months. Mascara can become contaminated with skin bacteria transferred by the applicator.
- If you wear contact lenses, follow directions for wearing, cleaning and disinfecting them.

▍Floaters (Specks in the Eye)

The jellylike substance behind your lens (vitreous) is supported and distributed evenly within your eyeball by a fibrous framework. As you age, the fibers thicken and gather in bundles, creating the appearance of specks, hairs, or strings that move in and out of your vision. Floaters that appear gradually and become less noticeable over time are usually harmless and require no treatment. However, floaters that appear suddenly may indicate a more serious eye disorder such as hemorrhage or retinal detachment. The retina is the light-sensitive layer of tissue at the back of the eye which transmits visual images to the brain.

Medical Help
If you see a cloud of spots or a spider web, especially accompanied by flashes of light, see your eye doctor (ophthalmologist). These symptoms can indicate a retinal tear or retinal detachment, which requires prompt surgery to prevent vision loss.

Common Problems

■ Pinkeye or Red Eye

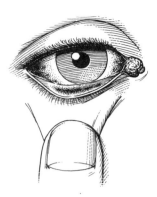

One or both eyes are red and itchy. There may be blurred vision and sensitivity to light. You may have a gritty feeling in the eye or a discharge in the eye which forms a crust during the night.

All of these are signs of a bacterial or viral infection commonly known as pink-eye. The medical term is "conjunctivitis." It is an inflammation of the membrane called the conjunctiva, which lines the eyelids and part of the eyeball.

The inflammation makes pinkeye an irritating condition, but it is usually harmless to sight. However, because it can be highly contagious, it must be diagnosed and treated early. Occasionally, pinkeye can cause eye complications.

Both viral and bacterial conjunctivitis are common among children and also affect adults. They are very contagious. Viral conjunctivitis usually produces a watery discharge, whereas bacterial conjunctivitis often produces a good deal of thick, yellow-green matter.

Allergic conjunctivitis is a response to an allergen (such as pollen) rather than an infection. In addition to intense itching, tearing and inflammation of the eye, you also may experience some degree of itching, sneezing and watery discharge from the nose.

Self-Care

- Apply a warm compress to the affected eye or eyes. Soak a clean, lint-free cloth in warm water, squeeze it dry and apply it over your gently closed eyelids.
- Allergic conjunctivitis is often effectively soothed with cool compresses.
- Try specially formulated eyedrops that contain both an antihistamine and an agent that constricts blood vessels, such as Naphcon-A, Opcon-A or a generic brand.

Prevention

Because pinkeye spreads easily and quickly, good hygiene is the most useful method for control. Once the infection has been diagnosed in you or a family member, the following steps may be useful to contain it:

- Keep hands away from your eyes.
- Wash hands frequently.
- Change towel and washcloth daily; don't share them.
- Wear clothes only once before washing.
- Change pillowcase each night.
- Discard eye cosmetics, particularly mascara, after a few months.
- Don't use other people's eye cosmetics, handkerchiefs or other personal items.

Medical Help

If you have any of the symptoms of pinkeye, see your physician. Your physician may culture the eye secretions to determine which form of infection you have. The physician may prescribe antibiotic eyedrops or ointments if the infection is bacterial. Viral conjunctivitis disappears on its own.

Kids' Care

Because the condition is contagious, keep your child away from other children. Many schools will send children with pinkeye home.

■ Sensitivity to Glare

Glare may result when light is scattered within the eyeball. Glare may be especially bothersome in low light when your pupils are dilated (enlarged) because light is allowed into your eyes at a wider angle. Sensitivity to glare may mean a developing cataract (see page 76). To evaluate your symptoms, your health-care provider may measure your vision under low, medium and high levels of glare.

Self-Care

- Reduce daytime glare by wearing polarized sunglasses with wide frames that follow your brow and opaque side shields.
- Have accurate correction for your distance vision to help minimize glare.

■ Other Eye Problems

Drooping Eyelid

Your upper eyelid may droop if the muscles responsible for raising your eyelid weaken. Normal aging, trauma or disorders of the nerves and muscles can lead to drooping eyelid. If your eyelid interferes with vision, your ophthalmologist may recommend surgery to strengthen supporting muscles. **Caution:** A drooping eyelid that develops suddenly needs immediate evaluation and treatment. It may be associated with stroke or other acute problems of your nervous system.

Inflamed (Granulated) Eyelid

A chronic inflammation along the edges of your eyelids is called blepharitis. It may accompany dry eyes. Some people produce excess oil in glands near their eyelashes. Oil encourages growth of bacteria and causes your skin to be irritated, itchy and red. Tiny scales form along the edges of your eyelids, further irritating your skin. **Self-Care:** Apply a warm compress over your gently closed eyelids two to four times a day for 10 minutes. Immediately afterward, wash away the scales with warm water or diluted baby shampoo. If the condition is caused by an infection, your health-care provider may prescribe a medicated ointment or an oral antibiotic.

Twitching Eyelid

Your eyelid takes on a life of its own—twitching at random, driving you crazy. The involuntary quivering of the eyelid muscle usually lasts less than a minute. The cause is unknown, but some people report that the painless twitching is brought on by nervous tension and fatigue. Rarely, it can be a symptom of muscle or nerve disease. Twitching eyelid is usually harmless and needs no treatment. **Self-Care:** Gentle massaging over the eyelid may help relieve the twitching.

Sty

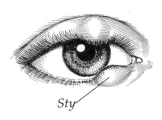

Sty

A sty is a red, painful lump on the edge of your eyelid. It is usually caused by bacterial infection in an eyelash follicle. Sties usually fill with pus and then burst in about a week. For persistent infections, your health-care provider might prescribe an antibiotic cream. **Self-Care:** Apply a clean, warm compress four times a day for 10 minutes to relieve the pain and help the sty come to a point sooner. Let the sty burst on its own, then rinse your eye thoroughly.

Common Problems

■ Common Eye Diseases

Cataract

A cataract is a clouding of the normally clear lens of your eye. Lens clouding impairs vision. Some degree of cataract formation is normal as you grow older, but some exposures or conditions can accelerate the process. Long-term exposure to ultraviolet light (UV), diabetes, a previous eye injury, exposure to X-rays and prolonged use of corticosteroid drugs increase your risk. Smoking may increase your risk for cataracts, and aspirin may decrease the risk. If cataracts interfere with your daily activities, your lens can be surgically replaced. **Self-Care:** Reduce glare. Prevent or slow cataracts by wearing UV-blocking sunglasses when outside in bright sun. Ensure adequate lighting.

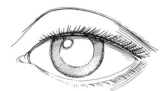 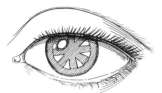

There are several forms of cataracts. Left: A nuclear cataract. Right: A wheel-spoke pattern cataract.

Glaucoma

Glaucoma involves damage to the eye (optic) nerve caused by increased pressure within the eyeball. Pressure increases when tiny pores that normally allow fluid to drain from inside your eye become blocked. Damage to the optic nerve causes your side vision to diminish slowly. Untreated, glaucoma can lead to blindness. **Caution:** Because the early symptoms can be subtle, it's important to have regular eye examinations. If diagnosed and treated early, chronic glaucoma usually can be controlled with eyedrops, oral medications or surgery. If you have symptoms such as a severe headache or pain in your eye or brow, nausea, blurred vision or rainbows around lights at night, seek immediate evaluation. Treatment may require emergency laser surgery.

Macular Degeneration

Macular degeneration blurs central vision and reduces your ability to see fine detail. It doesn't affect side vision and usually doesn't lead to total blindness. The condition occurs when tissue in the center of the retina (called the macula) deteriorates. The vision impairment is irreversible. However, when the condition is diagnosed early, laser treatment may help reduce or slow the loss of vision.

Transportation Advice for the Vision-Impaired

- Avoid stressful driving conditions—at night, in heavy traffic, in bad weather or on a freeway.
- Use public transportation or ask family members to help with night driving.
- Contact your local area agency on aging for a list of vans and shuttles, volunteer driver networks or ride-shares.
- Optimize the vision you have with the right glasses; keep an extra pair in the car.

■ Problems Related to Glasses, Contact Lenses

Many people begin to notice a change in their vision around age 40. Close-up objects that were once easy to see become blurred. The print in newspapers and books begins to seem smaller, and you instinctively hold reading material farther away from your eyes. The condition is presbyopia. It refers to the difficulty with near vision that develops as the lenses in your eyes become thicker and more rigid. Another symptom is eyestrain, which may include a feeling of tired eyes and a headache.

If you are already farsighted, you may notice the changes somewhat earlier and will need to have stronger corrective lenses. Even if you are nearsighted, you will experience the effects of presbyopia, and you may find yourself taking off your glasses to read small print. You may find that your eyes seem increasingly tired after reading.

Before trying over-the-counter reading glasses, first see an eye specialist to rule out other problems.

Medical Help

If you experience frequent headaches, see your ophthalmologist or optometrist, who will test your eyes and prescribe appropriate lenses, if needed.

Respond to warnings such as blurring of vision, yellowing of colors, increased sensitivity to light or loss of side vision, which could indicate cataracts or glaucoma.

Contact Lenses Versus Glasses

Contacts or glasses—which is better? Contact lenses are improving, but they are not for everyone. Certain diseases of the eye (dry eyes, previous corneal ulcers or corneas that have a loss of sensation) make wearing contact lenses inadvisable. Insertion, removal and care of contacts may be impractical for persons with arthritis of the hands, tremor from Parkinson's disease and physical disabilities from other disorders. However, contacts are preferable to glasses in some cases. For example, contact lenses offer markedly improved vision to people who are born with a malformation of the cornea. Contact lenses also offer advantages over glasses if you did not receive an artificial lens at the time of cataract removal.

Self-Care for Contact Lens Wearers
- Keep your contacts clean.
- Wash your hands before handling contacts.
- Use only commercial contact lens wetting and cleaning solutions.
- Have a pair of glasses as backup in case a problem requires you to stop wearing your contacts for a while.

Extended-Wear and Disposable Soft Contact Lenses
If you use extended-wear contact lenses, remove and sterilize them most nights. If you wear disposable lenses, do not wear them beyond the time recommended by your eye specialist. Wearing contact lenses too long without removing them may deprive your corneas of oxygen. Lack of oxygen can cause blurred vision, pain, tearing, redness and sensitivity to light. Remove your lenses at once if any of these symptoms occur. Have regular eye examinations to avoid problems that may result from extended contact wear.

FOR MORE INFORMATION
- The National Eye Institute, 2020 Vision Place, Bethesda, MD 20892-3655; (301) 496-5248; Internet address: www.nei.nih.gov.
- The Lighthouse Inc., 3620 Northern Blvd., Long Island City, NY 11101-1614; (800) 829-0500; Internet address: www.lighthouse.org.
- The local chapter of your State Society for the Blind and Visually Impaired.

Common Problems

Headache

Brain tissue can't ache. It doesn't have pain receptors. This seems incredible when your head hurts.

Headaches are the most common reported medical complaint. They may point to a serious medical problem. But that situation is rare.

About 95 percent of all headaches have no underlying disease. These so-called primary headaches differ greatly. Researchers aren't sure what happens physically when you get a headache, but research is under way to find out.

Types of Headaches

We divide primary headaches into three categories, although you may have a combination.

Tension Headaches
- Include 9 of 10 primary headaches
- Affect men and women equally
- Gradually produce a dull pain, knot or pressure in your neck, forehead or scalp

Migraine Headaches
- Total about 6 percent of primary headaches
- Affect three times as many women as men
- May begin in your teens, rarely after 40
- May be preceded by a visual change, tingling on one side of your face or body or a specific food craving

Cluster Headaches
- Produce steady, boring pain in and around one eye, occurring in episodes that often begin at the same time of day or night
- Cause watering and redness of an eye and nasal stuffiness on the same side of the face
- May occur like clockwork and be linked to light or seasonal changes
- Frequently affect men, especially heavy smokers and drinkers
- May be misdiagnosed as a sinus infection or dental problem

New Headache Theory

Researchers are focusing on the trigeminal nerve pathway and the brain chemical serotonin as possible culprits in severe headache pain.
Pain may result from an imbalance of chemicals in your brain. During a headache, serotonin levels drop. As a result, an impulse moves along the trigeminal nerve to blood vessels in your brain's outer covering (meninges). Here blood vessels relax and become inflamed and swollen. Your brain receives the pain message. The result: headache.

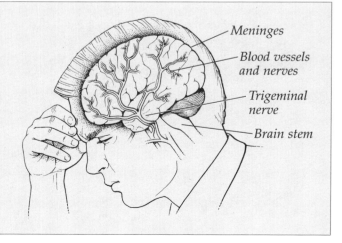

Meninges

Blood vessels and nerves

Trigeminal nerve

Brain stem

Self-Care	**For Occasional Tension-Type Headaches** First, try massage, hot or cold packs, a warm shower, rest or relaxation techniques. If these measures don't work, try a low dose of aspirin (adults only), acetaminophen or ibuprofen. Moderate exercise may help.

For Recurrent Headaches

- Keep a headache diary. Include these factors:
  - *Severity.* Is it disabling pain, or merely annoying?
  - *Frequency and duration.* When does the headache start? Does it begin gradually or strike rapidly? Does it occur at a certain time of day? In monthly or seasonal cycles? How long does it last? What makes it stop?
  - *Related symptoms.* Can you tell it's coming? Are you nauseated or dizzy? Do you see sparkling colors or blank spots? Do you have specific hungers beforehand?
  - *Location.* Is the pain usually on one side of your head? In your neck muscles? Around one eye?
  - *Family history.* Do other family members have similar headaches?
  - *Triggers.* Can you link your headache to any particular food, activity, weather, time frame or environmental factors? (See Avoiding Headache Triggers, page 80.)
- Avoid triggers, as possible. To do so may require lifestyle changes.
- Get adequate sleep and exercise.
- Use aspirin (adults only), acetaminophen or ibuprofen for pain relief.

Special Migraine Self-Care

Begin treatment when you feel a migraine coming. This approach is your best chance to stop it early. Use acetaminophen, ibuprofen or aspirin (adults only) at the recommended dosage for pain relief. Some people can abort an attack by going to sleep in a darkened room or consuming caffeine (coffee or cola).

Medical Help	If self-care doesn't help after 1 or 2 days, see your health-care provider. He or she will try to determine the type and cause of your headache, will try to exclude other possible sources of pain and may do tests. Your physician may prescribe one of many pain medications. Different medications are used for different types of headaches. For severe migraines, your physician may prescribe sumatriptan (Imitrex) or another medication. Sumatriptan mimics serotonin, a nerve chemical in your body. For frequent migraine attacks, your physician may prescribe a preventive medication to use on a daily basis.
Caution	Don't ignore unexplained headaches. Get medical attention right away if your headache: • Strikes suddenly and severely • Accompanies a fever, stiff neck, rash, mental confusion, seizures, double vision, weakness, numbness or speaking difficulties • Follows a recent sore throat or respiratory infection • Worsens after a head injury, fall or bump • Is a new pain, and you're over 55

Common Problems

Avoiding Headache Triggers

Does a particular food, drink or activity trigger your headaches? Some people can eliminate headaches by avoiding triggers. Triggers vary among individuals. Here are some common ones:

- Alcohol, red wine
- Smoking
- Stress or fatigue
- Eye strain
- Physical or sexual activity
- Poor posture
- Changing sleeping patterns or mealtimes

- Certain foods, such as:
  - fermented, pickled or marinated food
  - bananas
  - caffeine
  - aged cheeses
  - chocolate
  - citrus fruits
  - food additives (sodium nitrite in hot dogs, sausages or lunch meat, or monosodium glutamate in processed or Chinese foods) and seasonings
  - nuts or peanut butter
  - pizza
  - raisins
  - sourdough bread
- Weather, altitude or time zone changes
- Hormonal changes during your menstrual cycle or menopause, oral contraceptive use or hormone replacement therapy
- Strong or flickering lights
- Odors, including perfumes, flowers or natural gas
- Polluted air or stuffy rooms
- Excessive noise

Kids' Care

Recurrent headaches are common during late childhood and adolescence. They rarely represent a serious problem.

Headache is associated with many viral illnesses. However, if your child frequently complains of headache, even during times when he is otherwise well, consult your physician.

Migraine headaches may occur in children and may be suspected if there is a family history of migraine. In children, this type of headache often is accompanied by vomiting, light sensitivity and sleep. Recovery follows within a few hours.

A headache may indicate stress with school, friends or family. It may be a reaction to a medication, particularly a decongestant.

If you think it's a tension-type headache, try the nonmedicating tips listed on page 79. If it occurs frequently, help your child keep a headache diary. Use acetaminophen or ibuprofen sparingly and briefly to avoid missing serious problems that the pain reliever may be masking.

If your child's headache persists, comes suddenly without explanation or gets steadily worse, call your health-care provider. Also call about headaches that follow recent ear infections, toothaches, strep throat or other infections.

Be sure to tell your physician if there is any family history of migraines. That information could help lead to a diagnosis.

The Link Between Caffeine and Headaches

That morning caffeine headache can be very real, especially if you consume 4 or more cups of caffeinated drinks during the day. It may be a withdrawal headache after a night without caffeine.

But, for some headaches, caffeine may be a cure. Some kinds of headaches cause blood vessels to widen. Caffeine temporarily causes them to narrow.

So, for adults, if simple aspirin or acetaminophen doesn't help, you can use a medicine that includes caffeine. But don't overdo. Some of caffeine's side effects aren't helpful: jitteriness, rapid heart rate, sweating and, yes, withdrawal headaches.

Limbs, Muscles, Bones and Joints

Your body is amazingly intricate. You don't think about your body much when it's working fine. Somehow, everything holds together and you move about easily. But you usually do notice when there's a problem.

This chapter focuses on problems related to your limbs. Some conditions are common to many areas of your body, such as strains, sprains, broken bones, bursitis, tendinitis, fibromyalgia and gout. We address these conditions on pages 83 to 88. The remainder of the chapter provides additional information about problems related to specific limbs: shoulder; elbow; wrist, hand and fingers; hip; leg; knee; and ankle and foot. But first, here is some general information on anatomy.

Anatomy

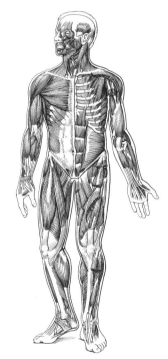

Many of your skeletal muscles are paired, enabling your body to move. Tendons connect these muscles to your bones.

Muscles and Tendons

Many of your 650 muscles help you move. Each skeletal muscle is attached to bones by bands called tendons. Pairs of muscles work together to move your bones. One muscle relaxes as its partner contracts.

If you are active, your muscles enable you to run, walk, swim, jump, climb stairs, bike, dance or mow the lawn. However, your muscles let you know when you've overdone it. They become sore and stiff.

Common causes of muscle injuries include accidents; strains; sudden, off-balance movements; overuse; and inflammation.

You can avoid many muscle and tendon aches by:
- Exercising regularly and moderately. Build up your activity gradually. You're not ready to run a marathon if you're not regularly running more than a few miles.
- Stretching your muscles gently before and after you exercise. For some people it's also helpful to use heat and massage to loosen their muscles before activity.
- Drinking plenty of water. Drinking 6 to 8 glasses of water a day maintains good hydration. But you'll need more than that when you're active, especially in the heat of summer.
- Conditioning your muscles gradually. Increase activity a little at a time.
- Strengthening your muscles with resistance exercise.
- Supporting previously injured areas with elastic tape or a brace.
- Avoiding stressing your muscles when you are tired.

Bones—Rigid, But Alive

You can't see it, but the 206 bones in your body change constantly. Proteins form the framework. Minerals, especially calcium and phosphate, fill in to give the bones strength. Because of this need for minerals, it's a good idea to consume mineral-rich milk and leafy green vegetables.

Common bone conditions include the following:
- Breaks, resulting from stress on a bone greater than it can withstand
- Bruising, usually from trauma
- Weakening through loss of minerals (osteoporosis)

A child's bones are more pliable than an adult's. When under strain or pressure, they are less likely to break. As you mature, your bones become more rigid.

Growing Pains Are Real

So-called growing pains can be very real during growth spurts. They usually occur in children's legs, often at night. They last a few hours and then go away. Growing pains usually don't hamper normal light activity.

If your child has growing pains:

- Use a warm heating pad for relief.
- Use recommended child's doses of acetaminophen or ibuprofen for pain. Don't give aspirin to children unless advised by your doctor to do so.
- Seek medical care if the area becomes swollen, hot and tender, or if your child develops a limp or unexplained fever.

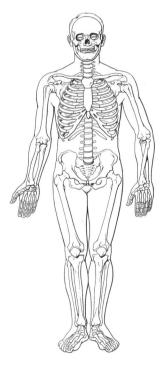

Your bones are living tissue and are always changing. They provide support for your body and function as your body's depository for important minerals.

Joints—Mechanical Masterpieces

Your bones come together at your joints. The end of each bone is covered by a layer of cartilage that glides smoothly and acts as a shock absorber. Tough bands of tissue (ligaments) hold your joints together.

Your body has several types of joints. This chapter discusses the following types:

- Hinge joints—in the ends of your fingers or your knees, for example. They allow one kind of back-and-forth movement.
- Ball and socket joints—in your shoulder or hip, for example. They allow a wide range of movement.

Causes of joint pain covered in this chapter include:

- Traumatic injuries or dislocation (when a joint is pushed out of place)
- Bursitis
- Fibromyalgia
- Gout
- Sprains

If your child has specific joint pain, you should be concerned. Call your health-care provider if your child has joint pain along with:

- A fever and rash
- Swelling, stiffness, abdominal pain or unexplained weight loss
- Enlarged and tender lymph glands in the neck
- Limping or impaired normal activity

Nerves—Lines of Communication

Most of this chapter focuses on bones, muscles and joints. However, all of your limbs are wired with nerves that carry messages to and from your brain. They sense pain and also help you locate its source. They direct your movement. They let you know when your muscles are tired or injured. They may keep a muscle from working properly.

Nerves help coordinate your movement. When your body is working properly, they are in constant contact with your brain. They also help you avoid many injuries.

It's easier for you or your health-care provider to identify and treat pain if you can tell how it happened. Did it follow:

- An accident
- Prolonged overuse or repetitive motions
- Inflammation
- An illness or condition elsewhere in your body

Muscle Strains: When You've Overdone It

A muscle becomes strained or "pulled"—or may even tear—when it stretches unusually far or abruptly. This type of injury often occurs when muscles suddenly and powerfully contract. A slip on the ice or lifting in an awkward position may cause a muscle strain.

Muscle strains vary in severity:

- **Mild:** causes pain and stiffness when you move and lasts a few days.
- **Moderate:** causes small muscle tears and more extensive pain, swelling and bruising. The pain may last 1 to 3 weeks.
- **Severe:** muscle becomes torn apart or ruptured. You may have significant internal bleeding, swelling and bruising around the muscle. Your muscle may not function at all. Seek medical attention immediately.

Self-Care

- Follow the instructions for P.R.I.C.E. (see below). The earlier the treatment, the speedier and more complete your recovery.
- For extensive swelling, use cold packs several times each day throughout your recovery.
- Do not apply heat when the area is still swollen.
- Avoid the activity that caused the strain while the muscle heals.
- Use over-the-counter pain medications as needed (see page 231). Avoid using aspirin in the first few hours after the strain because aspirin may make bleeding more extensive. Don't give aspirin to children.

Medical Help

Seek medical help immediately if the area quickly becomes swollen and is intensely painful. Call your health-care provider if the pain, swelling and stiffness don't improve much in 2 to 3 days or if you suspect a ruptured muscle or broken bone.

P.R.I.C.E.: Your Best Tool for Muscle or Joint Injury

We refer to this information frequently throughout this section.

- **P: Protect** the area from further injury. Use an elastic wrap, a sling, splint, cane, crutches or an air cast.
- **R: Rest** to promote tissue healing. Avoid activities that cause pain, swelling or discomfort.
- **I: Ice** the area immediately, even if you're seeking medical help. Use an ice pack or slush bath for about 15 minutes each time you apply the ice. Repeat every 2 to 3 hours while you're awake for the first 48 to 72 hours. Cold reduces pain, swelling and inflammation in injured muscles, joints and connecting tissues. It also may slow bleeding if a tear has occurred.
- **C: Compress** the area with an elastic bandage until the swelling stops. Don't wrap it tightly or you may hinder circulation. Begin wrapping at the end farthest from your heart. Loosen the wrap if the pain increases, the area becomes numb or swelling is occurring below the wrapped area.
- **E: Elevate** the area above your heart, especially at night. Gravity helps reduce swelling by draining excess fluid.
- After 48 hours, if the swelling is gone, you may apply warmth or gentle heat. Heat can improve the blood flow and speed healing.
- Apply cold to sore areas after a workout, even if you are not injured, to prevent inflammation and swelling.

■ Sprains: Damage to Your Ligaments

Strictly speaking, a sprain occurs when you overextend or tear a ligament. Ligaments are the tough, elastic-like bands that attach to your bones and hold your joints in place.

Sometimes we use the term "sprain" any time your joint moves outside its normal range of movement. Sprains frequently are caused by twisting. They occur most often in your ankles, knees or the arches of your feet. Sprains cause rapid swelling. Generally, the greater the pain, the more severe the injury. Sprains vary in severity:

- **Mild:** your ligament stretches excessively or tears slightly. The area is somewhat painful, especially with movement. It's tender. There is not a lot of swelling. You can put weight on the joint.
- **Moderate:** the fibers in your ligament tear, but they don't rupture completely. The joint is tender, painful and difficult to move. The area is swollen and discolored from bleeding in the area.
- **Severe:** one or more ligaments tear completely. The area is painful. You can't move your joint normally or put weight on it. It becomes very swollen and discolored. The injury may be difficult to distinguish from a fracture or dislocation, which requires medical care. You may need a cast to hold the joint motionless, or an operation, if torn ligaments cause joint instability.

Self-Care

- Follow the instructions for P.R.I.C.E. (see page 83).
- Use over-the-counter pain medications (see page 231).
- Gradually test and use the joint after 2 days. Mild to moderate sprains usually improve significantly in a week, although full healing may take 6 weeks.
- Avoid activities that stress your joint. Repeated minor sprains will weaken it.

Medical Help

Seek medical care immediately if:

- You hear a popping sound when your joint is injured and you can't use it. On the way to your health-care provider, apply cold.
- You have a fever and the area is red and hot. You may have an infection.
- You have a severe sprain, as described above. Inadequate or delayed treatment may cause long-term joint instability or chronic pain.

See your doctor if you are unable to bear weight on the joint after 2 to 3 days of self-care or if you don't experience much improvement in a week.

Preventing Sports Injuries

- Select your sport carefully. Don't jog if you have chronic back pain or sore knees.
- Warm up. Loosen, stretch and gradually increase your activity over 5 to 10 minutes. If you are prone to muscle pain, apply heat before you exercise.
- After exercising, cool down with muscle stretches.
- Begin a new sport gradually. Increase your level of exertion over several weeks.
- Use pain relievers with caution. It's easier to overexert and damage tissue without realizing it.
- Stop participating immediately if you think you may be injured, you become disoriented or dizzy or you lose consciousness, even briefly.
- Return gradually to full activity or switch sports until injuries heal.

■ Broken Bones (Fractures)

If you suspect a bone is broken, get medical care. A broken bone may or may not poke through your skin. Open fractures break through the skin. Simple fractures do not. Simple fractures are classified according to the way the bone breaks. Several varieties of simple fractures are included in the illustrations below.

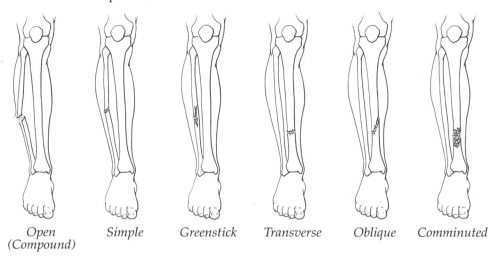

| *Open* | *Simple* | *Greenstick* | *Transverse* | *Oblique* | *Comminuted* |
| *(Compound)* | | | | | |

Emergency Treatment

After injury or trauma, seek medical care immediately if:
- The person is unconscious or can't be moved. Call 911.
- The person is not breathing or doesn't have a pulse. Begin CPR (see page 2).
- There is heavy bleeding.
- Even gentle pressure or movement produces pain.
- The limb or joint appears deformed or the bone has pierced the skin.
- The part farthest from the heart is numb or bluish at the tip.

Self-Care

Take these precautions immediately, and seek medical care:
- Protect the area from further damage.
- If there is bleeding, try to stop it. Press directly on the wound with a sterile bandage, clean cloth or piece of clothing. If nothing else is available, use your hand. Keep pressing until the bleeding stops.
- Use a splint or sling to hold the area still. You can make a splint from wood, plastic or rolled newspaper. Place it on both sides of the bone, extending beyond the ends of the bone. Hold it firmly in place with gauze, cloth strips, tape or string, but not tight enough to stop the blood flow.
- Do not try to set the bone yourself.
- If ice is available, wrap the ice in cloth and apply it to the splinted limb.
- Try to elevate the injured area above the heart to reduce bleeding and swelling.
- If the person becomes faint or is breathing in short breaths, he or she may be in shock. Lay the person down with his or her head slightly lower than the rest of the body.

Kids' Care

The bones in your child's arms and legs have growth plates near the ends that allow bones to lengthen. If growth plates become damaged, the bone may not grow properly. Check out any possible fractures with your doctor.

Common Problems

■ Bursitis

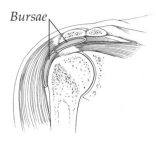

Bursae

You have more than 150 bursae in your body. These tiny, fluid-filled sacs lubricate and cushion pressure points for your bones, tendons and muscles near your joints. They help you move without pain. When they become inflamed, movement or pressure is painful. This condition is called bursitis. Bursitis is commonly caused by overuse, trauma, repeated bumping or prolonged pressure such as kneeling for an extended period. It may even result from an infection, arthritis or gout. Most often, bursitis affects the shoulder, elbow or hip joint. But you also can have bursitis at your knee, heel and even in the base of your big toe.

Self-Care

- Use over-the-counter pain medications (see page 231).
- Keep pressure off the joint. Use an elastic bandage, sling or soft foam pad to protect it until the swelling goes down.
- Simple cases of bursitis usually disappear within 2 weeks. Ease the area back into activity slowly.

Prevention

- Strengthen your muscles to help protect the joint. Don't start exercising a joint that has bursitis until the pain and inflammation are gone.
- Take frequent breaks from repetitive tasks. Alternate the repetitive task with rest or other activities, even briefly.
- Cushion the joint before applying pressure (such as with kneeling or elbow pads).

Medical Help

Seek medical care if the area becomes red and hot or doesn't improve, or if you also have a fever or rash.

■ Tendinitis

Tendinitis produces pain and tenderness near a joint. You can usually associate it with a specific movement (grasping, for example). It usually means you have an inflammation or a small tear of the tendon. Tendinitis is usually the result of overuse or a minor injury. It's most common around the shoulders, elbows and knees.

Pain may cause you to limit movement. Rest is important, but so is maintaining a full range of movement. If you don't treat tendinitis carefully, tendons and ligaments around your joint may gradually stiffen over several weeks. Movement may become limited and difficult.

Self-Care

- Follow the instructions for P.R.I.C.E. (see page 83).
- Gently move the joint through its full range four times a day. Otherwise rest it. A sling or elastic bandage may help.
- If soreness doesn't greatly improve in 2 weeks, see your health-care provider.

Prevention

- Use warm-up and cool-down exercises and strengthening exercises.
- If you are prone to tendinitis, apply heat to the area before you exercise and then apply cold afterward.
- Don't exercise every day when starting an exercise program.

Medical Help	Seek medical help immediately if you have a fever and the area is inflamed.

Sometimes doctors inject a drug into tissue around a tendon to relieve tendinitis. Cortisone injections reduce inflammation and can give rapid relief of pain. These injections must be used with care, however, because repeated injections may weaken the tendon or cause undesirable side effects.

■ Fibromyalgia

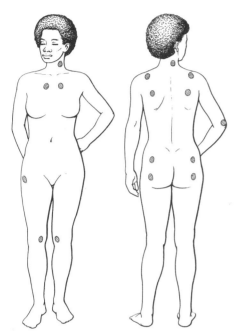

Common locations of fibromyalgia.

Persistent pain and stiffness in your muscles may have many causes. In recent years, health-care providers have increasingly diagnosed a condition called fibromyalgia.

Common symptoms that lead to the diagnosis include general aches and pain and stiffness in joints and muscles. The type of pain can vary. It often affects areas where tendons attach muscles to bones. Symptoms frequently include the following:

- Widespread aching, lasting more than 3 months
- Fatigue and non-restful, non-restorative sleep
- Morning stiffness
- Tender points on the body, usually at sites of muscle attachment (see illustration)
- Associated problems such as headaches (see page 87), irritable bowel syndrome (see page 61) and pelvic pain

Fibromyalgia is a "diagnosis of exclusion." Currently, there are no laboratory tests that can be used to help make the diagnosis. Your doctor will make the diagnosis after considering other causes for your symptoms.

Emotional tension or stress may increase your likelihood of having fibromyalgia. It is more frequent in women than in men. This difference may be partially due to the fact that men may be more reluctant to see a doctor about their symptoms.

Self-Care	

- Pace yourself. Reduce your stress and avoid long hours of repetitive activity. Develop a routine that alternates work with rest.
- Develop a regular, low-impact exercise program such as walking, biking, swimming and plenty of stretching exercises. Improve your posture by strengthening supportive muscles, especially abdominal muscles (see page 51).
- Improve your sleep naturally with daily physical activity. To avoid undesirable side effects, use sleep medications sparingly, if at all.
- If necessary, use over-the-counter pain medications occasionally (see page 231).

Prevention

The best thing you can do to avoid or minimize fibromyalgia is to keep yourself in good physical condition, reduce stress and get adequate sleep.

- Try not to quit your job. Fibromyalgia seems to worsen in people who go on disability and eliminate activity entirely.
- Learn relaxation techniques. Try massage and warm baths.
- Find a support group that emphasizes maintaining health.
- Ask your family and friends for support.

Common Problems

◼ Gout

Gout produces a sudden pain in a single joint, usually at the base of your big toe, although it may affect joints in your feet, ankles, knees, hands and wrists as well. The joint becomes swollen and red. Gout occurs most often in men older than 40. A fourth of persons with gout have a family history of the condition. Gout occurs when crystals of uric acid collect at a joint. Your risk of having gout increases if you are obese or have high blood pressure. Blood pressure medications that reduce your body's water content may provoke gout. Self-care measures include maintaining a reasonable weight, drinking plenty of water and avoiding heavy alcohol consumption. Seek medical care immediately if you have a fever and your joint is hot and inflamed. For more information, see page 158.

◼ Shoulder Pain

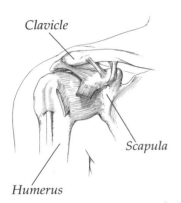

Clavicle

Scapula

Humerus

Treatment of shoulder pain depends on its cause. Bursitis and tendinitis are common causes of shoulder pain (see page 86), as are acute injury and rotator cuff tears (see page 89). Take note of how the pain began and what makes the pain worse. This information can be helpful if you need medical care.

Most shoulder pain is not life-threatening. Occasionally, however, shoulder pain signals a heart attack. Call 911 or your local rescue system right away if your pain:
- Starts as chest pain or pressure. The pain may occur suddenly or gradually. It may radiate to your shoulder, back, arms, jaw and neck.
- Is accompanied by excessive sweating, shortness of breath, faintness or nausea and vomiting.
- Is new and you have a known heart condition.

◼ Acute Painful Shoulder

Acute shoulder pain centers on your upper arm and neck. Pain may suddenly limit arm movement. Possible causes include overuse or trauma. Your shoulder may become inflamed and swollen at the tip. It may be very painful to put on a coat or extend your arm straight out from your side.

Self-Care
- Use over-the-counter pain medications (see page 231).
- If the bone isn't broken or dislocated, it's important to move the joint through it's full range four times a day to avoid stiffening or a permanent condition called "frozen shoulder." If necessary, ask a friend to help you move your arm gently through its full range.
- Once pain has resolved, exercise your arm daily.

Medical Help
Seek medical care if:
- Your shoulders appear uneven or you cannot raise the affected arm
- You have extreme tenderness at the end of your collarbone
- An injury causes you to wonder if a bone is broken
- You have redness, swelling or fever
- Your shoulder is not improving after a week of self-care

Rotator Cuff Injury

The rotator cuff is formed by the attachment of several tendons to the shoulder. Because of the shoulder's complexity, many problems are simply diagnosed as rotator cuff injuries. The tendons in your shoulder may have tiny tears, be irritated or pinched between your bones (called impingement). Pain may be more severe at night. This type of injury usually results from repetitive overhead motions (such as painting a ceiling, swimming, playing a racket sport or throwing a baseball or softball) or from trauma, such as falling on your shoulder.

Self-Care

- Follow the instructions for P.R.I.C.E. (see page 83).
- Take anti-inflammatory medicines (see page 231).
- Do stretching exercises and put the shoulder through its full range of motion four times daily.
- Wait until the pain is gone before gradually returning to the activity that caused the injury. You may have to wait 3 to 6 weeks.
- Alter your technique in racket sports, pitching or golf.

Medical Help

Seek medical care if the area is hot and inflamed and you have a fever, if your shoulders are uneven or if you can't move your arm at all.

If the pain hasn't diminished in 1 week despite the use of self-care measures, see your doctor.

Elbow and Forearm Pain

Bursitis and tendinitis are common sources of pain in your elbow (see page 86). Bursitis may produce a small, egg-shaped, fluid-filled sac at the tip of your elbow. If the pain hasn't improved after a few days of treatment and the area is still very sensitive to pressure, seek medical care. You may need an X-ray to determine whether a bone is broken.

A **dislocated elbow** may occur in a child if an adult suddenly pulls or jerks the child's arm. The elbow of a child—especially if younger than 6 years—cannot withstand this stress. Dislocation is very painful and limits movement. Seek medical treatment immediately. Your health-care provider will return the bones to their proper position, which usually relieves the pain. An X-ray can rule out other problems. Use a sling for 2 weeks or as directed to stabilize the joint.

A **hyperextended elbow** occurs when your elbow is pushed beyond its normal range of motion, often as a result of a fall or misplay during a tennis swing. Pain and swelling occur in your elbow and in the tissues beneath your elbow. Try P.R.I.C.E. (see page 83) and support your elbow with a splint or sling until the pain stops. If the pain has not improved in a week, see your health-care provider.

Medical Help

Seek medical care immediately if:

- Your elbow seems deformed
- Your elbow is very stiff and has limited range of motion after a fall
- The pain in your arm is severe

Common Problems

■ Tennis Elbow or Little League Elbow

This recurrent pain is actually a form of tendinitis (called epicondylitis). It affects the outside or inside of your forearm, just below your elbow. Pain may extend down toward your wrist. It's caused by repeated tiny tears in tendons that attach muscles of your lower arm to your elbow. Common causes include swinging a racket, baseball pitching, painting a house, using a screwdriver or hammer or any movement requiring twisting arm motions.

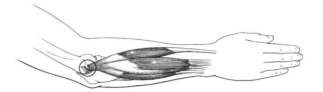

Tennis elbow produces pain on the outside or inside of your forearm near your elbow (see circle) when you exercise the joint. Tiny tears or inflammation causes the discomfort.

Self-Care

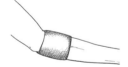

- Follow the instructions for P.R.I.C.E. (see page 83).
- Massage may speed healing by improving circulation in the area.
- Splinting your elbow and forearm at night may reduce pain.
- It may take 6 to 12 weeks of treatment for the pain to disappear.

Prevention
- Prepare for any sport season with appropriate preseason conditioning. Do strengthening exercises with a hand weight by flexing and extending the wrists.
- Wear forearm support bands just below your elbow.
- Warm up properly. Gently stretch the forearm muscles before and after use.
- Try applying a warm pack for 5 minutes before activity and an ice pack after heavy use.

Medical Help

Seek medical care immediately if:
- Your elbow is hot and inflamed and you have a fever
- You can't bend your elbow at all or it looks deformed
- A fall or injury causes you to wonder if a bone is broken

If the pain doesn't improve in a week or so, see your doctor to rule out other complications.

■ Wrist, Hand and Finger Pain

Think of all the things you do each day with your wrists, hands and fingers. You may not consider the many nerves, blood vessels, muscles and small bones that work together as you turn a key in the door—until the movement becomes painful.

Pain and swelling in your wrists, hands and fingers can result from injury or overuse. They can begin gradually or rapidly. They may be due to the following:

- A strain or sprain (see pages 83 and 84)
- Fracture, bursitis, tendinitis or gout (see pages 85, 86 and 88)
- Arthritis or fibromyalgia (see page 157 and page 87).

Self-Care

- Follow the instructions for P.R.I.C.E. (see page 83).
- Take over-the-counter pain medicines (see page 231).
- If an initial X-ray doesn't show a fracture and it's still quite painful a week later, ask your health-care provider to check again. Some fractures may require special X-ray views or be invisible in the first few days.
- If pain continues, you may need further testing, rest in a splint or cast or physical therapy.

Prevention

- Remove your rings before manual labor. If you injure your hand, remove your rings before your fingers become swollen.
- Take frequent breaks to rest muscles you've used steadily. Vary your activities.
- Use flexibility and strengthening exercises.

Medical Help

Seek medical care immediately if:

- You suspect a fracture
- A fall or accident has caused rapid swelling and moving the area is painful
- The area is hot and inflamed and you have a fever
- Your fingers suddenly become blue and numb

■ Common Problems

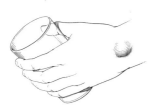

A ganglion is a swelling beneath the skin. It's a fluid-filled cyst lined with tissue bulging from a joint or tendon sheath.

Ganglions are fluid-filled lumps that usually appear on the back of the wrist, but they may be in the front, in the palm or over finger joints. They're filled with jelly-like material leaking from a joint or tendon, although they feel firm or solid. Ganglions are sometimes painful and, if bothersome, may require treatment. Seek medical care immediately if the lump becomes painful and inflamed or if the cyst breaks through the skin and drains (usually at the end of the fingers).

A **jammed finger** commonly occurs during sports activities. Pain may be caused by a sprain (stretched ligaments) or a fracture involving the joint surface. Follow the P.R.I.C.E. guidelines on page 83. To protect it during use, "buddy tape" the injured finger to an adjacent finger. Seek medical care immediately if:

- Your finger appears deformed
- You cannot straighten your finger
- The area becomes hot and inflamed and you have a fever
- Swelling and pain are significant or persistent

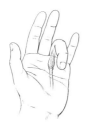

A **trigger finger** (called Dupuytren's contracture) is a condition that causes the finger to lock or catch in a bent position. It will straighten with a visible sudden "snap," and if it is severe, the finger may not fully straighten. Triggering is more pronounced in the morning and after firmly grasping an object. It is caused by a binding "knot" in the palm which prevents smooth tendon motion. Change your habits to avoid overuse. Seek medical care immediately if your finger is hot and inflamed and you have a fever.

■ Carpal Tunnel Syndrome

A narrow tunnel through your wrist (the carpal tunnel) protects your median nerve, which provides sensation to your fingers. When swelling occurs in the tunnel, the median nerve can become compressed, and pain is produced.

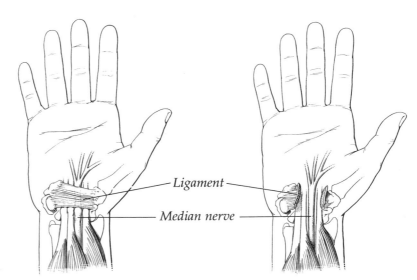

Ligament

Median nerve

Finger-bending (flexor) tendons and an important nerve pass through a tight space (the carpal tunnel) as they enter the hand. Swelling in the tunnel may squeeze the nerve. Most problems occur without a clear cause. Swelling is more common in women than in men, and it occurs more commonly in people who have hand-intensive occupations or hobbies, such as knitting, repetitive keyboarding, heavy lifting or grasping activities. It also may occur with pregnancy, thyroid conditions, diabetes and arthritis. Children who frequently play computer games may develop hand or wrist pain.

Symptoms include the following:
- Tingling or numbness in your fingers or hand (but not your little finger). It often occurs while sleeping, driving or holding the phone or newspaper.
- Pain radiating or extending from your wrist into your forearm or down into your palm or fingers.
- A sense of weakness; dropping objects.
- If the condition is advanced, a constant loss of feeling in some fingers.

Self-Care
- Take frequent breaks, even if for just a minute or two.
- Vary your activities. Stretch your wrists and hands at least once every hour.
- Try wearing a wrist splint at night. It should be snug but not tight.
- If you use a computer most of the day, refer to page 221 for additional tips.
- If the symptoms continue or worsen, see your health-care provider.

■ Thumb Pain

Pain at the base of your thumb may be the first sign of wear-and-tear arthritis in your hands (see page 157). You may notice pain and swelling at the base of your thumb when you write, open jars, turn your key in the door or ignition or try to hold small objects. It may be limited to one joint or extend to many. It's most common in women older than 55. In addition to arthritis, the pain can be caused by a previous injury, repetitive activity (such as screwing bolts) and heredity.

Self-Care

- Avoid activities that cause pain.
- Rest your thumb. Use a splint to stabilize the wrist and thumb. Remove the splint at least four times a day to move and stretch the joints to maintain flexibility.
- Use over-the counter pain medications (see page 231).
- Exercise your thumb daily while your hands are warm. Move your thumb in wide circles. Bend it to touch each of the other fingers on your hand.
- Use tools specially designed for people with arthritis.

Medical Help

Seek medical care immediately if pain limits activities or is too severe to tolerate most days. Cortisone injections, arthritis medicine and, occasionally, an operation are effective in alleviating pain.

■ Hip Pain

Hip pain frequently follows a fall or accident. It also may occur after vigorous speed walking or aerobics. Common causes include bursitis, tendinitis and arthritis (see pages 86 and 157, respectively) or strains and sprains (see pages 83 and 84). Only rarely is hip pain caused by having one leg shorter than the other, and differences in leg length of half an inch or more (1 to 2 cm) are common and normal.

Self-Care

- Follow the instructions for P.R.I.C.E. (see page 83).
- Avoid activities that aggravate the pain.
- Take over-the-counter pain medicines (see page 231).
- Strengthen the hip group muscles (especially the hip abductors, which move the leg out from the body) to relieve pain and improve function in an arthritic hip.

Medical Help

Seek medical care immediately if:
- You have fallen or had an accident and wonder if your hip may be broken
- You have followed the self-care instructions above after an accident or fall and your hip is more painful the following day
- You have osteoporosis and have injured your hip in a fall

Common Problems

■ Leg Pain

Many leg difficulties result from a combination of overuse, deconditioning (poor strength and flexibility), being overweight, trauma and poor circulation. Lifestyle changes may improve your legs' comfort.

Use the following exercises to strengthen your muscles and avoid injuries:
- Walk. Begin with short strides. Lengthen your stride as your muscles loosen.
- Bike. Gradually increase your distance and speed over weeks.
- Swim. Stretch and tone your muscles.
- Work paired muscles equally. For example, exercise the quadriceps (the muscles on the front of the thigh) equally with the hamstrings (muscles on the back of the thigh).

■ Pulled Hamstring Muscle

Athletes often bruise or strain hamstring muscles, especially during sports such as soccer or track-and-field activities. You may suspect such an injury if you experience pain after a slip or rigorous activity.

Self-Care

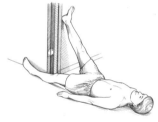

- Follow the instructions for P.R.I.C.E. (see page 83). If symptoms don't begin to improve after a week of P.R.I.C.E. treatment, see your health-care provider.

To avoid hamstring injury, do this simple exercise called the "doorframe stretch":
- Lie on the floor in front of a doorway and extend your left leg straight ahead across the threshold. Slide into the doorframe with the leg to be stretched up against the wall and straighten the leg. Hold for 30 seconds. Repeat, reversing leg positions. Do not lock your knee.
- As you get better, strive to bring your leg position perpendicular to your body.

■ Pain, Cramps and Charley Horses

A cramp, sometimes called a charley horse, is actually a muscle spasm. Cramps commonly occur in an athlete who is overfatigued and dehydrated during sports, especially in warm weather. However, almost everyone experiences a muscle cramp at some time. For most people, cramps are only an occasional inconvenience.

Self-Care

- Gently stretch and massage a cramping muscle.
- For lower leg (calf) cramps, put your weight on the leg and bend your knee slightly, or do the calf stretch outlined on page 102.
- For upper leg (hamstring) cramps, straighten your legs and lean forward at your waist. Steady yourself with a chair. Or do the hamstring stretch described above.
- Apply heat to relax tense, tight muscles.
- Apply cold to sore or tender muscles.
- Drink plenty of water. Fluid helps your muscles function normally.
- If you have troublesome leg cramps, ask your health-care provider about possible medication options.

Self-Care *(continued)*

Prevention

Stretch your leg muscles daily, using the following stretch for the Achilles tendon and calf (see the illustration on page 102):

- Stand an arm's length from a wall. Lean forward, resting your hands and forearms on the wall.
- Bend one leg at the knee and bring it toward the wall. Keep the other leg stiff. Keep both heels on the floor. Keep your back straight and move your hips toward the wall. Hold for 30 seconds.
- Repeat with the other leg. Repeat five times per leg.
- Stretch your muscles carefully and warm up before exercising vigorously.
- Stop exercising if a cramp begins.

Shin Splint

When pain occurs on the front, inside portion of the large bone of your lower leg (the tibia), it may be the result of a shin splint. Shin splints occur when tiny fibers of the membrane that attaches muscle to the tibia are irritated and inflamed, producing pain and sometimes swelling. Shin splits commonly occur in runners, basketball and tennis players and army recruits.

Self-Care

- Follow the instructions for P.R.I.C.E. (see page 83).
- Apply ice massage to the painful area.
- Try over-the-counter pain relievers (see page 231).
- Wait until the pain leaves before resuming the activity that caused it. The pain may last several weeks or even months. Meanwhile, bike or swim to maintain flexibility and strength.

Prevention

- Use stretching exercises before running to loosen the muscles in your legs and feet. Tap your foot up and down and side to side.
- A soft shoe insert may help cushion your leg.
- You may need a specially made insert (orthotic) to wear in your shoes, especially if you have flatfeet.
- A trainer can help evaluate and adjust your running style.

Medical Help

Seek medical care immediately if:

- Pain in your shin follows a fall or accident and is severe
- Your shin is hot and inflamed
- You have pain in your shin at rest or at night

Special X-rays may be used to look for a stress fracture.

Swollen Legs

Occasional swelling in your legs is a common problem and has many causes, including being overweight, sitting or standing for a long time, retaining fluids (common in pregnant or menstruating women), varicose veins, an allergic reaction and too much sun exposure.

Common Problems

Serious and ongoing swelling can be caused by the following medical conditions, which require medical attention:

- An *inflamed vein (phlebitis)*: Phlebitis can be dangerous if a blood clot develops and breaks loose. It usually occurs in the lower portion of one leg. The leg becomes sore, red and swollen. It often follows a period of inactivity—a long car or plane ride or after an operation, for example. See your health-care provider immediately.
- *Poor circulation (claudication)*: A cramping pain occurs at about the same point each time you walk. It goes away when you stop and rest. It's caused by a narrowed or blocked area in your leg arteries. See your health-care provider.
- *Heart failure*: If your heart is unable to keep up with the demands on it, you may retain fluid in your legs. This condition affects both legs at the same time and is not painful. See your health-care provider.

Self-Care

For Occasional Swelling

- Lose weight and limit salt intake.
- Elevate your legs to a level above your heart for 15 to 20 minutes every few hours to let gravity help move fluid toward your heart.
- For prolonged sitting and travel, walk around frequently and stretch your legs.

For Conditions That Cause Swelling

Although you cannot treat these conditions yourself, you can lower your risk if you do the following:

- Stop smoking.
- Control blood pressure.
- Exercise moderately and regularly.
- Attain a desirable weight.

Medical Help

Seek medical care immediately if you have unexplained, painful swelling in your legs or if a swollen leg becomes hot and inflamed.

Knee Pain

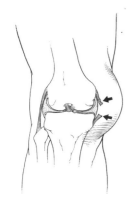

Arrows point to a torn ligament, a common form of knee injury. Swelling occurs and the joint becomes unstable.

Your knee is the largest joint in your body and is quite complex. The parts of your knee work together to support you each day as you bend, straighten and twist.

Your knee is very susceptible to injury because of its exposed location. It's not designed to handle sideways stress, and it carries a lot of weight.

Knee injuries are often complex. Many are sports-related or result from trauma. Sometimes pain is simply a matter of wear and tear. You cannot accurately tell how severe a knee injury is by the extent of pain and swelling. It's more important that your knee can bear weight, feels stable and has its full range of motion.

Pain can be due to the following:

- Strains and sprains (see pages 83 and 84), often from sudden twists or blows to your knee. A sprain will be on the opposite side of your knee from the side that took the blow. It may take days for swelling to develop fully around a knee strain or sprain.
- Tendinitis (see page 86), possibly as a result of intense bicycling or stair climbing. Runner's knee is a form of tendinitis. This overuse injury produces pain at the front of your knee. Your tendons become inflamed and it hurts to move your knee.

- Bursitis (see page 86).
- Osteoarthritis (see page 157). Arthritis often causes pain when you move or put weight on your knees.
- Torn cartilage or ligaments in your knee caused by twisting or impact. These are common injuries for skiers and basketball players who trip or fall.
- Loose pieces of your kneecap or cartilage floating around your joint. They may become pinched in your knee joint. This condition is painful and can cause your joint to lock.
- A tender, bulging cyst behind your knee (popliteal or Baker's cyst). It hurts to bend, squat or kneel.

Self-Care

- Follow the instructions for P.R.I.C.E. (see page 83).
- Take an anti-inflammatory medicine (see page 159). Remember that you may not feel injury-alerting pain after you take pain medicine.
- Flex and straighten your leg gently every day. If it's difficult for you to move your knee, someone can help move it for you at first. Try to straighten it and keep it straight.
- If you use a cane, carry it on the side that's not injured.
- Avoid strenuous activity until your knee heals. Start non-impact exercises slowly.
- Avoid squatting, kneeling or walking up and down hills.

Prevention

- Exercise regularly to strengthen your knee muscles. Bend your knee only to 90° during exercise. Don't do deep knee bends.

Medical Help

Seek medical care immediately if:

- The injury produces intense, immediate pain and your knee doesn't function properly.
- Your knee is very painful, even when you're not putting weight on it.
- The pain follows a popping sound or snapping sensation. Torn knee ligaments may need surgical repair. Delay reduces the likelihood of success.
- Your knee locks rigidly in one position, or your kneecap is visibly deformed (dislocated).
- Your knee seems unusually loose or unstable.
- You have rapid, unexplained swelling or a fever.

If pain is not improving after 1 week of home treatment, see your health-care provider.

Knee Supports and Braces

If your knees are unstable, try a brace or support bandage such as:

- A rubbery, neoprene sleeve. This slips over your knee and has a hole over your kneecap.
- An inexpensive, nonprescription knee brace. This may be hinged on the outer side or on both sides of your knee.

Caution: These devices appear to offer more support than they actually do. Although they don't protect your knee from injury, they may make it feel warm and secure and will protect it from scrapes. Use braces or supports under the direction of your doctor or therapist.

■ Ankle and Foot Pain

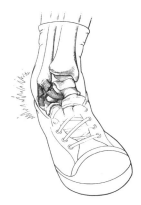

An ankle sprain occurs when ligaments that support your ankle are stretched or torn.

Your ankle is one of the most commonly injured joints. The ankle, where three bones meet, allows a wide-ranging foot movement and bears your full body weight. Common causes of foot or ankle pain include the following:

- Strains or sprains (see pages 83 and 84).
- Fractures (see page 85). High-impact activities such as basketball or aerobics can cause stress fractures. Stress fractures are really hairline cracks. They're often invisible on an X-ray for up to 6 weeks after the injury.
- Bursitis or tendinitis (see page 86).
- Achilles tendinitis occurs when the tendon that links your leg muscles to the bone at the back of your heel becomes inflamed. The tiny tears in the tendon may follow strenuous exercise. You'll feel a dull ache or pain, especially when you run or jump. The tendon also may be mildly swollen or tender.
- Bunion. Ill-fitting footwear is often the cause of this condition. Your big toe bends toward or overlaps the next toe. The base of your big toe extends beyond your foot's normal profile. That bump is called the bunion. The rubbing of shoes may cause corns, calluses and joint pain.

Self-Care

- Follow the instruction for P.R.I.C.E. (see page 83).
- Walking on an unstable joint may increase the damage, unless you stabilize it with an ankle brace, air splint or high, laced boots.

If you suspect a **fracture,** see your health-care provider. If you have a stress fracture:
- Allow at least 1 month for healing. You usually won't need a cast.
- Avoid high-impact activities for 3 to 6 weeks.

If you have **Achilles tendinitis:**
- Wear soft-soled running shoes, and avoid running or walking up or down hills.
- Avoid any impact on your heel for several days.
- Use gentle calf stretches daily (see pages 95 and 102).

If you have **bunions:**
- Wear shoes with adequate toe width. Wear sandals or go barefoot in the summer. Larger deformities may require special shoes.

Prevention
- Choose well-fitting, good-quality footwear. Shoes with a wider toe box will eliminate pressure on your toes. Avoid tight, thin-soled, high-heeled shoes.
- Stretch your Achilles tendon. Before exercise, follow the calf stretches outlined on pages 95 and 102.

Medical Help

Seek medical care immediately if:
- Your foot pain is severe and the area is swollen after an accident or injury
- Your foot is hot and inflamed or you have a fever
- Your foot or ankle is deformed or bent in an abnormal position
- The pain is so severe that you can't move your foot
- You can't bear weight 72 hours after any injury

◼ Flatfeet

All babies appear to have flatfeet. By the time we're teens, most of us develop arched feet. Arches go both from side to side and lengthwise and help distribute weight evenly across our feet.

Some people never develop arches. Others become flatfooted after they put many miles on their feet. But that isn't necessarily a problem. People with flatfeet sometimes have fewer lower back, leg or foot injuries.

Flatfeet can be a problem when:
- They place pressure on your foot's nerves and blood vessels
- They cause imbalance and joint problems in your ankles, knees, hips or lower back
- You carry excess body weight

Self-Care
- Arch supports in well-fitting shoes may give you a better weight-bearing position.
- See your health-care provider if your flatfeet are continually painful.

Kids' Care

Baby fat may make your infant's feet look flat. At about age 5 years, your child may begin to develop an arch. One in seven children never develops well-formed arches.

There are two kinds of flatfeet:
- *Flexible flatfeet* look flat only when your child stands up. Arches reappear if your child stands on tiptoe or takes weight off the foot. Flatfeet are painless and tend to run in families. There's usually no need to treat them. Some health-care providers recommend arch supports in firm shoes for increased comfort.
- *Fixed flatfeet* can be more difficult. If your child's feet are painful, stiff or extremely flat, special footwear or an operation may help.

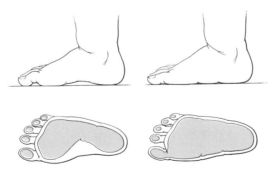

Flatfeet are feet that have little or no arch. Above at left (top and bottom) is a normal foot and footprint. If your child's foot and footprint more nearly resemble the illustrations at right, then he or she has flatfeet.

Common Problems

Burning Feet

Pain may be mild or severe burning or stinging. It may be constant or temporary. This condition is especially common in people older than 65 years. The cause may be difficult to pinpoint and may include the following:
- Irritating fabrics
- Poorly fitting shoes
- Athlete's foot (a fungal infection) (see page 118)
- Exposure to a toxic substance like poison ivy

Suspect a nerve or blood vessel disorder if you have:
- Burning with prickling, weakness or a change of sensation in your legs
- Burning with nausea, diarrhea, loss of urine or bowel control or impotence
- Other family members with the problem
- A persistent condition
- Diabetes mellitus

Self-Care
- Wear nonirritating cotton or cotton-synthetic blend socks and shoes of natural materials that breathe. A specially fitted insole may help, if it's in good condition.
- Eliminate activities that aggravate your condition.
- Soak your feet in cool tap water for 15 minutes twice each day.
- Reduce your stress and get adequate sleep.
- Use over-the-counter pain medications (see page 231).

Hammertoe and Mallet Toe

Unlike a bunion, which affects the big toe, hammertoe may occur in any toe (most commonly the second toe). The toe becomes bent and painful. Generally, both joints in a toe are affected, giving it a clawlike appearance. Hammertoe can result from wearing shoes that are too short, but the deformity also occurs in persons with long-term diabetes who have muscle and nerve damage as a result of the disease. A mallet toe is deformed at the end of the toe.

Self-Care
- A specially designed insert (orthotic) that fits into your shoe may help.
- Be sure your shoes fit well (that is, they accommodate your foot length and width).

Tips for Proper Shoe Fit

You can avoid many foot, heel and ankle problems with shoes that fit properly. Here's what to look for:
- Adequate toe room. Avoid shoes with pointed toes.
- Low heels will help you avoid back problems.
- Laced shoes are roomier and adjustable.
- Select comfortable athletic shoes, strapped sandals or soft, roomy pumps with cushioned insoles.
- Avoid vinyl and plastic shoes. They don't breathe when your feet perspire.
- Buy shoes at midday. Your feet are smaller in the morning and swell throughout the day. Measure both feet.
- As you age, your shoe size may change (especially the width).
- Have your shoe store stretch shoes in tight spots.

■ Swelling

Most people have swollen feet occasionally. Causes include all of those noted in Swollen Legs on page 95.

Self-Care
- Exercise your legs. Elevate your legs above your heart.
- Reduce your salt intake.

Prevention
- Wear support stockings. They apply constant pressure and reduce foot and ankle swelling. Poorly fitting stockings (too tight in the calf) can cause swelling.
- Maintain a regular exercise program.

Medical Help
Seek medical care immediately if one foot becomes swollen rapidly, your foot is inflamed and you have a fever.

■ Morton's Neuroma

Morton's neuroma causes a sharp, burning pain in the ball of your foot. It may feel like you're walking on stones. Your toes may sting, burn or feel numb. Soft tissue grows around a nerve in your foot (called a neuroma), often between your third and fourth toes. It may not hurt early in the day, but only after you stand or walk in tight shoes.

Self-Care
- Wear well-fitting shoes with enough room in the toe box, or wear sandals.
- Shoe supports (orthotics) or a foot pad may help.
- Reduce high-impact activities for a few weeks.

Medical Help
- A cortisone injection may reduce pain.
- The growth may be surgically removed if pain is chronic and severe.

■ Heel Pain

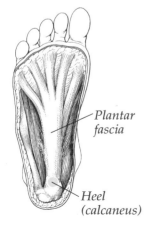

Plantar fascia

Heel (calcaneus)

Heel pain often results from stress on the plantar fascia.

Heel pain is irritating, but rarely serious. Although it can result from a pinched nerve or a chronic condition, such as arthritis or bursitis, the most common cause is plantar fasciitis. This is an inflammation of the plantar fascia, the fibrous tissue along the bottom of your foot which connects to your heel bone (calcaneus) and toes.

The pain usually develops gradually, but it can come on suddenly and severely. It tends to be worse when you are getting out of bed in the morning, when the fascia is stiff. Although both feet can be affected, it usually occurs in only one foot.

The pain generally goes away once your foot limbers up. It can recur if you stand or sit for a long time. Climbing stairs or standing on tiptoes also can produce pain. A bone spur (usually painless) may form from tension on your heel bone.

Plantar fasciitis can affect people of all ages. Factors that increase your risk include excess weight, improperly fitting shoes, foot abnormalities and activities that place added pressure on your feet.

Treatment involves simple steps to relieve the pain and inflammation. Don't expect a quick cure. It can take 6 months or longer before your heel is back to normal.

Self-Care

- Cut back on jogging or walking. Substitute exercises that put less weight on your heel, such as swimming or bicycling.
- Apply ice to the painful area for up to 20 minutes after activity.
- Stretching increases flexibility in your plantar fascia, Achilles' tendon and calf muscles. Stretching in the morning before you get out of bed helps reverse the tightening of the plantar fascia which occurs overnight.
- Strengthening muscles in your foot can help support your arch.
- Buy shoes with a low to moderate heel (1 to 2 inches) and good arch support and shock absorbency.
- Over-the-counter medications may ease the pain (see page 231).
- If you're overweight, shed excess pounds.
- Try heel pads or cups. They help cushion and support your heel.

These exercises stretch or strengthen your plantar fascia, Achilles' tendon and calf muscles. Hold each for 20 or 30 seconds, and do one or two repetitions two or three times a day.

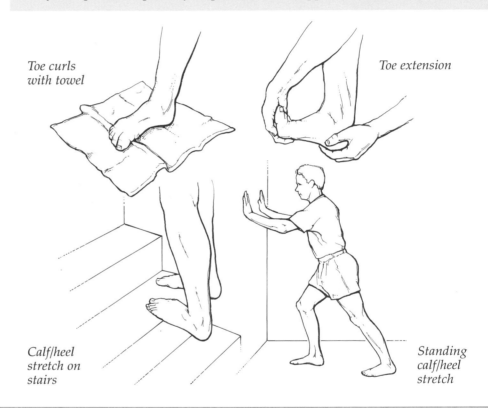

Toe curls with towel

Toe extension

Calf/heel stretch on stairs

Standing calf/heel stretch

Medical Help

If the self-care measures aren't effective, or if you believe your condition is due to a foot abnormality, see your doctor. Treatment options include the following:

- Custom orthotics.
- Night splints to keep tension on the tissue so it heals in a stretched position.
- Deep heat, which increases blood flow and promotes healing.
- A cortisone injection in your heel often can help relieve the inflammation when other steps aren't successful. But multiple injections aren't recommended because they can weaken and rupture your plantar fascia, as well as shrink the fat pad covering your heel bone.
- Doctors can detach your plantar fascia from your heel bone, but this is recommended only when all other treatments have failed.

Lungs, Chest and Breathing

Breathing is one of our most basic reflexes. We do it thousands of times a day. When we breathe in (inhale), we draw fresh oxygen into our lungs and bloodstream. When we breathe out (exhale), we remove the air from our lungs which contains carbon dioxide, a waste product of our bodies' activities. Breathing is something that most of us take for granted—until we have trouble with it.

■ Coughing: A Natural Reflex

A cough is a reflex—just like breathing. It's actually a way of protecting your lungs against irritants. When your breathing passages, called bronchi, have secretions in them, you cough to clear the passages so you can breathe more easily. A small amount of coughing is ordinary and even healthy as a way to maintain clear breathing passages.

However, strong or persistent coughing can be an irritant to your breathing passages. Repeated coughing causes your bronchi to contract and narrow, and these changes can irritate the membranes (the interior "walls" of your breathing passages).

What Causes Coughing? Coughing is frequently a symptom of a viral upper respiratory tract infection, which is an infection of your nose, sinuses and airways. A cold and influenza are common examples. Your voice box may become inflamed (a condition called laryngitis), causing hoarseness, which could affect your ability to speak. Coughing also may result from throat irritation caused by the drainage of mucus down the back of your throat (a condition called postnasal drainage).

The Cough

A cough begins when an irritant reaches one of the cough receptors in your nose, throat or chest (see dots). The receptor sends a message to the cough center in your brain, signaling your body to cough. After you inhale, your epiglottis and vocal cords close tightly, trapping air within your lungs. Your abdominal and chest muscles contract forcefully, pushing against your diaphragm. Finally, your vocal cords and epiglottis open suddenly, allowing trapped air to explode outward.

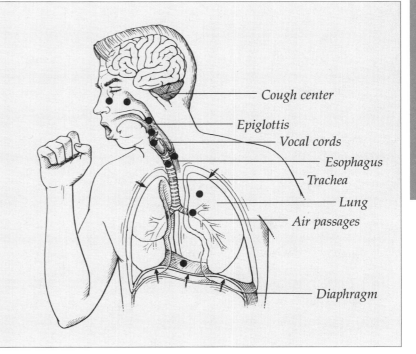

Cough center
Epiglottis
Vocal cords
Esophagus
Trachea
Lung
Air passages
Diaphragm

Coughing also occurs with chronic disorders. People with allergies and asthma have bouts of involuntary coughing, as do people who smoke. Irritants in the environment such as smog, dust, secondhand smoke and cold or dry air can cause coughing.

Sometimes coughing is caused by stomach acid that backs up into your esophagus or, in rare cases, your lungs. This condition is called gastroesophageal reflux (see page 60). Some people also develop a "habit" cough.

Self-Care	● **Drink plenty of fluids.** They help keep your throat clear. Drink water or fruit juices—not pop or coffee.
	● **Use a humidifier.** The air in your home can get very dry, especially during the winter. Dry air irritates your throat when you have a cold. Using a humidifier to moisturize the air will make breathing easier (see below).
	● **Honey, hard candy or medicated throat lozenges** may help to soothe a simple throat irritation and may help prevent coughing if your throat is dry or sore. Try drinking a cup of tea sweetened with honey.
	● **Try expectorants,** medications that help you to clear your throat of mucus. ("To expectorate" means "to spit.") Expectorants may increase the flow of normal fluids in your throat and help relieve some of the pain.
	● **Use cough suppressants,** available in both liquid and solid form. They act on the portion of your brain that controls your cough reflex. Mild over-the-counter versions are available. Stronger versions are available only by prescription.
	● If your cough is caused by a backup of stomach acids, try sleeping with the head of your bed elevated 4 to 6 inches. Also avoid food and drink within 2 to 3 hours of bedtime.
Medical Help	Contact a doctor if your cough lasts more than 2 or 3 weeks, or if it is accompanied by fever, increased shortness of breath or bloody phlegm. Managing a chronic cough requires careful evaluation.

Home Humidifiers—Help or Hazard?

When breathing dry indoor air makes you cough, increase the humidity. But don't let the remedy to one problem create another. Dirty humidifiers can be a source of bacteria and fungi. To minimize growth, the U.S. Consumer Product Safety Commission suggests the following:

● **Change the water every day.** Empty the tank and dry the surfaces with a soft towel. Then refill with clean water.

● **Some products recommend use of distilled water.** Tap water contains minerals that can create bacteria-friendly deposits. When released into the air, these minerals often appear as white dust on your furniture.

● **Sanitize the humidifier every 1 to 2 weeks.** Empty the tank. Fill it with a solution of 1 teaspoon bleach to 1 gallon water. Let the solution soak for 20 minutes and then empty the tank. Rinse the tank until you can no longer smell bleach.

● **Keep the humidity between 30 and 50 percent.** Levels higher than 60 percent may create a buildup of moisture. When moisture condenses on surfaces, bacteria and fungi can grow. Periodically check the humidity with a hygrometer, available at your local hardware store.

● **Follow the manufacturer's instructions** for regularly cleaning the humidifier to avoid a buildup of bacteria.

Bronchitis

Bronchitis is a common condition, much like the common cold. It usually is caused by a viral infection that spreads to the bronchi, producing a deep cough that, in turn, brings up yellowish gray matter from your lungs. The bronchi are the main air passages of your lungs. When the walls that line the bronchi become inflamed, this condition is called bronchitis.

Self-Care

- Get plenty of rest. Drink lots of fluids. Use a humidifier in your room.
- Take a nonprescription cough medicine (see page 232). Adults can take aspirin, NSAIDS or acetaminophen for a fever. Children should take only acetaminophen or ibuprofen.
- Avoid irritants to your airways, such as tobacco smoke.

Medical Help

Acute bronchitis usually disappears in a matter of days. Contact a doctor if you experience shortness of breath or a high temperature for more than 3 days. If your cough lasts for more than 10 days and your sputum (the matter you spit up from your lungs) becomes yellow, gray or green, the doctor may prescribe an antibiotic.

Croup

Croup is caused by a virus that infects the voice box (larynx), windpipe (trachea) and bronchial tubes. Croup occurs most often in children between the ages of 3 months and 5 years, and it more often affects boys than girls. Because of a narrowing of the airway, a child with croup has a tight, brassy cough that may resemble the barking of a seal. The child's voice becomes hoarse, and it is difficult for the child to breathe. The child may become agitated and begin crying, actions that make breathing even more difficult. Croup typically lasts 5 or 6 days. During this period, it may go from mild to severe several times. The symptoms are usually worse at night.

Self-Care

- Reassure your child. Cuddle, read a book or play a game for distraction.
- Give clear, warm fluids to help loosen thickened secretions.
- Keep the child away from smoke (it aggravates the symptoms).
- Expose the child to warm, humid air. Try one of the following methods:
  - Lay a wet washcloth loosely over your child's nose and mouth so that air moves easily in and out. (Do not do this if your child is in respiratory distress.)
  - Fill a humidifier with warm water and have your child put his or her face in or near the mist and breathe deeply through the mouth.
  - Have your child sit in a steamy bathroom for at least 10 minutes. Return as often as needed. (Try one trip outside if the weather is cool or cold.)
- Sleep in the same room as your child so you will be alert to any worsening of the condition.

Medical Help

Occasionally, croup may cause nearly complete blockage of the airway. Get emergency help if you notice any of the following symptoms: drooling or difficulty swallowing, difficulty bending the neck forward, blue or dusky lips, worsening cough and more difficulty with breathing and high-pitched noises when inhaling.

■ Wheezing

Wheezing occurs when you hear a high-pitched whistling sound coming from your chest as you breathe out. It is caused by a narrowing of the airways in the lungs and indicates breathing difficulty. Also, your chest may feel tight.

Wheezing is a common symptom of asthma, bronchitis, smoking, allergies, pneumonia, emphysema, lung cancer and heart failure. It also can be caused by environmental factors, such as chemicals or air pollution. Wheezing requires medical attention. See a doctor if you have difficulty breathing and are wheezing.

■ Shortness of Breath

In general, unexpected shortness of breath is a symptom that needs medical attention. Shortness of breath can be caused by illnesses ranging from heart attacks to blood clots in the lung to pneumonia. It also can be caused by pregnancy.

In its chronic form, shortness of breath is a symptom of illnesses such as asthma, emphysema, other lung diseases and heart disease. All of these chronic conditions also require medical attention. There are, however, some exercises you can do to help relieve shortness of breath if you have chronic lung disease (see below).

Simple Exercises Can Improve Your Breathing

Some simple breathing exercises may help you if you have emphysema or another chronic lung disorder. They help you control the emptying of your lungs by using your abdominal muscles. You also can increase the efficiency of your lungs. Ask your physician about them. Do them two to four times daily.

Diaphragmatic Breathing

Lie on your back with your head and knees supported by pillows. Begin by breathing in and out slowly and smoothly in a rhythmic pattern. Relax.

Place your fingertips on your abdomen, just below the base of your rib cage. As you inhale slowly, you should feel your diaphragm lifting your hand.

Practice pushing your abdomen against your hand as your chest becomes filled with air. Make sure your chest remains motionless. Try this while inhaling through your mouth and counting slowly to 3. Then purse your lips and exhale through your mouth while counting slowly to 6.

Practice diaphragmatic breathing on your back until you can take 10 to 15 consecutive breaths in one session without tiring. Then practice it on one side and then on the other. Progress to doing the exercise while sitting erect in a chair, standing up, walking and, finally, climbing stairs.

Pursed-Lip Breathing

Try the diaphragmatic breathing exercises with your lips pursed as you exhale, that is, with your lips puckered (the flow of air should make a soft "sssss" sound). Inhale deeply through your mouth and exhale. Repeat 10 times at each session.

Deep-Breathing Exercise

While sitting or standing, pull your elbows firmly backward as you inhale deeply. Hold the breath in, with your chest arched, for a count to 5 and then force the air out by contracting your abdominal muscles. Repeat the exercise 10 times.

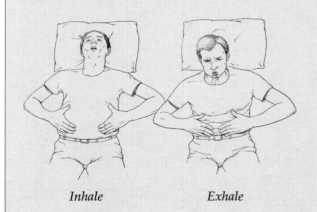

Inhale   *Exhale*

Chest Pain

Pain in your chest can be strong and severe, but it also can be difficult to interpret. The pain could be caused by something as simple as indigestion, or it could be the result of a serious medical situation.

Emergency Care

If pain in your chest persists and you suspect it is serious, contact a health-care provider immediately!

Heart attack: In addition to pain or pressure in your chest, you could experience pain or numbness in your face, arms, neck or back. Other symptoms of a heart attack may include shortness of breath, sweating, dizziness, nausea and vomiting. If you think you are having a heart attack, seek medical help or call 911 immediately. If you go to a hospital, *do not drive yourself!*

Other Causes of Chest Pain

Listed below are some of the common forms of chest pain which do not require immediate medical attention.

Chest wall pain: This is one of the most common forms of harmless chest pain. If probing the tender area with your finger causes the pain to return, then serious conditions, such as heart attack, are less likely. Chest wall pain usually lasts only a few days, and it can be treated with aspirin in adults. For children, treat with ibuprofen or acetaminophen. Apply low and intermittent heat to the area to help reduce the pain.

Heartburn: Symptoms are a warm or burning discomfort in the upper part of your abdomen and under your breastbone. You also may have an acid or sour taste in your mouth. Heartburn sometimes can be so painful that the symptoms are confused with the onset of a heart attack. Chest pain from heartburn usually can be relieved by belching or by taking an antacid.

Precordial catch: This is a condition that occurs most often in young adults. The symptom is a brief, sharp pain under the left breast which makes breathing difficult. There are no self-care measures. The condition goes away momentarily. The cause of this common condition is unknown, although it is apparently harmless.

Angina: Angina is the term used for the chest pain, or pressure, of heart disease. It is caused by a lack of oxygen reaching the heart muscle. When you've been diagnosed as having heart disease, develop a treatment plan with your doctor.

- You should not try to "work through" an episode of angina. Stop and treat it.
- It is usually treated with rest and a medication such as nitroglycerin.
- If you have a change in your pattern of angina, such as increased frequency or nightime attacks, see your doctor immediately.
- If you've tried measures to stop an angina attack but it lasts longer than 15 minutes or you're also having light-headedness or palpitations, seek emergency medical help.

Palpitations

A palpitation is the feeling you have in your chest when it feels as if your heart "skips a beat." Many people experience heart palpitations from time to time, and they are usually not dangerous. Palpitations can be caused by stress or by external factors such as consumption of caffeine and alcohol. Frequently, changes in lifestyle relieve the symptoms.

Common Problems

Nose and Sinuses

Your nose is the main gateway to your respiratory system. Normally, your nose filters, humidifies and warms the air you breathe as it moves from your nasal passage into your throat and lungs, 12 to 15 times a minute.

Occasionally, your nose is the site of conditions such as a nosebleed, cold, hay fever or a sinus infection. Luckily, most disorders of the nose and sinuses are temporary and easy to cure.

The following pages address the common disorders of the nose and its adjacent cavities, the sinuses. For information on respiratory allergies, see page 154.

■ Foreign Objects in the Nose

If a foreign object becomes lodged in the nose, follow these steps:
- Do not probe at the foreign object with a cotton swab or other tool. Do not try to inhale the object by forcefully breathing in; breathe through the mouth until the object is removed.
- Blow your nose gently to try to free the object, but do not blow hard or repeatedly.
- If the object protrudes from the nose and can be easily grasped with tweezers, gently remove it.

If these methods fail, seek emergency medical assistance.

■ Loss of Sense of Smell

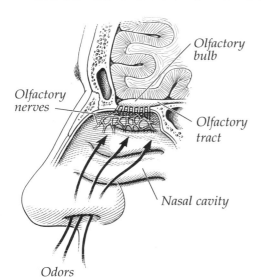

Olfactory bulb

Olfactory nerves

Olfactory tract

Nasal cavity

Odors

Your sense of smell and, to a large degree, your sense of taste begin with the olfactory nerve endings, which are found in the upper portion of your nose. The olfactory nerves contain very fine and sensitive fibers that transmit signals from the olfactory bulb to your brain.

Most people temporarily lose their sense of smell when they have a head cold. Usually, the sense of smell returns once the infection is gone.

However, when the sense of smell is lost without an apparent cause, the condition is called anosmia. Anosmia occurs from either an obstruction in your nose or nerve damage. An obstruction prevents odors from reaching the delicate nerve fibers in your nose. These nerves carry messages or signals to your brain. Nasal polyps, tumors, neurologic conditions or swelling of the mucous membrane can cause obstruction. Viral infections, chronic nasal infections or allergies also can damage the nerves that allow you to smell.

Medical Help

If you lose your sense of smell and you do not have a cold, consult your physician. Your physician will check for polyps or tumors of the nasal passages. When the problem is caused by a virus, the sense of smell usually returns when the tissues of the olfactory area heal.

■ Nosebleeds

Nosebleeds—almost all of us have had one. Most often they are a nuisance and not a true medical problem. But they can be both. Why do they start, and how can they be stopped?

Among children and young adults, nosebleeds usually begin on the septum, just inside the nose. The septum separates your nasal chambers.

In middle age and older, nosebleeds can begin on the septum, but they also may begin deeper in the nose's interior. This form of nosebleed is much less common. It may be caused by hardened arteries or high blood pressure. These nosebleeds begin spontaneously and are often difficult to stop. They require a specialist's help.

Self-Care

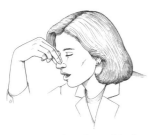

Use your thumb and index finger to squeeze together the soft portion of your nose, located between the end of your nose and the hard, bony ridge.

- **Sit or stand up.** By remaining upright, you reduce blood pressure in the veins of your nose. This action will discourage further bleeding.
- **Pinch your nose** with your thumb and index finger and breathe through your mouth. Continue the pinch for 5 or 10 minutes. This maneuver sends pressure to the bleeding point on the nasal septum and often stops the flow of blood.
- **Don't apply ice to the nose.** This is of little or no benefit. The cold only tightens blood vessels on the surface of the nose and does not penetrate deeply enough to help.
- **To prevent bleeding,** increase the humidity of the air you breathe in your home. A humidifier or vaporizer can help keep your nasal membranes moist. Lubricating your nose with Vaseline or other lubricants is often helpful.
- **To prevent rebleeding after bleeding has stopped,** do not pick or blow your nose until several hours after the bleeding episode, and do not bend down. Keep your head higher than the level of your heart.
- **If rebleeding occurs,** sniff in forcefully to clear your nose of blood clots, spray both sides of your nose with a decongestant nasal spray such as Afrin, Dristan or Neosynephrine. Pinch your nose again in the technique described above and call your doctor.

Medical Help

Seek medical care immediately if:
- The bleeding lasts for more than 15 to 30 minutes
- You feel weak or faint, which can result from the blood loss
- The bleeding is rapid or if the amount of blood loss is great
- Bleeding begins by trickling down the back of your throat

If you experience frequent nosebleeds, make an appointment with your physician. You may need to have the blood vessel that is causing your problem cauterized. Cautery is a technique in which the blood vessel is burned with electric current, silver nitrate or a laser.

Kids' Care

Frequent nosebleeds in children can be a sign of a benign tumor. It occurs at puberty in boys and rarely in girls. It may shrink on its own after puberty, but it can grow rapidly, produce obstruction of nasal passages and sinuses and cause frequent and often severe nosebleeds. If the tumor does not shrink, the physician may suggest a procedure to remove it surgically.

Common Problems

■ Stuffy Nose

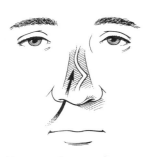

Your nasal septum separates your nasal chambers. A deviated septum may cause nasal obstruction.

One of our most common medical complaints is a "stuffy" nose. A stuffy nose usually means nasal congestion or an obstruction that causes difficulty breathing. In most cases, a stuffy nose is a mere nuisance. Other causes of nasal obstruction are nasal polyps, tumors, enlarged adenoids and foreign objects in the nose.

Four causes of nasal obstruction and congestion are outlined below.

Common cold: See Aaachoo! Is It a Cold or the Flu? on page 111.

Deformities of the nose and nasal septum (the cartilage and bony partition separating your two nasal chambers) are usually due to an injury. The injury may have occurred years earlier, even in childhood. Deformities of the nose such as a deviated septum are fairly common problems. The deviation also can cause nosebleeds or sinusitis. For many people, a deviated septum poses few problems. However, if the condition makes breathing difficult, a surgical procedure may be the answer. The surgery, called septoplasty, realigns your septum.

Allergies: Allergic rhinitis (which means nasal inflammation from allergies) is the medical term for hay fever, rose fever, grass fever and other seasonal allergies. The allergic reaction is an inflammatory response to specific foreign substances that enter the nose, such as pollen, mold or house dust.

Vasomotor rhinitis: This form of inflammation is often episodic and associated with triggers such as smoke, air conditioning or vigorous exercise.

Self-Care

- For colds, see Aaachoo! Is It a Cold or the Flu? on page 111.
- Regularly and gently blow your nose if mucus or debris is present.
- Breathing steam can loosen the mucus and clear your head.
- Take a warm shower or sit in the bathroom with the shower running.
- Drink plenty of liquids.
- Use nonprescription nasal sprays or nose drops for no more than 3 or 4 days. Nonprescription oral decongestants (liquid and pills) may be helpful.
- Try saline drops.

Medical Help

If nose congestion persists for more than 1 to 2 weeks, consult your physician, who will examine your nose for the cause of the obstruction, such as polyps or tumors. If the physician determines you have an allergy, he or she may prescribe a course of therapy that may include antihistamines and inhaled anti-inflammatory medications.

Beware of Nose Drop Addiction

Frequent use of decongestant drops and sprays can result in a condition called nose drop addiction. This is a vicious cycle requiring more frequent use of nose spray to keep your nasal passages clear.

Prolonged use of nasal sprays and drops can cause irritation of your mucous membrane, a stinging or burning in your nose and a chronic inflammation.

The only way to treat the problem is to stop using nose drops. You may want to take an oral decongestant instead. Your condition may become worse for a while, but over a period of weeks your breathing should become nearly normal as the ill effects of the nose drops wear off.

Remember, use decongestant drops or sprays for no more than 3 or 4 days.

■ Runny Nose

Runny nose commonly occurs early in a cold and in allergic irritation. Gently blowing the nose may be all the self-care you need. If the discharge is persistent and watery, an over-the-counter antihistamine may be helpful. If the discharge is thick, follow the recommendations for stuffy nose on page 110.

Aaachoo! Is It a Cold or the Flu?
Both are viral, upper respiratory tract infections

	Cold	Flu, Influenza
Usual symptoms	<ul><li>Runny nose, sneezing, nasal congestion</li><li>Sore throat (usually scratchy)</li><li>Cough</li><li>No fever or low fever</li><li>Mild fatigue</li></ul>	<ul><li>Runny nose and sneezing</li><li>Sore throat and headache</li><li>Cough</li><li>Fever (usually more than 101 F) and chills</li><li>Moderate to severe fatigue and weakness</li><li>Achy muscles</li></ul>
Cause	One of more than 200 viruses typically causes 2 to 4 colds a year in adults and 4 to 8 a year in kids	One of a few viruses from the influenza A or influenza B family. On average, adults have less than one infection a year
Seriousness	Usually not serious except in people with lung disease or other serious illness	Can be serious. A special concern in the elderly and people with chronic health conditions.
Can I work?	Often. Use care to avoid spreading a cold to others. Wash hands frequently.	No, not until fever, fatigue and all but the mild symptoms have resolved
Preventable?	Possibly, through careful handwashing, not sharing food, towels or handkerchiefs and getting good nutrition and enough rest	Usually, through vaccination. You need to be immunized every fall (see page 205)
Do antibiotics help?	No, not unless you also have a bacterial infection	Sometimes. Two antiviral antibiotics are available, but they work for only influenza A
Self-care	<ul><li>Drink plenty of warm liquids. Homemade chicken soup can help clear mucus</li><li>Increase sleep and rest</li><li>Use cold remedies cautiously, see page 232</li><li>Try zinc gluconate lozenges (13.3 mg, one every 2 hours while awake). For adult use only during a cold. Don't use if you are pregnant or immunocompromised (have cancer, AIDS or a chronic disease)</li></ul>	<ul><li>Drink plenty of fluids to avoid dehydration</li><li>Increase sleep and rest</li><li>Use over-the-counter pain relievers cautiously, as needed (see page 231)</li></ul>
Seek medical help	<ul><li>If you have difficulty breathing, faintness, change in alertness, severe sore throat, cough producing a lot of sputum or mucus (especially if green or yellow), pain in the face or a chronic health condition</li><li>If symptoms have not resolved in 10 days</li></ul>	

A word about pneumonia
Pneumonia can occur after a cold or flu or on its own. Pneumonia can be caused by viruses, bacteria or other organisms. Typically, you will have a prominent cough that brings up a lot of phlegm. A fever is common. You may experience a sharp pain when you breathe deeply, called pleurisy. If you are concerned about pneumonia, see your healthcare provider. You may need a chest X-ray and antibiotics.

Common Problems

■ Sinusitis

Signs of sinusitis include pain about your eyes or cheeks, fever and difficulty breathing through your nose. Occasionally, tooth pain occurs with the condition, or it may mimic a migraine headache.

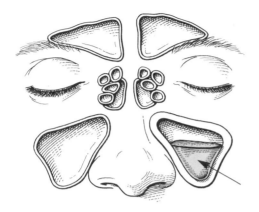

An infected maxillary sinus (arrow) is the most common site of sinusitis.

Your sinuses are cavities in the bones around your nose. They are connected to your nasal cavities by small openings. Normally, air passes in and out of your sinuses and mucus drains through these openings into your nose.

Sinusitis is an infection of the lining of one or more of these cavities. Usually, when your sinus is infected, the membranes of your nose also swell and cause a nasal obstruction. Swelling of the membranes of your nose may close off the opening of your sinus and thus prevent draining of pus or mucus. Pain in your sinus may result from inflammation itself or from the pressure as secretions build up in your sinus.

The infection can be bacterial, viral or fungal. A common cold is the most frequent cause. Allergies also can cause sinusitis.

Self-Care

- Stay indoors in an even temperature.
- Refrain from bending over with your head down—this movement usually increases the pain.
- Try applying warm facial packs, or cautiously inhale steam from a kettle or basin of boiling water.
- Drink plenty of liquids to help dilute the secretions.
- Gently and regularly blow your nose.
- Take pain relievers for discomfort.
- Use over-the-counter (OTC) decongestants and short-term decongestant sprays.
- Try OTC saltwater nose drops.
- If you are using OTC antihistamines, take care. They can do more harm than good by drying out your nose too much and thickening secretions. Use them only on the recommendation of your physician, and follow instructions carefully.

Medical Help

See your physician if you have a fever of more than 101 F, if the pain does not resolve in 24 hours or if the pain occurs repeatedly. X-rays and other examinations may be performed to discover the seriousness of the infection. If the infection is bacterial, your physician will prescribe a course of oral antibiotics to be taken for 7 to 14 days.

Skin, Hair and Nails

Because your skin, hair and nails are an integral part of your appearance, changes and problems involving them are often distressing. External irritants, infections, aging and even emotional stress can affect your skin, hair and nails in many ways. More rarely, underlying medical conditions and allergies to foods or medications trigger abnormalities.

Fortunately, many of these problems are not serious and respond well to self-care measures. The following pages explain some of the more common disorders and offer some self-care tips to help you find relief. But first, here are some general guidelines for proper skin care.

■ Proper Skin Care

Regardless of your skin color or type or your age, monitoring your exposure to the sun—and its ultraviolet rays—can help prevent unnecessary damage and, eventually, skin cancer.

Dark skin can tolerate more sun than fair skin. However, any skin can become blotchy, leathery and wrinkled from continued overexposure to the sun. Protective clothing, sunscreen preparations and daily lubrication or moisturizing can help.

Proper cleansing is another important strategy in protecting your skin. The best procedures and cleansing ingredients vary according to the type of skin you have— oily, dry, balanced or a combination of these.

Self-Care

- When washing your face, use tepid (never hot) water and a facecloth or sponge to remove dead cells. Use a mild soap. A superfatted soap, such as Basis or Dove, may be better for dry skin. You may need to clean oily skin two or three times each day.
- In general, avoid washing your body with very hot water or strong soaps. Bathing dries your skin. If you have dry skin, use soap only on your face, underarms, genital areas, hands and feet. After bathing, pat (rather than wipe) your skin dry, then immediately lubricate it with an oil or cream. Use a heavy, water-in-oil moisturizer rather than a light "disappearing" cream that contains mostly water, and avoid creams or lotions that contain alcohol. Keep the air in your home somewhat cool and humid.
- Shaving can be hard on a man's skin. If you shave with a blade razor, always use a sharp blade. Soften your beard by applying a warm facecloth for a few seconds; then use plenty of shaving cream. Pass the blade over your beard only once, in the direction of hair growth. Reversing the stroke to obtain a close shave can cause a skin irritation. Electric razors also may irritate your skin. Skin preparations are available to treat skin irritation.
- Match cosmetics to your skin type: an oil base is suitable for dry skin, and a water base is suitable for oily skin.
- For women, remove eye makeup before facial cleansing. Use cotton balls to avoid damaging the delicate tissue around your eyes.

Common Problems

■ Acne

It's a fear and frustration for teens, but acne can affect adults too. Acne is caused by plugged pores and bacteria in the skin. Oil from glands combines with dead skin to plug the pores, also called follicles. Follicles bulge, producing pimples and other types of blemishes:

- Whiteheads: clogged pores that have no opening
- Blackheads: pores that are open and have a dark surface
- Pimples: reddish spots that signal an infection by bacteria in plugged pores
- Cysts: thick lumps beneath the surface of your skin, formed by the buildup of secretions

Three of four teenagers have some acne. It is most prevalent in adolescence because hormonal changes stimulate the sebaceous glands during these years. The sebaceous glands secrete a fatty oil called sebum, which lubricates your hair and skin. Menstrual periods, the use of birth control pills or cortisone medications and stress may aggravate acne in later life.

Although a chronic problem for many people from puberty through early adulthood, acne eventually clears in most cases.

Self-Care

- Identify factors that aggravate your acne. Avoid oily or greasy cosmetics, sunscreens, hair styling products or acne coverups. Use products labeled "water-based" or "noncomedogenic."
- Wash problem areas daily with a cleanser that gently dries your skin and causes follicles to flake.
- Try over-the-counter acne lotion (containing benzoyl peroxide, resorcinol or salicylic acid as the active ingredient) to dry excess oil and promote peeling.
- Moderate exposure to the sun or careful use of a sun lamp may help. However, too much sun may cause wrinkles and skin cancer later in life.
- Keep your hair clean and off the face.
- Watch for signs of spreading infection beyond the edges of a pimple.
- Unless a food is clearly aggravating your acne, you don't need to eliminate it. Foods like chocolate, once thought to be a cause of acne, generally aren't the culprit.
- Don't pick or squeeze blemishes. These actions can cause infection or scarring.

Medical Help

Persistent pimples or inflamed cysts may need medical attention and treatment with prescription drugs. In rare cases, a sudden onset of severe acne in an older adult may signal an underlying disease requiring medical attention.

Physicians may use cosmetic surgery to diminish scars left by acne. The main procedures are dermabrasion or peeling by freezing or chemicals. However, if your skin tends to form scar tissue, these procedures can make your complexion much worse.

Peeling procedures eliminate superficial scars. Dermabrasion, usually reserved for more severe scarring, consists of abrading the skin with a rapidly rotating wire brush. Your physician will use a local anesthetic or topical freezing of your skin during the procedure. General anesthesia and hospitalization ordinarily are not required.

■ Boils

Boils are pink or red, very tender bumps under your skin which occur when bacteria infect one or more of your hair follicles. The bumps are usually larger than 1/2 inch in diameter. They typically grow rapidly, fill with pus and then burst, drain and heal. Although some boils resolve a few days after they appear, most burst and heal within about 2 weeks.

Boils can occur anywhere on your skin, but most often on the face, neck, armpits, buttocks or thighs. Poor health, clothing that binds or chafes and disorders such as acne, dermatitis, diabetes and anemia can increase your risk of infection.

Self-Care

To avoid spreading this infection and to minimize discomfort, follow these measures:
- Soak the area with a warm washcloth or compress for about 30 minutes every few hours. Doing so may help the boil burst and drain much sooner. Use warm saltwater. (Add 1 teaspoon of salt to 1 quart of boiling water and let it cool.)
- Gently wash the sore twice a day with antibacterial soap. Cover the sore with a bandage to prevent spreading.
- Apply an over-the-counter antibiotic ointment such as bacitracin.
- Never squeeze or lance a boil, because you might spread the infection.
- Launder towels, compresses or clothing that has touched the infected area.

Medical Help

Contact your health-care provider if the infection is located on your spine or on your face, worsens rapidly or causes severe pain, has not disappeared within 2 weeks or is accompanied by fever or reddish lines radiating from the boil. In some cases, antibiotics or surgical drainage may be necessary to clear your infection.

■ Cellulitis

Cellulitis may appear gradually over a couple of days or rapidly over a few hours. It begins as a localized area of red, painful, warm skin. It may be accompanied by fever and swelling. This fairly common infection occurs when bacteria or fungus enters your body through a break in the skin and infects the deeper layers of your skin.

Good hygiene and proper wound care can help prevent this type of infection. However, bacteria can enter your skin through even tiny cuts or abrasions, such as a crack around your nostrils or a simple puncture wound.

Self-Care

To prevent cellulitis and other wound infections, follow these measures:
- Keep skin wounds clean.
- Apply an antibiotic cream or ointment. If a rash develops, stop using the ointment and talk to your doctor or pharmacist. Ingredients in these ointments can cause a mild rash in some people.
- Cover the area with a bandage to help keep it clean and keep harmful bacteria out. Keep draining blisters covered until a scab forms.
- Change the bandage daily or whenever it becomes wet or dirty.

Medical Help

Contact your doctor if you suspect you have cellulitis. Antibiotics are usually necessary to prevent this infection from spreading and causing severe damage.

Common Problems

■ Corns and Calluses

These thickened, hardened layers of skin commonly appear on your hands and feet. Corns often appear as raised bumps of hardened skin less than ¼-inch long. Calluses vary in size and shape. Corns and calluses are your skin's attempt to protect itself. Although they can be unsightly, treatment may be necessary only if they cause discomfort. For most people, eliminating the source of friction or pressure will help corns and calluses disappear.

Self-Care

- Wear properly fitted shoes, with adequate toe room. Have your shoe shop stretch your shoes at any point that rubs or pinches. Place pads under your heels if your shoes rub. Try over-the-counter remedies to cushion or soften the corn while wearing shoes.
- Wear padded gloves when using hand tools, or try padding your tool handles with cloth tape or covers.
- Rub your skin with a pumice stone or washcloth during or after bathing to gradually thin some of the thickened skin. This advice is not recommended if you have diabetes or poor circulation.
- Try over-the-counter corn dissolvers containing salicylic acid (available in plaster-pad disks or solutions containing a thickener called collodion).
- Do not cut or shave corns or calluses with a sharp edge.

Medical Help

If a corn or callus becomes very painful or inflamed, contact your health-care provider.

■ Dandruff

Everyone has some degree of the scaling of the skin on his or her scalp. It is the normal process of the shedding of the dead, outer layer of cells. If the flaking becomes obvious on your hair and clothing, the condition is called dandruff. The problem often is worse in winter, perhaps because of lower indoor humidity and lack of ultraviolet exposure from the sun. Although 20 percent of adults have dandruff, it is not a contagious condition. Dandruff is rarely serious, but the skin may be more susceptible to infection.

Self-Care

- Shampoo regularly. Start with a mild, nonmedicated shampoo. Gently massage your scalp to loosen flakes. Rinse thoroughly.
- Use medicated shampoo for stubborn cases. Look for those containing zinc pyrithione, salicylic acid, coal tar or selenium sulfide in brands such as Head & Shoulders, Denorex, Selsun Blue, Tegrin or Neutrogena T/Gel and T/Sal. Use a dandruff shampoo each time you shampoo, if necessary, to control flaking.
- Use tar-based shampoos carefully. They can leave a brownish stain on light-colored or gray hair and make your scalp more sensitive to the sun.
- Use a conditioner regularly. For mild cases of dandruff, alternate dandruff shampoo with your regular shampoo.

Medical Help

If dandruff persists or if your scalp becomes irritated or severely itchy, you may need a prescription shampoo. A steroid lotion to suppress the flaking or a stronger medication may loosen the scales so you can wash them away more easily.

Dryness

This is by far the most common cause of itching, flaking skin. Although dryness can be a problem any time of the year, cold air and low humidity can be especially tough on your skin. Dry skin due to the weather depends on where you live (for example, the Minnesota "winter itch" and the Arizona "summer itch").

Self-Care

- Take fewer baths or showers. Keep them short and use lukewarm water and minimal amounts of soap. Mild superfatted soaps such as Basis or Dove will dry skin less. Add Aveno oatmeal powder or other bath oils to your bath.
- Pat (rather than wipe) your skin dry after bathing.
- Apply an oil or cream to your skin immediately after drying. Use a heavy, water-in-oil moisturizer, not a light "disappearing" cream that contains mostly water.
- Avoid creams or lotions containing alcohol.
- Use a humidifier and keep room temperatures cool.

Eczema (Dermatitis)

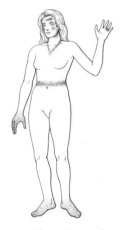

Frequent locations of irritation from contact dermatitis, the most common form of dermatitis.

The terms eczema and dermatitis are both used to describe irritated and inflamed (swollen or reddened) skin. Patches of dry, reddened and itchy skin are the major symptoms. Patches can thicken and develop blisters or weeping sores in severe cases.

Contact dermatitis results from direct contact with one of many irritants that can trigger this reaction. Common culprits include poison ivy (see Poisonous Plants, page 25), laundry and cleaning products, rubber, metals, jewelry, perfume or cosmetics.

Neurodermatitis can occur when something such as a tight garment rubs or scratches (or causes you to rub or scratch) your skin.

Seborrheic dermatitis (cradle cap in infants, see Baby Rashes, page 120) can appear as a stubborn, itchy dandruff. You may notice greasy, scaling areas at the sides of your nose, between your eyebrows, behind your ears or over your breastbone.

Stasis dermatitis may cause the skin at your ankles to become discolored (red or brown), thickened and itchy. It can occur when fluid accumulates in the tissues just beneath your skin.

Atopic dermatitis causes itchy, thickened, fissured skin, most often in the folds of the elbows or backs of the knees. It frequently runs in families and is often associated with allergies.

Self-Care

- Try to identify and avoid direct contact with irritants.
- Follow the self-care tips to prevent dry skin (see above).
- Soak in water for 20 to 30 minutes per day.
- After moisturizing, apply a cream containing 0.5 to 1 percent hydrocortisone.
- Avoid scratching whenever possible. Cover the itchy area with a dressing if you can't keep from scratching it. Trim nails and wear gloves at night.
- Shampoo with an antidandruff product if your scalp is affected.
- Support hose may help relieve stasis dermatitis.
- Dress appropriate to conditions to help avoid excessive sweating.
- Wear smooth-textured cotton clothing.
- Avoid wool carpeting, bedding and clothes and harsh soaps and detergents.
- Occasional use of over-the-counter antihistamines can reduce itching.

■ Fungal Infections

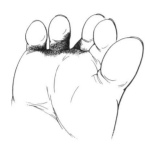

Typical pattern of athlete's foot.

Fungal infections are caused by microscopic organisms that become parasites on your body. Mold-like fungi called dermatophytes cause athlete's foot, jock itch and ringworm of the skin or scalp. These fungi live on dead tissues of your hair, nails and the outer layer of your skin. Poor hygiene, continually moist skin and minor skin or nail injuries increase your susceptibility to fungal infections.

Athlete's foot usually begins between your toes, causing your skin to itch, burn and crack. Sometimes the sole and sides of the foot are affected, becoming thickened and leathery in texture. Although locker rooms and public showers are often blamed for spreading athlete's foot, the environment *inside* your shoes is probably more important. It is also more common as we age.

Jock itch causes an itching or burning sensation around your groin. In addition to the itching, you will usually notice a red rash that may spread to the inner thighs, anal area and buttocks. This infection is mildly contagious. It can be spread by contact or sharing towels.

Ringworm often affects children. Symptoms are itchy, red, scaly, slightly raised, expanding rings on the trunk, face or groin and thigh fold. The rings grow outward as the infection spreads, and the central area begins to look like normal skin. This infection is passed from shared clothing, combs and barber tools. Pets also can transmit the fungus to humans.

Self-Care

General
● Practice good personal hygiene to prevent all forms of fungal infections.
● Use antifungal creams or drying powder two or three times a day until the rash disappears. Use medications that contain miconazole (Zeasorb-AF, Micatin), clotrimazole (Lotrimin AF, Mycelex OTC) or undecylenic acid (Desenex, Cruex).

For Athlete's Foot
● Keep your feet dry, particularly the area between your toes.
● Wear well-ventilated shoes. Avoid shoes made of synthetic materials.
● Don't wear the same shoes every day, and don't store them in plastic.
● Change socks (cotton or polypropylene) twice a day if your feet sweat a lot.
● Wear waterproof sandals or shoes around public pools, showers and locker rooms.

For Jock Itch
● Keep your groin clean and dry.   ● Shower and change clothes after exercise.
● Avoid clothes that chafe, and launder athletic supporters frequently.

For Ringworm
● Thoroughly clean brushes, combs or headgear that may have been infected.
● Wash hands before and after examining your child.
● Keep your child's linens separate from the rest of the family's.

Medical Help

See your health-care provider if symptoms last longer than 4 weeks or if you notice increased redness, drainage or fever. You may require treatment with prescription medications.

Hives

Hives are raised, red, often itchy welts of various sizes that appear and disappear on the skin. They are more common on areas of the body where clothes rub your skin. Hives tend to occur in batches and last anywhere from a few minutes to several days.

Angioedema, a similar swelling, causes large welts below your skin, especially near the eyes and lips but also on your hands and feet and inside your throat.

Hives and angioedema result when your body releases a natural chemical called histamine in your skin. Allergies to foods, drugs, pollen, insect bites, infections, illness, cold and heat and emotional distress can trigger a reaction. In most cases, hives and angioedema are harmless and leave no lasting marks. However, serious angioedema can cause your throat or tongue to block your airway and cause loss of consciousness.

Self-Care

- Avoid substances that have triggered past attacks.
- Take cool showers. Apply cool compresses. Wear light clothing. Minimize vigorous activity.
- Use calamine lotion or over-the-counter antihistamines such as diphenhydramine hydrochloride (Benadryl) or chlorpheniramine maleate (Chlor-Trimeton) to help relieve the itching.
- If foods are suspected of causing the problem, keep a food diary.

Medical Help

Seek emergency care if you feel light-headed or have difficulty breathing or if hives continue to appear for more than a couple days.

Impetigo

Impetigo is a common skin infection that usually appears on the face. The infection begins when bacteria (streptococci) penetrate your skin through a cut, scratch or insect bite. Impetigo is highly contagious and easily spread by contact.

The infection starts as a red sore that blisters briefly, oozes for a few days and forms a sticky crust. Scratching or touching the sores can spread this contagious infection to other people and other parts of your body.

Impetigo is more common among young children. In adults, it appears mostly as a complication of other skin problems such as dermatitis.

Self-Care

Good hygiene is essential for preventing impetigo and limiting its spread. For limited or minor infections that have not spread to other areas, try the following:

- Keep the sores and skin surrounding them clean.
- Soak the area of the rash with a solution of 1 tablespoon of liquid bleach to 1 quart of water for 20 minutes. This will make it easier to remove the scabs.
- After washing with the bleach solution, apply an antibiotic ointment three or four times daily. Wash the skin before each application, and pat the skin dry.
- Avoid scratching or touching the sores unnecessarily until they heal. Wash your hands after any contact with them. Children's fingernails should be trimmed.
- Do not share towels, clothing or razors with others. Replace linens often.

Medical Help

If the infection spreads, your health-care provider may prescribe oral antibiotics such as penicillin or erythromycin or an ointment of mupirocin (Bactroban).

Common Problems

◼ Itching and Rashes

Because so many things can cause itching and rashes, pinpointing the source of the problem can be difficult. For information about specific problems that cause itching and rashes, see the following segments in this book: Allergic Reactions, page 8; Lice, page 122; Insect Bites and Stings, page 11; Baby Rashes, see below; Common Childhood Rashes, page 121; Hives, page 119; Dryness, page 117; and Eczema (Dermatitis), page 117.

◼ Baby Rashes

Cradle cap: crusty, scaly skin on your baby's scalp. Wash your baby's hair only once a week with a mild shampoo and lukewarm water. Apply baby oil to the crusty areas and gently scrape off the scales with a soft brush after bathing. If the rash is red and irritated, apply a 0.5 percent hydrocortisone cream once a week.

Heat rash: fine red spots or bumps, usually on the neck or the upper back, chest or arms. This harmless rash often develops during hot, humid weather, especially if your baby is dressed too warmly. It also can occur if your baby has a fever.

Milia: tiny (pinpoint) white spots on the nose and cheeks. It is usually present at birth. The spots eventually disappear without treatment.

Infant acne: red bumps that can appear during the first few months after birth. Gently wash your baby's face daily with plain water and once or twice weekly with a mild soap. Do not use acne creams or lotions on an infant or young child.

Drool rash: a red rash on the cheeks and chin that comes and goes. This rash is caused by contact with food and sputum. Cleaning your baby's skin after feeding or spitting up usually helps clear this rash.

Diaper rash: reddish, puffy skin in the diaper area, especially in the folds of the skin. This irritation usually is caused by moisture, the acid in urine or stool and chafing of diapers. Some babies also get a rash from detergent used to wash cloth diapers, plastic pants, elastic or certain types of disposable diapers and diaper wipes. Sometimes a yeast infection is the cause.

Self-Care for Recurrent Diaper Rash	<ul><li>Change your baby's diapers frequently, placing the diaper loosely around the child, and expose the skin to air whenever possible. Avoid using plastic pants.</li><li>Use cloth diapers or disposable diapers without gathers. Wash cloth diapers in mild soap (Dreft or Ivory), and 1 cup of white vinegar should be added to the rinse cycle to help rid the diapers of bacteria. Avoid fabric softeners.</li><li>Wash and pat dry the area at each diaper change, using plain water or a mild soap and water.</li><li>Apply a thin layer of protective cream or ointment such as Desitin or A & D Ointment.</li><li>Try switching to a different brand of diapers if you use disposable diapers.</li><li>Avoid diaper wipes because many contain perfume and alcohol.</li><li>If the rash is particularly difficult to cleanse, place the baby in a sink of warm water with 2 ounces of white vinegar mixed in.</li><li>Do not apply cornstarch or talcum powder; they could worsen the condition.</li></ul>
Medical Help	See your health-care provider if the above tips don't help; if the rash is purple or bruised-looking, crusty, blistered or weepy; or if the baby has a fever.

Common Childhood Rashes

Chickenpox

Itchy, red spots on the face or chest which spread to the arms and legs. Spots quickly fill with a clear fluid to form blisters, rupture and turn crusty. New spots generally continue appearing over 4 to 5 days. Fever, a runny nose or cough often accompanies chickenpox. Chickenpox seldom lasts for more than 2 weeks after the first spot appears. Symptoms usually appear 14 to 21 days after exposure. The child is contagious until the rash crusts

- Give the child cool baths every 3 or 4 hours to reduce the itching. Sprinkle baking soda in the bath water for added relief
- Apply calamine lotion to the rash
- Switch to a bland diet of soft foods, and avoid citrus fruits if blisters are present in the mouth
- Trim fingernails. Put gloves on the child at night to prevent scratching

- If the rash involves the eyes, or if you develop a cough or shortness of breath
- If you are an older adult, have an impaired immune system or are pregnant and have not been previously exposed
- Doctors may prescribe a drug called acyclovir in severe cases. A vaccine is available for children ages 12 months or older and adults who have not yet had the virus

Roseola

Often begins with a high fever lasting about 3 days. When it subsides, a rash appears on the trunk and neck and lasts a few hours to a few days. Virus typically affects children, especially between ages 6 months and 3 years

The rash causes little discomfort and disappears on its own without treatment. Acetaminophen and tepid sponge baths may help relieve the discomfort caused by the fever

- If the rash lasts longer than 3 days. Young children may experience convulsions triggered by the high fever

Measles

Typically begins with fever, often as high as 104 to 105 F, and a cough, sneezing, sore throat and inflamed, watery eyes. Two to 4 days later, a rash appears. It often begins as fine red spots on the face and spreads to the trunk, arms and legs. Spots may become larger and usually last about a week. Small white spots may appear on inside lining of the cheek

- Bed rest, acetaminophen and an over-the-counter cough medication may help relieve the discomfort
- Lukewarm baths, calamine lotion or Benadryl solution will relieve itching

- If you suspect that you or a family member has measles. Measles has uncommon but potentially serious complications, such as pneumonia, encephalitis or a bacterial infection
- A vaccine to prevent measles is given to children between 12 and 15 months and between 4 and 12 years of age

Fifth disease

Bright red, raised patches appear on both cheeks. During the next few days, a pink, lacy, slightly raised rash develops on the arms, trunk, thighs and buttocks. Rash may come and go for up to 3 weeks. Often, there are no symptoms, or only mild, cold-like symptoms

No specific treatment. Use acetaminophen to relieve the fever and any discomfort

- If you aren't sure whether a rash is fifth disease or if you are pregnant and suspect that you've been exposed

Lice

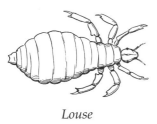

Louse

Lice are tiny parasitic insects. *Head lice* often are spread among children by contact, clothing or hairbrushes. *Body lice* are generally spread through clothing or bedding. *Pubic lice* (commonly called "crabs") can be spread by sexual contact, clothing, bedding or even toilet seats.

The first sign of lice is intense itching. With body lice, some people have hives and others have abrasions from scratching. Head lice are found on the scalp and are easiest to see at the nape of the neck and over the ears. Small nits (eggs) that resemble tiny pussy willow buds can be found on the hair shafts. Body lice are difficult to find on the body because they burrow into the skin, but they usually can be detected in the seams of underwear. Pubic lice are found on the skin and hair of the pubic areas. Lice live only 3 days off the body; eggs hatch in about 1 week.

Self-Care

- Several lotions and shampoos, both prescription and over-the-counter, are available. Apply the product to all infected and hair parts of the body. Any remaining nits can be removed with tweezers or a fine comb. Repeat treatment with the lotion or shampoo in 7 to 10 days.
- Your sexual partner should be examined and treated if infected.
- Keep infected children home until you complete this first treatment.
- Wash sheets, clothing and hats with hot, soapy water and dry them at high heat. Soak combs and brushes in very hot, soapy water for at least 5 minutes.
- Vacuum carpets, mattresses, pillows, upholstered furniture and car seats.

Medical Help

Consult your physician before using products in a child younger than 2 months or if you are pregnant.

Scabies

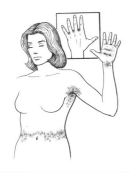

Almost impossible to see without a magnifying glass, scabies mites cause itching by burrowing under the skin. Itching is usually worse at night. The burrowing leaves tiny bumps and thin, irregular, pencil-like marks or tracks on your skin. They appear most often in the following areas: between your fingers, in your armpits, around your waist, along the insides of your wrists, on the back of your elbows, on your ankles and soles of your feet, around your breasts and genitals and on your buttocks. However, almost any part of the skin may be involved.

Close physical contact and, less often, sharing clothing or bedding with an infected person can spread these tiny mites. Often an entire family or members of a day-care group or school class will experience scabies.

Self-Care

Bathing and over-the-counter preparations will not eliminate scabies. Talk to your health-care provider if you have symptoms or if you believe you had contact with someone who has scabies.

Medical Help

Your doctor may prescribe a cream or lotion that you must apply all over your body and leave on overnight. All family members and sexual partners may require treatment. Also, all clothing and bedding that you used before treatment must be washed with hot, soapy water and dried with high heat.

Psoriasis

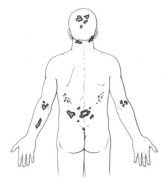

Some of the most common locations of psoriasis.

For some, psoriasis brings little more than recurrent bouts of mild itching, but for others, it's a lifetime of discomfort and unsightly skin changes.

Most often, psoriasis causes dry, red patches covered with thick, silvery scales. You may see a few spots of scaling or large areas of damaged skin. Knees, elbows, trunk and scalp are the most common locations. Patches on your scalp can shed large quantities of silvery-white scales resembling severe dandruff.

In more severe cases, pustules, cracked skin, itching, minor bleeding or aching joints also may develop. In addition, your fingernails and toenails may lose their normal luster and develop pits or ridges.

These skin eruptions are due to overly rapid growth of cells in your skin's outer layer. Many people also inherit a tendency toward psoriasis. Dry skin, skin injuries, infections, certain drugs, obesity, stress and lack of sunlight can all aggravate your symptoms. This condition is not contagious. You cannot spread it to other parts of your own body, or to other people, simply by touching it. Psoriasis typically goes through cycles. The symptoms can persist for weeks or months, followed by a break.

Self-Care

- Maintain good general health: a balanced diet, adequate rest and exercise.
- Maintain a normal weight. Psoriasis occurs often in skin creases or folds.
- Avoid scratching, rubbing or picking at the patches of psoriasis.
- Bathe daily to soak off the scales. Avoid hot water or harsh soap.
- Keep your skin moist (see Dryness, page 117).
- Use soaps, shampoos, cleansers or ointments containing coal tar or salicylic acid.
- Expose your skin to moderate sunlight, but avoid sunburn.
- Apply over-the-counter cortisone creams, 0.5 or 1 percent, for a few weeks when symptoms are especially bad.

Medical Help

If self-care remedies don't help, stronger cortisone-type creams or various forms of phototherapy may be prescribed. Phototherapy involves a combination of medications and ultraviolet light. Skin ointments containing a form of vitamin D (Dovenex) also may offer some relief. In severe cases, an anticancer drug called methotrexate or a drug used to prevent rejection in organ transplant recipients (cyclosporine) is sometimes prescribed.

Moles

Sometimes called "beauty marks," moles are usually harmless collections of pigment cells. They may contain hairs, stay smooth, become raised or wrinkled and even fall off in old age.

In rare cases, a mole can become cancerous. Talk to your health-care provider if pain, bleeding or inflammation occurs or if you notice a change in a mole (see Signs of Skin Cancer, page 125). Keep an eye on moles located around your nails or genitals, and those that have been present since birth. Giant moles, present at birth, are a special problem, and they may need to be removed to avoid the risk of cancer.

Self-Care

Healthy moles usually don't require special care unless they become cut or irritated. Your normal skin care routine will suffice.

■ Shingles

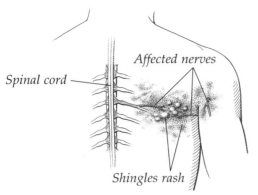

Spinal cord —

Affected nerves

Shingles rash

The shingles rash is associated with an inflammation of nerves beneath the skin.

Shingles (also known as herpes zoster) emerges when the virus that causes chickenpox (varicella zoster) reactivates after lying dormant within your nerve cells.

As this virus reactivates, you may notice pain or tingling in a limited area, usually on one side of your body or face. This pain occurs as the virus spreads along one of the nerves that spread outward on your face or from your spine. This pain or tingling can continue for several days or longer.

Subsequently, a rash with small blisters may appear. The rash may continue to spread over the next 3 to 5 days, often forming a band-like pattern on one side of your body. The blisters usually dry up in a few days, forming crusts that fall off over the next 2 to 3 weeks. The blisters contain a virus that is contagious, so avoid physical contact with others, especially pregnant women. Chickenpox in a newborn can be deadly.

Self-Care

You can relieve some of the discomfort by doing the following:
- Soak your blisters with cool, wet compresses (aluminum acetate solution).
- Wash blisters gently, and don't bandage them.
- Apply a soothing lotion such as calamine (Caladryl) lotion.
- Take over-the-counter pain relievers to alleviate pain.
- Over-the-counter analgesic creams also may alleviate your pain.

Medical Help

Contact your health-care provider promptly in the following situations:
- If the pain and rash occur near your eyes. If left untreated, this infection can lead to permanent eye damage.
- If you or someone in your family has a weakened immune system (due to cancer, medications or a chronic medical condition).
- If the rash is widespread and painful.
- If you are older than 60 years.

Acyclovir (Zovirax) and famciclovir (Famvir) are now available to hasten healing and reduce the severity of some complications caused by shingles.

When the Pain Persists After Shingles

Pain persisting for months or even years after a bout with shingles is called postherpetic neuralgia (PHN). It occurs in 50 percent of people older than 60 who have had shingles.

PHN is as individual as you are, and effective treatment for you may be useless for someone else. But new treatments show promise, and new findings support the benefit of early treatment of the acute viral infection that precedes PHN.

Because the pain of PHN tends to lessen as time passes, it's difficult to tell whether a medication is effective or the pain is subsiding on its own.

Several treatments may provide relief. They include analgesic medications, electrical stimulation, tricyclic antidepressants, certain anticonvulsant medications and neurosurgery in severe cases.

Most people are free of pain after 5 years.

■ Signs of Skin Cancer

Each year, skin cancer is diagnosed in approximately 1 million people, and about 10,000 people die each year of the disease. More than 90 percent of skin cancers occur on areas regularly exposed to ultraviolet radiation (from sunlight or tanning lights), and this exposure is considered to be the chief cause. Other factors include a genetic tendency, chemical pollution and X-ray radiation.

Here are the signs of the three most common types of skin cancer:

Basal cell cancer, by far the most common skin cancer, usually appears as a smooth, waxy or pearly bump that grows slowly and rarely spreads and causes death.

Squamous cell cancer causes a firm, nodular or flat growth with a crusted, ulcerated or scaly surface on the face, ears, neck, hands or arms.

Melanoma is the most serious but least common skin cancer.

The ABCD rule (see below) can help you tell a normal mole from one that could be melanoma. In addition, rapid growth, bleeding and nonhealing sores could be symptoms.

A

Asymmetry. Half of the lesion is unlike the other half.

B

Border irregular (ragged, notched or blurred).

C
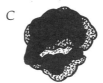
Color varies from one area to another. Different shades of tan and brown, black, red, white or blue.

D

Diameter is larger than the head of a pencil, about 1/4 of an inch.

Self-Care

- Avoid exposure to the sun to the point of a sunburn or a dark suntan. Both result in sun damage. Skin damage accumulates over time. Minimize your time in the sun and wear tightly woven clothing and a broad-brimmed hat. Remember, snow, water and ice reflect the sun's harmful rays.
- Use sunscreen as part of your daily outdoor routine. Apply a broad-spectrum sunscreen with a sun protection factor (SPF) of at least 15. (Broad-spectrum means it provides protection against ultraviolet A and B radiation.) Use sunscreen on all exposed skin, including your lips. Apply sunscreen 30 minutes before sun exposure.
- Avoid tanning salons.
- Check your skin at least every 3 months for the development of new skin growths or changes in existing moles, freckles, bumps and birthmarks.

Medical Help

If you notice a new growth, change in skin or sore that doesn't heal in 2 weeks, see your physician. Don't wait for pain; skin cancers are usually not painful. The cure rate for skin cancer is high if you receive treatment early.

If you have a family history of melanoma and many moles on your body (especially on the trunk), regular examination by a dermatologist may be appropriate.

Kids' Care

Getting severe, blistering sunburns as a child increases one's risk for the development of melanoma as an adult. Set time limits for your child when at the pool or beach. Remember, ultraviolet rays are strongest between 10 a.m. and 3 p.m. Clouds block only a small portion of ultraviolet rays.

Common Problems

■ Warts

Warts are skin growths caused by a common virus, but they can be painful and disfiguring and can spread to others.

There are more than 50 types of warts. They can appear on any part of your body, but they are most common on the hands or feet. Warts found on the feet, called plantar warts, can be painful because they press inward as you stand on them.

You can acquire warts through direct contact with an infected person or surface, such as a shower floor. The virus that causes them stimulates the rapid growth of cells on the outer layer of your skin.

Each person's immune system responds to warts differently. Most warts are not a serious health hazard and disappear without treatment. Because warts are more common among children than adults, some believe that many adults develop immunity to them. In many adults, warts eventually disappear within 2 years.

Certain warts trigger or signal more serious medical problems. Genital warts (see page 178) require treatment to avoid spreading them through sexual contact. Some strains of the papilloma virus increase a woman's risk for cervical cancer. Women also can pass this virus to their babies during birth, causing some complications.

Self-Care

- Over-the-counter topical medications may remove warts. Look for products containing salicylic acid, which peels off the infected skin. They require daily use, often for a few weeks. **Caution:** The acid can irritate or damage normal skin.
- To avoid spreading warts to other parts of your body, avoid brushing, combing or shaving over areas where there are warts.

Medical Help

You may want to see your health-care provider if your warts are tender or a cosmetic nuisance or interfere with your activities. Common treatments for warts include freezing with liquid nitrogen or dry ice, electrical burning, laser surgery or minor surgery.

■ Wrinkled Skin

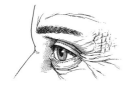

Common facial skin wrinkles.

As much as we try to hide the fact that we're aging, wrinkles or "character lines" are an inevitable part of this process. As you grow older, your skin gets thinner, drier and less elastic. Sagging and wrinkling begin because the connective tissue in your skin deteriorates. Some people don't seem to age as quickly as others. This difference is typically due to heredity or skin color. People with fair skin age faster because they have more severe damage from the sun. Cosmetic products that promise a fountain of youth are often expensive and fail to deliver real improvements.

Self-Care

There is no cure for wrinkled skin. These commonsense measures for good skin care may help slow the process:

- Maintain good general health.
- Don't smoke cigarettes.
- Avoid prolonged exposure to the sun. Use sunscreens when you are outdoors.
- Avoid harsh soaps and hot water when bathing.

Medical Help

Prescription medical treatments such as retinoic acid creams may work if used for a long time. Cosmetic procedures such as chemical peels, dermabrasion or lasers can alter your skin's appearance if it disturbs you.

Hair Loss

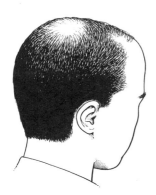

Male-pattern baldness typically appears first at the hairline or crown.

Healthy, lustrous hair has long been a symbol of youth and beauty. As a result, many people cringe at the first signs of hair thinning or baldness.

If your hair seems to be thinning, take comfort in the fact that it's normal to lose between 50 and 100 strands a day. Like your nails and skin, your hair goes through a cycle of growth and rest. Gradual thinning occurs as a normal part of the aging process.

Common baldness accounts for 99 percent of hair loss in both men and women and is genetic. Male-pattern baldness usually begins with thinning at your hairline, followed by moderate to extensive hair loss on the crown of your head. Bald patches rarely develop in women with common baldness. Instead, their hair becomes thinner all over the head. Heredity, hormones and age all play important roles in common baldness, so the best way to know what you will look like later in life is to look at your parents' families.

Gradual hair loss also can occur any time your hair's delicate growth cycle is upset. Diet, medications, hormones, pregnancy, improper hair care, poor nutrition, underlying diseases and other factors can cause too many follicles to rest at once, producing bald patches or diffuse thinning.

Sudden hair loss is usually due to a condition called alopecia areata. This fairly rare condition causes smooth, circular bald patches, up to 3 inches across, that may overlap. Stress and heredity may play a role in this disorder. About 90 percent of the time, the hair grows back within 6 to 24 months with no treatment.

Self-Care

There is no "magic bullet" to prevent hair loss or encourage new growth. However, the following tips can help keep your hair healthy.

- Eat a well-rounded diet.
- Handle your hair gently. When possible, allow your hair to dry naturally in the air.
- Avoid tight hairstyles such as braids, buns or ponytails.
- Avoid compulsively twisting, rubbing or pulling your hair.
- Check with hair care experts about hairpieces or styling techniques that help minimize the effects of common baldness.
- An over-the-counter medication called minoxidil can promote new hair growth in a small percentage of people, but the drug eventually loses its effectiveness and can be costly. Other hair growth products for baldness are of no proven benefit.

Medical Help

Although there is no cure for common genetic baldness, you may want to ask your health-care provider about medical treatments or hair replacement surgery. Because sudden hair loss can signal an underlying medical condition that may require treatment, contact your physician for evaluation.

Kids' Care

If your child has patches of broken hairs on the scalp or eyebrows, he or she may be rubbing or pulling out the hair. This signals a behavioral disorder called trichotillomania. Contact your health-care provider for evaluation.

Common Problems

■ Nail Fungal Infections

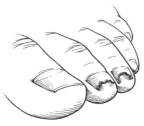

Typical fungal infection.

This stubborn, but harmless, problem often begins as a tiny white or yellow spot on your nail. Fungal infections can develop on your nails or under their outer edges if you continually expose them to a warm, moist environment. Depending on the type of fungus, your nails may discolor, thicken and develop crumbling edges or cracks.

Fungal infections usually affect your toenails more frequently than your fingernails and are more common among the elderly. Your risk for a toenail fungal infection is greater if your feet perspire heavily, and if you wear socks and shoes that hinder ventilation and don't absorb perspiration. You also can contract this infection by walking barefoot in public places and as a complication of other infections.

Fingernail fungal infections often result from overexposure to water and detergents. Moisture caught under artificial nails also can encourage fungus growth.

Self-Care

To help prevent fungal infections, try the following:
- Keep your nails dry and clean. Dry your feet thoroughly after bathing.
- Change your socks often and wear leather-soled shoes.
- Use an antifungal spray or powder on your feet and inside your shoes.
- Don't pick at or trim the skin around your nails.
- Avoid walking barefoot around public pools, showers and locker rooms.

Medical Help

Self-care measures usually fail to prevent the infection. Topical antifungal creams or oral antifungal medications such as griseofulvin, itraconazole, terbinafine hydrochloride and fluconazole are effective. In severe cases, surgical removal may be required.

■ Ingrown Toenails

Pain and tenderness in your toe often signal that you have an ingrown toenail. This common condition occurs when the sharp end or side of your toenail grows into the flesh of your toe. It affects your big toe most often, especially if you have curved toenails, if your shoes fit poorly or if you cut your nails improperly.

Self-Care

- Trim your toenails straight across and not too short.
- Wear socks and shoes that fit properly, and don't place excessive pressure on your toes. Wear open-toe shoes, if necessary, or try sandals.
- Soak your feet in warm salt water (1 tablespoon per quart) for 30 minutes four times a day to reduce swelling and relieve tenderness.
- After soaking, put tiny bits of sterile cotton under the ingrown edge. This will help the nail eventually grow above the skin edge. Change the cotton daily until the pain and redness subside.
- Apply an antibiotic ointment to the tender area.
- If there is severe pain, apply cotton saturated with an over-the-counter ingrown toenail reliever to the area. It will provide temporary relief.

Medical Help

If you experience severe discomfort or pus or redness that seems to be spreading, seek medical attention. Your doctor may need to remove the ingrown portion of the nail and prescribe antibiotics.

Throat and Mouth

■ Sore Throat

The tight, scratchy feeling in our throats is a familiar sign that a cold or flu is on the way. Most sore throats run their course in a few days, sometimes needing over-the-counter lozenges or gargles.

Most sore throats are caused by two types of infections—*viral* and *bacterial*—but they also can be caused by allergies and dry air. When a sore throat involves enlarged, tender tonsils, it's somtimes called tonsillitis.

Viral infections usually are the source of common colds and the flu and the sore throat that accompanies them. Colds usually go away on their own in about a week, once your system has built up antibodies that destroy the virus. Antibiotic medications are *not* effective in treating viral infections. The common symptoms are as follows:

- Sore or scratchy, dry feeling
- Coughing and sneezing
- Mild fever or no fever
- Hoarseness
- Runny nose and postnasal dripping

Bacterial infections are not as common as viral infections, but they can be more serious. "Strep throat" is the most common bacterial infection. Often a person with strep was exposed to someone else with strep throat in the past 2 to 7 days. Children ages 5 to 15 who are in a classroom or other group setting are most likely to get strep throat. It generally is spread by nose or throat secretions. Less commonly, infection may be transmitted through food, milk or water contaminated with streptococci, the bacterial agent. Strep throats require medical treatment. Common symptoms are:

- Swollen tonsils and neck glands
- Back of throat is bright red with white patches
- Fever, often more than 101 F, and often accompanied by chills
- Pain when swallowing

Most sore throat "bugs" are passed by direct contact. Mucus and saliva from one person's hands are transferred to objects, doorknobs and other surfaces, then to your hands and eventually to your mouth or nose.

Mononucleosis: A Tiresome Illness

Infectious mononucleosis. You've probably heard it called the "kissing disease." It's also known as mono, and it can be spread by kissing or, more commonly, through exposure resulting from coughing, sneezing or sharing a glass or cup.

Mono is caused by the Epstein-Barr virus. Anyone can get mono. By some estimates, 50 percent of the population has had mono by age 5. Most people older than 35 already have been exposed to the Epstein-Barr virus and have built up antibodies. They're immune and won't get it again. Full-blown mono is common in people age 7 to 35, especially teenagers.

Most people with mono experience fatigue and weakness. Other symptoms include a sore throat, fever, swollen lymph nodes in the neck and armpits, swollen tonsils, headache, rash and loss of appetite. Most symptoms abate within 10 days, but you shouldn't expect to return to your normal activities or contact sports for 3 weeks (your liver or spleen may be enlarged and at risk of injury). It may be 2 to 3 months before you feel completely normal. Rest and a healthful diet are the only treatments.

If symptoms linger more than a week or two or if they recur, see a doctor.

Self-Care

- Double your fluid intake. Fluids help keep your mucus thin and easy to clear.
- Gargle with warm salt water. Mix about a teaspoon of salt with a glass of warm water to gargle and spit. This will soothe and help clear your throat of mucus.
- Suck on a lozenge or hard candy, or chew sugarless gum. Chewing and sucking stimulate saliva production, which bathes and cleanses your throat.
- Take pain relievers. Over-the-counter medications, such as acetaminophen, ibuprofen and aspirin, relieve sore throat pain for 4 to 6 hours. Don't give aspirin to children or teenagers (see page 231).
- Rest your voice. If your sore throat has inflamed your larynx (voice box), talking may lead to more irritation and temporary loss of your voice, called laryngitis.
- Humidify the air. Adding moisture to the air prevents your mucous membranes from drying out (which causes irritation and makes it harder to sleep). Saline nasal sprays are also helpful.
- Avoid smoke and other air pollutants. Smoke irritates a sore throat. Stop smoking, and avoid all smoke and fumes from household cleaners or paint. Keep children away from secondhand smoke exposure.

Prevention

- Wash your hands frequently, especially during the cold and flu season.
- Keep your hands away from your face to avoid getting bacteria and viruses into your mouth or nose.

Medical Help

Serious throat infections, such as epiglottitis, can cause swelling that closes your airway. Seek emergency care if your sore throat is accompanied by any of the following symptoms:

- Drooling or difficulty swallowing or breathing
- A stiff, rigid neck and severe headache
- A fever of more than 102 F (103 F for children) or a fever that lasts for more than 48 hours
- A rash
- Persistent hoarseness or mouth ulcers lasting 2 weeks or more
- Recent exposure to strep throat

If the doctor suspects strep throat, a test will be ordered. You may learn the results before leaving the doctor's office, usually within 1 hour. Because this test misses about 20 percent of strep throats, many clinics do both the rapid test and a 24-hour throat culture. The rapid strep test also gives inaccurate results if you have recently been taking antibiotics. If the test result is positive, your doctor will prescribe an antibiotic, usually penicillin or a related medication.

Tonsils are rarely removed, except when recurrent infections cause serious problems.

Caution

If your doctor does prescribe a medication, take it for the full time indicated. Stopping use of the medication early can allow some bacteria to remain in the throat, potentially leading to a recurrence and complications such as rheumatic fever or a blood infection.

If your child has been taking antibiotics for at least 24 hours, has no fever and feels better, he or she may return to school or day care.

Lump in Your Throat

The expressions "all choked up" and "the words stuck in my throat" are a reflection of the relationship between your throat and your emotional system. That "lump" in your throat that you feel is muscle tension.

When you are anxious, depressed or under stress, the small muscular opening in the lower part of your throat (the pharynx) begins to tense. This muscle may tighten without your being aware of it. When the muscle tightens, it sends a signal to your brain saying that something is in your throat, even when nothing is there.

This condition is so common it has its own name (globus syndrome), and although it is unpleasant, it usually resolves in a matter of days.

Other causes of a lump in your throat include side effects of medications, such as antihistamines or medications for high blood pressure and depression; recent cold or cough; hiatal hernia; being overweight; and acid indigestion (especially if you overeat at night).

Self-Care

- Drink plenty of fluids.
- Chew gum or suck on lozenges to stimulate saliva, which will soothe your throat.
- Avoid heartburn (stomach acid may be slipping up your food pipe and into your throat). Take antacids at bedtime, and don't go to bed on a full stomach.
- Avoid chocolate, fatty meals, alcohol and overeating.

Medical Help

If the lump in your throat does not go away after a few days, see your health-care provider. Your doctor will perform tests to determine the exact cause of the lump and may adjust your medications to see if that will solve the problem.

Bad Breath

Everyone would like to have breath that always is "kissing sweet." Because fresh breath is important to us, makers of mints and mouthwashes sell millions of dollars worth of products every year. However, these products are only temporarily helpful for controlling bad breath. They actually may be less effective than simply rinsing your mouth with water and brushing and flossing your teeth.

There are many causes of bad breath. First, your mouth itself may be the source. Bacterial breakdown of food particles and other debris in and around your teeth can cause a foul odor. A dry mouth, such as occurs during sleep or as the result of some drugs or smoking, enables dead cells to accumulate on your tongue, gums and cheeks. As a result, they decompose and cause odor.

Eating foods containing oils with a strong odor causes bad breath. Onions and garlic are the best examples, but other vegetables and spices also may cause bad breath.

Lung disease can cause bad breath. Chronic infections in the lungs can produce very foul-smelling breath. Usually, much sputum (the mucus you cough up) is produced by these conditions. Several illnesses can cause a distinctive breath odor. Kidney failure can cause a urine-like odor, and liver failure may cause an odor described as "fishy." People with diabetes often have a fruity breath odor. This smell is also common in ill children who have eaten poorly for a few days. Bad breath in these situations can be corrected by treatment of the underlying condition.

Self-Care	For most people, bad breath can be improved by following a few simple steps: ● Brush your teeth after every meal. ● Brush your tongue to remove dead cells. ● Floss once a day to remove food particles from between your teeth. ● Drink plenty of water (not coffee, pop or alcohol) to keep your mouth moist. ● Avoid strong foods that cause bad breath. Toothbrushing or use of mouthwashes only partially disguises odors of garlic or onion which come from your lungs. ● Change your toothbrush every 2 to 3 months. ● Rinse your mouth after using inhaler medications.

■ Hoarseness or Loss of Voice

Loss of voice (laryngitis) or hoarseness occurs when your vocal cords become swollen or inflamed and no longer vibrate normally. They produce an unnatural sound, or they may not produce any sound at all.

Your speaking voice is formed when your diaphragm (the muscle above your stomach) pushes air from your lungs through your vocal cords. Air pressure forces your vocal cords to open and close, and the controlled escape of air vibrates the vocal cords, producing the sound that is your voice.

In addition to hoarseness, you may feel pain when speaking or have a raw and scratchy throat. Sometimes, your voice sounds higher or lower than normal.

The common causes of hoarseness or loss of voice are infections (as a result, you frequently lose your voice when you have a cold or flu), allergies, vocal strain (talking too loudly for too long or yelling), smoking and chronic esophageal reflux. Reflux, the backwash of acidic stomach contents into the food pipe, can sometimes spill over into the voice box.

Self-Care	● Limit your talking and whispering. (Whispering strains your vocal cords as much as talking.) ● Drink lots of warm, noncaffeinated fluids to keep your throat moist. ● Avoid clearing your throat. ● Stop smoking, and avoid exposure to smoke. Smoke dries your throat and irritates your vocal cords. ● Stop drinking alcohol, which also dries your throat and irritates your vocal cords. ● Use a humidifier to moisturize the air you breathe. (Follow the manufacturer's instructions to clean the humidifier and prevent bacterial buildup.)
Medical Help	If hoarseness lasts for more than 2 weeks, seek medical help. Your doctor may prescribe medications for infection or allergy. Take them just as prescribed. Hoarseness is rarely caused by cancer.

■ Mouth Sores

Irritating, painful and repetitive. That's how many people describe canker sores and cold sores. But the terminology can be confusing. Cold sores have nothing to do with the common cold. What's more, the cause, appearance, symptoms and treatments of canker sores and cold sores are very different. There are other mouth sores and conditions that are often mistaken for canker sores and cold sores.

■ Canker Sores

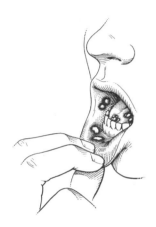

A canker sore is an ulcer on the soft tissue inside your mouth—on the tongue, soft palate and inside the cheeks. Typically, you notice a burning sensation and a round whitish spot with a red edge or halo. Pain lessens in a few days.

Despite a great deal of research into the problem, the cause of canker sores remains a mystery. Current thinking suggests that stress or tissue injury may cause the eruption of common canker sores. Some researchers think certain foods (for example, citrus fruits, tomatoes and some nuts) may complicate the problem. A minor injury, such as biting the inside of your mouth, may trigger a canker sore.

There are two types of canker sores: simple and complex. The simple type of canker sore may appear three or four times a year and last 4 to 7 days. The first occurrence is usually between the ages of 10 and 20, but it can occur in younger children. As a person reaches adulthood, the sores occur less frequently and may stop developing altogether. Women seem to get them more often than men, and they seem to run in families.

Complex canker sores are less common but much more of a problem. People with this condition may have sores 50 percent of the time—as old sores heal, new ones appear.

Self-Care

There is no cure for either simple or complex canker sores, and effective treatments are limited. However, the following practices may provide temporary relief:
- Avoid abrasive, acidic or spicy foods, which may increase the pain.
- Apply ice to the canker sore.
- Brush your teeth carefully to avoid irritating the sore.
- Use a topical ointment containing phenol.
- Rinse your mouth with over-the-counter preparations: try diluted hydrogen peroxide or elixir of Benadryl.
- Use an over-the-counter pain reliever.

Medical Help

For severe attacks of canker sores, your dentist or physician may recommend a prescription mouthwash, a corticosteroid salve or an anesthetic solution called viscous lidocaine.

Contact your physician in any of the following situations:
- New high fever with canker sores
- Spreading sores or signs of spreading infection
- Pain that is not controlled with the measures listed above
- Sores that do not heal completely within a week

See your dentist if you have sharp tooth surfaces or dental appliances that are causing the sores.

Common Problems

■ Cold Sores (Fever Blisters)

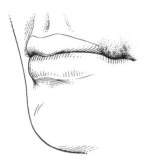

Also known as fever blisters, cold sores are very common. They may appear on your mouth, lips, nose, cheeks or fingers.

The herpes simplex virus causes cold sores. Herpes simplex virus type 1 usually causes cold sores. Herpes simplex virus type 2 is usually responsible for genital herpes. However, either form of the virus can cause sores in the facial area or on the genitals. You get cold sores from another person who has an active condition. Eating utensils, razors, towels or direct skin contact are common means of spreading this infection.

Symptoms may not start for as long as 20 days after you were exposed to the virus. Small, fluid-filled blisters develop on a raised, red, painful area of skin. Pain or tingling often precedes blisters by 1 to 2 days. Symptoms usually last 7 to 10 days.

After the first infection, the virus periodically reemerges at or near the original site. Fever, menstruation and exposure to the sun may trigger a recurrence.

The herpes simplex virus can be transmitted even when blisters aren't present. But the greatest risk of infection is from the time the blister appears until it has completely crusted over. Cold sores occur most often in adolescents and young adults, but they can occur at any age. Outbreaks decrease after age 35.

Self-Care

Cold sores generally clear up without treatment. The following steps may provide relief:

- Rest, take over-the-counter pain relievers (if you have a fever) or use over-the-counter creams for comfort (they won't speed healing). Children should avoid aspirin use.
- Do not squeeze, pinch or pick at any blister.
- Avoid kissing and skin contact with people while blisters are present.
- Wash your hands carefully before touching another person.
- Use sunblock on your lips and face before prolonged exposure to the sun— during both the winter and the summer to prevent cold sores.

Medical Help

If you experience frequent bouts of cold sores, the drug acyclovir may be the answer. The drug requires a prescription. It is available as pills and as an ointment. This drug inhibits the growth of the herpes virus. Studies of skiers who use sunscreen with and without acyclovir indicate that the drug offers significant additional protection.

You may feel a tingling sensation before the outbreak of a cold sore. This is called the prodrome. Many physicians recommend using acyclovir as soon as the prodrome begins.

Caution

- If you have a cold sore, take special care to avoid contact with infants or anyone who has a skin condition known as eczema (see page 117). They're more susceptible to infection. Also, avoid people who are taking medications for cancer and organ transplantation because they have decreased immunity. The virus can cause a life-threatening condition in them.
- Pregnant women and nursing mothers should avoid using acyclovir for treatment of cold sores unless specifically advised by their doctor to use it.
- Herpes simplex virus infections have potentially serious complications. The virus can spread to your eye. This is the most frequent cause of corneal blindness in the United States. If you have a burning pain in the eye or a rash near the eye or on the tip of your nose, see your doctor immediately.

■ Other Oral Infections and Disorders

Gingivostomatitis (also called trenchmouth): This is an oral infection that is common among children. It's caused by a virus and often accompanies a cold or flu. The infection generally lasts about 2 weeks and ranges from mild to severe. If your child has sores on the gums or on the inside of the cheeks, has bad breath, has a fever and feels generally unwell, consult your dentist or physician. Treatment of any underlying infection will help clear the mouth infection. A medicated oral rinse may help relieve the pain and promote healing. Practice good oral hygiene and eat a nutritious diet of soft foods and drink plenty of fluids. Use a mouthwash made of half a teaspoon of salt dissolved in 8 ounces of water, or use an over-the-counter mouthwash.

Oral thrush: This is caused by a fungus. There will be creamy-white soft patches in the mouth or throat. It often occurs when your body has been weakened by illness or when your mouth's natural balance of microbes has been upset by medications. Many people will experience an outbreak of oral thrush at some point in their lives. It is most common among babies, young children and the elderly. Although painful, oral thrush is not a serious disorder. However, it can interfere with eating and impair your nutrition. There is no self-care for this condition, but a dentist or physician can prescribe an oral medication that is taken for 7 to 10 days. Thrush tends to recur.

Leukoplakia: Thickened, white patches on a cheek or the tongue are often signs of leukoplakia. Leukoplakia is the mouth's reaction to chronic irritation. It may be caused by ill-fitting dentures or a rough tooth rubbing against the cheek or gum. When white patches develop in the mouths of smokers, the condition is called "smoker's keratosis." Snuff and chewing tobacco also produce chronic irritation. You can have leukoplakia at any time during your life, but it is most common among the elderly. Treatment involves removing the source of irritation. Once the source of irritation has been removed, the patch may clear up, usually within weeks or months. A doctor or dentist should evaluate white patches in the mouth. Tobacco use can lead to cancer of the lip, tongue or lungs.

Oral cancer: Cancer of the mouth is common. It usually occurs along the side or the bottom of the tongue or on the floor of the mouth. The tumors usually are painless at first and often are visible or can be felt with a finger. Regular examination of the soft tissues of the mouth is essential for early diagnosis. If you notice any persistent change from the usual appearance or feel of the soft tissues in your mouth, consult your dentist or physician. Early detection is important for successful treatment. Almost 25 percent of people with oral cancer die because of delayed discovery and treatment.

Routine self-examination of your mouth and tongue may enable you to see or feel an oral cancer when it is small and treatment may be most effective.

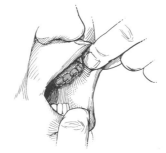
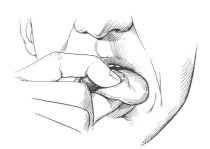

Men's Health

Testicular Pain

Any sharp and sudden pain in your testicles should be treated carefully, because it can be a symptom of a serious medical condition. Seek medical help if you have sudden pain in your testicles that does not go away in 10 or 15 minutes or if you have pain that recurs. Some causes of sudden testicular pain are discussed below.

Testicular torsion is caused when the *spermatic cord*, which carries blood to and from the testicle, gets twisted. This twisting cuts off the blood supply to the testicle, causing sharp and sudden pain. Testicular torsion sometimes occurs after strenuous physical activity, but it can happen with no apparent cause, even during sleep. This condition can occur at any age, but it usually occurs in boys. Symptoms include sudden and severe pain, which can cause fever, nausea and vomiting. You also may notice the elevation of one testicle within the scrotum.

Epididymitis occurs when the *epididymis*, a coiled tube that carries sperm from the testicles to the spermatic cord, becomes inflamed, usually by a bacterial infection. Symptoms include aching to moderately severe pain in the scrotum, which develops gradually over several hours or days; fever and swelling may occur. Epididymitis is occasionally caused by chlamydia, a sexually transmitted disease (see page 177). In these cases, your sexual partner may be infected and should also receive a medical examination.

Orchitis is an inflammation of the testicle, usually due to an infection. Orchitis frequently occurs with epididymitis (see above). Orchitis may occur when you have the mumps, or it may develop if you have a prostate infection. Orchitis is rare, but it could cause infertility if left untreated. Symptoms include pain in the scrotum, swelling (usually on one side of the scrotum only) and a feeling of weight in the scrotum.

Screening for Cancer of the Testicle

Testicular cancer is rare. It occurs most often in young men age 15 to 35. The major symptom is a lump, swelling or "heavy feeling" in a testicle.

A simple 2-minute self-examination each month could save the life of a man with early signs of testicular cancer. Perform the examination after a shower or warm bath, when the skin of your scrotum is loose and relaxed. Examine one testicle at a time. Roll it gently between your thumbs and forefingers, feeling for any lump on the surface of the testicle. You also should notice whether the testicle is enlarged, hardened or otherwise in a different condition than during the last examination. If you notice anything unusual, it may not necessarily mean cancer, but you should contact your physician.

Do not be alarmed if you feel a small, firm area near the rear of the testicle and a tube leading up from the testicle. This is normal. These are the *epididymis* and the *spermatic cord*, which store and transport sperm.

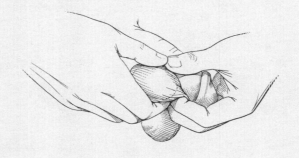

■ Enlarged Prostate

The *prostate* is a walnut-sized gland that is located just below the bladder and is present only in males. The prostate produces most of the fluids in the semen. Testosterone, the male sex hormone, causes the prostate to slowly enlarge with age. As the prostate enlarges, it can restrict the flow of urine through the *urethra* (the tube that passes urine from your bladder), causing slow or difficult urination. The symptoms can be mild and cause little difficulty with urinating, or they can be very painful if complete blockage occurs. Other symptoms may include more frequent nighttime voiding, dribbling after voiding or voiding twice in a row within 10 to 15 minutes.

Prostate enlargement can start as men reach their late 40s. Four of five men experience prostate enlargement by the time they reach age 80. From 25 to 30 percent of men will have some kind of procedure performed on their prostates to correct symptoms during their lifetime.

An enlarged prostate can produce difficulty with urination because the flow of urine is restricted.

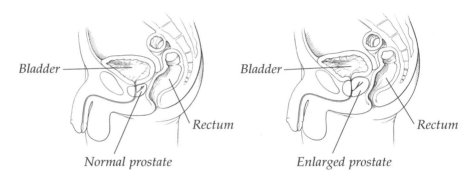

Bladder — Normal prostate — Rectum

Bladder — Enlarged prostate — Rectum

Medical Help

Your health-care provider will ask you detailed questions about your symptoms and may do tests on urine and blood samples. Using a gloved, lubricated finger, your health-care provider may examine your prostate for enlargement and lumps. Called the "digital rectal examination," this procedure causes only mild discomfort.

Initial treatment for an enlarged prostate may be medications that reduce the size of the prostate gland or improve urine flow by relaxing the tissues in the area of the prostate gland. If medications do not relieve the symptoms, surgery can be performed to reduce the size of the prostate or to remove it completely.

Screening for Prostate Cancer

Cancer of the prostate is the second leading cause of cancer death in American men. Prostate cancer occurs most frequently in men older than 60.

Screening for prostate cancer is controversial. Some doctors believe that many men will have unnecessary surgery or radiation because of screening. Others believe that screening is essential. The American Cancer Society recommends yearly screening for prostate cancer in men 50 or older. This involves digital rectal examination and a blood test for PSA (prostate-specific antigen). Ultrasound examination is another way to detect cancer. If detected early, prostate cancer can be cured. Symptoms are the same as those for prostate enlargement unless cancer has spread to the bone.

Common Problems

■ Painful Urination

Painful urination is usually caused by a *urinary tract infection* (UTI). UTIs are more common in women, but they also occur in men. Other symptoms include frequent or urgent urination, an inability to release more than a small amount of urine (followed by an urgent need to urinate again) and a burning sensation while urinating.

If your kidney also is infected, you may experience pain in your abdomen or back, chills, a fever or vomiting. A kidney infection is a serious condition that requires immediate medical attention.

Common Causes

E. coli bacteria: E. coli bacteria are common in the bowel. If E. coli bacteria enter the urethra (the tube through which urine passes), and then enter your urine or bladder, a UTI can result.

Chlamydia: One of several sexually transmitted organisms that can infect the urethra, causing penile drainage and painful urination.

Prostate problems: An enlarged prostate gland can restrict the flow of urine, causing urine retention and UTIs. Also, if your prostate gland produces fewer proteins as you age, the absence of these proteins may make you more susceptible to UTIs. (See Enlarged Prostate, page 137.)

Medical procedures: A urinary catheter or medical instruments can introduce bacteria into your urethra and bladder, causing a UTI.

Narrowed urethra: Injury to or frequent inflammation of the urethra can cause a narrowing (called a stricture) of the urethra. Strictures restrict urine flow and can cause UTIs.

Dehydration: Lack of fluids can lead to stagnant urine, which can cause a UTI.

Medical Help

See your health-care provider, who will take a urine sample and perform tests to determine whether you have a UTI. Do not force fluids just before you give a urine sample because your urine may be diluted and the results may be inaccurate. In most instances, UTIs can be treated with medications. Be sure to take all the medication, even if your symptoms go away after a few days. Failure to take all the medication can lead to a recurrence of the UTI.

■ Impotence

Occasional episodes of impotence are common in men. When impotence is a recurring problem, however, it can harm a man's self-image and affect his relationships. Fortunately, impotence often can be cured. Impotence is defined as an inability to achieve or maintain an erection adequate for sexual intercourse.

The causes of impotence can be psychological or physical. Stress, anxiety or depression can lead to impotence. Impotence also can be a side effect of alcohol use and some medications (such as some drugs used to treat high blood pressure). Impotence can be caused by diseases such as diabetes or multiple sclerosis or other chronic diseases. Impotence may be the result of a direct injury to the genitals or an injury that affects the spinal cord or nervous system. Radiation treatments or major pelvic surgeries, such as those performed for cancer of the prostate, bladder or rectum, also may result in impotence.

Self-Care	If you can still get an erection at certain times of the day, such as the morning, you may benefit from the following advice:
	• Limit alcohol consumption, especially before sexual activity.
	• Quit smoking.
	• Exercise regularly.
	• Reduce stress.
	• Work with your partner to create an atmosphere conducive to lovemaking.

Medical Help

Psychological treatment: If stress, anxiety or depression is the cause of impotence, you may want to seek counseling with a mental health professional or a sex therapist (either alone or with your partner).

Medications: Male hormone shots or pills may be prescribed by your doctor.

Penile injections: If impotence is caused by a decreased blood supply to the penis, medications that increase blood flow are prescribed. They are injected into the penis, and the injections can be performed at home after training by your physician.

Vacuum constriction device: A tube is placed over the penis, and air is withdrawn; as a result, blood flows to the penis and causes an erection. A rubber constricting band is placed around the base of the penis to prolong the erection. This low-cost device is available at most drugstores with a doctor's prescription.

Surgery: Surgery can be performed to increase blood flow to the penis or to implant devices to assist in achieving an erection.

Intraurethral medication: A small suppository (half the size of a grain of rice) is slid into the opening of the penis.

■ Male Birth Control

Vasectomy involves cutting and sealing the *vas deferens*, the tube that carries sperm. The procedure does not interfere with a man's ability to maintain an erection or reach orgasm, nor does it stop the production of male hormones or of sperm in the testicles. The only change is that the sperm's link to the outside is severed permanently. After a vasectomy, you continue to ejaculate about the same amount of semen because sperm account for only a small part of the ejaculate.

Before your vasectomy, you will be given an injection of anesthetic in the scrotum to numb the area so you will not feel pain. After your physician has located the vas deferens, a pair of small cuts are made in the skin of the scrotum. Each vas deferens is then pulled through the opening until it forms a loop. Approximately a half inch is cut out of each vas deferens and removed. The two ends of each vas deferens are closed by stitches or cauterization (or both) and are placed back in the scrotum. The incisions are closed with stitches.

The operation takes about 20 minutes. After a vasectomy, refrain from any strenuous activity, including intercourse, for at least 2 weeks. The stitches are generally of a type that dissolves in 2 to 3 weeks. You may notice some swelling and minor discomfort in the scrotum for several weeks. However, if the pain becomes severe or if fever develops, call your physician.

The failure rate for a vasectomy is less than 1 percent. Until your physician has determined that your ejaculate does not contain sperm, you should continue to use alternative contraception. This typically takes several months and several ejaculations.

Women's Health

■ Lumps in the Breast

Most breast lumps are not cancerous. However, because of the risk of cancer, all lumps should be carefully assessed. Many breast lumps are fluid-filled cysts that enlarge near the end of your monthly cycle. The lumps may or may not be painful. Perform a breast self-examination each month after your period to check for lumps and any other changes in your breasts (see below).

Self-Care

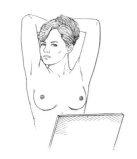
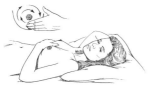
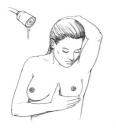

- Do a breast self-examination each month so you'll know whether a lump is new.
- Examine your breasts on the same day each month if you are past menopause. If you are still menstruating, the best time to examine your breasts is 7 to 10 days after your last period started. Breast cancer lumps usually aren't painful. Use your eyes and hands to search for lumps, thickened areas or swelling in your breasts. Notify your health-care provider of any changes.
- Refer to the illustrations at left.
  - Look into a mirror with your arms at your sides. Elevate your arms and thoroughly examine the skin on your breasts for puckering, dimples or changes in their size or shape. Look for changes in the natural symmetry of both breasts. Check to see whether your nipples are pushed in (inverted). Also note any unusual discharge from your nipples. Check for the same signs while you rest your hands on your hips and again with your hands behind your head.
  - Examine your breasts while standing in the shower and while lying on your back. Hold one hand behind your head and use a circular massaging motion with the other hand to check the tissue over the entire opposite breast, including the nipple and the tissue under your armpit. Repeat the procedure on the other side. Soap and water during a shower can make the procedure easier.
  - Check for lumps that don't disappear or change. Abnormal lumps may seem to appear suddenly and remain. They vary in size and firmness and often feel hard with irregular edges. Sometimes they just feel like thickened areas without distinct outlines. Cancerous lumps usually aren't painful.
- If the lump causes discomfort, take a mild pain medication (see page 231) or eliminate caffeine from your diet.

Medical Help

See your doctor if a lump in your breast doesn't go away after your menstrual cycle. A fluid-filled cyst may be drained with a needle after an injection of a local anesthetic. If you have a breast infection, your doctor will prescribe an antibiotic. Lumps that are not filled with fluid may require a biopsy (surgical removal and examination under a microscope) to determine whether they are cancerous.

Postmenopausal women should see their doctor if a lump lasts more than a week or becomes reddened, painful or enlarged.

Mammograms: Who Should Have Them?

A mammogram is a special breast X-ray that can detect tumors so small that your physician cannot even feel them. Mammography saves lives by identifying breast cancer at a stage when it is potentially curable. However, the test is not perfect. Occasionally it fails to show a tumor, and at other times it indicates a problem when there is not one. Screening by mammography is best combined with regular breast examinations.

There is controversy within the medical profession about the age at which you should begin to have regular mammograms. The breasts of young women are often too dense to x-ray well. Fortunately, young women rarely develop breast cancer. Because every woman's risk of cancer, preferences and concerns are different, the final decision about screening needs to be made by you and your doctor. Here are some guidelines.

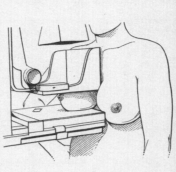
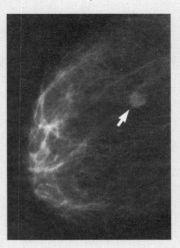

Mammograms are produced by a special X-ray device that can detect tumors before you or your physician can feel them.

Age	Expert Opinion	What to Do
Younger than 40	Experts agree generally	Monthly breast self-exam No mammogram
Younger than 40 at high risk (sister or mother with breast cancer at a young age)	Talk to your doctor for an individualized program	Monthly breast self-exam Annual physical exam Mammogram, often beginning 5-10 years before age at which mother or sister had cancer
40-50 not at high risk	Disagreement among experts	Monthly breast self-exam Physical exam every 1-3 years Mammogram, not at all to yearly
40-50 at high risk	Some disagreement	Monthly breast self-exam Physical exam every 1-3 years Mammogram, not at all to yearly
50-74 at normal or high risk	General agreement	Monthly breast self-exam Annual physical exam Annual mammogram
75 or older	Some disagreement	Monthly breast self-exam Annual physical exam Annual mammogram

Note: Risk factors for breast cancer include prior breast cancer, breast cancer in mother or sister, never pregnant or first pregnancy when older than 35, early onset of menses or late menopause. Your doctor also may consider other risk factors.

Common Problems

■ Pain in the Breast

The most common cause of pain in the breast is mastitis, which is caused by an infection or inflammation. It usually occurs in only one breast. Generalized tenderness in both breasts is common, especially during the week before a menstrual period, and it is also a symptom of premenstrual syndrome (see page 143). Exercises, such as jogging and aerobics, can cause breast tenderness. Tenderness also may be caused by an inflamed cyst. If fever and redness are present, infection is a concern. Infections, although not common, can occur with breast-feeding.

Self-Care

- Wear a comfortable and supportive bra.
- Take an over-the-counter pain reliever (see page 231).
- Reduce the salt in your diet before your period.
- Avoid sugar, caffeine, alcohol and chocolate.
- If pain is due to high-impact exercises, switch to a low-impact workout such as biking, walking or swimming and use an athletic bra.
- See other tips in the section on premenstrual syndrome (page 143).

Medical Help

If you have fever or redness along with the pain, see your doctor. You probably need an antibiotic. If pain is associated with a lump or a change in the texture of your breast, see your doctor.

■ Painful Menses

Most women are familiar with menstrual cramps. During menstruation, you may feel pain in the lower abdomen, possibly extending to the hips, lower back or thighs. Some women also have nausea, vomiting, diarrhea or general aching. It is normal to have mild abdominal cramps on the first day or two of your period (more than half of women do). However, about 10 percent of women experience pain so severe that they can't manage their normal routine unless they take medication.

If there is not an underlying gynecologic disorder, the pain is called primary dysmenorrhea. It is caused by high levels of prostaglandin (a substance that makes the muscles of the uterus contract and shed its lining). Although painful, primary dysmenorrhea is not harmful. It often disappears by your mid-20s or after you have a baby.

Pain that is caused by an underlying gynecologic disorder is called secondary dysmenorrhea. It may be due to a fibroid tumor (a benign tumor in the wall of your uterus), a sexually transmitted disease, endometriosis, pelvic inflammatory disease or an ovarian cyst or tumor.

Self-Care

- Nonsteroidal anti-inflammatory drugs or aspirin (see page 231) relieves pain in about 80 percent of women.
- Try soaking in a warm tub or exercising.

Medical Help

Treatment of the underlying cause should relieve the pain. If no cause for the pain is found, birth control pills may relieve the discomfort.

Talk to your health-care provider if the menstrual pain is severe or is associated with fever; if you have unusual nausea, vomiting or abdominal pain; or if the pain lasts beyond the third day of menstrual flow.

■ Irregular Periods

It is common for women to experience unexplained irregularities in their periods. Irregular periods are due to changes in hormone levels, which can be affected by stress or other emotional experiences, significant changes in the amount of aerobic exercise or dramatic decreases in the calories you consume. High levels of exercise in a woman with an excessively lean body may stop periods altogether.

Self-Care

- Keep a menstrual calendar for at least three cycles. Record the first day of flow, the day of maximal flow, the day that flow stops and times of intercourse to help evaluate menstrual changes.
- If your periods are irregular for more than three cycles, talk to your doctor.
- If you miss a period and have had intercourse, look for symptoms of pregnancy.

■ Bleeding Between Periods

Many women occasionally experience bleeding from the vagina between periods. Isolated episodes may be caused by intercourse or foreplay. Uterine fibroid tumors (noncancerous lumps in the wall of your uterus) also may cause bleeding. If bleeding continues for more than 4 days, soaks through a pad or tampon in less than 1 hour or recurs in three cycles over a 6-month period, talk to your health-care provider. If possible, keep a menstrual calendar (see above).

■ Premenstrual Syndrome

If you experience a predictable pattern of physical and emotional changes in the days before your period, you may have premenstrual syndrome (PMS). PMS is related to the normal hormone cycles and occurs with normal hormone levels. One clue to its cause may lie in a woman's response to serotonin. Serotonin is a substance in the brain which has been associated with clinical depression and other emotional disorders. Sometimes an underlying psychological condition such as depression is aggravated by the hormonal changes before a period.

Common Problems

Symptoms of PMS

Physical Changes	Emotional Changes
Fluid retention, bloating	Depression and sadness
Weight gain	Irritability
Frequent urination	Anxiety
Breast soreness	Tension
Aching, swollen hands and feet	Mood swings
Fatigue, nausea, vomiting	Difficulty in concentrating
Diarrhea, constipation	Lethargy
Aches: head, back, stomach	Food cravings
Skin problems	Forgetfulness

Self-Care

You can usually manage PMS with a combination of education and lifestyle changes.

- Maintain your weight at a healthy level.
- Eat smaller, more frequent meals. Don't skip meals. Eat at the same time every day if possible.
- Avoid salt for 1 to 2 weeks before your period to reduce bloating and fluid retention.
- Avoid caffeine (coffee, tea and some sodas) to reduce irritability, tension and breast soreness. See page 180 for the caffeine content of popular beverages.
- Avoid alcohol before your period to minimize depression and mood swings.
- Eat plenty of complex carbohydrates (breads, potatoes, cereals, vegetables, rice).
- Eat fewer foods containing simple sugars (table sugar, syrup, brown sugar, honey, candy, sweetened soda).
- Eat fewer foods containing fat. In particular, avoid heavily marbled meats, cold cuts, butter, whole milk, ice cream, cream and other foods that contain high levels of saturated fat.
- Reduce stress (see page 210). Stress can aggravate PMS.
- Walk, jog, bike, swim or perform some other aerobic exercise at least three times a week.
- Record your symptoms for a few months. You may find that PMS is more tolerable if you see that your symptoms are predictable and short-lived.

Medical Help

There are no physical findings or lab tests for diagnosing PMS. Instead, doctors rely on careful evaluation of your medical history. As part of the diagnostic process, women are asked to record the onset, duration, nature and severity of symptoms for at least two menstrual cycles.

If your PMS symptoms seriously affect your life and the suggestions listed above don't help, your doctor may recommend the following medications:

- Nonsteroidal anti-inflammatory drugs (NSAIDs) can ease cramps and breast discomfort (see page 231).
- Birth control pills often relieve symptoms by stopping ovulation.
- An injection of medroxyprogesterone acetate (Depo-Provera) can be used to temporarily stop ovulation and menstruation in severe cases.
- Antidepressants help about 60 percent of women who have severe emotional symptoms from PMS. Examples of these antidepressants are fluoxetine (Prozac), sertraline (Zoloft), paroxetine (Paxil), fluvoxamine (Luvox) and venlafaxine (Effexor). These drugs can be used in doses lower than those usually prescribed for depression and may be effective when taken only during the week or two before menstruation.
- If antidepressants are not effective, the antianxiety drug alprazolam (Xanax) may help, but it is a powerful and potentially addictive medication that should not be used long-term.

■ Menopause

Menopause is a natural stage of life which begins in most women between ages 40 and 55 years. The average age at onset has been increasing over the years and is currently about 51 years.

During menopause, the ovaries gradually stop producing estrogen. Your periods become irregular. The process may last several months to several years. Eventually, your menstrual periods stop, and you can no longer become pregnant.

As a woman's ovaries produce fewer hormones, various changes occur, although they vary a great deal from person to person. The uterus atrophies (shrinks), and the lining of her vagina becomes thin. The vagina also may become dry, making intercourse painful. Hot flashes cause flushing or sweating that may last from several minutes to more than an hour and may interrupt sleep and produce night sweats.

During and after menopause, a woman's body fat typically is redistributed as metabolism changes. Bones lose density and strength. Osteoporosis may occur (see below).

Some women develop emotional problems during menopause which seem to be related to hormonal changes. Some of these problems may be due to the stresses of midlife that affect both men and women. Many women find that menopause can have a positive effect on their physical and emotional health.

Self-Care

- Accept the changes as normal and healthy.
- Eat a balanced diet, exercise regularly and dress in layers.
- Use a water-soluble lubricating jelly if intercourse is painful.

Medical Help

Your doctor may prescribe estrogen replacement therapy to relieve hot flashes, halt the thinning of vaginal tissue, prevent or delay the progression of osteoporosis and possibly prevent or delay heart disease.

Estrogen replacement therapy does not affect mood swings. However, estrogen replacement therapy may increase the risk of breast or endometrial cancer. Therefore, if you still have your uterus, you generally should be given progesterone as well as estrogen.

Another hormone, megestrol acetate, can reduce the frequency and severity of hot flashes in women who can't use estrogens. If hormones are prescribed, you may resume menstrual bleeding.

How to Prevent Osteoporosis

The loss of estrogen after menopause greatly increases the likelihood of osteoporosis, a disorder in which your bones become porous and brittle. The most effective way to manage osteoporosis is to prevent it by maximizing your bone density when you are young.

- Eat enough calcium (1,200 to 1,500 mg per day) throughout adulthood to help prevent osteo-porosis. Foods rich in calcium include milk, yogurt, cheese, salmon and broccoli. Just 1 glass of milk is about 300 mg of calcium.
- If you are at an increased risk, your physician may suggest calcium tablets. Calcium, however, may be harmful for certain conditions. See your physician before taking a high-calcium supplement.
- Participate in weight-bearing exercises such as walking, dancing, swimming and jogging.

■ Urination Problems

Urinary tract infections (UTIs) are common among women. With the beginning of sexual activity, women have a marked increased in the number of infections. Sexual intercourse, pregnancy and urinary obstruction all contribute to the likelihood of such an infection. Symptoms of UTI include pain or a burning sensation during urination, increased frequency of urination and a feeling of urgency every time you need to urinate. If you have an infection, your doctor will prescribe an antibiotic.

Urinary incontinence is the involuntary loss or leakage of urine. The condition is often divided into "urge" and "stress" incontinence. Urge incontinence means that you leak urine when your bladder is full. It is often caused by a mild UTI or by excessive use of bladder stimulants such as caffeine. **Stress incontinence** is the loss of urine when you exert pressure on your bladder by coughing, laughing, jumping or lifting something heavy. It usually is caused by weakening of the muscles that support your bladder. These muscles can weaken because of childbirth, being overweight or aging.

Self-Care for Urine Leakage

- Try Kegel exercises. Begin by contracting your pelvic muscle, as you would to prevent a bowel movement or to stop urine flow. Relax, and then repeat the contraction. Do this 20 or 30 times. Rest 10 seconds between contractions. Repeat the exercise several times a day. Don't do it in the bathroom while urinating.
- Empty your bladder more often.
- Lean forward when urinating to empty your bladder more completely.
- Decrease your intake of caffeine-containing foods and beverages (see page 180).
- Use a pad to protect against small leaks. Change it every couple of hours.
- Try tampons while exercising.

■ Vaginal Discharge

Vaginal discharge is one symptom of vaginitis. Vaginitis is an inflammation of your vagina. It usually is caused by an infection or an alteration in the normal vaginal bacteria. In addition to vaginal discharge, you may have itching, irritation, pain during intercourse, pain in your lower abdomen, vaginal bleeding and odor.

There are three common types of vaginitis: trichomoniasis, yeast infections and bacterial vaginosis. Trichomoniasis is caused by a parasite. It may cause a smelly, greenish yellow, sometimes frothy discharge. You usually develop this infection as a result of sexual intercourse. Trichomonal vaginitis usually is treated with metronidazole tablets. Your partner also should be treated. Yeast infections are caused by a fungus. You are more susceptible to a yeast infection if you are pregnant or have diabetes; if you are taking antibiotics, cortisone or birth control pills; or if you have an iron deficiency. The main symptom is itching, but a white discharge also may be present.

Self-Care

- Use an over-the-counter antifungal cream or suppository for suspected yeast infections.
- Abstain from intercourse or have your partner use a condom for a week after beginning treatment.
- See your health-care provider if symptoms persist after 1 week.

■ Cancer Screening

See page 141 for breast cancer screening recommendations. Screening tests for cervical cancer include a Pap smear and a pelvic examination. The Pap smear detects 95 percent of cervical cancers at a curable stage.

Cervical cancer develops slowly, often over 10 to 20 years. It begins with changes in cells on the surface of the cervix. Doctors refer to these abnormal cells as precancerous. They may become cancerous with time.

Early changes in the size, shape or number of surface cells are called dysplasia or squamous intraepithelial lesions. Some of these abnormalities go away on their own, but others become larger or more abnormal. Precancerous conditions generally do not cause any symptoms, including pain.

Because doctors aren't in agreement about how often the Pap smear should be done, discuss with your physician what's best for you. Guidelines for a cost-effective screening strategy suggest the following:

- An initial Pap test at age 18 or with the beginning of sexual activity
- Subsequent Pap tests every 1 to 3 years
- After three consecutive Pap tests with normal results, a woman and her doctor may opt for less frequent testing
- For women who've had a total hysterectomy for a benign disease, routine Pap tests are no longer necessary
  Women at high risk should have more frequent testing.

You are at high risk if:

- You began sexual activity as a teenager, especially if you had multiple sex partners
- You currently have more than one sex partner
- You have had a sexually transmitted disease, including genital warts
- You have had an abnormal Pap test or a prior cancer
- You use tobacco

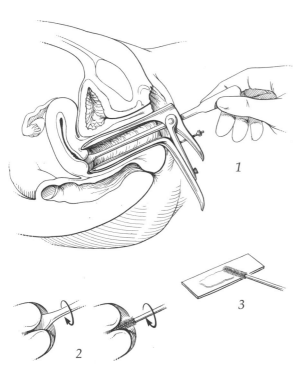

With speculum in place, your physician rotates a wooden spatula and then a brush to remove a sample of cells (1 and 2). The cells are smeared onto a glass slide (3) for examination under a microscope.

The Reliability of Pap Tests

The Pap test is a screening test and is not perfect. It may miss abnormal cells, causing a false negative result. That's why it's important to get regular Pap smears. A result could be inaccurate for these reasons:

- The patient washes away abnormal cells through sexual activity or douching before her examination.
- The doctor doesn't collect cells from the entire cervical area, missing abnormal cells; doesn't smear the sample onto the slide properly; or doesn't "fix" the cells immediately and correctly.
- The laboratory technician or pathologist fails to identify abnormal cells. A technician who screens more than 70 slides a day may make mistakes because the work requires intense concentration, which can lead to fatigue.

Common Problems

Contraception

Method	How It Works	Effectiveness*	Cautions
Natural family planning (rhythm method)	Relies on a woman's menstrual cycle to determine which days are safe for intercourse	Less than 80 percent	Works best with very regular periods. Do not have intercourse for 3 days before ovulation and 3 days after
Oral contraceptives (birth control pills)	Synthetic hormones prevent ovulation and impair fertilization. They are usually a combination of an estrogen and a progestin	More than 99 percent	Take pill at the same time every day. Do not smoke, especially after age 35. If you miss two periods in a row, consult your health-care provider
Contraceptive implants	Match-sized hormone sticks that are implanted under the skin of your upper arm	More than 95 percent	Sometimes difficult to remove
Intrauterine device (IUD)	Inserted into the uterus. Inhibits sperm migration and fertilization. Two are in use: one with progesterone and one with copper	95 to 98 percent	Increased tubal pregnancy; increase in menstrual blood loss with copper device. Check the string regularly to be sure that the device is still in place
Diaphragm	A rubber cap is inserted into vagina to cover the cervix. It must be fitted	About 95 percent when used consistently and correctly with a spermicide	May cause cervical irritation and increased risk of urinary tract infections. Must be inserted before intercourse
Cervical cap	The plastic cervical cap must be fitted by your health-care provider to cover your cervix	85 percent	May cause cervical irritation. Difficult to fit. Pap smear abnormalities. Must be inserted before intercourse
Female condom	Several different forms. Extends to the outside of the vagina	90 percent	Difficult to insert for some people
Depo-Provera shots	Shot in the arm or buttock every 2 to 3 months	More than 95 percent	May cause menstrual irregularities, headache, acne and weight gain
Tubal ligation (female sterilization)	Fallopian tubes are tied and cut or cauterized, thus preventing the egg from traveling down the tube and sperm from moving up the tube	More than 99 percent	Requires surgery, usually as an outpatient

*Effectiveness is defined as preventing pregnancy during 1 year of typical use.

■ Pregnancy

Although pregnancy is a natural state, you want to take especially good care of your health to help ensure that your baby will have the best possible start in life. It's a good idea to see your health-care provider for a complete physical examination before you become pregnant. You will be checked for several conditions that may not cause symptoms but can complicate pregnancy. These include diabetes, high blood pressure, pelvic tumors and anemia. If there is a health problem, your health-care provider will want to control the condition, ideally before you become pregnant. Your health-care provider will also review your immunizations to be sure you're immune to rubella (a viral infection).

Self-Care

To Prepare for Pregnancy
- If you are overweight, reduce your weight before you become pregnant. Do not begin a diet if you are pregnant.
- If you smoke, stop. And, if possible, avoid secondhand smoke (see page 209).
- Don't drink alcohol if you are trying to become pregnant.
- Take a multivitamin daily. Make sure it contains folic acid, which decreases the risk of neural tube defects (birth defects of the spinal column).
- Check with your health-care provider about taking over-the-counter or prescription medicines.

During Pregnancy
Once you are pregnant, the best ways to ensure a healthy baby are to:
- Obtain a book on pregnancy. Understand the changes your body is experiencing.
- Make regular visits to your health-care provider.
- Eat a healthful diet. Allow for appropriate weight gain.
- Avoid harmful substances such as cigarettes, alcohol and some medications and chemicals.
- Take a prenatal vitamin with folic acid. Your pharmacist can assist you.
- **Caution:** Bleeding from your vagina during pregnancy may indicate that something is wrong. Call your health-care provider immediately. Although some harmless spotting and bleeding occur in many women during early pregnancy, your health-care provider will want to rule out miscarriage, ectopic (tubal) pregnancy or other conditions such as a cervical lesion.

Home Pregnancy Tests

Home pregnancy tests provide a private way to find out whether you are pregnant. Most tests use a wand or stick placed into a urine stream or a collected urine specimen to detect the hormone hCG (human chorionic gonadotropin). The placenta begins to produce this hormone soon after conception. When performed correctly, the tests are 95 percent accurate 10 days after a missed period.

Home pregnancy tests can help you get your pregnancy off to a good nutritional start by using prenatal vitamin supplements early. They also help you avoid things that could harm the fetus such as alcohol and smoking and also some medications or chemicals at home or work. Home pregnancy tests also provide early warning for women who have had tubal pregnancy or early miscarriage so they can see their health-care provider as soon as possible.

Common Problems

Common Problems During Pregnancy

Common but bothersome concerns you may have during pregnancy are morning sickness, heartburn, backache and other problems. These may make you uncomfortable, but usually they do not threaten your health or the health of your developing baby. If they are severe or persist despite self-care measures, see your doctor.

Morning Sickness

About half of all pregnant women experience morning sickness during the first 12 weeks of pregnancy. Although it doesn't always happen during the morning, the term is used to describe nausea, queasiness or vomiting. It is usually harmless. If you have problems with morning sickness:

- Munch a few crackers before arising in the morning.
- Eat several small meals a day so that your stomach is never empty.
- Avoid smelling or eating foods that trigger the nausea, and avoid spicy, rich and fried foods if you are nauseated.
- Drink plenty of liquids, especially if you are vomiting. Try crushed ice, fruit juice or frozen ice pops if water upsets your stomach.
- Try using acupressure or motion-sickness bands to combat nausea.

Anemia

Some pregnant women develop anemia (an inadequate level of hemoglobin in the blood) because of an iron deficiency or an inadequate supply of folic acid. Symptoms of anemia include fatigue, breathlessness, fainting, palpitations and pale skin. This condition can be risky for both you and your baby. It is easily diagnosed with a blood test. If you are anemic:

- Eat a diet rich in iron (such as liver, eggs, dried fruit, whole grains and beef).
- Eat plenty of leafy green vegetables, liver, lentils, black-eyed peas, kidney beans and other cooked dried beans, oranges and grapefruit.
- Follow your health-care provider's recommendations.

Edema (Swelling)

When you are pregnant, your body tissues accumulate more fluid, and swelling is common. Warm weather may aggravate the condition. If you have problems with edema:

- Use cold-water compresses to help relieve swelling.
- Eat a low-salt diet.
- Lie down and elevate your legs for an hour in the middle of the afternoon to help relieve swelling in your legs.
- If your face becomes swollen, especially around the eyes, it may be a sign of a serious condition called preeclampsia. See your doctor right away.

Varicose Veins

About 20 percent of all pregnant women have varicose veins. Pregnancy increases the volume of blood in your body but decreases the flow of blood from your legs to your pelvis. This change causes the veins in your legs to become swollen and sometimes painful. If you have problems with varicose veins:

- Stay off your feet as much as possible, and elevate them as often as you can.
- Wear loose clothing around your legs and waist.
- Wear support stockings from the time you awaken until you go to bed.

Constipation

Constipation may worsen during pregnancy. Bowel activity may be slowed because of the increased pressure on the bowels from the growing baby inside the uterus.

- Drink plenty of liquids—at least 2 to 3 quarts per day.
- Exercise moderately every day.
- Eat several servings of fruits, vegetables and grains.
- Try taking a bulk-former that contains psyllium (available without a prescription). Do not take a laxative without discussing it with your health-care provider.

Heartburn

Heartburn is a burning sensation in the middle of your chest, often with a bad taste in your mouth. It is caused by reflux—stomach acid flowing up into your food pipe (esophagus). It has nothing to do with your heart. During the later part of pregnancy, your expanding uterus pushes the stomach out of position, which slows the rate that food empties from the stomach.

- Eat smaller meals more often, but eat slowly.
- Avoid greasy foods.
- Don't drink coffee. Both regular and decaffeinated coffee may worsen heartburn.
- Don't eat for 2 to 3 hours before you go to bed, and raise the head of your bed 4 to 6 inches. Reflux is worse when you lie flat.
- If these steps don't work, consult your health-care provider, who may recommend an antacid.

Backache

Backache is common in pregnancy and may worsen if you bend, lift, walk too much or are fatigued. Pain may be in the lower back, or it may radiate down your legs. Your abdomen also may hurt because of the stretching of ligaments. During pregnancy your ligaments are more elastic and so your joints are more prone to strain and injury. Your center of balance also changes during pregnancy. This puts more strain on your back.

- Don't gain more weight than your health-care provider recommends.
- Eliminate as much strain as possible. Try wearing a maternity girdle.
- Your health-care provider may recommend exercises to relieve the pain.

Hemorrhoids

Hemorrhoids are enlarged veins at the anal opening. They become enlarged from increased pressure. They are often worse during pregnancy and often accompany constipation.

- Avoid becoming constipated.
- Don't strain during bowel movements.
- Take frequent warm-water baths.
- Apply a cotton pad soaked with cold witch hazel cream to the area.

Sleeping Problems

Your sleep may be disturbed during the later stages of pregnancy because of the frequent need to urinate, the movements of your baby or the many things on your mind.

- Avoid caffeine.
- Do not eat a large meal right before bedtime; take a warm bath before going to bed.
- Exercise more during the day.
- If you can't sleep, get out of bed and do something else.
- Do not take any medicines unless recommended by your health-care provider.

Common Problems

■ Other Common Medical Conditions

Endometriosis

Endometriosis is a disorder of the reproductive system in which small pieces of the endometrium (the lining of the uterus) are thought to migrate out of the uterus through the fallopian tubes. The pieces implant on other pelvic organs, the pelvic walls and the outside of the ovaries or the fallopian tubes. During menstruation, blood from these patches is absorbed by the surrounding organs, which can cause inflammation. This process can create adhesions (scar tissue, which causes organs to stick together) on the ovaries and fallopian tubes, which can prevent pregnancy. Symptoms include painful periods, worsening of cramping during periods, pain deep in the pelvis during intercourse and pain during bowel movements or urination. The condition causes severe pain in some women, but others have no symptoms.

Endometriosis is diagnosed with laparoscopy (surgery in which a small viewing instrument is passed through a small incision near the navel). Treatment with hormones helps relieve the symptoms, stop the progression and prevent infertility. Sometimes more extensive surgery is needed.

Hysterectomy

Each year, half a million women have a hysterectomy (removal of all or a portion of the uterus). After a hysterectomy, you no longer menstruate, and you can no longer become pregnant.

A *vaginal hysterectomy* is removal of the uterus through an incision in the vagina. An *abdominal hysterectomy* is removal of the uterus through an incision in your abdomen. Abdominal hysterectomy is performed if you have suspected or confirmed uterine or ovarian cancer, extensive endometriosis or scarring in the pelvis, a history of pelvic infection or a uterus that's too large to remove vaginally.

Here's what you can expect during your recuperation:
- After a *vaginal hysterectomy*, you may feel pulling in your groin or have low back pain for a day or two. You may have a discharge for about 3 weeks as the stitches at the top of the vagina dissolve. An *abdominal hysterectomy* may cause more discomfort because the incision goes through the abdominal wall.

Toxic Shock Syndrome

Toxic shock syndrome (TSS) is a reaction to poisons produced by bacteria in the vagina. It typically occurs during menstruation and more frequently in tampon users. The symptoms of TSS develop suddenly, and the disease is serious. Your blood pressure can drop, and you may go into shock. Sometimes kidney failure results. TSS requires immediate medical attention.

Symptoms include a fever of 102 F or higher, vomiting, diarrhea, weakness, dizziness, fainting, disorientation and a rash resembling a sunburn, especially on your palms and soles.

If you use tampons, avoid superabsorbent brands. Change tampons at least every 8 hours. If you have ever had TSS, do not wear tampons at all.

Specific Conditions

- Respiratory Allergies
- Arthritis
- Asthma
- Cancer
- Diabetes
- Heart Disease
- High Blood Pressure
- Sexually Transmitted Diseases

Asthma, arthritis, serious respiratory allergies, cancer, diabetes, high blood pressure, heart disease and sexually transmitted diseases are common and costly medical conditions in which the normal rules of self-assessment and self-care may not apply. You should be examined by a physician for correct diagnosis and treatment of your condition.

In this section, we offer general guidelines on the prevention and management of these diseases. In some cases, we explain new developments that may be helpful to you. You should discuss new treatments with your doctor to determine their appropriateness to your condition.

Respiratory Allergies

Do you develop itchy, watery eyes or a stuffy, runny nose during the same season every year? Do you sneeze frequently when you're around animals or at work? If you answered "yes" to either of these questions, you may be 1 of 50 million Americans with an allergy (see Allergic Reactions, page 8, and Hives, page 119).

Allergic Reactions and Immune Response

An allergy is an overreaction by your immune system to an otherwise harmless substance, such as pollen or pet dander. Contact with this substance, called an allergen, triggers production of the antibody immunoglobulin E (IgE). IgE causes immune cells in the lining of your eyes and airways to release inflammatory substances, including histamine.

When these chemicals are released, they produce the familiar symptoms of allergy—itchy, red and swollen eyes, a stuffy or runny nose, frequent sneezing and cough, hives or bumps on the skin. This allergic reaction causes or aggravates some forms of asthma (see page 161).

Substances found outdoors, indoors and in the foods you eat can cause allergic reactions. The most common allergens are inhaled:

- **Pollen:** Spring, summer and autumn are the pollen-producing seasons in most climates. During these seasons, exposure to airborne pollen from trees, grasses and weeds is inevitable.
- **Dust mites:** House dust harbors all kinds of potential allergens, including pollen and molds. But the main allergy trigger is the dust mite. Thousands of these microscopic spider-like insects are contained in a pinch of house dust. House dust is a cause of year-round allergy symptoms.
- **Pet dander:** Dogs and especially cats are the most common animals to cause allergic reactions. The animal's dander (skin flakes), saliva, urine and sometimes hair are the main culprits.
- **Molds:** Many people are sensitive to airborne mold spores. Outdoor molds produce spores mostly in the summer and early autumn. Indoor molds shed spores all year long.

Discovering Causes

It's not clear why some people become sensitive to allergens such as pollen. But doctors know the tendency to develop allergies is inherited. If you're bothered by allergies, chances are someone in your immediate family also copes with allergic reactions.

Yet, you and your relatives won't necessarily be sensitive to the same allergens. You're less likely to inherit a sensitivity to a specific substance than you are to inherit the general tendency to develop allergies.

If your symptoms are mild, over-the-counter allergy medicines (usually a combination of an antihistamine and decongestant) may be all the treatment you need. But if your symptoms are persistent or bothersome, a trip to the doctor may bring you relief.

To diagnose allergies accurately, your doctor will need to know about your:

- Symptoms
- Past medical problems
- Past and current living conditions
- Possible exposure to allergens
- Family's medical history
- Diet, lifestyle and recreational habits

Mayo HealthQuest Guide to Self-Care

The next steps are typically a physical examination and skin tests. During a skin test, tiny, dilute drops of suspected allergens are applied to your skin. Then small pricks or punctures are made through the droplets. If your response to an allergen is positive, a skin reaction like a mosquito bite or small hive (called a wheal and flare) appears at the test site within about 20 minutes.

A positive result of a skin test means only that you might be allergic to a particular substance. To pinpoint the cause of your symptoms, your doctor considers the results of your skin test in addition to your history and physical examination.

The Difference Between Colds and Allergies

Because allergies often cause symptoms similar to those of a cold—congested head and chest, stuffy or runny nose, coughing and sneezing—many people mistake allergies for colds. With a cold, however, symptoms usually go away in a few days. If you have allergies, symptoms may flare under certain conditions or may seem never-ending.

Hay fever (medically referred to as allergic rhinitis) is a common respiratory allergy. The symptoms often appear during pollen season — spring, summer or autumn. Hay fever generally refers to seasonal allergic rhinitis due to pollen. It's not due to hay and there is no fever.

Some people have allergy symptoms mainly in the winter when their homes are closed to ventilation, allowing greater exposure to dust mites and molds. Others may experience symptoms when they enter a room with a cat. Still others find they have symptoms randomly occurring all year long.

Signs and symptoms of hay fever include the following:
- Stuffy or runny nose
- Itchy eyes, nose, throat or roof of your mouth
- Frequent sneezing
- Cough

Myths About Allergy

Allergies often seem vague in origin and unpredictable in response. So it's not surprising that several misconceptions about their causes and cure exist. Three common myths about allergies are described below.

- **Allergies are psychosomatic.** Although hay fever affects your eyes and nose, allergies aren't "all in your head." An allergy is a real medical condition involving your immune system. Stress or emotions may bring on or worsen symptoms, but emotions don't cause allergies.
- **Moving to Arizona will cure allergies.** Some people who are bothered by allergies to pollens and molds believe moving to the Southwest, where the foliage and climate are different, will cause their allergies to disappear. The desert may lack maple trees and ragweed, but it does have other plants that produce pollen such as sagebrush, cottonwood, ash and olive trees. People who are sensitive to some pollens and molds may become sensitive to the pollens and molds found in new environments.
- **Short-haired pets don't cause allergies.** An animal's fur (regardless of its length) isn't the culprit in allergies. The cause is the dander and sometimes saliva and urine. If you're allergic to furry pets, safer pets include fish and reptiles.

Specific Conditions

Self-Care

The best approach for managing allergies is to know and avoid your triggers:

Pollen
- Stay indoors when the pollen count is highest, between 5 a.m. and 10 a.m. Use an air conditioner with a good filter. Change it often.
- Wear a pollen mask when outdoors and for yard work.
- Vacation out of the region during the height of the pollen season.

Dust or Molds
- Limit your exposure by cleaning your home at least once a week. Wear a mask while cleaning, or have someone else clean for you.
- Encase mattresses, pillows and box springs in dustproof covers.
- Consider replacing upholstered furniture with leather or vinyl, carpeting with wood, vinyl or tile (particularly in the bedroom).
- Maintain indoor humidity between 30 and 50 percent. Use exhaust fans in your bathrooms and kitchen and a dehumidifier in your basement.
- Routinely change furnace filters according to the manufacturer's instructions. Also, consider installing a high-efficiency particulate-arresting (HEPA) filter in your heating system.
- Clean humidifiers frequently to prevent growth of molds and bacteria (see page 104).

Pets
- Avoid pets with fur or feathers. If you choose to keep a furry animal, wash it once a week with soap and water. Keep your animal outside as much as possible, and don't let it in your bedroom.

Medical Help

Antihistamines are widely used to control sneezing, runny nose and itchy eyes or throat. Antihistamines block the action of histamine, one of the irritating chemicals that are largely responsible for symptoms. **Caution:** Some antihistamines can cause drowsiness.

Decongestants relieve some allergy symptoms by reducing congestion or swelling in your nasal membranes. This allows you to breathe more easily. Many over-the-counter medications for allergies and colds combine decongestants with antihistamines.

Nasal sprays, available over-the-counter and by prescription, also can be part of your defense against allergies. The different forms are described here.
- *Corticosteroids:* Available by prescription, they relieve congestion when used daily but take at least a week to become fully effective.
- *Cromolyn sodium:* Nasal sprays containing cromolyn sodium prevent sneezing and an itchy, runny nose caused by mild to moderate allergies.
- *Saline:* Nonprescription nasal sprays containing a saltwater solution relieve mild congestion, loosen mucus and prevent crusting. You can use them safely as needed until symptoms improve.
- *Decongestants:* These sprays aren't intended for relief of chronic allergy symptoms. Avoid them or use sparingly for no more than 3 to 4 days.

Allergy shots (immunotherapy) involve injecting tiny amounts of known allergens into your system. After several injections, usually weekly, you may build up tolerance to the allergen. Then you may need monthly injections for up to several years.

Arthritis

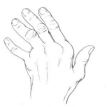

Rheumatoid arthritis can lead to a deformity in the fingers, commonly affecting the knuckles nearest the hand.

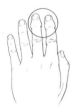

Heberden's nodes are bony lumps at the ends of fingers. They occur most often in women and may be a sign of osteoarthritis.

Arthritis is one of the most common medical problems in the United States. It strikes one person in seven. There are more than 100 forms of arthritis, and they have varying causes, symptoms and treatments. Refer to the chart on page 158 for a summary of symptoms of the major forms of arthritis.

The warning signs of arthritis include the following:
- Swelling in one or more joints
- Prolonged early-morning stiffness
- Recurring pain or tenderness in any joint
- Inability to move a joint normally
- Obvious redness and warmth in a joint
- Unexplained fevers, weight loss or weakness associated with joint pain

Any of these signs, when new, that last for more than 2 weeks require prompt medical evaluation. Distinguishing arthritis from simple aches and pains (rheumatism) is important for treating the problem correctly.

Arthritis can result from the normal wear and tear of the joints (as with osteoarthritis) or from an injury, inflammation, infection or some unknown cause. Most joint ailments caused by inflammation are termed arthritis, from the Greek words *arthron*, for "joint," and *itis*, for "inflammation."

The remainder of this chapter focuses on the management of osteoarthritis, which is the most common form of arthritis. Some of the self-care tips may apply to the other forms. Consult your physician regarding management of other forms of arthritis.

■ Exercise

Over time, exercise is probably the one therapy that will do the most good for managing your arthritis. Exercise must be done regularly to produce improvements. That's why you should check with your doctor and begin a regular exercise program for your specific needs.

Overall, you want to be in good general physical condition. This means maintaining flexibility, strength and endurance. Together, these will protect your joints against further damage, keep them aligned, reduce stiffness and minimize pain.

Different types of exercise achieve different goals. For flexibility, range-of-motion exercises (gentle stretching) move the joint from one end position to the other. In severe osteoarthritis, range-of-motion exercises may cause pain. Do not continue exercise beyond the point that is painful without the advice of your doctor or physical therapist.

Moving large muscle groups for 15 to 20 minutes is the primary way of exercising aerobically to strengthen muscles and build endurance. Walking, bicycling, swimming and dancing are good examples of aerobic-type exercises with low to moderate stress on the joint.

If you're carrying a lot of extra weight, moving around is more difficult. You're putting stress on your back, hips, knees and feet—all common places to have osteoarthritis. There's no positive evidence that excess weight causes osteoarthritis, but obesity clearly makes the symptoms worse.

Common Forms of Arthritis

Cause and Frequency	Key Symptoms	How Serious Is It?

Osteoarthritis

Cause and Frequency	Key Symptoms	How Serious Is It?
Normal wear and tear on the joints. Common in people older than 50; rare in young people unless a joint is injured	• Pain in a joint after use • Discomfort in a joint before or during a change in weather • Swelling and a loss of flexibility in a joint • Bony lumps at finger joints • Aching is common. Redness and warmth are less common	Usually not serious. It doesn't go away, although the pain may come and go. The effects are crippling in only rare cases. Joints such as the hip and knee may deteriorate to the point of needing replacement surgery. Age is the most significant factor.

Rheumatoid arthritis

Cause and Frequency	Key Symptoms	How Serious Is It?
The most common form of inflammatory arthritis.* Most often develops between ages 20 and 50. Caused by the body's immune system attacking joint-lining tissue	• Pain and swelling in the small joints of hands and feet • Overall aching or stiffness, especially first thing in the morning or after periods of rest • Affected joints are swollen, painful and warm during initial attack and flare-ups	It is the most debilitating form of arthritis. Disease frequently causes deformed joints. Some people experience sweats and fever along with the loss of strength in muscles attached to affected joints. Often chronic, although it can come and go

Infectious arthritis

Cause and Frequency	Key Symptoms	How Serious Is It?
Infectious agents include bacteria, fungus and viruses. Can be complication of sexually transmitted diseases. Can occur in anyone	• Pain and stiffness in one joint, typically a knee, shoulder, hip, ankle, elbow, finger or wrist • Surrounding tissues are warm and red • Chills, fever and weakness • May be associated with a rash	In most cases, prompt diagnosis and treatment of a joint infection result in rapid and complete recovery

Gout

Cause and Frequency	Key Symptoms	How Serious Is It?
Uric acid crystals form in joint. Most patients are men older than 40	• Severe pain that strikes suddenly in a single joint, often at the base of the big toe • Swelling and redness	An acute attack can be treated effectively. After an attack has run its course, the affected joint usually returns to normal. Attacks can recur and may require preventive treatment to lower uric acid levels in the blood

*Other types of inflammatory arthritis include *psoriatic arthritis,* which occurs in people with psoriasis, especially in the finger and foot joints; *Reiter's syndrome,* which often is transmitted by sexual contact and is characterized by pain in the joints, penile discharge, painful inflammation of the eye and a rash; *ankylosing spondylitis,* which affects the joints of the spine and, in advanced cases, causes a very stiff, inflexible backbone.

■ Medications Control Discomfort

The most common over-the-counter and prescription drugs used for osteoarthritis are described below. (See page 231 for more information on the use of these medications.)

- **Aspirin:** Dosage makes a difference, so your physician needs to specify the amount that's right for you. Pain may be relieved with 2 tablets every 4 hours. You might need to take this dosage for a week or two for inflammation.
- **Acetaminophen:** This nonprescription product relieves pain as well as aspirin and is less likely to upset your stomach. It doesn't help inflammation, but because joints often are not inflamed in osteoarthritis, it's a good choice most of the time.
- **NSAIDs:** The acronym stands for nonsteroidal anti-inflammatory drugs. NSAIDs work as well as aspirin and may have fewer side effects, but they cost more. You may need to take fewer doses daily than you would aspirin.
- **Corticosteroids:** These are like a hormone made in the adrenal gland of your body. They decrease inflammation. About 20 types are available; the most common is prednisone. Doctors do not prescribe oral corticosteroids for osteoarthritis, but they may occasionally inject a cortisone drug into an acutely inflamed joint. Because frequent use of this drug may accelerate joint disease, injections may be limited to no more than two or three annually.

Caution

Consult your physician if you are using NSAIDS or aspirin regularly for more than 2 weeks to treat joint pain.

■ Other Methods to Relieve Pain

Ask your doctor or your physical or occupational therapist about the therapies described below.

- **Heat** can relax muscles around a painful joint. You can apply heat superficially with warm water, a paraffin bath, electric pad, hot pack or heat lamp; but be careful to avoid a burn. For deep penetration, a physical therapist can use ultrasound or short-wave diathermy.
- **Cold** acts as a local anesthetic. It also decreases muscle spasms. Cold packs may help when you ache from holding muscles in the same position to avoid pain.
- **Splints** support and protect weak, painful joints during activity and provide proper positioning at night, which promotes restful sleep. Constant splinting, however, can weaken muscles and decrease flexibility.
- **Relaxation** techniques, including hypnosis, visualization, deep breathing, muscle relaxation, and other techniques may decrease pain.
- **Other techniques,** such as low-impact exercise, weight management, orthotics (such as shoe inserts) and gait aids (canes and walking sticks), strengthen muscles and reduce pressure on joints and thus decrease pain.

Specific Conditions

■ Joint Protection

Correct "body mechanics" help you move with minimal strain. A physical or occupational therapist can suggest techniques and equipment that protect your joints while decreasing stress and conserving energy.

Modifications you can make include:

- Avoid grasping actions that strain your finger joints. For example, instead of a clutch-style purse, select one with a shoulder strap. Use hot water to loosen a jar lid and pressure from your palm to open it, or use a jar opener. Don't twist or use your joints forcefully.
- Spread the weight of an object over several joints. Use both hands, for example, to lift a heavy pan. Try using a walking stick or cane.
- Take a break periodically to relax and stretch.
- Poor posture causes uneven weight distribution and may strain ligaments and muscles.
- Throughout the day, use your strongest muscles, and favor large joints. Don't push open a heavy glass door. Lean into it. To pick up an object, bend your knees and squat while keeping your back straight.
- Special tools that make gripping easier are available for buttoning shirts and kitchen use. Contact your pharmacy or health-care provider for information on ordering these items.

Don't Be Duped by Unproven Cures

One person in 10 who tries an unproven arthritis remedy reports harmful side effects. Here are some popular, but false, nutrition claims:

- **Cod liver oil "lubricates" stiff joints.** It may sound logical, but your body treats cod liver oil like any other fat; it provides no special help for joints. Large amounts of cod liver oil can lead to vitamin A and D toxicity.
- **Some foods cause "allergic arthritis."** There's no proof that food allergy causes arthritis. Also,

you can't relieve arthritis by avoiding tomatoes or other foods.

- **Fish oils reduce inflammation.** Research on rheumatoid arthritis suggests that omega-3 fatty acids in fish oils may give modest, temporary relief of inflammation. This finding is valid, but we don't advise fish oil supplements. You'd need about 15 capsules a day—and doctors don't know whether that's a safe amount. A lower dose won't help.

FOR MORE INFORMATION

- Arthritis Foundation, 1330 West Peachtree Street, Atlanta, GA 30309; (800) 283-7800; Internet address: http://www.arthritis.org.
- National Arthritis, Musculoskeletal and Skin Diseases Information Clearinghouse, National Institutes of Health, 1 AMS Circle, Bethesda, MD 20892-3675; (301) 495-4484; Internet address: http://www.nih.gov/niams.
- American College of Rheumatology, 60 Executive Park South, Suite 150, Atlanta, GA 30329; (404) 633-1870; Internet address: http://www.acr@rheumatology.org.

Asthma

Asthma occurs when the main air passages of your lungs, called the bronchial tubes, become inflamed. The muscles of bronchial walls tighten, and extra mucus is produced. Airflow out of your lungs is diminished, often causing wheezing.

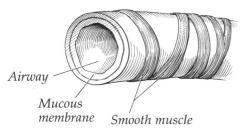

Normal airways in your lungs.

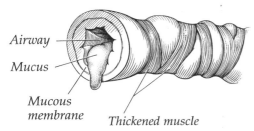

In asthma, airways in your lungs are inflamed and swollen.

Common symptoms are wheezing, difficulty breathing, "tightness" in the chest and coughing. In emergencies, the person will have extreme difficulty in breathing, bluish lips and nails, severe breathlessness, increased pulse rate, sweating and severe coughing.

Asthma is a serious medical condition, but with proper care and treatment you usually can control your symptoms and lead a normal life.

Approximately 10 percent of children and 5 percent of adults in the United States have asthma. About half of the children who have asthma develop the condition before age 10. Asthma is usually an inherited condition, and it is not contagious.

There are many causes, or "triggers," of asthma attacks. They can be triggered by an allergic reaction to dust mites, cockroaches, chemicals, pollen, mold or animal dander (dead skin cells that fall off animals). They can be triggered by exposure to substances in the home or workplace. Some people are more prone to suffer an asthma attack after exercise, especially if they exercise in cold air.

Respiratory infections caused by colds and the flu can aggravate the symptoms of asthma. (Adults with chronic asthma should get a yearly flu shot. Pregnant women and children, however, should check with their health-care provider before receiving flu shots.) Some additional triggers of asthma include sulfites, which are sprayed on vegetables and fruits by restaurants and stores to keep them from turning brown. Other foods or beverages, such as wine, also may contain sulfites as a preservative. Aspirin and other nonsteroidal anti-inflammatory drugs (NSAIDS) may trigger an asthma attack in some people.

Asthma attacks can range from very mild to life-threatening (see below). Asthma attacks can last for just a few minutes, or they can go on for hours and even days. If you have asthma, you should be receiving treatment from a health-care provider. Your health-care provider will work with you to identify the triggers that cause your asthma attacks. Together, you will devise a strategy to limit your exposure to these triggers, help control your symptoms and make sure your breathing is not severely obstructed.

Recognizing a Life-Threatening Attack

Prevent fatal attacks by treating symptoms early. Don't wait for wheezing as a sign of severity; wheezing may disappear when airflow is severely restricted. Get emergency care if:
- Breathing becomes difficult and your neck, chest or ribs pull in with each breath
- Nostrils flare

- Walking or talking becomes difficult
- Fingernails or lips turn blue
- Peak airflow (measured with a handheld meter you can use at home) reading decreases 50 percent below your normal level or keeps decreasing even after you take your medication

Specific Conditions

Self-Care

The following tips help control symptoms by "trigger-proofing" your environment.

- **Educate yourself about asthma.** The more you know, the easier it is to control.
- **Avoid allergens that might trigger your symptoms.** If you are allergic to cats or dogs, remove these pets from your home and avoid contact with other people's pets. Avoid buying clothing, furniture or rugs made from animal hair.
- **If you are allergic to airborne pollens and molds, use air-conditioning at home, at work and in your car.** (If temperature changes irritate your symptoms, you may not be able to do this.) Keep doors and windows closed to limit exposure to airborne pollens and molds.
- **Avoid activities that might contribute to your symptoms.** For example, home improvement projects might expose you to triggers that lead to an asthma attack, such as paint vapors, wood dust or similar irritants.
- **Check your furnace.** If you have a forced-air heating system and you are allergic to dust, use a filter for dust control. Change or clean filters on heating and cooling units frequently. (The best filter is a high-efficiency particulate-arresting filter, referred to as a HEPA filter.) Wear a mask when you remove dirty filters.
- Install an electrostatic filter on your vacuum cleaner (or use a two-ply microfiltration bag).
- Avoid projects that raise dust. If you cannot, then use a dust mask, which is available at drugstores and hardware stores.
- Review exercise habits and consider adjusting your routine (see below). Consider exercising indoors, which may limit your exposure to asthma triggers.
- Avoid all types of smoke, even smoke from a fireplace or burning leaves. Smoke irritates the eyes, nose and bronchial tubes. If you have asthma, you should not smoke and people should never smoke in your presence.
- Reduce stress and fatigue.
- Read labels carefully.
- If sensitive to aspirin, avoid other medications termed nonsteroidal anti-inflammatory agents (ibuprofen such as Motrin, Advil, Nuprin; naproxen such as Naprosyn, Anaprox, Aleve; and piroxicam such as Feldene).

Staying Active With Well-Planned Workouts

Years ago if you had asthma, doctors told you not to exercise. Now they believe well-planned regular workouts are beneficial, especially if you have mild to moderate disease. If you're fit, your heart and lungs don't have to work as hard to expel air.

But, because vigorous exercise can trigger an attack, be sure to discuss an exercise program with your doctor. In addition, follow these guidelines:

- **Know when not to exercise.** Avoid exercise when you have a viral infection, when the pollen count is more than 100 or in below-zero or extremely hot and humid conditions. In cold temperatures, wear a face mask to warm the air you breathe.
- **Medicate first.** Use your inhaled short-acting beta agonist 15 to 60 minutes before exercise.
- **Start slowly.** Five to 10 minutes of warm-up exercises may relax your chest muscles and widen your airways to ease breathing. Gradually work up to your desired pace.
- **Choose the type of exercise wisely.** Cold-weather activities such as skiing and long-distance, nonstop activities such as running most often cause wheezing. Exercise that requires short bursts of energy, such as walking, golf and leisure bicycling, may be better tolerated.

Medical Help

Testing for allergies: Your health-care provider may perform some tests to try to determine the triggers of your asthma attacks. A skin test or blood test may be performed. The blood test is more expensive and is less sensitive than skin tests, but it is sometimes preferable when the person being tested has a skin disease or is taking medications that might affect the test results.

Medications: Your doctor may prescribe some of the medications listed below to prevent or treat your asthma attacks. Take all the medications as prescribed, even if you are not experiencing any symptoms. Do not take more than the prescribed amount (excessive use of medications can be dangerous). These medications can be taken using an inhaler, or they may come in liquid, capsule or tablet form.

Preventers (anti-inflammatory medications): These medications reduce the inflammation in your airways and also help reduce the production of mucus. The result is a reduction of the spasms in your breathing passages. Take the daily dose of these medications as prescribed to prevent asthma attacks from occurring. Preventers include inhaled steroids, cromolyn sodium and nedocromil sodium.

Relievers (also called "bronchodilators"): Unlike preventers, these medications are taken once you are experiencing an asthma attack. Relievers help open narrow airways to allow you to breathe more easily during an attack. Relievers include beta agonists and theophylline.

Self-monitoring with peak flowmeter: You may be trained to use a peak flowmeter, a tube that measures how well you are breathing. The flowmeter acts like a gauge for your lungs, giving you a number that helps evaluate lung function. A low reading means your air passages are narrow and is an early warning that you may experience an asthma attack.

Inhalers: Risks of Misuse

Inhaling a bronchodilator (see Medical Help above) helps you breathe better immediately during an attack. But the drug doesn't correct inflammation.

Maximal daily use of a brochodilator is 2 puffs every 4 to 6 hours. If you use one more frequently to control symptoms, you need a more effective medication.

Fast relief may make it difficult to recognize worsening symptoms. Once the medication wears off, asthma returns with more severe wheezing.

You're then tempted to take another dose of the medication, delaying adequate treatment with anti-inflammatory medications.

Overuse also risks toxic drug levels that may lead to an irregular heartbeat, especially if you have a heart condition.

Over-the-counter inhalers also can relieve symptoms quickly—but temporarily. Relying on inhalers can mask a worsening attack and delay treatment with anti-inflammatory medications.

FOR MORE INFORMATION

- Asthma and Allergy Foundation of America, 1125 15th St. N.W., Suite 502, Washington, D.C. 20005; (800) 727-8462.
- American Lung Association, 1740 Broadway, New York, NY 10019; (800) 586-4872; Internet address: http://www.lungusa.org.
- National Institute of Allergy and Infectious Disease (NIH), Building 31, Room 7A50, 31 Center Drive, MSC 2520, Bethesda, MD 20892-2520; (301) 496-5717; Internet address: http://www.niaid.nih.gov.

Mayo HealthQuest Guide to Self-Care

Specific Conditions

Cancer

The day your cancer is diagnosed becomes a major event in your life. You see everything that follows in the context of your cancer diagnosis and treatment. That's a normal reaction.

There are many different kinds of cancer. We're constantly finding new ways to detect and treat it. Recently, survival rates for some cancers have improved dramatic-ally. Now, we talk of "living with cancer," rather than "dying of cancer" or becoming a "victim of cancer."

Incidence of cancer by site and sex. The statistics are 1997 estimates by the American Cancer Society. Figures exclude basal and squamous cell skin cancers and superficial cancers (in situ carcinoma), except bladder. (By permission of the American Cancer Society.)

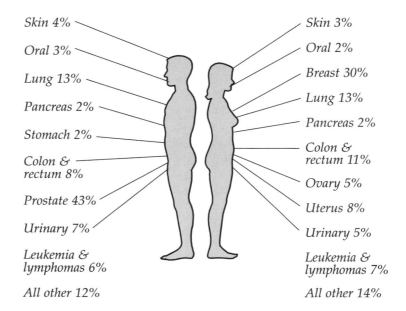

Skin 4%
Oral 3%
Lung 13%
Pancreas 2%
Stomach 2%
Colon & rectum 8%
Prostate 43%
Urinary 7%
Leukemia & lymphomas 6%
All other 12%

Skin 3%
Oral 2%
Breast 30%
Lung 13%
Pancreas 2%
Colon & rectum 11%
Ovary 5%
Uterus 8%
Urinary 5%
Leukemia & lymphomas 7%
All other 14%

The diagram shows the incidence of various kinds of cancer, according to the affected body part. The remainder of this chapter includes some advice for you or a family member with cancer.

For specific information on various types of cancer, refer to Index page 237.

■ Responding to the Cancer Diagnosis

As with any crisis or difficult time in life, you need healthful and effective coping strategies. Here are some suggestions:

1. **Get the facts.** Try to obtain as much basic, useful information as possible. Consider bringing a family member or friend with you to doctor appointments. Write down your questions and concerns beforehand. This approach helps you organize your thoughts, obtain accurate information, understand your cancer and treatment and participate in decision making. But remember, the answers are frequently educated guesses or statistics. Everyone is different. Questions often include the following:
   - Is my cancer curable?

- What are my treatment options?
- What can I expect during treatment?
- Will my treatments be painful?
- When do I need to call my doctor?
- What can I do to prevent cancer from recurring?
- What are the risk factors for my family members (especially children)?

2. **Develop your own coping strategy.** Just as each person's cancer treatment is individualized, so is the coping strategy that you must follow. Here are some ideas:
   - Learn relaxation techniques (see page 211).
   - Share feelings honestly with family, friends, a pastor or counselor.
   - Keep a journal to help organize your thoughts.
   - When faced with a difficult decision, list pros and cons for each choice.
   - Find a source of strength in your faith.
   - Find time to be alone.
   - Remain involved with work and leisure activities.

3. **Keep communication open** between you and your loved ones, health-care providers and others. You may feel particularly isolated if people try to protect you by keeping disappointing news from you or trying to put up a strong front. If you and others feel free to express your emotions, you can gain strength from each other.

4. **Your self-image is important.** Although some people may not notice physical changes, you will. Insurance will often help pay for wigs, prostheses and special adaptive devices.

5. **A healthful lifestyle** can improve your energy level and promote healthy cell growth. This includes adequate rest, good nutrition, exercise and fun activities.

6. **Let friends and family help you.** Often they can run errands, drive the carpool, prepare meals and help with household chores. Learn to accept help. Accepting help also gives those who care about you a sense of purpose at a difficult time.

7. **Review your goals and priorities.** Consider what's really important in your life. Reduce unnecessary activities. Find a new openness with loved ones. Share your thoughts and feelings with them. Cancer affects all of your relationships. Communication can help reduce the anxiety and fear that cancer can cause.

8. **Try to maintain your normal lifestyle.** Take each day one at a time. It's easy to overlook this simple strategy during stressful times. When the future is uncertain, organizing and planning for it can suddenly become overwhelming.

9. **Maintain a positive attitude.** Celebrate each day. If a day is difficult, let go of it and move on. Don't let cancer control your life.

10. **Fight stigmas.** Many of the old stigmas associated with cancer still exist. Your friends may wonder if cancer is contagious. Coworkers may doubt you're healthy enough to do your job and think you'll drain their health benefits. Reassure others that research shows cancer survivors are just as productive as other workers and don't miss work any more often. Remind friends that even if cancer has been a frightening part of your life, it shouldn't scare them to be near you.

11. **Look into insurance options.** If you're employed, you may feel "trapped," unable to change jobs for fear of not being eligible for new insurance. If you're retired, you may have difficulty purchasing supplemental insurance. Find out whether your state provides health insurance for people who are difficult to insure. Look into group insurance options through professional, fraternal or political organizations.

Specific Conditions

■ Good Nutrition: A Big "Plus"

There is no conclusive evidence that avoiding or overeating any specific food helps treat cancer. However, good nutrition is important to living with cancer. Your cancer treatment may reduce your appetite and change the flavor of foods. It also may interfere with absorption of nutrients in foods. Studies show that good nutrition can:

● Improve your chances of tolerating your treatment successfully
● Improve your sense of well-being
● Enhance your tissue and immune system functions
● Help you meet increased demands for calories and proteins in rebuilding damaged tissues

A new medicine, megestrol acetate (available in pill or liquid form), taken several times a day may help maintain or increase your weight.

Self-Care

Here are some specific tips for good nutrition:

● Mild-tasting dairy products such as cottage cheese and yogurt are good sources of protein. Try eating a peanut butter sandwich or peanut butter spread on fruit. Legumes such as kidney beans, chickpeas and black-eyed peas are good sources of protein, especially when combined with grains such as rice, corn or bread.
● Pack as many calories as possible into the foods you eat. Warm your bread, and spread it with butter, margarine, jam or honey. Sprinkle foods with chopped nuts.
● Fresh fruits and many vegetables are easy to eat and digest. Lightly seasoned dishes made with milk products, eggs, poultry, fish and pasta often are well tolerated.
● If you have trouble eating an adequate amount of food at a single sitting, eat smaller amounts more frequently. Chew your food slowly. Drink liquids at other times.
● If the aroma of food being prepared makes you feel ill, use a microwave or choose foods that require little cooking or foods that can be warmed at a low temperature.

■ What About Pain?

Pain is a big fear among people with cancer, but it need not be. More than half of all people who have cancer don't have notable pain. In fact, patients with cancer often experience less pain than people with arthritis or nerve disorders. Pain is almost always controllable. Pain control medications include the following:

● **Nonnarcotic drugs:** Aspirin is highly effective, and it often provides relief equivalent to more powerful painkillers. Acetaminophen and nonsteroidal anti-inflammatory drugs are equally effective and may require fewer doses per day than aspirin (see page 231). Antidepressants also are helpful pain relievers.
● **Narcotic drugs** such as morphine and codeine, used for severe pain, may be given by mouth (pills or liquid), injections, pumps you control or a slow-release skin patch.
● **Tranquilizers** may improve your comfort level when used with pain medications.

Nondrug pain control measures include radiation to shrink a tumor and lessen pain; injection or surgery to block pathways of nerves carrying pain messages to your brain; biofeedback, behavior modification, hypnosis, breathing and relaxation exercises, massage, transcutaneous electrical nerve stimulation (TENS) or hot and cold packs.

Self-Care

- Don't wait for the pain to become severe before taking a pain medication. Take pain medicines on a schedule.
- Don't be concerned about addiction. When used properly, the chance for addiction to narcotics is very small. Besides, if a narcotic is needed for a long time to relieve severe pain, the comfort it provides is often more important than any possibility of addiction.
- Develop a strategy for dealing with emotions such as anxiety and depression. They can make the pain seem worse.

■ Cancer in Children

Cancer in children is uncommon, but when it happens parents face special issues and problems. Researchers have made great strides in finding effective treatments for childhood cancers. Today, more than 70 percent of American children with cancer survive.

Self-Care

If your child has cancer, it's important to:

- Carefully choose the person who will treat your child. Look for a medical center with the latest treatments for childhood cancers. It also should provide emotional support for your family.
- Try to maintain as normal a lifestyle as possible. Keeping schedules, rules and previous expectations in place will help your child cope and plant the idea of a long future.
- Talk to your child's teachers to establish behavioral and academic expectations.
- Do your best to deal with the possibility of death in an honest, straightforward manner. Children need to be told as much as they can understand. There is no single "right" way to tell children about death. Encourage them to ask questions. Give them simple answers. Their fears may keep them from asking questions, so start by asking how they feel. Never lie, make promises you may not be able to keep or be afraid to say, "I don't know."
- Promote activities that reduce anxiety (such as drawing) and express feelings (role-playing or puppets).
- Don't ignore the needs of your other children. Siblings can be very supportive to their ill brother or sister, but they must know that their special place in the family is secure.
- Read "Talking With Your Child About Cancer," from the National Institutes of Health (Pamphlet #91-2761, available from the National Cancer Institute) (see below).

FOR MORE INFORMATION

- The National Cancer Institute Information Service, (800) 4-CANCER; CancerFax (800) 624-2511 (24 hours); Internet address: http://cancernet.nci.nih.gov.
- The American Cancer Society, 1599 Clifton Road NE, Atlanta GA 30329-4251; (800) ACS-2345; Internet address: http://www.cancer.org.

Specific Conditions

Diabetes

Diabetes is a disorder of your metabolism—the way your body uses digested food for energy and growth. Normally, your digestive system converts a portion of the food you eat into a sugar called glucose. That sugar then enters your bloodstream, ready to fuel your cells.

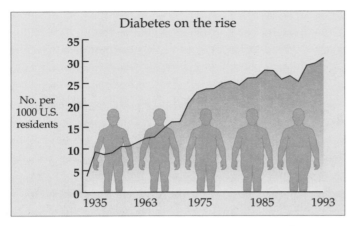

Diabetes on the rise

Diabetes has increased dramatically as obesity has become more common in the United States. The number of Americans diagnosed with any form of diabetes was just 3.7 per 1,000 U.S. residents in 1935. In 1993, it was 30.7 per 1,000 residents.

In order for your cells to receive the sugar, insulin, a hormone produced by your pancreas, must "escort" it in. Normally, your pancreas produces enough insulin to handle all the sugar that is present. There are two types of diabetes, both of which disrupt this process.

In type I diabetes, your pancreas produces reduced amounts of insulin. In type II diabetes, your body doesn't respond normally to the insulin that is made. In both types of diabetes, sugar enters body cells only in limited amounts. Some of the sugar then builds up in your blood, overflows into your urine and passes from your body unused.

Both types of diabetes can cause long-term complications such as heart disease, kidney failure, nerve damage, blindness and deterioration of blood vessels and nerves. Damage to your body's small and large blood vessels is at the root of most of these complications.

Type I and Type II: What's the Difference?

Type I diabetes affects 1 in 10 people with diabetes. It is also known as insulin-dependent diabetes mellitus (IDDM) or juvenile-onset diabetes and usually develops before age 30. If you have type I diabetes, you must receive insulin daily for the rest of your life. The symptoms can develop abruptly and include the following:

- Excessive thirst
- Frequent urination
- Extreme hunger
- Unexplained weight loss
- Weakness and fatigue

Type II diabetes is the most common form of diabetes. It is also called non-insulin-dependent diabetes mellitus (NIDDM) or adult-onset diabetes. Type II most often occurs after age 40 in overweight people. Balanced diet, moderate weight loss and exercise often can control it. If diet and exercise aren't effective, you may need oral medication or insulin injections. Many people with type II diabetes have few or no symptoms. These symptoms can develop slowly and include the following:

- Excessive thirst
- Frequent urination
- Blurred vision
- Recurring bladder, vaginal and skin infections
- Slow-healing sores
- Irritability
- Tingling or loss of feeling in your hands or feet

Self-Care

Managing diabetes is a balancing act. Illness, eating too much or too little, a change in exercise, travel and stress all affect your blood sugar level. Here are some tips to help you gain tighter control of your blood sugar level.

Diet

A well-balanced diet is the cornerstone of diabetes management. Remember to:

- **Stick to a schedule.** Eat three meals a day. Be consistent in the amount of food you eat and the timing of eating. If you take insulin or an oral diabetes medication, you may need to eat a bedtime snack.
- **Focus on fiber.** Eat a variety of fresh fruits, vegetables, legumes and whole-grain foods. These are low-fat and rich sources of vitamins and minerals.
- **Limit foods that are high in fat or cholesterol** to less than 30 percent of your total calorie intake. Choose lean cuts of meats and use low-fat dairy products.
- **Don't push proteins.** Too much protein can take its toll on your kidneys. Eat smaller portions (3 ounces) of meat, poultry or fish.
- **Avoid "empty" calories.** Candy, cookies and other sweets are not forbidden. But because they have little nutritional value, eat them in moderation and count them in your total carbohydrate intake.
- **Use alcohol in moderation.** If your doctor says it's safe, choose drinks that are low in sugar and alcohol, such as light beer and dry wines. Count alcoholic drinks in your total carbohydrate intake and do not drink on an empty stomach.
- **Watch your weight.** If you're overweight, losing even a few pounds may help.

Exercise

Regular exercise helps maintain overall health, benefits your heart and blood vessels and may improve circulation. It helps control your blood sugar level and may help prevent type II diabetes. If you have type II diabetes, regular exercise and a healthful diet may reduce or even eliminate your need for injected insulin or an oral medication.

Exercise alone is not enough to achieve good control of your blood sugar level if you have type I diabetes. However, it may enhance the effects of insulin that you take. You may need to eat additional food just before or during exercise to prevent sudden changes in your blood sugar level. Follow your doctor's advice on exercise.

Monitoring Your Blood Sugar

Checking your blood sugar level regularly is an essential part of managing your diabetes. How often you need to perform this test depends on the type of diabetes you have, how stable your blood sugar levels are and other factors. Your health-care team can help you determine reasonable goals for your blood sugar level. In addition to sticking with a proper diet and exercise, you also may need to learn how to adjust your medications, especially insulin, to keep your blood sugar level near normal.

Today, blood tests are the most accurate way to check your blood sugar level. To do so, you put a drop of fingertip blood onto a chemically treated test strip. The test strip reacts to the amount of glucose in your blood by changing color. You can read the blood glucose level by holding the test strip next to a color guide chart or by having an electronic glucose monitor read it. Reliable monitors cost between $40 and $120.

Specific Conditions

Self-Care *(continued)*

Medications

You may need medications to control your blood sugar level. But even with medication, exercise and diet are integral to managing your diabetes.

If you have type I diabetes, you must take insulin by injection. Insulin can't be taken by mouth because it breaks down in your digestive tract. The number of daily injections and type of insulin prescribed (short-, intermediate- or long-lasting) depend on your individual needs. If your blood sugar level is hard to control, your health-care provider may prescribe frequent injections or an insulin pump.

If you have type II diabetes and have trouble controlling your blood sugar with diet and exercise alone, your doctor may prescribe one of several oral medications. These medications can help your pancreas produce more insulin or help insulin to work better in your body. If oral medications aren't working well, insulin injections are best. Good control of the blood sugar level is key to avoiding complications.

Caution

Diabetes can cause one or more of the following emergencies:

Insulin reaction: This is also called hypoglycemia (low blood sugar). It can occur when excess insulin, excess exercise or too little food causes a decreased blood sugar level. Symptoms usually appear several hours after eating and include trembling, weakness and drowsiness followed by confusion, dizziness and double vision. If untreated, a low blood sugar level may cause seizures or loss of consciousness.

If you are concerned that you are having an insulin reaction, try eating something containing sugar, such as fruit juices, candy or soft drinks containing sugar, and check your blood sugar level. If you are helping someone in this condition, seek emergency medical care if the person vomits or is unable to cooperate, or if symptoms persist beyond 30 minutes after treatment. Remain with the person for an hour after recovery to ensure that he or she is thinking clearly.

Diabetic coma: Also called diabetic ketoacidosis or DKA, this complication develops more slowly than an insulin reaction, often over hours or days. DKA occurs when the blood sugar level is too high (hyperglycemia). Nausea, vomiting, abdominal pain, weakness, thirst, sweet-smelling breath and deeper and more rapid breathing all can precede gradual confusion and loss of consciousness. This reaction is most likely to occur in persons with type I diabetes who are ill or skip an insulin dose. It can be the first symptom of previously undiagnosed diabetes.

Foot Care Reduces the Risk of Injury and Infection

Diabetes can impair the circulation and nerve supply to your feet. Foot care is essential:

- Inspect your feet daily. Look for sores, color changes or altered sensation. Get help or a mirror to view all surfaces.
- Bathe your feet daily. Use warm (not hot) soapy water. Dry them thoroughly.
- Trim nails straight across, file rough edges.

- Don't use wart removers or trim calluses and corns yourself. See your doctor or a podiatrist.
- Wear cushioned, well-fitted shoes. Check inside shoes daily for sharp edges. Don't walk barefoot.
- Avoid tight clothing around your legs or ankles. Don't smoke; smoking can make bad circulation worse.

FOR MORE INFORMATION

- The American Diabetes Association, 1660 Duke Street, Alexandria, VA 22314; (800) DIABETES; Internet address: http://www.diabetes.org.

Heart Disease

Your heart pumps blood to every tissue in your body through a 60,000-mile network of blood vessels. Blood supplies the tissues with oxygen and nutrients that are essential for good health.

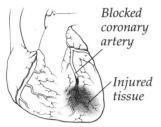

Blocked coronary artery

Injured tissue

A heart attack occurs when arteries supplying your heart with blood and oxygen become blocked.

Problems can arise in the heart muscle, the heart valves, the electrical conduction system, the pericardium (the sac that surrounds the heart) or the coronary arteries (the arteries that supply blood to the heart muscle itself). This chapter focuses on problems in the coronary arteries. Coronary artery problems cause "heart attacks," which kill 500,000 Americans annually.

As you age, fatty deposits may form in the coronary arteries in your heart, creating a condition called coronary artery disease. This condition is called atherosclerosis—often called "hardening of the arteries"—and it can occur in arteries in other areas of your body as well. As the coronary arteries become narrowed or blocked, blood flow to your heart muscle is reduced or stopped.

When your heart muscle doesn't receive enough blood, you may feel chest pain or pressure (angina). If the blood flow is blocked long enough in a coronary artery (about 30 minutes to 2 hours), the portion of the heart muscle that is supplied by that artery will die. Heart muscle death is known as a myocardial infarction (MI) or heart attack.

A heart attack usually is caused by sudden blockage of a heart artery by a blood clot. The clot usually forms in an artery that has been narrowed by fatty deposits.

Heart Attack: Reacting Promptly May Save a Life

A heart attack generally causes chest pain for more than 15 minutes. But a heart attack also can be "silent" and have no symptoms. About half of heart attack victims have warning symptoms hours, days or weeks in advance.

The American Heart Association lists the following warning signs of a heart attack. Be aware that you may not have them at all and that symptoms may come and go.

● Uncomfortable pressure, fullness or squeezing pain in the center of your chest, lasting more than a few minutes.
● Pain spreading to your shoulders, neck or arms.

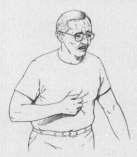

The pain of heart attack varies from person to person, but typically there is a profound squeezing sensation in the chest, accompanied by profuse perspiration. Pain may radiate to the left shoulder and arm, to the back and even to the jaw.

● Light-headedness, fainting, sweating, nausea or shortness of breath.

The more of these symptoms you have, the more likely it is that you are having a heart attack. Whether you suspect a heart attack or think it's just indigestion, act immediately:

● Call 911 first.
● Sit quietly or lie down if you are feeling faint. Breathe slowly and deeply.
● Chew an aspirin, unless you are allergic to it. Aspirin thins the blood and can decrease death rates significantly.

If you observe someone with chest pain, follow the above steps. If the person faints or loses consciousness, begin CPR (see page 2).

Once the heart attack victim arrives at a medical center, he or she may be given clot-dissolving drugs or undergo a procedure called angioplasty, which involves widening blocked arteries to let blood flow more freely to the heart. If the use of clot-dissolving drugs or angioplasty is delayed beyond 2 hours, benefits are substantially reduced.

What Is Your Risk of Heart Disease?

Cigarette smoking, high blood pressure and high blood cholesterol are some of the major risk factors for coronary artery disease. Your chances of having a heart attack or dying of heart disease within the next 8 years increase with each risk factor you have. Estimate your risk by adding up the points shown in the yellow-shaded areas.

If you're a man:

1. Do you smoke? No = 0 Yes = 3
2. Find your systolic blood pressure (top number in your reading) and circle the points directly below.

Blood pressure

100	110	120	130	140	150	160	170	180	190	200
1	2	4	5	6	7	8	9	10	12	13

3. Circle the number where your approximate age and blood cholesterol level meet.

Age

Total cholesterol	40	50	60	70
165	4	12	18	21
180	5	13	19	21
195	7	14	19	21
210	8	15	20	21
225	9	16	20	22
240	11	17	21	22
255	12	18	22	22
270	13	19	22	23
285	15	20	23	23
300	16	21	24	23
315	17	22	24	23

If you're a woman:

1. Do you smoke? No = 0 Yes = 1
2. Find your systolic blood pressure (top number in your reading) and circle the points directly below.

Blood pressure

100	110	120	130	140	150	160	170	180	190	200
1	2	3	4	5	6	7	8	9	10	11

3. Circle the number where your approximate age and blood cholesterol level meet.

Age

Total cholesterol	40	50	60	70
165	4	12	18	23
180	5	13	19	23
195	5	13	19	23
210	6	14	20	24
225	7	15	20	24
240	8	15	21	24
255	8	16	21	25
270	9	16	22	25
285	10	17	22	25
300	11	18	23	25
315	11	18	23	26

4. Record Your Points

☐	cigarette smoking
☐	systolic blood pressure
☐	age/blood cholesterol
☐	sex Male = 5 Female = 0
☐	TOTAL POINTS

5. Estimate Your Risk
   Find your total points to determine your chances (out of 100) of having heart disease within the next 8 years.

Total points	Chances (out of 100)	Total points	Chances (out of 100)
1-10	<1	35	17
11-13	1	36	19
14-17	2	37	21
18-21	3	38	24
22-23	4	39	26
24	5	40	28
25-26	6	41	31
27	7	42	34
28	8	43	36
29	9	44	39
30	10	45	42
31	11	46	46
32	13	47	49
33	14	48	52
34	16	49	55

Note: In this table, the effect on risk from blood cholesterol is limited to total cholesterol. If the assessment also reflected a low level of high-density lipoprotein (HDL) cholesterol, the estimated risk would be higher. This assessment also omits the effects of diabetes mellitus and an abnormal electrocardiogram indicating left ventricular hypertrophy. Women who have diabetes should add 6 points to the total score, and add 4 points if an electrocardiogram shows left ventricular hypertrophy. Men who have diabetes should add 3 points to the total score, and add 2 points for an electrocardiogram that shows left ventricular hypertrophy. (Tables are based on data from the Framingham Heart Study.)

■ Lowering Your Risk of Heart Disease

Several risk factors for coronary artery disease can be modified through lifestyle changes or medications. Here's what you can do to reduce your risk:

- Stop smoking. If you smoke, your risk of heart disease is at least two times higher than that of a person who doesn't smoke. For more information on smoking and ways to stop, see page 206.
- Reduce high blood pressure. See page 175.
- Reduce your cholesterol level. See page 201.
- Control diabetes. See pages 169 and 170.
- Maintain proper weight. See page 195.
- Exercise. See page 202.
- Reduce stress. See page 211.

The risk factors listed above may interact with each other to affect your total risk of developing coronary artery disease. The more risk factors you have, the greater your risk of a heart attack.

Controlling these risk factors often involves using medications. But you can usually lower your risk significantly through a careful diet and regular exercise; these efforts sometimes prevent the need for medications.

In addition to a good diet and regular exercise, studies have shown that the following also may lower your risk of heart attack. Discuss with your doctor how each of these factors fits in to lowering your risk.

Aspirin is often recommended to prevent heart attacks. Aspirin reduces the tendency of blood to clot by weakening the activity of platelets (small cell fragments in the blood that stick to each other to form a clot). It may help reduce a clot or even prevent a clot from causing a heart attack. It is inexpensive, generally safe and easy to take. One baby aspirin (which equals one-fourth of a regular-strength adult aspirin) is enough to reduce the risk of a heart attack substantially. In one study, aspirin cut the risk of heart attacks in half. Aspirin does increase the risk of bleeding if an artery to your brain ruptures. Ask your doctor about the risks and benefits of taking aspirin regularly.

Vitamins: Experts also recommend taking 1 or 2 tablets (400 International Units each) of vitamin E each day to help prevent heart attacks. Vitamin E is an antioxidant that blocks the buildup of LDL cholesterol (see page 200) in your vessel walls. Nurses who used 400 International Units of vitamin E had 25 percent fewer heart attacks. The value of taking vitamin C to reduce your risk of heart attack has not been clearly shown. However, if you have a family history of heart disease at an early age, your health-care provider may recommend that you take 1 mg of folic acid (another vitamin) every day.

Estrogen: If you are a woman past menopause, your risk of heart attack increases. Talk to your doctor about your overall risk. Evidence suggests that taking estrogen replacement after menopause will lower your risk of having a heart attack as well as prevent osteoporosis.

Risk-lowering prescription medications: If you've had a heart attack or you have been told by your doctor that you have coronary artery disease, other medicines may lower your risk of heart disease or heart attack. Talk with your doctor about cholesterol-lowering medicines, beta blockers and ACE inhibitors. These medicines, like aspirin, have been shown to lower your risk of heart attack and may be appropriate for you.

Specific Conditions

High Blood Pressure

High blood pressure (hypertension) is called the "silent killer." Most people with high blood pressure have no symptoms. One-third of the 50 million Americans with the condition are unaware of their risk. The risk lies in the long-term damage the ailment can cause to your heart, brain, kidneys and eyes.

High blood pressure is more common as we get older. In addition, high blood pressure is more common in blacks than in whites. More men than women have high blood pressure in young adulthood and early middle age, but rates are about equal for ages 55 to 64. Rates for women surpass those for men at age 65 or older.

What Is Blood Pressure?

Have you ever had your blood pressure taken, then wondered what the numbers mean? Knowing and understanding your numbers, then taking steps to control your blood pressure, are critical. Being informed and taking the proper steps can mean the difference between good health and hypertensive heart disease, stroke and kidney disease.

Blood pressure is determined by the amount of blood your heart pumps and the resistance to blood flow in the arteries. Small arteries limit blood flow. In general, the more blood the heart pumps and the smaller the arteries, the higher the blood pressure (that is, your heart must work harder to pump the same amount of blood).

A typical "normal" blood pressure reading is 120/80 mm Hg (millimeters of mercury). The top number (120), systolic pressure, is the amount of pressure your heart generates when pumping blood out through your arteries. The bottom number (80), diastolic pressure, is the amount of pressure in the arteries when the heart is at rest between beats.

Your blood pressure normally varies during the day. It rises during activity. It decreases with rest.

In general, the diagnosis of high blood pressure is made if your resting blood pressure is consistently 140/90 mm Hg or higher. Why it reaches or exceeds this level is not always known. In fact, a specific disease or cause is identified in fewer than 1 case in 20. When a cause cannot be determined, high blood pressure is called **essential** or **primary hypertension**.

When a cause is determined, the term **secondary hypertension** is used because the increased pressure is the result of another condition. These specific causes may include medications such as oral contraceptives and kidney disorders such as renal failure, glomerulonephritis and certain adrenal gland problems.

Hypotension (Low Blood Pressure)

Hypotension is low blood pressure. If blood pressure falls to dangerously low levels (shock), the situation can be life-threatening. Shock may result from significant loss of fluid or blood and rarely from serious infections.

Postural hypotension is one potentially dangerous manifestation of low blood pressure. Dizziness or faintness that occurs on standing up quickly from a seated position is the key symptom. (See Dizziness and Fainting, page 30.) It can be caused by medications, pregnancy or illnesses.

Classifying Blood Pressure

Here's the newest way to classify high blood pressure for healthy adults at least 18 years old.

Condition	Systolic (Top Number)	Diastolic (Bottom Number)	What to Do
Normal	Less than 130	Less than 85	Recheck in 2 years
High-normal	130-139	85-89	Recheck in 1 year
Hypertension			
Stage 1	140-159	90-99	Confirm within 2 months
Stage 2	160-179	100-109	See doctor within month
Stage 3	180-209	110-119	See doctor within week
Stage 4	210 or higher	120 or higher	See doctor immediately

Note: Blood pressure conditions are diagnosed based on the average of two or more readings taken at two different visits to your doctor, in addition to the original screening visit. (From The Fifth Report of the Joint National Committee on Detection, Evaluation, and Treatment of High Blood Pressure. Archives of Internal Medicine 153:154-185, 1993. By permission of the American Medical Association.)

Self-Care

The best strategy is to begin with lifestyle changes such as weight control, diet changes and exercise. If, after 3 to 6 months, your blood pressure has not decreased, your physician may prescribe a medication. Here's what you can do to help yourself:

- **Diet:** Reduce your intake of saturated fat and cholesterol.
- **Salt restriction:** Salt causes the body to retain fluids and thus, in many people, can cause high blood pressure. Don't add salt to food. Avoid salty foods such as cured meat, snack foods and canned or prepared foods.
- **Weight reduction:** If you are more than 10 percent above your ideal body weight, shed those extra pounds. A loss of as few as 10 pounds may reduce your blood pressure significantly. In some people, weight loss alone is sufficient to avoid the need to take antihypertensive drugs.
- **Exercise:** Regular aerobic exercise alone seems to lower blood pressure in some people, even without weight loss.
- **Stop smoking:** The use of tobacco can accelerate the process of atherosclerosis (narrowing of vessels) in people with high blood pressure. Smoking in combination with high blood pressure greatly increases your risk of artery damage.
- **Limit alcohol consumption:** Drinking more than 2 ounces of 100-proof liquor, 8 ounces of wine or 24 ounces of beer a day can increase your blood pressure.

The Use of Medications

Your physician will determine which drug or combination of drugs may be best for you. Some drugs work better than others at different ages or in certain races. Your doctor may consider the cost, side effects, the interaction between multiple drugs and how the drugs affect other illnesses. There may be several steps in the process to select medication because the first drug may not lower your blood pressure. A second, third or even fourth drug may be tried either as a substitute or as an additional drug.

Specific Conditions

Sexually Transmitted Diseases

Sexually transmitted disease (STD) is increasing in the United States. Most STDs are treatable, but human immunodeficiency virus (HIV), the cause of acquired immuno-deficiency syndrome (AIDS), has no "current" cure, and death eventually occurs in most cases.

Although HIV can be spread through use of contaminated needles or, rarely, through blood transfusion, it usually is transmitted by sexual contact. The virus is present in semen and vaginal secretions and enters a person's body through small tears that can develop in the vaginal or rectal tissues during sexual activity. Transmission of the virus occurs only after intimate contact with infected blood, semen or vaginal secretions. There have been cases of HIV being passed to health-care workers through needlesticks.

STDs such as chlamydia infections, gonorrhea, herpes, venereal warts and syphilis are highly contagious. Many of them can be spread through only one sexual contact. The microorganisms that cause STDs, including HIV, all die within hours once they are outside the body. However, none of these infections are spread through casual contact such as handshaking or sitting on a toilet seat.

The only sure way of preventing STDs and AIDS is through sexual abstinence or a relationship exclusively between two uninfected people. If you have several sexual partners or an infected partner, you place yourself at high risk of contracting an STD.

The Use of Condoms

Correct and consistent use of a latex condom and avoidance of certain sexual practices can decrease the risk of contracting AIDS and other STDs, although condoms do not completely eliminate the risk. Condoms sometimes are made of animal membrane, and the pores in such natural "skin" condoms may allow the AIDS virus to pass through. The use of latex condoms is recommended.

To be effective, a condom must be undamaged, applied before genital contact and remain intact until removed on completion of sexual activity. Extra lubrication (even with lubricated condoms) can help prevent the condom from breaking. Use only water-based lubricants. Oil-based lubricants can cause a condom to break down.

A new condom for females can help reduce the risk of contracting an STD. Most forms of female-directed contraception (for example, the pill) do not provide protection against STDs, although studies indicate that use of the spermicide nonoxynol-9 decreases the frequency of gonorrhea and chlamydial infection. Spermicides in conjunction with a diaphragm also may help kill bacteria.

Risky Behaviors

Different sexual practices carry different degrees of risk of contracting HIV infection. Receptive (passive) anal intercourse is the riskiest because damage to the anal and rectal membranes allows HIV to enter the bloodstream. The passive partner is at much higher risk of contracting HIV than is the active partner, although gonorrhea and syphilis can be acquired from the passive partner's rectum.

Heterosexual vaginal intercourse, particularly with multiple partners, carries a risk of contracting HIV. The virus is believed to be transmitted more easily from the man to the woman than vice versa.

Oral-genital sex is also a possible means of transmission of HIV, gonorrhea, herpes, syphilis and other STDs.

Sexually Transmitted Diseases

If you think you have a sexually transmitted disease (STD), see a physician immediately. If an STD is diagnosed, it is important that you share the information of a confirmed STD with your sexual partner(s). In all cases of STD, abstain from sexual contact until the infection is eliminated completely.

Signs and Symptoms	About the Disease	How Serious Is It?	Medical Treatment

AIDS

Signs and Symptoms	About the Disease	How Serious Is It?	Medical Treatment
• Persistent, unexplained fatigue • Soaking night sweats • Shaking chills or fever higher than 100 F for several weeks • Swelling of lymph nodes for more than 3 months • Chronic diarrhea • Persistent headaches • Dry cough and shortness of breath	AIDS, caused by HIV. Unfortunately, an HIV test is not accurate immediately after exposure, because it takes time for your body to develop or make antibodies. It can take up to 6 months to detect this antibody response	HIV weakens the immune system to the point that opportunistic diseases (ones that your body would normally fight off) begin to affect you. AIDS is a fatal illness, although there have been significant recent advances in the treatment of AIDS	There is no vaccine for AIDS. Treatment includes use of antiviral drugs, immune system boosters and medications to help prevent or treat opportunistic infections. A new class of drugs, called protease inhibitors, has shown promise

Chlamydia infection

Signs and Symptoms	About the Disease	How Serious Is It?	Medical Treatment
• Painful urination • Vaginal discharge in women • Urethral discharge in men • Infection may have no symptoms	Can cause scarring of fallopian tubes in women and prostatitis or epididymitis in men	Touching your eye with infectious secretions can cause eye infection. A mother can pass the infection to her child during delivery, causing pneumonia or eye infection	Antibiotics are prescribed. The infection should disappear within 1 to 2 weeks. All sexual partners must be treated, even though they may not have symptoms. Otherwise, they will pass the disease back and forth between them

Genital herpes

Signs and Symptoms	About the Disease	How Serious Is It?	Medical Treatment
• Pain or itching in the genital area • Water blisters or open sores • Genital sores may be present but invisible inside the vagina (women) or urethra (men) • Recurrent outbreaks	Caused by the herpes simplex virus, usually type 2. Symptoms begin 2 to 7 days after exposure. Itching or burning is followed by blisters and sores. They erupt in the vagina or on the labia, buttocks and anus. In men, on the penis, scrotum, buttocks, anus and thighs. Virus remains dormant in the infected areas and periodically reactivates, causing symptoms	There is no cure or vaccine. The disease is very contagious whenever sores are present. Newborn infants can become infected as they pass through the birth canal of mothers with open sores	Self-care consists of keeping sores clean and dry. The prescription antiviral drug acyclovir helps speed healing. If recurrences are frequent, oral acyclovir can be taken daily to suppress the virus. Another antiviral drug, famciclovir, also is available by prescription

Signs and Symptoms	About the Disease	How Serious Is It?	Medical Treatment

Genital warts

Signs and Symptoms	About the Disease	How Serious Is It?	Medical Treatment
• Warty growths on the genitals, anus, groin, urethra	Venereal warts or genital warts are caused by the human papilloma virus (HPV). They affect both men and women. Persons with impaired immune systems and pregnant women are more susceptible	Generally not serious, but contagious. Women with a history of genital warts have a higher risk of cervical cancer and should get yearly Pap smear	Warts are removed with medication, cryosurgery (freezing), lasers or electrical current. These procedures may require local or general anesthesia

Gonorrhea

Signs and Symptoms	About the Disease	How Serious Is It?	Medical Treatment
• Thick, pus-like discharge from urethra • Burning, frequent urination • Slight increase in vaginal discharge and inflammation in women • Anal discharge or irritation • Occasionally fever and abdominal pain	Gonorrhea is caused by bacteria. In men, first symptoms appear between 2 days and 2 weeks after exposure. In women, symptoms may not appear for 1 to 3 weeks. Infection usually affects the cervix and sometimes the fallopian tubes	Highly contagious, acute infection that may become chronic. In men, it may lead to epididymitis. In women, it can spread to fallopian tubes and cause pelvic inflammatory disease. May result in scarring of the tubes and infertility. Rarely causes joint or throat infection	Many antibiotics are safe and effective for treating gonorrhea. Although treatable, gonorrhea is becoming resistant to some antibiotics. It may be cured with a single injection of ceftriaxone. Oral antibiotics (cefixime, ciprofloxacin) also are effective

Hepatitis B

Signs and Symptoms	About the Disease	How Serious Is It?	Medical Treatment
• Skin and eyes are yellowish • Urine is tea-colored • Flu-like illness • Fatigue and achiness • Fever	Hepatitis B is caused by a virus. Some carriers never have symptoms but are capable of passing the virus to others	A pregnant woman may pass the virus to her developing fetus. Rarely causes liver failure and death	No antiviral treatment. Bed rest is not essential, although it may help you feel better. Maintain good nutrition. Abstain from alcohol use because of damage to the liver. Preventable by vaccination

Syphilis

Signs and Symptoms	About the Disease	How Serious Is It?	Medical Treatment
• Painless sores on the genitals, rectum, tongue or lips • Enlarged lymph nodes in the groin • Rash over any area of the body, especially on palms and soles • Fever • Headache • Soreness and aching in bones or joints	Syphilis is a complex disease caused by a bacterium. Primary stage, painless sores appear in the genital area, rectum or mouth 10 days to 6 weeks after exposure. Second stage, 1 week to 6 months later; red rash may appear anywhere on skin. Third stage, often after years-long latent period; heart disease, mental deterioration	It can be completely cured if the diagnosis is made early and the infection is treated. Left untreated, the disease can lead to death. In pregnant women, it can be transmitted to the fetus, causing deformities and death	Usually treated with penicillin. Other antibiotics can be used for patients allergic to penicillin. A person usually can no longer transmit syphilis 24 hours after beginning therapy. Some people do not respond to the usual doses of penicillin. They must get periodic blood tests to make sure the infectious agent has been destroyed

Mental Health

- **Addictive Behavior**
- **Alcohol Abuse and Alcoholism**
- **Anxiety and Panic Disorders**
- **Depression and the "Blues"**
- **Domestic Abuse**
- **Memory Loss**

In this section, we discuss a range of topics that affect the mental health of millions of Americans and their families. We offer helpful information on how to deal with addictive behavior (including drug use and alcoholism), depression, anxiety, domestic abuse and memory loss.

Addictive Behavior

You can be addicted to many substances and practices. The main trait of addictive behavior is a compelling need to engage in the activity or to use the addictive substance. In this chapter, we discuss caffeine addiction, drug dependency and compulsive gambling. In the next chapter, we discuss use and abuse of alcohol. See page 206 for information on nicotine addiction.

■ Caffeine Addiction

Caffeine occurs naturally in coffee, tea and chocolate. Caffeine frequently is added to soft drinks and over-the-counter drugs, including headache and cold tablets, stay awake medications and allergy remedies.

Although relying on caffeine is not recognized medically as a drug addiction, you still may feel "hooked." You may feel a "caffeine high" and you don't feel right until you've reached your high. When you try to give up caffeine, you get a headache and often feel drowsy. Other signs that you may be using too much caffeine include tiredness, irritability, nervousness, vague depression or frequent yawning.

Self-Care

If caffeine is bothering you, or you feel "hooked," try the following:
- If you drink more than 4 servings per day of caffeine-containing beverages, decrease your intake gradually (1 serving per day).
- When you are thirsty, drink decaffeinated beverages or water.
- Mix decaffeinated coffee in with your regular coffee before brewing.
- Substitute regular instant coffee, which contains less caffeine than brewed coffee.
- Switch to tea or other beverages. Be careful when switching to herb teas, however. Some types, particularly homemade varieties, can have the same effects as coffee, or worse.
- Symptoms should begin clearing in 4 to 10 days.

Caffeine Content of Common Beverages, Foods and Medications

	Milligrams of Caffeine*		Milligrams of Caffeine*		Milligrams of Caffeine*
Coffee, 5 ounces		Coca-Cola	46	Semisweet chocolate,	
Brewed, percolator	115	Diet Coke	46	1 ounce	6
Brewed, drip method	80	Shasta Cola	44	Chocolate syrup, 1 ounce	4
Instant	65	Mr. Pibb	41	OTC† medications	
Tea, 5 ounces		Dr. Pepper	40	Vivarin (1 tablet)	200
Brewed, imported	60	Pepsi Cola	38	No-Doz (maximum	
Brewed, U.S. brands	40	Diet Pepsi	36	strength, 1 tablet)	200
Instant	30	RC Cola	36	Excedrin‡ (aspirin-free	
Iced (12 ounces)	70	7-Up, Sprite, Crush and		extra strength, 1 tablet)	65
Soft drinks, 12 ounces		A&W Root Beer	0	Midol‡ (maximum	
Mountain Dew	55	Cocoa, 5 ounces	4	strength, 1 tablet)	60
Mellow Yellow	53	Chocolate milk, 8 ounces	5	Vanquish‡ (1 tablet)	33

*Average amounts, except for medications.
†OTC, Over-the-counter.
‡Excedrin, Midol and Vanquish also contain other active ingredients.

■ Drug Dependency

Dependency on drugs, whether prescription or illegal, is dangerous because of its long-term physical effects, its disruptive effect on family and work and the risks associated with sudden withdrawal. Illegal drugs are hazardous not only by their nature but also because of the risk of contamination with toxic or infectious substances. In most cases, help is essential to quitting.

Common Drugs of Abuse

Glue: Young children may sniff glue, which is a central nervous system depressant. At first, a few sniffs may give a "high," but the child develops a tolerance in a matter of weeks. The initial symptoms mimic alcoholic inebriation, including slurred speech, dizziness, breakdown of inhibitions, drowsiness and amnesia. The child may have hallucinations, lose weight and lose consciousness.

Central nervous system stimulants (amphetamines and cocaine): Known as "uppers," amphetamines produce an extraordinarily strong psychological addiction that amounts to a compulsion. Abusers develop a high degree of tolerance to the euphoric effects, which last for several hours. Cocaine triggers the release of chemicals in your body which stimulate your heart to pump faster and harder. These reactions result in the rush of euphoria, the illusion of control and heightened sexual drive. Even a modest dose of cocaine can kill you. Injecting or smoking cocaine (called "crack") can be more dangerous because a greater amount of it goes into your bloodstream.

Opioids: Opium is produced from the milky discharge from seeds of the poppy plant. Opioids include opiates (substances naturally produced from opium, such as heroin and morphine) and synthetic substances that have morphine-like action. Physicians may prescribe them as pain relievers, anesthetics or cough suppressants (such as codeine and methadone). Signs of abuse include depression, anxiety, impulsiveness, low frustration tolerance and the need for immediate gratification.

Marijuana and hashish: Marijuana is made from the leaves and flowers of the hemp plant, *Cannabis sativa.* Hashish comes from the concentrated resin of the same plant. Your body absorbs the psychoactive substances in these drugs. If you are acutely intoxicated with marijuana or hashish, you feel relaxed and euphoric. These compounds affect your concentration and perceptual and motor functions. Chronic users have an increased heart rate, redness of the eyes and a decrease in lung function. Withdrawal symptoms include sweating, tremors, nausea, vomiting, diarrhea, irritability and difficulty sleeping.

Hallucinogens: LSD (lysergic acid diethylamide) produces profound changes in mood and thought processes, resulting in hallucinations and a state resembling acute psychosis. Acute panic reactions may occur, as may rapid heart rate, hypertension and tremors. The most common street preparation of PCP (phencyclidine) is called "angel dust," a white granular powder. In low doses (5 mg), PCP produces excitement, incoordination and absence of sensation (analgesic). In high doses, it can cause drooling, vomiting, stupor or coma. When there is acute psychosis associated with PCP, the person is at high risk for suicide or violence toward others.

Designer drugs have become increasingly popular in the '90s. They are formulated to achieve specific effects and to chemically modify existing drugs to avoid criminal prosecution under existing laws. Common names include "ecstasy," "Adam," "Eve" and "China white." Use of these drugs produces intoxication and has caused serious medical conditions, including movement disorders and death.

Medical Help

Drug users may require an intervention on the part of family and friends. The drug user may require hospitalization for detoxification. Follow-up outpatient programs (support groups, day care or residential) lasting weeks or months may be necessary to prevent a relapse.

FOR MORE INFORMATION
- National Institute of Drug Abuse Hotline, (800) 662-HELP.
- Narcotics Anonymous (NA), World Office, P.O. Box 9999, Van Nuys, CA 91409-9999; (818) 773-9999.

How to Identify Drug Use Among Teenagers

These clues are only possible indications that your teenager is using drugs:
- **School:** The child suddenly shows an active dislike of school and looks for excuses to stay home. Contact school officials to see if your child's attendance record matches what you know about his or her absent days. An A or B student who suddenly begins to fail courses or receives only minimally passing grades may be using drugs.
- **Physical health:** Listlessness and apathy are possible indications of drug use.
- **Appearance** is extremely important to adolescents. A significant warning sign can be a sudden lack of interest in clothing or looks.
- **Personal behavior:** Teenagers enjoy their privacy. However, be wary of exaggerated efforts to bar you from going into their bedrooms or knowing where they go with their friends.
- **Money:** Sudden requests for more money without a reasonable explanation for its use may be an indication of drug use.

What can you do?

Adolescents need to feel that there is an open line of communication with their parents. Even in the face of your child's reluctance to share feelings, continue to express an interest in listening to your child talk about his or her experiences.

■ Compulsive Gambling

Pathologic gambling tends to be a more common compulsion among men than among women. It often goes hand-in-hand with excessive drinking. It is serious to the extent that it disrupts your personal life and may cause financial ruin.

Some experts warn that an increasing number of teenagers are addicted to gambling. Signs and symptoms include the following:
- Progressive gambling proceeds from occasional to habitual, usually with higher and higher stakes. Family, work and other interests may be neglected.
- Craving for the tension derived from the risk of gambling.
- Guilt feelings over lost money and concealment of losses.
- Lying to conceal losses.
- Gambling, whether winning or losing, until the place closes or no money is left.
- Resorting to unlawful activities in order to afford the habit and pay debts.

Medical Help

Alert your physician or a mental health professional if you or a family member needs help. Treatment includes psychotherapy and support groups such as Gamblers Anonymous.

Alcohol Abuse and Alcoholism

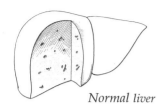

Normal liver

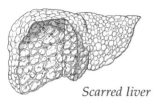

Scarred liver

Excessive alcohol intake can damage body tissues, particularly the liver. Excess use can cause scarring, called cirrhosis.

Alcoholism and alcohol abuse cause major social, economic and public health problems. Each year, more than 100,000 people die of alcohol-related causes. The annual cost of lost productivity and health expenses related to alcoholism is more than $100 billion. According to the National Council on Alcoholism and Drug Dependence, more than 13 million Americans abuse alcohol.

How Alcohol Works in Your Body

The form of alcohol in the beverages we drink is ethyl alcohol (ethanol), a colorless liquid that in its pure form has a burning taste. Ethanol is produced by the fermentation of sugars, which occur naturally in grains and fruits such as barley and grapes.

When you drink alcohol, it depresses your central nervous system by acting as a sedative. In some people, the initial reaction may be stimulation, but as drinking continues, sedating or calming effects occur. By depressing the control centers of your brain, it relaxes you and reduces your inhibitions. The more you drink, the more you are sedated. Initially, alcohol affects areas of thought, emotion and judgment. In sufficient amounts, alcohol impairs speech and muscle coordination and produces sleep. Taken in large enough quantities, alcohol is a lethal poison—it can cause life-threatening coma by severely depressing the vital centers of your brain.

Excessive use of alcohol can produce several harmful effects on your brain and nervous system. It also can severely damage your liver, pancreas and cardiovascular system. Alcohol use in pregnant women can damage the fetus.

Alcohol Intoxication

The intoxicating effects of alcohol relate to the concentration of alcohol in the blood. For example, if you are not a regular drinker and your blood alcohol concentration is more than 100 mg/dL (milligrams of alcohol per deciliter of blood), you may be quite intoxicated and have difficulty speaking, thinking and moving around. As your blood alcohol concentration increases, mild confusion may give way to stupor and, ultimately, coma. Alcoholics and regular drinkers develop a tolerance for alcohol.

How much food you have eaten and how recently you ate before drinking affect how you respond to alcohol. Size, body fat and tolerance to the effects of alcohol also play significant roles. Drinking equal amounts of alcohol may have a greater effect on a woman than on a man. Women generally have a higher blood alcohol concentration per drink because of their smaller size and less dilution of the alcohol. They also may metabolize alcohol more slowly than men.

Most states define legal intoxication as a blood alcohol concentration of at least 70 to 100 mg/dL, or 0.1 percent. Even at concentrations much lower than the legal limit, some people lose coordination and reaction time.

What Is Alcohol Abuse?

Drinking problems in people who do not have all the characteristics of alcoholism are often referred to as "alcohol abuse" or "problem drinking." These individuals engage in excessive drinking that results in health or social problems but are not dependent on alcohol and have not fully lost control over the use of alcohol.

Self-Administered Alcoholism Screening Test

To screen for alcoholism, Mayo Clinic developed the Self-Administered Alcoholism Screening Test (SAAST) in 1982. The SAAST consists of 37 questions. The test can identify 95 percent of alcoholics who are ill enough to be hospitalized.

The SAAST tries to identify behaviors, medical symptoms and consequences of drinking in the alcoholic. Here is a sample of questions from the test:

1. Do you have a drink now and then?
2. Do you feel you are a normal drinker (that is, drink no more than average)?
3. Have you ever awakened the morning after drinking the previous evening and found that you could not remember a part of the evening?
4. Do close relatives ever worry or complain about your drinking?
5. Can you stop drinking without a struggle after one or two drinks?
6. Do you ever feel guilty about your drinking?
7. Do friends or relatives think you are a normal drinker?
8. Are you always able to stop drinking when you want to?
9. Have you ever attended a meeting of Alcoholics Anonymous (AA) because of your drinking?
10. Have you gotten into physical fights when drinking?

These responses suggest you are at risk for alcoholism: 1. Yes; 2. No; 3. Yes; 4. Yes; 5. No; 6. Yes; 7. No; 8. No; 9. Yes; 10. Yes.

If you answered three or four of the questions with the responses listed, you likely have a drinking problem and need professional evaluation.

What Is Alcoholism?

Alcoholism is a chronic disease. It is often progressive and fatal. It is characterized by periods of preoccupation with alcohol and impaired control over alcohol intake. There is continued use despite adverse consequences and distortion in thinking. Most alcoholics deny there is a problem. Other signs include:

- Drinking alone or in secret
- Not remembering conversations or commitments
- Making a ritual of having drinks before, with or after dinner and becoming annoyed when this ritual is disturbed or questioned
- Losing interest in activities and hobbies that used to bring pleasure
- Irritability as usual drinking time nears, especially if alcohol isn't available
- Keeping alcohol in unlikely places at home, at work or in the car
- Gulping drinks, ordering doubles, becoming intoxicated intentionally to feel good or drinking to feel "normal"
- Having problems with relationships, employment or finances or legal problems

■ Treating Alcoholism and Alcohol Abuse

Most alcoholics, and alcohol abusers, enter treatment reluctantly because they deny the problem. They often must be pressured. Health or legal problems may prompt treatment.

Intervention is a process that helps an alcoholic recognize and accept the need for treatment. If you're concerned about a friend or family member, discuss intervention with a professional. The following suggestions may help an intervention:

- **Choose the right time to talk.** A good time is right after recovering from a drinking incident, *not* while the person is drinking or intoxicated.
- **Involve multiple people** who are concerned about the individual.
- **Have an assessment and treatment plan** ready as part of the intervention.

■ Individualized Treatment

A wide range of treatments are available to help people with alcohol problems. Treatment should be tailored to the individual. Treatment may involve an evaluation, a brief intervention, an outpatient program or counseling or a residential inpatient stay.

It is important to first determine whether you are alcohol-dependent. If you have not lost control over your use of alcohol, your treatment may involve reducing your drinking. If you are an alcohol abuser, you may be able to modify your drinking. If you have alcoholism, cutting back is ineffective and inappropriate. Abstinence must be a part of the alcoholic's treatment goal.

For people who are not dependent on alcohol but are experiencing the adverse effects of drinking, the goal of treatment is reduction of alcohol-related problems, often by counseling or a brief intervention. A brief intervention usually involves alcohol-abuse specialists who can establish a specific treatment plan. Interventions may include goal setting, behavioral modification techniques, use of self-help manuals, counseling and follow-up care at a treatment center.

The most common residential alcoholism treatment programs in the United States are based on the "Minnesota Model." This includes abstinence, individual and group therapy, participation in Alcoholics Anonymous, educational lectures, family involvement, work assignments, activity therapy and use of counselors (many of whom are recovering alcoholics) and multiprofessional staff. (Contact your insurance provider to determine whether residential treatment is included in your coverage.)

In addition to residential treatment, there are many other approaches including acupuncture, biofeedback, motivational enhancement therapy, cognitive-behavioral therapy and aversion therapy. Aversion therapy involves pairing the drinking of alcohol with a strong aversive response such as nausea or vomiting induced by a medication. After repeated pairing, the alcohol itself causes the aversive response and that decreases the likelihood of relapse. For obvious reasons, aversion therapy tends to be unappealing, although it is often effective.

Coping With Teenage Drinking

Although it may take years for many adults to develop alcohol dependence, teenagers can become addicted in months. Use among teens increases dramatically during the 10th and 11th grades. Each year in the United States, more than 2,000 young people between the ages of 15 and 20 die in alcohol-related automobile accidents, and many more are left disabled. Alcohol also is often implicated in other teenage deaths, including drownings, suicides and fires.

For young people, the likelihood of addiction depends on the influence of parents, peers and other role models, susceptibility to advertising, how early in life they begin to use alcohol, their psychological need for alcohol and genetic factors (family or parental alcoholism) that may predispose them to addiction.

Look for these signs:
● Loses interest in activities and hobbies
● Appears anxious, irritable
● Has difficulties or changes in relationships with friends; joins a new crowd
● Grades drop

To prevent teenage alcohol use:
● Set a good example regarding alcohol use.
● Communicate with your children.
● Discuss the legal and medical consequences of drinking.

The Minnesota Model

Here is what you might expect from a typical residential treatment program based in part on the "Minnesota Model."

- **Detoxification and withdrawal:** Treatment may begin with a program of detoxification. This usually takes about 4 to 7 days. Medications may be necessary to prevent delirium tremens (DTs) or other withdrawal seizures.
- **Medical assessment and treatment:** Common medical problems related to alcoholism are high blood pressure, increased blood sugar and liver and heart disease.
- **Psychological support and psychiatric treatment:** Group and individual counseling and therapy support recovery from the psychological aspects of alcoholism. Sometimes, emotional symptoms of the disease may mimic psychiatric disorders.
- **Recovery programs:** Detoxification and medical treatment are only the first steps for most people in a residential treatment program.
- **Acceptance and abstinence are emphasized:** Effective treatment is impossible unless you can accept that you are addicted and unable to control your drinking.
- **Drug treatments:** An alcohol-sensitizing drug called disulfiram (Antabuse) may be useful. If you drink alcohol, the drug produces a severe physical reaction that includes flushing, nausea, vomiting and headaches. Disulfiram will not cure alcoholism nor can it remove the compulsion to drink. But it can be a strong deterrent. Naltrexone, a drug long known to block the narcotic "high," recently has been found to reduce the urge to drink in recovering alcoholics. Unlike disulfiram, however, naltrexone does not cause a reaction within a few minutes of taking a drink. Naltrexone can produce side effects, particularly liver damage.
- **Continuing support:** Aftercare programs and Alcoholics Anonymous help recovering alcoholics maintain abstinence from alcohol, help to manage any relapses and help with needed lifestyle changes.

FOR MORE INFORMATION

- Alcoholics Anonymous, General Service Office, 475 Riverside Drive, New York, NY 10115. (Refer to your telephone book for local phone number.)
- Al-Anon Family Group Headquarters, Inc., 1600 Corporate Landing Parkway, Virginia Beach, VA 23454-5617; (800) 356-9996.
- National Council on Alcoholism and Drug Dependence, 12 West 21st Street, New York, NY 10010; 24-hour referral (800) NCA-CALL.

Treatment for Hangover: Avoid Alcohol Altogether

Even small amounts of alcohol can cause unpleasant side effects. Some people develop a flushed feeling, whereas others are sensitive to the chemical tyramine found in red wines, brandy and cognac.

The classic hangover, although well-studied, isn't fully understood. It's probably due to dehydration, by-products from the breakdown of alcohol, liver injury, overeating and disturbed sleep.

The best treatment for hangovers is to avoid alcohol altogether. The next best thing is to drink in moderation.

But if you have a hangover, it's too late to do much to improve your health and function. A lot of hangover remedies have been tried, but there isn't much evidence that they help—and they may hurt.

If you have a hangover, follow this advice:
- Rest and rehydrate. Drink bland liquids (water, soda, some fruit juices or broth). Avoid acidic, caffeinated or alcohol-containing beverages.
- Use over-the-counter pain medication with care. See page 231.

Anxiety and Panic Disorders

It can happen at any time. Suddenly, your heart begins to race, your face flushes and you have trouble breathing. You feel dizzy, nauseated, out of control—some people even feel like they are dying. Each year, thousands of Americans have an experience like this. Many, thinking they're having a heart attack, go to an emergency room. Others try to ignore it, not realizing that they've experienced a panic attack.

Panic attacks are sudden episodes of intense fear that prompt physical reactions in your body. Ten to 20 percent of Americans will have an attack like this at some time in their lives. Once dismissed as "nerves" or stress, a panic attack is now recognized as a potentially disabling but treatable condition.

Tripping an Alarm System

Panic attacks typically begin in young adulthood and can happen throughout your life. An episode usually begins abruptly, peaks within 10 minutes and lasts about half an hour. Symptoms can include a rapid heart rate, sweating, trembling and shortness of breath. You may have chills, hot flashes, nausea, abdominal cramping, chest pain and dizziness. Tightness in your throat or trouble swallowing is common.

If panic attacks are frequent, or if fear of having them affects your activities, you may have a condition called panic disorder. Women are more likely than men to have panic attacks. Researchers aren't sure why or what causes panic attacks. Heredity may play a role—your chance of having panic attacks increases if you have a close family member who has had them.

Many researchers believe your body's natural fight-or-flight response to danger is involved. For example, if a grizzly bear came after you, your body would react instinctively. Your heart and breathing would speed up as your body readied itself for a life-threatening situation. Many of the same reactions occur in a panic attack. No obvious stressor is present, but something trips your body's alarm system.

Other health problems—such as an impending heart attack, hyperthyroidism or drug withdrawal—can cause symptoms similar to panic attacks. If you have symptoms of a panic attack, seek medical care.

Treatment Options

Fortunately, treatment for panic attacks and panic disorder is very effective. Most people are able to resume everyday activities. Treatment may involve:

- **Education:** Knowing what you experienced is the first step in learning to manage it. Your doctor may give you information and teach you coping techniques.
- **Medication:** Your doctor may prescribe an antidepressant, which usually is effective for preventing future attacks. In some cases, a tranquilizer may be given alone or with other medications. Effectiveness varies. The duration of treatment depends on the severity of your disorder and your response to treatment.
- **Therapy:** During sessions with a psychiatrist or psychologist, coping skills and management of anxiety triggers are taught. Most people need only 8 to 10 sessions. Long-term psychotherapy usually isn't necessary.
- **Relaxation techniques:** See page 211.

FOR MORE INFORMATION

National Mental Health Association, 1021 Prince Street, Alexandria, VA 22314-2971; (800) 969-6642; Internet address: http://www.nmha.org.

Depression and the "Blues"

We've all had the blues from time to time—a period of several days or a week in which we seem to be in a "funk." This condition usually goes away and we resume our normal patterns. Nevertheless, having the blues is troublesome, and there are some things we can do to avoid having them.

Having the blues is not the same as having clinical depression. The blues are temporary and usually go away after a short time.

Depression is a persistent medical problem, but one that can be treated. It may improve eventually, but leaving it untreated typically means it will persist for many months or longer. A depressed person finds little, if any, joy in life. Someone who is depressed may have no energy, feel unworthy or guilty for no reason, find it difficult to concentrate or be irritable. A depressed person may wake up after only a few hours of sleep. He or she may have changes in appetite—eating less than usual or eating too much. Someone who is depressed may experience a sense of hopelessness or even consider suicide (see page 190). A person with depression may have some, most or all of these symptoms.

The following list shows the different signs for depression and the blues.

Signs of depression
- Persistent lack of energy
- Lasting sadness
- Irritability and mood swings
- Recurring sense of hopelessness
- Continual negative view of the world and others
- Overeating or loss of appetite
- Feelings of unworthiness or guilt
- Inability to concentrate, poor memory
- Recurrent early morning awakening or other changes in sleep patterns
- Inability to enjoy pleasurable activities

Signs of the blues
- Feeling down for a few days but still able to function normally in daily activities
- Occasional lack of energy, or a mild change in sleeping patterns
- Ability to enjoy some recreational activities
- Stable weight
- A quickly passing feeling of hopelessness

Self-Care for the Blues

If your mood falls into the "blues" column, try these things:
- Share your feelings. Talk to a trusted friend, spouse, family member or your pastor, priest or rabbi. They can offer you support, guidance and perspective.
- Spend time with other people.
- Engage in activities that have interested you in the past, particularly activities that you have enjoyed.
- Regular moderate exercise may lift your mood.
- Get adequate rest and eat balanced meals.
- Don't undertake too much at one time. If you have large tasks to do, break them into smaller ones. Set goals you can accomplish.
- Look for small opportunities to be helpful to someone less fortunate.

Causes of Depression

Every year in the United States, more than 17 million adults have a depressive illness. Occasionally, it is a side effect of a prescription drug, illness or poor diet. Imbalances of certain brain chemicals may be a factor. But often the cause is unclear.

You are at a higher risk for depression if a blood relative has had it. Depression also may recur. If you've had it once, you're at a higher risk to develop it again. Don't let these factors control your life. But be aware of them in assessing your mood. And don't delay seeking medical attention if you notice recurrent depressive symptoms. Also, if you're being treated for depression by one clinician, let your other health-care providers know so confusion and medication interactions can be avoided.

Depression also may be preceded by a severe shock or stress in life, such as the death of a loved one (see below) or the loss of a job, or it can arise when things are going very well. Certainly it's normal to feel sad after losses or setbacks. But if that sadness doesn't stop fairly quickly, a serious depression likely has developed.

Depression may not go away by itself. Don't expect to snap out of it all of a sudden or expect to be able to beat your depression through sheer determination. If depressive symptoms last more than a few weeks, or if you're feeling hopeless or suicidal, it's time to seek help. Don't blame yourself for feeling depressed. It's not your fault, and it's not a sign of weakness.

Contact your family doctor or ask for a referral to a psychiatrist. A psychiatrist, just as your family physician, is trained as a medical doctor and can help you exclude significant medical illnesses that might be contributing to your symptoms.

If your symptoms have been mild—but persistent—a psychologist (who is trained in various types of "talking therapy" but does not have a medical degree) may be very helpful. Discussing feelings with a family member or close friend is helpful, but it's no substitute for seeking professional help.

If you know someone who is depressed, invite him or her to take part in normal social activities. Gently but firmly encourage participation. But don't overdo it. The role of friends and family in helping people with depression is to encourage and support professional care. The problem shouldn't be trivialized, but rather it should be viewed as an opportunity to help, because depression can be treated successfully in most cases. Offer reassurance that things will get better, but don't expect a depressed person to improve suddenly. Don't minimize a depressed person's feelings. Instead, listen carefully to what he or she says.

Seasonal affective disorder, another form of depression, seems to be related to light exposure. It occurs more in northern climates in winter, when days are shorter. It affects women more than men and sometimes is treated with increased light exposure during the day, obtained with a light box (a source of bright broad-spectrum light).

Coping With Loss: Practical Suggestions

- **Express your feelings.** Write a book of memories, or even a letter to the person who died.
- **Ask for help.** When we experience sudden loss, our friends may not know how to respond. We can relieve others and help ourselves by asking for specific kinds of help.

- **Stay involved.** People who grieve may need to remind themselves about exercise, diet and rest.
- **When indicated, evaluate for depression.** If the grief is extremely severe in the short run or persistent over the long run (6 months or more), then consider depression as a possible cause.

■ Treatment Options

Most people who have depression improve a great deal when treated with antidepressant medicines. There are more than a dozen such medicines, some of which work in different ways. A physician, frequently a psychiatrist or family doctor, will select a medicine likely to be helpful. Discuss potential side effects with your physician. If you experience symptoms that concern you, call the physician who prescribed the medication. Common side effects may include dry mouth, rash, dizziness, constipation or jitteriness.

Other treatment methods include psychotherapy—talking about your feelings—and programs with a psychiatrist, psychologist or other qualified professional. There are various kinds of psychotherapy, some involving just the patient and the therapist, others involving a group of people with the same general problem who meet to discuss their situation under the guidance of a therapist.

Treatment takes time. Although some signs of change may be evident in as little as 2 weeks, full benefit may require 6 weeks or more. That lengthy process can be discouraging, so it's important for friends and family to provide support and encouragement during this time when medications may need ongoing adjustment.

Someone who is being treated should not expect a sudden dramatic change in mood and activity. Look for gradual improvement in sleep and a slow improvement in appetite and level of energy. The person's mood and overall sense of well-being will also show gradual positive shifts.

Aside from making sure that the person providing the treatment is qualified, it's important to feel comfortable with your clinician. He or she should listen to you describe your problem, ask questions, discuss findings and recommendations and explain possible risks and alternatives to the treatments being recommended.

Warning Signs of Potential Suicide

It is important to keep in mind that these warning signs are only guidelines. There is no one type of suicidal person. If you are concerned, seek help immediately.

- **Withdrawal:** Unwilling to communicate and appears to have an overwhelming urge to be alone.
- **Moodiness:** An emotional high one day followed by being down in the dumps. Sudden, inexplicable calm.
- **Life crisis or trauma:** Divorce, death, an accident or the loss of self-esteem that may occur after loss of a job or a financial setback may produce suicidal thinking.
- **Personality change:** A change in attitude, personal appearance or activities. An introvert suddenly becomes an extrovert.
- **Threats:** The popular assumption that people who threaten suicide don't do it is not true.
- **Gift giving:** The person "bequeaths" cherished belongings to friends and loved ones.
- **Depression:** The person appears to be physically depressed and may be unable to function socially or in the workplace.
- **Risk taking:** The suicidal urge may be manifested in sudden participation in high-speed driving or unsafe sex.

FOR MORE INFORMATION

- National Mental Health Association, 1021 Prince Street, Alexandria, VA 22314-2971; (800) 969-6642; Internet address: http://www.nmha.org.

Domestic Abuse

Beatings, forced sex, being afraid of violence from a spouse or partner or living in fear that your spouse or partner will harm or abuse your children: all of these situations are examples of domestic abuse.

Women predominantly, but not exclusively, suffer domestic abuse. Between 2 million and 4 million women are battered and 1,500 women are murdered annually by a husband, ex-husband or partner. Domestic violence can happen among all races, ages, income and religious groups.

Battering is the use of physical force to control and maintain power over another person. Domestic abuse also may involve intimidation, psychological abuse, harassment, humiliation and threats.

Symptoms of Abusive Behavior

You may be in an abusive relationship if you:

- Have ever been hit, kicked, shoved or threatened with violence
- Feel that you have no choice about how you spend your time, where you go or what you wear
- Have been accused by your partner of things you've never done
- Must ask your partner for permission to make everyday decisions
- Go along with your partner's decisions because you're afraid of his anger

Self-Care

How to Respond

- If you are concerned about the potential for physical abuse, talk to someone as soon as possible. Local crisis hotlines are one option. Social service agencies are another. Confide in a friend, physician or member of the clergy.
- If you are in an abusive relationship, have a flight plan. Be prepared to take your children, house keys and important papers. It's important to be alert. Be ready to leave at a moment's notice.
- Keep cash on hand in case of an emergency.
- Keep a list of phone numbers of friends who may be able to help you.
- Know the number of a women's shelter.

Professional Help

Some people are reluctant to discuss these issues because it's embarrassing to talk openly about such matters with strangers. But by calling a social service agency or confiding in a counselor, feelings of embarrassment or shame can be discussed.

If police are called, request a timely and serious response. Some jurisdictions have a mandatory arrest law, which means that an abuser will be removed from the home while the case is adjudicated.

If you go to a shelter, expect to be safe and to receive counseling. You should also inquire about legal assistance (for instance, the possibility of obtaining a restraining order that would legally bar the abuser from having contact with you).

Counseling also should be available as a means to provide support and discussion of your feelings. Counselors should discuss with you the decision as to whether to pursue legal action.

FOR MORE INFORMATION

- National Domestic Violence Hotline, (800) 799-7233.
- National Organization for Victim Assistance, (202) 232-6682.

Memory Loss

All of us experience short-term memory loss. We can't remember where we put the car keys, or we forget the name of a person we just met. This is normal. But if memory loss is persistent, you need to see a health-care professional.

We were born with billions of brain cells. As we age, some of these brain cells die and are not replaced. As we grow older, our bodies also produce less of the chemicals that our brain cells need to work. Although short-term and long-term memory aren't usually affected, recent memory can deteriorate with age.

The three types of memory are described below:
- **Short-term memory:** This is your temporary memory. You may look up a number in the phone book, but after you dial the number you forget it. Once you've finished using the information, it vanishes.
- **Recent memory:** This is memory that preserves the recent past, such as what you ate for breakfast today or what you wore yesterday.
- **Long-term memory:** This is memory that preserves the distant past, such as recollections from childhood.

Memory loss can be caused by many things: a side effect of medications, a head injury, alcoholism or a stroke. Hearing and vision problems can affect memory. Pregnant women sometimes have short-term memory problems. *Dementia* (what used to be referred to as being senile) also causes memory loss.

Alzheimer's disease is the most common form of dementia. Symptoms include gradual loss of memory for recent events and inability to learn new information; a growing tendency to repeat oneself, misplace objects, become confused and get lost; a slow disintegration of personality, judgment and social graces; and increasing irritability, anxiety, depression, confusion and restlessness.

Self-Care to Improve Your Memory

- **Establish a routine.** Managing your daily activities is easier when you follow a routine. (Choose a set time to do household chores: clean the bathroom on Saturday; water the plants on Sunday.)
- **Exercise your "mental muscles."** Play word games, crossword puzzles or other activities that challenge your mental abilities.
- **Practice.** When you walk into a room, make a mental inventory of people you recognize. When you meet someone, repeat his or her name in conversation.
- **Nudge the numbers.** For example, if your wife's birthday is October 3, do something to remind you, such as hum the song "Three Coins in a Fountain."
- **Make associations.** When driving, look for landmarks to associate with your route and name them out loud to imprint them on your memory ("turn at the high school to get to Bob's house").
- **Try not to worry.** Fretting about memory loss can make it worse.
- **Write lists.** Keep track of important tasks and appointments. For example, pay the water bill on a certain day each month.

Medical Help

Consult a health-care provider if you are concerned about memory loss.

FOR MORE INFORMATION
- The Alzheimer's Association, 919 N. Michigan Ave., Suite 1000, Chicago IL 60611-1676; (800) 272-3900; Internet address: http://www.alz.org.

Staying Healthy

- **Weight: What's Right for You?**
- **Eating Well**
- **Lowering Your Cholesterol**
- **Exercise and Fitness**
- **Screening and Immunizations**
- **Smoking and Tobacco Use**
- **Keeping Stress Under Control**
- **Protecting Yourself**

This section is filled with practical information designed to help you maintain and improve your health by establishing and sustaining a healthful lifestyle. You'll find tips on topics such as proper nutrition, weight control, exercise, stress management and prevention of injury and illness.

We also include a lengthy chapter on kicking the smoking habit. Smoking causes more deaths than any other human behavior. As soon as you stop smoking, you reduce your risk of dying from tobacco-related diseases—no matter how long you've smoked.

Weight: What's Right for You?

Many overweight people are stymied by trying to lose weight. We're all bombarded by diets and schemes. Weight loss sells! Being significantly overweight has risks. Success at weight loss requires the key ingredients of knowledge, committment, reasonable eating and regular exercise.

For most overweight Americans, weight loss is a healthy goal. Losing weight often means a reduced risk of heart disease, diabetes and high blood pressure. However, many people, often women, who aren't fat are trying to lose pounds. For them, losing weight offers no healthful benefits and may even be detrimental.

The Risks of Being Overweight

Your desirable weight is the weight at which you're as healthy as possible. And your weight is only one part of the lifestyle picture that contributes to your long-term health.

Being overweight may place you at risk for:

- Increased blood pressure
- Heart disease
- Non-insulin-dependent diabetes mellitus
- Deteriorating joints
- Chronic low back pain
- Gallstones
- Respiratory problems

Anyone who wants to be thinner meets a challenge. Of people who lose weight, as many as 95 percent regain the weight within 5 years. So, what should you do? First, determine whether you are really overweight. If so, develop a safe and healthful weight loss program.

Your body has a nearly unlimited capacity to store fat. Losing weight reduces crowding of your organs and the strain on your lower back, hips and knees.

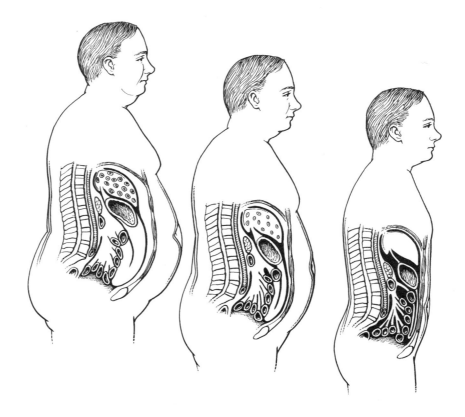

■ What Is Your "Desirable" Weight?

For more than 50 years, insurance companies have related weight to health risk. They evaluate their data to discover the weight of the healthiest people. This chart shows so-called desirable weights. This means that the incidence of health problems is lowest in people whose weight falls within these guidelines.

Because people are all different, desirable weight varies a lot. Take into consideration your body size and shape, how fit you are and whether you have medical conditions. Don't compare yourself to seemingly perfect bodies you see on television and on exercise videos.

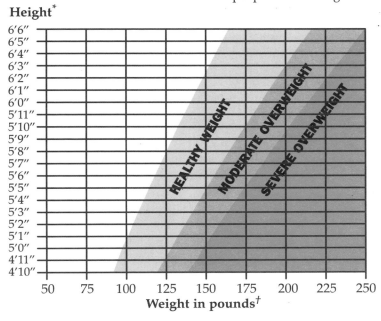

Height*

Heights listed: 6'6", 6'5", 6'4", 6'3", 6'2", 6'1", 6'0", 5'11", 5'10", 5'9", 5'8", 5'7", 5'6", 5'5", 5'4", 5'3", 5'2", 5'1", 5'0", 4'11", 4'10"

HEALTHY WEIGHT   MODERATE OVERWEIGHT   SEVERE OVERWEIGHT

Weight in pounds listed: 50, 75, 100, 125, 150, 175, 200, 225, 250

Weight in pounds†

*Without shoes.
†Without clothes. The higher weights apply to people with more muscle and bone, such as many men.
(From Report of the Dietary Guidelines Advisory Committee on the Dietary Guidelines for Americans, 1995, pages 23-24.)

Staying Healthy

Are You a Pear or an Apple?

Extra weight that settles around your waist (apple-shaped body) puts you at higher risk for heart disease, high blood pressure, stroke and diabetes. However, your health risks may be fairly average if the extra fat is on your hips and thighs (pear-shaped body).

The waist-to-hip ratio helps you evaluate the distribution of body fat:

1. Measure your waist at the narrowest point and your hips at the widest point (over your buttocks).
2. Divide your waist measurement by the number of inches around your hips (for example, 30-inch waist/40-inch hip = 0.75). If you're a woman, your health risks are higher if the number is more than 0.85. If you're a man, your health risks increase with a ratio of more than 1.

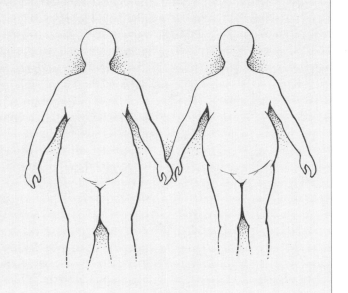

Body Mass Index: A Better Indicator

Recently, we've learned that body fat is a better predictor of health. Chances are, if you're overweight, you're also "overfat." However, highly muscular people weigh more, because muscle weighs more (is denser) than fat.

Body mass index (BMI) is a better indicator of body fat than weight alone, and it helps assess your risk for disease. A lower BMI is better. To calculate your body mass:

1. Multiply your weight in pounds by 0.45 (for example, 150 pounds x 0.45 = 68).
2. Multiply your height in inches by 0.025 (5 feet 10 inches = 70 inches x 0.025 = 1.75).
3. Square your answer from step 2 (1.75 x 1.75 = 3.0).
4. Divide your answer from step 1 by the answer from step 3 (68/3.0 = 22.6). Your estimated BMI is 22.6.

Generally, a healthful BMI ranges from 19 to 25. If your BMI is more than 28, talk with your health-care provider about a weight-control program.

Caution

Weight numbering systems such as the BMI and the waist-to-hip ratio are helpful but don't tell the whole story. Use them as a general guideline. If they don't seem right to you, talk to your health-care provider.

■ Tips on Losing Weight

To lose weight, you need to alter your lifestyle. You will need healthful dietary changes and physical activity in your weight control program. Commit to losing weight, lose weight slowly and work to gradually change your eating habits. It's long-term changes that spell success.

Self-Care

- **Set reasonable weight loss goals** (long- and short-term). If you want to lose 40 pounds, start with a goal of losing 5 pounds.
- **Check your food intake carefully.** Most adults underestimate how many calories they are eating. It's usually reasonable to cut 500 to 1,000 calories per day from what you're currently eating to produce a weight loss of 1 to 2 pounds per week. Diets that restrict you to fewer than 1,000 calories per day seldom meet your daily nutritional needs. Refer to Eating Well, page 198.
- **Keep diet records.** People who write down everything they eat are more successful at long-term weight maintenance.
- **Record the factors that influence your weight control efforts.** Note when you have the urge to eat. Is it tied to your mood, time of day, varieties of food available, a certain activity? Do you eat without thinking much about what you're doing, such as while watching television or reading a newspaper?
- **Learn to enjoy more healthful foods.** See the food pyramid for healthful diet recommendations, page 199.
- **Limit fat to less than 30 percent of your diet**—20 percent if possible. But don't overdo it. Your body needs some fats. You can lower your fat intake dramatically by eating less meat and avoiding fried foods, fat-laden desserts and fatty add-ons such as margarine, mayonnaise and salad dressing.
- **Don't skip meals.** Eating at established times keeps your appetite and food selections under better control. Eating breakfast helps increase your metabolism early in the day, and thus you burn more calories.
- **Try to consume more of your calories earlier in the day.**

Self-Care *(continued)*

- **Limit regular soft drinks and fruit juices.** They can add a lot of calories to your diet. Drink water instead. A moderate intake of diet soft drinks is okay.
- **Use a daily multivitamin** if you're dieting, especially if you limit your calories to 1,000 per day. Avoid expensive, high-dose or "weight-loss formulas."
- **Limit sugar and alcohol.** Both are high in calories and low in other nutrients. Alcohol can increase your appetite and decrease your willpower.
- **Eat slowly.** You'll eat less, because you'll feel fuller.
- **Focus on eating.** Don't do anything else while you eat (such as reading or watching television).
- **Serve yourself and other family members from the stove,** rather than placing the entire dish of food on the table.
- **Use a smaller plate,** serve yourself smaller portions and put down your fork or spoon between bites.
- **Try to ride out food cravings** when they hit. They usually pass in minutes.
- **Keep healthful foods on hand,** both for meals and snacking. Plan snacks.
- **Don't weigh yourself too often**—weekly is fine.
- **Don't start a weight-control program when you're depressed** or going through major life changes. Such ventures are often doomed to failure from the outset.

The health of some people is greatly affected as a result of being overweight (morbidly obese). For them, radical steps, such as medications to suppress appetite (Redux, Pondimin or Fenteramin), fasting or surgery, may be necessary to prevent premature death. Any of these approaches must always be done under the careful supervision of a physician. But, without a change in eating habits, even these radical steps may fail.

■ Physical Activity: The Key to Burning Calories

Exercise is an important part of any weight loss program. But make any changes gradually, especially if you are out-of-shape. If you're older than 40 or a smoker or have had a heart attack or have diabetes, consult your physician before you start a new exercise program. An exercise stress test may be necessary to assess your risks and limitations.

Self-Care

- **Try to find one or more activities that you enjoy** and can do regularly. Begin slowly, and increase gradually to your goal. Your goal is to maintain moderate activity for 30 minutes or more every day.
- **Your activity does not need to be overly strenuous** to produce positive results. You can achieve your goal through moderate, regular exercise like walking.
- **Vary your exercises** to improve overall fitness and to keep it interesting.
- **Find an exercise buddy.** It may help you stick to your schedule.
- **Little things can add up.** Park at the far end of the parking lot. Take the stairs rather than the elevator. Get off the bus a stop or two early and walk.
- **Keep a log of your activity.**
- **Stick with your exercise schedule.** Don't eliminate time for exercise.
- Refer to the chapter Exercise and Fitness, page 202, for more information.

Eating Well

The food we eat is the source of energy and nutrition for our bodies. And, of course, eating is a pleasurable experience for most people. Getting enough food is rarely a problem for most Americans, but getting good nutrition can be a challenge. To feel well, ward off disease and perform at a peak level, you need balanced nutrition.

Many chronic diseases (heart disease, cancer and stroke) are, in part, caused by eating too much of the wrong kinds of food. For most people, the best approach to good nutrition is to follow the principles of food selection advised by the government. The latest revision of the Dietary Guidelines for Americans advises you to do the following:

- **Eat a variety of foods** and consume plenty of vegetables, fruits and grain products.
- **Maintain a healthful weight** (see page 194).
- **Choose a diet low in fat and cholesterol** (see page 201).
- **Limit simple sugars** (sweets) in the diet. Although they don't cause hyperactivity or diabetes, they do add calories that lack other vital nutrients (vitamins and minerals). In addition, they often contribute to obesity, and obesity can cause diabetes. High sugar foods are usually low in other nutrients and contribute to obesity.
- **Limit salt** (sodium) intake by not adding salt to foods and by eating foods that are already salty sparingly. Sodium affects the body's fluid balance and can increase blood pressure.
- **Drink alcohol in moderation**. If you choose to drink, drink moderately. Moderate consumption is defined as no more than one drink per day for non-pregnant women and no more than two drinks per day for men. (One drink is 12 ounces of regular beer, 5 ounces of wine or 1.5 ounces of 80-proof distilled spirits.)

How Much Fat Should You Eat?

You may have noticed that you don't find a Recommended Dietary Allowance (RDA) for fat listed on nutritional labels. Actually, as little as 1 tablespoon of vegetable oil per day fills your need for essential fatty acids. Too much fat provides excess calories, can increase your weight and increases your risk of heart disease and some cancers.

Health experts recommend that you limit fat to 20 to 30 percent of your calories. Because saturated fat increases blood cholesterol levels, no more than one-third of your fat intake should be saturated. Foods with saturated fat include meats, milk (skim milk does not), cheese, ice cream and coconut and palm oil (found in nondairy creamers). Margarine and shortening that contain hydrogenated vegetable oils also increase blood cholesterol levels.

Use the "Nutrition Facts" labels on packaging to guide your food selections and to keep track of the fat you eat. If you are not overweight and are healthy—and don't have high blood cholesterol—the U.S. Departments of Agriculture and Health and Human Services suggest you limit your fat intake as follows:

	Total Grams of Fat	Grams of Saturated Fat
Most women and older adults	53	16
Most men, active women, teenage girls and children	73	22
Active men and teenage boys	93	28

The Food Guide Pyramid

The Food Guide Pyramid was developed by the U.S. Department of Agriculture. The pyramid incorporates many principles that add up to a plan for eating low-fat foods that are high in fiber and rich in important vitamins, minerals and other nutrients. All of these factors contribute to optimal health and energy, help you control your weight and reduce your risk of heart disease and some types of cancer. The arrangement of the food groups in a pyramid emphasizes the kinds of foods to eat more of and those to limit.

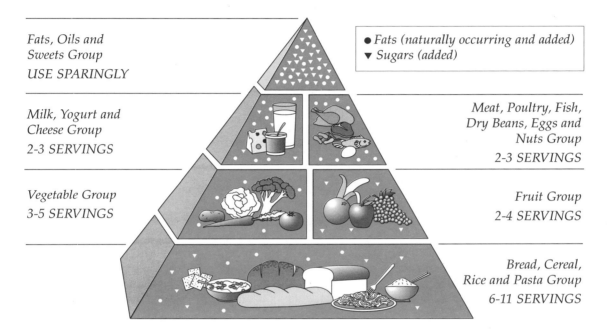

Fats, Oils and Sweets Group
USE SPARINGLY

● *Fats (naturally occurring and added)*
▼ *Sugars (added)*

Milk, Yogurt and Cheese Group
2-3 SERVINGS

Meat, Poultry, Fish, Dry Beans, Eggs and Nuts Group
2-3 SERVINGS

Vegetable Group
3-5 SERVINGS

Fruit Group
2-4 SERVINGS

Bread, Cereal, Rice and Pasta Group
6-11 SERVINGS

How Many Servings Do You Need Each Day?

	Women and Some Older Adults	Children, Teenage Girls, Active Women, Most Men	Teenage Boys, Active Men	Pregnant and Breast-Feeding Women
Calorie level*	About 1,600	About 2,200	About 2,800	About 1,800-2,800
Bread group	6	9	11	9
Vegetable group	3	4	5	4
Fruit group	2	3	4	3
Milk group	2-3†	2-3†	2-3†	3
Meat group	2 for a total of 5 oz	2 for a total of 6 oz	3 for a total of 7 oz	3 for a total of 7 oz

*These are the calorie levels if you choose low-fat, lean foods from the five major food groups and use foods from the fats, oils and sweets group sparingly.

†Teenagers and young adults to age 24 need 3 servings.

From Mayo Clinic Diet Manual, seventh edition, 1994. Also from the U.S. Department of Agriculture Food Guide Pyramid.

Lowering Your Cholesterol

Cardiovascular disease remains the leading cause of death in this country. Many of the 1 million deaths occur because of narrowed or blocked arteries (atherosclerosis). Cholesterol plays a significant role in this largely preventable condition.

Atherosclerosis is a silent, painless process in which cholesterol-containing fatty deposits accumulate in the walls of your arteries. These accumulations occur as bumps called plaques. As plaque builds up, the interior of your artery narrows and the flow of blood is reduced.

What Is Cholesterol?

Cholesterol is a waxy, fat-like substance (lipid). Although it's often discussed as if it were a poison, you can't live without it. Cholesterol is essential to your body's cell membranes, to the insulation of your nerves and to the production of certain hormones. It's used by your liver to make bile acids, which help digest your food.

The confusion that clouds cholesterol is partly due to the way some people use the word. "Cholesterol" is often a catch-all term for both the cholesterol you eat and the cholesterol in your blood.

- **Dietary cholesterol:** Cholesterol exists in your food as a dietary lipid. You'll find cholesterol only in animal products, such as meat and dairy foods.
- **Blood cholesterol:** Cholesterol exists in a different way as a natural component of your blood lipids.

The cholesterol in your blood comes both from your liver and from the foods you eat. Your liver makes about 80 percent of your blood cholesterol. About 20 percent comes from your diet. The amount of fat, especially saturated fat, and cholesterol you eat influences your blood cholesterol level.

Normal artery

Damaged artery

Athero-sclerotic plaque

An excess of LDL cholesterol particles in your blood increases your risk for a buildup of cholesterol within the wall of your arteries. Eventually, bumps called plaques may form, narrowing or even blocking your artery.

Blood Cholesterol—the Good, the Bad and the Ugly

For cholesterol to be carried in your blood, your body coats it with proteins called apoproteins. Once coated, they form a package called lipoproteins.

Lipoproteins carry both cholesterol and triglycerides (another blood lipid) in your blood. Some of your lipoproteins are called low-density lipoproteins (LDLs). They contain lots of cholesterol. Others are called high-density lipoproteins (HDLs). They contain mostly protein. Some people call LDL "bad cholesterol" and HDL "good cholesterol." Here's why:

Cholesterol serves as a building material in cells throughout your body. LDL particles, which carry cholesterol, attach themselves to receptors on cell surfaces and are then received into your cells.

If there are too many LDL particles in your blood, if your liver cells do not receive LDL particles normally or if there are too few LDL receptors in your liver, excess cholesterol is deposited in your artery walls.

At this point your high-density lipoproteins (HDLs) play their "good" role. They actually pick up cholesterol deposited in your artery walls and transport it to your liver for disposal. The situation can turn ugly if too much cholesterol from LDL particles remains deposited in your artery walls. Your arteries will develop plaques and begin to narrow. This process is atherosclerosis. Therefore, a high HDL level is good. It can help protect you from developing atherosclerosis.

Your Blood Test: What Do Those Numbers Mean?

Use this table as a general guide. The importance of each number varies somewhat for men and women and according to the individual's health status. For example, if you already have heart disease, you will want even lower LDL cholesterol levels—in the range of 100. Your health-care provider can clarify your specific risk.

Test	Your Level (in mg/dL)		
	Desirable	Borderline	Undesirable
Total cholesterol: accumulation of all forms	Less than 200	200-240	More than 240
HDL cholesterol: considered "good"— the higher the better	More than 45	35-45	Less than 35
LDL cholesterol*: considered "bad"— the lower the better	Less than 130	130-160	More than 160
Cholesterol/HDL ratio	Less than 4.5	4.5-5.5	More than 5.5
LDL/HDL ratio	Less than 3	3-5	More than 5
Triglycerides: other lipids in blood	Less than 200	200-400	More than 400

*LDL is not measured directly but is calculated from the other numbers. If you know your total cholesterol (TC) and your triglycerides (TG) and your HDL, you can calculate it yourself using this equation: LDL = TC - (HDL + TG/5).

■ Reducing Cholesterol Levels

Diet and exercise are your first lines of defense against high cholesterol. Decreasing cholesterol and saturated fats in your diet lowers your cholesterol level. A few people don't respond to diet and require medication. To reduce cholesterol through diet:

- **Lower your weight by reducing calories and increasing exercise.** Limit all types of fat to no more than 30 percent of your total daily calories (see chart on page 198).
- **Decrease saturated fat.** No more than one-third of the fat you eat should be saturated. Read labels carefully.
- **Reduce dietary cholesterol.** Your daily limit for dietary cholesterol is 300 milligrams. Avoid dairy products made with whole milk and cream and organ meats such as liver and tongue. Choose lean cuts of meat; trim fat and drain fat from browned meats. Reduce your intake of red meat. Limit egg yolks to three or four per week.
- **Eat more grain products, fruit and vegetables.**
- **Select a cookbook that includes vegetarian diets**.

If you've carried out these lifestyle changes and your total cholesterol, especially your LDL level, remains high, your doctor may recommend a medication. Your LDL cholesterol level is usually the deciding factor. If you have no risk factors for cardiovascular disease, an LDL level more than 190 generally requires medication. With two or more risk factors, an LDL level more than 160 may require medication. If you have heart disease already, your doctor may use a medication if your LDL is more than 130.

Exercise and Fitness

Regular exercise three or four times a week reduces risk of death from all causes, including heart disease and cancer, by about 70 percent. With routine exercise, you may reach a level of fitness comparable to an inactive person 10 to 20 years younger.

The benefits of exercise include the following:

- **Heart:** Exercise increases your heart's ability to pump blood and decreases your resting heart rate. Your heart can pump more blood with less effort.
- **Cholesterol:** Exercise improves cholesterol levels.
- **Blood pressure:** Exercise can lower blood pressure and is especially helpful if you have mild hypertension. Regular exercise also can help prevent as well as reduce high blood pressure.
- **Diabetes:** If you have diabetes, exercise can lower your blood sugar. Exercise can help prevent adult-onset diabetes.
- **Bones:** Women who exercise have a better chance of avoiding osteoporosis, provided that they do not become so active that menstruation stops.
- **General:** Regular exercise also relieves stress, improves your overall sense of well-being, helps you sleep better and improves concentration.

■ Aerobic vs. Anaerobic Exercise

Aerobic exercise (which literally means "to exercise with oxygen") occurs when you continuously move large muscle groups such as your leg muscles. This exercise places increased demands on the heart, lungs and muscle cells. It is not so intense, however, that it causes pain (from lactic acid buildup). If you're exercising in a good aerobic range, you should be breaking a sweat and breathing faster but still be able to exercise comfortably for 20 to 40 minutes. Aerobic exercise improves your overall endurance. Walking, biking, jogging and swimming are familiar aerobic exercises.

Anaerobic exercise ("to exercise without oxygen") occurs when the demands made on a muscle are great enough that it uses up all of the available oxygen and starts to burn stored energy without oxygen. This alternate path for burning energy produces lactic acid. As lactic acid builds up in muscles it causes pain. That's one reason why you can't carry on anaerobic exercises very long. Weight lifting is a classic example. Anaerobic exercise can be healthful but it builds strength more than endurance. If you are just starting an exercise program, supplement your aerobic exercise with light anaerobic exercises. Work with light weights or set machines at light resistance to avoid injuries.

What It Means to Be Fit

You're fit if you can:

- Carry out daily tasks without fatigue and have ample energy to enjoy leisure pursuits
- Walk a mile or climb a few flights of stairs without becoming "winded" or feeling heaviness or fatigue in your legs
- Carry on a conversation during light to moderate exercise such as brisk walking

If you sit most of the day, you're probably not fit. Signs of deconditioning include feeling tired most of the time, being unable to keep up with others your age, avoiding physical activity because you know you'll quickly tire and becoming short of breath or fatigued when walking a short distance.

■ Starting a Fitness Program

Consult your health-care provider before you begin an exercise program if you smoke, are overweight, are older than 40 years and have never exercised or have a chronic condition such as heart disease, diabetes, high blood pressure, lung disease or kidney disease. The risks of exercise stem from doing too much, too vigorously, with too little previous activity.

If you are medically able to begin a program, here are some helpful hints:

- **Begin gradually**. Don't overdo it. If you have trouble talking to a companion during your workout, you probably are pushing too hard.
- **Select the exercise that is right for you.** It should be something you enjoy—or at least find tolerable. Otherwise, in time you will avoid it.
- **Do it regularly but moderately** and never exercise to the point of nausea, dizziness or extreme shortness of breath. Your goals should be:
  - *Frequency:* Exercise at least three or four times a week.
  - *Intensity:* Aim for about 60 percent of your maximal aerobic capacity. For most people, 60 percent capacity means moderate exertion with deep breathing, but short of panting or becoming overheated.
  - *Time:* Set a goal of at least 20 to 30 minutes a session. If time is a factor, three 10-minute sessions can be as beneficial as one 30-minute workout. If you're not used to exercise, start at a comfortable length of time and gradually work up to your goal.
- **Always warm up and cool down.** Stretch in warm-up to help loosen muscles; stretch in cool-down to increase flexibility.

How Many Calories Does It Use Up?

Exercise that's equivalent to burning about 1,000 calories a week significantly lowers your overall risk of a heart attack. The chart shows the range of energy used while performing various activities for 1 hour. The more you weigh, the more calories you use.

Activity (1-Hour Duration)	Calories Used* 120- to 130- lb Person	Calories Used* 170- to 180- lb Person	Activity (1-Hour Duration)	Calories Used* 120- to 130- lb Person	Calories Used* 170- to 180- lb Person
Aerobic dancing	290-575	400-800	Racquetball	345-690	480-690
Backpacking	29-630	400-880	Rope skipping	345-690	480-960
Badminton	230-515	320-720	Running, 8 mph	745	1,040
Bicycling (outdoor)	170-800	240-1,120	Skating, ice or roller	230-460	320-640
Bicycling (stationary)	85-800	120-1,120	Skiing (cross-country)	290-800	400-1,120
Bowling	115-170	160-240	Skiing (downhill)	170-460	240-640
Canoeing	170-460	240-640	Stair climbing	230-460	320-640
Dancing	115-400	160-560	Swimming	230-690	320-900
Gardening	115-400	160-560	Tennis	230-515	320-720
Golfing (carrying bag)	115-400	160-560	Volleyball	170-400	240-560
Hiking	170-690	240-960	Walking, 2 mph	150	210
Jogging, 5 mph	460	640			

For other body weights, you can calculate approximate calories used by selecting the numbers of calories used from the second column. Multiply it by your weight and divide by 175. For example, if you weigh 220 lb, jogging uses

$\frac{640 \times 220}{175} = 804$ calories/hour.

Screening and Immunizations

■ Adult Screening Tests and Procedures

Test or Procedure	Purpose	Recommendation
Blood cholesterol test	Detect people at high risk of coronary artery disease	● Baseline test in your 20s. If values are within desirable ranges, every 5 years. See page 201
Blood pressure measurement	Early detection of high blood pressure	● Every 2 years or as your health-care provider recommends
Colon cancer screening (several tests are available)	Detect cancers and growths (polyps) on the inside wall of the colon which may become cancerous	● Flexible sigmoidoscopy, every 3 to 5 years after age 50. Occasionally, proctoscopy (a less extensive scoping) ● Colon X-ray, every 3 to 5 years after age 50, in combination with proctoscopy or sigmoidoscopy ● Colonoscopy, every 5 years after age 50. Replaces the need for other tests and is the most definitive method, but it also has more risk and is the most expensive
Complete physical examination*	Detect conditions before symptoms develop Preventive care reduces. your risk of developing certain diseases	● Twice in your 20s ● Three times in your 30s ● Four times in your 40s ● Five times in your 50s ● Annually after 60 ● More frequently if you have a chronic medical condition or take medications
Dental checkup	Detect cavities of teeth and problems of the gums, tongue and mouth	● At least once a year or as your dentist recommends
Electrocardiogram (ECG)	Identify injury to heart or irregular rhythms	● Baseline by age 40. As needed or recommended thereafter
Eye examination	Detect vision problems	● Every 4 to 5 years, or as recommended by your doctor
Mammogram (breast X-ray)	Early detection of breast cancer	● Yearly in women older than 50. Yearly in women in their 40s may be appropriate. See page 141
Pap smear	Detect abnormal cells that could develop into cancer	● Every 1 to 3 years based on your risk and as recommended by your health-care provider. See page 147
Prostate-specific antigen (PSA)	Measure amount of a protein secreted by the prostate gland. High levels can indicate prostate cancer	● Consider the test if you have a strong family history of prostate cancer and as recommended by your health-care provider. The PSA level also can be increased if the prostate is enlarged or inflamed but not cancerous

*Components of a "complete physical" depend on your age, sex, past illnesses, your risks based on your behavior and your family history of diseases.

Adult Immunization Schedule

Vaccine	Recommendation
Diphtheria/tetanus booster	● Every 10 years. After a deep or dirty wound if the most recent booster was more than 5 years ago. Boosters should be given within 2 days of the injury
Hepatitis A (2-shot series)	● Travelers and people in high-risk groups (chronic liver disease, men with male sex partners, intravenous drug users, people who have had contact with someone who has hepatitis A)
Hepatitis B (3-shot series)	● Health-care workers, high-risk groups (persons with multiple sexual partners, sexual partner who is a carrier, diabetics)
Influenza	● Every year for persons 65 or older, others at high risk, all health-care workers
Measles/mumps/rubella (2 shots recommended)	● Adults born after 1956 without proof of previous immunization or immunity
Pneumonia vaccination	● Age 65 or older or any adult with a medical condition that increases the risk of infection. One shot lasts a lifetime for most people
Varicella (chickenpox)	● Susceptible adults (health-care workers without immunity or adults without known disease who are exposed to chickenpox)

Well-Child Immunization Schedule

In the past few years, several new vaccines have become available for children. The recommendations are still being discussed and updated by medical organizations. The following chart includes the recommended schedule of vaccines used at the Mayo Clinic; it is a modification of recommendations endorsed in November 1996 by the American Academy of Family Physicians and the federal Centers for Disease Control. You should check with your personal physician or health-care provider regarding the timing of immunizations for your child.

Age	Vaccine	Age	Vaccine
Birth	HBV	9 months	HBV
2 months	HBV, DTP, HIB, OPV	15 months	MMR, VZV, DTP, HIB
4 months	DTP, HIB, OPV	5 years	DTaP, OPV
6 months	DTP, HIB, OPV	11 years	MMR, Td (HBV and VZV if not given previously)

Abbreviations

DTP	-	Diphtheria/tetanus/pertusis	MMR -	Measles, mumps, rubella
DTaP	-	A slightly different formula of DTP	OPV -	Oral polio virus
HBV	-	Hepatitis B	VZV -	Varicella-zoster virus (chickenpox)
HIB	-	Haemophilus influenza B	Td -	Tetanus/diphtheria/pertussis (booster shot)

Smoking and Tobacco Use

When you inhale the smoke of a cigarette, you're letting loose a chemical parade that will march through some of your body's vital organs—brain, lungs, heart and blood vessels. Your body is exposed to chemicals that cause cancer and addiction.

Although the link between smoking and lung cancer is well known, smoking harms other organs and tissues. Approximately one-fifth of all deaths in the United States are due to smoking.

Nicotine, one of the key ingredients in tobacco, stimulates brain chemicals that can lead to addiction. It triggers your adrenal glands to produce hormones that stress your heart by increasing blood pressure and heart rate.

The carbon monoxide you inhale from tobacco smoke replaces oxygen in your blood cells, robbing your heart, brain and the rest of your body of this life-giving element. Smoking also deadens your senses of taste and smell so food isn't as appetizing as it once was.

Cigarette smoke delivers more than 40 known cancer-causing chemicals, tiny amounts of poisons such as arsenic and cyanide and more than 4,000 other substances to your body. One of the most powerful chemicals is nicotine. It's the nicotine that keeps you smoking. Nicotine is addictive; it can be as addictive as cocaine. It increases the amount of a brain chemical called dopamine, which makes you feel good. Getting that "dopamine boost" is part of the addiction process.

■ How to Stop Smoking

Many smokers yearn to stop, but find it hard because of nicotine's powerful addictive hold. In fact, most people will need more than one attempt before they successfully stop. Here are some suggestions to help you stop smoking:

Do your homework. Examine the wide range of self-help materials available from the American Cancer Society, the American Lung Association, your physician and your library. Look into smoking-cessation programs. Talk to ex-smokers. Find out how they stopped and what they found helpful.

Make small changes. Limit places where you smoke by smoking in only one room in your home or even outside. Practice not smoking by not smoking in the car. Begin an exercise program if you are capable (see page 202).

Pay attention to your smoking. As you prepare to stop smoking, pay attention to your behavior. When do you smoke? Where? With whom do you smoke? List your key triggers to smoking. Plan to cope with them when you stop. Practice coping with these situations without smoking.

Seek help. Participate in a formal program. The more help you get, the better your chance of success. Studies show that people who try to stop through formal programs are up to 8 times more likely to succeed than those who try on their own.

Be motivated. The key to stopping is commitment. When Mayo Clinic studied the results of its own programs, it found that smokers who were more motivated to stop were twice as likely to be successful in stopping as those who were less motivated. List your reasons for stopping. To increase your motivation, add to the list regularly.

Set a stop date. Make it a day with low stress. Tell your friends, spouse and coworkers your intention. They can provide support through trying times.

Nicotine Replacement Therapy

The best tested treatments currently available to help people stop smoking are based on delivering nicotine to the brain—by means other than smoking. The theory is that nicotine replacement therapy helps relieve the symptoms of nicotine withdrawal experienced when smokers stop lighting up. Various over-the-counter and prescription medications can help in your attempt to stop smoking.

Over-the-Counter

Nicotine patch: The patch delivers nicotine through your skin and into your bloodstream. Until recently, it has been a prescription medication. Studies have shown that people who properly use the patch are twice as likely to succeed. To use the patch, place it on the least hairy areas of your body in the morning. Rotate locations. Remove the old patch before putting on a new one. Length of use varies with individual needs. Usually 6 to 8 weeks is necessary to learn how to change behavior associated with smoking. Strengths vary by brand; read label instructions carefully. Heavier smokers may need to start with a large patch and taper the size gradually. Caution: About 10 to 20 percent of people get a rash at the site of the patch. If it is a minor redness, use a small amount of hydrocortisone cream on the area after the patch is removed. If it is irritated, you will need to stop using the patch or switch to another brand. Do not smoke while wearing a patch.

Nicotine gum: This is not chewing gum. It is a gum-like resin that delivers nicotine to the blood through the lining of your mouth. Studies show that people who properly use the gum are more successful than those who try to stop smoking without nicotine replacement. Two strengths are available: 2 and 4 milligrams. Heavier smokers may need the higher dose. To use the gum, put a piece in your mouth and bite it gently a few times until its unusual taste is released. Then park the gum between your cheek and gum. Repeat the process every few minutes. A piece should last about 30 minutes. Use the gum when you feel the urge to smoke or in situations when you know the urge will be present. Initially, you may use up to 10 to 12 pieces a day. Gradually decrease the number over a period of weeks as you develop ways to deal with smoking triggers. **Caution:** Rapid chewing and swallowing inactivate the nicotine and may cause nausea. Read labels carefully.

Prescription Medications

Nicotine nasal spray: The nicotine in Nicotrol NS, sprayed directly into each nostril, is absorbed through nasal membranes into veins, transported to the heart and then sent to the brain. It is believed to be a quicker delivery system than the gum or patch, although it is not nearly as quick as a cigarette. The usual dose—one spray into each nostril—is 1 milligram. People typically are directed to start with 1 to 2 doses per hour; the minimum is 8 doses per day and the maximum is 40 doses per day. For most people, use of the spray should be reduced 6 to 8 weeks into the treatment. During the early days of treatment, the spray can be irritating to the nose, causing a hot, peppery feeling along with coughing and sneezing.

The nicotine inhaler (Nicotrol Inhaler) is shaped something like a cigarette. You puff on it and it gives off nicotine vapors in your mouth. The nicotine is absorbed through the lining of the mouth and into your bloodstream and goes to the brain, relieving withdrawal symptoms.

Bupropion (Wellbutrin) is an antidepressant drug. Bupropion tablets increase the level of dopamine, the chemical that is also boosted by nicotine, in the brain. As with many medications, it has side effects, including headache and dry mouth. If you have a history of seizures, do not use this drug.

Smokers who combine nicotine replacement therapy with follow-up visits to a health-care provider for support and counseling are much more successful than those who try to quit on their own. Only about 5 percent of smokers stop without help. The success rate averages closer to 30 percent for people receiving nicotine replacement therapy along with support and counseling.

■ Coping With Nicotine Withdrawal

Below is a list of common withdrawal symptoms and some suggestions for coping with them. Withdrawal can last from a few days to a few weeks. It's important to try new behaviors.

Problem	Solutions
Craving	● Distract yourself ● Do deep-breathing exercises (see page 211) ● Realize that the urge will pass
Irritability	● Take a few slow, deep breaths ● Image an enjoyable outdoor scene and take a mini-vacation ● Soak in a hot bath
Insomnia	● Take a walk several hours before going to bed ● Unwind by reading ● Take a warm bath ● Eat a banana or drink warm milk ● Avoid beverages with caffeine after noon ● See chapter on sleeping disorders, page 40
Increased appetite	● Make a personal survival kit. Include straws, cinnamon sticks, coffee stirrers, licorice, toothpicks, gum or fresh vegetables ● Drink lots of water or low-calorie liquids
Inability to concentrate	● Drink lots of water ● Take a brisk walk—outside if possible ● Simplify your schedule for a few days ● Take a break
Fatigue	● Get more exercise ● Get an adequate amount of sleep ● Take a nap ● Try not to push yourself for 2 to 4 weeks
Constipation, gas, stomach pain	● Drink plenty of fluids ● Add roughage to your diet: fruit, raw vegetables, whole-grain cereals ● Gradually change your diet ● See constipation, page 54; gas, page 56

Source: Mayo Nicotine Dependence Center.

Teenage Smoking: What Can Be Done?

What's the harm in children "experimenting" with cigarettes?

Cigarette smoking is addictive. Most teenagers underestimate the health risks of smoking and overestimate their ability to stop once they start. Many teenagers believe that they can stop smoking anytime they choose. The reality is that among high school seniors who smoke from one to five cigarettes a day, 70 percent will still be smoking 5 years later. More than half of those who smoke in high school have unsuccessfully tried to stop.

Teenagers start smoking earlier than many parents realize. Ten percent of current adult smokers began when they were between 9 and 10 years old and half of teenagers who start to smoke begin by 14 years of age. Almost 20 percent of eighth graders have smoked in the past 30 days. Among high school seniors, the rate is 30 percent. The younger a child begins smoking, the greater the chance that he or she will become a heavy smoker as an adult. Also, teenagers who smoke are more likely to experiment with marijuana and other illegal drugs.

Here are some strategies parents might try:

- **Talk with your teenagers. Ask whether their friends smoke.** The risk of your child smoking is 13 times higher if his or her best friends smoke. Most teenagers smoke their first cigarette with a friend who already smokes.
- **Learn what your children think about smoking.** Ask them to read this information so you can discuss it together.
- **Help your child explore personal feelings about peer pressures and smoking.** Use nonjudgmental questions and rehearse with them how they could handle tough situations.
- **Encourage your teenager to enjoy maximal energy and health.** The active, vivacious lifestyles portrayed in many cigarette advertisements are actually more representative of nonsmokers. People who smoke have colds and other respiratory infections more frequently.
- **Note the social repercussions.** Smoking gives you bad breath and makes your hair and clothes smell.
- **Set a personal example of not smoking.** If you currently smoke, one of the best reasons to stop is for the sake of your children.
- **Work with your schools.**

The Dangers of Secondhand Smoke

The health threat to the nonsmoker from exposure to tobacco smoke is well documented. Secondhand smoke exposure is associated with lung cancer and heart disease in nonsmokers. As a result, most states have enacted laws limiting smoking in public places.

Clearly, people with respiratory or heart conditions and the elderly in general are at special health risk when exposed to secondhand smoke.

Infants are three times more likely to die from sudden infant death syndrome if their mothers smoke during and after pregnancy.

Children younger than 1 year who are exposed to smoke have a higher frequency of admissions to hospitals for respiratory illness than children of parents who do not smoke. Secondhand smoke increases a child's risk of getting ear infections, pneumonia, bronchitis or tonsillitis.

Keeping Stress Under Control

Many factors can cause stress, often because they are related to changes in our lives. These changes can be events that we consider happy, such as a vacation or a job promotion, as well as negative changes, such as the death of a loved one or the loss of a job.

When we respond to stress with anxiety, tension or worry, that response is not just "mental." When we feel threatened in some way, chemical "messengers" are released, producing physical changes such as rapid pulse, quick breathing and dry mouth. These changes prepare the body for "fight or flight." If we react to stress for long periods, it may contribute to physical or emotional illness.

■ Signs and Symptoms of Stress

Physical	Psychological	Behavioral
Headaches	Anxiety	Overeating/loss of appetite
Grinding teeth	Irritability	Impatience
Tight, dry throat	Feeling of impending danger or doom	Argumentative
Clenched jaws	Depression	Procrastination
Chest pain	Slowed thinking	Increased use of alcohol or drugs
Shortness of breath	Racing thoughts	Increased smoking
Pounding heart	Feeling of helplessness	Withdrawal or isolation
High blood pressure	Feeling of hopelessness	Avoiding or neglecting
Muscle aches	Feeling of worthlessness	responsibility
Indigestion	Feeling of lack of direction	Poor job performance
Constipation/diarrhea	Feeling of insecurity	Burnout
Increased perspiration	Sadness	Poor personal hygiene
Cold, sweaty hands	Defensiveness	Change in religious practices
Fatigue	Anger	Change in family or close relationships
Insomnia	Hypersensitivity	
Frequent illness	Apathy	

Self-Care

- **Learn to relax.** Techniques such as guided imagery, meditation, muscle relaxation and relaxed breathing can help you relax (see page 211). Your goal is to lower your heart rate and blood pressure while reducing muscle tension.
- **Discuss your concerns** with a trusted friend. Talking helps to relieve strains and put things in perspective, and it may lead to a healthy plan of action.
- **Plan your work** in a step-by-step manner. Accomplish small tasks.
- **Deal with your anger.** Anger needs to be expressed, but carefully. "Count to 10," compose yourself and respond to the anger in a more effective manner.
- **Get away.** A change of pace can help develop a new outlook.
- **Be realistic.** Set realistic goals. Prioritize. Concentrate on what's important. Setting our goals unrealistically high invites failure. Decide on your priorities and concentrate on the things of most importance to you.

Self-Care *(continued)*

- **Avoid self-medication.** At times we may seek to use medication or alcohol for a feeling of relief. Such substances only mask the problem.
- **Get plenty of sleep, exercise and nutritious food.** A healthy body promotes good mental health. Sleep helps us tackle problems in a refreshed state. Exercise helps burn off the excess energy that stress can produce.
- **Seek help.** Contact your physician or a mental health professional if stress is building or you're not functioning well.

Relaxation Techniques to Reduce Stress

Progressive Muscle Relaxation

- Sit or lie in a comfortable position and close your eyes. Allow your jaw to drop and your eyelids to be relaxed but not tightly closed.
- Mentally scan your body, starting with your toes and working slowly to your head. Focus on each part individually; imagine tension melting away.
- Tighten the muscles in one area of your body and hold them for a count of 5, relax and move on to the next area.

Visual Imagery

- Allow thoughts to flow through your mind but do not focus on any of them. Suggest to yourself that you are relaxed and calm, that your hands are warm (or cool if you are hot) and heavy, that your heart is beating calmly.
- Breathe slowly, regularly and deeply.
- Once you are relaxed, imagine you are in a favorite place or in a spot of great beauty.
- After 5 or 10 minutes, rouse yourself from the state gradually.

Relaxed Breathing

With practice, you can breathe in a deep and relaxing way. At first, practice lying on your back while wearing clothing that is loose around your waist and abdomen. Once you have learned this position, practice while sitting and then while standing.

- Lie on your back on a bed.
- Place your feet slightly apart. Rest one hand comfortably on your abdomen near your navel. Place the other hand on your chest.
- Inhale through your nose. Exhale through your mouth.
- Concentrate on your breathing for a few minutes and become aware of which hand is rising and falling with each breath.
- Gently exhale most of the air in your lungs.
- Inhale while slowly counting to 4, about 1 second per count. As you inhale gently, slightly extend your abdomen, causing it to rise about 1 inch. (You should be able to feel the movement with your hand.) Do not pull your shoulders up or move your chest.
- As you breathe in, imagine the warmed air flowing into all parts of your body.
- Pause 1 second after inhaling.
- Slowly exhale to a count of 4. While you are exhaling, your abdomen will slowly fall.
- As air flows out, imagine that tension also is flowing out.
- Pause 1 second after exhaling.
- If it is difficult to inhale and exhale to a count of 4, shorten the count slightly and later work up to 4. If you feel light-headed, slow your breathing or breathe less deeply.
- Repeat the slow inhaling, pausing, slow exhaling and pausing 5 to 10 times. Exhale. Inhale slowly: 1, 2, 3, 4. Pause. Exhale slowly: 1, 2, 3, 4. Pause. Inhale: 1, 2, 3, 4. Pause. Exhale: 1, 2, 3, 4. Pause. Continue on your own.

If it's difficult to make your breathing regular, take a slightly deeper breath, hold it for a second or two and then let it out slowly through pursed lips for about 10 seconds. Repeat this once or twice and return to the other procedure.

Protecting Yourself

Nearly 1 in every 20 deaths in the United States results from accidents. Accidents are the most common cause of death in people younger than 35. Half of all childhood deaths are due to accidents. Many of these accidents could be avoided. In the following pages, we offer various safety tips. This information is not comprehensive, but it may alert you to other potentially dangerous circumstances in your everyday life. For a discussion of workplace safety, see page 224.

■ Reduce Your Risk on the Road

Approximately 50,000 people die on our roads and highways every year. Many more are severely injured. To reduce your risk, follow these suggestions:

- **Always wear a seat belt,** even if you are traveling only a short distance. Most accidents occur within a few miles of home.
- **Place children in car seats.** (See the article below.)
- **Drive defensively.** Be aware of other cars at all times.
  - Don't tailgate. Allow 1 car length of space for every 10 miles per hour of speed.
  - Keep windows and mirrors clean. Keep all lines of vision clear. Don't rely on mirrors—turn your head and check blind spots.
- **Consider the weather.** Carry food, blankets and protective clothing. Keep your gas tank as full as possible. Do not leave your car in an emergency. If your engine is running, roll windows down an inch or two to avoid a buildup of carbon monoxide.
- **Don't drive while impaired.** Don't drive after consuming alcohol or when you have taken medications that make you drowsy or impair your reaction time.
- **Avoid distractions.** Keep children in their seatbelts. Do not let the radio, a conversation on a cellular phone or a roadside attraction distract you.
- **Keep your car properly serviced** at the recommended intervals (at least every 6 months or 7,500 miles, whichever comes first) and before extended traveling.
- **Carry an emergency kit** (flashlight, first-aid supplies, jumper cable, a quarter for a phone call, flares, candle and matches).

Airbags and Infant Car Safety Seats Don't Mix

The force of an air bag's deployment can kill or severely injure infants or small children. Seat them all in back. Here's some advice for safely transporting your children:

- For infants who weigh less than 20 pounds or are younger than 1 year of age, use infant car safety seats—or convertible infant-toddler safety seats. In a collision, the rigid seat supports your baby's back, neck and head. Secure your infant's child safety seat properly in the back seat of your car.

- For children who weigh 20 to 40 pounds or are younger than 4 years, use a child safety seat, anchored correctly, in the back seat. The safety seat's straps should hold the upper third of your child's chest securely.

  For children who weigh more than 40 pounds but who are too small to wear a lap and shoulder belt properly, use a car booster seat to obtain correct positioning of the lap and shoulder belt.

Preventing Falls

Trips and falls pose a danger to young children and the elderly. In fact, falls are the leading cause of accidental death among people older than 65. Falls may be caused by faulty balance, poor vision, illness, medications and other factors. The best self-care is to develop a plan that reduces risk and prevents injury in the first place.

Self-Care

Here are some tips to prevent falls:

- **Have your vision and hearing checked regularly.** If vision and hearing are impaired, you lose important cues that help you maintain balance.
- **Exercise regularly.** Exercise improves your strength, muscle tone and coordination. This not only helps prevent falls but also reduces the severity of injury if you do fall.
- **Be wary of drugs.** Ask your doctor about the drugs you take. Some drugs may affect balance and coordination.
- **Avoid alcohol.** Even a little alcohol can cause falls, especially if your balance and reflexes are already impaired.
- **Get up slowly.** A momentary decrease in blood pressure, due to drugs or aging, can cause dizziness if you stand up too quickly.
- **Maintain balance and footing.** If you feel dizzy, use a cane or walker. Wear sturdy, low-heeled shoes with wide, nonslip soles.
- **Eliminate loose rugs or mats.**
- **Install adequate lighting,** especially night lighting.
- Block steps for infants and toddlers; install handrails for elderly.

Lead Exposure

One of every 11 children in the United States has dangerous levels of lead in his or her bloodstream, according to the U.S. Environmental Protection Agency (EPA). Children are more sensitive to lead poisoning than adults. The federal Centers for Disease Control and Prevention recommends having your child tested for lead poisoning at age 1, or at 6 months if you think your home has high levels of lead. Children older than 1 year should be tested every couple of years, or every year if the residence contains lead paint or you use lead in your job or hobby.

Here are some potential sources of lead poisoning:

- **Soil:** Lead particles that settle on the soil from paint or gasoline used years ago can stay there for many years. High concentrations of lead in soil can be found around old homes and in some urban settings.
- **Household dust:** This can contain lead from paint chips or soil brought in from outside.
- **Water:** Lead pipes, brass plumbing fixtures and copper pipes soldered with lead can release lead particles into tap water. If you have such plumbing, let cold water run 30 to 60 seconds before drinking it. Hot water absorbs more lead than cold water. The EPA warns against making baby formula from hot tap water in old plumbing systems.
- **Lead paint:** Although now outlawed, lead paint is still on walls and woodwork in many older homes. When sanding or stripping in an older home, wear a mask and keep children away from dust and chips.

Carbon Monoxide Poisoning

Carbon monoxide is a poisonous gas produced by incomplete burning of fuel. It has no color, taste or odor. Carbon monoxide builds up in red blood cells, preventing oxygen from being carried and starving your body of oxygen.

An estimated 10,000 people are affected by carbon monoxide poisoning each year in the United States. However, a few simple measures can help prevent poisoning.

- **Know the signs and symptoms.** They include headache, fever, red-appearing skin, dizziness, weakness, fatigue, nausea, vomiting, shortness of breath, chest pain and trouble thinking. Symptoms of carbon monoxide poisoning often come on slowly and may be mistaken for a cold or the flu. Clues include similar symptoms being experienced by everyone in the same building or improvement of symptoms when you leave the building for a day or more and then a return of the symptoms when you come back to the building.
- **Be aware of possible sources.** The most common sources are gas and oil furnaces, wood stoves, gas appliances, pool heaters and engine exhaust fumes. Cracked heat exchangers on furnaces, blocked chimneys, flues or appliance vents can allow carbon monoxide to reach living areas. An inadequate supply of fresh air to a furnace also can allow carbon monoxide to build up in living spaces. Tight home construction also may increase your risk because less fresh air gets in.
- **Get a detector.** The detectors sound a warning when carbon monoxide builds up. Look for UL 2034 on the package.
- **Know when to take action.** If the alarm sounds, ventilate the area by opening doors and windows. If anyone is experiencing poisoning symptoms, evacuate immediately and call 911 from a nearby phone. If no one is experiencing symptoms, continue to ventilate, turn off all fuel-burning appliances and have a qualified technician inspect your home.

Indoor Air Pollution

The U.S. Environmental Protection Agency (EPA) rates indoor air pollution among the top four environmental health risks. (Others are outdoor air pollution, toxic chemicals in the workplace and contaminated drinking water.)

Indoor air's most dangerous pollutants include the following:

- **Tobacco smoke:** Smoking causes lung cancer. Even if you don't smoke but live with someone who does, you have a 30 percent higher risk of lung cancer than someone who lives in a smoke-free home. Air-filtering devices help, but remove mainly smoke's solid particles, not the gases.
- **Radon:** This naturally occurring gas is made by the radioactive decay of uranium in rocks and soil. You can easily overlook radon because you can't see, taste or smell it. Yet, radon can seep into your home and other buildings through basement cracks, sewer openings and joints between walls and floors. After chronic exposure at high levels, radon may lead to lung cancer. To check your home's radon level, buy a radon detector. If your radon level is high, call the EPA radon hot line: (800) SOS-RADON.

Your Health and the Workplace

- **Avoiding Stress in the Workplace**

- **Commonly Asked Questions**

- **Drugs, Alcohol and Work**

- **Ergonomics**

- **Exercises for "Office Potatoes"**

- **Pregnancy and Work**

- **Safety in the Workplace**

This section focuses on ways to improve your health and well-being in the work environment. We suggest practical tips on reducing stress and job burnout and how to avoid strain-related injuries. We describe simple exercises for workers who are confined to offices. We offer some general guidelines for women who work while they are pregnant. We also discuss safety issues and the potential dangers posed by workers who abuse alcohol and drugs in the workplace. The chapter "Commonly Asked Questions" addresses various topics, ranging from going to work with a cold to returning to work after a back injury.

Avoiding Stress in the Workplace

We've all seen people at work who look "burned-out" or stressed, and we may have even had such feelings ourselves. Those feelings are usually temporary and may go away after a well-timed vacation or some private time to collect our thoughts.

But if you feel burned-out or stressed every day, you are facing a situation that could affect your health and productivity. The most common symptoms of stress are overwhelming frustration and indifference toward your job, persistent irritability, anger, sarcasm and a quickness to argue.

Self-Care

- **Take care of yourself.** Eat regular, balanced meals; get adequate sleep; and exercise.
- **Develop friendships** at work and outside the office. Share feelings with people you trust. Also, end relationships with "negative" friends who reinforce bad feelings.
- **Take time off.** Take a vacation or a long weekend. Plan private time each week when you do not answer calls or pages. During the work day, take short breaks.
- **Manage your time.** Set realistic goals and deadlines, and plan your projects accordingly. Do "must-do" tasks first. Schedule difficult tasks for the time of day when you are most productive. Tackle easy or "mindless" tasks when you feel low on energy or motivation.
- **Set limits.** When necessary, learn to say "no" in a friendly but firm manner.
- **Choose battles wisely.** Don't rush to argue every time someone disagrees with you. Keep a cool head, and save your argument for things that really matter. (Better yet, try not to argue at all.)
- **Use calming skills.** Don't act on your first impulse. Give your anger time to subside. See page 211 for relaxation techniques.
- **If appropriate, look at other job options.** But first, ask yourself whether you gave your job a fair chance.
- **Seek help.** If none of these steps relieve your feelings of stress or burnout, ask an employee assistance counselor or another professional for advice.

Dealing With Coworker Conflict

Although conflict usually is viewed as a negative situation, it can be an opportunity for growth. Perhaps the best way to deal with differences is directly. Talk with the person with whom you have a conflict. The manner of that discussion is crucial. Here are some helpful tips:

- **Discuss the matter privately** and, if possible, on neutral territory, at a time that each can agree on. Be specific in setting the time. Approach the other person in a nonthreatening manner. "I would like to talk something over with you. I'm feeling . . . ." Another opening line is, "I would like to check something out with you when you have a chance to talk."
- **Do not blame the other person.** Emphasize "I" statements. It will make the other person feel less defensive or angry.
- **Listen closely to the other person.** Understanding the other person's point of view may help you feel less stressed or angry.
- **Focus on ways to resolve the problem.**
- **Seek help.** Talk with an employee assistance counselor who can help develop ground rules for such discussions and promote respectful communication.

Commonly Asked Questions

Your ability to work with certain medical conditions depends on many factors: your underlying health, your particular job activities and the severity of your illness. Use the answers to the following questions as a general guide. It's always wise to consult with your physician or health-care provider before returning to work after a serious illness or injury. Your company may have a physician or nurse who knows your job requirements and can advise you on returning to work and specific ways your job might be modified to meet your health needs.

QUESTION: Can I work with low back pain?

Answer: The answer depends on the severity of the pain and your job function. In most cases, if you don't have numbness or weakness in your legs and you aren't having new problems with controlling your bowel or bladder, the answer is "yes." Recent studies have shown that if you remain active after a back injury, you recover more quickly. If your job involves a lot of bending or lifting, you should limit or avoid these activities. You should speak with your company nurse or your health-care provider about how to modify your job until your back recovers.

Do Back Belts Prevent Injury?

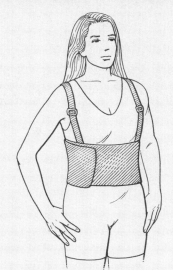

There's still debate on the question. Until recently, the consensus of experts was to avoid using them. Then a study by researchers at the University of California Los Angeles concluded that flexible back supports help to reduce back injury in the workplace. After studying more than 36,000 employees of the Home Depot discount chain during a 6-year period, the researchers reported that flexible back supports reduced injuries by 34 percent. Workers considered at highest risk of back injury (men 25 or younger or men older than 55 who had worked for the company for 1 to 2 years and had jobs that required the most lifting) seemed to benefit the most from using support belts, the researchers said.

Earlier studies had questioned the effectiveness of back belts for preventing injury, and many experts still believe the supports provide limited value. A health-care provider with special expertise in occupational medicine can help you decide if a back belt is right for you.

QUESTION: Can I go to work with a cold?

Answer: If you have a common cold, the answer is generally "yes." The viruses that cause the common cold usually are spread by direct contact. Careful hand washing and avoiding coughing or sneezing on people will prevent spread. If you have influenza or a more serious respiratory infection, you should not go to work. Influenza may be spread through airborne particles as well as direct contact. Signs of influenza include a fever of more than 100 F, chills, muscle aches, light-headedness and significant fatigue. (See page 111 for care of colds and flu.)

QUESTION: Can I go to work with a strep throat?

Answer: It depends on how you feel. You can go back to work after you've been taking antibiotics for 24 hours. If you had a fever of more than 100 F, wait until it has resolved. (See page 129 for information on strep throat.)

QUESTION: How long do I need to be off work after surgery?

Answer: Surgical methods have changed dramatically in the past 20 years. Recovery time depends on how physically demanding your job is and what surgical procedure was performed. If surgery was performed through a scope (called minimally invasive surgery), you may be able to return to an office job in 1 to 2 weeks, or even after a few days in some cases. If you have large abdominal or chest surgical incisions and your job involves heavy lifting, you may need to be away from work for 6 weeks or more, or you may need to return to work with restricted activity.

QUESTION: Are there some people who can't do shift work?

Answer: Most people can adjust to shift-work schedules (see page 224). However, shift work may be undesirable for some people with certain medical conditions. Diabetics who use insulin, for example, may have difficulty balancing blood sugars, and some people with major depression may not be able to do shift work. Some medical conditions, such as seizure disorders, produce or are worsened by fatigue and may make shift work difficult.

QUESTION: Are there prescription medicines that might interfere with my work?

Answer: "Yes." Some prescription and over-the-counter medicines cause drowsiness or impair judgment. These include some cold medicines (see page 232), some prescription pain killers, sleeping medicines, muscle relaxants, antidepressants and medicines with the "PM" added to the name (such as Tylenol PM). If you operate heavy equipment, work at heights or perform tasks that involve the safety of yourself, coworkers or the public, check with your doctor or pharmacist about the safety of using these medicines at work.

QUESTION: What are the risks of video display terminals (VDTs)?

Answer: More than 15 million Americans use VDTs for hours each day. Concerns include the potential risk of exposure to electrical and magnetic fields and radiation produced by screens of VDTs. To date, however, these risks appear to be insignificant. The exposure levels from the screens are well below currently acceptable levels. Although no major health risks from VDTs have been found, eye and hand strains have been reported with computer use. If you work at a VDT daily, refer to tips in the Ergonomics chapter, page 221.

QUESTION: When can I return to work after a heart attack?

Answer: Years ago, people would rest for weeks after a heart attack. Today, you are advised to become active as soon as possible after receiving appropriate medical treatment and clearance from your doctor. Your level of activity depends on many factors, including the severity of your heart attack, the type of treatment, your medications and your previous level of activity.

Exactly when you can return to work depends on these and other factors, including the specific demands of your job. Some people are able to return to work in a week, whereas for others the recovery period is 6 weeks or longer. Discuss your job activities with your doctor, who may order a stress test to determine how well your heart functions under physical demands.

QUESTION: Can I work with pinkeye?

Answer: Pinkeye (see page 74) is contagious. It usually is caused by a germ (virus or bacteria) and is spread by direct contact with the germ. In theory, you should be able to go to work if you wash your hands frequently and keep them away from your face in order to minimize spread of the germ. However, in practice, touching one's face is a common, often unnoticed habit. If the risk of infection is a particular concern in your job, such as in a hospital or day care, you should wait until signs of infection have cleared before you have contact with people. Talk with your manager about alternative activities at which your risk of infecting others is less.

QUESTION: Are there jobs I shouldn't do when I'm pregnant?

Answer: "Yes," but not many. Pregnancy raises many issues regarding home (see page 150) and work (see page 223). Several chemicals, such as lead and benzene, are suspected to pose a risk to the fetus during pregnancy. Significant levels of radiation are a concern, and certain infections can cause problems. Temperature extremes, heavy lifting and time on your feet also may cause problems. Fortunately, protective shielding and modifications to work areas may allow continued work during pregnancy. Companies are required to have available Material Safety Data Sheets that identify potentially harmful chemicals. If you are concerned about your pregnancy in the work environment, talk with your manager and your doctor.

QUESTION: How can I find out more about workplace health and safety?

Answer: The Occupational Safety and Health Administration (OSHA) offers free booklets and fact sheets. Contact the OSHA Publications Office, U.S. Department of Labor, 200 Constitution Avenue NW, Room N3101, Washington, D.C. 20210; Internet address: http://www.osha.gov. Another source is the National Institute for Occupational Safety and Health (NIOSH), 4676 Columbia Parkway, Cincinnati, OH 45226; phone: (800) 35-NIOSH; Internet address: http://www.cdc.gov/niosh/homepage.

Drugs, Alcohol and Work

Illegal street drugs and alcohol can affect your health and safety in the workplace, as well as the safety of your coworkers. Consider the following statistics:

- Drug- and alcohol-related problems are one of the four top reasons for workplace violence.
- The risk of an accident is five times greater in people who go to work under the influence of drugs or alcohol.
- People using drugs or alcohol miss nearly 10 times as much work as coworkers who do not use drugs or alcohol.
- Drug users, as a group, use medical benefits at a rate eight times higher than non-users.
- A Gallup poll of employees found that 97 percent agreed that workplace drug testing is appropriate under certain circumstances, and 85 percent believed that urine testing may deter illicit drug use.

Self-Assessment

To determine if you have a problem with alcohol or drugs, ask yourself the following questions:

- Have you used an illegal drug in the past 6 months?
- Have you misused a prescription drug because of its effect?
- Have you done something unsafe or taken risks while under the influence of alcohol or drugs, such as driving a car or operating heavy equipment?
- Have you used alcohol within 12 hours of going to work?
- Has your drug or alcohol use negatively affected your relationships, your health or your ability to work?

    If you answered "yes" to any of these questions, you are showing signs of substance abuse and should take action.

Self-Care

- If you or a family member is dependent on alcohol, refer to page 183.
- If you or a family member has problems with drug addiction, refer to page 181.
- Many large corporations offer confidential employee assistance programs to help workers deal with drug and alcohol abuse. Inquire about their availability through your personnel or human resources department.
- If your company does not offer an alcohol or drug rehabilitation program, contact your health-care provider or a mental health professional for a confidential referral.

Drug Testing in the Workplace

Drug testing programs are usually part of a comprehensive program to create a drug-free workplace. Drug testing in the workplace remains controversial. It is opposed by some employees and is touted by some companies as a strong message for a drug-free work environment.

    Workplace drug testing is used in several different ways:

- Pre-employment or applicant testing
- Post-accident or for-cause testing
- Scheduled testing (used during routine physical examinations, for example)
- Random testing (used for job categories involving public safety or security)
- Treatment follow-up testing to monitor an employee's success in remaining drug-free

Ergonomics

Ergonomics, fitting workplaces to workers, is a relatively new field of study. While research continues on ways to make the office a healthier place in which to work, there are some guidelines for reducing or avoiding work-related injury.

Remember, work is only part of the ergonomic equation. Problems outside the work environment may aggravate workplace strain. Review other activities, including driving, sleeping position, hobbies and other activities, including exercise habits.

Self-Care

- Use adjustable office equipment. Seek comfortable (rather than extreme) positions. Keep knees and elbows in a comfortable "mid" position.
- Avoid excessive repetition. Take frequent, short breaks, perhaps 30 seconds every 10 to 15 minutes.
- Change tasks frequently.
- Stand to answer your phone.
- Gently stretch hands, arms, shoulders and neck.
- Avoid holding one position for long periods (including "mousing" or extended telephone use).
- Participate in regular aerobic activities; you are less likely to experience strain.

Improving Your Posture

- Avoid tensing your shoulders. Your arms should rest comfortably at your sides.
- Your back should be well supported, and the chair should be adjusted so you are not reaching up or leaning forward.
- The position of your chair should allow your feet to rest on the floor or a footrest. Change leg positions frequently.

Computer Use

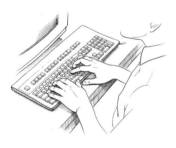

- Place your monitor as far away as possible for you to still see clearly. If your shoulders or back aches, try different monitor heights and distances. Your eyes should be level with the top line of copy on the monitor.
- If you have eye fatigue, have your eyes checked. Reading glasses for computer use are available. You may need a larger screen. If you wear bifocals, you may need high bifocal lenses to avoid holding your head in an awkward position.
- Place your keyboard at elbow height or lower (you may need to raise your chair or find a lower work surface).
- Don't rest your wrists or elbows on anything hard or sharp. Your arms should rest comfortably at your sides without reaching, with forearms roughly parallel to the floor. Don't reach for your keyboard or mouse.
- If you don't have a mouse table, place your mouse by your keyboard, at the same level. Keep your arms near your body as you use the mouse. A wrist rest, track ball or a different-shaped mouse may help; but if possible, try these changes awhile before deciding. If possible, learn to use the mouse with either hand.
- Type with your fingers gently curled and wrists straight. Have a "light" touch— use only enough pressure to depress the keys.

Caution

Advertisers promote many so-called ergonomic products to office workers. Experts warn: buyer beware. Everyone is different, and these products may or may not help you. One size does not fit all! Whenever possible, try a product before you switch.

Exercises for "Office Potatoes"

Sitting at work for 8 hours a day can cause office workers' syndrome—fatigue, stress, back pain, even blood clots—but it doesn't have to. These stretches will help (and may even improve your job performance).

Three 5-minute stretch breaks a day will perk you up, relax your muscles and enhance your flexibility. Here are six exercises you can do without leaving your desk. (Note: Hold each stretch for 10 to 20 seconds. Repeat each exercise once or twice on both sides.)

1. Stretch your fingers out as far as you can. Hold for 10 seconds. Relax. Now bend your fingers at the knuckles and squeeze.
2. Hold your left arm just above the elbow with your right hand. Gently pull your elbow across your chest toward the right shoulder while turning your head to look over the left shoulder.
3. Hold your left leg with both arms just below the knee. Gently pull your bent leg toward your chest. Step two: Hold it with your right arm and pull it toward your right shoulder.
4. Slowly tilt your head to the left until you feel a stretch on the side of your neck. Repeat to the right and forward.
5. Hold your left elbow with your right hand. Gently pull your elbow behind your head and toward your right shoulder until you feel a nice stretch in your shoulder or upper arms.
6. Cross your left leg over your right leg. Cross your right elbow over your left thigh. Gently press your leg with your elbow to twist your hip and lower and middle parts of your back. Look over your left shoulder to complete the stretch.

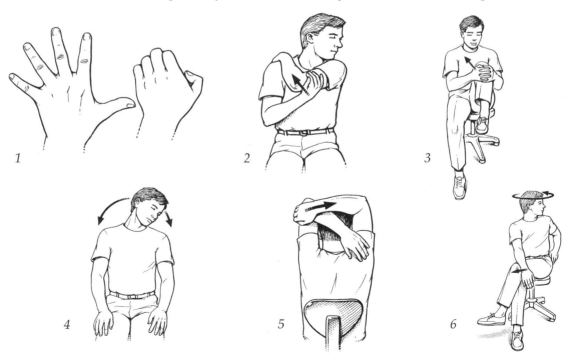

Pregnancy and Work

Job conditions may require modification during pregnancy. Pregnancy affects a woman's heat tolerance, stamina and balance.

If your work involves one or more of the conditions listed below, you may need to modify your job duties after discussions with your physician, your manager and your company's doctor or nurse:

- Heavy, repetitive lifting
- Prolonged standing
- Heavy vibration (such as that from large machines)
- Long, stressful commutes to and from work

The risk from prolonged standing may not seem obvious at first. However, during pregnancy there is increased dilatation of blood vessels and pooling of blood in the legs with standing. These effects may cause dizziness and even fainting, which could lead to accidents and injuries.

Exposure to Harmful Substances

Certain substances in the workplace are known to be harmful to the developing fetus. These include lead, mercury, X-rays and drugs used to treat cancer. Anesthetic gases and organic solvents such as benzene are suspected to be harmful, although results of studies are inconclusive.

Fortunately, few birth defects are caused by environmental agents. Of the 4 to 6 percent of birth defects that can be traced to an environmental cause, most involve alcohol, tobacco or drugs used during pregnancy — not substances in the workplace. Nevertheless, exposure to potentially harmful substances should be avoided.

Tell your doctor about your exposure to chemicals, drugs or radiation on the job as well as the use of equipment in the workplace designed to minimize exposure, such as ventilation systems. Your physician will determine whether a risk exists and, if so, what can be done to eliminate or reduce it. When these conditions exist, work with your manager to see what changes can be made.

Industries in the United States are required by federal law to have Material Safety Data Sheets on file to report hazardous substances in the workplace. This information must be made available to employees and can be helpful to your doctor and manager.

Infections

Health-care and child-care workers, schoolteachers, veterinary workers and meat handlers may be exposed to infections in the course of their jobs. Infections of greatest concern for pregnant women are rubella (German measles), chickenpox, fifth disease, cytomegalovirus, toxoplasmosis, herpes simplex, hepatitis B and AIDS.

You may already be immune to some of these diseases. If not, you should avoid situations in which you are exposed to the infection, such as close contact with a person who has the illness.

Health-care workers practice infection-control procedures such as wearing gloves, washing their hands and avoiding eating on the job. Child-care workers should wash their hands before eating and after changing diapers or helping children use the bathroom. Avoid contact with saliva, which means not kissing your young charges or sharing food with them.

If you are concerned about exposure to infection at work, speak with your doctor. Depending on your health, immune status and job duties, you may be told to take special precautions.

Safety in the Workplace

Protect yourself and others by following these safety rules and guidelines:

Protective eyewear: If your job carries a risk of eye injury, your employer is required by law to provide you with protective glasses, and you are required to wear them. If they interfere with your efficiency, try another design.

Protection from noise: In conditions of excessively loud noise, your employer should regularly measure noise levels or provide protective devices. Specially designed earmuffs are available. Some types close out all sound from the outside; others are fitted with earphones and a microphone that enable you to communicate with other workers. Commercially available earplugs made of foam, plastic or rubber or custom-molded plugs also effectively decrease your exposure to excessive noise. Don't use cotton balls. They can get stuck deep in your ear canal and don't block out noise very well.

Fumes, smoke, dust and gas hazards: Many respiratory symptoms can result from exposure to toxic fumes, gases, particles and smoke in the workplace. The exposure may be long-term with low levels of chemicals; accidental exposure also may occur in which high levels of industrial toxic chemicals are inhaled for a short time. Governmental agencies have established safety guidelines for exposures in the workplace. Wear proper clothing, air-filtration masks, eye gear and other appropriate protection. Be sure ventilation is adequate.

If you suspect that there may be dangerous smoke, fumes, dust or chemical exposure in your workplace, discuss the matter with your physician and your company's safety officer.

Shift work: If your job requires constant changing of shifts, your body will have more difficulty adjusting and readjusting as you get older. Some studies suggest that too frequent shift changes over a lengthy period increase the risk of coronary artery disease or peptic ulcer. Here are some strategies to try:

- Work a shift for 3 weeks rather than rotating to a different schedule every week.
- Change the sequence. A more normal sleep pattern results when the shift sequence is day-evening-night rather than the day-night-evening sequence.

Sleeping Hints for Shift Workers

About 20 percent of employed Americans have nontraditional schedules. Many have problems getting enough sleep and so are more prone to sleepiness on the job than the 9-to-5 worker. Employees on an 11 p.m. to 7 a.m. shift and those who rotate shifts are more likely to have sleep problems than other shift workers. Naps may help offset the sleep loss, but they are not a substitute for a regular schedule of quality sleep.

Here are some helpful hints:

- Maintain your workday sleep schedule on your days off.
- Sleep in dark, quiet rooms. Cover windows with opaque curtains or wear eyeshades.
- Talk with your family members about your sleep schedule.
- Turn off the phone, disconnect the doorbell or put up a "Do Not Disturb" sign.
- Don't go to bed hungry or immediately after eating a large meal.

The Healthy Consumer

- **You and Your Personal Physician**

- **Home Medical Testing Kits**

- **Your Family Medical Tree**

- **Medications and You**

- **The Healthy Traveler**

In this section, we answer questions related to the healthy consumer, such as, How can you best communicate and work with your physician? What can you learn from your family's medical history? How effective are home medical testing kits? What should you include in the family's home medicine chest and first aid kit? What are the potential health risks associated with travel? We also discuss proper use of medications and include easy-to-understand descriptions of cold remedies and over-the-counter pain medications that are mentioned throughout this book.

You and Your Personal Physician

Building a good relationship with your doctor is extremely important. Good communication is part of that relationship. Let your provider know when you are dissatisfied, but if necessary explore your options for making a change.

What to Expect From Your Doctor

You're more likely to be satisfied with your health care if you have realistic expectations about your doctor. You can't always expect a cure. You can expect your doctor to give you:

- **Time to ask questions and discuss concerns.** If you have a sore throat or ear pain, you may expect adequate care during a 10- to 15-minute appointment. Symptoms such as chronic stomach pain or stress or a complex problem takes more time. To reduce frustration caused by lack of time, try to anticipate when you may need more time and schedule appropriately.
- **Information.** Ask for a clear explanation of your illness.
- **Cost estimates of your care.** Your doctor should be willing to discuss fees for major tests and procedures before they are scheduled.
- **Consultation.** You're entitled to reasonable access to your doctor. This doesn't mean middle-of-the-night home visits, but it does mean contact as your medical condition dictates and as your doctor's schedule permits.
- **Emergency contacts.** In case you can't reach your own doctor, ask for a contact you can call.
- **Decision-making ability.** You should participate in decisions about your care.
- **Confidentiality.** The privacy of information contained in your medical records is protected by your doctor and other health-care professionals. For some conditions, such as certain infectious diseases, your doctor is required by law to notify government authorities. In general, however, your records can't be released to insurance companies, employers or other individuals unless you approve.
- **Appropriate referrals.** If you have an unusual or puzzling problem, referral to another doctor may be appropriate. You also can expect prompt transfer of your medical records if you move or change physicians.

Medical Office Visits

To get the most out of the time you spend with your doctor or health-care provider:

- **Before the visit,** jot down one to three main problems you're concerned about. Briefly describe your symptoms and when they occur.
- **Schedule appropriately.** If you feel your questions or concerns can't be covered in a typical 10- to 15-minute appointment, make that known when scheduling your visit.
- **Be prompt.** If you can't keep an appointment, cancel it, at least 24 hours ahead if possible.
- **Bring your medicines** in the original bottles.

- **Answer questions accurately and completely.** List all your prescription and over-the-counter medications, vitamins or herbal remedies. Be candid about alcohol and tobacco use and about other physicians or practitioners you see.
- **Listen carefully.** Repeat what you heard. Ask your doctor to clarify in understandable terms.
- **Follow instructions.** Studies show only one-third of all people follow their doctors' instructions.
- **Speak up.** If you have questions or doubts about your diagnosis or treatment, say so.

Home Medical Testing Kits

Your pharmacy or drugstore has kits that can be used to perform medical tests at home, without the involvement of a physician or health-care provider.

Like most tests in a laboratory, home tests use urine, blood or stool. Some of them are relatively inexpensive. Some contain enough supplies to perform the test more than once. The advantages of doing a test with a kit are convenience and a reduced cost over a medical laboratory. However, there are several disadvantages.

Types of Kits

- **Pregnancy tests** to determine whether you are pregnant.
- **Ovulation prediction tests** to help determine the best time for intercourse that may lead to conception.
- **Sugar tests,** of either urine or blood, to determine whether diabetes is present or well controlled.
- **Other urine tests**, such as for excess protein, which may signal a kidney problem.
- **Tests to detect blood** in the stool, which may indicate a tumor in the colon.
- **Human immunodeficiency virus (HIV) tests** check for antibodies to HIV, the virus that causes AIDS. The test involves placing a drop of blood on a test card with an identification number. You mail the card to the designated certified laboratory, then call for results in about 1 week.

Disadvantages of Home Tests

- **There is the risk of simply doing the test wrong** and, therefore, getting a misleading result. You must follow the instructions exactly or the test will not work properly. Professionals in a medical laboratory are less likely to make a mistake because they have more experience and better equipment.
- **Medical tests do not always work correctly.** This is true for tests done at home and for tests performed in a medical laboratory. A certain percentage of test results suggest that something is present when it is not (false positive). For example, a false-positive test result would indicate that you do have hidden blood in the stool when in fact you do not, or that you are pregnant when you are not.
- **False-negative results** can be found. A certain percentage of test results indicate that something is not present when it is, which is called a false negative. For example, a false-negative test result would indicate that your blood glucose concentration is normal when it is not, or that you are not pregnant when you are. A physician is in a better position to judge false-negative and false-positive test results on the basis of other medical evidence, training and experience.
- **You may interpret the result incorrectly.** Changes in the appearance of the test result, such as the color, may be confusing. Often, you need to see your physician or have the test repeated by a medical laboratory no matter what the result.
- **Indecision** is a factor. After performing the test, it is often difficult to decide what to do next. For example, if you are certain there is blood in your stool but the test indicates otherwise, should you still see your physician?

Caution

When used appropriately, many home testing kits can be accurate. Nevertheless, use them carefully. They are not a substitute for appropriate medical care, especially when you think you may be at risk of a serious medical condition. Follow up worrisome, unexpected test results with your health-care provider.

Healthy Consumer

Your Family Medical Tree

Family gatherings are an ideal time to catch up on family news. They are also an opportunity to learn more about your family health history.

Some 10 to 15 percent of people with colon cancer have a family history of the disease. Up to one-fourth of children of alcoholics are themselves likely to become alcoholics. And a family history of high blood pressure, diabetes, some cancers and certain psychiatric disorders significantly increases all family members' odds of developing the condition.

If blood relatives have had a particular disease or condition, are you destined to get it? Usually not. But it may mean you are at an increased risk.

Many major diseases have a hereditary component. But when you know you are at increased risk for a disease, you may be able to take steps to prevent it—or at least detect it early, when the odds for a cure may be in your favor.

Medical trees reveal patterns of hereditary illness. With this kind of information, your doctor may prescribe tests or recommend lifestyle changes. In fact, one study showed that 25,000 medical trees identified 43,000 people who were at risk for hereditary illnesses. And the people who were evaluated proved to be excellent candidates for preventive treatment.

Creating a Family Medical Tree

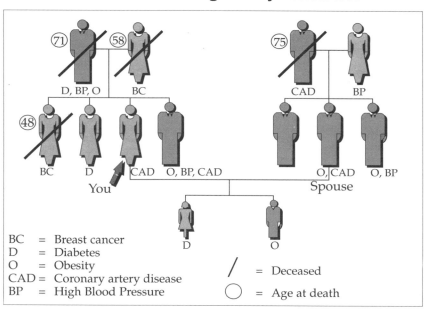

BC = Breast cancer
D = Diabetes
O = Obesity
CAD = Coronary artery disease
BP = High Blood Pressure

/ = Deceased
◯ = Age at death

A family tree showing how you can chart a family medical history.

- **Learn who's who.** Research your parents, siblings and children. Then add information about grandparents, aunts and uncles, cousins and nieces and nephews. The more relatives you include, the better.
- **Dig for details.** Interview relatives by phone, or mail them questionnaires.
- **Look into the past.** Information about any ailment—from allergies to limps—could prove helpful. Pay special attention to serious but potentially preventable conditions, such as cancer, high blood pressure, heart disease, diabetes, depression and alcoholism. Note the age of the relative when the illness was diagnosed. What kind of lifestyle did the person lead (smoker? activity level?).
- **Put it all together.** Organize your chart so you can view the health histories of several relatives at once (see the illustration). Assign each medical condition a letter, and then write this letter next to the person's name or figure. Note the person's age when he or she died.
- **Talk it over.** Ask your physician to review your medical tree.

Medications and You

No matter what your age or condition, there are fundamental rules to follow when taking medications.

- **Advise your physician about any over-the-counter drugs** you are taking, including laxatives or antacids; aspirin or acetaminophen; cough, cold or hay fever medicines; or mineral and vitamin supplements. Nonprescription drugs can be potent, and some can cause serious reactions when mixed with prescription drugs.
- **Read labels carefully.** Ask your physician and pharmacist about potential side effects, about any dietary restrictions you should follow, whether you should avoid alcohol while taking the drug or about other concerns you have. If you get a prescription refilled and it appears different from what you had been taking, ask your pharmacist why.
- **Follow instructions.** Anyone who uses more than the recommended dosage is in danger of an overdose. The "more is better" theory does not apply to drugs.
- **Do not stop taking a prescribed drug** just because your symptoms seem to lessen. Take your medication for the entire length of time prescribed, even if symptoms have disappeared, unless instructed otherwise by your physician.
- **Keep a record** of what you take if you are taking numerous medications on a daily basis. Carry it in your purse or wallet. Also, list your allergies and any intolerance to drugs.
- **Inform your physician of side effects.** Be alert to headache, dizziness, blurred vision, ringing in your ears, shortness of breath, hives and other unexpected effects.
- **Have prescriptions filled at one pharmacy.** Using one pharmacy can help you avoid problems with drug interactions. Your pharmacist can help monitor the mix of medications, even if they are prescribed by different physicians.
- **Properly store medications.** Most require a dry, secure place at room temperature and out of direct sunlight. Some drugs need refrigeration. A bathroom cabinet is often a poor place to store medications because of temperature and moisture variations.
- **Discard outdated drugs.** Medicine deteriorates over time and can sometimes become toxic. Never take leftover medicine.
- **Be concerned for children.** Keep prescription and nonprescription drugs safely away from the reach of children. Buy childproof packages, especially if you have young children, grandchildren or very young guests.
- **Keep medicines in their original containers.** If the label gets separated from a medicine container and there is any doubt as to its contents, discard the medicine immediately. Prescription containers are designed to protect medications from light and moisture.
- **If you have trouble opening a container** with a safety cap, ask your pharmacist for a special nonsafety cap.
- **Don't lend or share prescription drugs.** What helps you might harm others.
- **Don't take a medication in the dark.**
- **Avoid mixing medications and alcohol.** This combination can cause a harmful interaction.

Healthy Consumer

■ Pain Relievers: Matching the Pill to the Pain

Although the packaging and promises are different, all nonprescription pain relievers contain one of these five chemicals—aspirin, acetaminophen, ibuprofen, naproxen sodium and, most recently, ketoprofen. For pain relief, the differences among products are more subtle than significant.

Pain relievers are called analgesics (from the Greek words *an*, meaning "without," and *algos*, meaning "pain"). Over-the-counter (OTC) analgesics relieve mild to moderate pain associated with headache, colds, toothache, muscle ache, backache, arthritis and menstrual cramps. They also reduce fever. OTC analgesics fall into two main categories: those that also decrease inflammation and those that don't.

- **NSAIDS:** Aspirin, ibuprofen, naproxen sodium and ketoprofen reduce inflammation and are called nonsteroidal anti-inflammatory drugs (NSAIDs). They're most helpful when a painful condition also involves inflammation (some forms of arthritis, tendinitis). Common side effects include stomach upset, ulcer and bleeding (see page 231).
- **Acetaminophen** doesn't relieve inflammation. Because it's relatively free of side effects at recommended doses, it may be a good alternative for long-term use or when taking NSAIDs presents a risk.

All regular-strength doses of OTC pain relievers provide comparable relief for everyday pain such as headache or sore muscles. For menstrual pain, ibuprofen, naproxen sodium and ketoprofen may offer better relief.

Separating Help From Hype

OTC pain medications come in a great variety of forms. Often, the least expensive generic form is all you need. If you have questions, ask a pharmacist or your doctor.

Here's a guide for sorting through different forms of drug delivery:

- **Buffered:** A buffered analgesic contains an antacid to reduce acidity. It's controversial whether these products actually protect your stomach.
- **Enteric-coated:** A special coating allows pills to pass through your stomach and dissolve in the small intestine. This helps reduce stomach irritation. Consider an enteric-coated product if you need daily relief for chronic pain. Because the coating delays absorption, it's not the best choice for quick relief (such as for a headache).
- **Timed-release:** Also called extended-release and sustained-release, these products dissolve slowly. They prolong relief by maintaining a constant level of analgesic in your blood. Use them if you need lasting, not immediate, relief.
- **Extra-strength:** A single dose of these preparations contains more pain-relieving medicine than regular-strength products—typically 500 milligrams of aspirin or acetaminophen vs. 325 milligrams. They're more convenient when it takes more than one regular-strength dose to improve your symptoms, but you should take them less often.
- **Combination formulas:** Some products are paired with caffeine or an antihistamine to boost their effect. Studies show that the addition of caffeine to aspirin or acetaminophen does improve pain relief.
- **Tablet, caplet, gelcap, gum or liquid:** If you have trouble swallowing a round tablet or oval caplet, a smooth gelcap might work better. Other options include taking aspirin as an effervescing pain reliever plus antacid (Alka-Seltzer) or chewing aspirin as a gum (Aspergum).
- **Generic:** Generic pain relievers almost always cost less than brand name drugs, but they're just as effective.

- **Know your special risks.** In general, don't take NSAIDs if you also take a blood thinner, or if you have kidney disease, ulcers, a bleeding disorder or an allergy to aspirin.
- **Avoid drug interactions.** If you take other OTC or prescription medications, talk with your doctor or pharmacist about which pain reliever is best.
- **Don't exceed the recommended dose**—unless your doctor advises it.
- **Avoid alcohol.** Mixing alcohol with aspirin, ibuprofen or naproxen sodium increases the chance of stomach upset and bleeding. In combination with higher-than-recommended doses of acetaminophen, alcohol increases the risk of serious damage to your liver.
- **Take NSAIDs with milk and food** to help minimize stomach upset.
- **Don't take longer than necessary**. Periodically reevaluate your need for pain relievers.
- Always read and follow label instructions.

Over-the-Counter Pain Relievers

	Aspirin	Acetaminophen	Ibuprofen	Naproxen Sodium	Ketoprofen
Sampling of brand names	Anacin, Ascriptin, Bayer, Bufferin, Ecotrin, Empirin	Excedrin (Aspirin Free), Panadol, Tylenol	Advil, Ibuprin, Motrin-IB, Nuprin	Aleve	Orudis KT, Actron
Reduces pain and fever	Yes	Yes	Yes	Yes	Yes
Reduces inflammation	Yes	No	Yes	Yes	Yes
Side effects	Gastrointestinal (GI) bleeding, stomach upset and ulceration	None when taken as directed for short periods (days to weeks)	GI bleeding, stomach upset, ulceration and pain	GI bleeding, stomach upset, bloating and dizziness	GI bleeding, ulceration
Special cautions	Don't take if you have allergy to aspirin, asthma, bleeding disorder, gout or ulcers	Overdoses can be toxic to the liver. Alcohol enhances toxic effects of high doses	Don't take if you have allergy to aspirin, asthma, heart failure, kidney problems, ulcers	Don't take if you have allergy to aspirin, asthma, heart failure, kidney problems, ulcers	Don't take if you have allergy to aspirin, asthma, heart failure, kidney problems, ulcers
Children's use	Can cause Reye's syndrome* in children with chickenpox, the flu or other viral illness	Available for children. Dosages based on age and weight. Consult your physician	Available for children. Dosages based on age and weight. Consult your physician	Do not give to children younger than 12 except on advice of a doctor	Not recommended. Safety and effectiveness have not been studied

*Reye's syndrome is a potentially fatal swelling of brain tussues. Note: This list is not comprehensive and is not an endorsement. We have not tested these products but rely on data supplied by the manufacturers.

■ Cold Remedies: What They Can and Cannot Do

There is no cure for the common cold. Yet drugs used to treat the effects of the common cold—runny nose, fever, congestion and cough—are the largest segment of the over-the-counter market for America's pharmaceutical industry. Some of these medications also are formulated as allergy medicines to treat itchy eyes and sneezing.

Most people don't need any medication for a cold. With the possible exception of zinc lozenges (see page 111), none of the various cold remedies will make your cold heal more quickly. But if your cold symptoms are particularly bothersome, careful use of over-the-counter cold medicines may provide some relief. If used at the wrong time, they can make you feel worse.

Cold Remedies

	Antihistamines	Decongestants	Cough Medicines	Cough/Cold Combinations

Products and brand names	Benadryl
	Chlor-Trimeton
	Tavist
	Teldrin
	Generics
		Neo-Synephrine
		Afrin
		Propagest
		Sudafed
		Generics
			Expectorants
			  Robitussin
			  Generics that
			  contain
			  guaifenesin
			Antitussives
			  Robitussin-DM
			  Generics that
			  contain
			  dextromethorphan
				Actifed
				Chlor-Trimeton D
				Contac
				Dimetapp
				Drixoral
				Sudafed Plus
				Tavist D
				Generics

Symptoms relieved	Sneezing, runny nose, itchy eyes, congestion due to allergies	Congestion, stuffiness	*Expectorants* loosen mucus in the chest, making it easier to cough *Antitussives* reduce the frequency of coughing	Cough, stuffy nose, general discomfort
Side effects and cautions	Drowsiness, dry mouth, may dry secretions making mucus harder to clear, may increase the effects of alcohol	Insomnia, jitters, palpitations, may raise blood pressure	Antitussives may have a sedating effect because some include narcotic-like substances	Many do not contain enough antihistamine for significant benefit, may combine three or more products
Time of maximal benefit	Early in a cold when sneezing and watery, runny nose are common	When nose is stuffed up. Use for only a few days; the effect often wears off after 3 to 4 days of use	When mucus is thick and cough is prominent	Use individual products instead, when they will have the most benefit

Self-Care

Here's some helpful advice on the use of cold medicines:

- **Always read the labels** to determine the active ingredients and side effects of the particular medicine.
- **A single-symptom medicine is often better** than a combination medication.
- **Most combination cold medications contain some form of analgesic** such as aspirin, ibuprofen or acetaminophen (see page 231). Therefore, you don't need to take a separate analgesic.
- **Don't mix** various cold medications or take with other medications without consulting your physician or pharmacist.
- **Avoid alcohol** when taking cold medications.
- **Consult your physician** before giving any cold medicine to a child.

Home Medical Supplies

When an emergency or medical problem occurs in the home, you often don't have time to search for supplies. Keep your medical supplies in a place that is easily accessible to adults but out of the reach of children. And remember to replace items after their use to make sure the kit is always complete. Here's what you need to be properly prepared for accidents and common illnesses that are mentioned in this book:

- **For cuts:** Bandages of various sizes, gauze, adhesive tape, an antiseptic solution to clean wounds and an antiseptic cream to prevent infection.
- **For burns:** Cold packs, gauze, burn spray and an antiseptic cream.
- **For aches, pain and fever:** Aspirin (for adults only) or another nonsteroidal anti-inflammatory drug, and acetaminophen for children or adults.
- **For eye injuries:** Eyewash, an eyewash cup and eye patches.
- **For sprains, strains and fractures:** Cold packs, elastic wraps for wrapping injuries and a triangular bandage for making an arm sling.
- **For insect bites and stings:** A tweezers to remove stingers and hydrocortisone cream to relieve itching. If a family member is allergic to insect stings, also include a kit containing a syringe and epinephrine (adrenaline).
- **For ingestion of poisons:** Syrup of ipecac to induce vomiting. Use it only after contacting a poison control center or medical professional (keep the number of your local poison control center on a sticker on your telephone).
- **For general care:** Thermometer, sharp scissors, cottons swabs, tissues, soap or cleansing pads, gloves for use if blood or body fluids are present and a first aid manual.

The Healthy Traveler

Becoming ill away from home poses a special set of problems. This chapter suggests ways to deal with common conditions that plague travelers. For people with chronic health problems, it's always a good idea to talk with your physician before you leave home.

■ Air Travel Hazards

The fastest way to travel—by airplane—is also one of the safest. Yet by placing you thousands of feet in the air, moving at a speed of hundreds of miles per hour, air travel does subject your body to special challenges. Here are common problems that you might experience during air travel:

Dehydration
The pressurized cabin of an airplane has extremely low humidity, only 5 to 10 percent. This may cause you to become dehydrated. To prevent dehydration, drink liquids such as water and fruit juices during your flight. Avoid alcohol and caffeine.

Blood Clots
Sitting during a long flight causes fluid to accumulate in the soft tissues in your legs. This increases your risk of a blood clot (thrombophlebitis). To improve circulation back to your heart:
- Stand up and stretch periodically after the "wear your seat belt" sign is turned off. Take a walk through the cabin once an hour or so.
- Flex your ankles or press your feet against the floor or seat mountings in front of you.
- If you're prone to swollen ankles or have varicose veins, consider wearing support hose.

Ear Pain
To avoid ear pain during ascent or descent, try this exercise to equalize the pressure in your ears:
- Take a deep breath; hold it for 2 seconds.
- Slowly exhale about 20 percent of the air while gradually pursing your lips.
- With your lips tightly closed, try to gently blow air as though you were playing a trumpet. Don't blow too hard.
- After about 2 seconds, exhale normally.
- To avoid light-headedness, limit your pressure breaths to no more than 10.
- Yawning, chewing gum and swallowing also help during ascent or descent.

Jet Lag
If you've ever traveled by air to a different time zone, you're probably familiar with what it's like to get jet lag—that dragged-out, out-of-sync feeling. Not all jet lag is the same. Flying eastward—and therefore resetting your body clock forward—is often more difficult than flying westward and adding hours to your day. Most peoples' bodies adjust at the rate of about 1 hour a day. Thus, after a change of four time zones, your body will require about 4 days to resynchronize its usual rhythms.

- **Reset your body's clock.** Begin resetting your body's clock several days in advance of your departure by adopting a sleep-wake pattern similar to the day-night cycle at your destination.
- **Drink plenty of fluids and eat lightly.** Drink extra liquids during your flight to avoid dehydration, but limit beverages with alcohol and caffeine. They increase dehydration and may disrupt your sleep. Limit your intake of salty or fatty food.

Motion Sickness

Any type of transportation can cause motion sickness. It can strike suddenly, progressing from a feeling of restlessness to a cold sweat, dizziness and then vomiting and diarrhea. Motion sickness usually quiets down as soon as the motion stops. The more you travel, the more easily you'll adjust to being in motion.

You may escape motion sickness by planning ahead.

- If you're traveling by ship, request a cabin in the middle of the ship, near the waterline. If you're on a plane, ask for a seat over the front edge of a wing. Once aboard, direct the air vent at your face. On a train, take a seat near a window, and face forward. In an automobile, drive or sit in the front passenger's seat.

If you're susceptible to motion sickness:

- Focus on the horizon or a distant, stationary object. Don't read.
- Keep your head still, rested against a seat back.
- Don't smoke or sit near smokers.
- Avoid spicy foods and alcohol. Don't overeat.
- Take an over-the-counter antihistamine such as meclizine or dimenhydrinate before you feel sick. Expect drowsiness as a side effect.
- Consider scopolamine, available in a prescription adhesive patch. Several hours before you're in motion, apply the patch behind your ear for 72-hour protection. Talk to your doctor before using the medication if you have health problems such as asthma, glaucoma or urine retention.
- If you become ill, eating dry crackers or drinking a carbonated beverage may help settle your stomach.

Traveler's Diarrhea

Traveler's diarrhea may be attributed to several causes, including unaccustomed food and drink, change in living habits and bacterial and viral infections due to poor sanitation. Symptoms generally subside in 3 or 4 days.

To avoid the problem:

- **Use proper water sources.** Drink only water that has been properly chlorinated or boiled. Factory-bottled water should be safe. Beware of beverages that contain ice as well as fruit juices because they often are diluted with tap water.
- **Eat safe foods.** Do not eat raw foods, especially salads that contain lettuce or raw vegetables. Avoid fruit and vegetables that are already peeled and unpasteurized milk and dairy products.
- **Drink plenty of safe liquids.** Do not become dehydrated.

Index

D O I N G
E T H I C S

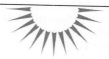

Moral Reasoning and Contemporary Issues

Fourth Edition

Lewis Vaughn

W. W. NORTON & COMPANY Independent and Employee-Owned New York · London

W. W. Norton & Company has been independent since its founding in 1923, when William Warder Norton and Mary D. Herter Norton first published lectures delivered at the People's Institute, the adult education division of New York City's Cooper Union. The firm soon expanded its program beyond the Institute, publishing books by celebrated academics from America and abroad. By midcentury, the two major pillars of Norton's publishing program—trade books and college texts—were firmly established. In the 1950s, the Norton family transferred control of the company to its employees, and today—with a staff of four hundred and a comparable number of trade, college, and professional titles published each year—W. W. Norton & Company stands as the largest and oldest publishing house owned wholly by its employees.

Editor: Peter J. Simon
Project Editor: Rachel Mayer
Assistant Editor: Gerra Goff
Manuscript Editor: Barbara Curialle
Managing Editor, College: Marian Johnson
Managing Editor, College Digital Media: Kim Yi
Production Manager: Ben Reynolds
Media Editor: Erica Wnek
Assistant Media Editor: Cara Folkman
Marketing Manager, Philosophy: Michael Moss
Design Director: Rubina Yeh
Permissions Manager: Megan Jackson
Permissions Clearer: Elizabeth Trammell
Composition: Jouve International—Brattleboro, VT
Manufacturing: LSC Crawfordsville

Permission to use copyrighted material is included as a footnote on the first page of each reading.

ISBN 978-0-393-26541-5

W. W. Norton & Company, Inc., 500 Fifth Avenue, New York, NY 10110-0017

wwnorton.com

W. W. Norton & Company Ltd., 15 Carlisle Street, London W1D 3BS

4 5 6 7 8 9 0

CONTENTS

PREFACE xv

PART 1: FUNDAMENTALS

PART 2: MORAL REASONING

This fourth edition of *Doing Ethics* brings another set of substantial improvements to a text that had already been greatly expanded and improved. The aims that have shaped this text from the beginning have not changed: to help students (1) see why ethics matters to society and to themselves; (2) understand core concepts (theories, principles, values, virtues, and the like); (3) be familiar with the background (scientific, legal, and otherwise) of contemporary moral problems; and (4) know how to apply critical reasoning to those problems—to assess moral judgments and principles, construct and evaluate moral arguments, and apply and critique moral theories. This book, then, tries hard to provide the strongest possible support to teachers of applied ethics who want students, above all, to think for themselves and competently do what is often required of morally mature persons—that is, to do *ethics*.

These goals are reflected in the book's extensive introductions to concepts, cases, and issues; its large collection of readings and exercises; and its chapter-by-chapter coverage of moral reasoning—perhaps the most thorough introduction to these skills available in an applied-ethics text. This latter theme gets systematic treatment in five chapters, threads prominently throughout all the others, and is reinforced everywhere by "Critical Thought" text boxes prompting students to apply critical thinking to real debates and cases. The point of all this is to help students not just to study ethics but to become fully involved in the ethical enterprise and the moral life.

NEW FEATURES

- A new chapter on the morality of personal use of illicit drugs and the laws and policies that pertain to that use: Chapter 12, Drug Use, Harm, and Personal Liberty. It includes three new readings by major figures in the debates on illegal drugs.

- A new chapter on the moral permissibility of affirmative action: Chapter 18, Equality and Affirmative Action. It includes four readings by prominent commentators on the issue.

- A revamped chapter on sexual morality that includes two new readings on pornography: Chapter 13, Sexual Morality.

- Six new readings to supplement the already extensive collection of essays.

ORGANIZATION

Part 1 ("Fundamentals") prepares students for the tasks enumerated above. Chapter 1 explains why ethics is important and why thinking critically about ethical issues is essential to the examined life. It introduces the field of moral philosophy, defines and illustrates basic terminology, clarifies the connection between religion and morality, and explains why moral reasoning is crucial to moral maturity and personal freedom. Chapter 2 investigates a favorite doctrine of undergraduates—ethical relativism—and examines its distant cousin, emotivism.

Part 2 ("Moral Reasoning") consists of Chapter 3, which starts by reassuring students that moral reasoning is neither alien nor difficult but is simply ordinary critical reasoning applied to ethics. They've seen this kind of reasoning before and done it before. Thus, the chapter focuses on identifying, devising, diagramming, and evaluating moral arguments and encourages practice and competence in finding implied premises, testing moral premises, assessing nonmoral premises, and dealing with common argument fallacies.

Part 3 ("Theories of Morality") is about applying critical reasoning to moral theories. Chapter 4 explains how moral theories work and how they are related to other important elements in moral experience: considered judgments, moral arguments, moral principles and rules, and cases and issues. It reviews major theories and shows how students can evaluate them by applying plausible criteria. The rest of Part 3 (Chapters 5 through 7) covers key theories in depth—utilitarianism, ethical egoism, Kant's theory, natural law theory, and the ethics of virtue. Students see how each theory is applied to moral issues and how those issues' strengths and weaknesses are revealed by applying the criteria of evaluation.

In Part 4 ("Ethical Issues"), each of twelve chapters explores a timely moral issue through discussion and relevant readings: abortion, genetic manipulation and human cloning, euthanasia and physician-assisted suicide, drug use, capital punishment, sexual morality, same-sex marriage, environmental ethics, animal rights, affirmative action, political violence, and global economic justice. Every chapter supplies legal, scientific, and other background information on the issue; discusses how major theories have been applied to the problem; examines arguments that have been used in the debate; and includes additional cases for analysis with questions. The readings are a mix of well-known essays and surprising new voices, both classic and contemporary.

PEDAGOGICAL FEATURES

In addition to the "Critical Thought" boxes and "Cases for Analysis," there are other pedagogical devices:

- "Quick Review" boxes that reiterate key points or terms mentioned in previous pages
- Text boxes that discuss additional topics or issues related to main chapter material
- End-of-chapter review and discussion questions
- Chapter summaries
- Suggestions for further reading for each issues chapter
- Glossary

ACKNOWLEDGMENTS

Many people have helped make this third edition a great deal better than its previous incarnations. Among these I think first of my editor at W. W. Norton, Pete Simon, who believed in the project from the outset and helped me shape and improve it. Others at Norton also gave their time and talent to this text: Marian Johnson, managing editor; Rachel Mayer, project editor; Barbara Curialle, copy editor; Benjamin Reynolds, production manager; Megan Jackson, permissions manager; and Gerra Goff, assistant editor.

The silent partners in this venture are the many reviewers who helped in countless ways to make the book better. They include Harry Adams (Prairie View A&M University), Alex Aguado (University of North Alabama), Edwin Aiman (University of Houston), Daniel Alvarez (Colorado State University), Peter Amato (Drexel University), Robert Bass (Coastal Carolina University), Ken Beals (Mary Baldwin College), Helen Becker (Shepherd University), Paul Bloomfield (University of Connecticut), Robyn Bluhm (Old Dominion University), Vanda Bozicevic (Bergen Community College), Brent Braga (Northland Community and Technical College), Mark Raymond Brown (University of Ottawa), Matthew Burstein (Washington and Lee University), Gabriel R. Camacho (El Paso Community College), Jay Campbell (St. Louis Community College at Meramec), Jeffrey Carr (Illinois State University), Alan Clark (Del Mar College), Andrew J. Cohen (Georgia State University), Elliot D. Cohen (Indian River State College), Robert Colter (Centre College), Timothy Conn (Sierra College), Guy Crain (University of Oklahoma), Sharon Crasnow (Norco College), Kelso Cratsley (University of Massachusetts, Boston), George Cronk (Bergen Community College), Kevin DeCoux (Minnesota West Community and Technical College), Lara Denis (Agnes Scott College), Steve Dickerson (South Puget Sound Community College), Nicholas Diehl (Sacramento City College), Robin S. Dillon (Lehigh University), Peter Dlugos (Bergen Community College), Matt Drabek (University of Iowa), David Drebushenko (University of Southern Indiana), Clint Dunagan (Northwest Vista College), Paul Eckstein (Bergen Community College), Andrew Fiala (California State University, Fresno), Stephen Finlay (University of Southern California), Matthew Fitzsimmons (University of North Alabama), Tammie Foltz (Des Moines Area Community College), Tim Fout (University of Louisville), Dimitria Gatzia (University of Akron), Candace Gauthier (University of North Carolina, Wilmington), Mark Greene (University of Delaware), Kevin Guilfoy (Carroll University), Katherine Guin (The College at Brockport: SUNY), Don Habibi (University of North Carolina, Wilmington), Barbara M. Hands (University of North Carolina, Greensboro), Craig Hanks (Texas State University), Jane Haproff (Sierra College), Ed Harris (Texas A&M University), Blake Heffner (Raritan Valley Community College), Marko Hilgersom (Lethbridge Community College), John Holder III (Pensacola Junior College), Mark Hollifield (Clayton College and State University), Margaret Houck (University of South Carolina), Michael Howard (University of Maine, Orono), Frances Howard-Snyder (Western Washington University), Kenneth Howarth (Mercer County Community College), Louis F. Howe, Jr. (Naugatuck Valley Community College), Kyle Hubbard (Saint Anselm College), Robert Hull (Western Virginia Wesleyan College), Amy Jeffers (Owens Community College), Timothy Jessen (Ivy Tech Community College, Bloomington), John Johnston (College of the Redwoods), Marc Jolley (Mercer University), Frederik Kaufman (Ithaca College), Thomas D. Kennedy (Berry College), W. Glenn Kirkconnell (Santa Fe College), Donald Knudsen (Montgomery County Community College), Gilbert Kohler (Shawnee Community College), Thomas Larson (Saint Anselm College), Matt Lawrence (Long Beach City College), Clayton Littlejohn (Southern Methodist University), Jessica Logue (University of Portland), Ian D. MacKinnon (The University of Akron), Tim Madigan (St. John Fisher College), Ernâni Magalhães (West Virginia University), Daniel Malotky (Greensboro College), Ron Martin (Lynchburg College), Michael McKeon (Barry University), Katherine Mendis (Hunter College, CUNY), Joshua Mills-Knutsen (Indiana University Southeast), Michael Monge (Long Beach City College), Eric Moore (Longwood University), Jon S. Moran (Southwest Missouri State University), Dale Murray (Virginia Commonwealth University), Elizabeth Murray (Loyola Marymount University), Thomas Nadelhoffer (Dickinson College), Jay Newhard (East Carolina University), Charles L. North (Southern New Hampshire University), Robert F. O'Connor (Texas State University), Jeffrey P. Ogle (Metropolitan State University of Denver), Don Olive (Roane State Community College), Leonard Olson (California State University, Fresno), Jessica Payson (Bryn Mawr College), Gregory E. Pence (University of Alabama), Donald Petkus (Indiana University School of Public and Environmental Affairs), Trisha Philips (Mississippi State University), Thomas M. Powers (University of Delaware), Marjorie Price (University of Alabama), Netty Provost (Indiana University, Kokomo), Elisa Rapaport (Molloy College), Michael Redmond (Bergen Community College), Daniel Regan (Villanova University), Joseph J. Rogers (University of Texas, San Antonio), John Returra (Lackawanna College), Robert M. Seltzer (Western Illinois University), Edward Sherline (University of Wyoming), Aeon J. Skoble (Bridgewater Community College), Eric Snider (Lansing Community College), Eric Sotnak (University of Akron), Piers

H.G. Stephens (University of Georgia), Grant Sterling (Eastern Illinois University), John Stilwell (University of Texas at Dallas), Tyler Suggs (Virginia Tech), Michele Svatos (Eastfield College), David Svolba (Fitchburg State University), Allen Thompson (Virginia Commonwealth University), Peter B. Trumbull (Madison College), Donald Turner (Nashville State Community College), Julie C. Van Camp (California State University, Long Beach), Michelle Rehwinkel Vasilinda (Tallahassee Community College), Kris Vigneron (Columbus State Community College), Christine Vitrano (Brooklyn College, CUNY), Mark Vopat (Youngstown State University), Matt Waldschlagel (University of North Carolina, Wilmington), Steve Wall (Hillsborough Community College), Bill Warnken (Granite State College), Jamie Carlin Watson (Young Harris College), Rivka Weinberg (Scripps College), Cheryl Wertheimer (Butler Community College), Monique Whitaker (Hunter College, CUNY) Phillip Wiebe (Trinity Western University), Jonathan Wight (University of Richmond), John Yanovitch (Molloy College), Steven Zusman (Waubonsee Community College), and Matt Zwolinski (University of San Diego). Thank you all.

Fundamentals

thing as *desirable*? How can a moral principle be justified? Is there such a thing as moral truth? To do normative ethics, we must assume certain things about the meaning of moral terms and the logical relations among them. But the job of metaethics is to question all these assumptions, to see if they really make sense.

Finally, there is **applied ethics**—the application of moral norms to specific moral issues or cases, particularly those in a profession such as medicine or law. Applied ethics in these fields goes under names such as medical ethics, journalistic ethics, and business ethics. In applied ethics we study the results derived from applying a moral principle or theory to specific circumstances. The purpose of the exercise is to learn something important about either the moral characteristics of the situation or the adequacy of the moral norms. Did the doctor do right in performing that abortion? Is it morally permissible for scientists to perform experiments on people without their consent? Was it right for the journalist to distort her reporting to aid a particular side in the war? Questions like these drive the search for answers in applied ethics.

In every division of ethics, we must be careful to distinguish between *values* and *obligations*. Sometimes we may be interested in concepts or judgments of *value*—that is, about what is morally *good*, *bad*, *blameworthy*, or *praiseworthy*. We properly use these kinds of terms to refer mostly to persons, character traits, motives, and intentions. We may say "She is a good person" or "He is to blame for that tragedy." Other times, we may be interested in concepts or judgments of *obligation*—that is, about what is obligatory or a duty or what we should or ought to do. We use these terms to refer to *actions*. We may say "She has a duty to tell the truth" or "What he did was wrong."

When we talk about value in the sense just described, we mean *moral* value. If she is a good person, she is good in the moral sense. But we can also talk about *nonmoral* value. We can say that things such as televisions, rockets, experiences, and artwork (things other than persons, intentions, etc.) are good, but we mean "good" only in a nonmoral way. It makes no sense to assert that in themselves televisions or rockets are morally good or bad. Perhaps a rocket could be used to perform an action that is morally wrong. In that case, the action would be immoral, while the rocket itself would still have nonmoral value only.

Many things in life have value for us, but they are not necessarily valuable in the same way. Some things are valuable because they are a means to something else. We might say that gasoline is good because it is a means to make a gas-powered vehicle work, or that a pen is good because it can be used to write a letter. Such things are said to be **instrumentally,** or **extrinsically, valuable**—they are valuable as a means to something else. Some things, however, are valuable in themselves or for their own sakes. They are valuable simply because they are what they are, without being a means to something else. Things that have been regarded as valuable in themselves include happiness, pleasure, virtue, and beauty. These are said to be **intrinsically valuable**—they are valuable in themselves.

THE ELEMENTS OF ETHICS

We all do ethics, and we all have a general sense of what is involved. But we can still ask, What are the elements of ethics that make it the peculiar enterprise that it is? We can include at least the following factors:

The Preeminence of Reason

Doing ethics typically involves grappling with our feelings, taking into account the facts of the situation (including our own observations and relevant knowledge), and trying to understand the ideas that bear on the case. But above all, it involves, even requires, critical reasoning—the consideration of reasons for whatever statements

PART
1

Fundamentals

CHAPTER 1

Ethics and the Examined Life

Ethics, or **moral philosophy,** is the philosophical study of morality. **Morality** refers to beliefs concerning right and wrong, good and bad—beliefs that can include judgments, values, rules, principles, and theories. They help guide our actions, define our values, and give us reasons for being the persons we are. (*Ethical* and *moral,* the adjective forms, are often used to mean simply "having to do with morality," and *ethics* and *morality* are sometimes used to refer to the moral norms of a specific group or individual, as in "Greek ethics" or "Russell's morality.") Ethics, then, addresses the powerful question that Socrates formulated twenty-four hundred years ago: how ought we to live?

The scope and continued relevance of this query suggest something compelling about ethics: you cannot escape it. You cannot run away from all the choices, feelings, and actions that accompany ideas about right and wrong, good and bad—ideas that persist in your culture and in your mind. After all, for much of your life, you have been assimilating, modifying, or rejecting the ethical norms you inherited from your family, community, and society. Unless you are very unusual, from time to time you deliberate about the rightness or wrongness of actions, embrace or reject particular moral principles or codes, judge the goodness of your character or intentions (or someone else's), perhaps even question (and agonize over) the soundness of your own moral outlook when it conflicts with that of others. In other words, you are involved in ethics—you *do ethics.*

Even if you try to remove yourself from the ethical realm by insisting that all ethical concepts are irrelevant or empty, you assume a particular view, a theory in the broadest sense, about morality and its place in your life. If at some point you are intellectually brave enough to wonder whether your moral beliefs rest on some coherent supporting considerations, you will see that you cannot even begin to sort out such considerations without—again—doing ethics. In any case, in your life you must deal with the rest of the world, which turns on moral conflict and resolution, moral decision and debate.

What is at stake when we do ethics? In an important sense, the answer is *everything we hold dear.* Ethics is concerned with values—specifically, *moral values.* Through the sifting and weighing of moral values we determine what the most important things are in our lives, what is worth living for and what is worth dying for. We decide what is the greatest good, what goals we should pursue in life, what virtues we should cultivate, what duties we should or should not fulfill, what value we should put on human life, and what pain and perils we should be willing to endure for notions such as the common good, justice, and rights.

Does it matter whether the state executes a criminal who has the mental capacity of a ten-year-old? Does it matter who actually writes the term paper you turn in and represent as your own? Does it matter whether we can easily save a drowning child but casually decide not to? Does it matter whether young girls in Africa undergo painful

3

genital mutilation for reasons of custom or religion? Do these actions and a million others just as controversial matter at all? Most of us—regardless of our opinion on these issues—would say that they matter a great deal. If they matter, then ethics matters, because these are ethical concerns requiring careful reflection using concepts and reasoning peculiar to ethics.

But even though in life ethics is inescapable and important, you are still free to take the easy way out, and many people do. You are free *not* to think too deeply or too systematically about ethical concerns. You can simply embrace the moral beliefs and norms given to you by your family and your society. You can just accept them without question or serious examination. In other words, you can try *not* to do ethics. This approach can be simple and painless—at least for a while—but it has some drawbacks.

First, it undermines your personal freedom. If you accept and never question the moral beliefs handed to you by your culture, then those beliefs are not really yours—and they, not you, control the path you take in life. Only if you critically examine these beliefs *yourself* and decide for *yourself* whether they have merit will they be truly yours. Only then will you be in charge of your own choices and actions.

Second, the no-questions-asked approach increases the chances that your responses to moral dilemmas or contradictions will be incomplete, confused, or mistaken. Sometimes in real life, moral codes or rules do not fit the situations at hand, or moral principles conflict with one another, or entirely new circumstances are not covered by any moral policy at all. Solving these problems requires something that a hand-me-down morality does not include: the intellectual tools to critically evaluate (and reevaluate) existing moral beliefs.

Third, if there is such a thing as intellectual moral growth, you are unlikely to find it on the safe route. To not do ethics is to stay locked in a kind of intellectual limbo, where exploration in ethics and personal moral progress are barely possible.

The philosopher Paul Taylor suggests that there is yet another risk in taking the easy road. If someone blindly embraces the morality bequeathed to him by his society, he may very well be a fine embodiment of the rules of his culture and accept them with certainty. But he also will lack the ability to defend his beliefs by rational argument against criticism. What happens when he encounters others who also have very strong beliefs that contradict his? "He will feel lost and bewildered," Taylor says, and his confusion might leave him disillusioned about morality. "Unable to give an objective, reasoned justification for his own convictions, he may turn from dogmatic certainty to total skepticism. And from total skepticism it is but a short step to an 'amoral' life. . . . Thus the person who begins by accepting moral beliefs blindly can end up denying all morality."[1]

There are other easy roads—roads that also bypass critical and thoughtful scrutiny of morality. We can describe most of them as various forms of subjectivism, a topic that we closely examine in the next chapter. You may decide, for example, that you can establish all your moral beliefs by simply consulting your feelings. In situations calling for moral judgments, you let your emotions be your guide. If it feels right, it *is* right. Alternatively, you may come to believe that moral realities are relative to each person, a view known as *subjective relativism* (also covered in the next chapter). That is, you think that what a person believes or approves of determines the rightness or wrongness of actions. If you believe that abortion is wrong,

[1]Paul W. Taylor, *Principles of Ethics: An Introduction* (Encino, CA: Dickenson, 1975), 9–10.

then it *is* wrong. If you believe it is right, then it *is* right.

But these facile ways through ethical terrain are no better than blindly accepting existing norms. Even if you want to take the subjectivist route, you still need to critically examine it to see if there are good reasons for choosing it—otherwise your choice is arbitrary and therefore not really yours. And unless you thoughtfully consider the merits of moral beliefs (including subjectivist beliefs), your chances of being wrong about them are substantial.

Ethics does not give us a royal road to moral truth. Instead, it shows us how to ask critical questions about morality and systematically seek answers supported by good reasons. This is a tall order because, as we have seen, many of the questions in ethics are among the toughest we can ever ask—and among the most important in life.

THE ETHICAL LANDSCAPE

The domain of ethics is large, divided into several areas of investigation and cordoned off from related subjects. So let us map the territory carefully. As the term *moral philosophy* suggests, ethics is a branch of philosophy. A very rough characterization of philosophy is the systematic use of critical reasoning to answer the most fundamental questions in life. Moral philosophy, obviously, tries to answer the fundamental questions of morality. The other major philosophical divisions address other basic questions; these are *logic* (the study of correct reasoning), *metaphysics* (the study of the fundamental nature of reality), and *epistemology* (the study of knowledge). As a division of philosophy, ethics does its work primarily through critical reasoning. Critical reasoning is the careful, systematic evaluation of statements, or claims—a process used in all fields of study, not just in ethics. Mainly this process includes both the evaluation of logical arguments and the careful analysis of concepts.

Science also studies morality, but not in the way that moral philosophy does. Its approach is known as **descriptive ethics**—the *scientific* study of moral beliefs and practices. Its aim is to describe and explain how people actually behave and think when dealing with moral issues and concepts. This kind of empirical research is usually conducted by sociologists, anthropologists, and psychologists. In contrast, the focus of moral philosophy is not what people actually believe and do, but what they *should* believe and do. The point of moral philosophy is to determine what actions are right (or wrong) and what things are good (or bad).

Philosophers distinguish three major divisions in ethics, each one representing a different way to approach the subject. The first is **normative ethics**—the study of the principles, rules, or theories that guide our actions and judgments. (The word *normative* refers to norms, or standards, of judgment—in this case, norms for judging rightness and goodness.) The ultimate purpose of doing normative ethics is to try to establish the soundness of moral norms, especially the norms embodied in a comprehensive moral system, or theory. We do normative ethics when we use critical reasoning to demonstrate that a moral principle is justified, or that a professional code of conduct is contradictory, or that one proposed moral theory is better than another, or that a person's motive is good. Should the rightness of actions be judged by their consequences? Is happiness the greatest good in life? Is utilitarianism a good moral theory? Such questions are the preoccupation of normative ethics.

Another major division is **metaethics**—the study of the meaning and logical structure of moral beliefs. It asks not whether an action is right or whether a person's character is good. It takes a step back from these concerns and asks more fundamental questions about them: What does it mean for an action to be *right*? Is *good* the same thing as *desirable*? How can a moral principle be justified? Is there such a thing as moral truth? To do normative ethics, we must assume certain things about the meaning of moral terms and the logical relations among them. But the job of metaethics is to question all these assumptions, to see if they really make sense.

Finally, there is **applied ethics**—the application of moral norms to specific moral issues or cases, particularly those in a profession such as medicine or law. Applied ethics in these fields goes under names such as medical ethics, journalistic ethics, and business ethics. In applied ethics we study the results derived from applying a moral principle or theory to specific circumstances. The purpose of the exercise is to learn something important about either the moral characteristics of the situation or the adequacy of the moral norms. Did the doctor do right in performing that abortion? Is it morally permissible for scientists to perform experiments on people without their consent? Was it right for the journalist to distort her reporting to aid a particular side in the war? Questions like these drive the search for answers in applied ethics.

In every division of ethics, we must be careful to distinguish between *values* and *obligations*. Sometimes we may be interested in concepts or judgments of *value*—that is, about what is morally *good, bad, blameworthy,* or *praiseworthy*. We properly use these kinds of terms to refer mostly to persons, character traits, motives, and intentions. We may say "She is a good person" or "He is to blame for that tragedy." Other times, we may be interested in concepts or judgments of *obligation*—that is, about what is obligatory or a duty or what we should or ought to do. We use these terms to refer to *actions*. We may say "She has a duty to tell the truth" or "What he did was wrong."

When we talk about value in the sense just described, we mean *moral* value. If she is a good person, she is good in the moral sense. But we can also talk about *nonmoral* value. We can say that

things such as televisions, rockets, experiences, and artwork (things other than persons, intentions, etc.) are good, but we mean "good" only in a nonmoral way. It makes no sense to assert that in themselves televisions or rockets are morally good or bad. Perhaps a rocket could be used to perform an action that is morally wrong. In that case, the action would be immoral, while the rocket itself would still have nonmoral value only.

Many things in life have value for us, but they are not necessarily valuable in the same way. Some things are valuable because they are a means to something else. We might say that gasoline is good because it is a means to make a gas-powered vehicle work, or that a pen is good because it can be used to write a letter. Such things are said to be **instrumentally,** or **extrinsically, valuable**—they are valuable as a means to something else. Some things, however, are valuable in themselves or for their own sakes. They are valuable simply because they are what they are, without being a means to something else. Things that have been regarded as valuable in themselves include happiness, pleasure, virtue, and beauty. These are said to be **intrinsically valuable**—they are valuable in themselves.

THE ELEMENTS OF ETHICS

We all do ethics, and we all have a general sense of what is involved. But we can still ask, What are the elements of ethics that make it the peculiar enterprise that it is? We can include at least the following factors:

The Preeminence of Reason
Doing ethics typically involves grappling with our feelings, taking into account the facts of the situation (including our own observations and relevant knowledge), and trying to understand the ideas that bear on the case. But above all, it involves, even requires, critical reasoning—the consideration of reasons for whatever statements

QUICK REVIEW

ethics (or moral philosophy)—The philosophical study of morality.

morality—Beliefs concerning right and wrong, good and bad; they can include judgments, rules, principles, and theories.

descriptive ethics—The scientific study of moral beliefs and practices.

normative ethics—The study of the principles, rules, or theories that guide our actions and judgments.

metaethics—The study of the meaning and logical structure of moral beliefs.

applied ethics—The application of moral norms to specific moral issues or cases, particularly those in a profession such as medicine or law.

instrumentally (or extrinsically) valuable—Valuable as a means to something else.

intrinsically valuable—Valuable in itself, for its own sake.

(moral or otherwise) are in question. Whatever our view on moral issues and whatever moral outlook we subscribe to, our commonsense moral experience suggests that if a moral judgment is to be worthy of acceptance, it must be supported by good reasons, and our deliberations on the issue must include a consideration of those reasons.

The backbone of critical reasoning generally and moral reasoning in particular is logical argument. This kind of argument—not the angry-exchange type—consists of a statement to be supported (the assertion to be proved, the conclusion) and the statements that do the supporting (the reasons for believing the statement, the premises). With such arguments, we try to show that a

moral judgment is or is not justified, that a moral principle is or is not sound, that an action is or is not morally permissible, or that a moral theory is or is not plausible.

Our use of critical reasoning and argument helps us keep our feelings about moral issues in perspective. Feelings are an important part of our moral experience. They make empathy possible, which gives us a deeper understanding of the human impact of moral norms. They also can serve as internal alarm bells, warning us of the possibility of injustice, suffering, and wrongdoing. But they are unreliable guides to moral truth. They may simply reflect our own emotional needs, prejudices, upbringing, culture, and self-interests. Careful reasoning, however, can inform our feelings and help us decide moral questions on their merits.

The Universal Perspective

Logic requires that moral norms and judgments follow the *principle of universalizability*—the idea that a moral statement (a principle, rule, or judgment) that applies in one situation must apply in all other situations that are relevantly similar. If you say, for example, that lying is wrong in a particular situation, then you implicitly agree that lying is wrong for anyone in relevantly similar situations. If you say that killing in self-defense is morally permissible, then you say in effect that killing in self-defense is permissible for everyone in relevantly similar situations. It cannot be the case that an action performed by A is *wrong* while the same action performed by B in relevantly similar circumstances is *right*. It cannot be the case that the moral judgments formed in these two situations must differ just because two different people are involved.

This point about universalizability also applies to reasons used to support moral judgments. If reasons apply in a specific case, then those reasons also apply in all relevantly similar cases. It cannot be true that reasons that apply in a specific case do not apply to other cases that are similar in all relevant respects.

The Principle of Impartiality

From the moral point of view, all persons are considered equal and should be treated accordingly. This sense of impartiality is implied in all moral statements. It means that the welfare and interests of each individual should be given the same weight as the welfare and interests of all others. Unless there is a morally relevant difference between people, we should treat them the same: we must treat equals equally. We would think it outrageous for a moral rule to say something like "Everyone must refrain from stealing food in grocery stores—except for Mr. X, who may steal all he wants." Imagine that there is no morally relevant reason for making this exception to food stealing; Mr. X is exempted merely because, say, he is a celebrity known for outrageous behavior. We not only would object to this rule, we might even begin to wonder if it was a genuine moral rule at all since it lacks impartiality. Similarly, we would reject a moral rule that says something like "Everyone is entitled to basic human rights—except Native Americans." Such a rule would be a prime example of unfair discrimination based on race. We can see this blatant partiality best if we ask what morally relevant difference there is between Native Americans and everyone else. Differences in income, social status, skin color, ancestry, and the like are not morally relevant. Apparently there are no morally relevant differences. Because there are none, we must conclude that the rule sanctions unfair discrimination.

We must keep in mind, however, that sometimes there are good reasons for treating someone differently. Imagine a hospital that generally gives equal care to patients, treating equals equally. But suppose a patient comes to the hospital in an ambulance because she has had a heart attack and will die without immediate care. The hospital staff responds quickly, giving her faster and more sophisticated care than other patients receive. The situation is a matter of life and death—a good reason for *not* treating everyone the same and for providing the heart attack patient with special consideration. This instance of discrimination is justified.

The Dominance of Moral Norms

Not all norms are moral norms. There are legal norms (laws, statutes), aesthetic norms (for judging artistic creations), prudential norms (practical considerations of self-interest), and others. Moral norms seem to stand out from all these in an interesting way: they dominate. Whenever moral principles or values conflict in some way with nonmoral principles or values, the moral considerations usually override the others. Moral considerations seem more important, more critical, or more weighty. A principle of prudence such as "Never help a stranger" may be well justified, but it must yield to any moral principle that contradicts it, such as "Help a stranger in an emergency if you can do so without endangering yourself." An aesthetic norm that somehow involved violating a moral principle would have to take a backseat to the moral considerations. A law that conflicted with a moral principle would be suspect, and the latter would have to prevail over the former. Ultimately the justification for civil disobedience is that specific laws conflict with moral norms and are therefore invalid. If we judge a law to be bad, we usually do so on moral grounds.

RELIGION AND MORALITY

Many people believe that morality and religion are inseparable—that religion is the source or basis of morality and that moral precepts are simply what God says should be done. This view is not at all surprising, since all religions imply or assert a perspective on morality. The three great religions in the Western tradition—Christianity, Judaism, and

Islam—provide to their believers commandments or principles of conduct that are thought to constitute the moral law, the essence of morality. For millions of these adherents, the moral law is the will of God, and the will of God is the moral law. In the West at least, the powerful imprint of religion is evident in secular laws and in the private morality of believers and unbelievers alike. Secular systems of morality—for example, those of the ancient Greek philosophers, Immanuel Kant, the utilitarians, and others—have of course left their mark on Western ethics. But they have not moved the millions who think that morality is a product exclusively of religion.

So what is the relationship between religion and morality? For our purposes, we should break this question into two parts: (1) what is the relationship between religion and *ethics* (the philosophical study of morality), and (2) what is the relationship between religion and *morality* (beliefs about right and wrong)? The first question asks about how religion relates to the kind of investigation we conduct in this book—the use of experience and critical reasoning to study morality. The key point about the relationship is that whatever your views on religion and morality, an open-minded expedition into ethics is more useful and empowering than you may realize, especially now at the beginning of your journey into moral philosophy. You may believe, for example, that God determines what is right and wrong, so there is no need to apply critical reasoning to morality—you just need to know what God says. But this judgment—and similar dismissals of ethics—would be premature. Consider the following:

Believers Need Moral Reasoning

It is difficult—perhaps impossible—for most people to avoid using moral reasoning. Religious people are no exception. One reason is that religious moral codes (such as the Ten Command-

ments) and other major religious rules of conduct are usually vague, laying out general principles that may be difficult to apply to specific cases. (Secular moral codes have the same disadvantage.) For example, we may be commanded to love our neighbor, but what neighbors are included—people of a different religion? people who denounce our religion? the gay or lesbian couple? those who steal from us? the convicted child molester next door? the drug dealers on the corner? the woman who got an abortion? Also, what does loving our neighbor demand of us? How does love require us to behave toward the drug dealers, the gay couple, or the person who denounces our religion? If our terminally ill neighbor asks us in the name of love to help him kill himself, what should we do? Does love require us to kill him—or to refrain from killing him? And, of course, commandments can conflict—as when, for example, the only way to avoid killing an innocent person is to tell a lie, or the only way to save the life of one person is to kill another. All these situations force the believer to interpret religious directives, to try to apply general rules to specific cases, to draw out the implications of particular views—in other words, to do ethics.

When Conflicts Arise, Ethics Steps In

Very often moral contradictions or inconsistencies confront the religious believer, and only moral reasoning can help resolve them. Believers sometimes disagree with their religious leaders on moral issues. Adherents of one religious tradition may disagree with those from another tradition on whether an act is right or wrong. Sincere devotees in a religious tradition may wonder if its moral teachings make sense. In all such cases, intelligent resolution of the conflict of moral claims can be achieved only by applying a neutral standard that helps sort out the competing viewpoints. Moral philosophy supplies the neutral standard in the form of critical thinking, well-made arguments,

CRITICAL THOUGHT: Ethics, Religion, and Tough Moral Issues

How can we hope to grapple with complex moral issues that have emerged only in recent years? Can religion alone handle the job? Consider the following case:

> According to a report by CNN, Jack and Lisa Nash made history when they used genetic testing to save the life of their six-year-old daughter, Molly, by having another child. Molly had a rare genetic disorder known as Fanconi anemia, which prevents the generation of bone marrow and produces a fatal leukemia. Molly's best chance to live was to get a transplant of stem cells from the umbilical cord of a sibling, and Molly's parents were determined to give her that sibling, brother Adam. Through genetic testing (and in vitro fertilization), Jack and Lisa were able to select a child who would not only be born without a particular disease (Fanconi anemia, in this case) but also would help a sibling combat the disease by being

the optimal tissue match for a transplant—a historic combination. As Lisa Nash said, "I was going to save Molly no matter what, and I wanted Molly to have siblings."*

Is it right to produce a child to save the life or health of someone else? More to the point, do the scriptures of the three major Western religions provide any guidance on this question? Do any of these traditions offer useful methods for productively discussing or debating such issues with people of different faiths? How might ethics help with these challenges? Is it possible to formulate a reasonable opinion on this case *without doing ethics*? Why or why not?

*"Genetic Selection Gives Girl a Brother and a Second Chance," *CNN.com*, 3 October 2000, http://archives.cnn.com/2000/HEALTH/10/03/testube.brother/index.html (8 December 2005).

and careful analysis. No wonder then that many great religious minds—Aquinas, Leibniz, Descartes, Kant, Maimonides, Averroës, and others—have relied on reason to examine the nature of morality. In fact, countless theists have regarded reason as a gift from God that enables human beings to grasp the truths of science, life, and morality.

Moral Philosophy Enables Productive Discourse

Any fruitful discussions about morality undertaken between people from different religious traditions or between believers and nonbelievers will require a common set of ethical concepts and a shared procedure for deciding issues and making judgments. Ethics provides these tools. Without them, conversations will resolve nothing, and participants will learn little. Without them, people

will talk past each other, appealing only to their own religious views. Furthermore, in a pluralistic society, most of the public discussions about important moral issues take place in a context of shared values such as justice, fairness, equality, and tolerance. Just as important, they also occur according to an unwritten understanding that (1) moral positions should be explained, (2) claims should be supported by reasons, and (3) reasoning should be judged by common rational standards. These skills, of course, are at the heart of ethics.

Now consider the second question from above: What is the relationship between religion and morality? For many people, the most interesting query about the relationship between religion and morality is this: Is God the maker of morality? That is, is God the author of the moral law? Those who answer yes are endorsing a theory of morality known as the *divine command theory*. It says that right actions are those that are willed by God, that God literally defines right and wrong. Something is right or good only because God makes it so. In the simplest version of the theory, God can determine right and wrong because he is omnipotent. He is all-powerful—powerful enough even to create moral norms. On this view, God is a divine lawgiver, and his laws constitute morality.

In general, believers are divided on whether the divine command theory gives an accurate account of the source of morality. Notable among the theory's detractors are the great theistic philosophers Gottfried Leibniz (1646–1716) and Thomas Aquinas (1225–74). And conversely, as odd as it may sound, some nonbelievers have subscribed to it. In *The Brothers Karamazov* (1879–80), the character Ivan Karamazov declares, "If God doesn't exist, everything is permissible." This very sentiment was espoused by, among others, the famous atheist philosopher Jean-Paul Sartre.

Both religious and secular critics of the divine command theory believe that it poses a serious dilemma, one first articulated by Socrates two and one-half millennia ago. In the dialogue *Euthyphro*, Socrates asks, Is an action morally right because God wills it to be so, or does God will it to be so because it is morally right? Critics say that if an action is right only because God wills it (that is, if right and wrong are dependent on God), then many heinous crimes and evil actions would be right if God willed them. If God willed murder, theft, or torture, these deeds would be morally right. If God has unlimited power, he could easily will such actions. If the rightness of an action depended on God's will alone, he could not have reasons for willing what he wills. No reasons would be available and none required. Therefore, if God commanded an action, the command would be without reason, completely arbitrary. Neither the believer nor the nonbeliever would think this state of affairs plausible. On the other

hand, if God wills an action because it is morally right (if moral norms are independent of God), then the divine command theory must be false. God does not create rightness; he simply knows what is right and wrong and is subject to the moral law just as humans are.

For some theists, this charge of arbitrariness is especially worrisome. Leibniz, for example, rejects the divine command theory, declaring that it implies that God is unworthy of worship:

In saying, therefore, that things are not good according to any standard of goodness, but simply by the will of God, it seems to me that one destroys, without realizing it, all the love of God and all his glory; for why praise him for what he has done, if he would be equally praiseworthy in doing the contrary? Where will be his justice and his wisdom if he has only a certain despotic power, if arbitrary will takes the place of reasonableness, and if in accord with the definition of tyrants, justice consists in that which is pleasing to the most powerful?[2]

Defenders of the divine command theory may reply to the arbitrariness argument by contending that God would never command us to commit heinous acts, because God is all-good. Because of his supreme goodness, he would will only what is good. Some thinkers, however, believe that such reasoning renders the very idea of God's goodness meaningless. As one philosopher says,

[O]n this view, the doctrine of the goodness of God is reduced to nonsense. It is important to religious believers that God is not only all-powerful and all-knowing, but that he is also good; yet if we accept the idea that good and bad are defined by reference to God's will, this notion is deprived of any meaning. What could it mean to say that God's commands are good? If "X is good" means "X is commanded by God," then "God's commands are

[2]G. W. von Leibniz, "Discourse on Metaphysics," in *Selections*, ed. Philip P. Wiener (New York: Scribner, 1951), 292.

good" would mean only "God's commands are commanded by God," an empty truism.[3]

In any case, it seems that through critical reasoning we can indeed learn much about morality and the moral life. After all, there are complete moral systems (some of which are examined in this book) that are not based on religion, that contain genuine moral norms indistinguishable from those embraced by religion, and that are justified not by reference to religious precepts but by careful thinking and moral arguments. As the philosopher Jonathan Berg says, "Those who would refuse to recognize as adequately justified any moral beliefs not derived from knowledge of or about God, would have to refute the whole vast range of arguments put by Kant and all others who ever proposed a rational basis for ethics!"[4] Moreover, if we can do ethics—if we can use critical reasoning to discern moral norms certified by the best reasons and evidence—then critical reasoning is sufficient to guide us to moral standards and values. Since we obviously can do ethics (as the following chapters demonstrate), morality is both accessible and meaningful to us whether we are religious or not.

SUMMARY

Ethics is the philosophical study of morality, and morality consists of beliefs concerning right and wrong, good and bad. These beliefs can include judgments, principles, and theories. Participating in the exploration of morality—that is, doing ethics—is inescapable. We all must make moral judgments, assess moral norms, judge people's character, and question the soundness of our moral outlooks. A great deal is at stake when we do ethics, including countless decisions that determine the quality of our lives.

[3]James Rachels, *The Elements of Moral Philosophy,* 4th ed. (Boston: McGraw-Hill, 2003), 51.

[4]Jonathan Berg, "How Could Ethics Depend on Religion?" in *A Companion to Ethics,* ed. Peter Singer, corr. ed. (Oxford: Blackwell, 1993), 525–33.

You can decide to forgo any ethical deliberations and simply embrace the moral beliefs and norms you inherited from your family and culture. But this approach undermines your freedom, for if you accept without question whatever moral beliefs come your way, they are not really yours. Only if you critically examine them for yourself are they truly yours.

The three main divisions of ethics proper are normative ethics (the study of the moral norms that guide our actions and judgments), metaethics (the study of the meaning and logical structure of moral beliefs), and applied ethics (the application of moral norms to specific moral issues or cases).

Ethics involves a distinctive set of elements. These include the preeminence of reason, the universal perspective, the principle of impartiality, and the dominance of moral norms.

Some people claim that morality depends on God, a view known as the divine command theory. Both theists and nontheists have raised doubts about this doctrine. The larger point is that doing ethics—using critical reasoning to examine the moral life—can be a useful and productive enterprise for believer and nonbeliever alike.

EXERCISES

Review Questions

1. When can it be said that your moral beliefs are not really yours? (p. 3)
2. In what ways are we forced to do ethics? What is at stake in these deliberations? (pp. 3–4)
3. What is the unfortunate result of accepting moral beliefs without questioning them? (pp. 4–5)
4. Can our feelings be our sole guide to morality? Why or why not? (pp. 4–5)
5. What are some questions asked in normative ethics? (p. 5)
6. What is the difference between normative ethics and metaethics? (pp. 5–6)
7. What is the dilemma about God and morality that Socrates posed in *Euthyphro*? (p. 11)
8. What kinds of moral contradictions or inconsistencies confront religious believers? (p. 9)

9. What are the premises in the arbitrariness argument against the divine command theory? (p. 11)
10. Does the principle of impartiality imply that we must always treat equals equally? Why or why not? (p. 8)

Discussion Questions

1. Do you think that morality ultimately depends on God (that God is the author of the moral law)? Why or why not?
2. Do you believe that you have absorbed or adopted without question most of your moral beliefs? Why or why not?
3. Formulate an argument against the divine command theory, then formulate one for it.
4. Give an example of how you or someone you know has used reasons to support a moral judgment.
5. Identify at least two normative ethical questions that you have wondered about in the past year.

6. Name two things (persons, objects, experiences, etc.) in your life that you consider intrinsically valuable. Name three that are instrumentally valuable.
7. How do your feelings affect the moral judgments you make? Do they *determine* your judgments? Do they inform them? If so, how?
8. What is the logic behind the principle of universalizability? Cite an example of how the principle has entered into your moral deliberations.
9. How does racial discrimination violate the principle of impartiality?
10. What is the "dominance of moral norms"? Does it strike you as reasonable? Or do you believe that sometimes nonmoral norms can outweigh moral ones? If the latter, provide an example.

READINGS

From *What Is the Socratic Method?*

CHRISTOPHER PHILLIPS

The Socratic method is a way to seek truths by your own lights.

It is a system, a spirit, a method, a type of philosophical inquiry, an intellectual technique, all rolled into one.

Socrates himself never spelled out a "method." However, the Socratic method is named after him because Socrates, more than any other before or since, models for us *philosophy practiced*—philosophy as deed, as way of living, as something that any of us can do. It is an *open system* of philosophical inquiry that allows one to interrogate from many vantage points.

Gregory Vlastos, a Socrates scholar and professor of philosophy at Princeton, described Socrates'

Although not specifically concerned with ethics, this short piece by Christopher Phillips makes a persuasive case for using the "Socratic method" to think through difficult philosophical issues. To see the Socratic method applied to ethics, read the excerpt from Plato's *Euthyphro* that follows on p. 16.

Christopher Phillips, from *Socrates Café*. Copyright © 2001 by Christopher Phillips. Used by permission of W. W. Norton & Company, Inc. and Felicia Eth Literary Representation.

method of inquiry as "among the greatest achievements of humanity." Why? Because, he says, it makes philosophical inquiry "a common human enterprise, open to every man." Instead of requiring allegiance to a specific philosophical viewpoint or analytic technique or specialized vocabulary, the Socratic method "calls for common sense and common speech." And this, he says, "is as it should be, for how many should live is every man's business."

I think, however, that the Socratic method goes beyond Vlastos' description. It does not merely call for common sense but examines what common sense *is*. The Socratic method asks: Does the common sense of our day offer us the greatest potential for self-understanding and human excellence? Or is the prevailing common sense in fact a roadblock to realizing this potential?

Vlastos goes on to say that Socratic inquiry is by no means simple, and "calls not only for the highest degree of mental alertness of which anyone is capable" but also for "moral qualities of a high order: sincerity, humility, courage." Such qualities "protect against the possibility" that Socratic dialogue, no matter how rigorous, "would merely grind out . . . wild conclusions with irresponsible premises." I agree, though I would replace the quality of sincerity with honesty, since one can hold a conviction sincerely without examining it, while honesty would require that one subject one's convictions to frequent scrutiny.

A Socratic dialogue reveals how different our outlooks can be on concepts we use every day. It reveals how different our philosophies are, and often how tenable—or untenable, as the case may be—a range of philosophies can be. Moreover, even the most universally recognized and used concept, when subjected to Socratic scrutiny, might reveal not only that there is *not* universal agreement, after all, on the meaning of any given concept, but that every single person has a somewhat different take on each and every concept under the sun.

What's more, there seems to be no such thing as a concept so abstract, or question so off base, that it can't be fruitfully explored [using the Socratic method]. In the course of Socratizing, it often turns out to be

the case that some of the most so-called abstract concepts are intimately related to the most profoundly relevant human experiences. In fact, it's been my experience that virtually any question can be plumbed Socratically. Sometimes you don't know what question will have the most lasting and significant impact until you take a risk and delve into it for a while.

What distinguishes the Socratic method from mere nonsystematic inquiry is the sustained attempt to explore the ramifications of certain opinions and then offer compelling objections and alternatives. This scrupulous and exhaustive form of inquiry in many ways resembles the scientific method. But unlike Socratic inquiry, scientific inquiry would often lead us to believe that whatever is not measurable cannot be investigated. This "belief" fails to address such paramount human concerns as sorrow and joy and suffering and love.

Instead of focusing on the outer cosmos, Socrates focused primarily on human beings and their cosmos within, utilizing his method to open up new realms of self-knowledge while at the same time exposing a great deal of error, superstition, and dogmatic nonsense. The Spanish-born American philosopher and poet George Santayana said that Socrates knew that "the foreground of human life is necessarily moral and practical" and that "it is so even so for artists"—and even for scientists, try as some might to divorce their work from these dimensions of human existence.

Scholars call Socrates' method the *elenchus*, which is Hellenistic Greek for *inquiry* or *cross-examination*. But it is not just any type of inquiry or examination. It is a type that reveals people to themselves, that makes them see what their opinions really amount to. C. D. C. Reeve, professor of philosophy at Reed College, gives the standard explanation of an elenchus in saying that its aim "is not simply to reach adequate definitions" of such things as virtues; rather, it also has a "moral reformatory purpose, for Socrates believes that regular elenctic philosophizing makes people happier and more virtuous than anything else. . . . Indeed philosophizing is so important for human welfare, on his view, that he is willing to accept execution rather than give it up."

Socrates' method of examination can indeed be a vital part of existence, but I would not go so far as to say that it *should* be. And I do not think that Socrates felt that habitual use of this method "makes people happier." The fulfillment that comes from Socratizing comes only at a price—it could well make us *unhappier,* more uncertain, more troubled, as well as more fulfilled. It can leave us with a sense that we *don't* know the answers after all, that we are much further from knowing the answers than we'd ever realized before engaging in Socratic discourse. And this is fulfilling—and exhilarating and humbling and perplexing.

* * *

There is no neat divide between one's views of philosophy and of life. They are overlapping and kindred views. It is virtually impossible in many instances to *know* what we believe in daily life until we engage others in dialogue. Likewise, to discover our philosophical views, we must engage with ourselves, with the lives we already lead. Our views form, change, evolve, as we participate in this dialogue. It is the only way truly to discover what philosophical colors we sail under. Everyone at some point preaches to himself and others what he does not yet practice; everyone acts in or on the world in ways that are in some way contradictory or inconsistent with the views he or she confesses or professes to hold. For instance, the Danish philosopher Søren Kierkegaard, the influential founder of existentialism, put Socratic principles to use in writing his dissertation on the concept of irony in Socrates, often using pseudonyms so he could argue his own positions with himself. In addition, the sixteenth-century essayist Michel de Montaigne, who was called "the French Socrates" and was known as the father of skepticism in modern Europe, would

write and add conflicting and even contradictory passages in the same work. And like Socrates, he believed the search for truth was worth dying for.

The Socratic method forces people "to confront their own dogmatism," according to Leonard Nelson, a German philosopher who wrote on such subjects as ethics and theory of knowledge until he was forced by the rise of Nazism to quit. By doing so, participants in Socratic dialogue are, in effect, "*forcing* themselves to be free," Nelson maintains. But they're not just confronted with their own dogmatism. In the course of a [Socratic dialogue], they may be confronted with an array of hypotheses, convictions, conjectures and theories offered by the other participants, and themselves—all of which subscribe to some sort of dogma. The Socratic method requires that—honestly and openly, rationally and imaginatively—they confront the dogma by asking such questions as: What does this mean? What speaks for and against it? Are there alternative ways of considering it that are even more plausible and tenable?

At certain junctures of a Socratic dialogue, the "forcing" that this confrontation entails—the insistence that each participant carefully articulate her singular philosophical perspective—can be upsetting. But that is all to the good. If it never touches any nerves, if it doesn't upset, if it doesn't mentally and spiritually challenge and perplex, in a wonderful and exhilarating way, it is not Socratic dialogue. This "forcing" opens us up to the varieties of experiences of others—whether through direct dialogue, or through other means, like drama or books, or through a work of art or a dance. It compels us to explore alternative perspectives, asking what might be said for or against each.

* * *

From *The Euthyphro*

PLATO

* * *

Euthyphro. Piety . . . is that which is dear to the gods, and impiety is that which is not dear to them.

Socrates. Very good, Euthyphro; you have now given me the sort of answer which I wanted. But whether what you say is true or not I cannot as yet tell, although I make no doubt that you will prove the truth of your words.

Euthyphro. Of course.

Socrates. Come, then, and let us examine what we are saying. That thing or person which is dear to the gods is pious, and that thing or person which is hateful to the gods is impious, these two being the extreme opposites of one another. Was not that said?

Euthyphro. It was.

Socrates. And well said?

Euthyphro. Yes, Socrates, I thought so; it was certainly said.

Socrates. And further, Euthyphro, the gods were admitted to have enmities and hatreds and differences?

Euthyphro. Yes, that was also said.

Socrates. And what sort of difference creates enmity and anger? Suppose for example that you and I, my good friend, differ about a number; do differences of this sort make us enemies and set us at variance with one another? Do we not go at once to arithmetic, and put an end to them by a sum?

Euthyphro. True.

Socrates. Or suppose that we differ about magnitudes, do we not quickly end the differences by measuring?

Euthyphro. Very true.

Socrates. And we end a controversy about heavy and light by resorting to a weighing machine?

Plato, *The Euthyphro*, translated by Benjamin Jowett.

Euthyphro. To be sure.

Socrates. But what differences are there which cannot be thus decided, and which therefore make us angry and set us at enmity with one another? I dare say the answer does not occur to you at the moment, and therefore I will suggest that these enmities arise when the matters of difference are the just and unjust, good and evil, honourable and dishonourable. Are not these the points about which men differ, and about which when we are unable satisfactorily to decide our differences, you and I and all of us quarrel, when we do quarrel?

Euthyphro. Yes, Socrates, the nature of the differences about which we quarrel is such as you describe.

Socrates. And the quarrels of the gods, noble Euthyphro, when they occur, are of a like nature?

Euthyphro. Certainly they are.

Socrates. They have differences of opinion, as you say, about good and evil, just and unjust, honourable and dishonourable: there would have been no quarrels among them, if there had been no such differences—would there now?

Euthyphro. You are quite right.

Socrates. Does not every man love that which he deems noble and good, and hate the opposite of them?

Euthyphro. Very true.

Socrates. But, as you say, people regard the same things, some as just and others as unjust,—about these they dispute; and so there arise wars and fightings among them.

Euthyphro. Very true.

Socrates. Then the same things are hated by the gods and loved by the gods, and are both hateful and dear to them?

Euthyphro. True.

Socrates. And upon this view the same things, Euthyphro, will be pious and also impious?

Euthyphro. So I should suppose.

Socrates. Then, my friend, I remark with surprise that you have not answered the question which I asked. For I certainly did not ask you to tell me what action is both pious and impious: but now it would seem that what is loved by the gods is also hated by them. And therefore, Euthyphro, in thus chastising your father you may very likely be doing what is agreeable to Zeus but disagreeable to Cronos or Uranus, and what is acceptable to Hephaestus but unacceptable to Hera, and there may be other gods who have similar differences of opinion.

Euthyphro. But I believe, Socrates, that all the gods would be agreed as to the propriety of punishing a murderer: there would be no difference of opinion about that.

Socrates. Well, but speaking of men, Euthyphro, did you ever hear any one arguing that a murderer or any sort of evil-doer ought to be let off?

Euthyphro. I should rather say that these are the questions which they are always arguing, especially in courts of law: they commit all sorts of crimes, and there is nothing which they will not do or say in their own defence.

Socrates. But do they admit their guilt, Euthyphro, and yet say that they ought not to be punished?

Euthyphro. No; they do not.

Socrates. Then there are some things which they do not venture to say and do: for they do not venture to argue that the guilty are to be unpunished, but they deny their guilt, do they not?

Euthyphro. Yes.

Socrates. Then they do not argue that the evil-doer should not be punished, but they argue about the fact of who the evil-doer is, and what he did and when?

Euthyphro. True.

Socrates. And the gods are in the same case, if as you assert they quarrel about just and unjust, and some of them say while others deny that injustice is done among them. For surely neither God nor man will ever venture to say that the doer of injustice is not to be punished?

Euthyphro. That is true, Socrates, in the main.

Socrates. But they join issue about the particulars—gods and men alike; and, if they dispute at all, they dispute about some act which is called in question, and which by some is affirmed to be just, by others to be unjust. Is not that true?

Euthyphro. Quite true.

Socrates. Well then, my dear friend Euthyphro, do tell me, for my better instruction and information, what proof have you that in the opinion of all the gods a servant who is guilty of murder, and is put in chains by the master of the dead man, and dies because he is put in chains before he who bound him can learn from the interpreters of the gods what he ought to do with him, dies unjustly; and that on behalf of such an one a son ought to proceed against his father and accuse him of murder. How would you show that all the gods absolutely agree in approving of his act? Prove to me that they do, and I will applaud your wisdom as long as I live.

Euthyphro. It will be a difficult task; but I could make the matter very clear indeed to you.

Socrates. I understand; you mean to say that I am not so quick of apprehension as the judges: for to them you will be sure to prove that the act is unjust, and hateful to the gods.

Euthyphro. Yes indeed, Socrates; at least if they will listen to me.

Socrates. But they will be sure to listen if they find that you are a good speaker. There was a notion that came into my mind while you were speaking; I said to myself: "Well, and what if Euthyphro does prove to me that all the gods regarded the death of the serf as unjust, how do I know anything more of the nature of piety and impiety? for granting that this action may be hateful to the gods, still piety and impiety are not adequately defined by these distinctions, for that which is hateful to the gods has been shown to be also pleasing and dear to them." And therefore, Euthyphro, I do not ask you to prove this; I will suppose, if you like, that all the gods condemn and abominate such an action. But I will amend the definition so far as to say that what all the gods hate is impious, and what they love pious or holy; and what some of them love and others hate is both or neither. Shall this be our definition of piety and impiety?

Euthyphro. Why not, Socrates?

Socrates. Why not! Certainly, as far as I am concerned, Euthyphro, there is no reason why not. But whether this admission will greatly assist you in the task of instructing me as you promised, is a matter for you to consider.

Euthyphro. Yes, I should say that what all the gods love is pious and holy, and the opposite which they all hate, impious.

Socrates. Ought we to enquire into the truth of this, Euthyphro, or simply to accept the mere statement on our own authority and that of others? What do you say?

Euthyphro. We should enquire; and I believe that the statement will stand the test of enquiry.

Socrates. We shall know better, my good friend, in a little while. The point which I should first wish to understand is whether the pious or holy is beloved by the gods because it is holy, or holy because it is beloved of the gods.

Euthyphro. I do not understand your meaning, Socrates.

Socrates. I will endeavour to explain: we speak of carrying and we speak of being carried, of leading and being led, seeing and being seen. You know that in all such cases there is a difference, and you know also in what the difference lies?

Euthyphro. I think that I understand.

Socrates. And is not that which is beloved distinct from that which loves?

Euthyphro. Certainly.

Socrates. Well; and now tell me, is that which is carried in this state of carrying because it is carried, or for some other reason?

Euthyphro. No; that is the reason.

Socrates. And the same is true of what is led and of what is seen?

Euthyphro. True.

Socrates. And a thing is not seen because it is visible, but conversely, visible because it is seen; nor is a thing led because it is in the state of being led, or carried because it is in the state of being carried, but the converse of this. And now I think, Euthyphro, that my meaning will be intelligible; and my meaning is, that any state of action or passion implies previous action or passion. It does not become because it is becoming, but it is in a state of becoming because it becomes; neither does it suffer because it is in a state of suffering, but it is in a state of suffering because it suffers. Do you not agree?

Euthyphro. Yes.

Socrates. Is not that which is loved in some state either of becoming or suffering?

Euthyphro. Yes.

Socrates. And the same holds as in the previous instances; the state of being loved follows the act of being loved, and not the act the state.

Euthyphro. Certainly.

Socrates. And what do you say of piety, Euthyphro; is not piety, according to your definition, loved by all the gods?

Euthyphro. Yes.

Socrates. Because it is pious or holy, or for some other reason?

Euthyphro. No, that is the reason.

Socrates. It is loved because it is holy, not holy because it is loved?

Euthyphro. Yes.

Socrates. And that which is dear to the gods is loved by them, and is in a state to be loved of them because it is loved of them?

Euthyphro. Certainly.

Socrates. Then that which is dear to the gods, Euthyphro, is not holy, nor is that which is holy loved of God, as you affirm; but they are two different things.

Euthyphro. How do you mean, Socrates?

Socrates. I mean to say that the holy has been acknowledged by us to be loved of God because it is holy, not to be holy because it is loved.

Euthyphro. Yes.

Socrates. But that which is dear to the gods is dear to them because it is loved by them, not loved by them because it is dear to them.

Euthyphro. True.

Socrates. But, friend Euthyphro, if that which is holy is the same with that which is dear to God, and is loved because it is holy, then that which is dear to God would have been loved as being dear to God; but if that which dear to God is dear to him because loved by him, then that which is holy would have been holy because loved by him. But now you see that the reverse is the case, and that they are quite different from one another. For one (Θεοφιλὲs) is of a kind to be loved because it is loved, and the other (oʹσιον) is loved because it is of a kind to be loved. Thus you appear to me, Euthyphro, when I ask you what is the essence of holiness, to offer an attribute only, and not the essence—the attribute of being loved by all the gods. But you still refuse to explain to me the nature of holiness. And therefore, if you please, I will ask you not to hide your treasure, but to tell me once more what holiness or piety really is, whether dear to the gods or not (for that is a matter about which we will not quarrel) and what is impiety?

Euthyphro. I really do not know, Socrates, how to express what I mean. For somehow or other our arguments, on whatever ground we rest them, seem to turn around and walk away from us.

* * *

CHAPTER 2

Subjectivism, Relativism, and Emotivism

Consider the following: Abdulla Yones killed his sixteen-year-old daughter Heshu in their apartment in west London. The murder was yet another example of an "honor killing," an ancient tradition still practiced in many parts of the world. Using a kitchen knife, Yones stabbed Heshu eleven times and slit her throat. He later declared that he *had* to kill her to expunge a stain from his family, a stain that Heshu had caused by her outrageous behavior. What was outrageous behavior to Yones, however, would seem to many Westerners to be typical teenage antics, annoying but benign. Heshu's precise offense against her family's honor is unclear, but the possibilities include wearing makeup, having a boyfriend, and showing an independent streak that would be thought perfectly normal throughout the West. In some countries, honor killings are sometimes endorsed by the local community or even given the tacit blessing of the state.

What do you think of this time-honored way of dealing with family conflicts? Specifically, what is your opinion regarding the *morality* of honor killing? Your response to this question is likely to reveal not only your view of honor killing but your overall approach to morality as well. Suppose your response is something like this: "Honor killing is morally *wrong*—wrong no matter where it's done or who does it." With this statement, you implicitly embrace moral **objectivism,** the doctrine that some moral norms or principles are valid for everyone—*universal,* in other words—regardless of how cultures may differ in their moral outlooks. However, you need not hold that

the objective principles are rigid rules that have no exceptions (a view known as *absolutism*) or that they must be applied in exactly the same way in every situation and culture.

On the other hand, let us say that you assess the case like this: "In societies that approve of honor killing, the practice is morally right; in those that do not approve, it is morally wrong. My society approves of honor killing, so it is morally right." If you believe what you say, then you are a cultural relativist. **Cultural relativism** is the view that an action is morally right if one's culture approves of it. Moral rightness and wrongness are therefore relative to cultures. So in one culture, an action may be morally right; in another culture, it may be morally wrong.

Perhaps you prefer an even narrower view of morality, and so you say, "Honor killing may be right for you, but it is most certainly not right for me." If you mean this literally, then you are committed to another kind of relativism called **subjective relativism**—the view that an action is morally right if one approves of it. Moral rightness and wrongness are relative not to cultures but to individuals. An action then can be right for you but wrong for someone else. Your approving of an action makes it right. There is therefore no objective morality, and cultural norms do not make right or wrong—individuals make right or wrong.

Finally, imagine that you wish to take a different tack regarding the subject of honor killing. You say, "I abhor the practice of honor killing"—but you believe that in uttering these words you are saying nothing that is true or false. You believe that despite what your statement seems to mean, you are simply expressing your emotions. You therefore hold to **emotivism**—the view that moral utterances are neither true nor false but are instead expressions of emotions or attitudes. So in your sentence about honor killing, you are not stating a fact—you are merely emoting and possibly trying to influence someone's behavior. Even when emotivists express a more specific preference regarding other people's behavior—by saying, for instance, "No one should commit an honor killing"—they are still not making a factual claim. They are simply expressing a preference, and perhaps hoping to persuade other people to see things their way.

These four replies represent four distinctive perspectives (though certainly not the *only* perspectives) on the meaning and import of moral judgments. Moreover, they are not purely theoretical but real and relevant. People actually live their lives (or try to) as moral objectivists, or relativists, or emotivists, or some strange and inconsistent mixture of these. (There is an excellent chance, for example, that you were raised as an objectivist but now accept some form of relativism—or even try to hold to objectivism in some instances and relativism in others.)

In any case, the question that you should ask (and that ethics can help you answer) is not whether you in fact accept any of these views, but whether you are justified in doing so. Let us see then where an examination of reasons for and against them will lead.

SUBJECTIVE RELATIVISM

What view of morality could be more tempting (and convenient) than the notion that an action is right if someone approves of it? Subjective relativism says that action X is right for Ann if she approves of it yet wrong for Greg if he disapproves of it. Thus action X can be both right and wrong—right for Ann but wrong for Greg. A person's approval of an action *makes it right* for that person. Action X is not *objectively* right (or wrong). It is

> ## QUICK REVIEW
>
> *objectivism*—The view that some moral principles are valid for everyone.
>
> *cultural relativism*—The view that an action is morally right if one's culture approves of it. *Implications:* that cultures are morally infallible, that social reformers can never be morally right, that moral disagreements between individuals in the same culture amount to arguments over whether someone disagrees with her culture, that other cultures cannot be legitimately criticized, and that moral progress is impossible.
>
> *subjective relativism*—The view that an action is morally right if one approves of it. *Implications:* that individuals are morally infallible and that genuine moral disagreement between individuals is nearly impossible.
>
> *emotivism*—The view that moral utterances are neither true nor false but are expressions of emotions or attitudes. *Implications:* that people cannot disagree over the moral facts because there are no moral facts, that presenting reasons in support of a moral utterance is a matter of offering nonmoral facts that can influence someone's attitude, and that nothing is actually good or bad.

right (or wrong) relative to individuals. In this way, moral rightness becomes a matter of personal taste. If to Ann strawberry ice cream tastes good, then it is good (for her). If to Greg strawberry ice cream tastes bad, then it is bad (for him). There is no such thing as strawberry ice cream tasting good objectively or generally. Likewise, the morality of an action depends on Ann and Greg's moral tastes.

Many people claim they are subjective relativists—until they realize the implications of the doctrine, implications that are at odds with

Judge Not?

Jesus said "Judge not that ye be not judged." Some have taken this to mean that we should not make moral judgments about others, and many who have never heard those words are convinced that to judge others is to be insensitive, intolerant, or absolutist. Professor Jean Bethke Elshtain examines this attitude and finds it both mistaken and harmful.

> I have also found helpful the discussion of the lively British philosopher, Mary Midgley. In her book *Can't We Make Moral Judgments?* Midgley notes our contemporary search for a nonjudgmental politics and quotes all those people who cry, in effect, "But surely it's always wrong to make moral judgments." We are not permitted to make anyone uncomfortable, to be "insensitive." Yet moral judgment of "some kind," says Midgley, "is a necessary element to our thinking." Judging involves our whole nature—it isn't just icing on the cake of self-identity. Judging makes it possible for us to "find our way through a whole forest of possibilities."

Midgley argues that Jesus was taking aim at sweeping condemnations and vindictiveness: he was not trashing the "whole faculty of judgment." Indeed, Jesus is making the "subtle point that while we cannot possibly avoid judging, we can see to it that we judge fairly, as we would expect others to do to us." This is part and parcel, then, of justice as fairness, as a discernment about a particular case and person and deed. Subjectivism in such matters—of the "I'm okay, you're okay," variety—is a cop-out, a way to stop forming and expressing moral judgments altogether. This strange suspension of specific moments of judgment goes hand-in-glove, of course, with an often violent rhetoric of condemnation of whole categories of persons, past and present—that all-purpose villain, the Dead White European Male, comes to mind.[*]

[*]Jean Bethke Elshtain, "Judge Not?" *First Things*, No. 46, pp. 36–40, October 1994. Reprinted by permission of the publisher.

our commonsense moral experience. First, subjective relativism implies that in the rendering of any moral opinion, each person is incapable of being in error. Each of us is *morally infallible*. If we approve of an action—and we are sincere in our approval—then that action is morally right. We literally cannot be mistaken about this, because our approval makes the action right. If we say that inflicting pain on an innocent child for no reason is right (that is, we approve of such an action), then the action is right. Our moral judgment is correct, and it cannot be otherwise. Yet if anything is obvious about our moral experience, it is that we are *not* infallible. We sometimes *are* mistaken in our moral judgments. We are, after all, not gods.

By all accounts, Adolf Hitler approved of (and ordered) the extermination of vast numbers of innocent people, including six million Jews. If so, by the lights of subjective relativism, his facilitating those deaths was morally right. It seems that the totalitar-

ian leader Pol Pot approved of his murdering more than a million innocent people in Cambodia. If so, it was right for him to murder those people. But it seems obvious that what these men did was wrong, and their approving of their actions did not make the actions right. Because subjective relativism suggests otherwise, it is a dubious doctrine.

Another obvious feature of our commonsense moral experience is that from time to time we have moral disagreements. Maria says that capital punishment is right, but Carlos says that it is wrong. This seems like a perfectly clear case of two people disagreeing about the morality of capital punishment. Subjective relativism, however, implies that such disagreements cannot happen. Subjective relativism says that when Maria states that capital punishment is right, she is just saying that she approves of it. And when Carlos states that capital punishment is wrong, he is just saying that he disapproves of it. But they are not really disagreeing, because they are merely describing their attitudes toward capital punishment. In effect, Maria is saying "This is my attitude on the subject," and Carlos is saying "Here is my attitude on the subject." But these two claims are not opposed to one another. They are about different subjects, so both statements could be true. Maria and Carlos might as well be discussing how strawberry ice cream tastes to each of them, for nothing that Maria says could contradict what Carlos says. Because genuine disagreement is a fact of our moral life, and subjective relativism is inconsistent with this fact, the doctrine is implausible.

In practice, subjective relativism is a difficult view to hold consistently. At times, of course, you can insist that an action is right for you but wrong for someone else. But you may also find yourself saying something like "Pol Pot committed absolutely heinous acts; he was evil" or "What Hitler did was wrong"—and what you mean is that what Pol Pot and Hitler did was objectively wrong, not just wrong relative to you. Such slides from subjective relativism to objectivism suggest a conflict between these two perspectives and the need to resolve it through critical reasoning.

CULTURAL RELATIVISM

To many people, the idea that morality is relative to culture is obvious. It seems obvious primarily because modern sociology has left no doubt that people's moral judgments differ from culture to culture. The moral judgments of people in other cultures are often shockingly different from our own. In some societies, it is morally permissible to kill infants at birth, burn widows alive with the bodies of their husbands, steal and commit acts of treachery, surgically remove the clitorises of young girls for no medical reason, kill one's elderly parents, have multiple husbands or wives, and make up for someone's death by murdering others. Among some people, it has been considered morally acceptable to kill those of a different sexual orientation, lynch persons with a different skin color, and allow children to die by refusing to give them available medical treatment. (These latter acts have all been practiced in subcultures within the United States, so not all such cultural differences happen far from home.) It is only a small step from acknowledging this moral diversity among cultures to the conclusion that cultures determine moral rightness and that objective morality is a myth.

The philosopher Walter T. Stace (1886–1967) illustrates how easily this conclusion has come to many in Western societies:

> It was easy enough to believe in a single absolute morality in older times when there was no anthropology, when all humanity was divided clearly into two groups, Christian peoples and the "heathen." Christian peoples knew and possessed the one true morality. The rest were savages whose moral ideas could be ignored. But all this changed. Greater knowledge has brought greater tolerance. We can no longer exalt our own moralities as alone true, while dismissing all other moralities as false or inferior. The investigations of anthropologists have shown that there exist side by side in the world a bewildering variety of moral codes. On this topic endless volumes have been written, masses of evidence piled up. Anthropologists have ransacked the Melanesian Islands, the jungles of New Guinea, the steppes of Siberia, the deserts of Australia, the forests of central Africa, and have brought back with them countless examples of weird, extravagant, and fantastic "moral" customs with which to confound us. We learn that all kinds of horrible practices are, in this, that, or the other place, regarded as essential to virtue. We find that there is nothing, or next to nothing, which has always and everywhere been regarded as morally good by all men. Where then is our universal morality? Can we, in face of all this evidence, deny that it is nothing but an empty dream?[1]

Here, Stace spells out in rough form the most common argument for cultural relativism, an inference from differences in the moral beliefs of cultures to the conclusion that cultures make morality. Before we conclude that objectivism is in

[1]Walter T. Stace, *The Concept of Morals* (1937; reprint, New York: Macmillan, 1965), 8–58.

fact an empty dream, we should state the argument more precisely and examine it closely. We can lay out the argument like this:

1. People's judgments about right and wrong differ from culture to culture.

2. If people's judgments about right and wrong differ from culture to culture, then right and wrong are relative to culture, and there are no objective moral principles.

3. Therefore, right and wrong are relative to culture, and there are no objective moral principles.

A good argument gives us good reason to accept its conclusion, and an argument is good if its logic is solid (the conclusion follows logically from the premises) *and* the premises are true. So is the foregoing argument a good one? We can see

right away that the logic is in fact solid. That is, the argument is valid: the conclusion does indeed follow from the premises. The question then becomes whether the premises are true. As we have seen, Premise 1 is most certainly true. People's judgments about right and wrong do vary from culture to culture. But what of Premise 2? Does the diversity of views about right and wrong among cultures show that right and wrong are determined by culture, that there are no universal moral truths? There are good reasons to think this premise false.

Premise 2 says that because there are disagreements among cultures about right and wrong, there must not be any universal standards of right and wrong. But even if the moral judgments of people in various cultures do differ, such difference in itself does not show that morality is relative to culture. Just because people in different cultures have different views about morality, their

---

CRITICAL THOUGHT: "Female Circumcision" and Cultural Relativism

In recent years many conflicts have flared between those who espouse universal human rights and those who embrace cultural relativism. One issue that has been a flashpoint in the contentious debates is a practice called *female genital cutting* (FGC). Other names include *female circumcision* and *female genital mutilation*.

In FGC, all or part of the female genitals are removed. The procedure, used mostly in Africa and the Middle East, is usually performed on girls between the ages of four and eight, but sometimes on young women. A report in the *Yale Journal of Public Health* states that in Sudan 89 percent of girls receive FGC and that the cutting tools "include knives, scissors, razors, and broken glass. The operation is typically performed by elderly women or traditional birth attendants, though increasing numbers of doctors are taking over these roles."* The practice occurs for various reasons, including religious and sociological, and is defended by some

who say that it prepares girls for their role in society and marriage and discourages illicit sex.

Public health officials regard FGC as a serious health problem. It can cause reproductive tract infections, pain during intercourse, painful menstruation, complications during childbirth, greater risk of HIV infection, bleeding, and even death. International health agencies denounce FGC, but many say that no one outside a culture using FGC has a right to criticize the practice.

Do you think that FGC is morally permissible? If you judge the practice wrong, are you appealing to some notion of objective morality? If you judge it permissible, are you doing so because you are a cultural relativist? In either case, explain your reasoning.

*Sarah Cannon and Daniel Berman, "Cut Off: The Female Genital-Cutting Controversy," *Yale Journal of Public Health* 1, no. 2 (2004).

disagreement does not prove that no view can be objectively correct—no more than people's disagreements about the size of a house show that no one's opinion about it can be objectively true. Suppose Culture A endorses infanticide, but Culture B does not. Such a disagreement does not demonstrate that both cultures are equally correct or that there is no objectively correct answer. After all, it is possible that infanticide is objectively right (or wrong) and that the relevant moral beliefs of either Culture A or Culture B are false.

Another reason to doubt the truth of Premise 2 comes from questioning how deep the disagreements among cultures really are. Judgments about the rightness of actions obviously do vary across cultures. But people can differ in their moral judgments not just because they accept different moral principles, but also because they have divergent *nonmoral* beliefs. They may actually embrace the *same* moral principles, but their moral judgments conflict because their nonmoral beliefs lead them to apply those principles in very different ways. If so, the diversity of moral judgments across cultures does not necessarily indicate deep disagreements over fundamental moral principles or standards. Here is a classic example:

> [T]he story is told of a culture in which a son is regarded as obligated to kill his father when the latter reaches age sixty. Given just this much information about the culture and the practice in question it is tempting to conclude that the members of that culture differ radically from members of our culture in their moral beliefs and attitudes. We, after all, believe it is immoral to take a human life, and regard patricide as especially wrong. But suppose that in the culture we are considering, those who belong to it believe (a) that at the moment of death one enters heaven; (b) one's physical and mental condition in the afterlife is exactly what it is at the moment of death; and (c) men are at the peak of their physical and mental powers when they are sixty. Then what appeared at first to be peculiarities in moral outlook on the part of the cultural group in question regarding the sanctity of life and respect for parents, turn

out to be located rather in a nonmoral outlook of the group. A man in that culture who kills his father is doing so out of concern for the latter's well-being—to prevent him, for example, from spending eternity blind or senile. It is not at all clear that, if we shared the relevant nonmoral beliefs of this other culture, we would not believe with them that sons should kill their fathers at the appropriate time.[2]

To find similar examples, we need not search for the exotic. In Western cultures we have the familiar case of abortion, an issue hotly debated among those who at first glance appear to be disagreeing about moral principles. But in fact the disputants agree about the moral principle involved: that murder (unjustly killing a person) is morally wrong. What they do disagree about is a nonmoral factual matter—whether the fetus is an entity that can be murdered (that is, whether it is a person). Disagreement over the nonmoral facts masks substantial agreement on fundamental moral standards.

The work of several anthropologists provides some evidence for these kinds of disagreements as well as for the existence of cross-cultural moral agreement in general. The social psychologist Solomon Asch, for instance, maintains that differing moral judgments among societies often arise when the same moral principles are operating but the particulars of cultural situations vary.[3] Other observers claim that across numerous diverse cultures we can find many common moral elements such as prohibitions against murder, lying, incest, and adultery and obligations of fairness, reciprocity, and consideration toward parents and children.[4]

---

[2]Phillip Montague, "Are There Objective and Absolute Moral Standards?" in *Reason and Responsibility: Readings in Some Basic Problems in Philosophy,* ed. Joel Feinberg, 5th ed. (Belmont, CA: Wadsworth, 1978), 490–91.

[3]Solomon Asch, *Social Psychology* (Englewood Cliffs, NJ: Prentice-Hall, 1952), 378–79.

[4]See, for example, Clyde Kluckhohn, "Ethical Relativity: Sic et Non," *Journal of Philosophy* 52 (1955): 663–77, and E. O. Wilson, *On Human Nature* (1978; reprint, New York: Bantam, 1979).

Some philosophers argue that a core set of moral values—including, for example, truth telling and prohibitions against murder—*must* be universal, otherwise cultures would not survive.

These points demonstrate that Premise 2 of the argument for cultural relativism is false. The argument therefore gives us no good reasons to believe that an action is right simply because one's culture approves of it.

For many people, however, the failure of the argument for cultural relativism may be beside the point. They find the doctrine appealing mainly because it seems to promote the humane and enlightened attitude of tolerance toward other cultures. Broad expanses of history are drenched with blood and marked by cruelty because of the evil of intolerance—religious, racial, political, and social. Tolerance therefore seems a supreme virtue, and cultural relativism appears to provide a justification and vehicle for it. After all, if all cultures are morally equal, does not cultural relativism both entail and promote tolerance?

We should hope that tolerance does reign in a pluralistic world, but there is no necessary connection between tolerance and cultural relativism. For one thing, cultural relativists cannot consistently advocate tolerance. To advocate tolerance is to advocate an objective moral value. But if tolerance is an objective moral value, then cultural relativism must be false, because it says that there are no objective moral values. So instead of justifying tolerance toward all, cultural relativism actually undercuts universal tolerance. Moreover, according to cultural relativism, intolerance can be justified just as easily as tolerance can. If a culture approves of intolerance, then intolerance is right for that culture. If a culture approves of tolerance, then tolerance is right for that culture. Cultural relativists are thus committed to the view that intolerance can in fact be justified, and they cannot consistently claim that tolerance is morally right everywhere.

At this point we are left with no good reasons to believe that cultural relativism is true. But the problems for the doctrine are deeper than that. Like subjective relativism, it has several implications that render it highly implausible.

First, as is the case with subjective relativism, cultural relativism implies moral infallibility. A culture simply cannot be mistaken about a moral issue. If it approves of an action, then that action is morally right, and there is no possibility of error as long as the culture's approval is genuine. But, of course, cultural infallibility in moral matters is flagrantly implausible, just as individual infallibility is. At one time or another, cultures have sanctioned witch burning, slavery, genocide, racism, rape, human sacrifice, and religious persecution. Does it make any sense to say that they could not have been mistaken about the morality of these actions?

Cultural relativism also has the peculiar consequence that social reformers of every sort would *always be wrong*. Their culture would be the ultimate authority on moral matters, so if they disagree with their culture, they could not possibly be right. If their culture approves of genocide, genocide would be right, and antigenocide reformers would be wrong to oppose the practice. In this upside-down world, the antigenocide reformers would be immoral and the genocidal culture would be the real paragon of righteousness. Reformers such as Martin Luther King Jr., Mahatma Gandhi, Mary Wollstonecraft (champion of women's rights), and Frederick Douglass (American abolitionist) would be great crusaders—for immorality. Our moral experience, however, suggests that cultural relativism has matters exactly backward. Social reformers have often been right when they claimed their cultures were wrong, and this fact suggests that cultural relativism is wrong about morality.

Where cultural relativism holds, if you have a disagreement with your culture about the rightness of an action, you automatically lose. You are in error by definition. But what about a disagreement among members of the same society? What would such a disagreement amount to? It amounts to something very strange, according to cultural relativism. When two people in the same culture disagree on a moral issue, what they are really disagreeing about—the only thing they can rationally disagree about—is whether their society endorses a particular view. After all, society makes actions right by approving or disapproving of them. According to cultural relativism, if René and Michel (both members of society X) are disagreeing about capital punishment, their disagreement must actually be about whether society X approves of capital punishment. Since right and wrong are determined by one's culture, René and Michel are disagreeing about what society X says. But this view of moral disagreement is dubious, to say the least. When we have a moral disagreement, we do not think that the crux of it is whether our society approves of an action. We do not think that deciding a moral issue is simply a matter of polling the public to see which way opinion leans. We do not think that René and Michel will ever find out whether capital punishment is morally permissible by consulting public opinion. Determining whether an action is right is a very different thing from determining what most people think. This odd consequence of cultural relativism suggests that the doctrine is flawed.

One of the more disturbing implications of cultural relativism is that cultures cannot be legitimately criticized from the outside. If a culture approves of the actions that it performs, then those actions are morally right regardless of what other cultures have to say about the matter. One society's practices are as morally justified as any other's, as long as the practices are socially sanctioned. This consequence of cultural relativism may not seem too worrisome when the societies in question are long dead. But it takes on a different tone when the societies are closer to us in time. Consider the 1994 genocide committed in Rwanda in which a million people died. Suppose the killers' society (their tribe) approved of the murders. Then the genocide was morally justified.

And what of Hitler's "final solution"—the murder of millions of Jews in World War II? Say that German society approved of Hitler's actions (and those of the men who carried out his orders). Then Hitler's final solution was morally right; engineering the Holocaust was morally permissible. If you are a cultural relativist, you cannot legitimately condemn these monstrous deeds. Because they were approved by their respective societies, they were morally justified. They were just as morally justified as the socially sanctioned activities of Albert Schweitzer, Jonas Salk, or Florence Nightingale. But all this seems implausible. We do in fact sometimes criticize other cultures and believe that it is legitimate to do so.

Contrary to the popular view, rejecting cultural relativism (embracing moral objectivism) does not entail intolerance. In fact, it provides a plausible starting point for tolerance. A moral objectivist realizes that she can legitimately criticize other cultures—and that people of other cultures can legitimately criticize her culture. A recognition of this fact together with an objectivist's sense of fallibility can lead her to an openness to criticism of her own culture and to acceptance of everyone's right to disagree.

We not only criticize other cultures, but we also compare the past with the present. We compare the actions of the past with those of the present and judge whether moral progress has been made. We see that slavery has been abolished, that we no longer burn witches, that we recognize racism as evil—then we judge that these changes represent moral progress. For moral relativists, however, there is no objective standard by which to compare the ways of the past with the ways of the present. Societies of the past approved or disapproved of certain practices, and contemporary societies approve or disapprove of them, and no transcultural moral assessments can be made. But if there is such a thing as moral progress, then there must be some cross-cultural moral yardstick by which we can evaluate actions. There must be objective standards by which we can judge that actions of the present are better than those of the past. If there are no objective moral standards, our judging that we are in fact making moral progress is hard to explain.

Finally, there is a fundamental difficulty concerning the application of cultural relativism to moral questions: the doctrine is nearly impossible to use. The problem is that cultural relativism applies to societies (or social groups), but we all belong to several societies, and there is no way to choose which one is the proper one. What society do you belong to if you are an Italian American Buddhist living in Atlanta, Georgia, who is a member of the National Organization for Women and a breast cancer support group? The hope of cultural relativists is that they can use the doctrine to make better, more enlightened moral decisions. But this society-identification problem seems to preclude any moral decisions, let alone enlightened ones.

What, then, can we conclude from our examination of cultural relativism? We have found that the basic argument for the view fails; we therefore have no good reasons to believe that the doctrine is true. Beyond that, we have good grounds for thinking the doctrine false. Its surprising implications regarding moral infallibility, moral reformers, moral progress, the nature of moral disagreements within societies, and the possibility of cross-cultural criticism show it to be highly implausible. The crux of the matter is that cultural relativism does a poor job of explaining some important features of our moral experience. A far better explanation of these features is that some form of moral objectivism is true.

EMOTIVISM

The commonsense view of moral judgments is that they ascribe moral properties to such things as actions and people and that they are therefore statements that can be true or false. This view of moral judgments is known as *cognitivism*. The

opposing view, called *noncognitivism,* denies that moral judgments are statements that can be true or false; they do not ascribe properties to anything. Probably the most famous noncognitivist view is emotivism, which says that moral judgments cannot be true or false because they do not make any claims—they merely express emotions or attitudes. For the emotivist, moral utterances are something akin to exclamations that simply express approving or disapproving feelings: "Violence against women—disgusting!" or "Shoplifting—love it!"

The English philosopher A. J. Ayer (1910–89), an early champion of emotivism, is clear and blunt about what a moral utterance such as "Stealing money is wrong" signifies. This sentence, he says,

> expresses no proposition which can be either true or false. It is as if I had written "Stealing money!!"— where the shape and thickness of the exclamation marks show, by a suitable convention, that a special sort of moral disapproval is the feeling which is being expressed. It is clear that there is nothing said here which can be true or false. . . . For in saying that a certain type of action is right or wrong, I am not making any factual statement, not even a statement about my own state of mind.[5]

If moral judgments are about feelings and not the truth or falsity of moral assertions, then ethics is a very different sort of inquiry than most people imagine. As Ayer says,

> [A]s ethical judgements are mere expressions of feeling, there can be no way of determining the validity of any ethical system, and, indeed, no sense in asking whether any such system is true. All that one may legitimately enquire in this connection is, What are the moral habits of a given person or group of people, and what causes them to have precisely those habits and feelings? And this enquiry falls wholly within the scope of the existing social sciences.[6]

---

[5]A. J. Ayer, "Critique of Ethics and Theology," in *Language, Truth and Logic* (1936; reprint, New York: Dover, 1952), 107.
[6]Ayer, 112.

The emotivist points out that while moral utterances express feelings and attitudes, they also function to influence people's attitudes and behavior. So the sentence "Stealing money is wrong" not only expresses feelings of disapproval, it also can influence others to have similar feelings and act accordingly.

Emotivists also take an unusual position on moral disagreements. They maintain that moral disagreements are not conflicts of beliefs, as is the case when one person asserts that something is the case and another person asserts that it is not the case. Instead, moral disagreements are *disagreements in attitude*. Jane has positive feelings or a favorable attitude toward abortion, but Ellen has negative feelings or an unfavorable attitude toward abortion. The disagreement is emotive, not cognitive. Jane may say "Abortion is right," and Ellen may say "Abortion is wrong," but they are not really disagreeing over the facts. They are expressing conflicting attitudes and trying to influence each other's attitude and behavior.

Philosophers have criticized emotivism on several grounds, and this emotivist analysis of disagreement has been a prime target. As you might suspect, their concern is that this notion of disagreement is radically different from our ordinary view. Like subjective relativism, emotivism implies that disagreements in the usual sense are impossible. People cannot disagree over the moral facts, because there are no moral facts. But we tend to think that when we disagree with someone on a moral issue, there really is a conflict of statements about what is the case. Of course, when we are involved in a conflict of beliefs, we may also experience conflicting attitudes. But we do not think that we are *only* experiencing a disagreement in attitudes.

Emotivism also provides a curious account of how reasons function in moral discourse. Our commonsense view is that a moral judgment is the kind of thing that makes a claim about moral properties and that such a claim can be supported by reasons. If someone asserts "Euthanasia is wrong," we may sensibly ask her what reasons she has for believing that claim. If she replies that there are no reasons to back up her claim or that moral utterances are not the kind of things that can be supported by reasons, we would probably think that she misunderstood the question or the nature of morality. For the emotivist, "moral" reasons have a very different function. Here reasons are intended not to support statements (since there are no moral statements) but to influence the emotions or attitudes of others. Since moral utterances express emotions or attitudes, "presenting reasons" is a matter of offering nonmoral facts that can influence those emotions and attitudes. Suppose A has a favorable attitude toward abortion, and B has an unfavorable one (that is, A and B are having a disagreement in attitude). For A, to present reasons is to provide information that might cause B to have a more favorable attitude toward abortion.

This conception of the function of reasons, however, implies that good reasons encompass *any* nonmoral facts that can alter someone's attitude. On this view, the relevance of these facts to the judgment at hand is beside the point. The essential criterion is whether the adduced facts are sufficiently influential. They need not have any logical or cognitive connection to the moral judgment to be changed. They may, for example, appeal to someone's ignorance, arrogance, racism, or fear. But we ordinarily suppose that reasons *should* be relevant to the cognitive content of moral judgments. Moreover, we normally make a clear distinction between influencing someone's attitudes and showing (by providing reasons) that a claim is true—a distinction that emotivism cannot make.

The final implication of emotivism is also problematic: there is no such thing as goodness or badness. We cannot legitimately claim that anything is good or bad, because these properties do not exist. To declare that something is good is just to express positive emotions or a favorable attitude toward it. We may say that pain is bad, but badness (or goodness) is not a feature of pain. Our saying that pain is bad is just an expression of our unfavorable attitude toward pain.

Suppose a six-year-old girl is living in a small village in Syria during the civil war between President Bashar al-Assad's Baathist government and rebel forces. Assad's henchmen firebomb the village, destroying it and incinerating everyone except the girl, who is burned from head to toe and endures excruciating pain for three days before she dies. Suppose that we are deeply moved by this tragedy as we consider her unimaginable suffering and we remark, "How horrible. The little girl's suffering was a very bad thing."[7] When we say something like this, we ordinarily mean that the girl's suffering had a certain moral property: that the suffering was bad. But according to emotivism, her suffering had no moral properties at all. When we comment on the girl's suffering, we are simply expressing our feelings; the suffering itself was neither good nor bad. But this view of things seems implausible. Our moral experience suggests that some things in fact are bad and some are good.

The philosopher Brand Blanshard (1892–1987) makes the point in the following way:

> [T]he emotivist is cut off by his theory from admitting that there has been anything good or evil in the past, either animal or human. There have been Black Deaths, to be sure, and wars and rumours of war; there have been the burning of countless women as witches, and the massacre in the Katyn forest, and Oswiecim, and Dachau, and an unbearable procession of horrors; but one cannot meaningfully say that anything evil has ever happened. The people who suffered from these things did indeed take up attitudes of revulsion toward them; we can now judge that they took them; but in such judgments we are not saying that anything evil occurred. . . . [Emotivism], when first presented, has some plausibility. But when this is balanced against the implied unplausibility of setting down as meaningless every suggestion that good or evil events have ever occurred, it is outweighed enormously.[8]

Obviously, emotivism does not fare well when examined in light of our commonsense moral experience. We must keep in mind, though, that common sense is fallible. On the other hand, we should not jettison common sense in favor of another view unless we have good reasons to do so. In the case of emotivism, we have no good reasons to prefer it over common sense—and we have good grounds for rejecting it.

SUMMARY

Subjective relativism is the view that an action is morally right if one approves of it. A person's approval makes the action right. This doctrine (as well as cultural relativism) is in stark contrast to *moral objectivism,* the view that some moral principles are valid for everyone. Subjective relativism, though, has some troubling implications. It implies that each person is morally infallible and that individuals can never have a genuine moral disagreement.

Cultural relativism is the view that an action is morally right if one's culture approves of it. The argument for this doctrine is based on the diversity of moral judgments among cultures: because people's judgments about right and wrong differ from culture to culture, right and wrong must be relative to culture, and there are no objective moral principles. This argument is defective, however, because the diversity of moral views does not imply that morality is relative to cultures. In addition, the alleged diversity of basic moral standards among cultures may be only apparent, not real. Societies whose moral judgments conflict may be differing not over moral principles but over nonmoral facts.

Some think that tolerance is entailed by cultural relativism. But there is no necessary connection

---

[7]This scenario is inspired by some of Brand Blanshard's examples from "Emotivism," in *Reason and Goodness* (1961; reprint, New York: G. Allen and Unwin, 1978).

[8]Blanshard, 204–5.

between tolerance and the doctrine. Indeed, the cultural relativist cannot consistently advocate tolerance while maintaining his relativist standpoint. To advocate tolerance is to advocate an objective moral value. But if tolerance is an objective moral value, then cultural relativism must be false, because it says that there are no objective moral values.

Like subjective relativism, cultural relativism has some disturbing consequences. It implies that cultures are morally infallible, that social reformers can never be morally right, that moral disagreements between individuals in the same culture amount to arguments over whether they disagree with their culture, that other cultures cannot be legitimately criticized, and that moral progress is impossible.

Emotivism is the view that moral utterances are neither true nor false but are expressions of emotions or attitudes. It leads to the conclusion that people can disagree only in attitude, not in beliefs. People cannot disagree over the moral facts, because there are no moral facts. Emotivism also implies that presenting reasons in support of a moral utterance is a matter of offering nonmoral facts that can influence someone's attitude. It seems that any nonmoral facts will do, as long as they affect attitudes. Perhaps the most far-reaching implication of emotivism is that nothing is actually good or bad. There simply are no properties of goodness and badness. There is only the expression of favorable or unfavorable emotions or attitudes toward something.

EXERCISES

Review Questions

1. Does objectivism entail intolerance? Why or why not? (p. 20)
2. Does objectivism require absolutism? Why or why not? (p. 20)
3. How does subjective relativism differ from cultural relativism? (p. 20)
4. What is emotivism? How does emotivism differ from objectivism? (p. 21)
5. How does subjective relativism imply moral infallibility? (p. 22)

6. According to moral subjectivism, are moral disagreements possible? Why or why not? (pp. 22–23)
7. What is the argument for cultural relativism? Is the argument sound? Why or why not? (pp. 23–26)
8. Does the diversity of moral outlooks in cultures show that right and wrong are determined by culture? Why or why not? (pp. 24–26)
9. According to the text, how is it possible for people in different cultures to disagree about moral judgments and still embrace the same fundamental moral principles? (pp. 25–26)
10. Is there a necessary connection between cultural relativism and tolerance? Why or why not? (p. 26)
11. What does cultural relativism imply about the moral status of social reformers? (p. 26)
12. What is the emotivist view of moral disagreements? (p. 28)
13. According to emotivism, how do reasons function in moral discourse? (p. 29)

Discussion Questions

1. Are you a subjective relativist? If so, how did you come to adopt this view? If not, what is your explanation for not accepting it?
2. Suppose a serial killer approves of his murderous actions. According to subjective relativism, are the killer's actions therefore justified? Do you believe a serial killer's murders are justified? If not, is your judgment based on a subjective relativist's perspective or an objectivist perspective?
3. Are you a cultural relativist? Why or why not?
4. Suppose a majority of the German people approved of Hitler's murdering six million Jews in World War II. Would this approval make Hitler's actions morally justified? If so, why? If not, why not—and what moral outlook are you using to make such a determination?
5. When cultural relativists say that every culture should embrace a policy of tolerance, are they contradicting themselves? If so, how? If

cultural relativism were true, would this fact make wars between societies less or more likely? Explain your answer.

6. If you traveled the world and saw that cultures differ dramatically in their moral judgments, would you conclude from this evidence that cultural relativism was true? Why or why not?

7. According to a cultural relativist, would the civil rights reforms that Martin Luther King Jr. sought be morally right or wrong? Do *you* think that his efforts at reform were morally wrong? What are your reasons for your decision?

8. Do you believe that there has been moral progress in the past thousand years of human history? Why or why not?

9. Suppose a deer that had been shot by a hunter writhed in agony for days before dying. You exclaim, "How she must have suffered! Her horrendous pain was a bad thing." In this situation, does the word *bad* refer to any moral properties? Is there really something *bad* about the deer's suffering—or is your use of the word just a way to express your horror without making any moral statement at all? Explain your answers.

READINGS

From *Anthropology and the Abnormal*

RUTH BENEDICT

Modern social anthropology has become more and more a study of the varieties and common elements of cultural environment and the consequences of these in human behavior. For such a study of diverse social orders primitive peoples fortunately provide a laboratory not yet entirely vitiated by the spread of a standardized worldwide civilization. Dyaks and Hopis, Fijians and Yakuts are significant for psychological and sociological study because only among these simpler peoples has there been sufficient isolation to give opportunity for the development of localized social forms. In the higher cultures the standardization of custom and belief over a couple of continents has given a false sense of the inevitability of the particular forms that have gained currency, and we need to turn to a wider survey in order to

Ruth Benedict, excerpts from "Anthropology and the Abnormal." *The Journal of General Psychology* 10 (1934), pp. 59–82. © 1934 Routledge. Reprinted by permission of the publisher (Taylor & Francis Ltd, http://www.tandfonline.com).

check the conclusions we hastily base upon this near-universality of familiar customs. Most of the simpler cultures did not gain the wide currency of the one which, out of our experience, we identify with human nature, but this was for various historical reasons, and certainly not for any that gives us as its carriers a monopoly of social good or of social sanity. Modern civilization, from this point of view, becomes not a necessary pinnacle of human achievement but one entry in a long series of possible adjustments.

These adjustments, whether they are in mannerisms like the ways of showing anger, or joy, or grief in any society, or in major human drives like those of sex, prove to be far more variable than experience in any one culture would suggest. In certain fields, such as that of religion or of formal marriage arrangements, these wide limits of variability are well known and can be fairly described. In others it is not yet possible to give a generalized account, but that does not absolve us of the task of indicating the significance of the work that has been done and of the problems that have arisen.

One of these problems relates to the customary modern normal-abnormal categories and our conclusions regarding them. In how far are such categories culturally determined, or in how far can we with assurance regard them as absolute? In how far can we regard inability to function socially as diagnostic of abnormality, or in how far is it necessary to regard this as a function of the culture?

As a matter of fact, one of the most striking facts that emerge from a study of widely varying cultures is the ease with which our abnormals function in other cultures. It does not matter what kind of "abnormality" we choose for illustration, those which indicate extreme instability, or those which are more in the nature of character traits like sadism or delusions of grandeur or of persecution, there are well-described cultures in which these abnormals function at ease and with honor, and apparently without danger or difficulty to the society.

The most notorious of these is trance and catalepsy. Even a very mild mystic is aberrant in our culture. But most peoples have regarded even extreme psychic manifestations not only as normal and desirable, but even as characteristic of highly valued and gifted individuals. This was true even in our own cultural background in that period when Catholicism made the ecstatic experience the mark of sainthood. It is hard for us, born and brought up in a culture that makes no use of the experience, to realize how important a rôle it may play and how many individuals are capable of it, once it has been given an honorable place in any society.

* * *

Cataleptic and trance phenomena are, of course, only one illustration of the fact that those whom we regard as abnormals may function adequately in other cultures. Many of our culturally discarded traits are selected for elaboration in different societies. Homosexuality is an excellent example, for in this case our attention is not constantly diverted, as in the consideration of trance, to the interruption of routine activity which it implies. Homosexuality poses the problem very simply. A tendency toward this trait in our culture exposes an individual to all the conflicts to which all aberrants are always exposed, and we tend to identify the consequences of this conflict with homosexuality. But these consequences are obviously local and cultural. Homosexuals in many societies are not incompetent, but they may be such if the culture asks adjustments of them that would strain any man's vitality. Wherever homosexuality has been given an honorable place in any society, those to whom it is congenial have filled adequately the honorable rôles society assigns to them. Plato's *Republic* is, of course, the most convincing statement of such a reading of homosexuality. It is presented as one of the major means to the good life, and it was generally so regarded in Greece at that time.

The cultural attitude toward homosexuals has not always been on such a high ethical plane, but it has been varied. Among many American Indian tribes there exists the institution of the berdache, as the French called them. These men-women were men who at puberty or thereafter took the dress and the occupations of women. Sometimes they married other men and lived with them. Sometimes they were men with no inversion, persons of weak sexual endowment who chose this rôle to avoid the jeers of the women. The berdaches were never regarded as of first-rate supernatural power, as similar men-women were in Siberia, but rather as leaders in women's occupations, good healers in certain diseases, or, among certain tribes, as the genial organizers of social affairs. In any case, they were socially placed. They were not left exposed to the conflicts that visit the deviant who is excluded from participation in the recognized patterns of his society.

* * *

No one civilization can possibly utilize in its mores the whole potential range of human behavior. Just as there are great numbers of possible phonetic articulations, and the possibility of language depends on a selection and standardization of a few of these in order that speech communication may be possible at all, so the possibility of organized behavior of every sort, from the fashions of local dress and houses to the dicta of a people's ethics and religion, depends upon a similar selection among the possible behavior traits. In the field of recognized economic obligations or sex tabus this selection is as nonrational and subconscious a process as it is in the field of phonetics. It is a process which goes on in the group for long periods of time and is historically conditioned by innumerable accidents of isolation or of contact of peoples. In any comprehensive study of psychology, the selection that different cultures have made in the course of history within the great circumference of potential behavior is of great significance.

Every society, beginning with some slight inclination in one direction or another, carries its preference farther and farther, integrating itself more and more completely upon its chosen basis, and discarding those types of behavior that are uncongenial. Most of these organizations of personality that seem to us most incontrovertibly abnormal have been used by different civilizations in the very foundations of their institutional life. Conversely the most valued traits of our normal individuals have been looked on in differently organized cultures as aberrant. Normality, in short, within a very wide range, is culturally defined. It is primarily a term for the socially elaborated segment of human behavior in any culture; and abnormality, a term for the segment that that particular civilization does not use. The very eyes with which we see the problem are conditioned by the long traditional habits of our own society.

It is a point that has been made more often in relation to ethics than in relation to psychiatry. We do not any longer make the mistake of deriving the morality of our own locality and decade directly from the inevitable constitution of human nature. We do not elevate it to the dignity of a first principle. We recognize that morality differs in every society, and is a convenient term for socially approved habits. Mankind has always preferred to say, "It is a morally good," rather than "It is habitual," and the fact of this preference is matter enough for a critical science of ethics. But historically the two phrases are synonymous.

The concept of the normal is properly a variant of the concept of the good. It is that which society has approved. A normal action is one which falls well within the limits of expected behavior for a particular society. Its variability among different peoples is essentially a function of the variability of the behavior patterns that different societies have created for themselves, and can never be wholly divorced from a consideration of culturally institutionalized types of behavior.

Each culture is a more or less elaborate working-out of the potentialities of the segment it has chosen. In so far as a civilization is well integrated and consistent within itself, it will tend to carry farther and farther, according to its nature, its initial impulse toward a particular type of action, and from the point of view of any other culture those elaborations will include more and more extreme and aberrant traits.

Each of these traits, in proportion as it reinforces the chosen behavior patterns of that culture, is for that culture normal. Those individuals to whom it is congenial either congenitally, or as the result of childhood sets, are accorded to prestige in that culture, and are not visited with the social contempt or disapproval which their traits would call down upon them in a society that was differently organized. On the other hand, those individuals whose characteristics are not congenial to the selected type of human behavior in that community are the deviants, no matter how valued their personality traits may be in a contrasted civilization.

* * *

I have spoken of individuals as having sets toward certain types of behavior, and of these sets as running sometimes counter to the types of behavior which are institutionalized in the culture to which they belong. From all that we know of contrasting cultures it seems clear that differences of temperament occur in every society. The matter has never been made the subject of investigation, but from the available material it would appear that these temperament types are very likely of universal recurrence. That is, there is an ascertainable range of human behavior that is found wherever a sufficiently large series of individuals is observed. But the proportion in which behavior types stand to one another in different societies is not universal. The vast majority of the individuals in any group are shaped to the fashion of that culture. In other words, most individuals are plastic to the moulding force of the society into which they are born. In a society that values trance, as in India, they will have supernormal experience. In a society that institutionalizes homosexuality, they will be homosexual. In a society that sets the gathering of possessions as the chief human objective, they will amass property. The deviants, whatever the type of behavior the culture has institutionalized, will remain few in number, and there seems no more difficulty in moulding the vast malleable majority to the "normality" of what we consider an aberrant trait, such as delusions of reference, than to the normality of such accepted behavior patterns as acquisitiveness. The small proportion of the number of the deviants in any culture is not a function of the sure instinct with which that society has built itself upon the fundamental sanities, but of the universal fact that, happily, the majority of mankind quite readily take any shape that is presented to them.

* * *

Trying Out One's New Sword

Mary Midgley

All of us are, more or less, in trouble today about trying to understand cultures strange to us. We hear constantly of alien customs. We see changes in our lifetime which would have astonished our parents. I want to discuss here one very short way of dealing with this difficulty, a drastic way which many people now theoretically favour. It consists in simply denying that we can ever understand any culture except our own well enough to make judgements about it. Those who recommend this hold that the world is sharply divided into separate societies, sealed units, each with its own system of thought. They feel that the respect and tolerance due from one system to another forbids us ever to take up a critical position to any other culture. Moral judgment, they suggest, is a kind of coinage valid only in its country of origin.

I shall call this position 'moral isolationism'. I shall suggest that it is certainly not forced upon us, and indeed that it makes no sense at all. People usually take it up because they think it is a respectful attitude to other cultures. In fact, however, it is not respectful. Nobody can respect what is entirely unin-

telligible to them. To respect someone, we have to know enough about him to make a *favourable* judgement, however general and tentative. And we do understand people in other cultures to this extent. Otherwise a great mass of our most valuable thinking would be paralysed.

To show this, I shall take a remote example, because we shall probably find it easier to think calmly about it than we should with a contemporary one, such as female circumcision in Africa or the Chinese Cultural Revolution. The principles involved will still be the same. My example is this. There is, it seems, a verb in classical Japanese which means 'to try out one's new sword on a chance wayfarer'. (The word is *tsujigiri,* literally 'crossroads-cut'.) A samurai sword had to be tried out because, if it was to work properly, it had to slice through someone at a single blow, from the shoulder to the opposite flank. Otherwise, the warrior bungled his stroke. This could injure his honour, offend his ancestors, and even let down his emperor. So tests were needed, and wayfarers had to be expended. Any wayfarer would do—provided, of course, that he was not another Samurai. Scientists will recognize a familiar problem about the rights of experimental subjects.

Now when we hear of a custom like this, we may well reflect that we simply do not understand it; and

Mary Midgley, "Trying out One's New Sword" in *Heart and Mind: The Varieties of Moral Experience* (Brighton, Sussex: Harvester Press, 1981), pp. 69–75. Reprinted by permission of David Higham Associates.

therefore are not qualified to criticize it at all, because we are not members of that culture. But we are not members of any other culture either, except our own. So we extend the principle to cover all extraneous cultures, and we seem therefore to be moral isolationists. But this is, as we shall see, an impossible position. Let us ask what it would involve.

We must ask first. Does the isolating barrier work both ways? Are people in other cultures equally unable to criticize *us*? This question struck me sharply when I read a remark in *The Guardian* by an anthropologist about a South American Indian who had been taken into a Brazilian town for an operation, which saved his life. When he came back to his village, he made several highly critical remarks about the white Brazilians' way of life. They may very well have been justified. But the interesting point was that the anthropologist called these remarks 'a damning indictment of Western civilization'. Now the Indian had been in that town about two weeks. Was he in a position to deliver a damning indictment? Would we ourselves be qualified to deliver such an indictment on the Samurai, provided we could spend two weeks in ancient Japan? What do we really think about this?

My own impression is that we believe that outsiders can, in principle, deliver perfectly good indictments— only, it usually takes more than two weeks to make them damning. Understanding has degrees. It is not a slapdash yes-or-no matter. Intelligent outsiders can progress in it, and in some ways will be at an advantage over the locals. But if this is so, it must clearly apply to ourselves as much as anybody else.

Our next question is this: Does the isolating barrier between cultures block praise as well as blame? If I want to say that the Samurai culture has many virtues, or to praise the South American Indians, am I prevented from doing *that* by my outside status? Now, we certainly do need to praise other societies in this way. But it is hardly possible that we could praise them effectively if we could not, in principle, criticize them. Our praise would be worthless if it rested on no definite grounds, if it did not flow from some understanding. Certainly we may need to praise things which we do not *fully* understand. We say 'there's something very good here, but I can't quite make out

what it is yet'. This happens when we want to learn from strangers. And we can learn from strangers. But to do this we have to distinguish between those strangers who are worth learning from and those who are not. Can we then judge which is which?

This brings us to our third question: What is involved in judging? Now plainly there is no question here of sitting on a bench in a red robe and sentencing people. Judging simply means forming an opinion, and expressing it if it is called for. Is there anything wrong about this? Naturally, we ought to avoid forming—and expressing—*crude* opinions, like that of a simple-minded missionary, who might dismiss the whole Samurai culture as entirely bad, because non-Christian. But this is a different objection. The trouble with crude opinions is that they are crude, whoever forms them, not that they are formed by the wrong people. Anthropologists, after all, are outsiders quite as much as missionaries. Moral isolationism forbids us to form *any* opinions on these matters. Its ground for doing so is that we don't understand them. But there is much that we don't understand in our own culture too. This brings us to our last question: If we can't judge other cultures, can we really judge our own? Our efforts to do so will be much damaged if we are really deprived of our opinions about other societies, because these provide the range of comparison, the spectrum of alternatives against which we set what we want to understand. We would have to stop using the mirror which anthropology so helpfully holds up to us.

In short, moral isolationism would lay down a general ban on moral reasoning. Essentially, this is the programme of immoralism, and it carries a distressing logical difficulty. Immoralists like Nietzsche are actually just a rather specialized sect of moralists. They can no more afford to put moralizing out of business than smugglers can afford to abolish customs regulations. The power of moral judgement is, in fact, not a luxury, not a perverse indulgence of the self-righteous. It is a necessity. When we judge something to be bad or good, better or worse than something else, we are taking it as an example to aim at or avoid. Without opinions of this sort, we would have no framework of comparison for our own policy, no chance of profiting by other people's insights or mistakes. In this vacuum, we could form no judgements on our own actions.

Now it would be odd if Homo sapiens had really got himself into a position as bad as this—a position where his main evolutionary asset, his brain, was so little use to him. None of us is going to accept this sceptical diagnosis. We cannot do so, because our involvement in moral isolationism does not flow from apathy, but from a rather acute concern about human hypocrisy and other forms of wickedness. But we polarize that concern around a few selected moral truths. We are rightly angry with those who despise, oppress or steamroll other cultures. We think that doing these things is actually *wrong*. But this is itself a moral judgement. We could not condemn oppression and insolence if we thought that all our condemnations were just a trivial local quirk of our own culture. We could still less do it if we tried to stop judging altogether.

Real moral scepticism, in fact, could lead only to inaction, to our losing all interest in moral questions, most of all in those which concern other societies. When we discuss these things, it becomes instantly clear how far we are from doing this. Suppose, for instance, that I criticize the bisecting Samurai, that I say his behaviour is brutal. What will usually happen next is that someone will protest, will say that I have no right to make criticisms like that of another culture. But it is most unlikely that he will use this move to end the discussion of the subject. Instead, he will justify the Samurai. He will try to fill in the background, to make me understand the custom, by explaining the exalted ideals of discipline and devotion which produced it. He will probably talk of the lower value which the ancient Japanese placed on individual life generally. He may well suggest that this is a healthier attitude than our own obsession with security. He may add, too, that the wayfarers did not seriously mind being bisected, that in principle they accepted the whole arrangement.

Now an objector who talks like this is implying that it *is* possible to understand alien customs. That is just what he is trying to make me do. And he implies, too, that if I do succeed in understanding them, I shall do something better than giving up judging them. He expects me to change my present judgement to a truer one—namely, one that is favourable. And the standards I must use to do this cannot just be Samurai standards. They have to be ones current in my own culture. Ideals like discipline and devotion will not move anybody unless he himself accepts them. As it happens, neither discipline nor devotion is very popular in the West at present. Anyone who appeals to them may well have to do some more arguing to make *them* acceptable, before he can use them to explain the Samurai. But if he does succeed here, he will have persuaded us, not just that there was something to be said for them in ancient Japan, but that there would be here as well.

Isolating barriers simply cannot arise here. If we accept something as a serious moral truth about one culture, we can't refuse to apply it—in however different an outward form—to other cultures as well, wherever circumstance admit it. If we refuse to do this, we just are not taking the other culture seriously. This becomes clear if we look at the last argument used by my objector—that of justification by consent of the victim. It is suggested that sudden bisection is quite in order, *provided* that it takes place between consenting adults. I cannot now discuss how conclusive this justification is. What I am pointing out is simply that it can only work if we believe that *consent* can make such a transaction respectable—and this is a thoroughly modern and Western idea. It would probably never occur to a Samurai; if it did, it would surprise him very much. It is *our* standard. In applying it, too, we are likely to make another typically Western demand. We shall ask for good factual evidence that the wayfarers actually do have this rather surprising taste—that they are really willing to be bisected. In applying Western standards in this way, we are not being confused or irrelevant. We are asking the questions which arise *from where we stand*, questions which we can see the sense of. We do this because asking questions which you can't see the sense of is humbug. Certainly we can extend our questioning by imaginative effort. We can come to understand other societies better. By doing so, we may make their questions our own, or we may see that they are really forms of the questions which we are asking already. This is not impossible. It is just very hard work. The obstacles which often prevent it are simply those of ordinary ignorance, laziness and prejudice.

If there were really an isolating barrier, of course, our own culture could never have been formed. It is no scaled box, but a fertile jungle of different influences—Greek, Jewish, Roman, Norse, Celtic and so forth, into which further influences are still pouring—American, Indian, Japanese, Jamaican, you name it. The moral isolationist's picture of separate, unmixable cultures is quite unreal. People who talk about British history usually stress the value of this fertilizing mix, no doubt rightly. But this is not just an odd fact about Britain. Except for the very smallest and most remote, all cultures are formed out of many streams. All have the problem of digesting and assimilating things which, at the start, they do not understand. All have the choice of learning something from this challenge, or, alternatively, of refusing to learn, and fighting it mindlessly instead.

This universal predicament has been obscured by the fact that anthropologists used to concentrate largely on very small and remote cultures, which did not seem to have this problem. These tiny societies, which had often forgotten their own history, made neat, self-contained subjects for study. No doubt it was valuable to emphasize their remoteness, their extreme strangeness, their independence of our cultural tradition. This emphasis was, I think, the root of moral isolationism. But, as the tribal studies themselves showed, even there the anthropologists were able to interpret what they saw and make judgements—often favourable—about the tribesmen. And the tribesmen, too, were quite equal to making judgements about the anthropologists—and about the tourists and Coca-Cola salesmen who followed them. Both sets of judgements, no doubt, were somewhat hasty, both have been refined in the light of further experience. A similar transaction between us and the Samurai might take even longer. But that is no reason at all for deeming it impossible. Morally as well as physically, there is only one world, and we all have to live in it.

PART

2

Moral Reasoning

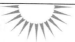

CHAPTER 3

Evaluating Moral Arguments

This much is clear: we cannot escape the ethical facts of life. We often must make moral judgments, assess moral principles or rules, contend with moral theories, and argue the pros and cons of moral issues. Typically we do all of these things believing that in one way or another they *really matter*.

Because we think that ethics (that is, moral *philosophy*) matters, it follows that moral *reasoning* matters, for we could make little headway in these difficult waters without the use of reasons and arguments. Along the way we may take into account our feelings, desires, beliefs, and other factors, but getting to our destination depends mostly on the quality of our moral reasoning. Through moral reasoning we assess what is right and wrong, good and bad, virtuous and vicious. We make and dismantle arguments for this view and for that. In our finest moments, we follow the lead of reason in the search for answers, trying to rise above subjectivism, prejudice, and confusion.

In this chapter you will discover (if you haven't already) that you are no stranger to moral reasoning. Moral reasoning is ordinary critical reasoning applied to ethics. Critical reasoning (or critical thinking) is the careful, systematic evaluation of statements or claims. We use critical reasoning every day to determine whether a statement is worthy of acceptance—that is, whether it is true. We harness critical reasoning to assess the truth of all sorts of claims in all kinds of contexts—personal, professional, academic, philosophical, scientific, political, and ethical. Moral reasoning, then, is not a type of reasoning that you have never seen before.

We therefore begin this chapter with the basics of critical reasoning. The focus is on the skills that are at the heart of this kind of thinking—the formulation and evaluation of logical arguments. The rest of the chapter is about applying critical reasoning to the claims and arguments of ethics.

CLAIMS AND ARGUMENTS

When you use critical reasoning, your ultimate aim is usually to figure out whether to accept, or believe, a statement—either someone else's statement or one of your own. A **statement,** or claim, is an assertion that something is or is not the case; it is either true or false. These are statements:

- The ship sailed on the wind-tossed sea.
- I feel tired and listless.
- Murder is wrong.
- 5 + 5 = 10.
- A circle is not a square.

These statements assert that something is or is not the case. Whether you accept them, reject them, or neither, they are still statements because they are assertions that can be either true or false.

The following, however, are not statements; they do not assert that something is or is not the case:

- Why is Anna laughing?
- Is abortion immoral?
- Hand me the screwdriver.
- Don't speak to me.

- Hello, Webster.
- For heaven's sake!

A fundamental principle of critical reasoning is that we should not accept a statement as true without good reasons. If a statement is supported by good reasons, we are entitled to believe it. The better the reasons supporting a statement, the more likely it is to be true. Our acceptance of a statement, then, can vary in strength. If a statement is supported by strong reasons, we are entitled to believe it strongly. If it is supported by weaker reasons, our belief should likewise be weaker. If the reasons are equivocal—if they do not help us decide one way or another—we should suspend judgment until the evidence is more definitive.

Reasons supporting a statement are themselves statements. To lend credence to another claim, these supporting statements may assert something about scientific evidence, expert opinion, relevant examples, or other considerations. In this way they provide reasons for believing that a statement is true, that what is asserted is actual. When this state of affairs exists—when at least one statement attempts to provide reasons for believing another statement—we have an **argument.** An argument is a group of statements, one of which is supposed to be supported by the rest. An argument in this sense, of course, has nothing to do with the common notion of arguments as shouting matches or vehement quarrels.

In an argument, the supporting statements are known as **premises;** the statement being supported is known as a **conclusion.** Consider these arguments:

Argument 1. Capital punishment is morally permissible because it helps to deter crime.

Argument 2. If John killed Bill in self-defense, he did not commit murder. He did act in self-defense. Therefore, he did not commit murder.

Argument 3. Telling a white lie is morally permissible. We should judge the rightness of an act by its impact on human well-being. If an act increases human well-being, then it is right. Without question, telling a white lie increases human well-being because it spares people's feelings; that's what white lies are for.

These arguments are fairly simple. In Argument 1, a single premise ("because it helps to deter crime") supports a straightforward conclusion—"Capital punishment is morally permissible." Argument 2 has two premises: "If John killed Bill in self-defense, he did not commit murder" and "He did act in self-defense." And the conclusion is "Therefore, he did not commit murder." Argument 3 has three premises: "We should judge the rightness of an act by its impact on human well-being," "If an act increases human well-being, then it is right," and "Without question, telling a white lie increases human well-being because it spares people's feelings." Its conclusion is "Telling a white lie is morally permissible."

As you can see, these three arguments have different structures. Argument 1, for example, has just one premise, but Arguments 2 and 3 have two and three premises. In Arguments 1 and 3, the conclusion is stated first; in Argument 2, last. Obviously, arguments can vary dramatically in their number of premises, in the placement of premises and conclusion, and in the wording of each of these parts. But all arguments share a common pattern: at least one premise is intended to support a conclusion. This pattern is what makes an argument an argument.

Despite the simplicity of this premise-conclusion arrangement, though, arguments are not always easy to identify. They can be embedded in long passages of nonargumentative prose, and nonargumentative prose can often look like arguments. Consider:

> The number of abortions performed in this state is increasing. More and more women say that they favor greater access to abortion. This is an outrage.

Do you see an argument in this passage? You shouldn't, because there is none. The first two sentences are meant to be assertions of fact, and the last one is an expression of indignation. There is no premise providing reasons to accept a conclusion. But what if we altered the passage to make it an argument? Look:

> The number of abortions performed in this state is increasing, and more and more women say that they favor greater access to abortion. Therefore, in this state the trend among women is toward greater acceptance of abortion.

This is now an argument. There is a conclusion ("Therefore, in this state the trend among women is toward greater acceptance of abortion") supported by two premises ("The number of abortions performed in this state is increasing, and more and more women say that they favor greater access to abortion"). We are given reasons for accepting a claim.

Notice how easy it would be to elaborate on the nonargumentative version, adding other unsupported claims and more expressions of the writer's attitude toward the subject matter. We would end up with a much longer passage piled high with more assertions—but with no argument in sight. Often those who write such passages believe that because they have stated their opinion, they have presented an argument. But a bundle of unsupported claims—however clearly stated—does not an argument make. Only when reasons are given for believing one of these claims is an argument made.

Learning to distinguish arguments from nonargumentative material takes practice. The job gets easier, however, if you pay attention to **indicator words.** Indicator words are terms that often appear in arguments and signal that a premise or conclusion may be nearby. Notice that in the argument about abortion, the word *therefore* indicates that the conclusion follows, and in Argument 1 the word *because* signals the beginning of a premise. In addition to *therefore*, common conclusion indicators include *consequently, hence, it follows that, thus, so, it must be that,* and *as a result.* Besides *because,* some common premise indicators are *since, for, given that, due to the fact that, for the reason that, the reason being, assuming that,* and *as indicated by.*

Understand that indicator words are not foolproof evidence that a premise or conclusion is near. Sometimes words that often function as indicators appear when no argument at all is present. Indicator words are simply hints that an argument may be close by.

Probably the most reliable way to identify arguments is to *always look for the conclusion first.* When you know what claim is being supported, you can more easily see what statements are doing the supporting. A true argument always has something to prove. If there is no statement that the writer is trying to convince you to accept, no argument is present.

Finally, understand that *argumentation* (the presentation of an argument) is not the same thing as *persuasion.* To offer a good argument is to present reasons why a particular assertion is true. To persuade someone of something is to influence her opinion by any number of means, including emotional appeals, linguistic or rhetorical tricks, deception, threats, propaganda, and more. Reasoned argument does not necessarily play any part at all. You may be able to use some of these ploys to persuade people to believe a claim. But if you do, you will not have established that the claim is worth believing. On the other hand, if you articulate a good argument, then you prove something—and others just might be persuaded by your reasoning.

ARGUMENTS GOOD AND BAD

A good argument shows that its conclusion is worthy of belief or acceptance; a bad argument fails to show this. A good argument gives you good reasons to accept a claim; a bad argument proves nothing. So the crucial question is, How can you tell which is which? To start, you can learn more about different kinds of arguments and how they get to be good or bad.

There are two basic types of arguments: **deductive** and **inductive.** Deductive arguments are supposed to give logically conclusive support to their

CRITICAL THOUGHT: The Morality of Critical Thinking

You might be surprised to learn that some philosophers consider reasoning itself a moral issue. That is, they think that believing a claim without good reasons (an unsupported statement) is immoral. Probably the most famous exposition of this point comes from the philosopher and mathematician W. K. Clifford (1845–79). He has this to say on the subject:

> It is wrong always, everywhere, and for anyone, to believe anything upon insufficient evidence. If a man, holding a belief which he was taught in childhood or persuaded of afterwards, keeps down and pushes away any doubts which arise about it in his mind . . . and regards as impious

those questions which cannot easily be asked without disturbing it—the life of that man is one long sin against mankind.[*]

Do you agree with Clifford? Can you think of a counterexample to his argument—that is, instances in which believing without evidence would be morally permissible? Suppose the power of reason is a gift from God to be used to help you live a good life. If so, would believing without evidence (failing to use critical thinking) be immoral?

*W. K. Clifford, "The Ethics of Belief," in *The Rationality of Belief in God*, ed. George I. Mavrodes (Englewood Cliffs, NJ: Prentice-Hall, 1970), 159–60.

---

conclusions. Inductive arguments, on the other hand, are supposed to offer only probable support for their conclusions.

Consider this classic deductive argument:

All men are mortal.

Socrates is a man.

Therefore, Socrates is mortal.

It is deductive because the support offered for the conclusion is meant to be absolutely unshakable. When a deductive argument actually achieves this kind of conclusive support, it is said to be **valid.** In a valid argument, if the premises are true, then the conclusion absolutely has to be true. In the Socrates argument, if the premises are true, the conclusion *must be true*. The conclusion follows inexorably from the premises. The argument is therefore valid. When a deductive argument does not offer conclusive support for the conclusion, it is said to be **invalid.** In an invalid argument, it is not the case that if the premises are true, the conclusion must be true. Suppose the first premise of the Socrates argument was changed to "All ducks

are mortal." Then the argument would be invalid because even if the premises were true, the conclusion would not necessarily be true. The conclusion would not follow inexorably from the premises.

Notice that the validity or invalidity of an argument is a matter of its *form*, not its content. The structure of a deductive argument renders it either valid or invalid, and validity is a separate matter from the truth of the argument's statements. Its statements (premises and conclusion) may be either true or false, but that has nothing to do with validity. Saying that an argument is valid means that it has a particular form that ensures that if the premises are true, the conclusion can be nothing but true. There is no way that the premises can be true and the conclusion false.

Recall that there are indicator words that point to the presence of premises and conclusions. There are also indicator words that suggest (but do not prove) that an argument is deductive. Some of the more common terms are *it necessarily follows that, it must be the case that, it logically follows that, conclusively,* and *necessarily.*

Now let us turn to inductive arguments. Examine this one:

Almost all the men at this college have high SAT scores.

Therefore, Julio (a male student at the college) probably has high SAT scores.

This argument is inductive because it is intended to provide probable, not decisive, support to the conclusion. That is, the argument is intended to show only that, at best, the conclusion is probably true. With any inductive argument, it is possible for the premises to be true and the conclusion false. An inductive argument that manages to actually give probable support to the conclusion is said to be **strong.** In a strong argument, if the premises are true, the conclusion is probably true (more likely to be true than not). The SAT argument is strong. An inductive argument that does not give probable support to the conclusion is said to be **weak.** In a weak argument, if the premises are true, the conclusion is not probable (not more likely to be true than not true). If we change the first premise in the SAT argument to "Twenty percent of the men at this college have high SAT scores," the argument would be weak.

Like deductive arguments, inductive ones are often accompanied by indicator words. These terms include *probably, likely, in all probability, it is reasonable to suppose that, odds are,* and *chances are.*

Good arguments provide you with good reasons for believing their conclusions. You now know that good arguments must be valid or strong. But they must also have true premises. Good arguments must both have the right form (be valid or strong) and have reliable content (have true premises). Any argument that fails in either of these respects is a bad argument. A valid argument with true premises is said to be **sound;** a strong argument with true premises is said to be **cogent.**

To evaluate an argument is to determine whether it is good or not, and establishing that requires you to check the argument's form and the truth of its premises. You can check the truth of premises in many different ways. Sometimes you can see immediately that a premise is true (or false). At other times you may need to examine a premise more closely or even do some research. Assessing an argument's form is also usually a very straightforward process. With inductive arguments, sometimes common sense is all that's required to see whether they are strong or weak (whether the conclusions follow from the premises). With deductive arguments, just thinking about how the premises are related to the conclusion is often sufficient. In all cases the key to correctly and efficiently determining the validity or strength of arguments is practice.

Fortunately, there are some techniques that can improve your ability to check the validity of deductive arguments. Some deductive forms are so common that just being familiar with them can give you a big advantage. Let's look at some of them.

To begin, understand that you can easily indicate an argument's form by using a kind of standard shorthand, with letters standing for statements. Consider, for example, this argument:

If Maria walks to work, then she will be late.

She is walking to work.

Therefore, she will be late.

Here's how we symbolize this argument's form:

If *p,* then *q.*

p.

Therefore, *q.*

We represent each statement with a letter, thereby laying bare the argument's skeletal form. The first premise is a compound statement, consisting of two constituent statements, *p* and *q.* This particular argument form is known as a *conditional.* A conditional argument has at least one conditional premise—a premise in an if-then pattern (If *p,* then *q*). The two parts of a conditional premise are known as the *antecedent* (which begins with *if*) and the *consequent* (which follows *then*).

This argument form happens to be very common—so common that it has a name, *modus ponens,* or affirming the antecedent. The first premise is conditional ("If Maria walks to work, then she will be late"), and the second premise affirms the antecedent of that conditional ("She is walking to work"). This form is *always valid:* if the premises are true, the conclusion *has to be true.* Any argument that has this form will be valid regardless of the subject matter.

Another frequently occurring form is known as *modus tollens,* or denying the consequent:

If Maria walks to work, then she will be late.

She will not be late.

Therefore, she will not walk to work.

Symbolized, *modus tollens* looks like this:

If *p,* then *q.*

Not *q.*

Therefore, not *p.*

Modus tollens is always valid, no matter what statements you plug into the formula.

Here are two more common argument forms. These, however, are *always invalid.*

Denying the antecedent:

If Maria walks to work, then she will be late.

She will not walk to work.

Therefore, she will not be late.

If *p,* then *q.*

Not *p.*

Therefore, not *q.*

Affirming the consequent:

If Maria walks to work, then she will be late.

She will be late.

Therefore, she will walk to work.

If *p,* then *q.*

q.

Therefore, *p.*

Do you see the problem with these two? In the first one (denying the antecedent), even a false antecedent (if Maria will not walk to work) doesn't mean that she will not be late. Maybe she will sit at home and be late, or be late for some other reason. When the antecedent is denied, the premises can be true and the conclusion false—clearly an invalid argument. In the second argument (affirming the consequent), even a true consequent (if Maria will be late) doesn't mean that she will walk to work. Some other factor besides her walking could cause Maria to be late. Again, the premises can be true while the conclusion is false—definitely invalid.

Consider one last form, the hypothetical syllogism (*hypothetical* means *conditional;* a *syllogism* is a three-statement deductive argument):

If Maria walks to work, then she will be late.

If she is late, she will be fired.

Therefore, if Maria walks to work, she will be fired.

If *p,* then *q.*

If *q,* then *r.*

Therefore, if *p,* then *r.*

The hypothetical syllogism is a valid argument form. If the premises are true, the conclusion must be true.

Obviously, if *modus ponens, modus tollens,* and the hypothetical syllogism are always valid, then any arguments you encounter that have the same form will also be valid. And if denying the antecedent and affirming the consequent are always invalid, any arguments you come across that have the same form will also be invalid. The best way to make use of these facts is to memorize each argument form so you can tell right away when an argument matches one of them—and thereby see immediately that it is valid (or invalid).

But what if you bump into a deductive argument that does not match one of these common forms? You can try the *counterexample method*. This approach is based on a fundamental fact that you already know: *it is impossible for a valid argument to have true premises and a false conclusion*. So to test the validity of an argument, you first invent a twin argument that has exactly the same form as the argument you are examining—but you try to give this new argument true premises and a false conclusion. If you can construct such an argument, you have proven that your original argument is invalid.

Suppose you want to test this argument for validity:

If capital punishment deters crime, then the number of death row inmates will decrease over time.

But capital punishment does not deter crime.

Therefore, the number of death row inmates will not decrease over time.

You can probably see right away that this argument is an example of denying the antecedent, an invalid form. But for the sake of example, let's use the counterexample method in this case. Suppose we come up with this twin argument:

If lizards are mammals, then they have legs.

But they are not mammals.

Therefore, they do not have legs.

We have invented a twin argument that has true premises and a false conclusion, so we know that the original argument is invalid.

IMPLIED PREMISES

Most of the arguments that we encounter in everyday life are embedded in larger tracts of nonargumentative prose—in essays, reports, letters to the editor, editorials, and the like. The challenge is to pick out the premises and conclusions and evaluate

the assembled arguments. In many cases, though, there is an additional obstacle: some premises may be implied instead of stated. Sometimes the premises are implicit because they are too obvious to

---

QUICK REVIEW

statement—An assertion that something is or is not the case.

argument—A group of statements, one of which is supposed to be supported by the rest.

premise—A supporting statement in an argument.

conclusion—The statement supported in an argument.

indicator words—Terms that often appear in arguments to signal the presence of a premise or conclusion, or to indicate that an argument is deductive or inductive.

deductive argument—An argument that is supposed to give logically conclusive support to its conclusion.

inductive argument—An argument that is supposed to offer probable support to its conclusion.

valid argument—A deductive argument that does in fact provide logically conclusive support for its conclusion.

invalid argument—A deductive argument that does not offer logically conclusive support for the conclusion.

strong argument—An inductive argument that does in fact provide probable support for its conclusion.

weak argument—An inductive argument that does not give probable support to the conclusion.

sound argument—A valid argument with true premises.

cogent argument—A strong argument with true premises.

mention; readers mentally fill in the blanks. But in most cases, implicit premises should not be left unstated. It is often unclear what premises have been assumed; and unless these are spelled out, argument evaluation becomes difficult or impossible. More to the point, unstated premises are often the most dubious parts of an argument. This problem is especially common in moral arguments, where the implicit premises are frequently the most controversial and the most in need of close scrutiny.

Here is a typical argument with an unstated premise:

> The use of condoms is completely unnatural. They have been manufactured for the explicit purpose of interfering with the natural process of procreation. Therefore, the use of condoms should be banned.

In this argument, the first two sentences constitute a single premise, the gist of which is that using condoms is unnatural. The conclusion is that the use of condoms should be banned. This conclusion, however, does not follow from the stated premise. There is a logical gap between premise and conclusion. The argument will work only if the missing premise is supplied. Here's a good possibility: "Anything that interferes with a natural process should not be allowed." The argument then becomes:

> The use of condoms is completely unnatural. They have been manufactured for the explicit purpose of interfering with the natural process of procreation. Anything that interferes with a natural process should not be allowed. Therefore, the use of condoms should be banned.

By adding the implicit premise, we have filled out the argument, making it valid and a little less mysterious. But now that the missing premise has been brought out into the open, we can see that it is dubious or, at least, controversial. Should everything that interferes with a natural process be banned? If so, we would have to ban antibiotics, anticancer drugs, deodorants, and automobiles.

(Later in this chapter, ways to judge the truth of moral premises are discussed.)

When you evaluate an argument, you should try to explicitly state any implied premise (or premises) when (1) there seems to be a logical gap between premises or between premises and the conclusion and (2) the missing material is not a commonsense assumption. In general, the supplied premise should make the argument valid (when the argument is supposed to be deductive) or strong (when the argument is supposed to be inductive). It should also be *plausible* (as close to the truth as possible) and *fitting* (coinciding with what you think is the author's intent). The point of these stipulations is that when you supply a missing premise, you should be fair and honest, expressing it in such a way that the argument is as solid as possible and in keeping with the author's purpose. Adding a premise that renders an argument ridiculous is easy, and so is distorting the author's intent—and with neither tack are you likely to learn anything or uncover the truth.

Be aware, though, that some arguments are irredeemably bad, and no supplied premise that is properly made can save them. They cannot be turned into good arguments without altering them beyond recognition or original intent. You need not take these arguments seriously, and the responsibility of recasting them lies with those who offer them.

DECONSTRUCTING ARGUMENTS

In the real world, arguments do not come neatly labeled, their parts identified and their relationships laid bare. So you have to do the labeling and connecting yourself, and that can be hard work. Where are the premises and the conclusion? Are there implied premises? What statements are irrelevant to the argument, just background or window dressing? How are all these pieces related? Fortunately there is a tool that can help you penetrate all the verbiage to uncover the essential argument (or arguments) within: *argument diagramming*.

So let's try to diagram the argument in this passage:

> In 2003 the United States attacked Iraq and thereby started a war. President Bush justified his decision to go to war by saying that the action was necessary to preempt Iraq from launching a military strike against the United States. But the obvious question about the war has hardly been addressed and rarely answered: Was the United States morally justified in going to war against Iraq? I think just war theory gives us an answer. The theory says a preemptive attack against a state is justified only if that state presents a substantial danger that is "immediate and imminent." That is, to meet this criterion, an attack by an aggressor nation must be in the final planning stages—an attack must not be merely feared, but about to happen. If invading Iraq were justified, there would have been clear indications of Iraq's final preparations to attack the United States. But there were no such indications. There was only a fantasy about Iraq's having weapons of mass destruction, and in the Bush administration, there was only the fear that the Iraqis were up to no good. In addition, because there was no serious attempt by the United States to try to find a peaceful solution, the war was premature and therefore unjust. Most news accounts at the time reveal that steps by the United States to head off war were halfhearted at best. Finally, the war was unjustified because it violated the moral standard that must be met by any war: The cause of the war must be just. Consequently we are forced to conclude that the war in Iraq was not morally justified.

The first step is to number all the statements for identification and underline any premise or conclusion indicator words. (Note: We count an if-then, or conditional, statement as one statement, and we count multiple statements in a compound sentence separately.) Next we search for the conclusion and draw a <u>double line</u> under it. Locating the conclusion can then help us find the premises, which we tag by <u>underlining</u> them. The marked-up passage then should look like this:

(1) In 2003 the United States attacked Iraq and thereby started a war. (2) President Bush justified his decision to go to war by saying that the action was necessary to preempt Iraq from launching a military strike against the United States. (3) But the obvious question about the war has hardly been addressed and rarely answered: Was the United States morally justified in going to war against Iraq? (4) I think just war theory gives us an answer. (5) The theory says a preemptive attack against a state is justified only if that state presents a substantial danger that is "immediate and imminent." (6) That is, to meet this criterion, an attack by an aggressor nation must be in the final planning stages—an attack must not be merely feared, but about to happen. (7) <u>If invading Iraq were justified, there would have been clear indications of Iraq's final preparations to attack the United States.</u> (8) <u>But there were no such indications.</u> (9) There was only a fantasy about Iraq's having weapons of mass destruction, (10) and in the Bush administration, there was only the fear that the Iraqis were up to no good. (11) <u>In addition, because there was no serious attempt by the United States to try to find a peaceful solution, the war was premature and therefore unjust.</u> (12) <u>Most news accounts at the time reveal that steps by the United States to head off war were halfhearted at best.</u> (13) <u>Finally, the war was unjustified because it violated the moral standard that must be met by any war: The cause of the war must be just.</u> (14) <u>Consequently we are forced to conclude that the war in Iraq was not morally justified.</u>

A key reason for diagramming is to distinguish the premises and conclusions from everything else: background information, redundancies, asides, clarifications, illustrations, and any other material that is logically irrelevant to the argument (or arguments). So the next step is to cross out these irrelevancies, like this:

(1) ~~In 2003 the United States attacked Iraq and thereby started a war that continues to this day.~~ (2) ~~President Bush justified his decision to go to war by saying that the action was necessary to preempt Iraq from launching a military strike against the United States.~~ (3) ~~But the obvious question about the war has hardly been addressed and rarely answered: Was the United States morally justified in going to war against Iraq?~~ (4) ~~I think just war theory gives us an answer.~~ (5) ~~The theory says a preemptive attack~~

against a state is justified only if that state presents a substantial danger that is "immediate and imminent." (6) That is, to meet this criterion, an attack by an aggressor nation must be in the final planning stages—an attack must not be merely feared, but about to happen. (7) If invading Iraq were justified, there would have been clear indications of Iraq's final preparations to attack the United States. (8) But there were no such indications. (9) There was only a fantasy about Iraq's having weapons of mass destruction, (10) and in the Bush administration, there was only the fear that the Iraqis were up to no good. (11) In addition, because there was no serious attempt by the United States to try to find a peaceful solution, the war was premature and therefore unjust. (12) Most news accounts at the time reveal that steps by the United States to head off war were halfhearted at best. (13) Finally, the war was unjustified because it violated the moral standard that must be met by any war: The cause of the war must be just. (14) Consequently we are forced to conclude that the war in Iraq was not morally justified.

We now can see that most of this passage is logically extraneous material. Statements 1 through 6 are background information and introductory remarks. Statement 3, for example, is an assertion of the issue to be addressed in the passage. Statements 9 and 10 are embellishments of Statement 8.

The premises and conclusion are asserted in Statements 7, 8, 11, 12, 13, and 14:

(7) If invading Iraq were justified, there would have been clear indications of Iraq's final preparations to attack the United States.
(8) But there were no such indications.
(11) In addition, because there was no serious attempt by the United States to try to find a peaceful solution, the war was premature and therefore unjust.
(12) Most news accounts at the time reveal that steps by the United States to head off war were halfhearted at best.
(13) Finally, the war was unjustified because it violated the moral standard that must be met by any war: The cause of the war must be just.
(14) Consequently we are forced to conclude that the war in Iraq was not morally justified.

But how are these statements related? To find out, we draw a diagram. Using the numbers to represent the premises and conclusion, we write down the number for the conclusion and place the numbers for the premises above it. Then to show how the premises support the conclusion, we draw arrows from the premises to the conclusion. Each arrow indicates the logical connection between premise and conclusion, representing such expressions as "Premise 11 supports the Conclusion (14)" or "the Conclusion (14) is supported by Premise 11." Here's the completed diagram:

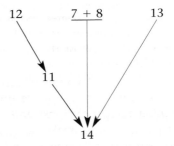

In the simplest relationship depicted here, Premise 13 provides direct support to the conclusion. Premise 11 also supplies direct support to the Conclusion (14), and this premise in turn is backed up by Premise 12. (See how an arrow goes from 11 to 14, and then from 12 to 11.) Premises 7 and 8 are linked to the conclusion in a different way, reflecting the fact that some premises are *dependent* and some are *independent*. An independent premise (such as Premise 13) supports a conclusion without relying on any other premises; a dependent premise gives little or no support on its own and requires the assistance of at least one other premise. Premises 7 and 8 are dependent premises and are joined by a plus sign to represent this fact. Together, Premises 7 and 8 provide support to the conclusion; they give a reason for accepting it. But if either premise is deleted, the remaining premise can provide no substantial support.

As you work through the diagramming exercises at the end of this chapter, you will come to understand why diagramming arguments can be so useful. You will learn a great deal about the structure of arguments—which is a prerequisite for being able to devise, deconstruct, and evaluate them.

MORAL STATEMENTS AND ARGUMENTS

When we deliberate about the rightness of our actions, make careful moral judgments about the character or behavior of others, or strive to resolve complex ethical issues, we are usually making or critiquing moral arguments—or trying to. And rightly so. To a remarkable degree, moral arguments are the vehicles that move ethical thinking and discourse along. The rest of this chapter should give you a demonstration of how far skill in devising and evaluating moral arguments can take you.

Recall that arguments are made up of statements (premises and conclusions), and thus moral arguments are too. What makes an argument a moral argument is that its conclusion is always a moral statement. A **moral statement** is a statement affirming that an action is right or wrong or that a person (or one's motive or character) is good or bad. These are moral statements:

- Capital punishment is wrong.
- Jena should not have lied.
- You ought to treat him as he treated you.
- Tania is a good person.
- Cruelty to animals is immoral.

Notice the use of the terms *wrong*, *should*, *ought*, *good*, and *immoral*. Such words are the mainstays of moral discourse, though some of them (for example, *good* and *wrong*) are also used in nonmoral senses.

Nonmoral statements are very different. They do not affirm that an action is right or wrong or that a person is good or bad. They assert that a state of affairs is actual (true or false) but do not assign a moral value to it. Most of the statements that we encounter every day are nonmoral. Of course, nonmoral statements may assert nonmoral normative judgments, such as "This is a good library" or "Jack ought to invest in stocks," but these are clearly not moral statements. They may also describe a state of affairs that touches on moral concerns—without *being* moral statements. For example:

- Many people think that capital punishment is wrong.
- Jena did not lie.
- You treated him as he treated you.
- Tania tries to be a good person.
- Animals are treated cruelly.

Now we can be more specific about the structure of moral arguments. A typical moral argument consists of premises and a conclusion, just as any other kind of argument does, with the conclusion being a moral statement, or judgment. The premises, however, are a combination of the moral and nonmoral. At least one premise must be a moral statement affirming a moral principle or rule (a general moral standard), and at least one premise must be a nonmoral statement about a state of affairs, usually a specific type of action. Beyond these simple requirements, the structure of moral arguments can vary in standard ways: there may be many premises or few; premises may be implicit not overt; and extraneous material may be present or absent. Take a look at this moral argument:

1. Committing a violent act to defend yourself against physical attack is morally permissible.
2. Assaulting someone who is attacking you is a violent act of self-defense.
3. Therefore, assaulting someone who is attacking you is morally permissible.

Premise 1 is a moral statement asserting a general moral principle about the rightness of a category of actions (violent acts in self-defense).

Premise 2 is a nonmoral statement about the characteristics of a specific kind of action (violent acts against someone who is attacking you). It asserts that a specific kind of action falls under the general moral principle expressed in Premise 1. Premise 3, the conclusion, is a moral judgment about the rightness of the specific kind of action in light of the general moral principle.

Why must we have at least one premise that is a moral statement? Without a moral premise, the argument would not get off the ground. We cannot infer a moral statement (conclusion) from a nonmoral statement (premise). That is, we cannot reason that a moral statement must be true because a nonmoral state of affairs is actual. Or as philosophers say, we cannot establish what *ought to be* or *should be* solely on the basis of on what *is*. What if our self-defense argument contained no moral premise? Look:

2. Assaulting a person who is attacking you is a violent act of self-defense.

3. Therefore, assaulting a person who is attacking you is morally permissible.

The conclusion no longer follows. It says something about the rightness of an action, but the premise asserts nothing about rightness—it just characterizes the nonmoral aspects of an action. Perhaps the action described is morally permissible, or perhaps it is not—Premise 2 does not say.

Another example:

1. Not using every medical means available to keep a seriously ill newborn infant alive is allowing the infant to die.

3. Therefore, not using every medical means available to keep a seriously ill newborn infant alive is wrong.

As it stands, this argument is seriously flawed. The conclusion (a moral statement) does not follow from the nonmoral premise. Even if we know that "not using every medical means" is equivalent to allowing a seriously ill newborn to die, we cannot then conclude that the action is wrong. We need a premise making that assertion:

2. Allowing terminally ill newborn infants to die is wrong.

Here's the complete argument:

1. Not using every medical means available to keep a seriously ill newborn infant alive is allowing the infant to die.

2. Allowing terminally ill newborn infants to die is wrong.

3. Therefore, not using every medical means available to keep a seriously ill newborn infant alive is wrong.

A nonmoral premise is also necessary in a moral argument. Why exactly? Recall that the conclusion of a typical moral argument is a moral judgment, or claim, about a particular kind of action. The moral premise is a general moral principle, or standard, concerning a wider category of actions. But we cannot infer a statement (conclusion) about a *particular kind of action* from a moral statement (premise) about a *broad category of actions*—unless we have a nonmoral premise to link the two. We saw, for example, that we cannot infer from the general principle that "committing a violent act to defend yourself . . . is morally permissible" the conclusion that "assaulting a person who is attacking you is morally permissible" unless a nonmoral premise tells us that assaulting a person who is attacking you is an instance of self-defense. (The nonmoral premise may seem obvious here, but not everyone would agree that violence against a person who is attacking you is an example of self-defense. Some might claim that such violence is an unnecessary act of retaliation or revenge.) The role of the nonmoral premise, then, is to affirm that the general moral principle does indeed apply to the particular case.

Unfortunately, both moral and nonmoral premises are often left unstated in moral arguments. As we noted earlier, making implicit premises explicit is always a good idea, but in moral arguments it is critical. The unseen premises (an argument may have several) are the ones most likely to be dubious or unfounded, a problem that can arise whether an argument is yours or someone else's. Too many times, unstated premises are assumptions that you may be barely aware of; they might be the true, unacknowledged source of disagreement between you and others. No premise should be left unexamined. (More about assessing the truth of premises in the next section.)

The general guidelines discussed earlier about uncovering unstated premises apply to moral arguments—but we need to add a proviso. Remember, in a moral argument, as in any other kind of argument, you have good reason to look for implicit premises if there is a logical gap between premises, and the missing premise is not simply common sense. And any premise you supply should be both plausible and fitting. But note: The easiest way to identify implied premises in a moral argument is to treat it as *deductive*. Approaching moral arguments this way helps you not only find implied premises but also assess the worth of *all* the premises.

For example:

1. The use of capital punishment does not deter crime.

2. Therefore, the use of capital punishment is immoral.

This is an invalid argument. Even if the premise is true, the conclusion does not follow from it. The argument needs a premise that can bridge the gap between the current premise and the conclusion. So we should ask, "What premise can we add that will be plausible and fitting *and* make the argument valid?" This premise will do: "Administering a punishment to criminals that does not deter crime is immoral." The argument then becomes:

1. Administering a punishment to criminals that does not deter crime is immoral.

2. The use of capital punishment does not deter crime.

3. Therefore, the use of capital punishment is immoral.

Now the argument is valid, and trying to make it valid has helped us find at least one premise that might work. Moreover, if we know that the argument is valid, we can focus our inquiry on the truth of the premises. After all, if there is something wrong with a valid argument (that is, if the argument is not sound), we know that the trouble is in the premises—specifically, that at least one premise must be false. To put it another way, whether or not such an argument is a good argument depends entirely on the truth of the premises.

As it turns out, our added premise is a general moral principle. And like many implied premises, it is questionable. Deterrence is not necessarily the only reason for administering punishment. Some would say that justice is a better reason; others, that rehabilitation is. (The second premise is also dubious, but we won't worry about that now.)

In any case, if the supplied premise renders the argument valid, and the premise is plausible and fitting, we can then conclude that we have filled out the argument properly. We can then examine the resulting argument and either accept or reject it. And if we wish to explore the issue at greater depth, we can overhaul the argument altogether to see what we can learn. We can radically change or add premises until we have a sound argument or at least a valid one with plausible premises.

TESTING MORAL PREMISES

But how can we evaluate moral premises? After all, we cannot check them by consulting a scientific study or opinion poll as we might when examining nonmoral premises. Usually the best approach is to use counterexamples.

If we want to test a universal generalization such as "All dogs have tails," we can look for counterexamples—instances that prove the generalization false. All we have to do to show that the statement "All dogs have tails" is false is to find one tailless dog. And a thorough search for tailless dogs is a way to check the generalization. Likewise, if we want to test a moral premise (a variety of universal generalization), we can look for counterexamples.

Examine this valid moral argument:

1. Causing a person's death is wrong.

2. Individuals in a deep, irreversible coma are incapacitated persons.

3. "Pulling the plug" on someone in a deep, irreversible coma is causing a person to die.

4. Therefore, "pulling the plug" on someone in a deep, irreversible coma is wrong.

Premise 1 is the moral premise, a general moral principle about killing. Premises 2 and 3 are non-moral premises. (Premise 2 is entailed by Premise 3, but we separate the two to emphasize the importance to this argument of the concept of personhood.) Statement 4, of course, is the conclusion, the verdict that causing someone in a deep coma to die is immoral.

Is Premise 1 true? It is at least dubious, because counterexamples abound in which the principle seems false. Is it wrong to kill one person to save a hundred? Is it wrong to kill a person in self-defense? Is it wrong to kill a person in wartime? As it stands, Premise 1 seems implausible.

To salvage the argument, we can revise Premise 1 (as well as Premise 3) to try to make it impervious to counterexamples. We can change it like this:

1. Causing the death of a person who is incapacitated is wrong.

2. Individuals in a deep, irreversible coma are persons.

3. "Pulling the plug" on someone in a deep, irreversible coma is causing an incapacitated person to die.

4. Therefore, "pulling the plug" on someone in a deep, irreversible coma is wrong.

Premise 1 now seems a bit more reasonable. In its current form, it rules out the counterexamples involving self-defense and war. But it does not escape the killing-to-save-lives counterexample. In some circumstances it may be morally permissible to kill someone to save many others, even if the person is incapacitated. To get around this problem, we can amend Premise 1 so the counterexample is no longer a threat (and make a corresponding change in the conclusion). For example:

1. Causing the death of a person who is incapacitated is wrong, except to save lives.

2. Individuals in a deep, irreversible coma are persons.

3. "Pulling the plug" on someone in a deep, irreversible coma is causing an incapacitated person to die.

4. Therefore, "pulling the plug" on someone in a deep, irreversible coma is wrong, except to save lives.

Premise 1 now seems much closer to being correct than before. It may not be flawless, but it is much improved. By considering counterexamples, we have made the whole argument better.

Checking a moral premise against possible counterexamples is a way to consult our considered moral judgments, a topic we broached in Chapter 1 and take up again in Part 3 (Theories of Morality). If our considered moral judgments are at odds with a moral premise that is based on a cherished moral principle or moral theory, we may have a prima facie (at first sight) reason to doubt not only the premise but also the principle or theory from which it is derived. We may then need to reexamine the claims involved and how they are related. If we do, we may find that our judgments are on solid ground and the premise, principle, or theory needs to be adjusted—or vice versa. If our purpose is solely to evaluate a moral premise in an argument, we need not carry our investigation this far. But we should understand that widening our investigation may sometimes be appropriate and that our moral beliefs are often more interconnected than we might realize. Our ultimate goal should be to ensure that all our moral beliefs are as logically consistent as we can make them.

ASSESSING NONMORAL PREMISES

Sometimes the sticking point in a moral argument is not a moral premise but a nonmoral one—a claim about a nonmoral state of affairs. Often people on both sides of a dispute may agree on a moral principle but differ dramatically on the nonmoral facts. Usually these facts concern the consequences of an action or the characteristics of the parties involved. Does pornography cause people to commit sex crimes? Does capital punishment deter crime? Is a depressed person competent to decide whether to commit suicide? When does a fetus become viable? Are African Americans underrepresented among executives in corporate America? Does gay marriage undermine the institution of heterosexual marriage? These and countless other questions arise—and must be answered—as we try to develop and analyze moral arguments.

The most important principle to remember is that nonmoral premises, like all premises, *must be supported by good reasons.* As we have already seen, simply believing or asserting a claim does not make it so. We should insist that our own nonmoral premises and those of others be backed by reliable scientific research, the opinions of trustworthy experts, pertinent examples and analogies, historical records, or our own background knowledge (claims that we have excellent reasons to believe).

Ensuring that nonmoral premises are supported by good reasons is sometimes difficult but always worth the effort. The process begins by simply asking, "Is this statement true?" and "What reasons do I have for believing this?"

QUICK REVIEW

- Look for an implicit premise when (1) there seems to be a logical gap between premises or between premises and the conclusion; and (2) the missing material is not a commonplace assumption.

- Any supplied unstated premise should be valid or strong, plausible, and fitting.

- A typical moral argument has at least one moral premise and at least one nonmoral premise.

- The easiest way to identify implied premises in a moral argument is to treat it as deductive.

- Test moral premises with counterexamples.

moral statement—A statement affirming that an action is right or wrong or that a person (or one's motive or character) is good or bad.

nonmoral statement—A statement that does not affirm that an action is right or wrong or that a person (or one's motive or character) is good or bad.

In your search for answers, keep the following in mind:

1. *Use reliable sources.* If you have reason to doubt the accuracy of a source, do not use it. Doubt it if it produces statements you know to be false, ignores reliable data (such as the latest scientific research), or has a track record of presenting inaccurate information or dubious arguments. Make sure that any experts you rely on are in fact experts in their chosen field. In general, true experts have the requisite education and training, the relevant experience in making reliable judgments, and a good reputation among peers.

Probably every major moral issue discussed in this book is associated with numerous advocacy groups, each one devoted to promoting its particular view of things. Too often the information coming from many of these groups is unreliable. Do not automatically assume otherwise. Double-check any information you get from them with sources you know are reliable and see if it is supported by scientific studies, expert opinion, or other evidence.

2. *Beware when evidence conflicts.* You have good reason to doubt a statement if it conflicts with other statements you think are well supported. If your nonmoral premise is inconsistent with another claim you believe is true, you cannot simply choose the one you like best. To resolve the conflict, you must evaluate them both by weighing the evidence for each one.

3. *Let reason rule.* Deliberating on moral issues is serious business, often involving the questioning of cherished views and the stirring of strong feelings. Many times the temptation to dispense with reason and blindly embrace a favorite outlook is enormous. This common—and very human—predicament can lead us to veer far from the relevant evidence and true nonmoral premises. Specifically, we may reject or disregard evidence that conflicts with what we most want to believe. We may even try to pretend that the conflicting evidence actually supports our preconceptions. Yet resisting the relevant evidence is just one side of the coin. We may also look for and find only evidence that supports what we want to believe, going around the world to confirm our prejudices.

Our best chance to avert these tendencies is to try hard to be both critical and fair—to make a deliberate effort to examine *all* the relevant evidence, the information both for and against our preferred beliefs. After all, the point of assessing a moral argument is to discover the truth. We must be brave enough to let the evidence point where it will.

AVOIDING BAD ARGUMENTS

Recall that a good argument has true premises plus a conclusion that follows from those premises. A bad argument fails at least one of these conditions—

it has a false premise or a conclusion that does not follow. This failure, however, can appear in many different argument forms, some of which are extremely common. These commonly bad arguments are known as *fallacies*. They are so distinctive and are used so often that they have been given names and are usually covered in courses on critical reasoning. Though flawed, fallacies are often persuasive and frequently employed to mislead the unwary—even in (or *especially* in) moral reasoning. The best way to avoid using fallacies—or being taken in by them—is to study them so you know how they work and can easily identify them. The following is a brief review of some fallacies that are most prevalent in moral argumentation.

Begging the Question

Begging the question is the fallacy of arguing in a circle—that is, trying to use a statement as both a premise in an argument and the conclusion of that argument. Such an argument says, in effect, *p* is true because *p* is true. That kind of reasoning, of course, proves nothing.

For example:

1. Women in Muslim countries, regardless of their social status and economic limitations, are entitled to certain rights, including but not necessarily limited to suffrage.

2. Therefore, all women in Muslim countries have the right to vote in political elections.

This argument is equivalent to saying "Women in Muslim countries have a right to vote because women in Muslim countries have a right to vote." The conclusion merely repeats the premise but in different words. The best protection against circular reasoning is a close reading of the argument.

Equivocation

The fallacy of **equivocation** assigns two different meanings to the same term in an argument. Here's an example that, in one form or another, is commonplace in the abortion debate:

1. A fetus is an individual that is indisputably human.

2. A human is endowed with rights that cannot be invalidated, including a right to life.

3. Therefore, a fetus has a right to life.

This argument equivocates on the word *human*. In Premise 1, the term means physiologically human, as in having human DNA. This claim, of course, is indeed indisputable. But in Premise 2, *human* is used in the sense of *person*—that is, an individual having full moral rights. Since the premises refer to two different things, the conclusion does not follow. If you are not paying close attention, though, you might not detect the equivocation and accept the argument as it is.

Appeal to Authority

This is the fallacy of relying on the opinion of someone thought to be an expert who is not. An expert, of course, can be a source of reliable information—but only if he really is an authority in the designated subject area. A true expert is someone who is both knowledgeable about the facts and able to make reliable judgments about them. Ulti-

mately, experts are experts because they carefully base their opinions on the available evidence.

We make a fallacious **appeal to authority** when we (1) cite experts who are not experts in the field under discussion (though they may be experts in some other field) or (2) cite nonexperts as experts. Expertise in one field does not automatically carry over to another, and even nonexperts who are prestigious and famous are still just nonexperts. In general, on subjects outside an expert's area of expertise, her opinions are no more reliable than those of nonexperts.

Two rules of thumb should guide your use of expert opinion. First, if a claim conflicts with the consensus of opinion among experts, you have good reason to doubt the claim. Second, if experts disagree about a claim, you again have good reason to doubt it.

Slippery Slope

Slippery slope is the fallacy of using dubious premises to argue that doing a particular action will inevitably lead to other actions that will result in disaster, so you should not do that first action. This way of arguing is perfectly legitimate if the

Appeal to Emotion

Emotions have a role to play in the moral life. In moral arguments, however, the use of emotions alone as substitutes for premises is a fallacy. We commit this fallacy when we try to convince someone to accept a conclusion not by providing them with relevant reasons but by appealing only to fear, guilt, anger, hate, compassion, and the like. For example:

> The defendant is obviously guilty of murder in this case. Look at him in the courtroom—he's terrifying and menacing. And no one can ignore the way

he stabbed that girl and mutilated her body. And her poor parents. . . .

The question here is whether the defendant committed the crime, and the feelings of fear and pity that he evokes are not relevant to it. But if the question were about the anguish or torment inflicted on the victim or her parents, then our feelings of empathy would indeed be relevant—and so would any pertinent moral principles or theories.

premises are solid—that is, if there are good reasons to believe that the first step really will lead to ruin. Consider:

1. Rampant proliferation of pornography on the Internet leads to obsession with pornographic materials.
2. Obsession with pornographic materials disrupts relationships, and that disruption leads to divorce.
3. Therefore, we should ban pornography on the Internet.

Perhaps the chain of events laid out here could actually occur, but we have been given no reason to believe that it would. (You can see that this argument is also missing a moral premise.) Scientific evidence showing that this sequence of cause and effect does occur as described would constitute good reason to accept Premises 1 and 2.

Faulty Analogy

The use of an analogy to argue for a conclusion is known, not surprisingly, as argument by analogy. It is a type of inductive argument that says because two things are alike in some ways, they must be alike in some additional way. For example:

1. Humans feel pain, care for their young, live in social groups, and understand nuclear physics.
2. Apes also feel pain, care for their young, and live in social groups.
3. Therefore, apes can understand nuclear physics.

In argument by analogy, the probability that the conclusion is true depends on the relevant similarities between the two things being compared. The greater the relevant similarities, the more likely the conclusion is true. Humans and apes are relevantly similar in several ways, but the question is, Are they relevantly similar enough to render the conclusion probable? In this case, though humans and apes are similar in some ways, they are not relevantly similar enough to adequately

support the conclusion. Humans and apes have many differences—the most relevant of which for this argument is probably in the physiology of their brains and in their capacity for advanced learning.

Arguments by analogy are common in moral reasoning. For example:

1. When a neighbor needs your help (as when he needs to borrow your garden hose to put out a fire in his house), it is morally permissible to lend the neighbor what he needs.
2. Britain is a neighbor of the United States, and it is in dire need of help to win the war against Germany.
3. Therefore, it is morally permissible for the United States to lend Britain the material and equipment it needs to defeat Germany.

This is roughly the moral argument that President Franklin Roosevelt made during World War II to convince Americans to aid Britain in its struggle. The strength of the argument depends on the degree of similarity between the two situations described. At the time, many Americans thought the argument strong.

The fallacy of **faulty analogy** is arguing by an analogy that is weak. In strong arguments by analogy, not only must the degree of similarity be great but also the similarities must be relevant. This means that the similarities must relate specifically to the conclusion. Irrelevant similarities cannot strengthen an argument.

Appeal to Ignorance

This fallacy consists of arguing that the *absence of evidence* entitles us to believe a claim. Consider these two arguments:

- No one has proven that the fetus is not a person, so it is in fact a person.
- It is obviously false that a fetus is a person, because science has not proven that it is a person.

Both these arguments are **appeals to ignorance.** The first one says that because a statement has not been proven false, it must be true. The second one has things the other way around: because a statement has not been proven true, it must be false. The problem in both these is that a *lack* of evidence cannot be evidence for anything. A dearth of evidence simply indicates that we are ignorant of the facts. If having no evidence could prove something, we could prove all sorts of outrageous claims. We could argue that because no one has proven that there are no space aliens controlling all our moral decisions, there are in fact space aliens controlling all our moral decisions.

Straw Man

Unfortunately, this fallacy is rampant in debates about moral issues. It amounts to misrepresenting someone's claim or argument so it can be more easily refuted. For example, suppose you are trying to argue that a code of ethics for your professional group should be secular so that it can be appreciated and used by as many people as possible, regardless of their religious views. Suppose further that your opponent argues against your claim in this fashion:

> X obviously wants to strip religious faith away from every member of our profession and to banish religion from the realm of ethics. We should not let this happen. We should not let X have his way. Vote against the secular code of ethics.

This argument misrepresents your view, distorting it so that it seems outrageous and unacceptable. Your opponent argues against the distorted version and then concludes that your (original) position should be rejected.

The **straw man** fallacy is not just a bad argument—it flies in the face of the spirit of moral reasoning, which is about seeking understanding through critical thinking and honest and fair exploration of issues. If you agree with this approach, then you should not use the straw man fallacy—and you should beware of its use by others.

Appeal to the Person

Appeal to the person (also known as *ad hominem*) is arguing that a claim should be rejected solely because of the characteristics of the person who makes it. Look at these:

- We should reject Alice's assertion that cheating on your taxes is wrong. She's a political libertarian.

- Jerome argues that we should all give a portion of our income to feed the hungry people of the world. But that's just what you'd expect a rich guy like him to say. Ignore him.

- Maria says that animals have rights and that we shouldn't use animal products on moral grounds. Don't believe a word of it. She owns a fur coat—she's a big hypocrite.

In each of these arguments, a claim is rejected on the grounds that the person making it has a particular character, political affiliation, or motive. Such personal characteristics, however, are irrelevant to the truth of a claim. A claim must stand or fall on its own merits. Whether a statement is true or false, it must be judged according to the quality of the reasoning and evidence behind it. Bad people can construct good arguments; good people can construct bad arguments.

Hasty Generalization

Hasty generalization is a fallacy of inductive reasoning. It is the mistake of drawing a conclusion about an entire group of people or things based on an undersized sample of the group.

- In this town three pro-life demonstrators have been arrested for trespassing or assault. I'm telling you, pro-lifers are lawbreakers.

- In the past thirty years, at least two people on death row in this state have been executed and later found to be innocent by DNA evidence. Why is the state constantly executing innocent people?

QUICK REVIEW

begging the question—The fallacy of arguing in a circle—that is, trying to use a statement as both a premise in an argument and the conclusion of that argument. Such an argument says, in effect, *p* is true because *p* is true.

equivocation—The fallacy of assigning two different meanings to the same term in an argument.

appeal to authority—The fallacy of relying on the opinion of someone thought to be an expert who is not.

slippery slope—The fallacy of using dubious premises to argue that doing a particular action will inevitably lead to other actions that will result in disaster, so you should not do that first action.

faulty analogy—The use of a flawed analogy to argue for a conclusion.

appeal to ignorance—The fallacy of arguing that the absence of evidence entitles us to believe a claim.

straw man—The fallacy of misrepresenting someone's claim or argument so it can be more easily refuted.

appeal to the person—The fallacy (also known as *ad hominem*) of arguing that a claim should be rejected solely because of the characteristics of the person who makes it.

hasty generalization—The fallacy of drawing a conclusion about an entire group of people or things based on an undersized sample of the group.

In the first argument, a conclusion is drawn about all people with pro-life views from a sample of just three people. When it is spelled out plainly, the leap in logic is clearly preposterous. Yet such preposterous leaps are extremely common. In the

second argument, the conclusion is that wrongful executions in the state happen frequently. This conclusion, though, is not justified by the tiny sample of cases.

WRITING AND SPEAKING ABOUT MORAL ISSUES

A common view about ethics is that arguing about morality is unproductive, unenlightening, frustrating, unsatisfying—and therefore pointless. A typical moral disagreement can go like this:

"The university should ban alcohol everywhere on campus," says X. "Drinking is immoral, whether on campus or off."

"You sound like the administration hacks. They're all idiots!" says Y.

X: "They're not *all* idiots. Some are nice."

Y: "Wrong. They're idiots, and they drink plenty of alcohol every day. Alcohol helps them forget they're idiots."

X: "What about Professor Jones? She doesn't drink."

Y: "Yeah, but she's boring. And for a college professor, being boring is the worst moral failing imaginable."

This exchange really *is* pointless; it's going nowhere. It's the kind of conversation that gives moral discourse a bad name. As we've seen, proper discussions about moral issues—whether in written or oral form—are not at all pointless. They are often productive, thought-provoking, even enlightening. You may not always like where the conversation ends up (what conclusions are arrived at), but you will likely think the trip is worthwhile.

Good moral essays or conversations have several essential elements, without which no progress could be made in resolving the issue at hand.

1. *A claim to be proved.* Almost always, the point of writing or speaking about a moral issue is to

resolve it—that is, to determine whether the central moral claim or statement (a judgment, principle, or theory) is true. Is it the case that same-sex marriage is wrong (or right)? Is it true that Maria's action is morally permissible (or impermissible)? Should actions always be judged right or wrong according to the consequences they produce? To answer such questions is to resolve the issue at hand, and resolving the issue at hand is the point of the written or spoken discourse. Without a clear idea of the claim in question, the essay or conversation will meander, as it does in the previous example.

In an essay, the claim should be spelled out (or sometimes implied) in the first one or two paragraphs. In a conversation, it is most often mentioned (or understood) at the beginning. In either case, it is by grasping the claim that we come to understand the point of it all and to follow the thread of the discussion.

In the most productive moral essays or conversations, something else is made apparent early on: the reason the claim is worth discussing in the first place. This means making sure the meaning of the claim is clear and its implications are apparent. Sometimes this step requires only a sentence or two, but usually much more explaining is necessary. Just as essential is ensuring that readers or listeners understand why anyone would *want* to address the issue—why the issue is deemed important enough to warrant an essay or serious conversation. Often all that's required is a brief explanation of how the issue directly affects people's lives. How, for example, might attitudes and lives change if everyone agreed that same-sex marriage was morally permissible? Or how differently might we view the world if all moral judgments were based on the consequences of actions?

Many times the best reason for dealing with a particular moral issue is that others have addressed it, and we want to disagree or agree with their response. So we might say, "Juan argues that using illicit drugs is morally right, but I think he's wrong

on several counts." Or, "In the debates over abortion, many commentators have asserted that a human fetus is a person with moral standing. But there are at least three reasons for rejecting this view." Or, "Does science prove that persons do not have free will? Some philosophers think so. But I, along with many astute commentators, beg to differ."

2. *An argument for or against the claim.* By now, you know that the essence of moral reasoning, the means for resolving (or trying to resolve) a moral issue, and the overall shape of an essay or conversation about a moral claim is the moral argument. The common pattern in an essay is to follow the introduction (where the moral claim is stated) with a moral argument. Likewise, in a truly rewarding conversation on a moral issue, the main event is the presentation of a moral argument and the ensuing discussion about the quality of that argument (whether the premises are true and the conclusion logically follows from them).

Setting forth the argument involves explaining and amplifying each premise and supporting them with evidence (expert opinion, studies, statistics), examples, or analogies. The aim is to demonstrate clearly and carefully that the conclusion follows from the premises and that the premises are true.

In a worthwhile oral debate, the elements are much the same. Enough time and attention must be allowed for giving and explaining an argument and for thoughtful responses to that argument.

3. *Consideration of Alternative Views.* In any good essay or conversation about moral issues, presenting an argument is not enough. There must be space or time to consider alternative views on the subject. Specifically, there should be an honest and thorough assessment of objections to your argument and its conclusion. Students are often reluctant to take this step because they think it will weaken their case. But the opposite is true. When you carefully consider contrary opinions, you gain credibility because you show that you are

fair-minded and careful. You demonstrate to readers or listeners that you are aware of possible objections and that you have good replies to them. Would you trust the assertions of someone who dogmatically pushes his own view and ignores or dismisses out of hand anyone who disagrees? Remember that a logical argument is not a quarrel or spat and that a truly productive debate is not a competition or shouting match. In ethics, written and oral approaches to moral issues are honest searches for truth and sincere exchanges of ideas.

In an essay, an assessment of objections can come early or late but usually appears after the presentation of the argument. In conversation, objections may be taken up throughout and be addressed as interlocutors raise them. Mutual respect and fairness is a necessity in oral debate. Speakers must be given a chance to have their say—to present arguments, raise objections, or respond to objections.

Handling objections properly involves both summarizing and examining them. We of course always should avoid the fallacies mentioned earlier, but in considering alternative views, we need to be especially alert to the *straw man*. Because the essence of the straw man fallacy is the misrepresenting of someone's claim or argument so it can be more easily refuted, inserting the fallacy into discussions is both dishonest and counterproductive. And by using it you miss an opportunity to spot weaknesses in your case, which means you also miss a chance to strengthen it.

SUMMARY

An argument is a group of statements, one of which is supposed to be supported by the rest. To be more precise, an argument consists of one or more premises and a conclusion. In a good argument, the conclusion must follow from the premises, and the premises must be true.

Arguments come in two basic types: deductive and inductive. Deductive arguments are meant to give logically conclusive support for their conclusions. A deductive argument that actually provides this kind of support is said to be valid. If it also has true premises, it is said to be sound. An inductive argument is meant to provide probable support for its conclusion. An inductive argument that actually provides this kind of support is said to be strong. If it also has true premises, it is said to be cogent.

Deductive arguments come in different forms. Some of these forms are known to be valid; some, invalid. Knowing these patterns helps you determine the validity of deductive arguments. Using the counterexample method can also aid your analysis.

The typical moral argument consists of at least one moral premise and at least one nonmoral premise. The best approach to evaluating moral arguments is to treat them as deductive. This tack enables you to uncover implicit premises. Implicit premises are often moral premises, which may be controversial or dubious. They can be tested through the use of counterexamples.

In moral reasoning, you frequently encounter fallacies—bad arguments that arise repeatedly. Some of those you are most likely to come across are begging the question, equivocation, appeal to authority, slippery slope, faulty analogy, appeal to ignorance, straw man, appeal to the person, and hasty generalization.

EXERCISES

Review Questions

1. Are all persuasive arguments valid? Recount a situation in which you tried to persuade someone of a view by using an argument. (p. 44)
2. Can a valid deductive argument ever have false premises? Why or why not? (p. 44)
3. Are the premises of a cogent argument always true? Is the conclusion always true? Explain. (p. 45)
4. What is the term designating a valid argument with true premises? a strong argument with true premises? (p. 45)

5. Is the following argument form valid or invalid? Why or why not? (p. 45)

    If p, then q.

    p.

    Therefore, q.

6. Is the following argument form valid or invalid? Why or why not? (p. 46)

    If p, then q.

    If q, then r.

    Therefore, if p, then r.

7. What is the counterexample method? (p. 47)
8. What kind of premises must a moral argument have? (p. 51)
9. What is the best method for evaluating moral premises? (pp. 53–55)
10. Explain the method for locating implied premises. (pp. 47–48)

Discussion Questions

1. Is it immoral to believe a claim without evidence? Why or why not?
2. If moral reasoning is largely about providing good reasons for moral claims, where do feelings enter the picture? Is it possible to present a good argument that you feel strongly about? If so, provide an example of such an argument.
3. Which of the following passages are arguments (in the sense of displaying critical reasoning)? Explain your answers.
   - If you harm someone, they will harm you.
   - Racial profiling is wrong. It discriminates against racial groups, and discrimination is wrong.
   - If you say something that offends me, I have the right to prevent you from saying it again. After all, words are weapons, and I have a right to prevent the use of weapons against me.
4. What is the difference between persuading someone to believe a claim and giving them reasons to accept it? Can a good argument be persuasive? Why or why not?

5. Why do you think people are tempted to use the straw man fallacy in disagreements on moral issues? How do you feel when someone uses this fallacy against you?

Argument Exercises

Diagram the following arguments. Exercises marked with an asterisk (*) have answers in Answers to Argument Exercises at the end of the text.

*1. If John works out at the gym daily, he will be healthier. He is working out at the gym daily. So he will be healthier.
2. If when you are in a coma you are no longer a person, then giving you a drug to kill you would not be murder. In a coma, you are in fact not a person. Therefore, giving you the drug is not murder.
*3. Ghosts do not exist. There is no reliable evidence showing that any disembodied persons exist anywhere.
4. If you smoke, your heart will be damaged. If your heart is damaged, your risk of dying due to heart problems will increase. Therefore, smoking can increase your risk of dying due to heart problems.
*5. The mayor is soft on crime. He cut back on misdemeanor enforcement and told the police department to be more lenient with traffic violators.
6. Grow accustomed to the belief that death is nothing to us, since every good and evil lie in sensation. However, death is the deprivation of sensation. Therefore, death is nothing to us.
*7. The president is either dishonest or incompetent. He's not incompetent, though, because he's an expert at getting self-serving legislation through Congress. I guess he's just dishonest.
8. Most Republicans are conservatives, and Kurt is a Republican. Therefore, Kurt is probably a conservative. Therefore Kurt is probably

opposed to increases in welfare benefits because most conservatives are opposed to increased welfare benefits.

*9. Can people without strong religious beliefs be moral? Countless people have been nonbelievers or nontheists and still behaved according to lofty moral principles; for example, the Buddhists of Asia and the Confucianists of China. Consider also the great secular philosophers from the ancient Greeks to the likes of David Hume and Bertrand Russell. So it's not true that those without strong religious beliefs cannot be moral.

10. Jan is a student at Harvard. No student at Harvard has won a Pulitzer prize. Therefore, Jan has not won a Pulitzer.

*11. We shouldn't pay the lawnmower guy so much money because he never completes the work, and he will probably just gamble the money away because he has no self-control.

12. Either Manny, Mo, or Jack crashed the car. Manny couldn't have done it because he was sleeping in his room and was observed the whole time. Mo couldn't have done it because he was out of town at the time and has witnesses to prove it. So the guy who crashed the car had to be Jack.

PART
3

Theories of Morality

PART

3

Theories of Morality

CHAPTER 4

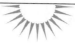

The Power of Moral Theories

Recall that Part 1 (Fundamentals) gave you a broad view of our subject, outlining the major concerns of moral philosophy, the function of moral judgments and principles, the nature of moral problems, the elements of our common moral experience, and the challenges of moral relativism and emotivism. Part 2 (Moral Reasoning) covered ethics at the ground level—the fundamentals of critical reasoning as applied to everyday moral claims, arguments, and conflicts. Here in Part 3 (Chapters 4–7) we touch again on a great deal of this previous material as we explore a central concern of contemporary ethics: moral theory.

THEORIES OF RIGHT AND WRONG

Whatever else the moral life entails, it surely has moral reasoning at its core. We act, we feel, we choose, and in our best moments, we are guided by the sifting of reasons and the weighing of arguments. Much of the time, we expect—and want—this process to yield plausible moral judgments. We confront the cases that unsettle us and hope to respond to them with credible assessments of the right and the good. In making these judgments, we may appeal to moral standards—principles or rules that help us sort out right and wrong, good and bad. Our deliberations may even work the other way around: moral judgments may help us mold moral principles. If we think carefully about our own deliberations, however, we will likely come to understand that this interplay between moral judgments and principles cannot be the whole story of moral reasoning. From time to time we step back from such considerations and ask ourselves if a trusted moral principle is truly sound, whether a conflict of principles can be resolved, or if a new principle can handle cases that we have never had to address before. When we puzzle over such things, we enter the realm of moral theory. We theorize—trying to use, make, or revise a moral theory or a piece of one.

A **moral theory** is an explanation of what makes an action right or what makes a person or thing good. Its focus is not the rightness or goodness of specific actions or persons but the very nature of rightness or goodness itself. Moral theories concerned with the goodness of persons or things are known as *theories of value*. Moral theories concerned with the rightness or wrongness of actions are called *theories of obligation*. In this text, we focus mostly on theories of obligation and, unless otherwise indicated, will use the more general term *moral theories* to refer to them. A moral theory in this sense, then, is an explanation of what makes an action right or wrong. It says, in effect, that a particular action is right (or wrong) because it has *this* property, or characteristic.

Moral theories and theorizing are hard to avoid. To wonder what makes an action right is to theorize. To try *not* to think much about morality but to rely on your default moral theory—the one you inherited from your family or culture—is of course to live by the lights of a moral theory. To reject all moral theories, to deny the possibility of objective morality, or to embrace a subjectivist view of right

Moral Theories versus Moral Codes

A moral theory explains what makes an action right; a moral code is simply a set of rules. We value a moral theory because it identifies for us the essence of rightness and thereby helps us make moral judgments, derive moral principles, and resolve conflicts between moral statements. A moral code, however, is much less useful than a moral theory. The rules in a moral code inevitably conflict but provide no means for resolving their inconsistencies. Rules saying both "Do not kill" and "Protect human life," for example, will clash when the only way to protect human life is to kill. Also, rules are always general—usually too general to cover many specific situations that call for a moral decision—yet not general enough (in the way that theories are) to help us deal with such an array of specifics. How does a rule insisting "Children must obey their parents" apply when the parents are criminally insane or under the influence of drugs, or when there are no parents, just legal guardians? To make the rule apply, we would have to interpret it—and that gets us back into the realm of moral theory.

The point is that moral codes may have their place in the moral life, but they are no substitute for a plausible moral theory. Rules are rules, but a moral theory can help us see beyond the rules.

and wrong is to have a particular overarching view of morality, a view that in the broadest sense constitutes a moral theory or part of one.

A moral theory provides us with very general norms, or standards, that can help us make sense of our moral experiences, judgments, and principles. (Some moral theories feature only *one* overarching standard.) The standards are meant to be general enough and substantial enough to inform our moral reasoning—to help us assess the worth of less general principles, to shed light on our moral judgments, to corroborate or challenge aspects of our moral experience, and even to generate new lower-level principles if need be.

Moral theories and moral arguments often work together. A statement expressing a moral theory may itself act as the moral premise in an argument. More often, an argument's moral premise is ultimately backed by a moral theory from which the moral premise (principle or rule) is derived. Testing the premise may require examining one or more supporting principles or perhaps the most general norm (the theory) itself.

Classic utilitarianism (covered in the next chapter) is an example of a simple moral theory, one based on a single, all-encompassing standard: right actions are those that directly produce the greatest overall happiness, everyone considered. What matters most are the consequences of actions. Thus in a particular situation, if there are only two possible actions, and action X produces, say, 100 units of overall happiness for everyone involved (early utilitarians were the first to use this strange-sounding notion of *units* of happiness) while action Y produces only 50 units, action X is the morally right action to perform. The theory therefore identifies what is thought to be the most important factor in the moral life (happiness) and provides a procedure for making judgments about right and wrong actions.

Should we therefore conclude that a moral theory is the final authority in moral reasoning? Not at all. A moral theory is not like a mathematical axiom. From a moral theory we cannot derive in strict logical fashion principles or judgments that will solve all the problems of our real-world cases. Because moral theories are by definition general and theoretical, they cannot by themselves give us precisely tailored right answers. But neither can we dispense with moral theories and rely solely on judgments about particular cases and issues. In the field of ethics, most philosophers agree that carefully made moral judgments about cases and issues are generally reliable data that we should take very seriously. Such opinions are called *considered moral judgments* because they are formed after careful deliberation that is as free of bias as possible. Our considered judgments (including the principles or rules sanctioned by those judgments) by themselves, however, are sometimes of limited use. They may conflict. They may lack sufficient justification. A moral theory provides standards that can help overcome these limitations.

So where does theory fit in our moral deliberations? Theory plays a role along with judgments and principles or rules. In trying to determine the morally right thing to do in a specific case, we may find ourselves reflecting on just one of these elements or on all of them at once. We may, for example, begin by considering the insights embodied in our moral theory, which give some justification to several relevant principles. In light of these principles, we may decide to perform a particular action. But we may also discover that our considered judgment in the case conflicts with the deliverances of the relevant principles or even with the overarching theory. Depending on the weight we give to the particular judgment, we may decide to adjust the principles or the theory so that it is compatible with the judgment. A moral theory can crystallize important insights in morality and thereby give us general guidance as we make judgments about cases and issues. But the judgments—if they are indeed trustworthy—can compel us to reconsider the theory.

The ultimate goal in this give-and-take of theory and judgment (or principle) is a kind of close coherence between the two—what has come to be known as *reflective equilibrium.*[1] They should fit together as closely as possible, with maximum agreement between them. This process is similar to the one used in science to reconcile theory and experimental data, a topic we address in more detail later in this chapter.

[1]John Rawls, *A Theory of Justice,* rev. ed. (Cambridge, MA: Harvard University Press, Belknap Press, 1999).

MAJOR THEORIES

Moral philosophers have traditionally grouped theories of morality into two major categories: consequentialist (or teleological) and nonconsequentialist (or deontological). In general, **consequentialist** moral theories say that what makes an action right is its *consequences.* Specifically, the rightness of an action depends on the amount of good it produces. A consequentialist theory may define the good in different ways—as, for example, pleasure, happiness, well-being, flourishing, or knowledge. But however good is defined, the morally right action is the one that results in the most favorable balance of good over bad.

Nonconsequentialist moral theories say that the rightness of an action does *not* depend entirely on its consequences. It depends primarily, or completely, on the nature of the action itself. To a nonconsequentialist, the balance of good over bad that results from an action may matter little or not at all. What is of primary concern is the *kind* of action in question. To a consequentialist, telling a lie may be considered wrong because it leads to more unhappiness than other actions do. To a nonconsequentialist, telling a lie may be considered wrong simply because it violates an exceptionless rule. Thus by nonconsequentialist lights, an action could be morally right—even though it produces less good than any alternative action.

Consequentialist Theories
There are several consequentialist theories, each differing on who is to benefit from the goods or what kinds of goods are to be pursued. But two theories have received the most attention from moral philosophers: utilitarianism and ethical egoism.

Utilitarianism says that the morally right action is the one that produces the most favorable balance of good over evil, everyone considered. That is, the right action maximizes the good (however *good* is defined) better than any alternative action, everyone considered. Utilitarianism insists that *everyone* affected by an action must be included in any proper calculation of overall consequences. The crucial factor is how much net good is produced when everyone involved is counted.

Moral philosophers distinguish two major types of utilitarianism, according to whether judgments of rightness focus on individual acts (without reference to rules) or on rules that cover various categories of acts. **Act-utilitarianism** says that right actions are those that *directly* produce the greatest overall good, everyone considered. The consequences that flow directly from a particular act are all that matter; rules are irrelevant to this calculation. In act-utilitarianism, each situation calling for a moral judgment is unique and demands a new calculation of the balance of good over evil. Thus, breaking a promise may be right in one situation and wrong in another, depending on the consequences. **Rule-utilitarianism,** on the other hand, says that the morally right action is the one *covered by a rule* that if generally followed would produce the most favorable balance of good over evil, everyone considered. The consequences of generally following a rule are of supreme importance—not the direct consequences of performing a particular action. Specific rules are justified because if people follow them all the time (or most of the time), the result will be a general maximization of good over evil. We are to follow such rules consistently even if doing so in a particular circumstance results in bad consequences.

Ethical egoism says that the morally right action is the one that produces the most favorable balance of good over evil *for oneself.* That is, in every situation the right action is the one that advances one's own best interests. In each circumstance, the ethical egoist must ask, Which action, among all possible actions, will result in the most good *for me?* Ironically, it may be possible for an ethical egoist to consistently practice this creed without appearing to be selfish or committing many selfishly unkind acts. The egoist may think that *completely* disregarding the welfare of others is not in

his or her best interests. After all, people tend to resent such behavior and may respond accordingly. Nevertheless, the bottom line in all moral deliberations is whether an action maximizes the good for the egoist. This approach to morality seems to radically conflict with commonsense moral experience as well as with the basic principles of most other moral theories.

Nonconsequentialist Theories

Nonconsequentialist (deontological) theories also take various forms. They differ on, among other things, the number of foundational principles or basic rules used and the ultimate basis of those principles.

By far the most influential nonconsequentialist theory is that of Immanuel Kant (1724–1804). Kant wants to establish as the foundation of his theory a single principle from which all additional maxims can be derived, a principle he calls the **categorical imperative.** One way that he states his principle is "Act only on that maxim through which you can at the same time will that it should become a universal law."[2] (Kant insists that he formulates just one principle but expresses it in several different forms; the forms, however, seem to be separate principles.) The categorical imperative, Kant says, is self-evident—and therefore founded on reason. The principle and the maxims derived from it are also universal (applying to all persons) and absolutist, meaning that they are moral laws that have no exceptions. **Kant's theory,** then, is the view that the morally right action is the one done in accordance with the categorical imperative.

For Kant, every action implies a rule or maxim that says, in effect, always do this in these circumstances. An action is right, he says, if and only if you could rationally will the rule to be universal— to have everyone in a similar situation always act

[2]Immanuel Kant, *Groundwork of the Metaphysic of Morals,* trans. H. J. Paton (1948; reprint, New York: Harper & Row, 1964), 88.

according to the same rule. Breaking promises is wrong because if the implied rule (something like "Break promises whenever you want") were universalized (if everyone followed the rule), then no promise anywhere could be trusted, and the whole convention of promise making would be obliterated—and no one would be willing to live in such a world. In other words, universalizing the breaking of promises would result in a logically contradictory state of affairs, a situation that makes no moral sense.

Notice again the stark contrast between utilitarianism and Kant's theory. For the former, the rightness of an action depends solely on its consequences, on what results the action produces for the individuals involved. For the latter, the consequences of actions for particular individuals never enter into the equation. An action is right if and only if it possesses a particular property—the property of according with the categorical imperative, of not involving a logical contradiction.

Another notable nonconsequentialist view is the theory of natural law. **Natural law theory** says that the morally right action is the one that follows the dictates of nature. What does nature have to do with ethics? According to the most influential form of this theory (traditional natural law theory), the natural world, including humankind, exhibits a rational order in which everything has its proper place and purpose, with each thing given a specific role to play by God. In this grand order, natural laws reflect how the world is as well as how it should be. People are supposed to live according to natural law—that is, they are to fulfill their rightful, *natural* purpose. To act morally, they must act naturally; they must do what they were designed to do by God. They must obey the absolutist moral rules that anyone can read in the natural order.

A natural law theorist might reason like this: Lying is immoral because it goes against human nature. Truth telling is natural for humans because they are social creatures with an inborn tendency

QUICK REVIEW

moral theory—An explanation of what makes an action right or what makes a person or thing good.

consequentialist theory—A theory asserting that what makes an action right is its consequences.

nonconsequentialist theory—A theory asserting that the rightness of an action does not depend on its consequences.

utilitarianism—A theory asserting that the morally right action is the one that produces the most favorable balance of good over evil, everyone considered.

act-utilitarianism—A utilitarian theory asserting that the morally right action is the one that directly produces the most favorable balance of good over evil, everyone considered.

rule-utilitarianism—A utilitarian theory asserting that the morally right action is the one covered by a rule that if generally followed would produce the most favorable balance of good over evil, everyone considered.

ethical egoism—A theory asserting that the morally right action is the one that produces the most favorable balance of good over evil for oneself.

categorical imperative—An imperative that we should follow regardless of our particular wants and needs; also, the principle that defines Kant's ethical system.

Kant's theory—A theory asserting that the morally right action is the one done in accordance with the categorical imperative.

natural law theory—A theory asserting that the morally right action is the one that follows the dictates of nature.

divine command theory—A theory asserting that the morally right action is the one that God commands.

to care about the welfare of others. Truth telling helps humans get along, maintain viable societies, and show respect for others. Lying is therefore unnatural and wrong. Another example: Some natural law theorists claim that "unnatural" sexual activity is immoral. They argue that because the natural purpose of sex is procreation, and such practices as homosexual behavior or anal sex have nothing to do with procreation, these practices are immoral.

Another critical aspect of the traditional theory is that it insists that humans can discover what is natural, and thus moral, through reason. God has created a natural order and given humans the gift of rationality to correctly apprehend this order. This means that any rational person—whether religious or not—can discern the moral rules and live a moral life.

One of the simplest nonconsequentialist theories is the **divine command theory,** a view discussed in Chapter 1. It says that the morally right action is the one that God commands. An action is right if and only if God says it is. The rightness of an action does not depend in any way on its consequences. According to the divine command theory, an action may be deemed right even though it does *not* maximize the good, or deemed wrong even if it does maximize the good. It may incorporate one principle only (the core principle that God makes rightness) or the core principle plus several subordinate rules, as is the case with divine command views that designate the Ten Commandments as a God-made moral code.

EVALUATING THEORIES

We come now to the question that moral philosophers have been asking in one way or another for centuries: Is this moral theory a *good* theory? That is, Is it true? Does it reliably explain what makes an action right? As we have seen, not all moral theories are created equal. Some are better than others; some are seriously flawed; and some, though imperfect,

have taught the world important lessons about the moral life.

The next question, of course, is, How do we go about answering the first question? At first glance, it seems that impartially judging the worth of a moral theory is impossible, since we all look at the world through our own tainted lens, our own moral theory or theory fragments. However, our review of subjectivism and relativism (Chapter 2) suggests that this worry is overblown. More to the point, there are plausible criteria that we can use to evaluate the adequacy of moral theories (our own and those of others), standards that moral philosophers and others have used to appraise even the most complex theories of morality. These are what we may call the *moral criteria of adequacy*.

The first step in any theory assessment (before using these criteria) is to ensure that the theory meets the minimum requirement of *coherence*. A moral theory that is coherent is *eligible* to be evaluated using the criteria of adequacy. A coherent theory is internally consistent, which means that its central claims are consistent with each other—they are not contradictory. An internally consistent theory would not assert, for example, both that (1) actions are right if and only if they are natural; and (2) it is morally right to use unnatural means to save a life. Contradictory claims assert both that something *is* and *is not* the case; one statement says X and another says not-X. When claims conflict in this way, we know that at least one of them is false. So if two substantial claims in a theory are contradictory, one of the claims must be false—and the theory is refuted. This kind of inconsistency is such a serious shortcoming in a moral theory that further evaluation of it would be unnecessary. It is, in fact, not eligible for evaluation. Ineligible theories would get low marks on each criterion of adequacy.

Eligible moral theories are a different matter. Unlike ineligible theories, they are not guaranteed to fare poorly when evaluated, and testing their mettle with the moral criteria of adequacy is almost always revealing. But how do we use these criteria? The answer is that we apply them in much the same way and for a few of the same reasons that scientists apply their criteria to scientific theories.

Scientific theories are introduced to explain data concerning the causes of events—why something happens as it does or why it is the way it is. Usually scientists devise several theories (explanations) of a phenomenon, ensuring that each one is minimally adequate for evaluation. Then they try to determine which of these is best, which offers the best explanation for the data in question, for they know that the best theory is the one most likely to be true. To discover which is the best, they must judge each theory according to some generally accepted standards—the scientific criteria of adequacy. One criterion, for example, is *conservatism:* how well a theory fits with what scientists already know. A scientific theory that conflicts with existing knowledge (well-established facts, scientific laws, or extensively confirmed theories) is not likely to be true. On the other hand, the more conservative a theory is (that is, the less it conflicts with existing knowledge), the more likely it is to be true. All things being equal, a conservative theory is better than one that is not conservative. Another criterion is *fruitfulness:* how many successful novel predictions the theory makes. The more such predictions, the more plausible the theory is.

Now consider the following criteria of adequacy for moral theories:

Criterion 1: Consistency with Considered Judgments

To be worth evaluating, a plausible scientific theory must be consistent with the data it was introduced to explain. A theory meant to explain an epidemic, for example, must account for the nature of the disease and the method of transmission. Otherwise it is a very poor theory. A moral theory must also be consistent with the data it was introduced to explain. A moral theory is supposed to explain what makes an action right, and the data relevant to that issue are our *considered moral judgments.*

Considered Moral Judgments

The philosopher John Rawls devised the notion of reflective equilibrium and put heavy emphasis on the quality of moral judgments in his own moral theory. This is what he has to say about the nature of considered moral judgments:

> Now, as already suggested, [considered judgments] enter as those judgments in which our moral capacities are most likely to be displayed without distortion. Thus in deciding which of our judgments to take into account we may reasonably select some and exclude others. For example, we may discard those judgments made with hesitation, or in which we have little confidence. Similarly, those given when we are upset or frightened, or when we stand to gain one way or the other can be left aside. All these judgments are likely to be erroneous or to be influenced by an excessive attention to our own interests. Considered judgments are simply those rendered under conditions favorable to the exercise of the sense of justice, and therefore in circumstances where the more common excuses and explanations for making a mistake do not obtain. The person making the judgment is presumed, then, to have the ability, the opportunity, and the desire to reach a correct decision (or at least, not the desire not to). Moreover, the criteria that identify these judgments are not arbitrary. They are, in fact, similar to those that single out considered judgments of any kind.*

*John Rawls, *A Theory of Justice,* rev. ed. (Cambridge, MA: Harvard University Press, Belknap Press, 1999), 42.

Recall that considered moral judgments are views that we form after careful deliberation under conditions that minimize bias and error. They are therefore thought to have considerable weight as reasons or evidence in moral matters, even though they can be mistaken and other considerations (such as an established moral principle or a well-supported theory) can sometimes overrule them.

A moral theory that is inconsistent with trustworthy judgments is at least dubious and likely to be false, in need of drastic overhaul or rejection. There is something seriously wrong, for example, with a theory that approves of the murder of innocent people, the wanton torture of children, or the enslavement of millions of men and women. As we will see in the next chapter, inconsistency with considered judgments can be the undoing of even the most influential and attractive moral theories.

Consider Theory X. It says that right actions are those that enhance the harmonious function-ing of a community. On the face of it, this theory appears to be a wise policy. But it seems to imply that certain heinous acts are right. It suggests, for example, that if killing an innocent person would enhance a community's harmonious functioning, killing that person would be right. This view con-flicts dramatically with our considered judgment that murdering an innocent person just to make a community happy is wrong. Theory X should be rejected.

Criterion 2: Consistency with Our Moral Experiences

As we saw earlier, a good scientific theory should be conservative. It should, in other words, be consistent with scientific background knowledge—with the many beliefs that science has already firmly estab-lished. Likewise, a plausible moral theory should be consistent with moral background knowledge—with what we take to be the fundamental facts of our

---

CRITICAL THOUGHT: A 100 Percent All-Natural Theory

Imagine that you come across a theory based on this moral standard: Only actions that are "natural" are morally right; "unnatural" actions are wrong. We can call it the all-natural theory. It defines nat-ural actions as (1) those done in accordance with the normal biological urges and needs of human beings, (2) those that reflect typically human psy-chological tendencies and patterns, and (3) those that help ensure the survival of the human species. (This approach should not be confused with the more sophisticated and historically important nat-ural law theory.) An all-natural theorist might view these actions as morally permissible: walking, talk-ing, eating, having sex, cooperating with others, caring for loved ones, teaching children, creating art, growing food, building shelters, going to war, solving problems, and protecting the environ-ment. Impermissible actions might include building spaceships, using birth control, using performance-enhancing drugs, being a loner or a hermit, and intervening in reproductive processes (as in cloning, abortion, fertility treatments, in vitro fertilization, and stem cell research).

Is this a good theory? Is it internally inconsis-tent? (For example, do the three definitions of nat-ural actions conflict? Would applying Definition 3 contradict the results of applying Definitions 1 and 2?) Is the all-natural theory consistent with our considered moral judgments? (Hint: Would it con-done murder? Would it conflict with our usual con-cepts of justice?) If it is not consistent, supply an example (a counterexample). Is the theory consis-tent with our moral experience? Give reasons for your answer. Is the theory useful? If not, why not?

moral experience. Whatever our views on morality, few of us would deny that we do in fact have these experiences:

- We sometimes make moral judgments.
- We often give reasons for particular moral beliefs.
- We are sometimes mistaken in our moral beliefs.
- We occasionally have moral disagreements.
- We occasionally commit wrongful acts.

As is the case with theories that conflict with considered judgments, a theory in conflict with these experiences is at least dubious and probably false. A moral theory is inconsistent with the moral life if it implies that we do not have one or more of these basic moral experiences.

Suppose Theory Y says that our feelings alone determine whether actions are right. If our feelings lead us to believe that an action is right, then it is right. But this theory suggests that we are *never* mistaken in our moral beliefs, for if our feelings determine what is right, we cannot be wrong. Whatever we happen to feel tells us what actions are right. Our moral experience, however, is good evidence that we are *not* morally infallible. Theory Y therefore is problematic, to say the least.

Could we possibly be mistaken about our moral experience? Yes. It is possible that our experience of the moral life is illusory. Perhaps we are morally infallible after all, or maybe we do not actually make moral judgments. But like our considered moral judgments, our commonsense moral experience carries weight as evidence—good evidence that the moral life is, for the most part, as we think it is. We therefore are entitled to accept this evidence as trustworthy unless we have good reason to think otherwise.

Criterion 3: Usefulness in Moral Problem Solving

Good scientific theories increase our understanding of the world, and greater understanding leads to greater usefulness—the capacity to solve problems and answer questions. The more useful a scientific theory is, the more credibility it acquires. A good moral theory is also useful—it helps us solve moral problems in real-life situations. It helps us make reliable judgments about moral principles and actions and resolve conflicts among conflicting judgments, principles, and the theory itself. A major reason for devising a moral theory is to obtain this kind of practical guidance.

Usefulness is a necessary, though not sufficient, characteristic of a good moral theory. This means that all good theories are useful, but usefulness alone does not make a moral theory good. It is possible for a bad theory to be useful as well (to be useful but fail some other criterion of adequacy). But any moral theory that lacks usefulness is a dubious theory.

Now we can be more specific about the similarities between science and ethics in handling theory and data. In science, the interaction between a theory and the relevant data is dynamic. The theory is designed to explain the data, so the data help shape the theory. But a plausible theory can give scientists good reasons to accept or reject specific data or to reinterpret them. Both the theory and the data contribute to the process of searching for the truth. Scientists work to get the balance between these two just right. They try to ensure a

---

QUICK REVIEW

The Moral Criteria of Adequacy

Criterion 1: Consistency with considered judgments.

Criterion 2: Consistency with our moral experiences.

Criterion 3: Usefulness in moral problem solving.

very close fit between them—so close that there is no need for major alterations in either the theory or the data. In ethics, the link between theory and data (considered judgments) is similar. Considered judgments help shape theory (and its principles or rules), and a good theory sheds light on judgments and helps adjudicate conflicts between judgments and other moral statements. As in science, we should strive for a strong logical harmony between theory, data, and subordinate principles.

Remember, though, theory evaluation is not a mechanical process, and neither is the application of theories to moral problems. There is no formula or set of instructions for applying our three criteria to a theory. Neither is there a calculating machine for determining how much weight to give each criterion in particular situations. We must make an informed judgment about the importance of particular criteria in each new instance. Nevertheless, applying the criteria is not a subjective, arbitrary affair. It is rational and objective—like, for example, the diagnosis of an illness, based on the educated judgment of a physician using appropriate guidelines.

Now suppose you apply the moral criteria of adequacy and reach a verdict on the worth of a theory: you reject it. Should this verdict be the end of your inquiry? In general, no. There is often much to be learned from even seriously defective theories. Many philosophers who reject utilitarianism, for example, also believe that it makes a valuable point that any theory should take into account: the consequences of actions do matter. Judiciously applying the criteria of adequacy to a theory can help us see a theory's strengths as well as its weakness. Such insights can inspire us to improve any moral theory—or perhaps create a new one.

You will get a chance to see firsthand how theory evaluation is done. In Chapters 5 and 6 we will apply the moral criteria of adequacy to several major moral theories.

SUMMARY

A moral theory is an explanation of what makes an action right or what makes a person or thing good. Theories concerned with the rightness or wrongness of actions are known as theories of obligation (or, in this text, simply moral theories). A moral theory is interconnected with considered judgments and principles. Considered judgments can shape a theory, and a theory can shed light on judgments and principles.

The two major types of theories are consequentialist and nonconsequentialist. Consequentialist theories say that what makes an action right is its consequences. Nonconsequentialist moral theories say that the rightness of an action does not depend entirely on its consequences. Consequentialist theories include utilitarianism (both act- and rule-utilitarianism) and ethical egoism; nonconsequentialist theories include Kant's theory, natural law theory, and divine command theory.

Since not all theories are of equal worth, we must try to discover which one is best—a task that we can perform by applying the moral criteria of adequacy to theories. The three criteria are (1) consistency with considered judgments, (2) consistency with our moral experiences, and (3) usefulness in moral problem solving.

EXERCISES

Review Questions

1. Is a moral theory the final authority in moral reasoning? Why or why not? (p. 68)
2. What is the difference between a moral theory and a moral code? (p. 68)
3. How can a moral theory be used in a moral argument? (p. 68)
4. What is a considered moral judgment? (p. 68)
5. What are the two main categories of moral theory? (p. 69)
6. What is utilitarianism? ethical egoism? (pp. 69–70)

7. According to Kant's moral theory, what makes an action right? (pp. 70–71)
8. What are the three moral criteria of adequacy? (pp. 73–76)

Discussion Questions

1. Do you try to guide your moral choices with a moral code or a moral theory or both? If so, how?
2. Suppose you try to use the Ten Commandments as a moral code to help you make moral decisions. How would you resolve conflicts between commandments? Does your approach to resolving the conflicts imply a moral theory? If so, can you explain the main idea behind the theory?
3. What considered moral judgments have you made or appealed to in the past month? Do you think that these judgments reflect a moral principle or moral theory you implicitly appeal to? If so, what is it?
4. Would you describe your approach to morality as consequentialist, nonconsequentialist, or some combination of both? What reasons do you have for adopting this particular approach?
5. Give an example of a possible conflict between a consequentialist theory and a considered moral judgment. (Show how these two may be inconsistent.)
6. Provide an example of a conflict between a nonconsequentialist theory and a moral judgment based on the consequences of an action.
7. Using the moral criteria of adequacy, evaluate act-utilitarianism.
8. Using the moral criteria of adequacy, evaluate natural law theory.

CHAPTER 5

Consequentialist Theories: Maximize the Good

There is something in consequentialist moral theories that we find appealing, something simple and commonsensical that jibes with everyday moral experience. This attractive core is the notion that right actions must produce the best balance of good over evil. Never mind (for now) how *good* and *evil* are defined. The essential concern is how much good can result from actions performed. In this chapter, we examine the plausibility of this consequentialist maxim and explore how it is worked out in its two most influential theories: ethical egoism and utilitarianism.

ETHICAL EGOISM

Ethical egoism is the theory that the right action is the one that advances one's own best interests. It is a provocative doctrine, in part because it forces us to consider two opposing attitudes in ourselves. On the one hand, we tend to view selfish or flagrantly self-interested behavior as wicked, or at least troubling. Self-love is bad love. We frown on people who trample others in life to get to the head of the line. On the other hand, sometimes we want to look out for number one, to give priority to our own needs and desires. We think, If we do not help ourselves, who will? Self-love is good love.

Ethical egoism says that one's only moral duty is to promote the most favorable balance of good over evil for oneself. Each person must put his or her own welfare first. Advancing the interests of others is part of this moral equation only if it helps promote one's own good. Yet this extreme self-

interest is not necessarily selfishness. Selfish acts advance one's own interests regardless of how others are affected. Self-interested acts promote one's own interests but not necessarily to the detriment of others. To further your own interests you may actually find yourself helping others. To gain some advantage, you may perform actions that are decidedly unselfish.

Just as we cannot equate ethical egoism with selfishness, neither can we assume it is synonymous with self-indulgence or recklessness. An ethical egoist does not necessarily do whatever she desires to do or whatever gives her the most immediate pleasure. She does what is in her best interests, and instant gratification may not be in her best interests. She may want to spend all her money at the casino or work eighteen hours a day, but over the long haul doing so may be disastrous for her. Even ethical egoists have to consider the long-term effects of their actions. They also have to take into account their interactions with others. At least most of the time, egoists are probably better off if they cooperate with others, develop reciprocal relationships, and avoid actions that antagonize people in their community or society.

Ethical egoism comes in two forms—one applying the doctrine to individual *acts* and one to relevant *rules*. **Act-egoism** says that to determine right action, you must apply the egoistic principle to individual acts. Act A is preferable to Act B because it promotes your self-interest better. **Rule-egoism** says that to determine right action, you must see if an act falls under a rule that if consistently followed would maximize your self-interest. Act A is preferable to Act B because it falls under a rule that maximizes your self-interest better than any other relevant rule applying to Act B. An ethical egoist can define self-interest in various ways. The Greek philosopher Epicurus (341–270 B.C.E.), a famous ethical egoist from whose name we derive the words *epicure* and *epicurean,* gave a hedonist answer: The greatest good is pleasure, and the greatest evil, pain. The duty of a good ethical egoist is to maximize pleasure for oneself. (Contrary to legend, Epicurus thought that wanton overindulgence in the delights of the senses was not in one's best interests. He insisted that the best pleasures were those of the contemplative life and that extravagant pleasures such as drunkenness and gluttony eventually lead to misery.) Other egoistic notions of the greatest good include self-actualization (fulfilling one's potential), security and material success, satisfaction of desires, acquisition of power, and the experience of happiness.

To many people, ethical egoism may sound alien, especially if they have heard all their lives about the noble virtue of altruism and the evils of self-centeredness. But consider that self-interest is a pillar on which the economic system of capitalism is built. In a capitalist system, self-interest is supposed to drive people to seek advantages for themselves in the marketplace, compelling them to compete against each other to build a better mousetrap at a lower price. Economists argue that the result of this clash of self-interests is a better, more prosperous society.

Applying the Theory

Suppose Rosa is a successful executive at a large media corporation, and she has her eye on a vice president's position, which has just become vacant. Vincent, another successful executive in the company, also wants the VP job. Management wants to fill the vacancy as soon as possible, and they are trying to decide between the two most qualified candidates—Rosa and Vincent. One day Rosa discovers some documents left near a photocopier and quickly realizes that they belong to Vincent. One of them is an old memo from the president of a company where Vincent used to work. In it, the president lambastes Vincent for botching an important company project. Rosa knows that despite what she reads in the memo, Vincent has had an exemplary professional career in which he has managed most of his projects extremely well. In fact, she believes that the two of them are about equal in professional skills and accomplishments. She also knows that if management saw the memo, they would almost certainly choose her over Vincent for the VP position. She figures that Vincent probably left the documents there by mistake and would soon return to retrieve them. Impulsively, she makes a copy of the memo for herself.

Now she is confronted with a moral choice. Let us suppose that she has only three options. First, she can destroy her copy of the memo and forget about the whole incident. Second, she can discredit Vincent by showing it to management, thereby securing the VP slot for herself. Third, she can achieve the same result by discrediting Vincent surreptitiously: she can simply leave a copy where management is sure to discover it. Let us also assume that she is an act-egoist who defines her self-interest as self-actualization. Self-actualization for her means developing into the most powerful, most highly respected executive in her profession while maximizing the virtues of loyalty and honesty.

So by the lights of her act-egoism what should Rosa do? Which choice is in her best interests? Option one is neutral regarding her self-interest. If she destroys her copy of the memo, she will neither gain nor lose an advantage for herself. Option two is more complicated. If she overtly discredits Vincent, she will probably land the VP spot—a feat that fits nicely with her desire to become a powerful executive. But such a barefaced sabotaging of someone else's career would likely trouble management, and their loss of some respect for

Rosa would impede future advancement in her career. They may also come to distrust her. Rosa's backstabbing would also probably erode the trust and respect of her subordinates (those who report to her). If so, their performance may suffer, and any deficiencies in Rosa's subordinates would reflect on her leadership skills. Over time, she may be able to regain the respect of management through dazzling successes in her field, but the respect and trust of others may be much harder to regain. Option two involves the unauthorized, deceitful use of personal information against another person—not an action that encourages the virtue of honesty in Rosa. In fact, her dishonesty may weaken her moral resolve and make similar acts of deceit more probable. Like option two, option three would likely secure the VP job for Rosa. But because the deed is surreptitious, it would probably not diminish the respect and trust of others. There is a low probability, however, that Rosa's secret would eventually be uncovered—especially if Vincent suspects Rosa, which is likely. If she is found out, the damage done to her reputation (and possibly her career) might be greater than that caused by the more up-front tactic of option two. Also like option two, option three might weaken the virtue of honesty in Rosa's character.

Given this situation and Rosa's brand of act-egoism, she should probably go with option three—but only if the risk of being found out is extremely low. Option three promotes her self-interest dramatically by securing the coveted job at a relatively low cost (a possible erosion of virtue). Option two would also land the job but at very high cost—a loss of other people's trust and respect, a possible decrease in her chances for career advancement, damage to her professional reputation, and a likely lessening of a virtue critical to Rosa's self-actualization (honesty).

If Rosa believes that the risks to her career and character involved in options two and three are too high, she should probably choose option one.

This choice would not promote her best interests, but it would not diminish them either.

Would Rosa's action be any different if judged from the perspective of rule-egoism? Suppose Rosa, like many other ethical egoists, thinks that her actions should be guided by this rule (or something like it): People should be honest in their dealings with others—that is, except in insignificant matters (white lies), they should not lie to others or mislead them. She believes that adhering to this prohibition against dishonesty is in her best interests. The rule, however, would disallow both options two and three, for they involve significant deception. Only option one would be left. But if obeying the rule would lead to a major setback for her interests, Rosa might decide to ignore it in this case (or reject it altogether as contrary to the spirit of ethical egoism). If so, she might have to fall back to act-egoism and decide in favor of option three.

Evaluating the Theory

Is ethical egoism a plausible moral theory? Let us find out by examining arguments in its favor and applying the moral criteria of adequacy.

The primary argument for ethical egoism depends heavily on a scientific theory known as **psychological egoism,** the view that the motive for all our actions is self-interest. Whatever we do, we do because we want to promote our own welfare. Psychological egoism, we are told, is simply a description of the true nature of our motivations. We are, in short, born to look out for number one.

Putting psychological egoism to good use, the ethical egoist reasons as follows: We can never be morally obligated to perform an action that we cannot possibly do. This is just an obvious fact about morality. Since we are *not able* to prevent a hurricane from blasting across a coastal city, we are *not morally obligated* to prevent it. Likewise, since we are not able to perform an action except out of self-interest (the claim of psychological egoism), we are not morally obligated to perform an action unless motivated by self-interest. That is, we are morally obligated to do only what our self-interest motivates us to do. Here is the argument stated more formally:

1. We are not able to perform an action except out of self-interest (psychological egoism).
2. We are not morally obligated to perform an action unless motivated by self-interest.
3. Therefore, we are morally obligated to do only what our self-interest motivates us to do.

Notice that even if psychological egoism is true, this argument does not establish that an action is right if and only if it promotes one's self-interest (the claim of ethical egoism). But it does demonstrate that an action cannot be right unless it at least promotes one's self-interest. To put it another way, an action that does not advance one's own welfare cannot be right.

Is psychological egoism true? Many people think it is and offer several arguments in its favor. One line of reasoning is that psychological egoism is true because experience shows that all our actions are in fact motivated by self-interest. All our actions—including seemingly altruistic ones—are performed to gain some benefit for ourselves. This argument, however, is far from conclusive. Sometimes people do perform altruistic acts because doing so is in their best interests. Smith may contribute to charity because such generosity furthers his political ambitions. Jones may do volunteer work for the Red Cross because it looks good on her résumé. But people also seem to do things that are *not* motivated by self-interest. They sometimes risk their lives by rushing into a burning building to rescue a complete stranger. They may impair their health by donating a kidney to prevent one of their children from dying. Explanations that appeal to self-interest in such cases seem implausible. Moreover, people often have self-destructive habits (for example, drinking excessively and driving recklessly)—habits that are unlikely to be in anyone's best interests.

Some ethical egoists may argue in a slightly different vein: People get satisfaction (or happiness or pleasure) from what they do, including their so-called unselfish or altruistic acts. Therefore, they perform unselfish or altruistic actions because doing so gives them satisfaction. A man saves a child from a burning building because he wants the emotional satisfaction that comes from saving a life. Our actions, no matter how we characterize them, are all about self-interest.

This argument is based on a conceptual confusion. It says that we perform selfless acts to achieve satisfaction. Satisfaction is the object of the whole exercise. But if we experience satisfaction in performing an action, that does not show that our goal in performing the action is satisfaction. A much more plausible account is that we desire something other than satisfaction and then experience satisfaction as a result of getting what we desired. Consider, for example, our man who saves the child from a fire. He rescues the child and feels satisfaction—but he could not have experienced that satisfaction unless he already had a desire to save the child or cared what happened to her. If he did not have such a desire or care about her, how could he have derived any satisfaction from his actions? To experience satisfaction he had to have a desire for something other than his own satisfaction. The moral of the story is that satisfaction is the result of getting what we want—not the object of our desires.

This view fits well with our own experience. Most often when we act according to some purpose, we are not focused on, or aware of, our satisfaction. We concentrate on obtaining the real object of our efforts, and when we succeed, we then feel satisfaction.

The philosopher Joel Feinberg makes a similar point about the pursuit of happiness. He asks us to imagine a person, Jones, who has no desire for much of anything—except happiness. Jones has no interest in knowledge for its own sake, the beauty of nature, art and literature, sports, crafts,

Can Ethical Egoism Be Advocated?

Some critics of ethical egoism say that it is a very strange theory because its adherents cannot urge others to become ethical egoists! The philosopher Theodore Schick Jr. makes the point:

> Even if ethical egoism did provide necessary and sufficient conditions for an action's being right, it would be a peculiar sort of ethical theory, for its adherents couldn't consistently advocate it. Suppose that someone came to an ethical egoist for moral advice. If the ethical egoist wanted to do what is in his best interest, he would not tell his client to do what is in her best interest because her interests might conflict with his. Rather, he would tell her to do what is in his best interest.

Such advice has been satirized on national TV. Al Franken, a former writer for *Saturday Night Live* and author of *Rush Limbaugh Is a Big Fat Idiot and Other Observations,* proclaimed on a number of *Saturday Night Live* shows in the early 1980s that whereas the 1970s were known as the "me" decade, the 1980s were going to be known as the "Al Franken" decade. So whenever anyone was faced with a difficult decision, the individual should ask herself, "How can I most benefit Al Franken?"*

*Theodore Schick Jr., in *Doing Philosophy: An Introduction through Thought Experiments*, by Schick and Lewis Vaughn, 2nd ed. (Boston: McGraw-Hill, 2003), 327.

or business. But Jones does have "an overwhelming passion for, a complete preoccupation with, his own happiness. The one desire of his life is to be happy."[1] The irony is that using this approach, Jones will *not* find happiness. He cannot pursue happiness directly and expect to find it. To achieve happiness, he must pursue other aims whose pursuit yields happiness as a by-product. We must conclude that it is not the case that our only motivation for our actions is the desire for happiness (or satisfaction or pleasure).

These reflections show that psychological egoism is a dubious theory, and if we construe self-interest as satisfaction, pleasure, or happiness, the theory seems false. Still, some may not give up the argument from experience (mentioned earlier), insisting that when properly interpreted, all our actions (including those that seem purely altruistic or unselfish) can be shown to be motivated by self-interest. All the counterexamples that seem to

suggest that psychological egoism is false actually are evidence that it is true. Smith's contributing to charity may look altruistic, but he is really trying to impress a woman he would like to date. Jones's volunteer work at the Red Cross may seem unselfish, but she is just trying to cultivate some business contacts. Every counterexample can be reinterpreted to support the theory.

Critics have been quick to charge that this way of defending psychological egoism is a mistake. It renders the theory untestable and useless. It ensures that no evidence could possibly count against it, and therefore it does not tell us anything about self-interested actions. Anything we say about such actions would be consistent with the theory. Any theory that is so uninformative could not be used to support another theory—including ethical egoism.

So far we have found the arguments for ethical egoism ineffective. Now we can ask another question: Are there any good arguments *against* ethical egoism? This is where the moral criteria of adequacy come in.

Recall that an important first step in evaluating a moral theory (or any other kind of theory) is to determine if it meets the minimum require-

[1] Joel Feinberg, "Psychological Egoism," in *Moral Philosophy: Selected Readings,* ed. George Sher (San Diego: Harcourt Brace Jovanovich, 1987), 11–12.

ment of coherence, or internal consistency. As it turns out, some critics of ethical egoism have brought the charge of logical or practical inconsistency against the theory. But in general these criticisms seem to fall short of a knockout blow to ethical egoism. Devising counterarguments that can undercut the criticisms seems to be a straightforward business. Let us assume, then, that ethical egoism is in fact eligible for evaluation using the criteria of adequacy.

We begin with Criterion 1, consistency with considered judgments. A major criticism of ethical egoism is that it is *not* consistent with many of our considered moral judgments—judgments that seem highly plausible and commonsensical. Specifically, ethical egoism seems to sanction actions that we would surely regard as abominable. Suppose a young man visits his elderly, bedridden father. When he sees that no one else is around, he uses a pillow to smother the old man in order to collect on his life insurance. Suppose also that the action is in the son's best interests; it will cause not the least bit of unpleasant feelings in him; and the crime will remain his own terrible secret. According to ethical egoism, this heinous act is morally right. The son did his duty.

An ethical egoist might object to this line by saying that *refraining* from committing evil acts is actually endorsed by ethical egoism—one's best interests are served by refraining. You should not murder or steal, for example, because it might encourage others to do the same to you, or it might undermine trust, security, or cooperation in society, which would not be in your best interests. For these reasons, you should obey the law or the rules of conventional morality (as the rule-egoist might do).

But following the rules is clearly not always in one's best interests. Sometimes committing a wicked act really does promote one's own welfare. In the case of the murdering son, no one will seek revenge for the secret murder, cooperation and trust in society will not be affected, and the mur-

derer will suffer no psychological torments. There seems to be no downside here—but the son's rewards for committing the deed will be great. Consistently looking out for one's own welfare sometimes requires rule violations and exceptions. In fact, some argue that the interests of ethical egoists may be best served when they urge everyone else to obey the rules while they themselves secretly break them.

If ethical egoism does conflict with our considered judgments, it is questionable at best. But it has been accused of another defect as well: it fails Criterion 2, consistency with our moral experiences.

One aspect of morality is so fundamental that we may plausibly view it as a basic fact of the moral life: moral impartiality, or treating equals equally. We know that in our dealings with the world, we are supposed to take into account the treatment of others as well as that of ourselves. The moral life is lived with the wider world in mind. We must give all persons their due and treat all equals equally, for in the moral sense we are all equals. Each person is presumed to have the same rights—and to have interests that are just as important—as everyone else, unless we have good reason for thinking otherwise. If one person is qualified for a job, and another person is equally qualified, we would be guilty of discrimination if we hired one and not the other based solely on race, sex, skin color, or ancestry. These factors are not morally relevant. People who do treat equals unequally in such ways are known as racists, sexists, bigots, and the like. Probably the most serious charge against ethical egoism is that it discriminates against people in the same fashion. It arbitrarily treats the interests of some people (oneself) as more important than the interests of all others (the rest of the world)—even though there is no morally relevant difference between the two.

The failure of ethical egoism to treat equals equally seems a serious defect in the theory. It conflicts with a major component of our moral

> ## QUICK REVIEW
>
> ***act-egoism***—The theory that to determine right action, you must apply the egoistic principle to individual acts.
>
> ***rule-egoism***—The theory that to determine right action, you must see if an act falls under a rule that if consistently followed would maximize your self-interest.
>
> ***psychological egoism***—The view that the motive for all our actions is self-interest.

existence. For many critics, this single defect is enough reason to reject the theory.

Recall that Criterion 3 is usefulness in moral problem solving. Some philosophers argue that ethical egoism fails this standard because the theory seems to lead to contradictory advice or conflicting actions. If real, this problem would constitute a significant failing of the theory. But these criticisms depend on controversial assumptions about ethical egoism or morality in general, so we will not dwell on them here. Our analysis of ethical egoism's problems using the first two criteria should be sufficient to raise serious doubts about the theory.

UTILITARIANISM

Are you a utilitarian? To find out, consider the following scenario: After years of research, a medical scientist—Dr. X—realizes that she is just one step away from developing a cure for all known forms of heart disease. Such a breakthrough would save hundreds of thousands of lives—perhaps millions. The world could finally be rid of heart attacks, strokes, heart failure, and the like, a feat as monumental as the eradication of deadly smallpox. That one last step in her research, however, is tech-

nologically feasible but morally problematic. It involves the killing of a single healthy human being to microscopically examine the person's heart tissue just seconds after the heart stops beating. The crucial piece of information needed to perfect the cure can be acquired only as just described; it cannot be extracted from the heart of a cadaver, an accident victim, someone suffering from a disease, or a person who has been dead for more than sixty seconds. Dr. X decides that the benefits to humanity from the cure are just too great to ignore. She locates a suitable candidate for the operation: a homeless man with no living relatives and no friends—someone who would not be missed. Through some elaborate subterfuge she manages to secretly do what needs to be done, killing the man and successfully performing the operation. She formulates the cure and saves countless lives. No one ever discovers how she obtained the last bit of information she needed to devise the cure, and she feels not the slightest guilt for her actions.

Did Dr. X do right? If you think so, then you may be a utilitarian. A utilitarian is more likely to believe that what Dr. X did was right, because it brought about consequences that were more good than bad. One man died, but countless others were saved. If you think that Dr. X did wrong, you may be a nonconsequentialist. A nonconsequentialist is likely to believe that Dr. X did wrong, because of the nature of her action: it was murder. The consequences are beside the point.

In this example, we get a hint of some of the elements that have made utilitarianism so attractive (and often controversial) to so many. First, whether or not we agree with the utilitarian view in this case, we can see that it has some plausibility. We tend to think it entirely natural to judge the morality of an action by the effects that it has on the people involved. To decide if we do right or wrong, we want to know whether the consequences of our actions are good or bad, whether they bring pleasure or pain, whether they enhance or diminish the welfare of ourselves and others. Second, the utilitarian formula for distinguishing right and wrong actions seems exceptionally straightforward. We simply calculate which action among several possible actions has the best balance of good over evil, everyone considered—and act accordingly. Moral choice is apparently reduced to a single moral principle and simple math. Third, at least sometimes, we all seem to be utilitarians. We may tell a white lie because the truth would hurt someone's feelings. We may break a promise because keeping it causes more harm than good. We may want a criminal punished not because he broke the law but because the punishment may deter him from future crimes. We justify such departures from conventional morality on the grounds that they produce better consequences.

Utilitarianism is one of the most influential moral theories in history. The English philosopher Jeremy Bentham (1748–1832) was the first to fill out the theory in detail, and the English philosopher and economist John Stuart Mill (1806–73) developed it further. In their hands utilitarianism became a powerful instrument of social reform. It provided a rationale for promoting women's rights, improving the treatment of prisoners, advocating animal rights, and aiding the poor—all radical ideas in Bentham's and Mill's day. In the twenty-first century, the theory still has a strong effect on moral and policy decision making in many areas, including health care, criminal justice, and government.

Classic utilitarianism—the kind of act-utilitarianism formulated by Bentham—is the simplest form of the theory. It affirms the principle that the right action is the one that directly produces the best balance of happiness over unhappiness for all concerned. Happiness is an intrinsic good—the *only* intrinsic good. What matters most is how much net happiness comes directly from performing an action (as opposed to following a

rule that applies to such actions). To determine the right action, we need only compute the amount of happiness that each possible action generates and choose the one that generates the most. There are no rules to take into account—just the single, simple utilitarian principle. Each set of circumstances calling for a moral choice is unique, requiring a new calculation of the varying consequences of possible actions.

Bentham called the utilitarian principle the **principle of utility** and asserted that all our actions can be judged by it. (Mill called it the **greatest happiness principle.**) As Bentham says,

> By the principle of utility is meant that principle which approves or disapproves of every action whatsoever, according to the tendency which it appears to have to augment or diminish the happiness of the party whose interest is in question: or, what is the same thing in other words, to promote or to oppose that happiness. . . .
>
> By utility is meant that property in any object, whereby it tends to produce benefit, advantage, pleasure, good, or happiness, (all this in the present case comes to the same thing) or (what comes again to the same thing) to prevent the happening of mischief, pain, evil, or unhappiness to the party whose interest is considered[.][2]

The principle of utility, of course, makes the theory consequentialist. The emphasis on happiness or pleasure makes it hedonistic, for happiness is the only intrinsic good.

As you can see, there is a world of difference between the moral focus of utilitarianism (in all its forms) and that of ethical egoism. The point of ethical egoism is to promote one's own good. An underlying tenet of utilitarianism is that you should promote the good of *everyone concerned* and that everyone *counts equally*. When deliberating

[2]Jeremy Bentham, "Of the Principle of Utility," in *An Introduction to the Principles of Morals and Legislation* (1789; reprint, Oxford: Clarendon Press, 1879), 1–7.

about which action to perform, you must take into account your own happiness as well as that of everyone else who will be affected by your decision—and no one is to be given privileged status. Such evenhandedness requires a large measure of impartiality, a quality that plays a role in every plausible moral theory. Mill says it best:

> [T]he happiness which forms the utilitarian standard of what is right in conduct, is not the agent's own happiness, but that of all concerned. As between his own happiness and that of others, utilitarianism requires him to be as strictly impartial as a disinterested and benevolent spectator.[3]

In classic act-utilitarianism, knowing how to tote up the amount of utility, or happiness, generated by various actions is essential. Bentham's answer to this requirement is the *hedonic calculus,* which quantifies happiness and handles the necessary calculations. His approach is straightforward in conception but complicated in the details: For each possible action in a particular situation, determine the total amount of happiness or unhappiness produced by it for one individual (that is, the *net* happiness—happiness minus unhappiness). Gauge the level of happiness with seven basic characteristics such as intensity, duration, and fecundity (how likely the pleasure or pain is to be followed by more pleasure or pain). Repeat this process for all individuals involved and sum their happiness or unhappiness to arrive at an overall net happiness for that particular action. Repeat for each possible action. The action with the best score (the most happiness or least unhappiness) is the morally right one.

Notice that in this arrangement, only the *total amount* of net happiness for each action matters. How the happiness is distributed among the persons involved does not figure into the calculations. This means that an action that affects ten

people and produces one hundred units of happiness is to be preferred over an action that affects those same ten people but generates only fifty units of happiness—even if most of the one hundred units go to just one individual, and the fifty units divide equally among the ten. The aggregate of happiness is decisive; its distribution is not. Classic utilitarianism, though, does ask that any given amount of happiness be spread among as many people as possible—thus the utilitarian slogan "The greatest happiness for the greatest number."

Both Bentham and Mill define happiness as pleasure. In Mill's words,

> The creed which accepts as the foundation of morals *utility,* or the *greatest happiness principle,* holds that actions are right in proportion as they tend to promote happiness, wrong as they tend to produce the reverse of happiness. By "happiness" is intended pleasure, and the absence of pain; by "unhappiness," pain, and the privation of pleasure.[4]

They differ, though, on the nature of happiness and how it should be measured. Bentham thinks that happiness varies only in quantity—different actions produce different amounts of happiness. To judge the intensity, duration, or fecundity of happiness is to calculate its quantity. Mill contends that happiness can vary in quantity *and* quality. There are lower pleasures, such as eating, drinking, and having sex, and there are higher pleasures, such as pursuing knowledge, appreciating beauty, and creating art. The higher pleasures are superior to the lower ones. The lower ones can be intense and enjoyable, but the higher ones are qualitatively better and more fulfilling. In this scheme, a person enjoying a mere taste of a higher pleasure may be closer to the moral ideal than a hedonistic glutton who gorges on lower pleasures. Thus Mill declared, "It is better to be a human being dissatisfied than a pig satisfied; better to be Socrates dissatisfied than a fool satisfied."[5] In Ben-

---

[3]John Stuart Mill, "What Utilitarianism Is," in *Utilitarianism,* 7th ed. (London: Longmans, Green, 1879), Chapter II.

[4]Mill, Chapter II.
[5]Mill, Chapter II.

tham's view, the glutton—who acquires a larger quantity of pleasure—would be closer to the ideal.

The problem for Mill is to justify his hierarchical ranking of the various pleasures. He tries to do so by appealing to what the majority prefers—that is, the majority of people who have experienced both the lower and higher pleasures. But this approach probably will not help, because people can differ drastically in how they rank pleasures. It is possible, for example, that a majority of people who have experienced a range of pleasures would actually disagree with Mill's rankings. In fact, any effort to devise such rankings using the principle of utility seems unlikely to succeed.

Many critics have argued that the idea of defining right action in terms of some intrinsic nonmoral good (whether pleasure, happiness, or anything else) is seriously problematic. Attempts to devise such a definition have been fraught with complications—a major one being that people have different ideas about what things are intrinsically valuable. Some utilitarians have tried to sidestep these difficulties by insisting that maximizing utility means maximizing people's *preferences,* whatever they are. This formulation seems to avoid some of the difficulties just mentioned but falls prey to another: some people's preferences may be clearly objectionable when judged by almost any moral standard, whether utilitarian or nonconsequentialist. Some people, after all, have ghastly preferences—preferences, say, for torturing children or killing innocent people for fun. Some critics say that repairing this preference utilitarianism to avoid sanctioning objectionable actions seems unlikely without introducing some nonutilitarian moral principles such as justice, rights, and obligations.

Like act-utilitarianism, rule-utilitarianism aims at the greatest good for all affected individuals, but it maintains that we travel an indirect route to that goal. In rule-utilitarianism, the morally right action is not the one that directly brings about the greatest good but the one covered by a rule that, if followed consistently, produces the great-

est good for all. In act-utilitarianism, we must examine each action to see how much good (or evil) it generates. Rule-utilitarianism would have us first determine what rule an action falls under, then see if that rule would likely maximize utility if everyone followed it. In effect, the rule-utilitarian asks, "What if everyone followed this rule?"

An act-utilitarian tries to judge the rightness of actions by the consequences they produce, occasionally relying on "rules of thumb" (such as "Usually we should not harm innocents") merely to save time. A rule-utilitarian, however, tries to follow every valid rule—even if doing so may not maximize utility in a specific situation.

In our example featuring Dr. X and the cure for heart disease, an act-utilitarian might compare the net happiness produced by performing the lethal operation and by not performing it, opting finally for the former because it maximizes happiness. A rule-utilitarian, on the other hand, would consider what moral rules seem to apply to the situation. One rule might be "It is permissible to conduct medical procedures or experiments on people without their full knowledge and consent in order to substantially advance medical science." Another one might say "Do not conduct medical procedures or experiments on people without their full knowledge and consent." If the first rule is generally followed, happiness is not likely to be maximized in the long run. Widespread adherence to this rule would encourage medical scientists and physicians to murder patients for the good of science. Such practices would outrage people and cause them to fear and distrust science and the medical profession, leading to the breakdown of the entire health care system and most medical research. But if the second rule is consistently adhered to, happiness is likely to be maximized over the long haul. Trust in physicians and medical scientists would be maintained, and promising research could continue as long as it was conducted with the patient's consent. The right action, then, is for Dr. X *not* to perform the gruesome operation.

Applying the Theory

Let us apply utilitarianism to another type of case. Imagine that for more than a year a terrorist has been carrying out devastating attacks in a developing country, killing hundreds of innocent men, women, and children. He seems unstoppable. He always manages to elude capture. In fact, because of his stealth, the expert assistance of a few accomplices, and his support among the general population, he will most likely never be captured or killed. The authorities have no idea where he hides or where he will strike next. But they are sure that he will go on killing indefinitely. They have tried every tactic they know to put an end to the slaughter, but it goes on and on. Finally, as a last resort, the chief of the nation's antiterrorist police orders the arrest of the terrorist's family—a wife and seven children. The chief intends to kill the wife and three of the children right away (to show that he is serious), then threaten to kill the remaining four unless the terrorist turns himself in. There is no doubt that the chief will make good on his intentions, and there is excellent reason to believe that the terrorist will indeed turn himself in rather than allow his remaining children to be executed.

Suppose that the chief has only two options: (1) refrain from murdering the terrorist's family and continue with the usual antiterrorist tactics (which have only a tiny chance of being successful); or (2) kill the wife and three of the children

---

Peter Singer, Utilitarian

The distinguished philosopher Peter Singer is arguably the most famous (and controversial) utilitarian of recent years. Many newspaper and magazine articles have been written about him, and many people have declared their agreement with, or vociferous opposition to, his views. This is how one magazine characterizes Singer and his ideas:

> *The New Yorker* calls him "the most influential living philosopher." His critics call him "the most dangerous man in the world." Peter Singer, the De Camp Professor of Bioethics at Princeton University's Center for Human Values, is most widely and controversially known for his view that animals have the same moral status as humans. . . .
>
> Singer is perhaps the most thoroughgoing philosophical utilitarian since Jeremy Bentham. As such, he believes animals have rights because the relevant moral consideration is not whether a being can reason or talk but whether it can suffer. Jettisoning the traditional distinction between humans and nonhumans, Singer distinguishes instead between persons and non-persons. Persons are beings that feel, reason, have self-awareness, and look forward to a future. Thus, fetuses and some very impaired human beings are not persons in his view and have a lesser moral status than, say, adult gorillas and chimpanzees.
>
> Given such views, it was no surprise that anti-abortion activists and disability rights advocates loudly decried the Australian-born Singer's appointment at Princeton last year. Indeed, his language regarding the treatment of disabled human beings is at times appallingly similar to the eugenic arguments used by Nazi theorists concerning "life unworthy of life." Singer, however, believes that only parents, not the state, should have the power to make decisions about the fates of disabled infants.[*]

*Ronald Bailey, excerpts from "The Pursuit of Happiness, Peter Singer Interviewed by Ronald Bailey." *Reason Magazine*, December 2000. Reprinted with permission from Reason Magazine and Reason.com.

and threaten to kill the rest (a strategy with a very high chance of success). According to utilitarianism, which action is right?

As an act-utilitarian, the chief might reason like this: Action 2 would probably result in a net gain of happiness, everyone considered. Forcing the terrorist to turn himself in would save hundreds of lives. His killing spree would be over. The general level of fear and apprehension in the country might subside, and even the economy—which has slowed because of terrorism—might improve. The prestige of the terrorism chief and his agents might increase. On the downside, performing Action 2 would guarantee that four innocent people (and perhaps eight) would lose their lives, and the terrorist (whose welfare must also be included in the calculations) would be imprisoned for life or executed. In addition, many citizens would be disturbed by the killing of innocent people and the flouting of the law by the police, believing that these actions are wrong and likely to set a dangerous precedent. Over time, though, these misgivings may diminish. All things considered, then, Action 2 would probably produce more happiness than unhappiness. Action 1, on the other hand, maintains the status quo. It would allow the terrorist to continue murdering innocent people and spreading fear throughout the land—a decidedly unhappy result. It clearly would produce more unhappiness than happiness. Action 2, therefore, would produce the most happiness and would therefore be the morally right option.

As a rule-utilitarian, the chief might make a different choice. He would have to decide what rules would apply to the situation then determine which one, if consistently followed, would yield the most utility. Suppose he must decide between Rule 1 and Rule 2. Rule 1 says, "Do not kill innocent people in order to prevent terrorists from killing other innocent people." Rule 2 says, "Killing innocent people is permissible if it helps to stop terrorist attacks." The chief might deliberate as follows: We can be confident that consis-

tently following Rule 2 would have some dire consequences for society. Innocent people would be subject to arbitrary execution, civil rights would be regularly violated, the rule of law would be severely compromised, and trust in government would be degraded. In fact, adhering to Rule 2 might make people more fearful and less secure than terrorist attacks would; it would undermine the very foundations of a free society. In a particular case, killing innocent people to fight terror could possibly have more utility than not killing them. But whether such a strategy would be advantageous to society over the long haul is not at all certain. Consistently following Rule 1 would have none of these unfortunate consequences. If so, a society living according to Rule 1 would be better off than one adhering to Rule 2, and therefore the innocent should not be killed to stop the terrorist.

Evaluating the Theory

Bentham and Mill do not offer ironclad arguments demonstrating that utilitarianism is the best moral theory. Mill, however, does try to show that the principle of utility is at least a plausible basis for the theory. After all, he says, humans by nature desire happiness and nothing but happiness. If so, happiness is the standard by which we should judge human conduct, and therefore the principle of utility is the heart of morality. But this kind of moral argument is controversial, because it reasons from what *is* to what *should be*. In addition, as pointed out in the discussion of psychological egoism, the notion that happiness is our sole motivation is dubious.

What can we learn about utilitarianism by applying the moral criteria of adequacy? Let us begin with classic act-utilitarianism and deal with rule-utilitarianism later. We can also postpone discussion of the minimum requirement of coherence, because critics have been more inclined to charge rule-utilitarianism than act-utilitarianism with having significant internal inconsistencies.

If we begin with Criterion 1 (consistency with considered judgments), we run into what some have called act-utilitarianism's most serious problem: It conflicts with commonsense views about justice. Justice requires equal treatment of persons. It demands, for example, that goods such as happiness be distributed fairly, that we not harm one person to make several other persons happy. Utilitarianism says that everyone should be included in utility calculations, but it does not require that everyone get an equal share. Consider this famous scenario from the philosopher H. J. McCloskey:

> While a utilitarian is visiting an area plagued by racial tension, a black man rapes a white woman. Race riots ensue, and white mobs roam the streets, beating and lynching black people as the police secretly condone the violence and do nothing to stop it. The utilitarian realizes that by giving false testimony, he could bring about the quick arrest and conviction of a black man whom he picks at random. As a result of this lie, the riots and the lynchings would stop, and innocent lives would be spared. As a utilitarian, he believes he has a duty to bear false witness to punish an innocent person.

If right actions are those that maximize happiness, then it seems that the utilitarian would be doing right by framing the innocent person. The innocent person, of course, would experience unhappiness (he might be sent to prison or even executed), but framing him would halt the riots and prevent many other innocent people from being killed, resulting in a net gain in overall happiness. Framing the innocent is unjust, though, and our considered moral judgments would be at odds with such an action. Here the commonsense idea of justice and the principle of utility collide. The conflict raises doubts about act-utilitarianism as a moral theory.

Here is another famous example:

> This time you are to imagine yourself to be a surgeon, a truly great surgeon. Among other things you do, you transplant organs, and you are such a great surgeon that the organs you transplant always take. At the moment you have five patients who need organs. Two need one lung each, two need a kidney each, and the fifth needs a heart. If they do not get those organs today, they will all die; if you find organs for them today, you can transplant the organs and they will all live. But where to find the lungs, the kidneys, and the heart? The time is almost up when a report is brought to you that a young man who has just come into your clinic for his yearly check-up has exactly the right blood type, and is in excellent health. Lo, you have a possible donor. All you need do is cut him up and distribute his parts among the five who need them. You ask, but he says, "Sorry. I deeply sympathize, but no." Would it be morally permissible for you to operate anyway?[6]

This scenario involves the possible killing of an innocent person for the good of others. There seems little doubt that carrying out the murder and transplanting the victim's organs into five other people (and thus saving their lives) would maximize utility (assuming, of course, that the

[6]Judith Jarvis Thomson, "The Trolley Problem," in *Rights, Restitution, and Risk: Essays in Moral Theory*, ed. William Parent (Cambridge, MA: Harvard University Press, 1986), 95.

surgeon's deed would not become public, he or she suffered no untoward psychological effects, etc.). Compared with the happiness produced by doing the transplants, the unhappiness of the one unlucky donor seems minor. Therefore, according to act-utilitarianism, you (the surgeon) should commit the murder and do the transplants. But this choice appears to conflict with our considered moral judgments. Killing the healthy young man to benefit the five unhealthy ones seems unjust.

Look at one final case. Suppose a tsunami devastates a coastal area of Singapore. Relief agencies arrive on the scene to distribute food, shelter, and medical care to 100 tsunami victims—disaster aid that amounts to, say, 1,000 units of happiness. There are only two options for the distribution of the 1,000 units. Option A is to divide the 1,000 units equally among all 100 victims, supplying 10 units to each person. Option B is to give 901 units to one victim (who happens to be the richest man in the area) and 99 units to the remaining victims, providing 1 unit per person. Both options distribute the same amount of happiness to the victims—1,000 units. Following the dictates of act-utilitarianism, we would have to say that the two actions (options) have equal utility and so are equally right. But this seems wrong. It seems unjust to distribute the units of happiness so unevenly when all recipients are equals in all morally relevant respects. Like the other examples, this one suggests that act-utilitarianism may be an inadequate theory.

Detractors also make parallel arguments against the theory in many cases besides those involving injustice. A familiar charge is that act-utilitarianism conflicts with our commonsense judgments both about people's rights and about their obligations to one another. Consider first this scenario about rights: Mr. Y is a nurse in a care facility for the elderly. He tends to many bedridden patients who are in pain most of the time, are financial and emotional burdens to their families, and are not expected to live more than a few weeks. Despite

their misery, they do not wish for death; they want only to be free of pain. Mr. Y, an act-utilitarian, sees that there would be a lot more happiness in the world and less pain if these patients died sooner rather than later. He decides to take matters into his own hands, so he secretly gives them a drug that kills them quietly and painlessly. Their families and the facility staff feel enormous relief. No one will ever know what Mr. Y has done, and no one suspects foul play. He feels no guilt—only immense satisfaction knowing that he has helped make the world a better place.

If Mr. Y does indeed maximize happiness in this situation, then his action is right, according to act-utilitarianism. Yet most people would probably say that he violated the rights of his patients. The commonsense view is that people have certain rights that should not be violated merely to create a better balance of happiness over unhappiness.

Another typical criticism of act-utilitarianism is that it appears to fly in the face of our considered judgments about our obligations to other people. Suppose Ms. Z must decide between two actions: Action A will produce 1,001 units of happiness; Action B, 1,000 units. The only other significant difference between them is that Action A entails the breaking of a promise. By act-utilitarian lights, Ms. Z should choose Action A because it yields more happiness than Action B does. But we tend to think that keeping a promise is more important than a tiny gain in happiness. We often try to keep our promises even when we know that doing so will result in a decrease in utility. Some say that if our obligations to others sometimes outweigh considerations of overall happiness, then act-utilitarianism must be problematic.[7]

What can an act-utilitarian say to rebut these charges about justice, rights, and obligations? One frequent response goes like this: The scenarios put

---

[7]This case is based on one devised by W. D. Ross in *The Right and the Good* (Oxford: Clarendon Press, 1930), 34–35.

forth by critics (such as the cases just cited) are misleading and implausible. They are always set up so that actions regarded as immoral produce the greatest happiness, leading to the conclusion that utilitarianism conflicts with commonsense morality and therefore cannot be an adequate moral theory. But in real life these kinds of actions almost never maximize happiness. In the case of Dr. X, her crime would almost certainly be discovered by physicians or other scientists, and she would be exposed as a murderer. This revelation would surely destroy her career, undermine patient-physician trust, tarnish the reputation of the scientific community, dry up funding for legitimate research, and prompt countless lawsuits. Scientists might even refuse to use the data from Dr. X's research because she obtained them through a heinous act. As one philosopher put it, "Given a clearheaded view of the world as it is and a realistic understanding of man's nature, it becomes more and more evident that injustice will never have, in the long run, greater utility than justice. . . . Thus injustice becomes, in actual practice, a source of great social disutility."[8]

The usual response to this defense is that the act-utilitarian is probably correct that most violations of commonsense morality do not maximize happiness—but at least some violations do. At least sometimes actions that have the best consequences do conflict with our credible moral principles or considered moral judgments. The charge is that the act-utilitarian cannot plausibly dismiss all counterexamples, and only one counterexample is required to show that maximizing utility is not a necessary and sufficient condition for right action.[9]

[8]Paul W. Taylor, *Principles of Ethics: An Introduction* (Encino, CA: Dickenson, 1975), 77–78.
[9]The points in this and the preceding paragraph were inspired by James Rachels, *The Elements of Moral Philosophy*, 4th ed. (Boston: McGraw-Hill, 2003), 111–12.

Unlike ethical egoism, act-utilitarianism (as well as rule-utilitarianism) does not fail Criterion 2 (consistency with our moral experiences), so we can move on to Criterion 3 (usefulness in moral problem solving). On this score, some scholars argue that act-utilitarianism deserves bad marks. Probably their most common complaint is what has been called the *no-rest problem*. Utilitarianism (in all its forms) requires that in our actions we *always* try to maximize utility, everyone considered. Say you are watching television. Utilitarianism would have you ask yourself, "Is this the best way to maximize happiness for everyone?" Probably not. You could be giving to charity or working as a volunteer for the local hospital or giving your coat to a homeless person or selling everything you own to buy food for hungry children. Whatever you are doing, there usually is something else you could do that would better maximize net happiness for everyone.

If act-utilitarianism does demand too much of us, then its usefulness as a guide to the moral life is suspect. One possible reply to this criticism is that the utilitarian burden can be lightened by devising rules that place limits on supererogatory actions. Another reply is that our moral common sense is simply wrong on this issue—we *should* be willing to perform, as our duty, many actions that are usually considered supererogatory. If necessary, we should be willing to give up our personal ambitions for the good of everyone. We should be willing, for example, to sacrifice a very large portion of our resources to help the poor.

To some, this reply seems questionable precisely because it challenges our commonsense moral intuitions—the very intuitions that we use to measure the plausibility of our moral judgments and principles. Moral common sense, they say, can be mistaken, and our intuitions can be tenuous or distorted—but we should cast them aside only for good reasons.

But a few utilitarians directly reject this appeal to common sense, declaring that relying so heavily on such intuitions is a mistake:

Admittedly utilitarianism does have consequences which are incompatible with the common moral consciousness, but I tended to take the view "so much the worse for the common moral consciousness." That is, I was inclined to reject the common methodology of testing general ethical principles by seeing how they square with our feelings in particular instances.[10]

These utilitarians would ask, Isn't it possible that in dire circumstances, saving a hundred innocent lives by allowing one to die would be the best thing to do even though allowing that one death would be a tragedy? Aren't there times when the norms of justice and duty *should* be ignored for the greater good of society?

To avoid the problems that act-utilitarianism is alleged to have, some utilitarians have turned to rule-utilitarianism. By positing rules that should be consistently followed, rule-utilitarianism seems to align its moral judgments closer to those of common sense. And the theory itself is based on ideas about morality that seem perfectly sensible:

> In general, rule utilitarianism seems to involve two rather plausible intuitions. In the first place, rule utilitarians want to emphasize that moral rules are important. Individual acts are justified by being shown to be in accordance with correct moral rules. In the second place, utility is important. Moral rules are shown to be correct by being shown to lead, somehow, to the maximization of utility. . . . Rule utilitarianism, in its various forms, tries to combine these intuitions into a single, coherent criterion of morality.[11]

But some philosophers have accused the theory of being internally inconsistent. They say, in other words, that it fails the minimum requirement of coherence. (If so, we can forgo discussion of our three criteria of adequacy.) They argue as follows: Rule-utilitarianism says that actions are right if they conform to rules devised to maximize utility. Rules with exceptions or qualifications, however, maximize utility better than rules without them. For example, a rule like "Do not steal except in these circumstances" maximizes utility better than the rule "Do not steal." It seems, then, that the best rules are those with amendments that make them as specific as possible to particular cases. But if the rules are changed in this way to maximize utility, they would end up mandating the same actions that act-utilitarianism does. They all would say, in effect, "do not do this except to maximize utility." Rule-utilitarianism would lapse into act-utilitarianism.

Some rule-utilitarians respond to this criticism by denying that rules with a lot of exceptions would maximize utility. They say that people might fear that their own well-being would be threatened when others make multiple exceptions to rules. You might be reassured by a rule such as "Do not harm others" but feel uneasy about the rule "Do not harm others except in this situation." What if you end up in that particular situation?

Those who criticize the theory admit that it is indeed possible for an exception-laden rule to produce more unhappiness than happiness because of the anxiety it causes. But, they say, it is also possible for such a rule to generate a very large measure of happiness—large enough to more than offset any ill effects spawned by rule exceptions. If so, then rule-utilitarianism could easily slip into act-utilitarianism, thus exhibiting all the conflicts with commonsense morality that act-utilitarianism is supposed to have.

LEARNING FROM UTILITARIANISM

Regardless of how much credence we give to the arguments for and against utilitarianism, we must admit that the theory seems to embody a large part of the truth about morality. First, utilitarianism

---

[10]J. J. C. Smart, *Utilitarianism: For and Against* (Cambridge: Cambridge University Press, 1973), 68.

[11]Fred Feldman, *Introductory Ethics* (Englewood Cliffs, NJ: Prentice-Hall, 1978), 77–78.

CRITICAL THOUGHT: Cross-Species Transplants: What Would a Utilitarian Do?

Like any adequate moral theory, utilitarianism should be able to help us resolve moral problems, including new moral issues arising from advances in science and medicine. A striking example of one such issue is cross-species transplantation, the transplanting of organs from one species to another, usually from nonhuman animals to humans. Scientists are already bioengineering pigs so their organs will not provoke tissue rejection in human recipients. Pigs are thought to be promising organ donors because of the similarities between pig and human organs. Many people are in favor of such research because it could open up new sources of transplantable organs, which are now in short supply and desperately needed by thousands of people whose organs are failing.

Would an act-utilitarian be likely to condone cross-species transplants of organs? If so, on what grounds? Would the unprecedented, "unnatural" character of these operations bother a utilitarian? Why or why not? Would you expect an act-utilitarian to approve of cross-species organ transplants if they involved the killing of one hundred pigs for every successful transplant? If only a very limited number of transplants could be done successfully each year, how do you think an act-utilitarian would decide who gets the operations? Would she choose randomly? Would she ever be justified (by utilitarian considerations) in, say, deciding to save a rich philanthropist while letting a poor person die for lack of a transplant?

begs us to consider that the consequences of our actions do indeed make a difference in our moral deliberations. Whatever factors work to make an action right (or wrong), surely the consequences of what we do must somehow be among them. Even if lying is morally wrong primarily because of the kind of act it is, we cannot plausibly think that a lie that saves a thousand lives is morally equivalent to one that changes nothing. Sometimes our considered moral judgments may tell us that an action is right regardless of the good (or evil) it does. And sometimes they may say that the good it does matters a great deal.

Second, utilitarianism—perhaps more than any other moral theory—incorporates the principle of impartiality, a fundamental pillar of morality itself. Everyone concerned counts equally in every moral decision. As Mill says, when we judge the rightness of our actions, utilitarianism requires us to be "as strictly impartial as a disinterested and benevolent spectator." Discrimination is forbidden, and equality reigns. We would expect no less from a plausible moral theory.

Third, utilitarianism is through and through a moral theory for promoting human welfare. At its core is the moral principle of beneficence—the obligation to act for the well-being of others. Beneficence is not the whole of morality, but to most people it is at least close to its heart.

SUMMARY

Ethical egoism is the theory that the right action is the one that advances one's own best interests. It promotes self-interested behavior but not necessarily selfish acts. The ethical egoist may define his self-interest in various ways—as pleasure, self-actualization, power, happiness, or other goods. The most important argument for ethical egoism relies on the theory known as psychological egoism, the view that the motive for all our actions is self-interest. Psychological egoism, however, seems to ignore the fact that people sometimes do things that are not in their best interests. It also seems to misconstrue the relationship between our actions and the satisfaction that often follows from them. We seem to desire something other than satisfaction and then experience satisfaction as a result of getting what we desire.

Utilitarianism is the view that the morally right action is the one that produces the most favorable balance of good over evil, everyone considered. Act-utilitarianism says that right actions are those that directly produce the greatest overall happiness, everyone considered. Rule-utilitarianism says that the morally right action is the one covered by a rule that if generally followed would produce the most favorable balance of good over evil, everyone considered.

Critics argue that act-utilitarianism is not consistent with our considered judgments about justice. In many possible scenarios, the action that maximizes utility in a situation also seems blatantly unjust. Likewise, the theory seems to collide with our notions of rights and obligations. Again, it seems relatively easy to imagine scenarios in which utility is maximized while rights or obligations are shortchanged. An act-utilitarian might respond to these points by saying that such examples are unrealistic—that in real life, actions thought to be immoral almost never maximize happiness.

Rule-utilitarianism has been accused of being internally inconsistent—of easily collapsing into act-utilitarianism. The charge is that the rules that maximize happiness best are specific to particular cases, but such rules would sanction the same actions that act-utilitarianism does.

Regardless of criticisms lodged against it, utilitarianism offers important insights about the nature of morality: The consequences of our actions surely do matter in our moral deliberations and in our lives. The principle of impartiality is an essential part of moral decision making. And any plausible moral theory must somehow take into account the principle of beneficence.

EXERCISES

Review Questions

1. What is ethical egoism? What is the difference between act- and rule-egoism? (p. 78)
2. What is psychological egoism? (p. 80)
3. What is the psychological egoist argument for ethical egoism? (p. 81)
4. Is psychological egoism true? Why or why not? (pp. 81–82)
5. In what way is ethical egoism not consistent with our considered moral judgments? (p. 83)
6. What is the principle of utility? (p. 85)
7. What is the main difference between the ways that Mill and Bentham conceive of happiness? Which view seems more plausible? (pp. 86–87)
8. What is the difference between act- and rule-utilitarianism? (p. 87)
9. How do act- and rule-utilitarians differ in their views on rules? (p. 87)
10. Is act-utilitarianism consistent with our considered moral judgments regarding justice? Why or why not? (pp. 90–91)

Discussion Questions

1. Is psychological egoism based on a conceptual confusion? Why or why not?
2. Why do critics regard ethical egoism as an inadequate moral theory? Are the critics right? Why or why not?
3. How would your life change if you became a consistent act-utilitarian?
4. How would your life change if you became a consistent rule-utilitarian?
5. To what was Mill referring when he said, "It is better to be a human being dissatisfied than a pig satisfied"? Do you agree with this statement? Why or why not?
6. If you were on trial for your life (because of an alleged murder), would you want the judge to be an act-utilitarian, a rule-utilitarian, or neither? Why?

7. If you were the surgeon in the example about the five transplants, what would you do? Why?

8. Does act-utilitarianism conflict with commonsense judgments about rights? Why or why not?

9. Is there such a thing as a supererogatory act—or are all right actions simply our duty? What

would an act-utilitarian say about supererogatory acts?

10. Suppose you had to decide which one of a dozen dying patients should receive a lifesaving drug, knowing that there was only enough of the medicine for one person. Would you feel comfortable making the decision as an act-utilitarian would? Why or why not?

READING

From *Utilitarianism*

JOHN STUART MILL

**CHAPTER II.
WHAT UTILITARIANISM IS**

* * *

The creed which accepts, as the foundation of morals, Utility, or the Greatest Happiness Principle, holds that actions are right in proportion as they tend to promote happiness, wrong as they tend to produce the reverse of happiness. By happiness is intended pleasure, and the absence of pain; by unhappiness, pain, and the privation of pleasure. To give a clear view of the moral standard set up by the theory, much more requires to be said; in particular, what things it includes in the ideas of pain and pleasure; and to what extent this is left an open question. But these supplementary explanations do not affect the theory of life on which this theory of morality is grounded—namely, that pleasure, and freedom from pain, are the only things desirable as ends; and that all desirable things (which are as numerous in the utilitarian as in any other scheme) are desirable either for the pleasure inherent in themselves, or as means to the promotion of pleasure and the prevention of pain.

Now, such a theory of life excites in many minds, and among them in some of the most estimable in feeling and purpose, inveterate dislike. To suppose that life has (as they express it) no higher end than pleasure—no better and nobler object of desire and pursuit—they designate as utterly mean and grovelling; as a doctrine worthy only of swine, to whom the followers of Epicurus were, at a very early period, contemptuously likened; and modern holders of the doctrine are occasionally made the subject of equally polite comparisons by its German, French, and English assailants.

When thus attacked, the Epicureans have always answered, that it is not they, but their accusers, who represent human nature in a degrading light; since the accusation supposes human beings to be capable of no pleasures except those of which swine are capable. If this supposition were true, the charge could not be gainsaid, but would then be no longer an imputation; for if the sources of pleasure were precisely the same to human beings and to swine, the rule of life which is good enough for the one would be good enough for the other. The comparison of the Epicurean life to that of beasts is felt as degrading, precisely because a beast's pleasures do not satisfy a human being's conceptions of happiness. Human beings have faculties more elevated than the animal

John Stuart Mill, *Utilitarianism*, Chapter II (edited).

appetites, and when once made conscious of them, do not regard anything as happiness which does not include their gratification. I do not, indeed, consider the Epicureans to have been by any means faultless in drawing out their scheme of consequences from the utilitarian principle. To do this in any sufficient manner, many Stoic, as well as Christian elements require to be included. But there is no known Epicurean theory of life which does not assign to the pleasures of the intellect, of the feelings and imagination, and of the moral sentiments, a much higher value as pleasures than to those of mere sensation. It must be admitted, however, that utilitarian writers in general have placed the superiority of mental over bodily pleasures chiefly in the greater permanency, safety, uncostliness, &c., of the former—that is, in their circumstantial advantages rather than in their intrinsic nature. And on all these points utilitarians have fully proved their case; but they might have taken the other, and, as it may be called, higher ground, with entire consistency. It is quite compatible with the principle of utility to recognise the fact, that some *kinds* of pleasure are more desirable and more valuable than others. It would be absurd that while, in estimating all other things, quality is considered as well as quantity, the estimation of pleasures should be supposed to depend on quantity alone.

If I am asked, what I mean by difference of quality in pleasures, or what makes one pleasure more valuable than another, merely as a pleasure, except its being greater in amount, there is but one possible answer. Of two pleasures, if there be one to which all or almost all who have experience of both give a decided preference, irrespective of any feeling of moral obligation to prefer it, that is the more desirable pleasure. If one of the two is, by those who are competently acquainted with both, placed so far above the other that they prefer it, even though knowing it to be attended with a greater amount of discontent, and would not resign it for any quantity of the other pleasure which their nature is capable of, we are justified in ascribing to the preferred enjoyment a superiority in quality, so far outweighing quantity as to render it, in comparison, of small account.

Now it is an unquestionable fact that those who are equally acquainted with, and equally capable of appreciating and enjoying, both, do give a most marked preference to the manner of existence which employs their higher faculties. Few human creatures would consent to be changed into any of the lower animals, for a promise of the fullest allowance of a beast's pleasures; no intelligent human being would consent to be a fool, no instructed person would be an ignoramus, no person of feeling and conscience would be selfish and base, even though they should be persuaded that the fool, the dunce, or the rascal is better satisfied with his lot than they are with theirs. They would not resign what they possess more than he, for the most complete satisfaction of all the desires which they have in common with him. If they ever fancy they would, it is only in cases of unhappiness so extreme, that to escape from it they would exchange their lot for almost any other, however, undesirable in their own eyes. A being of higher faculties requires more to make him happy, is capable probably of more acute suffering, and is certainly accessible to it at more points, than one of an inferior type; but in spite of these liabilities, he can never really wish to sink into what he feels to be a lower grade of existence. We may give what explanation we please of this unwillingness; we may attribute it to pride, a name which is given indiscriminately to some of the most and to some of the least estimable feelings of which mankind are capable; we may refer it to the love of liberty and personal independence, an appeal to which was with the Stoics one of the most effective means for the inculcation of it; to the love of power, or the love of excitement, both of which do really enter into and contribute to it: but its most appropriate appellation is a sense of dignity, which all human beings possess in one form or other, and in some, though by no means in exact, proportion to their higher faculties, and which is so essential a part of the happiness of those in whom it is strong, that nothing which conflicts with it could be, otherwise than momentarily, an object of desire to them. Whoever supposes that this preference takes place at a sacrifice of happiness—that the superior being, in anything like equal circumstances, is not happier than the inferior—confounds the two very different ideas, of happiness, and content. It is indisputable that the being whose capacities of enjoyment are low, has the greatest chance of having them fully satisfied; and a highly-endowed being will always feel that any happiness which he can look for, as the world is constitute, is imperfect. But he can learn to bear its imperfections, if they are at all bearable; and they will not make him envy the being who is indeed unconscious of the imperfections, but only because he feels not at all the good which those imperfections qualify. It is better to be a human being dissatisfied than a pig satisfied; better to be Socrates dissatisfied than a fool satisfied. And if the fool, or the pig, is of a different opinion, it is because they only know their own side of the question. The other party to the comparison knows both sides.

It may be objected, that many who are capable of the higher pleasures, occasionally, under the influence of temptation, postpone them to the lower. But this is quite compatible with a full appreciation of the intrinsic superiority of the higher. Men often, from infirmity of character, make their election for the nearer good, though they know it to be the less valuable; and this no less when the choice is between two bodily pleasures, than when it is between bodily and mental. They pursue sensual indulgences to the injury of health, though perfectly aware that health is the greater good. It may be further objected, that many who begin with youthful enthusiasm for everything noble, as they advance in years sink into indolence and selfishness. But I do not believe that those who undergo this very common change, voluntarily choose the lower description of pleasures in preference to the higher. I believe that before they devote themselves exclusively to the one, they have already become incapable of the other. Capacity for the nobler feelings is in most natures a very tender plant, easily killed, not only by hostile influences, but by mere want of sustenance; and in the majority of young persons it speedily dies away if the occupations to which their position in life has devoted them, and the society into which it has thrown them,

are not favourable to keeping that higher capacity in exercise. Men lose their high aspirations as they lose their intellectual tastes, because they have not time or opportunity for indulging them; and they addict themselves to inferior pleasures, not because they deliberately prefer them, but because they are either the only ones to which they have access, or the only ones which they are any longer capable of enjoying. It may be questioned whether any one who has remained equally susceptible to both classes of pleasures, ever knowingly and calmly preferred the lower; though many, in all ages, have broken down in an ineffectual attempt to combine both.

From this verdict of the only competent judges, I apprehend there can be no appeal. On a question which is the best worth having of two pleasures, or which of two modes of existence is the most grateful to the feelings, apart from its moral attributes and from its consequences, the judgment of those who are qualified by knowledge of both, or, if they differ, that of the majority among them, must be admitted as final. And there needs be the less hesitation to accept this judgment respecting the quality of pleasures, since there is no other tribunal to be referred to even on the question of quantity. What means are there of determining which is the acutest of two pains, or the intensest of two pleasurable sensations, except the general suffrage of those who are familiar with both? Neither pains nor pleasures are homogeneous, and pain is always heterogeneous with pleasure. What is there to decide whether a particular pleasure is worth purchasing at the cost of a particular pain, except the feelings and judgment of the experienced? When, therefore, those feelings and judgment declare the pleasures derived from the higher faculties to be preferable *in kind,* apart from the question of intensity, to those of which the animal nature, disjoined from the higher faculties, is susceptible, they are entitled on this subject to the same regard.

I have dwelt on this point, as being a necessary part of a perfectly just conception of Utility or Happiness, considered as the directive rule of human conduct. But it is by no means an indispensable condition to the acceptance of the utilitarian standard; for that standard is not the agent's own greatest happiness, but the greatest amount of happiness altogether; and if it may possibly be doubted whether a noble character is always the happier for its nobleness, there can be no doubt that it makes other people happier, and that the world in general is immensely a gainer by it. Utilitarianism, therefore, could only attain its end by the general cultivation of nobleness of character, even if each individual were only benefited by the nobleness of others, and his own, so far as happiness is concerned, were a sheer deduction from the benefit. But the bare enunciation of such an absurdity as this last, renders refutation superfluous.

According to the Greatest Happiness Principle, as above explained, the ultimate end, with reference to and for the sake of which all other things are desirable (whether we are considering our own good or that of other people), is an existence exempt as far as possible from pain, and as rich as possible in enjoyments, both in point of quantity and quality; the test of quality, and the rule for measuring it against quantity, being the preference felt by those who, in their opportunities of experience, to which must be added their habits of self-consciousness and self-observation, are best furnished with the means of comparison. This being, according to the utilitarian opinion, the end of human action, is necessarily also the standard of morality; which may accordingly be defined, the rules and precepts for human conduct, by the observance of which an existence such as has been described might be, to the greatest extent possible, secured to all mankind; and not to them only, but, so far as the nature of things admits, to the whole sentient creation.

* * *

I must again repeat, what the assailants of utilitarianism seldom have the justice to acknowledge, that the happiness which forms the utilitarian standard of what is right in conduct, is not the agent's own happiness, but that of all concerned. As between his own happiness and that of others, utilitarianism requires him to be as strictly impartial as a disinterested and benevolent spectator. In the golden rule of Jesus of Nazareth, we read the complete spirit of the ethics of utility. To do as one would be done by, and to love one's neighbour as oneself, constitute the ideal perfection of utilitarian morality. As the means of making the nearest approach to this ideal, utility would enjoin, first, that laws and social arrangements should place the happiness, or (as speaking practically it may be called) the interest, of every individual, as nearly as possible in harmony with the interest of the whole; and secondly, that education and opinion, which have so vast a power over human character, should so use that power as to establish in the mind of every individual an indissoluble association between his own happiness and the good of the whole; especially between his own happiness and the practice of such modes of conduct, negative and positive, as regard for the universal happiness prescribes: so that not only he may be unable to conceive the possibility of happiness to himself, consistently with conduct opposed to the general good, but also that a direct impulse to promote the general good may be in every individual one of the habitual motives of action, and the sentiments connected therewith may fill a large and prominent place in every human being's sentient existence. If the impugners of the utilitarian morality represented it to their own minds in this its true character, I know not what recommendation possessed by any other morality they could possibly affirm to be wanting to it: what more beautiful or more exalted developments of human nature any other ethical system can be supposed to foster, or what springs of action, not accessible to the utilitarian, such systems rely on for giving effect to their mandates.

* * *

It may not be superfluous to notice a few more of the common misapprehensions of utilitarian ethics, even those which are so obvious and gross that it might appear impossible for any person of candour and intelligence to fall into them: since persons, even of considerable mental endowments, often give themselves so little trouble to understand the bearings of any opinion against which they entertain a prejudice, and men are in general so little conscious of this voluntary ignorance as a defect, that the vulgarest misunderstandings of ethical doctrines are continually met with in the deliberate writings of persons of the greatest pretensions both to high principle and to philosophy. We not uncommonly hear the doctrine of utility inveighed against as a *godless* doctrine. If it be necessary to say anything at all against so mere an assumption, we may say that the question depends upon what idea we have formed of the moral character of the Deity. If it be a true belief that God desires, above all things, the happiness of his creatures, and that this was his purpose in their creation, utility is not only not a godless doctrine, but more profoundly religious than any other. If it be meant that utilitarianism does not recognise the revealed will of God as the supreme law of morals, I answer, that an utilitarian who believes in the perfect goodness and wisdom of God, necessarily believes that whatever God has thought fit to reveal on the subject of morals, must fulfil the requirements of utility in a supreme degree. But others besides utilitarians have been of opinion that the Christian revelation was intended, and is fitted, to inform the hearts and minds of mankind with a spirit which should enable them to find for themselves what is right, and incline them to do it when found, rather than to tell them, except in a very general way, what it is: and that we need a doctrine of ethics, carefully followed out, to *interpret* to us the will of God. Whether this opinion is correct or not, it is superfluous here to discuss; since whatever aid religion, either natural or revealed, can afford to ethical investigation, is as open to the utilitarian moralist as to any other. He can use it as the testimony of God to the usefulness or hurtfulness of any given course of action, by as good a right as others can use it for the indication of a transcendental law, having no connexion with usefulness or with happiness.

Again, Utility is often summarily stigmatized as an immoral doctrine by giving it the name of Expediency, and taking advantage of the popular use of that term to contrast it with Principle. But the Expedient, in the sense in which it is opposed to the Right, generally means that which is expedient for the particular interest of the agent himself: as when a minister sacrifices the interest of his country to keep himself in place. When it means anything better than this, it means that which is expedient for some immediate object, some temporary purpose, but which violates a rule whose observance is expedient in a much higher degree. The Expedient, in this sense, instead of being the same thing with the useful, is a branch of the hurtful. Thus, it would often be expedient, for the purpose of getting over some momentary embarrassment, or attaining some object immediately useful to ourselves or others, to tell a lie. But inasmuch as the cultivation in ourselves of a sensitive feeling on the subject of veracity, is one of the most useful, and the enfeeblement of that feeling one of the most hurtful, things to which our conduct can be instrumental; and inasmuch as any, even unintentional, deviation from truth, does that much towards weakening the trustworthiness of human assertion, which is not only the principal support of all present social well-being, but the insufficiency of which does more than any one thing that can be named to keep back civilisation, virtue, everything on which human happiness on the largest scale depends; we feel that the violation, for a present advantage, of a rule of such transcendent expediency, is not expedient, and that he who, for the sake of a convenience to himself or to some other individual, does what depends on him to deprive mankind of the good, and inflict upon them the evil, involved in the greater or less reliance which they can place in each other's word, acts the part of one of their worst enemies. Yet that even this rule, sacred as it is, admits of possible exceptions, is acknowledged by all moralists; the chief of which is when the withholding of some fact (as of information from a malefactor, or of bad news from a person dangerously ill) would preserve some one (especially a person other than oneself) from great and unmerited evil, and when the withholding can only be effected by denial. But in order that the exception may not extend itself beyond the need, and may have the least possible effect in weakening reliance on veracity, it ought to be recognized, and, if possible, its limits defined; and if the principle of utility is good for anything, it must be good for weighing these conflicting utilities against one another, and marking out the region within which one or the other preponderates.

* * *

CHAPTER 6

Nonconsequentialist Theories: Do Your Duty

For the consequentialist, the rightness of an action depends entirely on the effects of that action (or of following the rule that governs it). Good effects make the deed right; bad effects make the deed wrong. But for the nonconsequentialist (otherwise known as a *deontologist*), the rightness of an action can never be measured by such a variable, contingent standard as the quantity of goodness brought into the world. Rightness derives not from the consequences of an action but from its nature, its right-making characteristics. An action is right (or wrong) not because of what it produces but because of what it *is*. Yet for all their differences, both consequentialist and deontological theories contain elements that seem to go to the heart of morality and our moral experience. So in this chapter, we look at ethics through a deontological lens and explore the two deontological theories that historically have offered the strongest challenges to consequentialist views: Kant's moral system and natural law theory.

KANT'S ETHICS

The German philosopher Immanuel Kant (1724–1804) is considered one of the greatest moral philosophers of the modern era. Many scholars would go further and say that he is *the* greatest moral philosopher of the modern era. As a distinguished thinker of the Enlightenment, he sought to make reason the foundation of morality. For him, reason alone leads us to the right and the good. Therefore, to discover the true path we need not appeal to utility, religion, tradition, authority, hap-piness, desires, or intuition. We need only heed the dictates of reason, for reason informs us of the moral law just as surely as it reveals the truths of mathematics. Because of each person's capacity for reason, he or she is a sovereign in the moral realm, a supreme judge of what morality demands. What morality demands (in other words, our duty) is enshrined in the moral law—the changeless, necessary, universal body of moral rules.

In Kant's ethics, right actions have moral value only if they are done with a "good will"—that is, a will to do your duty for duty's sake. To act with a good will is to act with a desire to do your duty *simply because it is your duty*, to act out of pure reverence for the moral law. Without a good will, your actions have no moral worth—even if they accord with the moral law, even if they are done out of sympathy or love, even if they produce good results. Only a good will is unconditionally good, and only an accompanying good will can give your talents, virtues, and actions moral worth. As Kant explains,

> Nothing can possibly be conceived in the world, or even out of it, which can be called good without qual-ification, except a *good will*. Intelligence, wit, judge-ment, and the other *talents* of the mind, however they may be named, or courage, resolution, perse-verance, as qualities of temperament, are undoubt-edly good and desirable in many respects; but these gifts of nature may also become extremely bad and mischievous if the will which is to make use of them, and which, therefore, constitutes what is called *char-acter*, is not good. It is the same with the *gifts of fortune*. Power, riches, honour, even health, and the general well-being and contentment with one's condition

which is called *happiness,* inspire pride, and often presumption, if there is not a good will to correct the influence of these on the mind. . . . A good will is good not because of what it performs or effects, not by its aptness for the attainment of some proposed end, but simply by virtue of the volition—that is, it is good in itself, and considered by itself is to be esteemed much higher than all that can be brought about by it in favour of any inclination, nay, even of the sum-total of all inclinations.[1]

So to do right, we must do it for duty's sake, motivated solely by respect for the moral law. But how do we know what the moral law is? Kant sees the moral law as a set of principles, or rules, stated in the form of imperatives, or commands. Imperatives can be *hypothetical* or *categorical.* A **hypothetical imperative** tells us what we should do if we have certain desires: for example, "If you need money, work for it" or "If you want orange juice, ask for it." We should obey such imperatives only if we desire the outcomes specified. A **categorical imperative,** however, is not so iffy. It tells us that we should do something in all situations *regardless of our wants and needs.* A moral categorical imperative expresses a command like "Do not steal" or "Do not commit suicide." Such imperatives are universal and unconditional, containing no stipulations contingent on human desires or preferences. Kant says that the moral law consists entirely of categorical imperatives. They are the authoritative expression of our moral duties. Because they are the products of rational insight and we are rational agents, we can straightforwardly access, understand, and know them as the great truths that they are.

Kant says that all our duties, all the moral categorical imperatives, can be logically derived from a principle that he calls *the* categorical imperative. It tells us to "Act only on that maxim through which you can at the same time will that it should become a universal law."[2] (Kant actually devised three statements, or versions, of the principle, the one given here and two others; in the next few pages we will examine only the two most important ones.) Kant believes that every action implies a general rule, or maxim. If you steal a car, then your action implies a maxim such as "In this situation, steal a car if you want one." So the first version of the categorical imperative says that an action is right if you can will that the maxim of an action becomes a moral law applying to all persons. That is, an action is permissible if (1) its maxim can be universalized (if everyone can consistently act on the maxim in similar situations); and (2) you would be willing to let that happen. If you can so will the maxim, then the action is right (permissible). If you cannot, the action is wrong (prohibited). Right actions pass the test of the categorical imperative; wrong actions do not.

Some of the duties derived from the categorical imperative are, in Kant's words, perfect duties and some, imperfect duties. **Perfect duties** are those that absolutely must be followed without fail; they have no exceptions. Some perfect duties cited by Kant include duties not to break a promise, not to lie, and not to commit suicide. **Imperfect duties** are not always to be followed; they do have exceptions. As examples of imperfect duties, Kant mentions duties to develop your talents and to help others in need.

Kant demonstrates how to apply the first version of the categorical imperative to several cases, the most famous of which involves a lying promise. Imagine that you want to borrow money from someone, and you know you will not be able to repay the debt. You also know that you will get the loan if you falsely promise to pay the money back. Is such deceptive borrowing morally permissible? To find out, you have to devise a maxim for the action and ask whether you could consistently will

[1]Immanuel Kant, *Fundamental Principles of the Metaphysic of Morals,* trans. Thomas K. Abbott, 2nd ed. (London: Longmans, Green, 1879), 1–2.

[2]Kant, *Fundamental Principles of the Metaphysic of Morals,* 52.

CRITICAL THOUGHT: Sizing Up the Golden Rule

The Golden Rule—"Do unto others as you would have them do unto you"—has some resemblance to Kant's ethics and has been, in one form or another, implicit in many religious traditions and moral systems. Moral philosophers generally think that it touches on a significant truth about morality. But some have argued that taken by itself, without the aid of any other moral principles or theory, the Golden Rule can lead to implausible conclusions and absurd results. Here is part of a famous critique by Richard Whately (1787–1863):

> Supposing any one should regard this golden rule as designed to answer the purpose of a complete system of morality, and to teach us the difference of right and wrong; then, if he had let his land to a farmer, he might consider that the farmer would be glad to be excused paying any rent for it, since he would himself, if he were the farmer, prefer having the land rent-free; and that, therefore, the rule of doing as he would be done by requires him to give up all his property. So also the shopkeeper

might, on the same principle, think that the rule required him to part with his goods under prime cost, or to give them away, and thus to ruin himself. Now such a procedure would be *absurd*. . . .

> You have seen, then, that the golden rule was far from being designed to impart to men the first notions of justice. On the contrary, it *presupposes* that knowledge; and if we had *no* such notions, we could not properly apply the rule. But the real design of it is to put us on our guard against the danger of being blinded by self-interest.*

How does the Golden Rule resemble Kant's theory? How does it differ? Do you agree with Whately's criticism? Why or why not? How could the Golden Rule be qualified or supplemented to blunt Whately's critique? John Stuart Mill said that the Golden Rule was the essence of utilitarianism. What do you think he meant by this?

*Richard Whately, quoted in Louis P. Pojman and Lewis Vaughn, *The Moral Life* (New York: Oxford University Press, 2007), 353–54.

---

it to become a universal law. Could you consistently will everyone to act on the maxim "If you need money, make a lying promise to borrow some"? Kant's emphatic answer is no. If all persons adopted this rule, then they would make lying promises to obtain loans. But then everyone would know that such promises are false, and the practice of giving loans based on a promise would no longer exist, because no promises could be trusted. The maxim says that everyone should make a false promise in order to borrow money, but then no one would loan money on the basis of a promise. If acted on by everyone, the maxim would defeat itself. As Kant says, the "maxim would necessarily destroy itself as soon as it was made a universal law."[3] Therefore,

you cannot consistently will the maxim to become a universal law. The action, then, is not morally permissible.

Kant believes that besides the rule forbidding the breaking of promises, the categorical imperative generates several other duties. Among these he includes prohibitions against committing suicide, lying, and killing innocent people.

Some universalized maxims may fail the test of the categorical imperative (first version) not by being self-defeating (as in the case of a lying promise) but by constituting rules that you would not want everyone else to act on. (Remember that an action is permissible if everyone can consistently act on it in similar situations *and* you would be willing to let that happen.) Kant asks us to consider a maxim that mandates *not* contributing any-

[3]Kant, *Fundamental Principles of the Metaphysic of Morals*, 55.

thing to the welfare of others or aiding them when they are in distress. If you willed this maxim to become a universal moral law (if everyone followed it), no self-defeating state of affairs would obtain. Everyone could conceivably follow this rule. But you probably would not want people to act on this maxim because one day *you* may need *their* help and sympathy. Right now you may will the maxim to become universal law, but later, when the tables are turned, you may regret that policy. The inconsistency lies in wanting the rule to be universalized and not wanting it to be universalized. Kant says that this alternative kind of inconsistency shows that the action embodied in the maxim is not permissible.

Kant's second version of the categorical imperative is probably more famous and influential than the first. (Kant thought the two versions virtually synonymous, but they seem to be distinct principles.) He declares, "So act as to treat humanity, whether in thine own person or in that of any other, in every case as an end withal, never as means only."[4] This rule—the **means-end principle**—says that we must always treat people (including ourselves) as ends in themselves, as creatures of great intrinsic worth, never merely as things of instrumental value, never merely as tools to be used for someone else's purpose.

This statement of the categorical imperative reflects Kant's view of the status of rational beings, or persons. Persons have intrinsic value and dignity because they, unlike the rest of creation, are rational agents who are free to choose their own ends, legislate their own moral laws, and assign value to things in the world. Persons are the givers of value, so they must have ultimate value. They therefore must always be treated as ultimate ends and never merely as means.

Kant's idea is that people not only have intrinsic worth—they also have *equal* intrinsic worth.

Each rational being has the same inherent value as every other rational being. This equality of value cannot be altered by, and has no connection to, social and economic status, racial and ethnic considerations, or the possession of prestige or power. Any two persons are entitled to the same moral rights, even if one is rich, wise, powerful, and famous—and the other is not.

To treat people merely as a means rather than as an end is to fail to recognize the true nature and status of persons. Since people are by nature free, rational, autonomous, and equal, we treat them merely as a means if we do not respect these attributes—if we, for example, interfere with people's right to make informed choices by lying to them, inhibit their free and autonomous actions by enslaving or coercing them, or violate their equality by discriminating against them. For Kant, lying or breaking a promise is wrong because to do so is to use people merely as a means to an end, rather than as an end in themselves.

Sometimes we use people to achieve some end, yet our actions are not wrong. To see why, we must understand that there is a moral difference between treating persons as a means and treating them *merely*, or *only*, as a means. We may treat a mechanic as a means to repair our cars, but we do not treat him merely as a means if we also respect his status as a person. We do not treat him only as means if we neither restrict his freedom nor ignore his rights.

As noted earlier, Kant insists that the two versions of the categorical imperative are two ways of stating the same idea. But the two principles seem to be distinct, occasionally leading to different conclusions about the rightness of an action. The maxim of an action, for example, may pass the first version (be permissible) by being universalizable but fail the second by not treating persons as ends. A more plausible approach is to view the two versions not as alternative tests but as a single two-part test that an action must pass to be judged morally permissible. So before we can declare a

[4]Kant, *Fundamental Principles of the Metaphysic of Morals,* 66–67.

maxim a bona fide categorical imperative, we must be able to consistently will it to become a universal law *and* know that it would have us treat persons not only as a means but as ends.

Applying the Theory

How might a Kantian decide the case of the antiterrorist chief of police, discussed in Chapter 5, who considers killing a terrorist's wife and children? Recall that the terrorist is murdering hundreds of innocent people each year and that the chief has good reasons to believe that killing the wife and children (who are also innocent) will end the terrorist's attacks. Recall also the verdict on this case rendered from both the act- and rule-utilitarian perspectives. By act-utilitarian lights, the chief should kill some of the terrorist's innocent relatives (and threaten to kill others). The rule-utilitarian view, however, is that the chief should *not* kill them.

Suppose the maxim in question is "When the usual antiterrorist tactics fail to stop terrorists from killing many innocent people, the authorities should kill (and threaten to kill) the terrorists' relatives." Can we consistently will this maxim to become a universal law? Does this maxim involve treating persons merely as a means to an end rather than an end in themselves? To answer the first question, we should try to imagine what would happen if everyone in the position of the relevant authorities followed this maxim. Would any inconsistencies or self-defeating states of affairs arise? We can see that the consequences of universalizing the maxim would not be pleasant. The authorities would kill the innocent—actions that could be as gruesome and frightening as terrorist attacks. But our willing that everyone act on the maxim would not be self-defeating or otherwise contradictory. Would we nevertheless be willing to live in a world where the maxim was universally followed? Again, there seems to be no good reason why we could not. The maxim therefore passes the first test of the categorical imperative.

To answer the second (ends-means) question, we must inquire whether following the maxim would involve treating someone merely as a means. The obvious answer is yes. This antiterrorism policy would use the innocent relatives of terrorists as a means to stop terrorist acts. Their freedom and their rights as persons would be violated. The maxim therefore fails the second test, and the acts sanctioned by the maxim would not be permissible. From the Kantian perspective, using the innocent relatives would be wrong no matter what—regardless of how many lives the policy would save or how much safer the world would be. So in this case, the Kantian verdict would coincide with that of rule-utilitarianism but not that of act-utilitarianism.

Evaluating the Theory

Kant's moral theory meets the minimum requirement of coherence and is generally consistent with our moral experience (Criterion 2). In some troubling ways, however, it seems to conflict with our commonsense moral judgments (Criterion 1) and appears to have some flaws that restrict its usefulness in moral problem solving (Criterion 3).

As we saw earlier, some duties generated by the categorical imperative are absolute—they are, as Kant says, perfect duties, allowing no exceptions whatsoever. We have, for example, a perfect (exceptionless) duty not to lie—ever. But what should we do if lying is the only way to prevent a terrible tragedy? Suppose a friend of yours comes to your house in a panic and begs you to hide her from an insane man intent on murdering her. No sooner do you hide her in the cellar than the insane man appears at your door with a bloody knife in his hand and asks where your friend is. You have no doubt that the man is serious and that your friend will in fact be brutally murdered if the man finds her. Imagine that you have only two choices (and saying "I don't know" is not one of them): either you lie to the man and thereby save your friend's life, or you tell the man where

The Kantian View of Punishment

Kant's philosophical position on punishment is radically different from that of the utilitarians. Generally, they think that criminals should not be punished for purposes of justice or retribution. Criminals should be corrected or schooled so they do not commit more crimes, or they should be imprisoned only to protect the public. To them, the point of "punishment" is to promote the good of society. Kant thinks that criminals should be punished *only* because they perpetrated crimes; the public good is irrelevant. In addition, Kant thinks that the central principle of punishment is that the punishment should fit the crime. For Kant, this principle constitutes a solid justification for capital punishment: killers should be killed. As Kant explains,

Even if a civil society resolved to dissolve itself with the consent of all its members—as might be supposed in the case of a people inhabiting an island resolving to separate and scatter throughout the whole world—that last murderer lying in prison ought to be executed before the resolution was carried out. This ought to be done in order that every one may realize the desert of his deeds, and that blood-guiltiness may not remain on the people; for otherwise they will all be regarded as participants in the murder as a public violation of justice.*

*Immanuel Kant, *The Philosophy of Law*, trans. W. Hostie (Edinburgh: Clark, 1887), 198.

---

she is hiding and guarantee her murder. Kant actually considers such a case and renders this verdict on it: you should tell the truth though the heavens fall. He says, as he must, that the consequences of your action here are irrelevant, and not lying is a perfect duty. There can be no exceptions. Yet Kant's answer seems contrary to our considered moral judgments. Moral common sense seems to suggest that in a case like this, saving a life would be much more important than telling the truth.

Another classic example involves promise keeping, which is also a perfect duty. Suppose you promise to meet a friend for lunch, and on your way to the restaurant you are called upon to help someone injured in a car crash. No one else can help her, and she will die unless you render aid. But if you help her, you will break your promise to meet your friend. What should you do? Kant would say that come what may, your duty is to keep your promise to meet your friend. Under these circumstances, however, keeping the promise just seems wrong.

These scenarios are significant because, contrary to Kant's view, we seem to have no absolute, or exceptionless, moral duties. We can easily imagine many cases like those just mentioned. Moreover, we can also envision situations in which we must choose between two allegedly perfect duties, each one prohibiting some action. We cannot fulfill both duties at once, and we must make a choice. Such conflicts provide plausible evidence against the notion that there are exceptionless moral rules.[5]

Conflicts of duties, of course, are not just deficiencies regarding Criterion 1. They also indicate difficulties with Criterion 3. Like many moral theories, Kant's system fails to provide an effective means of resolving major conflicts of duties.

Some additional inconsistencies with our common moral judgments seem to arise from

[5]I owe this point to James Rachels, *The Elements of Moral Philosophy*, 4th ed. (Boston: McGraw-Hill, 2003), 126.

applications of the first version of the categorical imperative. Remember that the first version says that an action is permissible if everyone can consistently act on it and if you would be willing to have that happen. At first glance, it seems to guarantee that moral rules are universally fair. But it makes the acceptability of a moral rule depend largely on whether *you personally* are willing to live in a world that conforms to the rule. If you are not willing to live in such a world, then the rule fails the first version of the categorical imperative, and your conforming to the rule is wrong. But if you are the sort of person who would prefer such a world, then conforming to the rule would be morally permissible. This subjectivity in Kant's theory could lead to the sanctioning of heinous acts of all kinds. Suppose the rule is "Kill everyone with dark skin" or "Murder all Jews." Neither rule would be contradictory if universalized; everyone could consistently act on it. Moreover, if you were willing to have everyone act on it—even willing to be killed if *you* have dark skin or are a Jew—then acts endorsed by the rule would be permissible. Thus the first version seems to bless acts that are clearly immoral.

Critics say that another difficulty with Kant's theory concerns the phrasing of the maxims to be universalized. Oddly enough, Kant does not provide any guidance for how we should state a rule describing an action, an oversight that allows us to word a rule in many different ways. Consider, for example, our duty not to lie. We might state the relevant rule like this: "Lie only to avoid injury or death to others." But we could also say "Lie only to avoid injury, death, or embarrassment to anyone who has green eyes and red hair" (a group that includes you and your relatives). Neither rule would lead to an inconsistency if everyone acted on it, so they both describe permissible actions. The second rule, though, is obviously not morally acceptable. More to the point, it shows that we could use the first version of the categorical imperative to sanction all sorts of immoral acts if we state the rule *in enough detail*. This result suggests

not only a problem with Criterion 1 but also a limitation on the usefulness of the theory, a fault measured by Criterion 3. Judging the rightness of an action is close to impossible if the language of the relevant rule can change with the wind.

It may be feasible to remedy some of the shortcomings of the first version of the categorical imperative by combining it with the second. Rules such as "Kill everyone with dark skin" or "Lie only to avoid injury, death, or embarrassment to anyone who has green eyes and red hair" would be unacceptable because they would allow people to be treated merely as a means. But the means-ends principle itself appears to be in need of modification. The main difficulty is that our duties not to use people merely as a means can conflict, and Kant provides no counsel on how to resolve such dilemmas. Say, for example, that hundreds of innocent people are enslaved inside a brutal Nazi concentration camp, and the only way we can free them is to kill the Nazis guarding the camp. We must therefore choose between allowing the prisoners to be used merely as a means by the Nazis or using the Nazis merely as a means by killing them to free the prisoners.

Here is another example, a classic case from the philosopher C. D. Broad:

> Again, there seem to be cases in which you must either treat A or treat B, not as an end, but as a means. If we isolate a man who is a carrier of typhoid, we are treating him merely as a cause of infection to others. But, if we refuse to isolate him, we are treating other people merely as means to his comfort and culture.[6]

Kant's means-ends principle captures an important truth about the intrinsic value of persons. But we apparently cannot fully implement it, because sometimes we are forced to treat people merely as a means and not as an end in themselves.

---

[6]C. D. Broad, *Five Types of Ethical Theory* (1930; reprint, London: Routledge & Kegan Paul, 1956), 132.

LEARNING FROM KANT'S THEORY

Despite these criticisms, Kant's theory has been influential because it embodies a large part of the whole truth about morality. At a minimum, it promotes many of the duties and rights that our considered judgments lead us to embrace. More important, it emphasizes three of morality's most important features: (1) universality, (2) impartiality, and (3) respect for persons.

Kant's first version of the categorical imperative rests firmly on universality—the notion that the moral law applies to all persons in relevantly similar situations. Impartiality requires that the moral law apply to everyone in the same way, that no one can claim a privileged moral status. In Kantian ethics, double standards are inherently bad. Ethical egoism fails as a moral theory in large part because it lacks this kind of impartiality. The first version of the categorical imperative, in contrast, enshrines impartiality as essential to the moral life. Kant's principle of respect for persons (the means-ends imperative) entails a recognition that persons have ultimate and inherent value, that they should not be used merely as a means to utilitarian ends, that equals should be treated equally, and that there are limits to what can be done to persons for the sake of good consequences. To many scholars, the central flaw of utilitarianism is that it does not incorporate a fully developed respect for persons. But in Kant's theory, the rights and duties of persons override any consequentialist calculus.

So Kantian ethics has many of the most important qualities that we associate with adequate moral theories. And no one has explained better than Kant why persons deserve full respect and how we are to determine whether persons are getting the respect they deserve.

NATURAL LAW THEORY

The natural law theory of morality comes to us from ancient Greek and Roman philosophers (most notably, Aristotle and the Stoics) through the theologian and philosopher Thomas Aquinas (1225–74). Aquinas molded it into its most influential form and bequeathed it to the world and the Roman Catholic Church, which embraced it as its official system of ethics. To this day, the theory is the primary basis for the church's views on abortion, homosexuality, euthanasia, and other controversial issues.

Here we focus on the traditional version of the theory derived from Aquinas. This form is theistic, assuming a divine lawgiver that has given us the gift of reason to comprehend the order of nature. But there are other natural law theories of a more recent vintage that dispense with the religious elements, basing objective moral standards on human nature and the natural needs and interests of humans.

According to Aquinas, at the heart of the traditional theory is the notion that right actions are those that accord with the natural law—the moral principles that we can "read" clearly in the very structure of nature itself, including human nature. We can look into nature and somehow uncover moral standards because nature is a certain way: it is rationally ordered and teleological (goal-directed), with every part having its own purpose or end at which it naturally aims. From this notion about nature, traditional natural law theorists draw the following conclusion: How nature *is* reveals how it *should be*. The goals to which nature inclines reveal the values that we should embrace and the moral purposes to which we should aspire.

In conformity with an inherent, natural purpose or goal—that is, according to natural law—an acorn develops into a seedling, then into a sapling and finally into an oak. The end toward which the acorn strives is the good (for acorns)—that is, to be a well-formed and well-functioning oak. Natural law determines how an oak functions—*and* indicates how an oak should function. If the oak does not function according to its natural purpose (if, for example, it is deformed or weak), it fails to be as it should be, deviating from its proper path laid down in natural law. Likewise, humans have a nature—a natural function and purpose unique among all living things. In human nature, in the mandates of the natural law for humanity, are the aims toward which human life strives. In these teleological strivings, in these facts about what human nature *is,* we can perceive what it *should be.*

What is it, exactly, that human nature aims at? Aquinas says that humans naturally incline toward preservation of human life, avoidance of harm, basic functions that humans and animals have in common (sexual intercourse, raising offspring, and the like), the search for truth, the nurturing of social ties, and behavior that is benign and reasonable. For humans, these inclinations constitute the good—the good of human flourishing and well-being. Our duty then is to achieve the good, to fully realize the goals to which our nature is already inclined. As Aquinas says,

> [T]his is the first precept of law, that *good is to be done and promoted, and evil is to be avoided.* All other precepts of the natural law are based upon this; so that all things which the practical reason naturally apprehends as man's good belong to the precepts of the natural law under the form of things to be done or avoided.
>
> Since, however, good has the nature of an end, and evil, the nature of the contrary, hence it is that all those things to which man has a natural inclination are naturally apprehended by reason as good, and consequently as objects of pursuit, and their contraries as evil, and objects of avoidance. Therefore, the order of the precepts of the natural law is according to the order of natural inclinations.[7]

In this passage, Aquinas refers to the aspect of human nature that enables us to decipher and implement the precepts of natural law: reason. Humans, unlike the rest of nature, are rational creatures, capable of understanding, deliberation, and free choice. Since all of nature is ordered and

[7]Thomas Aquinas, *Summa Theologica,* in *Basic Writings of Saint Thomas Aquinas,* ed. and annotated by Anton C. Pegis (New York: Random House, 1945), First Part of the Second Part, Question 94, Article 2.

rational, only rational beings such as humans can peer into it and discern the inclinations in their nature, derive from the natural tendencies the natural laws, and apply the laws to their actions and their lives. Humans have the gift of reason (a gift from God, Aquinas says), and reason gives us access to the laws. Reason therefore is the foundation of morality. Judging the rightness of actions, then, is a matter of consulting reason, of considering rational grounds for moral beliefs.

It follows from these points that the natural (moral) laws are both objective and universal. The general principles of right and wrong do not vary from person to person or culture to culture. The dynamics of each situation may alter how a principle is applied, and not every situation has a relevant principle, but principles do not change with the tide. The natural laws are the natural laws. Further, they are not only binding on all persons, but they can be known by all persons. Aquinas insists that belief in God or inspiration from above is not a prerequisite for knowledge of morality. A person's effective use of reason is the only requirement.

Like Kant's categorical imperative, traditional natural law theory is, in the main, strongly absolutist. Natural law theorists commonly insist on several exceptionless rules. Directly killing the innocent is always wrong (which means that direct abortion is always wrong). Use of contraceptives is always wrong (on the grounds that it interferes with the natural human inclination toward procreation). Homosexuality is always wrong (again because it thwarts procreation). For Aquinas, lying, adultery, and blasphemy are always wrong.

As we have seen, moral principles—especially absolutist rules—can give rise to conflicts of duties. Kant's view on conflicting perfect duties is that such inconsistencies cannot happen. The natural law tradition gives a different answer: Conflicts between duties are possible, but they can be resolved by applying the **doctrine of double effect.** This principle pertains to situations in which an action has both good and bad effects. It says that performing a good action may be permissible even if it has bad effects, but performing a bad action for the purpose of achieving good effects is never permissible. More formally, in a traditional interpretation of the doctrine, an action is permissible if four requirements are met:

1. *The action is inherently (without reference to consequences) either morally good or morally neutral.* That is, the action itself must at least be morally permissible.

2. *The bad effect is not used to produce the good effect (though the bad may be a side effect of the good).* Killing a fetus to save the mother's life is never permissible. However, using a drug to cure the mother's life-threatening disease—even though the fetus dies as a side effect of the treatment—may be permissible.

3. *The intention must always be to bring about the good effect.* For any given action, the bad effect may occur, and it may even be foreseen, but it must not be intended.

4. *The good effect must be at least as important as the bad effect.* The good of an action must be proportional to the bad. If the bad heavily outweighs the good, the action is not permissible. The good of saving your own life in an act of self-defense, for example, must be at least as great as the bad of taking the life of your attacker.

The doctrine of double effect is surprisingly versatile. Natural law theorists have used it to navigate moral dilemmas in medical ethics, reproductive health, warfare, and other life-and-death issues. The next section provides a demonstration.

Applying the Theory

Traditional natural law theory and its double-effect doctrine figure prominently in obstetrics cases in which a choice must be made between harming a pregnant woman or her fetus. A typical scenario goes something like this: A pregnant woman has cancer and will die unless she receives chemotherapy to destroy the tumors. If she does take the

QUICK REVIEW

hypothetical imperative—An imperative that tells us what we should do if we have certain desires.

categorical imperative—An imperative that we should follow regardless of our particular wants and needs; also, the principle that defines Kant's ethical system.

perfect duty—A duty that has no exceptions.

imperfect duty—A duty that has exceptions.

means-ends principle—The rule that we must always treat people (including ourselves) as ends in themselves, never merely as a means.

doctrine of double effect—The principle that performing a good action may be permissible even if it has bad effects, but performing a bad action for the purpose of achieving good effects is never permissible; any bad effects must be unintended.

chemotherapy, the fetus will die. Is it morally permissible for her to do so?

In itself, the act of taking the chemotherapy is morally permissible. There is nothing inherently wrong with using a medical treatment to try to cure a life-threatening illness. So the action meets Condition 1. We can also see that the bad effect (killing the fetus) is not used to produce the good effect (saving the woman's life). Receiving the chemotherapy is the method used to achieve the good effect. The loss of the fetus is an indirect, unintended result of the attempt to destroy the cancer. The action therefore meets Condition 2. The intention behind the action is to kill the cancer and thereby save the woman's life—not to kill the fetus. The woman and her doctors know that the unfortunate consequence of treating the cancer will be the death of the fetus. They foresee the

CRITICAL THOUGHT: Double Effect and the "Trolley Problem"

Consider the following thought experiment, first proposed by the philosopher Philippa Foot and set forth here by the philosopher Judith Jarvis Thomson:

> Suppose you are the driver of a trolley. The trolley rounds a bend, and there come into view ahead five track workmen, who have been repairing the track. The track goes through a bit of a valley at that point, and the sides are steep, so you must stop the trolley if you are to avoid running the five men down. You step on the brakes, but alas they don't work. Now you suddenly see a spur of track leading off to the right. You can turn the trolley onto it, and thus save the five men on the straight track ahead. Unfortunately, Mrs. Foot has arranged that there is one track workman on that spur of track. He can no more get off the track in

time than the five can, so you will kill him if you turn the trolley onto him. Is it morally permissible for you to turn the trolley?*

If you were the driver of the trolley, which option would you choose? Would you consider it morally permissible to turn the trolley onto the one workman to save the other five? Why or why not? What would the doctrine of double effect have you do in this case? Does your moral intuition seem to conflict with what the doctrine would have you do? What reasons can you give for the choice you make?

*Judith Jarvis Thomson, "Critical Thought: Double Effect and the 'Trolley Problem,'" *Yale Law Journal*, Vol. 94, No. 6, May 1985. Reprinted with permission from the Yale Law Journal.

death, but their intention is not to kill the fetus. Thus, the action meets Condition 3. Is the good effect proportional to the bad effect? In this case, a life is balanced against a life, the life of the woman and the life of the fetus. From the natural law perspective, both sides of the scale seem about equal in importance. If the good effect to be achieved for the woman was, say, a nicer appearance through cosmetic surgery, and the bad effect was the death of the fetus, the two sides would not have the same level of importance. But in this case, the action does meet Condition 4. Because the action meets all four conditions, receiving the chemotherapy is morally permissible for the woman.

Now let us examine a different kind of scenario. Remember that earlier in this chapter, we applied both utilitarianism and Kant's theory to the antiterrorism tactic of killing a terrorist's relatives. To stop the murder of many innocent people by a relentless terrorist, the authorities consider killing his wife and three of his children and

threatening to kill the remaining four children. What verdict would the doctrine of double effect yield in this case?

Here the action is the antiterrorist tactic just described. The good effect is preventing the death of innocent citizens; the bad effect is the killing of other innocents. Right away we can see that the action, in itself, is not morally good. Directly killing the innocent is never permissible, so the action does not meet Condition 1. Failing to measure up to even one condition shows the action to be prohibited, but we will continue our analysis anyway. Is the bad effect used to produce the good effect? Yes. The point of the action is to prevent further terrorist killings, and the means to that end is killing the terrorist's wife and children. The bad is used to achieve the good. So the action does not meet Condition 2, either. It does, however, meet Condition 3 because the intention behind the action is to bring about the good effect, preventing further terrorist killings. Finally, if we view the good effect (preventing the deaths of citizens) as comparable to the bad effect (the killing of the terrorist's wife and children), we should infer that the action meets Condition 4. In any case, since the action fails Conditions 1 and 2, we have to say that the action of the authorities in killing members of the terrorist's family is not permissible.

As suggested earlier, a Kantian theorist would likely agree with this decision, and a rule-utilitarian would probably concur. However, judging that the good consequences outweigh the bad, an act-utilitarian might very well say that killing the wife and children to prevent many other deaths would be not only permissible but obligatory.

Evaluating the Theory

Traditional natural law theory appears to contain no crippling internal inconsistencies, so we will regard it as an eligible theory for evaluation. But it does encounter difficulties with Criteria 1 and 3.

The theory seems to fall short of Criterion 1 (conflicts with commonsense moral judgments) in part because of its absolutism, a feature that also encumbers Kant's theory. As we have seen, natural law theorists maintain that some actions are *always* wrong: for example, intentionally killing the innocent, impeding procreation (through contraception, sterilization, or sexual preferences), or lying. Such absolutes, though, can lead to moral judgments that seem to diverge from common sense. The absolute prohibition against directly killing the innocent, for example, could actually result in great loss of life in certain extreme circumstances. Imagine that a thousand innocent people are taken hostage by a homicidal madman, and the only way to save the lives of nine hundred and ninety-nine is to intentionally kill one of them. If the one is not killed, all one thousand will die. Most of us would probably regard the killing of the one hostage as a tragic but necessary measure to prevent a massive loss of life. The alternative—letting them all die—would seem a much greater tragedy.

But many natural law theorists would condemn the killing of the one innocent person even if it would save the lives of hundreds.

Similarly, suppose a pregnant woman will die unless her fetus is aborted. Would it be morally permissible for her to have the abortion? Given the natural law prohibition against killing the innocent, many natural law theorists would say no. Aborting the fetus would be wrong, even to save the mother's life. But most people would probably say that this view contradicts our considered moral judgments.

The absolutism of natural law theory arises from the notion that nature is authoritatively teleological. Nature aims toward particular ends that are ordained by the divine, and the values inherent in this arrangement cannot and must not be ignored or altered. How nature *is* reveals how it *should be*. Period. But the teleological character of nature has never been established by logical argument or empirical science—at least not to the satisfaction of most philosophers and scientists. In fact, science (including evolutionary theory) suggests that nature is not teleological at all but instead random and purposeless, changing and adapting according to scientific laws, blind cause and effect, chance mutation, and competition among species. Moreover, the idea that values can somehow be extracted from the facts of nature is as problematic for natural law theory as it is for ethical egoism and utilitarianism. From the fact that humans have a natural inclination toward procreation it does not follow that discouraging procreation through contraception is morally wrong.

Natural law theory seems to falter on Criterion 3 (usefulness) because, as just mentioned, discovering what values are inscribed in nature is problematic. The kind of moral principles that we might extract from nature depends on our conception of nature, and such conceptions can vary. Taking their cue from Aquinas, many natural law theorists see the inclinations of human nature as benign; others, as fundamentally depraved. Historically, humans have shown a capacity for both great good and monstrous evil. Which inclination is the true one? And even if we could accurately identify human inclinations, there seems to be no reliable procedure for uncovering the corresponding moral values or telling whether moral principles should be absolutist.

LEARNING FROM NATURAL LAW

Like Kantian ethics, natural law theory is universalist, objective, and rational, applying to all persons and requiring that moral choices be backed by good reasons. The emphasis on reason makes morality independent of religion and belief in God, a distinction also found in Kant's ethics. At the heart of natural law theory is a strong respect for human life, an attitude that is close to, but not quite the same thing as, Kant's means-ends principle. Respect for life or persons is, of course, a primary concern of our moral experience and seems to preclude the kind of wholesale end-justifies-the-means calculations that are a defining characteristic of many forms of utilitarianism.

Natural law theory emphasizes a significant element in moral deliberation that some other theories play down: intention. In general, intention plays a larger role in natural law theory than it does in Kant's categorical imperative. To many natural law theorists, the rightness of an action often depends on the intentions of the moral agent performing it. In our previous example of the pregnant woman with cancer, for example, the intention behind the act of taking the chemotherapy is to kill the cancer, not the fetus, though the fetus dies because of the treatment. So the action is thought to be morally permissible. If the intention had been to directly kill the fetus, the action would have been deemed wrong. In our everyday moral experience, we frequently take intentions into account in evaluating an action. We usually would think that there must be some morally rele-

vant difference between a terrorist's intentionally killing ten people and a police officer's accidentally killing those same ten people while chasing the terrorist, though both scenarios result in the same tragic loss of life.

SUMMARY

Kant's moral theory is perhaps the most influential of all nonconsequentialist approaches. In his view, right actions have moral value only if they are done with a "good will"—for duty's sake alone. The meat of Kant's theory is the categorical imperative, a principle that he formulates in three versions. The first version says that an action is right if you can will that the maxim of an action becomes a moral law applying to all persons. An action is permissible if (1) its maxim can be universalized (if everyone can consistently act on it) and (2) you would be willing to have that happen. The second version of the categorical imperative says that we must always treat people as ends in themselves and never merely as a means to an end.

Kant's theory seems to conflict with our common-sense moral judgments (Criterion 1) and has flaws that limit its usefulness in moral problem solving (Criterion 3). The theory falters on Criterion 1 mainly because some duties generated by the categorical imperative are absolute. Absolute duties can conflict, and Kant provides no way to resolve the inconsistencies, a failure of Criterion 3. Furthermore, we seem to have no genuine absolute duties.

Natural law theory is based on the notion that right actions are those that accord with natural law— the moral principles embedded in nature itself. How nature *is* reveals how it *should be*. The inclinations of human nature reveal the values that humans should live by. Aquinas, who gave us the most influential form of natural law theory, says that humans naturally incline toward preservation of human life, procreation, the search for truth, community, and benign and reasonable behavior. Like Kant's theory, traditional natural law theory is absolutist, maintaining that some actions are always wrong. These immoral actions include directly killing the innocent, interfering with procreation, and lying. The theory's absolutist rules do occasionally conflict, and the proposed remedy for any such inconsistencies is the doctrine of double effect. The principle applies to situations in which an action produces both good and bad effects. It says that performing a good action may be permissible even if it has bad effects, but performing a bad action for the purpose of achieving good effects is never permissible. Despite the double-effect doctrine, the theory's biggest weakness is still its absolutism, which seems to mandate actions that conflict with our considered moral judgments. In some cases, for example, the theory might require someone to allow hundreds of innocent people to die just to avoid the direct killing of a single person.

EXERCISES

Review Questions

1. What is the significance of a "good will" in Kant's ethics? (pp. 102–3)
2. What is the difference between a hypothetical and a categorical imperative? (p. 103)
3. What is the moral principle laid out in the first version of Kant's categorical imperative? (p. 103)
4. What is the difference between perfect and imperfect duties? (p. 103)
5. How does Kant distinguish between treating someone as a means and treating someone *merely* as a means? (p. 105)
6. How can the absolutism of Kant's theory lead to judgments that conflict with moral common sense? (pp. 106–7)
7. How might the subjectivity of Kant's theory lead to the sanctioning of heinous acts? (p. 108)
8. What is natural law theory? (pp. 109–10)
9. According to natural law theorists, how can nature reveal anything about morality? (pp. 109–10)
10. According to Aquinas, what is the good that human nature aims at? (p. 110)
11. According to natural law theory, how are moral principles objective? How are they universal? (p. 110)
12. What is the doctrine of double effect? (pp. 110–11)
13. How can the absolutism of natural law theory lead to moral judgments that conflict with moral common sense? (p. 113)

Discussion Questions

1. Which moral theory—Kant's or natural law— seems more plausible to you? Why?
2. What elements of Kant's theory do you think could or should be part of any viable moral theory?
3. In what way is Kant's ethics independent of (not based on) religious belief? Is natural law theory independent of religious belief? Why or why not?
4. According to Kant, why is breaking a promise or lying immoral? Do you agree with Kant's reasoning? Why or why not?
5. How might your life change if you completely embraced Kant's theory of morality?
6. How might your life change if you adopted the natural law theory of morality?
7. Would a Kantian and a natural law theorist agree on whether having an abortion is moral? Why or why not?
8. Do you believe, as Kant does, that there are perfect (absolute) duties? Why or why not?
9. According to the textbook, natural law theory generates judgments that conflict with commonsense morality. Do you agree with this assessment? Why or why not?
10. Is natural law theory more plausible than utilitarianism? Why or why not?

READINGS

From *Fundamental Principles of the Metaphysic of Morals*

IMMANUEL KANT

* * *

Nothing can possibly be conceived in the world, or even out of it, which can be called good, without qualification, except a *good will*. Intelligence, wit, judgement, and the other talents of the mind, however, they may be named, or courage, resolution, perseverance, as qualities of temperament, are undoubtedly good and desirable in many respects; but these gifts of nature may also become extremely bad and mischievous if the will which is to make use of them, and which, therefore, constitutes what is called *character*, is not good. It is the same with the *gifts of fortune.* Power, riches, honour, even health, and the general well-being and contentment with one's condition which is called *happiness*, inspire pride, and often presumption, if there is not a good will to correct the influence of these on the mind, and with this also to rectify the whole principle of acting and adapt it to its end. The sight of a being who is not adorned with a single feature of a pure and good will, enjoying unbroken prosperity, can never give pleasure to an impartial rational spectator. Thus a good will appears to constitute the indispensable condition even of being worthy of happiness.

There are even some qualities which are of service to this good will itself and may facilitate its action, yet which have no intrinsic unconditional value, but always presuppose a good will, and this qualifies the esteem that we justly have for them and does not permit us to regard them as absolutely good. Moderation in the affections and passions, self-control, and calm deliberation are not only good in many respects, but even seem to constitute part of the intrinsic worth of the person; but they are far from deserving to be called good without qualification, although they have been so unconditionally praised by the ancients. For without the principles of a good will, they may become extremely bad, and the coolness of a villain not only makes him far more dangerous, but also directly makes him more abominable in our eyes than he would have been without it.

A good will is good not because of what it performs or effects, not by its aptness for the attainment of some proposed end, but simply by virtue of the volition—that is, it is good in itself, and considered by itself is to be esteemed much higher than all that can be brought about by it in favour of any inclination, nay, even of the sum-total of all inclinations. Even if it should happen that, owing to special disfavour of fortune, or the niggardly provision of a step-motherly nature, this will should wholly lack power to accomplish its purpose, if with its greatest efforts it should yet achieve nothing, and there should remain only the good will (not, to be sure, a mere wish, but the summoning of all means in our power), then, like a jewel, it would still shine by its own light, as a thing which has its whole value in itself. Its usefulness or fruitfulness can neither add nor take away anything from this value. It would be, as it were, only the setting to enable us to handle it the more conveniently in common commerce, or to attract to it the attention of those who are not yet connoisseurs, but not to recommend it to true connoisseurs, or to determine its value.

There is, however, something so strange in this idea of the absolute value of the mere will, in which no account is taken of its utility, that notwithstanding the thorough assent of even common reason to the idea, yet a suspicion must arise that it may perhaps really be the product of mere high-flown fancy, and that we may have misunderstood the purpose of nature in assigning reason as the governor of our

Immanuel Kant, *Fundamental Principles of the Metaphysic of Morals*, trans. Thomas K. Abbott (edited).

will. Therefore we will examine this idea from this point of view.

* * *

To be beneficent when we can is a duty; and besides this, there are many minds so sympathetically constituted that, without any other motive of vanity or self-interest, they find a pleasure in spreading joy around them and can take delight in the satisfaction of others so far as it is their own work. But I maintain that in such a case an action of this kind, however proper, however amiable it may be, has nevertheless no true moral worth, but is on a level with other inclinations, e.g., the inclination to honour, which, if it is happily directed to that which is in fact of public utility and accordant with duty and consequently honourable, deserves praise and encouragement, but not esteem. For the maxim lacks the moral import, namely, that such actions be done from duty, not from inclination. Put the case that the mind of that philanthropist were clouded by sorrow of his own, extinguishing all sympathy with the lot of others, and that, while he still has the power to benefit others in distress, he is not touched by their trouble because he is absorbed with his own; and now suppose that he tears himself out of this dead insensibility, and performs the action without any inclination to it, but simply from duty, then first has his action its genuine moral worth. Further still, if nature has put little sympathy in the heart of this or that man; if he, supposed to be an upright man, is by temperament cold and indifferent to the sufferings of others, perhaps because in respect of his own he is provided with the special gift of patience and fortitude and supposes, or even requires, that others should have the same—and such a man would certainly not be the meanest product of nature—but if nature had not specially framed him for a philanthropist, would he not still find in himself a source from whence to give himself a far higher worth than that of a good-natured temperament could be? Unquestionably. It is just in this that the moral worth of the character is brought out which is incomparably the highest of all, namely, that he is beneficent, not from inclination, but from duty.

* * *

Thus the moral worth of an action does not lie in the effect expected from it, nor in any principle of action which requires to borrow its motive from this expected effect. For all these effects—agreeableness of one's condition and even the promotion of the happiness of others—could have been also brought about by other causes, so that for this there would have been no need of the will of a rational being; whereas it is in this alone that the supreme and unconditional good can be found. The pre-eminent good which we call moral can therefore consist in nothing else than the conception of law in itself, which certainly is only possible in a rational being, in so far as this conception, and not the expected effect, determines the will. This is a good which is already present in the person who acts accordingly, and we have not to wait for it to appear first in the result.

* * *

But what sort of law can that be, the conception of which must determine the will, even without paying any regard to the effect expected from it, in order that this will may be called good absolutely and without qualification? As I have deprived the will of every impulse which could arise to it from obedience to any law, there remains nothing but the universal conformity of its actions to law in general, which alone is to serve the will as a principle, i.e., I am never to act otherwise than so that I could also will that my maxim should become a universal law. Here, now, it is the simple conformity to law in general, without assuming any particular law applicable to certain actions, that serves the will as its principle and must so serve it, if duty is not to be a vain delusion and a chimerical notion. The common reason of men in its practical judgements perfectly coincides with this and always has in view the principle here suggested. Let the question be, for example: May I when in distress make a promise with the intention not to keep it? I readily distinguish here between the two significations which the question may have: Whether it is prudent, or whether it is right, to make a false promise? The former may undoubtedly often be the case. I see clearly indeed that it is not enough to extricate myself from a present difficulty by means of this subterfuge, but it must be well considered whether there may not hereafter spring from this lie much greater inconvenience than that from which I now free myself, and as, with all my supposed cunning, the consequences cannot be so easily foreseen but that credit once lost may be much more injurious to me than any mischief which I seek to avoid at present, it should be considered whether it would not be more prudent to act herein according to a universal maxim and to make it a habit to promise nothing except with the intention of keeping it. But it is soon clear to me that such a maxim will still only be based on the fear of consequences. Now it is a wholly different thing to be truthful from duty, and to be so from apprehension of injurious consequences. In the first case, the very notion of the action already implies a law for me; in the second case, I must first look about elsewhere to see what results may be combined with it which would affect myself. For to deviate from the principle of duty is beyond all doubt wicked; but to be unfaithful to my maxim of prudence may often be very advantageous to me, although to abide by it is certainly safer. The shortest way, however, and an unerring one, to discover the answer to this question whether a lying promise is consistent with duty, is to ask myself, "Should I be content that my maxim (to extricate myself from difficulty by a false promise) should hold good as a universal law, for myself as well as for others?" and should I be able to say to myself, "Every one may make a deceitful promise when he finds himself in a difficulty from which he cannot otherwise extricate himself?" Then I presently become aware that while I can will the lie, I can by no means will that lying should be a universal law. For with such a law there would be no promises at all, since it would be in vain to allege my intention in regard to my future actions to those who would not believe this allegation, or if they over hastily did so would pay me back in my own coin. Hence my maxim, as soon as it should be made a universal law, would necessarily destroy itself.

I do not, therefore, need any far-reaching penetration to discern what I have to do in order that my will may be morally good. Inexperienced in the course of the world, incapable of being prepared for all its contingencies, I only ask myself: Canst thou also will that thy maxim should be a universal law? If not, then it must be rejected, and that not because of a disadvantage accruing from it to myself or even to others, but because it cannot enter as a principle into a possible universal legislation, and reason extorts from me immediate respect for such legislation. I do not indeed as yet discern on what this respect is based (this the philosopher may inquire), but at least I understand this, that it is an estimation of the worth which far outweighs all worth of what is recommended by inclination, and that the necessity of acting from pure respect for the practical law is what constitutes duty, to which every other motive must give place, because it is the condition of a will being good in itself, and the worth of such a will is above everything.

* * *

Nor could anything be more fatal to morality than that we should wish to derive it from examples. For every example of it that is set before me must be first itself tested by principles of morality, whether it is worthy to serve as an original example, i.e., as a pattern; but by no means can it authoritatively furnish the conception of morality. Even the Holy One of the Gospels must first be compared with our ideal of moral perfection before we can recognise Him as such; and so He says of Himself, "Why call ye Me (whom you see) good; none is good (the model of good) but God only (whom ye do not see)?" But whence have we the conception of God as the supreme good? Simply from the idea of moral perfection, which reason frames a priori and connects inseparably with the notion of a free will. Imitation finds no place at all in morality, and examples serve only for encouragement, i.e., they put beyond doubt the feasibility of what the law commands, they make visible that which the practical rule expresses more generally, but they can never authorize us to set aside the true original which lies in reason and to guide ourselves by examples.

* * *

From what has been said, it is clear that all moral conceptions have their seat and origin completely a priori in the reason, and that, moreover, in the commonest reason just as truly as in that which is in the highest degree speculative; that they cannot be obtained by abstraction from any empirical, and therefore merely contingent, knowledge; that it is just this purity of their origin that makes them worthy to serve as our supreme practical principle, and that just in proportion as we add anything empirical, we detract from their genuine influence and from the absolute value of actions; that it is not only of the greatest necessity, in a purely speculative point of view, but is also of the greatest practical importance, to derive these notions and laws from pure reason, to present them pure and unmixed, and even to determine the compass of this practical or pure rational knowledge, i.e., to determine the whole faculty of pure practical reason; and, in doing so, we must not make its principles dependent on the particular nature of human reason, though in speculative philosophy this may be permitted, or may even at times be necessary; but since moral laws ought to hold good for every rational creature, we must derive them from the general concept of a rational being. In this way, although for its application to man morality has need of anthropology, yet, in the first instance, we must treat it independently as pure philosophy, i.e., as metaphysic, complete in itself (a thing which in such distinct branches of science is easily done); knowing well that unless we are in possession of this, it would not only be vain to determine the moral element of duty in right actions for purposes of speculative criticism, but it would be impossible to base morals on their genuine principles, even for common practical purposes, especially of moral instruction, so as to produce pure moral dispositions, and to engraft them on men's minds to the promotion of the greatest possible good in the world.

But in order that in this study we may not merely advance by the natural steps from the common moral judgement (in this case very worthy of respect) to the philosophical, as has been already done, but also from a popular philosophy, which goes no further than it can reach by groping with the help of examples, to metaphysic (which does not allow itself to be checked by anything empirical and, as it must measure the whole extent of this kind of rational knowledge, goes as far as ideal conceptions, where even examples fail us), we must follow and clearly describe the practical faculty of reason, from the general rules of its determination to the point where the notion of duty springs from it.

Everything in nature works according to laws. Rational beings alone have the faculty of acting according to the conception of laws—that is, according to principles, that is, have a will. Since the deduction of actions from principles requires reason, the will is nothing but practical reason. If reason infallibly determines the will, then the actions of such a being which are recognised as objectively necessary are subjectively necessary also, that is, the will is a faculty to choose that only which reason independent of inclination recognises as practically necessary, that is, as good. But if reason of itself does not sufficiently determine the will, if the latter is subject also to subjective conditions (particular impulses) which do not always coincide with the objective conditions; in a word, if the will does not in itself completely accord with reason (which is actually the case with men), then the actions which objectively are recognised as necessary are subjectively contingent, and the determination of such a will according to objective laws is obligation, that is to say, the relation of the objective laws to a will that is not thoroughly good is conceived as the determination of the will of a rational being by principles of reason, but which the will from its nature does not of necessity follow.

The conception of an objective principle, in so far as it is obligatory for a will, is called a command (of reason), and the formula of the command is called an imperative.

All imperatives are expressed by the word ought [or shall], and thereby indicate the relation of an objective law of reason to a will, which from its subjective constitution is not necessarily determined by it (an obligation). They say that something would be good to do or to forbear, but they say it to a will which does not always do a thing because it is conceived to be good to do it. That is practically good, however, which determines the will by means of the conceptions of reason, and consequently not from subjective causes, but objectively, that is, on principles which are valid for every rational being as such.

It is distinguished from the pleasant, as that which influences the will only by means of sensation from merely subjective causes, valid only for the sense of this or that one, and not as a principle of reason, which holds for every one.

* * *

Now all imperatives command either hypothetically or categorically. The former represent the practical necessity of a possible action as means to something else that is willed (or at least which one might possibly will). The categorical imperative would be that which represented an action as necessary of itself without reference to another end, that is, as objectively necessary.

Since every practical law represents a possible action as good and, on this account, for a subject who is practically determinable by reason, necessary, all imperatives are formulae determining an action which is necessary according to the principle of a will good in some respects. If now the action is good only as a means to something else, then the imperative is hypothetical; if it is conceived as good in itself and consequently as being necessarily the principle of a will which of itself conforms to reason, then it is categorical.

Thus the imperative declares what action possible by me would be good and presents the practical rule in relation to a will which does not forthwith perform an action simply because it is good, whether because the subject does not always know that it is good, or because, even if it know this, yet its maxims might be opposed to the objective principles of practical reason.

Accordingly the hypothetical imperative only says that the action is good for some purpose, possible or actual. In the first case it is a problematical, in the second an assertorial practical principle. The categorical imperative which declares an action to be objectively necessary in itself without reference to any purpose, i.e., without any other end, is valid as an apodeictic (practical) principle.

* * *

Finally, there is an imperative which commands a certain conduct immediately, without having as its condition any other purpose to be attained by it. This imperative is categorical. It concerns not the matter of the action, or its intended result, but its form and the principle of which it is itself a result; and what is essentially good in it consists in the mental disposition, let the consequence be what it may. This imperative may be called that of morality.

* * *

[The] question how the imperative of morality is possible, is undoubtedly one, the only one, demanding a solution, as this is not at all hypothetical, and the objective necessity which it presents cannot rest on any hypothesis, as is the case with the hypothetical imperatives. Only here we must never leave out of consideration that we cannot make out by any example, in other words empirically, whether there is such an imperative at all, but it is rather to be feared that all those which seem to be categorical may yet be at bottom hypothetical. For instance, when the precept is: "Thou shalt not promise deceitfully"; and it is assumed that the necessity of this is not a mere counsel to avoid some other evil, so that it should mean: "Thou shalt not make a lying promise, lest if it become known thou shouldst destroy thy credit," but that an action of this kind must be regarded as evil in itself, so that the imperative of the prohibition is categorical; then we cannot show with certainty in any example that the will was determined merely by the law, without any other spring of action, although it may appear to be so. For it is always possible that fear of disgrace, perhaps also obscure dread of other dangers, may have a secret influence on the will. Who can prove by experience the non-existence of a cause when all that experience tells us is that we do not perceive it? But in such a case the so-called moral imperative, which as such appears to be categorical and unconditional, would in reality be only a pragmatic precept, drawing our attention to our own interests and merely teaching us to take these into consideration.

We shall therefore have to investigate a priori the possibility of a categorical imperative, as we have not in this case the advantage of its reality being given in experience, so that [the elucidation of] its possibility should be requisite only for its explanation, not for its establishment. In the meantime it may be discerned beforehand that the categorical imperative alone has the purport of a practical law; all the rest may indeed be called principles of the will but not laws, since whatever is only necessary for the attainment of some arbitrary purpose may be considered as in itself contingent, and we can at any time be free from the precept if we give up the purpose; on the contrary, the unconditional command leaves the will no liberty to choose the opposite; consequently it alone carries with it that necessity which we require in a law.

Secondly, in the case of this categorical imperative or law of morality, the difficulty (of discerning its possibility) is a very profound one. It is an a priori synthetical practical proposition; and as there is so much difficulty in discerning the possibility of speculative propositions of this kind, it may readily be supposed that the difficulty will be no less with the practical.

* * *

In this problem we will first inquire whether the mere conception of a categorical imperative may not perhaps supply us also with the formula of it, containing the proposition which alone can be a categorical imperative; for even if we know the tenor of such an absolute command, yet how it is possible will require further special and laborious study, which we postpone to the last section.

When I conceive a hypothetical imperative, in general I do not know beforehand what it will contain until I am given the condition. But when I conceive a categorical imperative, I know at once what it contains. For as the imperative contains besides the law only the necessity that the maxims shall conform to this law, while the law contains no conditions restricting it, there remains nothing but the general statement that the maxim of the action should conform to a universal law, and it is this conformity alone that the imperative properly represents as necessary.

* * *

There is therefore but one categorical imperative, namely, this: Act only on that maxim whereby thou canst at the same time will that it should become a universal law.

Now if all imperatives of duty can be deduced from this one imperative as from their principle, then, although it should remain undecided what is called

duty is not merely a vain notion, yet at least we shall be able to show what we understand by it and what this notion means.

Since the universality of the law according to which effects are produced constitutes what is properly called nature in the most general sense (as to form), that is the existence of things so far as it is determined by general laws, the imperative of duty may be expressed thus: Act as if the maxim of thy action were to become by thy will a universal law of nature.

We will now enumerate a few duties, adopting the usual division of them into duties to ourselves and to others, and into perfect and imperfect duties.

* * *

1. A man reduced to despair by a series of misfortunes feels wearied of life, but is still so far in possession of his reason that he can ask himself whether it would not be contrary to his duty to himself to take his own life. Now he inquires whether the maxim of his action could become a universal law of nature. His maxim is: "From self-love I adopt it as a principle to shorten my life when its longer duration is likely to bring more evil than satisfaction." It is asked then simply whether this principle founded on self-love can become a universal law of nature. Now we see at once that a system of nature of which it should be a law to destroy life by means of the very feeling whose special nature it is to impel to the improvement of life would contradict itself and, therefore, could not exist as a system of nature; hence that maxim cannot possibly exist as a universal law of nature and, consequently, would be wholly inconsistent with the supreme principle of all duty.

2. Another finds himself forced by necessity to borrow money. He knows that he will not be able to repay it, but sees also that nothing will be lent to him unless he promises stoutly to repay it in a definite time. He desires to make this promise, but he has still so much conscience as to ask himself: "Is it not unlawful and inconsistent with duty to get out of a difficulty in this way?" Suppose however that he resolves to do so: then the maxim of his action would be expressed thus: "When I think myself in want of money, I will borrow money and promise to repay it,

although I know that I never can do so." Now this principle of self-love or of one's own advantage may perhaps be consistent with my whole future welfare; but the question now is, "Is it right?" I change then the suggestion of self-love into a universal law, and state the question thus: "How would it be if my maxim were a universal law?" Then I see at once that it could never hold as a universal law of nature, but would necessarily contradict itself. For supposing it to be a universal law that everyone when he thinks himself in a difficulty should be able to promise whatever he pleases, with the purpose of not keeping his promise, the promise itself would become impossible, as well as the end that one might have in view in it, since no one would consider that anything was promised to him, but would ridicule all such statements as vain pretences.

3. A third finds in himself a talent which with the help of some culture might make him a useful man in many respects. But he finds himself in comfortable circumstances and prefers to indulge in pleasure rather than to take pains in enlarging and improving his happy natural capacities. He asks, however, whether his maxim of neglect of his natural gifts, besides agreeing with his inclination to indulgence, agrees also with what is called duty. He sees then that a system of nature could indeed subsist with such a universal law although men (like the South Sea islanders) should let their talents rest and resolve to devote their lives merely to idleness, amusement, and propagation of their species—in a word, to enjoyment; but he cannot possibly will that this should be a universal law of nature, or be implanted in us as such by a natural instinct. For, as a rational being, he necessarily wills that his faculties be developed, since they serve him and have been given him, for all sorts of possible purposes.

4. A fourth, who is in prosperity, while he sees that others have to contend with great wretchedness and that he could help them, thinks: "What concern is it of mine? Let everyone be as happy as Heaven pleases, or as he can make himself; I will take nothing from him nor even envy him, only I do not wish to contribute anything to his welfare or to his assistance in distress!" Now no doubt if such a mode of thinking

were a universal law, the human race might very well subsist and doubtless even better than in a state in which everyone talks of sympathy and goodwill, or even takes care occasionally to put it into practice, but, on the other side, also cheats when he can, betrays the rights of men, or otherwise violates them. But although it is possible that a universal law of nature might exist in accordance with that maxim, it is impossible to will that such a principle should have the universal validity of a law of nature. For a will which resolved this would contradict itself, inasmuch as many cases might occur in which one would have need of the love and sympathy of others, and in which, by such a law of nature, sprung from his own will, he would deprive himself of all hope of the aid he desires.

These are a few of the many actual duties, or at least what we regard as such, which obviously fall into two classes on the one principle that we have laid down. We must be able to will that a maxim of our action should be a universal law. This is the canon of the moral appreciation of the action generally. Some actions are of such a character that their maxim cannot without contradiction be even conceived as a universal law of nature, far from it being possible that we should will that it should be so. In others this intrinsic impossibility is not found, but still it is impossible to will that their maxim should be raised to the universality of a law of nature, since such a will would contradict itself. It is easily seen that the former violate strict or rigorous (inflexible) duty; the latter only laxer (meritorious) duty. Thus it has been completely shown how all duties depend as regards the nature of the obligation (not the object of the action) on the same principle.

* * *

Now I say: man and generally any rational being exists as an end in himself, not merely as a means to be arbitrarily used by this or that will, but in all his actions, whether they concern himself or other rational beings, must be always regarded at the same time as an end. All objects of the inclinations have only a conditional worth, for if the inclinations and the wants founded on them did not exist, then their object would be without value. But the inclinations, themselves being sources of want, are so far from having an absolute worth for which they should be desired that on the contrary it must be the universal wish of every rational being to be wholly free from them. Thus the worth of any object which is to be acquired by our action is always conditional. Beings whose existence depends not on our will but on nature's, have nevertheless, if they are irrational beings, only a relative value as means, and are therefore called things; rational beings, on the contrary, are called persons, because their very nature points them out as ends in themselves, that is as something which must not be used merely as means, and so far therefore restricts freedom of actions (and is an object of respect). These, therefore, are not merely subjective ends whose existence has a worth for us as an effect of our action, but objective ends, that is, things whose existence is an end in itself; an end moreover for which no other can be substituted, which they should subserve merely as means, for otherwise nothing whatever would possess absolute worth; but if all worth were conditioned and therefore contingent, then there would be no supreme practical principle of reason whatever.

If then there is a supreme practical principle or, in respect of the human will, a categorical imperative, it must be one which, being drawn from the conception of that which is necessarily an end for everyone because it is an end in itself, constitutes an objective principle of will, and can therefore serve as a universal practical law. The foundation of this principle is: rational nature exists as an end in itself. Man necessarily conceives his own existence as being so; so far then this is a subjective principle of human actions. But every other rational being regards its existence similarly, just on the same rational principle that holds for me: so that it is at the same time an objective principle, from which as a supreme practical law all laws of the will must be capable of being deduced. Accordingly the practical imperative will be as follows: So act as to treat humanity, whether in thine own person or in that of any other, in every case as an end withal, never as means only. We will now inquire whether this can be practically carried out.

* * *

To abide by the previous examples:

Firstly, under the head of necessary duty to oneself: He who contemplates suicide should ask himself whether his action can be consistent with the idea of humanity as an end in itself. If he destroys himself in order to escape from painful circumstances, he uses a person merely as a mean to maintain a tolerable condition up to the end of life. But a man is not a thing, that is to say, something which can be used merely as means, but must in all his actions be always considered as an end in himself. I cannot, therefore, dispose in any way of a man in my own person so as to mutilate him, to damage or kill him. (It belongs to ethics proper to define this principle more precisely, so as to avoid all misunderstanding, for example, as to the amputation of the limbs in order to preserve myself as to exposing my life to danger with a view to preserve it, etc. This question is therefore omitted here.)

Secondly, as regards necessary duties, or those of strict obligation, towards others: He who is thinking of making a lying promise to others will see at once that he would be using another man merely as a mean, without the latter containing at the same time the end in himself. For he whom I propose by such a promise to use for my own purposes cannot possibly assent to my mode of acting towards him and, therefore, cannot himself contain the end of this action. This violation of the principle of humanity in other men is more obvious if we take in examples of attacks on the freedom and property of others. For then it is clear that he who transgresses the rights of men intends to use the person of others merely as a means, without considering that as rational beings they ought always to be esteemed also as ends, that is, as beings who must be capable of containing in themselves the end of the very same action.

* * *

Thirdly, as regards contingent (meritorious) duties to oneself: It is not enough that the action does not violate humanity in our own person as an end in itself, it must also harmonize with it. Now there are in humanity capacities of greater perfection, which belong to the end that nature has in view in regard to humanity in ourselves as the subject: to neglect these might perhaps be consistent with the maintenance of humanity as an end in itself, but not with the advancement of this end.

* * *

Looking back now on all previous attempts to discover the principle of morality, we need not wonder why they all failed. It was seen that man was bound to laws by duty, but it was not observed that the laws to which he is subject are only those of his own giving, though at the same time they are universal, and that he is only bound to act in conformity with his own will; a will, however, which is designed by nature to give universal laws. For when one has conceived man only as subject to a law (no matter what), then this law required some interest, either by way of attraction or constraint, since it did not originate as a law from his own will, but this will was according to a law obliged by something else to act in a certain manner. Now by this necessary consequence all the labour spent in finding a supreme principle of duty was irrevocably lost. For men never elicited duty, but only a necessity of acting from a certain interest. Whether this interest was private or otherwise, in any case the imperative must be conditional and could not by any means be capable of being a moral command. I will therefore call this the principle of autonomy of the will, in contrast with every other which I accordingly reckon as heteronomy.

The conception of the will of every rational being as one which must consider itself as giving in all the maxims of its will universal laws, so as to judge itself and its actions from this point of view—this conception leads to another which depends on it and is very fruitful, namely that of a kingdom of ends.

By a kingdom I understand the union of different rational beings in a system by common laws. Now since it is by laws that ends are determined as regards their universal validity, hence, if we abstract from the personal differences of rational beings and likewise from all the content of their private ends, we shall be able to conceive all ends combined in a systematic whole (including both rational beings as ends in themselves, and also the special ends which each

may propose to himself), that is to say, we can conceive a kingdom of ends, which on the preceding principles is possible.

For all rational beings come under the law that each of them must treat itself and all others never merely as means, but in every case at the same time as ends in themselves. Hence results a systematic union of rational being by common objective laws, that is, a kingdom which may be called a kingdom of ends, since what these laws have in view is just the relation of these beings to one another as ends and means. It is certainly only an ideal.

A rational being belongs as a member to the kingdom of ends when, although giving universal laws in it, he is also himself subject to these laws. He belongs to it as sovereign when, while giving laws, he is not subject to the will of any other.

A rational being must always regard himself as giving laws either as member or as sovereign in a kingdom of ends which is rendered possible by the freedom of will. He cannot, however, maintain the latter position merely by the maxims of his will, but only in case he is a completely independent being without wants and with unrestricted power adequate to his will.

Morality consists then in the reference of all action to the legislation which alone can render a kingdom of ends possible. This legislation must be capable of existing in every rational being and of emanating from his will, so that the principle of this will is never to act on any maxim which could not without contradiction be also a universal law and, accordingly, always so to act that the will could at the same time regard itself as giving in its maxims universal laws. If now the maxims of rational beings are not by their own nature coincident with this objective principle, then the necessity of acting on it is called practical necessitation, that is, duty. Duty does not apply to the sovereign in the kingdom of ends, but it does to every member of it and to all in the same degree.

* * *

From Summa Theologica, First Part of the Second Part

St. Thomas Aquinas

QUESTION 91.
OF THE VARIOUS KINDS OF LAW.

* * *

First Article.
Whether There Is an Eternal Law?

Objection 1. It would seem that there is no eternal law. Because every law is imposed on someone. But there was not someone from eternity on whom a law could be imposed: since God alone was from eternity. Therefore no law is eternal.

Obj. 2. Further, promulgation is essential to law. But promulgation could not be from eternity: because there was no one to whom it could be promulgated from eternity. Therefore no law can be eternal.

Obj. 3. Further, a law implies order to an end. But nothing ordained to an end is eternal: for the last end alone is eternal. Therefore no law is eternal.

On the contrary, Augustine says: *That Law which is the Supreme Reason cannot be understood to be otherwise than unchangeable and eternal.*

I answer that . . . a law is nothing else but a dictate of practical reason emanating from the ruler who governs a perfect community. Now it is evident, granted that the world is ruled by Divine Providence . . . that the whole community of the universe is governed by Divine Reason. Wherefore the very Idea of the government of things in God the Ruler of the universe, has the nature of a law. And since the Divine Reason's conception of things is not subject to time but is eternal, according to Proverbs 8.23, therefore it is that this kind of law must be called eternal.

Reply Obj. 1. Those things that are not in themselves, exist with God, inasmuch as they are foreknown and preordained by Him, according to

Thomas Aquinas, *Summa Theologica*, First Part of the Second Part, Questions 91 and 94 (edited). Translated by Fathers of the English Dominican Province, 1911.

Romans 4:17: *Who calls those things that are not, as those that are.* Accordingly the eternal concept of the Divine law bears the character of an eternal law, in so far as it is ordained by God to the government of things foreknown by Him.

Reply Obj. 2. Promulgation is made by word of mouth or in writing; and in both ways the eternal law is promulgated: because both the Divine Word and the writing of the Book of Life are eternal. But the promulgation cannot be from eternity on the part of the creature that hears or reads.

Reply Obj. 3. The law implies order to the end actively, in so far as it directs certain things to the end; but not passively—that is to say, the law itself is not ordained to the end—except accidentally, in a governor whose end is extrinsic to him, and to which end his law must needs be ordained. But the end of the Divine government is God Himself, and His law is not distinct from Himself. Wherefore the eternal law is not ordained to another end.

Second Article.
Whether There Is in Us a Natural Law?

Objection 1. It would seem that there is no natural law in us. Because man is governed sufficiently by the eternal law: for Augustine says that *the eternal law is that by which it is right that all things should be most orderly.* But nature does not abound in superfluities as neither does she fail in necessaries. Therefore no law is natural to man.

Obj. 2. Further, by the law man is directed, in his acts, to the end . . . But the directing of human acts to their end is not a function of nature, as is the case in irrational creatures, which act for an end solely by their natural appetite; whereas man acts for an end by his reason and will. Therefore no law is natural to man.

Obj. 3. Further, the more a man is free, the less is he under the law. But man is freer than all the animals, on account of his free-will, with which he is endowed above all other animals. Since therefore other animals are not subject to a natural law, neither is man subject to a natural law.

On the contrary, A gloss on Romans 2.14: *When the Gentiles, who have not the law, do by nature those things that are of the law,* comments as follows: *Although they have no written law, yet they have the natural law, whereby each one knows, and is conscious of, what is good and what is evil.*

I answer that . . . law, being a rule and measure, can be in a person in two ways: in one way, as in him that rules and measures; in another way, as in that which is ruled and measured, since a thing is ruled and measured, in so far as it partakes of the rule or measure. Wherefore, since all things subject to Divine providence are ruled and measured by the eternal law . . . ; it is evident that all things partake somewhat of the eternal law, in so far as, namely, from its being imprinted on them, they derive their respective inclinations to their proper acts and ends. Now among all others, the rational creature is subject to Divine providence in the most excellent way, in so far as it partakes of a share of providence, by being provident both for itself and for others. Wherefore it has a share of the Eternal Reason, whereby it has a natural inclination to its proper act and end: and this participation of the eternal law in the rational creature is called the natural law. Hence the Psalmist after saying (Psalms 4.6): *Offer up the sacrifice of justice,* as though someone asked what the works of justice are, adds: *Many say, Who showeth us good things?* in answer to which question he says: *The light of Thy countenance, O Lord, is signed upon us:* thus implying that the light of natural reason, whereby we discern what is good and what is evil, which is the function of the natural law, is nothing else than an imprint on us of the Divine light. It is therefore evident that the natural law is nothing else than the rational creature's participation of the eternal law.

Reply Obj. 1. This argument would hold, if the natural law were something different from the eternal law: whereas it is nothing but a participation thereof, as stated above.

Reply Obj. 2. Every act of reason and will in us is based on that which is according to nature . . . : for every act of reasoning is based on principles that are known naturally, and every act of appetite in respect of the means is derived from the natural appetite in respect of the last end. Accordingly the first direction of our acts to their end must needs be in virtue of the natural law.

Reply Obj. 3. Even irrational animals partake in their own way of the Eternal Reason, just as the rational creature does. But because the rational creature partakes thereof in an intellectual and rational manner, therefore the participation of the eternal law in the rational creature is properly called a law, since a law is something pertaining to reason . . . Irrational creatures, however, do not partake thereof in a rational manner, wherefore there is no participation of the eternal law in them, except by way of similitude.

Third Article.
Whether There Is a Human Law?

Objection 1. It would seem that there is not a human law. For the natural law is a participation of the eternal law . . . Now through the eternal law *all things are most orderly,* as Augustine states. Therefore the natural law suffices for the ordering of all human affairs. Consequently there is no need for a human law.

Obj. 2. Further, a law bears the character of a measure. . . . But human reason is not a measure of things, but vice versa. . . . Therefore no law can emanate from human reason.

Obj. 3. Further, a measure should be most certain. . . . But the dictates of human reason in matters of conduct are uncertain, according to Book of Wisdom 9.14: *The thoughts of mortal men are fearful, and our counsels uncertain.* Therefore no law can emanate from human reason.

On the contrary, Augustine distinguishes two kinds of law, the one eternal, the other temporal, which he calls human.

I answer that . . . a law is a dictate of the practical reason. Now it is to be observed that the same procedure takes place in the practical and in the speculative reason: for each proceeds from principles to conclusions . . . Accordingly we conclude that just as, in the speculative reason, from naturally known indemonstrable principles, we draw the conclusions of the various sciences, the knowledge of which is not imparted to us by nature, but acquired by the efforts of reason, so too it is from the precepts of the natural law, as from general and indemonstrable principles, that the human reason needs to proceed to the more particular determination of certain matters. These particular determinations, devised by human reason, are called human laws, provided the other essential conditions of law be observed . . . Wherefore Tully [Cicero] says in his *Rhetoric* that *justice has its source in nature; thence certain things came into custom by reason of their utility; afterwards these things which emanated from nature and were approved by custom, were sanctioned by fear and reverence for the law.*

Reply Obj. 1. The human reason cannot have a full participation of the dictate of the Divine Reason, but according to its own mode, and imperfectly. Consequently, as on the part of the speculative reason, by a natural participation of Divine Wisdom, there is in us the knowledge of certain general principles, but not proper knowledge of each single truth, such as that contained in the Divine Wisdom; so too, on the part of the practical reason, man has a natural participation of the eternal law, according to certain general principles, but not as regards the particular determinations of individual cases, which are, however, contained in the eternal law. Hence the need for human reason to proceed further to sanction them by law.

Reply Obj. 2. Human reason is not, of itself, the rule of things: but the principles impressed on it by nature, are general rules and measures of all things relating to human conduct, whereof the natural reason is the rule and measure, although it is not the measure of things that are from nature.

Reply Obj. 3. The practical reason is concerned with practical matters, which are singular and contingent: but not with necessary things, with which the speculative reason is concerned. Wherefore human laws cannot have that inerrancy that belongs to the demonstrated conclusions of sciences. Nor is it necessary for every measure to be altogether unerring

and certain, but according as it is possible in its own particular genus.

Fourth Article.
Whether There Was Any Need for a Divine Law?

Objection 1. It would seem that there was no need for a Divine law. Because . . . the natural law is a participation in us of the eternal law. But the eternal law is a Divine law . . . Therefore there was no need for a Divine law in addition to the natural law, and human laws derived therefrom.

Obj. 2. Further, it is written (Ecclesiasticus 15.14) that *God left man in the hand of his own counsel.* Now counsel is an act of reason . . . Therefore man was left to the direction of his reason. But a dictate of human reason is a human law . . . Therefore there is no need for man to be governed also by a Divine law.

Obj. 3. Further, human nature is more self-sufficing than irrational creatures. But irrational creatures have no Divine law besides the natural inclination impressed on them. Much less, therefore, should the rational creature have a Divine law in addition to the natural law.

On the contrary, David prayed God to set His law before him, saying (Psalms 118.33): *Set before me for a law the way of Thy justifications, O Lord.*

I answer that, Besides the natural and the human law it was necessary for the directing of human conduct to have a Divine law. And this for four reasons. First, because it is by law that man is directed how to perform his proper acts in view of his last end. And indeed if man were ordained to no other end than that which is proportionate to his natural faculty, there would be no need for man to have any further direction of the part of his reason, besides the natural law and human law which is derived from it. But since man is ordained to an end of eternal happiness which is inproportionate to man's natural faculty . . . therefore it was necessary that, besides the natural and the human law, man should be directed to his end by a law given by God.

Secondly, because, on account of the uncertainty of human judgment, especially on contingent and particular matters, different people form different judgments on human acts; whence also different and contrary laws result. In order, therefore, that man may know without any doubt what he ought to do and what he ought to avoid, it was necessary for man to be directed in his proper acts by a law given by God, for it is certain that such a law cannot err.

Thirdly, because man can make laws in those matters of which he is competent to judge. But man is not competent to judge of interior movements, that are hidden, but only of exterior acts which appear: and yet for the perfection of virtue it is necessary for man to conduct himself aright in both kinds of acts. Consequently human law could not sufficiently curb and direct interior acts; and it was necessary for this purpose that a Divine law should supervene.

Fourthly, because, as Augustine says, human law cannot punish or forbid all evil deeds: since while aiming at doing away with all evils, it would do away with many good things, and would hinder the advance of the common good, which is necessary for human intercourse. In order, therefore, that no evil might remain unforbidden and unpunished, it was necessary for the Divine law to supervene, whereby all sins are forbidden.

And these four causes are touched upon in Psalms 118.8, where it is said: *The law of the Lord is unspotted,* i.e. allowing no foulness of sin; *converting souls,* because it directs not only exterior, but also interior acts; *the testimony of the Lord is faithful,* because of the certainty of what is true and right; *giving wisdom to little ones,* by directing man to an end supernatural and Divine.

Reply Obj. 1. By the natural law the eternal law is participated proportionately to the capacity of human nature. But to his supernatural end man needs to be directed in a yet higher way. Hence the additional law given by God, whereby man shares more perfectly in the eternal law.

Reply Obj. 2. Counsel is a kind of inquiry: hence it must proceed from some principles. Nor is it enough for it to proceed from principles imparted by nature, which are the precepts of the natural law, for the reasons given above: but there is need for certain additional principles, namely, the precepts of the Divine law.

Reply Obj. 3. Irrational creatures are not ordained to an end higher than that which is proportionate to their natural powers: consequently the comparison fails.

Fifth Article.
Whether There Is But One Divine Law?

Objection 1. It would seem that there is but one Divine law. Because, where there is one king in one kingdom there is but one law. Now the whole of mankind is compared to God as to one king, according to Psalms 46.8: *God is the King of all the earth.* Therefore there is but one Divine law.

Obj. 2. Further, every law is directed to the end which the lawgiver intends for those for whom he makes the law. But God intends one and the same thing for all men; since according to 1 Timothy 2.4: *He will have all men to be saved, and to come to the knowledge of the truth.* Therefore there is but one Divine law.

Obj. 3. Further, the Divine law seems to be more akin to the eternal law, which is one, than the natural law, according as the revelation of grace is of a higher order than natural knowledge. Therefore much more is the Divine law but one.

On the contrary, The Apostle says (Hebrews 7.12): *The priesthood being translated, it is necessary that a translation also be made of the law.* But the priesthood is twofold, as stated in the same passage, viz. the levitical priesthood, and the priesthood of Christ. Therefore the Divine law is twofold, namely the Old Law and the New Law.

I answer that . . . distinction is the cause of number. Now things may be distinguished in two ways. First, as those things that are altogether specifically different, e.g., a horse and an ox. Secondly, as perfect and imperfect in the same species, e.g., a boy and a man: and in this way the Divine law is divided into Old and New. Hence the Apostle (Galatians 3:24, 25) compares the state of man under the Old Law to that of a child *under a pedagogue;* but the state under the New Law, to that of a full grown man, who is *no longer under a pedagogue.*

Now the perfection and imperfection of these two laws is to be taken in connection with the three conditions pertaining to law, as stated above. For, in the first place, it belongs to law to be directed to the common good as to its end . . . This good may be twofold. It may be a sensible and earthly good; and to this, man was directly ordained by the Old Law: wherefore, at the very outset of the law, the people were invited to the earthly kingdom of the Chananaeans (Exodus 3.8, 17). Again it may be an intelligible and heavenly good: and to this, man is ordained by the New Law. Wherefore, at the very beginning of His preaching, Christ invited men to the kingdom of heaven, saying (Matthew 4.17): *Do penance, for the kingdom of heaven is at hand.* Hence Augustine says that *promises of temporal goods are contained in the Old Testament, for which reason it is called old; but the promise of eternal life belongs to the New Testament.*

Secondly, it belongs to the law to direct human acts according to the order of righteousness: wherein also the New Law surpasses the Old Law, since it directs our internal acts, according to Matthew 5.20: *Unless your justice abound more than that of the Scribes and Pharisees, you shall not enter into the kingdom of heaven.* Hence the saying that *the Old Law restrains the hand, but the New Law controls the mind.*

Thirdly, it belongs to the law to induce men to observe its commandments. This the Old Law did by the fear of punishment: but the New Law, by love, which is poured into our hearts by the grace of Christ, bestowed in the New Law, but foreshadowed in the Old. Hence Augustine says that *there is little difference between the Law and the Gospel—fear and love.*

Reply Obj. 1. As the father of a family issues different commands to the children and to the adults, so also the one King, God, in His one kingdom, gave one law to men, while they were yet imperfect, and another more perfect law, when, by the preceding law, they had been led to a greater capacity for Divine things.

Reply Obj. 2. The salvation of man could not be achieved otherwise than through Christ, according to Acts 4:12: *There is no other name . . . given to men, whereby we must be saved.* Consequently the law that brings all to salvation could not be given until after the coming of Christ. But before His coming it was necessary to give to the people, of whom Christ was to be born, a law containing certain rudiments of righteousness unto salvation, in order to prepare them to receive Him.

Reply Obj. 3. The natural law directs man by way of certain general precepts, common to both the perfect and the imperfect: wherefore it is one and the same for all. But the Divine law directs man also in certain particular matters, to which the perfect and imperfect do not stand in the same relation. Hence the necessity for the Divine law to be twofold, as already explained.

* * *

QUESTION 94.
OF THE NATURAL LAW.

First Article.
Whether the Natural Law Is a Habit?

Objection 1. It would seem that the natural law is a habit. Because, as the Philosopher [Aristotle] says, *there are three things in the soul: power, habit, and passion.* But the natural law is not one of the soul's powers: nor is it one of the passions; as we may see by going through them one by one. Therefore the natural law is a habit.

Obj. 2. Further, Basil says that the conscience or *synderesis is the law of our mind;* which can only apply to the natural law. But the *synderesis* is a habit. . . . Therefore the natural law is a habit.

Obj. 3. Further, the natural law abides in man always . . . But man's reason, which the law regards, does not always think about the natural law. Therefore the natural law is not an act, but a habit.

On the contrary, Augustine says that *a habit is that whereby something is done when necessary.* But such is not the natural law: since it is in infants and in the damned who cannot act by it. Therefore the natural law is not a habit.

I answer that, A thing may be called a habit in two ways. First, properly and essentially: and thus the natural law is not a habit. For . . . the natural law is something appointed by reason, just as a proposition is a work of reason. Now that which a man does is not the same as that whereby he does it: for he makes a becoming speech by the habit of grammar. Since then a habit is that by which we act, a law cannot be a habit properly and essentially.

Secondly, the term habit may be applied to that which we hold by a habit: thus faith may mean that which we hold by faith. And accordingly, since the precepts of the natural law are sometimes considered by reason actually, while sometimes they are in the reason only habitually, in this way the natural law may be called a habit. Thus, in speculative matters, the indemonstrable principles are not the habit itself whereby we hold those principles, but are the principles the habit of which we possess.

Reply Obj. 1. The Philosopher [Aristotle] proposes to discover the genus of virtue; and since it is evident that virtue is a principle of action, he mentions only those things which are principles of human acts, viz. powers, habits and passions. But there are other things in the soul besides these three: there are acts; thus *to will* is in the one that wills; again, things known are in the knower; moreover its own natural properties are in the soul, such as immortality and the like.

Reply Obj. 2. *Synderesis* is said to be the law of our mind, because it is a habit containing the precepts of the natural law, which are the first principles of human actions.

Reply Obj. 3. This argument proves that the natural law is held habitually; and this is granted.

To the argument advanced in the contrary sense we reply that sometimes a man is unable to make use of that which is in him habitually, on account of some impediment: thus, on account of sleep, a man is unable to use the habit of science. In like manner, through the deficiency of his age, a child cannot use the habit of understanding of principles, or the natural law, which is in him habitually.

Second Article.
Whether the Natural Law Contains Several Precepts, or Only One?

Objection 1. It would seem that the natural law contains, not several precepts, but one only. For law

is a kind of precept. . . . If therefore there were many precepts of the natural law, it would follow that there are also many natural laws.

Obj. 2. Further, the natural law is consequent to human nature. But human nature, as a whole, is one; though, as to its parts, it is manifold. Therefore, either there is but one precept of the law of nature, on account of the unity of nature as a whole; or there are many, by reason of the number of parts of human nature. The result would be that even things relating to the inclination of the concupiscible faculty belong to the natural law.

Obj. 3. Further, law is something pertaining to reason . . . Now reason is but one in man. Therefore there is only one precept of the natural law.

On the contrary, The precepts of the natural law in man stand in relation to practical matters, as the first principles to matters of demonstration. But there are several first indemonstrable principles. Therefore there are also several precepts of the natural law.

I answer that . . . the precepts of the natural law are to the practical reason, what the first principles of demonstrations are to the speculative reason; because both are self-evident principles. Now a thing is said to be self-evident in two ways: first, in itself; secondly, in relation to us. Any proposition is said to be self-evident in itself, if its predicate is contained in the notion of the subject: although, to one who knows not the definition of the subject, it happens that such a proposition is not self-evident. For instance, this proposition, *Man is a rational being,* is, in its very nature, self-evident, since who says *man,* says *a rational being*: and yet to one who knows not what a man is, this proposition is not self-evident. Hence it is that, as Boethius says, certain axioms or propositions are universally self-evident to all; and such are those propositions whose terms are known to all, as, *Every whole is greater than its part,* and, *Things equal to one and the same are equal to one another.* But some propositions are self-evident only to the wise, who understand the meaning of the terms of such propositions: thus to one who understands that an angel is not a body, it is self-evident that an angel is not circumscriptively in a place: but this is not evident to the unlearned, for they cannot grasp it.

Now a certain order is to be found in those things that are apprehended universally. For that which, before aught else, falls under apprehension, is *being,* the notion of which is included in all things whatsoever a man apprehends. Wherefore the first indemon strable principle is that *the same thing cannot be affirmed and denied at the same time,* which is based on the notion of *being* and *not-being*: and on this principle all others are based . . . Now as *being* is the first thing that falls under the apprehension simply, so *good* is the first thing that falls under the apprehension of the practical reason, which is directed to action: since every agent acts for an end under the aspect of good. Consequently the first principle of practical reason is one founded on the notion of good, viz. that *good is that which all things seek after.* Hence this is the first precept of law, that *good is to be done and pursued, and evil is to be avoided.* All other precepts of the natural law are based upon this: so that whatever the practical reason naturally apprehends as man's good (or evil) belongs to the precepts of the natural law as something to be done or avoided.

Since, however, good has the nature of an end, and evil, the nature of a contrary, hence it is that all those things to which man has a natural inclination, are naturally apprehended by reason as being good, and consequently as objects of pursuit, and their contraries as evil, and objects of avoidance. Wherefore according to the order of natural inclinations, is the order of the precepts of the natural law. Because in man there is first of all an inclination to good in accordance with the nature which he has in common with all substances: inasmuch as every substance seeks the preservation of its own being, according to its nature: and by reason of this inclination, whatever is a means of preserving human life, and of warding off its obstacles, belongs to the natural law. Secondly, there is in man an inclination to things that pertain to him more specially, according to that nature which he has in common with other animals: and in virtue of this inclination, those things are said to

belong to the natural law, *which nature has taught to all animals,* such as sexual intercourse, education of offspring and so forth. Thirdly, there is in man an inclination to good, according to the nature of his reason, which nature is proper to him: thus man has a natural inclination to know the truth about God, and to live in society: and in this respect, whatever pertains to this inclination belongs to the natural law; for instance, to shun ignorance, to avoid offending those among whom one has to live, and other such things regarding the above inclination.

Reply Obj. 1. All these precepts of the law of nature have the character of one natural law, inasmuch as they flow from one first precept.

Reply Obj. 2. All the inclinations of any parts whatsoever of human nature, e.g. of the concupiscible and irascible parts, in so far as they are ruled by reason, belong to the natural law, and are reduced to one first precept, as stated above: so that the precepts of the natural law are many in themselves, but are based on one common foundation.

Reply Obj. 3. Although reason is one in itself, yet it directs all things regarding man; so that whatever can be ruled by reason, is contained under the law of reason.

Third Article.
Whether All Acts of Virtue Are Prescribed by the Natural Law?

Objection 1. It would seem that not all acts of virtue are prescribed by the natural law. Because . . . it is essential to a law that it be ordained to the common good. But some acts of virtue are ordained to the private good of the individual, as is evident especially in regards to acts of temperance. Therefore not all acts of virtue are the subject of natural law.

Obj. 2. Further, every sin is opposed to some virtuous act. If therefore all acts of virtue are prescribed by the natural law, it seems to follow that all sins are against nature: whereas this applies to certain special sins.

Obj. 3. Further, those things which are according to nature are common to all. But acts of virtue are not common to all: since a thing is virtuous in one, and vicious in another. Therefore not all acts of virtue are prescribed by the natural law.

On the contrary, Damascene says that *virtues are natural.* Therefore virtuous acts also are a subject of the natural law.

I answer that, We may speak of virtuous acts in two ways: first, under the aspect of virtuous; secondly, as such and such acts considered in their proper species. If then we speak of acts of virtue, considered as virtuous, thus all virtuous acts belong to the natural law. For it has been stated that to the natural law belongs everything to which a man is inclined according to his nature. Now each thing is inclined naturally to an operation that is suitable to it according to its form: thus fire is inclined to give heat. Wherefore, since the rational soul is the proper form of man, there is in every man a natural inclination to act according to reason: and this is to act according to virtue. Consequently, considered thus, all acts of virtue are prescribed by the natural law: since each one's reason naturally dictates to him to act virtuously. But if we speak of virtuous acts, considered in themselves, i.e. in their proper species, thus not all virtuous acts are prescribed by the natural law: for many things are done virtuously, to which nature does not incline at first; but which, through the inquiry of reason, have been found by men to be conducive to well-living.

Reply Obj. 1. Temperance is about the natural concupiscences of food, drink and sexual matters, which are indeed ordained to the natural common good, just as other matters of law are ordained to the moral common good.

Reply Obj. 2. By human nature we may mean either that which is proper to man—and in this sense all sins, as being against reason, are also against nature, as Damascene states: or we may mean that nature which is common to man and other animals; and in this sense, certain special sins are said to be against nature; thus contrary to sexual intercourse, which is natural to all animals, is unisexual lust, which has received the special name of the unnatural crime.

Reply Obj. 3. This argument considers acts in themselves. For it is owing to the various conditions of men, that certain acts are virtuous for some, as being proportionate and becoming to them, while they are vicious for others, as being out of proportion to them.

Fourth Article.
Whether the Natural Law Is the Same in All Men?

Objection 1. It would seem that the natural law is not the same in all. For it is stated in the Decretals that *the natural law is that which is contained in the Law and the Gospel.* But this is not common to all men; because, as it is written (Romans 10.16), *all do not obey the gospel.* Therefore the natural law is not the same in all men.

Obj. 2. Further, *Things which are according to the law are said to be just....* But ... nothing is so universally just as not to be subject to change in regard to some men. Therefore even the natural law is not the same in all men.

Obj. 3. Further... to the natural law belongs everything to which a man is inclined according to his nature. Now different men are naturally inclined to different things; some to the desire of pleasures, others to the desire of honors, and other men to other things. Therefore there is not one natural law for all.

On the contrary, Isidore says: *The natural law is common to all nations.*

I answer that ... to the natural law belongs those things to which a man is inclined naturally: and among these it is proper to man to be inclined to act according to reason. Now the process of reason is from the common to the proper ... The speculative reason, however, is differently situated in this matter, from the practical reason. For, since the speculative reason is busied chiefly with the necessary things, which cannot be otherwise than they are, its proper conclusions, like the universal principles, contain the truth without fail. The practical reason, on the other hand, is busied with contingent matters, about which human actions are concerned: and consequently, although there is necessity in the general principles, the more we descend to matters of detail, the more frequently we encounter defects. Accordingly then in speculative matters truth is the same in all men, both as to principles and as to conclusions: although the truth is not known to all as regards the conclusions, but only as regards the principles which are called common notions. But in matters of action, truth or practical rectitude is not the same for all, as to matters of detail, but only as to the general principles: and where there is the same rectitude in matters of detail, it is not equally known to all.

It is therefore evident that, as regards the general principles whether of speculative or of practical reason, truth or rectitude is the same for all, and is equally known by all. As to the proper conclusions of the speculative reason, the truth is the same for all, but is not equally known to all: thus it is true for all that the three angles of a triangle are together equal to two right angles, although it is not known to all. But as to the proper conclusions of the practical reason, neither is the truth or rectitude the same for all, nor, where it is the same, is it equally known by all. Thus it is right and true for all to act according to reason: and from this principle it follows as a proper conclusion, that goods entrusted to another should be restored to their owner. Now this is true for the majority of cases: but it may happen in a particular case that it would be injurious, and therefore unreasonable, to restore goods held in trust; for instance, if they are claimed for the purpose of fighting against one's country. And this principle will be found to fail the more, according as we descend further into detail, e.g. if one were to say that goods held in trust should be restored with such and such a guarantee, or in such and such a way; because the greater the number of conditions added, the greater the number of ways in which the principle may fail, so that it be not right to restore or not to restore.

Consequently we must say that the natural law, as to general principles, is the same for all, both as to rectitude and as to knowledge. But as to certain matters of detail, which are conclusions, as it were, of those general principles, it is the same for all in the majority of cases, both as to rectitude and as to knowledge; and yet in some few cases it may fail, both as to rectitude, by reason of certain obstacles (just as natures subject to generation and corruption

fail in some few cases on account of some obstacle), and as to knowledge, since in some the reason is perverted by passion, or evil habit, or an evil disposition of nature; thus formerly, theft, although it is expressly contrary to the natural law, was not considered wrong among the Germans, as Julius Caesar relates.

Reply Obj. 1. The meaning of the sentence quoted is not that whatever is contained in the Law and the Gospel belongs to the natural law, since they contain many things that are above nature; but that whatever belongs to the natural law is fully contained in them. Wherefore Gratian, after saying that *the natural law is what is contained in the Law and the Gospel,* adds at once, by way of example, *by which everyone is commanded to do to others as he would be done by.*

Reply Obj. 2. The saying of the Philosopher is to be understood of things that are naturally just, not as general principles, but as conclusions drawn from them, having rectitude in the majority of cases, but failing in a few.

Reply Obj. 3. As, in man, reason rules and commands the other powers, so all the natural inclinations belonging to the other powers must needs be directed according to reason. Wherefore it is universally right for all men, that all their inclinations should be directed according to reason.

Fifth Article.
Whether the Natural Law Can Be Changed?

Objection 1. It would seem that the natural law can be changed. Because on Eccliasticus 17.9, *He gave them instructions, and the law of life,* the gloss says: *He wished the law of the letter to be written, in order to correct the law of nature.* But that which is corrected is changed. Therefore the natural law can be changed.

Obj. 2. Further, the slaying of the innocent, adultery, and theft are against the natural law. But we find these things changed by God: as when God commanded Abraham to slay his innocent son (Genesis 22.2); and when he ordered the Jews to borrow and purloin the vessels of the Egyptians (Exodus 12.35); and when He commanded Osee to take to himself *a wife of fornications* (Hosea 1.2). Therefore the natural law can be changed.

Obj. 3. Further, Isidore says that *the possession of all things in common, and universal freedom, are matters of natural law.* But these things are seen to be changed by human laws. Therefore it seems that the natural law is subject to change.

On the contrary, It is said in the Decretals: *The natural law dates from the creation of the rational creature. It does not vary according to time, but remains unchangeable.*

I answer that, A change in the natural law may be understood in two ways. First, by way of addition. In this sense nothing hinders the natural law from being changed: since many things for the benefit of human life have been added over and above the natural law, both by the Divine law and by human laws.

Secondly, a change in the natural law may be understood by way of subtraction, so that what previously was according to the natural law, ceases to be so. In this sense, the natural law is altogether unchangeable in its first principles: but in its secondary principles, which, as we have said, are certain detailed proximate conclusions drawn from the first principles, the natural law is not changed so that what it prescribes be not right in most cases. But it may be changed in some particular cases of rare occurrence, through some special causes hindering the observance of such precepts.

Reply Obj. 1. The written law is said to be given for the correction of the natural law, either because it supplies what was wanting to the natural law; or because the natural law was perverted in the hearts of some men, as to certain matters, so that they esteemed those things good which are naturally evil; which perversion stood in need of correction.

Reply Obj. 2. All men alike, both guilty and innocent, die the death of nature: which death of nature is inflicted by the power of God on account of original sin, according to 1 Kings 2:6: *The Lord killeth and maketh alive.* Consequently, by the command of God, death can be inflicted on any man, guilty or innocent, without any injustice whatever. In like manner adultery is intercourse with another's wife; who is allotted to him by the law emanating from God. Consequently intercourse with any woman, by the com-mand of God, is neither adultery nor fornication. The same applies to theft, which is the taking of another's property. For whatever is taken by the command of God, to Whom all things belong, is not taken against the will of its owner, whereas it is in this that theft consists. Nor is it only in human things, that whatever is commanded by God is right; but also in natural things, whatever is done by God, is, in some way, natural . . .

Reply Obj. 3. A thing is said to belong to the natural law in two ways. First, because nature inclines thereto: e.g. that one should not do harm to another. Secondly, because nature did not bring in the contrary: thus we might say that for man to be naked is of the natural law, because nature did not give him clothes, but art invented them. In this sense, *the possession of all things in common and universal freedom* are said to be of the natural law, because, to wit, the distinction of possessions and slavery were not brought in by nature, but devised by human reason for the benefit of human life. Accordingly the law of nature was not changed in this respect, except by addition.

Sixth Article.
Whether the Law of Nature Can Be Abolished from the Heart of Man?

Objection 1. It would seem that the natural law can be abolished from the heart of man. Because on Romans 2.14, *When the Gentiles who have not the law,* etc. a gloss says that *the law of righteousness, which sin had blotted out, is graven on the heart of man when he is restored by grace.* But the law of righteousness is the law of nature. Therefore the law of nature can be blotted out.

Obj. 2. Further, the law of grace is more efficacious than the law of nature. But the law of grace is blotted out by sin. Much more therefore can the law of nature be blotted out.

Obj. 3. Further, that which is established by law is made just. But many things are enacted by men, which are contrary to the law of nature. Therefore the law of nature can be abolished from the heart of man.

On the contrary, Augustine says: *Thy law is written in the hearts of men, which iniquity itself effaces not.* But the law which is written in men's hearts is the natural law. Therefore the natural law cannot be blotted out.

I answer that ... there belong to the natural law, first, certain most general precepts, that are known to all; and secondly, certain secondary and more detailed precepts, which are, as it were, conclusions following closely from first principles. As to those general principles, the natural law, in the abstract, can nowise be blotted out from men's hearts. But it is blotted out in the case of a particular action, in so far as reason is hindered from applying the general principle to a particular point of practice, on account of concupiscence or some other passion ... But as to the other, i.e. the secondary precepts, the natural law can be blotted out from the human heart, either by evil persuasions, just as in speculative matters errors occur in respect of necessary conclusions; or by vicious customs and corrupt habits, as among some men, theft, and even unnatural vices, as the Apostle states, were not esteemed sinful.

Reply Obj. 1. Sin blots out the law of nature in particular cases, not universally, except perchance in regard to the secondary precepts of the natural law, in the way stated above.

Reply Obj. 2. Although grace is more efficacious than nature, yet nature is more essential to man, and therefore more enduring.

Reply Obj. 3. This argument is true of the secondary precepts of the natural law, against which some legislators have framed certain enactments which are unjust.

CHAPTER 7

Virtue Ethics: Be a Good Person

Consequentialist moral theories are concerned with the consequences of actions, for the consequences determine the moral rightness of conduct. The production of good over evil is the essence of morality. Nonconsequentialist moral theories are concerned with the moral nature of actions, for the right-making characteristics of actions determine the rightness of conduct. Virtue ethics, however, takes a different turn. **Virtue ethics** is a theory of morality that makes virtue the central concern. When confronted with a moral problem, a utilitarian or a Kantian theorist asks, "What should I *do*?" But a virtue ethicist asks, in effect, "What should I *be*?" For the former, moral conduct is primarily a matter of following or applying a moral principle or rule to a particular situation, and morality is mainly duty-based. For the latter, moral conduct is something that emanates from a person's moral virtues, from his or her moral character, not from obedience to moral laws. In this chapter we try to understand both the main attractions and the major criticisms of this virtue-centered approach to ethics and the moral life.

THE ETHICS OF VIRTUE

Most modern virtue ethicists trace their theoretical roots back to the ancients, most notably to Aristotle (384–322 B.C.E.). His ethics is a coherent, virtue-based view that interlocks with his broader philosophical concerns—his theories about causation, society, self, education, mind, and metaphysics. He says the moral life consists not in following moral rules that stipulate right actions but in striving to be a particular kind of person—a virtuous person whose actions stem naturally from virtuous character.

For Aristotle, every living being has an end toward which it naturally aims. Life is teleological; it is meant not just to *be* something but to *aspire toward* something, to fulfill its proper function. What is the proper aim of human beings? Aristotle argues that the true goal of humans—their greatest good—is **eudaimonia,** which means "happiness" or "flourishing" and refers to the full realization of the good life. To achieve *eudaimonia,* human beings must fulfill the function that is natural and distinctive to them: living fully in accordance with reason. The life of reason entails a life of virtue because the virtues themselves are rational modes of behaving. Thus Aristotle says, "Happiness is an activity of the soul in accordance with complete or perfect virtue." The virtuous life both helps human beings *achieve* true happiness and *is the realization of* true happiness. Virtues make you good, *and* they help you have a good life.

A **virtue** is a stable disposition to act and feel according to some ideal or model of excellence. It is a deeply embedded character trait that can affect actions in countless situations. Aristotle distinguishes between intellectual and moral virtues. Intellectual virtues include wisdom, prudence, rationality, and the like. Moral virtues include fairness, benevolence, honesty, loyalty, conscientiousness, and courage. He believes that intellectual virtues can be taught, just as logic and mathematics can be taught. But moral virtues can be learned only through practice:

CRITICAL THOUGHT: Learning Virtues in the Classroom

Years ago the *New York Times* reported that the teaching of traditional virtues such as honesty and civility was becoming more common in public schools. The article highlighted Paul Meck, an elementary school guidance counselor who spent much of his time teaching students about virtues and values. Meck's approach was to visit classrooms and lead discussions on such topics as honesty, friendship, and shoplifting. When he talked to younger students, he played his guitar and sang lyrics that underscored his points. "Whether through song, discussion or simply a straightfor-ward lecture," the reporter noted, "there is an effort afoot to awaken the interest of youngsters in these subjects."*

Would Aristotle approve of the methods cited here (song, discussion, lecture)? Why or why not? What type of virtue education would he approve of? Which approach—Aristotle's or the one mentioned in this news article—do you think would be most effective? Give reasons for your answer.

* Gene I. Maeroff, "About Education; Values Regain Their Popularity," *New York Times*, Science Desk, 10 April 1984.

[M]oral virtue comes about as a result of habit. . . . From this it is also plain that none of the moral virtues arises in us by nature. . . . [B]ut the virtues we get by first exercising them, as also happens in the case of the arts as well. For the things we have to learn before we can do them, we learn by doing them, e.g. men become builders by building and lyreplayers by playing the lyre; so too we become just by doing just acts, temperate by doing temperate acts, brave by doing brave acts.[1]

Aristotle's notion of a moral virtue is what he calls the "**Golden Mean,**" a balance between two behavioral extremes. A moral virtue (courage, for example) is the midpoint between excess (an excess of courage, or foolhardiness) and deficit (a deficit of courage, or cowardice). For Aristotle, then, the virtuous—and happy—life is a life of moderation in all things.

Modern virtue ethicists follow Aristotle's lead in many respects. Some thinkers take issue with his teleological theory of human nature and his concept of a virtue as a mean between opposing tendencies. And some have offered interesting alternatives to his virtue ethics. But almost all

[1] Aristotle, *Nicomachean Ethics,* trans. W. D. Ross, book II, chapter 1, eBooks@Adelaide, 2004.

virtue theories owe a debt to Aristotle in one way or another.

Like Aristotle, contemporary thinkers put the emphasis on quality of character and virtues (character traits), rather than on adherence to particular principles or rules of right action. They are of course concerned with doing the right thing, but moral obligations are derived from virtues. Virtue ethicists are, for example, less likely to ask whether lying is wrong in a particular situation than whether the action or person is honest or dishonest, or whether honesty precludes lying in this case, or whether an exemplar of honesty (say, Gandhi or Jesus) would lie in these circumstances.

Contemporary virtue ethicists are also Aristotelian in believing that a pure duty-based morality of rule adherence represents a barren, one-dimensional conception of the moral life. First, they agree with Aristotle that the cultivation of virtues is not merely a moral requirement—it is a way (some would say the *only* way) to ensure human flourishing and the good life. Second, they maintain that a full-blown ethics must take into account motives, feelings, intentions, and moral wisdom—factors that they think duty-based morality neglects. This view contrasts dramatically with

Kant's duty-based ethics. He argues that to act morally is simply to act out of duty—that is, to do our duty *because* it is our duty. We need not act out of friendship, loyalty, kindness, love, or sympathy. But in virtue ethics, acting from such motivations is a crucial part of acting from a virtuous character, for virtues are stable dispositions that naturally include motivations and feelings. Contrast the action of someone who methodically aids his sick mother solely out of a sense of duty with the person who tends to her mother out of sympathy, love, and loyalty (perhaps in addition to a sense of duty). Most people would probably think that the latter is a better model of the moral life, while the former seems incomplete.

Virtue in Action

If moral rules are secondary in virtue ethics, how does a virtue ethicist make moral decisions or guide his or her conduct or judge the behavior of others? Suppose Helen, a conscientious practitioner of Aristotelian virtue ethics, hears William lie to a friend to avoid paying a debt. She does not have to appeal to a moral rule such as "Do not lie" to know that William's action is an instance of dishonesty (or untruthfulness) and that William himself is dishonest. She can see by his actions that he lacks the virtue of honesty.

But to Helen, honesty is more than just a character trait: it is also an essential part of human happiness and flourishing. In her case, honesty is a virtue that she has cultivated for years by behaving honestly and truthfully in a variety of situations (not just in cases of lying). She has taken such trouble in part because cultivating this virtue has helped her become the kind of person she wants to be. She has developed the disposition to act honestly; acting honestly is part of who she is. She sometimes relies on moral rules (or moral rules of thumb) to make moral decisions, but she usually does not need them, because her actions naturally reflect her virtuous character.

In addition, Helen's trained virtues not only guide her actions, but they also inspire the motivations and feelings appropriate to the actions. Helen avoids dishonest dealings, and she does so because that is what a virtuous person would do, because she has compassion and sympathy for innocent people who are cheated, and because dishonesty is not conducive to human happiness and flourishing.

What guidance can Helen obtain in her strivings toward a moral ideal? Like most virtue ethicists, she looks to moral exemplars—people who embody the virtues and inspire others to follow in their steps. (For exemplars of honesty, Helen has several moral heroes to choose from—Socrates, Gandhi, Jesus, the Buddha, Thomas Aquinas, and many others.) As the philosopher Louis Pojman says of virtue systems,

> The primary focus is not on abstract reason but on ideal types of persons or on actual ideal persons. Discovering the proper moral example and imitating that person or ideal type thus replace casuistic reason as the most significant aspects of the moral life. Eventually, the apprentice-like training in virtue gained by imitating the ideal model results in a virtuous person who spontaneously does what is good.[2]

Evaluating Virtue Ethics

A case can be made for virtue ethics based on how well it seems to explain important aspects of the moral life. Some philosophers, for example, claim that the virtue approach offers a more plausible explanation of the role of motivation in moral actions than duty-based moral systems do. By Kantian lights your conduct may be morally acceptable even if you, say, save a friend's life out of a sense of duty alone (that is, without any sincere regard for your friend). But this motivation—your calculating sense of duty—seems a very cold and anemic motivation indeed. Virtue theorists

---

[2]Louis P. Pojman, *Ethics: Discovering Right and Wrong*, 4th ed. (Belmont, CA: Wadsworth, 2002), 165.

would say that a more natural and morally appropriate response would be to save your friend primarily out of compassion, love, loyalty, or something similar—and these motives are just what we would expect from a virtuous person acting from fully developed virtues.

Some philosophers also remind us that virtue ethics puts primary emphasis on being a good person and living a good life, a life of happiness and flourishing. They say that these aims are obviously central to the moral life and should be part of any adequate theory of morality. Duty-based moral systems, however, pay much less attention to these essential elements.

Many duty-based theorists are willing to concede that there is some truth in both these claims. They believe that motivation for moral action cannot be derived entirely from considerations of duty, just as appropriate motivation cannot be based solely on virtuous character. And they recognize that the moral life involves more than merely honoring rules and principles. As Aristotle insists, there should be room for moral achievement in morality, for striving toward moral ideals. But even if these claims of the virtue ethicist are true, it does not follow that traditional virtue ethics is the best moral theory or that an ethics without duties or principles is plausible.

Virtue-based ethics seems to meet the minimum requirement of coherence, and it appears to be generally consistent with our commonsense moral judgments and moral experience. Nevertheless critics have taken it to task, with most of the strongest criticisms centering on alleged problems with applying the theory—in other words, with usefulness (Criterion 3).

The critics' main contention is that appeals to virtues or virtuous character without reference to principles of duty cannot give us any useful guidance in deciding what to do. Suppose we are trying to decide what to do when a desperately poor stranger steals money from us. Should we have him arrested? Give him even more money? Ignore

the whole affair? According to virtue ethics, we should do what a virtuous person would do, or do what moral exemplars such as Jesus or Buddha would do, or do what is benevolent or conscientious. But what exactly *would* a virtuous person do? Or what precisely *is* the benevolent or conscientious action? As many philosophers see it, the problem is that virtue ethics says that the right action is the one performed by the virtuous person and that the virtuous person is the one who performs the right action. But this is to argue in a circle and to give us no help in figuring out what to do. To avoid this circularity, they say, we must appeal to some kind of moral standard or principle to evaluate the action itself. Before we can decide if a person is virtuous, we need to judge if her actions are right or wrong—and such judgments take us beyond virtue ethics.

Some argue in a similar vein by pointing out that a person may possess all the proper virtues and still be unable to tell right from wrong actions. Dr. Green may be benevolent and just and still not know if stem cell research should be continued or stopped, or if he should help a terminal patient commit suicide, or if he should perform a late-term abortion. Likewise, we know that it is possible for a virtuous person to act entirely from virtue—and still commit an immoral act. This shows, critics say, that the rightness of actions does not necessarily (or invariably) depend on the content of one's character. We seem to have independent moral standards—independent of character considerations—by which we judge the moral permissibility of actions.

The virtue theorist can respond to these criticisms by asserting that there actually is plenty of moral guidance to be had in statements about virtues and vices. According to the virtue ethicist Rosalind Hursthouse,

[A] great deal of specific action guidance could be found in rules employing the virtue and vice terms ("v-rules") such as "Do what is honest/charitable; do not do what is dishonest/uncharitable." (It is a

CRITICAL THOUGHT: Warrior Virtues and Moral Disagreements

A 2005 report from *Voice of America* told of a dispute over the war in Iraq among highly regarded war veterans. Democratic Representative John Murtha, a decorated Marine Corps veteran who fought in Vietnam, was a strong supporter of the military—but thought the war in Iraq was a disaster and demanded that U.S. forces be withdrawn from Iraq within six months. Democratic Senator John Kerry, also a decorated veteran of the Vietnam War, disagreed with Murtha's timetable for troop withdrawal. He proposed that troops start to leave Iraq later, in early 2007. Republican Senator John McCain, a former Navy fighter pilot and POW in the Vietnam conflict, supported the president's view that the troops should stay in Iraq until the job was done.*

Assume that all these men were honorable and had all the appropriate warrior virtues such as courage and loyalty. If they were then comparably virtuous in the ways indicated, how could they have disagreed about the conduct of the war? Suppose they all possessed exactly the same virtues to exactly the same degree and had access to the same set of facts about the war. Would it still have been possible for them to disagree? Why or why not? Do you think that any of these considerations suggest that virtue ethics may be a flawed moral theory? Why or why not?

*Jim Malone, "Waning US Iraq War Support Stirs New Comparisons to Vietnam Conflict," *VOANews.com* (22 November 2005), http://www.51voa.com/VOA_Standard _English/VOA_Standard_3636.html (9 January 2015).

noteworthy feature of our virtue and vice vocabulary that, although our list of generally recognised virtue terms is comparatively short, our list of vice terms is remarkably, and usefully, long, far exceeding anything that anyone who thinks in terms of standard deontological rules has ever come up with. Much invaluable action guidance comes from avoiding courses of action that would be irresponsible, feckless, lazy, inconsiderate, uncooperative, harsh, intolerant, selfish, mercenary, indiscreet, tactless, arrogant . . . and on and on.)[3]

Hursthouse believes we can discover our moral duties by examining terms that refer to virtues and vices, because moral guidance is implicit in these terms.

Another usefulness criticism crops up because of apparent conflicts between virtues. What should you do if you have to choose between performing or not performing a particular action, and each option involves the same two virtues but in contradictory ways? Suppose your best friend is on trial for murder, and under oath you must testify about what you know of the case—and what you know will incriminate her. The question is, Should you lie? If you lie to save your friend, you will be loyal but dishonest. If you tell the truth, you will be honest but disloyal. The virtues of loyalty and honesty conflict; you simply cannot be both loyal and honest. Virtue ethics says you should act as a virtuous person would. But such advice gives you no guidance on how to do that in this particular case. You need to know which virtue is more important in this situation, but virtue ethics does not seem to provide a useful answer.

The proponent of virtue ethics has a ready reply to this criticism: Some duty-based moral theories, such as Kantian ethics, are also troubled by conflicts (conflicts of rules or principles, for example). Obviously the existence of such conflicts is not a fatal flaw in duty-based ethics, and so it must not be in virtue approaches either. When principles seem to conflict, the duty-based theorist must

[3]Rosalind Hursthouse, "Virtue Ethics," *The Stanford Encyclopedia of Philosophy* (Fall 2003 ed.), ed. Edward N. Zalta, http://plato.stanford.edu/archives/fall2003/entries/ethics -virtue/ (9 January 2015).

determine if the conflict is real and, if so, if it can be resolved (by, say, weighting one principle more than another). Virtue ethics, the argument goes, can exercise the same kind of options. Some might observe, however, that incorporating a weighting rule or similar standard into virtue ethics seems to make the theory a blend of duty-based and virtue-based features.

THE ETHICS OF CARE

Associated with virtue ethics is an approach known as the **ethics of care.** The ethics of care is a perspective on moral issues that emphasizes close personal relationships and moral virtues such as compassion, love, and sympathy. It contrasts dramatically with traditional moral theories that are preoccupied with principles, rules, and legalistic moral reasoning. The ethics of care is probably best characterized as an important component of virtue ethics (or of *any* approach to morality), though some prefer to think of it as a full-fledged moral theory in its own right.

Much of the interest in the ethics of care was sparked by research done by the psychologist Carol Gilligan on how men and women think about moral problems.[4] She maintains that men and women think in radically different ways when making moral decisions. According to Gilligan, in moral decision making, men deliberate about rights, justice, and rules; women, on the other hand, focus on personal relationships, caring for others, and being aware of people's feelings, needs, and viewpoints. She dubbed these two approaches the *ethic of justice* and the *ethic of care*. Some feminist thinkers have used this gender distinction as a starting point to advance the new way of looking at ethics known as the ethics of care.

More recent research has raised doubts about whether there really is a gap between the moral

> ### QUICK REVIEW
>
> *virtue ethics*—A theory of morality that makes virtue the central concern.
>
> **eudaimonia**—Happiness, or flourishing.
>
> *virtue*—A stable disposition to act and feel according to some ideal or model of excellence.
>
> *Golden Mean*—Aristotle's notion of a virtue as a balance between two behavioral extremes.
>
> *ethics of care*—A perspective on moral issues that emphasizes close personal relationships and moral virtues such as compassion, love, and sympathy.

thinking styles of men and women. But these findings do not dilute the relevance of caring to ethics. The ethics of care, regardless of any empirical underpinnings, is a reminder that caring is a vital and inescapable part of the moral life—a conclusion that few philosophers would deny. If virtues are a part of the moral life (as they surely are), and if caring (or compassion, sympathy, or love) is a virtue, then there must be a place for caring alongside principles of moral conduct and moral reasoning. The philosopher Annette C. Baier, an early proponent of the ethics of care, makes a case for both care and justice: "It is clear, I think, that the best moral theory has to be a cooperative product of women and men, has to harmonize justice and care. The morality it theorizes about is after all for all persons, for men and women, and will need their combined insights."[5]

LEARNING FROM VIRTUE ETHICS

Why does the ancient moral tradition of virtue ethics persist—and not just persist but thrive, even enjoying a revival in modern times? Many

[4]Carol Gilligan, *In a Different Voice: Psychological Theory and Women's Development* (Cambridge, MA: Harvard University Press, 1982).

[5]Annette C. Baier, "The Need for More Than Justice," *Canadian Journal of Philosophy*, suppl. vol. 13 (1988): 56.

FEMINIST ETHICS

The ethics of care is an example of *feminist ethics*. Feminist ethics is not a moral theory so much as an alternative way of looking at the concepts and concerns of the moral life. It is an approach focused on women's interests and experiences and devoted to supporting the moral equality of women and men.

Feminists are a diverse group with contrasting viewpoints, so it should not be a surprise that they approach feminist ethics in different ways and arrive at different conclusions. Still, some generalizations are possible.

An emphasis on personal relationships. For the most part, traditional moral theories have been concerned with what we could call "public life"—the realm where unrelated individuals try to figure out how to behave toward one another and how to ensure that, among strangers, justice is done, rights are respected, and utility is maximized. The focus has been mostly on moral judgments and theories pertaining to people as separate members of the community, the polity, and the culture. But feminist ethics narrows the area of moral concern down to the interconnected and familiar small group—to the people with whom we have close personal relationships. The relationships of interest are the ties of kinship, the bonds of friendship, or the connections between caregivers and the cared for—the sphere of the domestic and the private. This is the realm of intimate relations, sexual behavior, child rearing, and family struggles—the place we all come from and perhaps never leave, and where we live a large part of our moral lives.

A suspicion of moral principles. Feminist philosophers resist the temptation to map out moral actions according to moral principles. Whereas Kant wants to reduce all moral deliberation to adherence to a single rule (the categorical imperative), feminists demur. They argue that principles such as autonomy, justice, and utility are too general and too unwieldy to be of much use in the complicated, multifaceted arena of the domestic, social, and personal. The principle of autonomy may tell a woman she has freedom of choice, but it has nothing to say about her particular situation and the restraints placed on her by her poverty, culture, religion, upbringing, male relatives, social expectations, financial dependence on her husband or other males, and overwhelming domestic duties.

The rejection of impartiality. Recall that the principle of impartiality is regarded as a defining characteristic of morality itself. Impartiality says that from the moral point of view, all persons are considered equal and should be treated accordingly. But in the domestic sphere we are anything but impartial. We are naturally partial to the people we care about—our family and friends. Typically we would not think of treating our spouse the same way we treat a store clerk or the bus driver. We have moral duties to the former that we do not have to the latter. Feminist ethics tries to take these duties into account instead of ignoring them, as Kant and Mill would have us do.

A greater respect for emotions. As we've seen, Kant has no place for emotions in his theory. Reading our moral duties off the categorical imperative is all that is required. But in feminist ethics, emotions play a larger role. Feminist ethics is more comfortable with moral guides in the form of virtues rather than rules, and the cornerstones of the ethics of care are not rules but feelings. Moral philosophers of all stripes recognize the importance of emotions. They understand that emotions can alert us to moral evil, provide the motivation to pursue the good, and enable us to empathize with the suffering of others. (Moral philosophers also caution that feelings without thinking are blind, and thinking without feelings makes for a sterile morality.)

thinkers would say that virtue ethics is alive and well because it is sustained by an important ethical truth: virtue and character are large, unavoidable constituents of our moral experience. As moral creatures, we regularly judge the moral permissibility of actions—*and* assess the goodness of character. If someone commits an immoral act (kills an innocent human being, for example), it matters to us whether the act was committed out of compassion (as in euthanasia), benevolence, loyalty, revenge, rage, or ignorance. The undeniable significance of virtue in morality has obliged many philosophers to consider how best to accommodate virtues into their principle-based theories of morality or to recast those theories entirely to give virtues a larger role.

The rise of virtue ethics has also forced many thinkers to reexamine the place of principles in morality. If we have virtues, do we need principles? Most philosophers would probably say yes and agree with the philosopher William Frankena that "principles without traits [virtues] are impotent and traits without principles are blind":

> To be or to do, that is the question. Should we construe morality as primarily a following of certain principles or as primarily a cultivation of certain dispositions and traits? Must we choose? It is hard to see how a morality of principles can get off the ground except through the development of dispositions to act in accordance with its principles, else all motivation to act on them must be of an *ad hoc* kind, either prudential or impulsively altruistic. Moreover, morality can hardly be content with a mere conformity to rules, however willing and self-conscious it may be, unless it has no interest in the spirit of its law but only in the letter. On the other hand, one cannot conceive of traits of character except as including dispositions and tendencies to act in certain ways in certain circumstances. Hating involves being disposed to kill or harm, being just involves tending to do just acts (acts that conform to the principle of justice) when the occasion calls. Again, it is hard to see how we could know what traits to encourage or inculcate if we did not subscribe to

principles, for example, to the principle of utility, or to those of benevolence and justice.[6]

Kant would have us act out of duty alone, granting no bonus points for acting from virtue. Utilitarianism doesn't require, but also doesn't reject, virtuous motives. Yet virtue seems to be as much a part of our moral experience as moral disagreements, moral errors, and moral reasoning. The question is not whether we should care about virtues but how much we should care and how we can incorporate them into our lives.

SUMMARY

Virtue ethics is a moral theory that makes virtue the central concern. In virtue ethics, moral conduct is supposed to radiate naturally from moral virtues. That is, moral actions are derived from virtues. A virtue is a stable disposition to act and feel according to an ideal or model of excellence.

Most modern virtue ethicists take their inspiration from Aristotle. He argues that humankind's greatest good is happiness, or *eudaimonia*. To achieve happiness, human beings must fulfill their natural function—to live fully in accordance with reason. To live this way is to cultivate the virtues, for they are rational ways of being and flourishing. Aristotle suggests that a moral virtue is a Golden Mean, a midpoint between two extreme ways of behaving. So he says that the good life is a life in the middle, a life of moderation.

Virtue theorists think that acting out of duty alone is a distortion of true morality. A full-blown morality, they insist, must include motives, emotions, intentions, and moral wisdom. Acting morally means acting from virtue—from the appropriate motives and feelings, taking all the factors of the situation into account.

Virtue-based ethics seems to meet the minimum requirement of coherence, and it fits with our

[6]William K. Frankena, *Ethics*, 2nd ed. (Englewood Cliff, NJ: Prentice-Hall, 1973), 65.

commonsense moral judgments and experience. But it has been accused of not being useful. The main criticism is that appeals to virtue alone (sans principles) give us little or no guidance about how to act. Critics argue that virtue ethics defines virtue in terms of right actions and defines right actions in terms of virtue. But this is circular reasoning and provides no help for making moral decisions. Virtue theorists, however, can reply that guidance in moral decision making is in fact available—it is inherent in statements about virtues and vices.

The ethics of care is a perspective on moral issues that emphasizes personal relationships and the virtues of compassion, love, sympathy, and the like. It can be thought of as an essential element in virtue ethics. The ethics of care is a reminder that caring is a crucial part of the moral life. Many philosophers have acknowledged this fact by trying to incorporate care into moral theories containing principles.

EXERCISES

Review Questions

1. How does virtue ethics differ from duty-based ethics? (p. 136)
2. In what way is Aristotle's virtue ethics considered teleological? (p. 136)
3. What, according to Aristotle, must humans do to achieve *eudaimonia?* (p. 136)
4. What is a virtue? Give three examples of moral virtues. Give two examples of intellectual virtues. (p. 136)
5. What important elements do virtue ethicists think are missing from traditional duty-based ethics? (p. 138)

6. How do virtue ethicists use moral exemplars? (p. 138)
7. Does virtue ethics seem to offer a more plausible explanation of the role of motivation in moral actions than does Kantian ethics? If so, how? (p. 139)
8. What is the chief argument against virtue ethics? How can the virtue ethicist respond? (p. 139)
9. What is the ethics of care? (p. 141)
10. According to Annette Baier, are justice and care compatible? Why or why not? (p. 141)

Discussion Questions

1. Critique Aristotle's virtue ethics theory. What are its strengths and weaknesses?
2. According to Aristotle, the virtuous life helps us *achieve* happiness and *is* happiness. What does this mean?
3. Is Aristotle's notion of the Golden Mean helpful in identifying the virtues in any situation? Why or why not?
4. Kant says that to act morally is to act out of duty. How does this differ from the virtue ethics approach? Are you likely to admire someone who always acts out of duty alone? Why or why not?
5. Compare the advantages and disadvantages of act-utilitarianism and virtue ethics. Which do you think is the better theory? How would you combine the two approaches to fashion a better theory?
6. William Frankena says that morality requires both principles and virtues. Do you agree? Why or why not?

READINGS

From *Nicomachean Ethics*

ARISTOTLE

BOOK I

1

Every art and every inquiry, and similarly every action and pursuit, is thought to aim at some good; and for this reason the good has rightly been declared to be that at which all things aim. But a certain difference is found among ends; some are activities, others are products apart from the activities that produce them. Where there are ends apart from the actions, it is the nature of the products to be better than the activities. Now, as there are many actions, arts, and sciences, their ends also are many; the end of the medical art is health, that of shipbuilding a vessel, that of strategy victory, that of economics wealth. But where such arts fall under a single capacity—as bridle-making and the other arts concerned with the equipment of horses fall under the art of riding, and this and every military action under strategy, in the same way other arts fall under yet others—in all of these the ends of the master arts are to be preferred to all the subordinate ends; for it is for the sake of the former that the latter are pursued. It makes no difference whether the activities themselves are the ends of the actions, or something else apart from the activities, as in the case of the sciences just mentioned.

2

If, then, there is some end of the things we do, which we desire for its own sake (everything else being desired for the sake of this), and if we do not choose everything for the sake of something else (for at that rate the process would go on to infinity, so that our desire would be empty and vain), clearly this must be the good and the chief good. Will not the knowledge of it, then, have a great influence on life? Shall we not, like archers who have a mark to aim at, be more

Aristotle, Books I and II of *Nicomachean Ethics*, trans. W. D. Ross (edited).

likely to hit upon what is right? If so, we must try, in outline at least, to determine what it is, and of which of the sciences or capacities it is the object. It would seem to belong to the most authoritative art and that which is most truly the master art. And politics appears to be of this nature; for it is this that ordains which of the sciences should be studied in a state, and which each class of citizens should learn and up to what point they should learn them; and we see even the most highly esteemed of capacities to fall under this, e.g. strategy, economics, rhetoric; now, since politics uses the rest of the sciences, and since, again, it legislates as to what we are to do and what we are to abstain from, the end of this science must include those of the others, so that this end must be the good for man. For even if the end is the same for a single man and for a state, that of the state seems at all events something greater and more complete whether to attain or to preserve; though it is worth while to attain the end merely for one man, it is finer and more godlike to attain it for a nation or for city-states. These, then, are the ends at which our inquiry aims, since it is political science, in one sense of that term.

3

* * *

Now each man judges well the things he knows, and of these he is a good judge. And so the man who has been educated in a subject is a good judge of that subject, and the man who has received an all-round education is a good judge in general. Hence a young man is not a proper hearer of lectures on political science; for he is inexperienced in the actions that occur in life, but its discussions start from these and are about these; and, further, since he tends to follow his passions, his study will be vain and unprofitable, because the end aimed at is not knowledge but action. It makes no difference whether he is young youthful in character; the defect does not depend on time, but on his living, and pursuing each successive object, as passion directs. For to such persons, as to the incontinent, knowledge brings no profit; but to those who desire and act in accordance with a rational principle knowledge about such matters will be of great benefit. These remarks about the student, the sort of treatment to be expected, and the purpose of the inquiry, may be taken as our preface.

4

Let us resume our inquiry and state, in view of the fact that all knowledge and every pursuit aims at some good, what it is that we say political science aims at and what is the highest of all goods achievable by action. Verbally there is very general agreement; for both the general run of men and people of superior refinement say that it is happiness, and identify living well and doing well with being happy; but with regard to what happiness is they differ, and the many do not give the same account as the wise. For the former think it is some plain and obvious thing, like pleasure, wealth, or honour; they differ, however, from one another—and often even the same man identifies it with different things, with health when he is ill, with wealth when he is poor; but, conscious of their ignorance, they admire those who proclaim some great ideal that is above their comprehension. Now some thought that apart from these many goods there is another which is self-subsistent and causes the goodness of all these as well. To examine all the opinions that have been held were perhaps somewhat fruitless; enough to examine those that are most prevalent or that seem to be arguable.

* * *

5

Let us, however, resume our discussion from the point at which we digressed. To judge from the lives that men lead, most men, and men of the most vulgar type, seem (not without some ground) to identify the good, or happiness, with pleasure; which is the reason why they love the life of enjoyment. For there are, we may say, three prominent types of life—that just mentioned, the political, and thirdly the con-

templative life. Now the mass of mankind are evidently quite slavish in their tastes, preferring a life suitable to beasts, but they get some ground for their view from the fact that many of those in high places share the tastes of Sardanapallus. A consideration of the prominent types of life shows that people of superior refinement and of active disposition identify happiness with honour, for this is, roughly speaking, the end of the political life. But it seems too superficial to be what we are looking for, since it is thought to depend on those who bestow honour rather than on him who receives it, but the good we divine to be something proper to a man and not easily taken from him. Further, men seem to pursue honour in order that they may be assured of their goodness; at least it is by men of practical wisdom that they seek to be honoured, and among those who know them, and on the ground of their virtue; clearly, then, according to them, at any rate, virtue is better. And perhaps one might even suppose this to be, rather than honour, the end of the political life. But even this appears somewhat incomplete; for possession of virtue seems actually compatible with being asleep, or with life-long inactivity, and, further, with the greatest sufferings and misfortunes; but a man who was living so no one would call happy, unless he were maintaining a thesis at all costs. But enough of this; for the subject has been sufficiently treated even in the current discussions. Third comes the contemplative life, which we shall consider later.

The life of money-making is one undertaken under compulsion, and wealth is evidently not the good we are seeking; for it is merely useful and for the sake of something else. And so one might rather take the aforenamed objects to be ends; for they are loved for themselves. But it is evident that not even these are ends; yet many arguments have been thrown away in support of them. Let us leave this subject, then.

* * *

7

Let us again return to the good we are seeking, and ask what it can be. It seems different in different actions and arts; it is different in medicine, in strategy, and in the other arts likewise. What then is the good of each? Surely that for whose sake everything else is done. In medicine this is health, in strategy victory, in architecture a house, in any other sphere something else, and in every action and pursuit the end; for it is for the sake of this that all men do whatever else they do. Therefore, if there is an end for all that we do, this will be the good achievable by action, and if there are more than one, these will be the goods achievable by action.

So the argument has by a different course reached the same point; but we must try to state this even more clearly. Since there are evidently more than one end, and we choose some of these (e.g. wealth, flutes, and in general instruments) for the sake of something else, clearly not all ends are final ends; but the chief good is evidently something final. Therefore, if there is only one final end, this will be what we are seeking, and if there are more than one, the most final of these will be what we are seeking. Now we call that which is in itself worthy of pursuit more final than that which is worthy of pursuit for the sake of something else, and that which is never desirable for the sake of something else more final than the things that are desirable both in themselves and for the sake of that other thing, and therefore we call final without qualification that which is always desirable in itself and never for the sake of something else.

Now such a thing happiness, above all else, is held to be; for this we choose always for self and never for the sake of something else, but honour, pleasure, reason, and every virtue we choose indeed for themselves (for if nothing resulted from them we should still choose each of them), but we choose them also for the sake of happiness, judging that by means of them we shall be happy. Happiness, on the other hand, no one chooses for the sake of these, nor, in general, for anything other than itself.

From the point of view of self-sufficiency the same result seems to follow; for the final good is thought to be self-sufficient. Now by self-sufficient we do not mean that which is sufficient for a man by himself, for one who lives a solitary life, but also for parents, children, wife, and in general for his friends and fellow citizens, since man is born for citizenship.

But some limit must be set to this; for if we extend our requirement to ancestors and descendants and friends' friends we are in for an infinite series. Let us examine this question, however, on another occasion; the self-sufficient we now define as that which when isolated makes life desirable and lacking in nothing; and such we think happiness to be; and further we think it most desirable of all things, without being counted as one good thing among others—if it were so counted it would clearly be made more desirable by the addition of even the least of goods; for that which is added becomes an excess of goods, and of goods the greater is always more desirable. Happiness, then, is something final and self-sufficient, and is the end of action.

Presumably, however, to say that happiness is the chief good seems a platitude, and a clearer account of what it is still desired. This might perhaps be given, if we could first ascertain the function of man. For just as for a flute-player, a sculptor, or an artist, and, in general, for all things that have a function or activity, the good and the 'well' is thought to reside in the function, so would it seem to be for man, if he has a function. Have the carpenter, then, and the tanner certain functions or activities, and has man none? Is he born without a function? Or as eye, hand, foot, and in general each of the parts evidently has a function, may one lay it down that man similarly has a function apart from all these? What then can this be? Life seems to be common even to plants, but we are seeking what is peculiar to man. Let us exclude, therefore, the life of nutrition and growth. Next there would be a life of perception, but it also seems to be common even to the horse, the ox, and every animal. There remains, then, an active life of the element that has a rational principle; of this, one part has such a principle in the sense of being obedient to one, the other in the sense of possessing one and exercising thought. And, as 'life of the rational element' also has two meanings, we must state that life in the sense of activity is what we mean; for this seems to be the more proper sense of the term. Now if the function of man is an activity of soul which follows or implies a rational principle, and if we say 'a so-and-so' and 'a good so-and-so' have a function which is the s' in kind, e.g. a lyre, and a good lyre-player, without qualification in all cases, eminence of goodness being added to the name of the function (for the function of a lyre-player is to play the lyre, and that of a good lyre-player is to do so well): if this is the case, and we state the function of man to be a certain kind of life, and this to be an activity or actions of the soul implying a rational principle, and the function of a good man to be the good and noble performance of these, and if any action is well performed when it is performed in accordance with the appropriate excellence: if this is the case, human good turns out to be activity of soul in accordance with virtue, and if there are more than one virtue, in accordance with the best and most complete.

But we must add 'in a complete life.' For one swallow does not make a summer, nor does one day; and so too one day, or a short time, does not make a man blessed and happy.

* * *

BOOK II
1

Virtue, then, being of two kinds, intellectual and moral, intellectual virtue in the main owes both its birth and its growth to teaching (for which reason it requires experience and time), while moral virtue comes about as a result of habit, whence also its name (ēthikē) is one that is formed by a slight variation from the word ethos (habit). From this it is also plain that none of the moral virtues arises in us by nature; for nothing that exists by nature can form a habit contrary to its nature. For instance the stone which by nature moves downwards cannot be habituated to move upwards, not even if one tries to train it by throwing it up ten thousand times; nor can fire be habituated to move downwards, nor can anything else that by nature behaves in one way be trained to behave in another. Neither by nature, then, nor contrary to nature do the virtues arise in us; rather we are adapted by nature to receive them, and are made perfect by habit.

Again, of all the things that come to us by nature we first acquire the potentiality and later exhibit the activity (this is plain in the case of the senses; for it was not by often seeing or often hearing that we got these senses, but on the contrary we had them before we

used them, and did not come to have them by using them); but the virtues we get by first exercising them, as also happens in the case of the arts as well. For the things we have to learn before we can do them, we learn by doing them, e.g. men become builders by building and lyre-players by playing the lyre; so too we become just by doing just acts, temperate by doing temperate acts, brave by doing brave acts.

This is confirmed by what happens in states; for legislators make the citizens good by forming habits in them, and this is the wish of every legislator, and those who do not effect it miss their mark, and it is in this that a good constitution differs from a bad one.

Again, it is from the same causes and by the same means that every virtue is both produced and destroyed, and similarly every art; for it is from playing the lyre that both good and bad lyre-players are produced. And the corresponding statement is true of builders and of all the rest; men will be good or bad builders as a result of building well or badly. For if this were not so, there would have been no need of a teacher, but all men would have been born good or bad at their craft. This, then, is the case with the virtues also; by doing the acts that we do in our transactions with other men we become just or unjust, and by doing the acts that we do in the presence of danger, and being habituated to feel fear or confidence, we become brave or cowardly. The same is true of appetites and feelings of anger; some men become temperate and good-tempered, others self-indulgent and irascible, by behaving in one way or the other in the appropriate circumstances. Thus, in one word, states of character arise out of like activities. This is why the activities we exhibit must be of a certain kind; it is because the states of character correspond to the differences between these. It makes no small difference, then, whether we form habits of one kind or of another from our very youth; it makes a very great difference, or rather all the difference.

2

Since, then, the present inquiry does not aim at theoretical knowledge like the others (for we are inquiring not in order to know what virtue is, but in order to become good, since otherwise our inquiry would have been of no use), we must examine the nature of actions, namely how we ought to do them; for these determine also the nature of the states of character that are produced, as we have said. Now, that we must act according to the right rule is a common principle and must be assumed—it will be discussed later, i.e. both what the right rule is, and how it is related to the other virtues. But this must be agreed upon beforehand, that the whole account of matters of conduct must be given in outline and not precisely, as we said at the very beginning that the accounts we demand must be in accordance with the subject-matter; matters concerned with conduct and questions of what is good for us have no fixity, any more than matters of health. The general account being of this nature, the account of particular cases is yet more lacking in exactness; for they do not fall under any art or precept but the agents themselves must in each case consider what is appropriate to the occasion, as happens also in the art of medicine or of navigation.

But though our present account is of this nature we must give what help we can. First, then, let us consider this, that it is the nature of such things to be destroyed by defect and excess, as we see in the case of strength and of health (for to gain light on things imperceptible we must use the evidence of sensible things); both excessive and defective exercise destroys the strength, and similarly drink or food which is above or below a certain amount destroys the health, while that which is proportionate both produces and increases and preserves it. So too is it, then, in the case of temperance and courage and the other virtues. For the man who flies from and fears everything and does not stand his ground against anything becomes a coward, and the man who fears nothing at all but goes to meet every danger becomes rash; and similarly the man who indulges in every pleasure and abstains from none becomes self-indulgent, while the man who shuns every pleasure, as boors do, becomes in a way insensible; temperance and courage, then, are destroyed by excess and defect, and preserved by the mean.

But not only are the sources and causes of their origination and growth the same as those of their destruction, but also the sphere of their actualization

will be the same; for this is also true of the things which are more evident to sense, e.g. of strength; it is produced by taking much food and undergoing much exertion, and it is the strong man that will be most able to do these things. So too is it with the virtues; by abstaining from pleasures we become temperate, and it is when we have become so that we are most able to abstain from them; and similarly too in the case of courage; for by being habituated to despise things that are terrible and to stand our ground against them we become brave, and it is when we have become so that we shall be most able to stand our ground against them.

* * *

4

The question might be asked, what we mean by saying that we must become just by doing just acts, and temperate by doing temperate acts; for if men do just and temperate acts, they are already just and temperate, exactly as, if they do what is in accordance with the laws of grammar and of music, they are grammarians and musicians.

Or is this not true even of the arts? It is possible to do something that is in accordance with the laws of grammar, either by chance or at the suggestion of another. A man will be a grammarian, then, only when he has both done something grammatical and done it grammatically; and this means doing it in accordance with the grammatical knowledge in himself.

Again, the case of the arts and that of the virtues are not similar; for the products of the arts have their goodness in themselves, so that it is enough that they should have a certain character, but if the acts that are in accordance with the virtues have themselves a certain character it does not follow that they are done justly or temperately. The agent also must be in a certain condition when he does them; in the first place he must have knowledge, secondly he must choose the acts, and choose them for their own sakes, and thirdly his action must proceed from a firm and unchangeable character. These are not reckoned in as conditions of the possession of the arts, except the bare knowledge; but as a condition of the possess of the virtues knowledge has little or no weight the other conditions count not for a little but for everything, i.e. the very conditions which result from often doing just and temperate acts.

Actions, then, are called just and temperate when they are such as the just or the temperate man would do; but it is not the man who does these that is just and temperate, but the man who also does them as just and temperate men do them. It is well said, then, that it is by doing just acts that the just man is produced, and by doing temperate acts the temperate man; without doing these no one would have even a prospect of becoming good.

But most people do not do these, but take refuge in theory and think they are being philosophers and will become good in this way, behaving somewhat like patients who listen attentively to their doctors, but do none of the things they are ordered to do. As the latter will not be made well in body by such a course of treatment, the former will not be made well in soul by such a course of philosophy.

5

Next we must consider what virtue is. Since things that are found in the soul are of three kinds—passions, faculties, states of character, virtue must be one of these. By passions I mean appetite, anger, fear, confidence, envy, joy, friendly feeling, hatred, longing, emulation, pity, and in general the feelings that are accompanied by pleasure or pain; by faculties the things in virtue of which we are said to be capable of feeling these, e.g. of becoming angry or being pained or feeling pity; by states of character the things in virtue of which we stand well or badly with reference to the passions, e.g. with reference to anger we stand badly if we feel it violently or too weakly, and well if we feel it moderately; and similarly with reference to the other passions.

Now neither the virtues nor the vices are passions, because we are not called good or bad on the ground of our passions, but are so called on the ground of our virtues and our vices, and because we are neither praised nor blamed for our passions (for the man who feels fear or anger is not praised, nor is the man who simply feels anger blamed, but the man who feels it in a certain way), but for our virtues and our vices we are praised or blamed.

Again, we feel anger and fear without choice, but the virtues are modes of choice or involve choice. Further, in respect of the passions we are said to be moved, but in respect of the virtues and the vices we are said not to be moved but to be disposed in a particular way.

For these reasons also they are not faculties; for we are neither called good nor bad, nor praised nor blamed, for the simple capacity of feeling the passions; again, we have the faculties by nature, but we are not made good or bad by nature; we have spoken of this before. If, then, the virtues are neither passions nor faculties, all that remains is that they should be states of character.

Thus we have stated what virtue is in respect of its genus.

6

We must, however, not only describe virtue as a state of character, but also say what sort of state it is. We may remark, then, that every virtue or excellence both brings into good condition the thing of which it is the excellence and makes the work of that thing be done well; e.g. the excellence of the eye makes both the eye and its work good; for it is by the excellence of the eye that we see well. Similarly the excellence of the horse makes a horse both good in itself and good at running and at carrying its rider and at awaiting the attack of the enemy. Therefore, if this is true in every case, the virtue of man also will be the state of character which makes a man good and which makes him do his own work well.

How this is to happen we have stated already, but it will be made plain also by the following consideration of the specific nature of virtue. In everything that is continuous and divisible it is possible to take more, less, or an equal amount, and that either in terms of the thing itself or relatively to us; and the equal is an intermediate between excess and defect. By the intermediate in the object I mean that which is equidistant from each of the extremes, which is one and the same for all men; by the intermediate relatively to us that which is neither too much nor too little—and this is not one, nor the same for all. For instance, if ten is many and two is few, six is the intermediate, taken in terms of the object; for it exceeds and is exceeded by an equal amount; this is intermediate according to arithmetical proportion. But the intermediate relatively to us is not to be taken so; if ten pounds are too much for a particular person to eat and two too little, it does not follow that the trainer will order six pounds; for this also is perhaps too much for the person who is to take it, or too little—too little for Milo, too much for the beginner in athletic exercises. The same is true of running and wrestling. Thus a master of any art avoids excess and defect, but seeks the intermediate and chooses this— the intermediate not in the object but relatively to us.

If it is thus, then, that every art does its work well—by looking to the intermediate and judging its works by this standard (so that we often say of good works of art that it is not possible either to take away or to add anything, implying that excess and defect destroy the goodness of works of art, while the mean preserves it; and good artists, as we say, look to this in their work), and if, further, virtue is more exact and better than any art, as nature also is, then virtue must have the quality of aiming at the intermediate. I mean moral virtue; for it is this that is concerned with passions and actions, and in these there is excess, defect, and the intermediate. For instance, both fear and confidence and appetite and anger and pity and in general pleasure and pain may be felt both too much and too little, and in both cases not well; but to feel them at the right times, with reference to the right objects, towards the right people, with the right motive, and in the right way, is what is both intermediate and best, and this is characteristic of virtue. Similarly with regard to actions also there is excess, defect, and the intermediate. Now virtue is concerned with passions and actions, in which excess is a form of failure, and so is defect, while the intermediate is praised and is a form of success; and being praised and being successful are both characteristics of virtue. Therefore virtue is a kind of mean, since, as we have seen, it aims at what is intermediate.

Again, it is possible to fail in many ways (for evil belongs to the class of the unlimited, as the Pythagoreans conjectured, and good to that of the limited), while to succeed is possible only in one way (for which reason also one is easy and the other difficult—to miss the mark easy, to hit it difficult); for these reasons also, then, excess and defect are characteristic of vice, and the mean of virtue;

For men are good in but one way, but bad in many.

Virtue, then, is a state of character concerned with choice, lying in a mean, i.e. the mean relative to us, this being determined by a rational principle, and by that principle by which the man of practical wisdom would determine it. Now it is a mean between two vices, that which depends on excess and that which depends on defect; and again it is a mean because the vices respectively fall short of or exceed what is right in both passions and actions, while virtue both finds and chooses that which is intermediate. Hence in respect of its substance and the definition which states its essence virtue is a mean, with regard to what is best and right an extreme.

But not every action nor every passion admits of a mean; for some have names that already imply badness, e.g. spite, shamelessness, envy, and in the case of actions adultery, theft, murder; for all of these and suchlike things imply by their names that they are themselves bad, and not the excesses or deficiencies of them. It is not possible, then, ever to be right with regard to them; one must always be wrong. Nor does goodness or badness with regard to such things depend on committing adultery with the right women, at the right time, and in the right way, but simply to do any of them is to go wrong. It would be equally absurd, then, to expect that in unjust, cowardly, and voluptuous action there should be a mean, an excess, and a deficiency; for at that rate there would be a mean of excess and of deficiency, an excess of excess, and a deficiency of deficiency. But as there is no excess and deficiency of temperance and courage because what is intermediate is in a sense an extreme, so too of the actions we have mentioned there is no mean nor any excess and deficiency, but however they are done they are wrong; for in general there is neither a mean of excess and deficiency, nor excess and deficiency of a mean.

7

We must, however, not only make this general st‾ ment, but also apply it to the individual fac‾ among statements about conduct those ⱱ‾

general apply more widely, but those which are particular are more genuine, since conduct has to do with individual cases, and our statements must harmonize with the facts in these cases. We may take these cases from our table. With regard to feelings of fear and confidence courage is the mean; of the people who exceed, he who exceeds in fearlessness has no name (many of the states have no name), while the man who exceeds in confidence is rash, and he who exceeds in fear and falls short in confidence is a coward. With regard to pleasures and pains—not all of them, and not so much with regard to the pains—the mean is temperance, the excess self-indulgence. Persons deficient with regard to the pleasures are not often found; hence such persons also have received no name. But let us call them 'insensible'.

With regard to giving and taking of money the mean is liberality, the excess and the defect prodigality and meanness. In these actions people exceed and fall short in contrary ways; the prodigal exceeds in spending and falls short in taking, while the mean man exceeds in taking and falls short in spending. (At present we are giving a mere outline or summary, and are satisfied with this; later these states will be more exactly determined.) With regard to money there are also other dispositions—a mean, magnificence (for the magnificent man differs from the liberal man; the former deals with large sums, the latter with small ones), an excess, tastelessness and vulgarity, and a deficiency, niggardliness; these differ from the states opposed to liberality, and the mode of their difference will be stated later. With regard to honour and dishonour the mean is proper pride, the excess is known as a sort of 'empty vanity', and the deficiency is undue humility; and as we said liberality was related to magnificence, differing from it by dealing with small sums, so there is a state similarly related to proper pride, being concerned with small honours while that is concerned with great. For it is possible to desire honour as one ought, and more than one ought, and less, and the man who exceeds in his desires is called ambitious, the man who falls short unambitious, while the intermediate person has no name. The dispositions also are nameless, except that that of the ambitious man is called ambition. Hence the people who are at the extremes lay claim to the middle place; and we ourselves sometimes call the intermediate person ambitious and sometimes unambitious, and sometimes praise the ambitious man and sometimes the unambitious. The reason of our doing this will be stated in what follows; but now let us speak of the remaining states according to the method which has been indicated.

With regard to anger also there is an excess, a deficiency, and a mean. Although they can scarcely be said to have names, yet since we call the intermediate person good-tempered let us call the mean good temper; of the persons at the extremes let the one who exceeds be called irascible, and his vice irascibility, and the man who falls short an inirascible sort of person, and the deficiency inirascibility.

There are also three other means, which have a certain likeness to one another, but differ from one another: for they are all concerned with intercourse in words and actions, but differ in that one is concerned with truth in this sphere, the other two with pleasantness; and of this one kind is exhibited in giving amusement, the other in all the circumstances of life. We must therefore speak of these two, that we may the better see that in all things the mean is praiseworthy, and the extremes neither praiseworthy nor right, but worthy of blame. Now most of these states also have no names, but we must try, as in the other cases, to invent names ourselves so that we may be clear and easy to follow. With regard to truth, then, the intermediate is a truthful sort of person and the mean may be called truthfulness, while the pretence which exaggerates is boastfulness and the person characterized by it a boaster, and that which understates is mock modesty and the person characterized by it mock-modest. With regard to pleasantness in the giving of amusement the intermediate person is ready-witted and the disposition ready wit, the excess is buffoonery and the person characterized by it a buffoon, while the man who falls short is a sort of boor and his state is boorishness. With regard to the remaining kind of pleasantness, that which is exhibited in life in general, the man who is pleasant in the right way is friendly and the mean is friendliness, while the man who exceeds is an obsequious person if he has no end in view, a flatterer if he is aiming at his own advantage, and the man who falls short and is unpleasant in all circumstances is a quarrelsome and surly sort of person.

* * *

9

That moral virtue is a mean, then, and in what sense it is so, and that it is a mean between two vices, the one involving excess, the other deficiency, and that it is such because its character is to aim at what is intermediate in passions and in actions, has been sufficiently stated. Hence also it is no easy task to be good. For in everything it is no easy task to find the middle, e.g. to find the middle of a circle is not for every one but for him who knows; so, too, any one can get angry—that is easy—or give or spend money; but to do this to the right person, to the right extent, at the right time, with the right motive, and in the right way, that is not for every one, nor is it easy; wherefore goodness is both rare and laudable and noble.

* * *

The Need for More Than Justice

ANNETTE C. BAIER

In recent decades in North American social and moral philosophy, alongside the development and discussion of widely influential theories of justice, taken as Rawls takes it as the 'first virtue of social institutions,'[1] there has been a counter-movement gathering strength, one coming from some interesting sources. For some of the most outspoken of the diverse group who have in a variety of ways been challenging the assumed supremacy of justice among the moral and social virtues are members of those sections of society whom one might have expected to be especially aware of the supreme importance of justice, namely blacks and women. Those who have only recently seen the correction or partial correction of long-standing racist and sexist injustices to their race and sex, are among the philosophers now suggesting that justice is only one virtue among many, and one that may need the presence of the others in order to deliver its own undenied value. Among these philosophers of the philosophical counterculture, as it were—but an increasingly large counterculture—I include Alasdair MacIntyre, Michael Stocker, Lawrence Blum, Michael Slote, Laurence Thomas, Claudia Card, Alison Jaggar, Susan Wolf and a whole group of men and women, myself included, who have been influenced by the writings of Harvard educational psychologist Carol Gilligan, whose book *In a Different Voice* (Harvard 1982; hereafter D.V.) caused a considerable stir both in the popular press and, more slowly, in the philosophical journals.

Let me say quite clearly at this early point that there is little disagreement that justice is *a* social value of very great importance, and injustice an evil. Nor would those who have worked on theories of justice want to deny that other things matter besides justice. Rawls, for example, incorporates the value of freedom into his account of justice, so that denial of basic freedoms counts as injustice. Rawls also leaves room for a wider theory of the right, of which the theory of justice is just a part. Still, he does claim that justice is the 'first' virtue of social institutions, and it is only that claim about priority that I think has been challenged. It is easy to exaggerate the differences of view that exist, and I want to avoid that. The differences are as much in emphasis as in substance, or we can say that they are differences in tone of voice. But these differences do tend to make a difference in approaches ʼ wide range of topics not just in moral theory ʼ areas like medical ethics, where the discussiᵓ

Annette C. Baier, "The Need for More Than Justice" in *Canadian Journal of Philosophy* Supplementary Vol. 13 (1988): 41–56. Published by University of Calgary Press. Reprinted with permission of University of Calgary Press.

be conducted in terms of patients' rights, of informed consent, and so on, but now tends to get conducted in an enlarged moral vocabulary, which draws on what Gilligan calls the ethics of *care* as well as that of *justice*.

For 'care' is the new buzz-word. It is not, as Shakespeare's Portia demanded, mercy that is to season justice, but a less authoritarian humanitarian supplement, a felt concern for the good of others and for community with them. The 'cold jealous virtue of justice' (Hume) is found to be too cold, and it is 'warmer' more communitarian virtues and social ideals that are being called in to supplement it. One might say that liberty and equality are being found inadequate without fraternity, except that 'fraternity' will be quite the wrong word, if as Gilligan initially suggested, it is *women* who perceive this value most easily. ('Sorority' will do no better, since it is too exclusive, and English has no gender-neuter word for the mutual concern of siblings.) She has since modified this claim, allowing that there are two perspectives on moral and social issues that we all tend to alternate between, and which are not always easy to combine, one of them what she called the justice perspective, the other the care perspective. It is increasingly obvious that there are many male philosophical spokespersons for the care perspective (Laurence Thomas, Lawrence Blum, Michael Stocker) so that it cannot be the prerogative of women. Nevertheless Gilligan still wants to claim that women are most unlikely to take *only* the justice perspective, as some men are claimed to, at least until some mid-life crisis jolts them into 'bifocal' moral vision (see D.V., ch. 6).

Gilligan in her book did not offer any explanatory theory of why there should be any difference between female and male moral outlook, but she did tend to link the naturalness to women of the care perspective with their role as primary care-takers of young children, that is with their parental and specifically maternal role. She avoided the question of whether it is their biological or their social parental role that is relevant, and some of those who dislike her book are worried precisely by this uncertainty. Some find it retrograde to hail as a special sort of moral wisdom an outlook that may be the product of the socially enforced restriction of women to domestic roles (and the reservation of such roles for them alone). For that might seem to play into the hands of those who still favor such restriction. (Marxists, presumably, will not find it so surprising that moral truths might depend for their initial clear voicing on the social oppression, and memory of it, of those who voice the truths.) Gilligan did in the first chapter of D.V. cite the theory of Nancy Chodorow (as presented in *The Reproduction of Mothering* [Berkeley 1978]) which traces what appears as gender differences in personality to early social development, in particular to the effects of the child's primary caretaker being or not being of the same gender as the child. Later, both in 'The Conquistador and the Dark Continent: Reflections on the Nature of Love' (*Daedalus* [Summer 1984]), and 'The Origins of Morality in Early Childhood' (in press), she develops this explanation. She postulates two evils that any infant may become aware of, the evil of detachment or isolation from others whose love one needs, and the evil of relative powerlessness and weakness. Two dimensions of moral development are thereby set—one aimed at achieving satisfying community with others, the other aiming at autonomy or equality of power. The relative predominance of one over the other development will depend both upon the relative salience of the two evils in early childhood, and on early and later reinforcement or discouragement in attempts made to guard against these two evils. This provides the germs of a theory about *why*, given current customs of childrearing, it should be mainly women who are not content with only the moral outlook that she calls the justice perspective, necessary though that was and is seen by them to have been to their hard won liberation from sexist oppression. They, like the blacks, used the language of rights and justice to change their own social position, but nevertheless see limitations in that language, according to Gilligan's findings as a moral psychologist. She reports their discontent with the individualist more or less Kantian moral framework that dominates Western moral theory and which influenced moral psychologists such as Lawrence Kohlberg, to whose conception of moral maturity she seeks an alternative. Since the target of Gilligan's criticism is the dominant Kantian tradition, and since that has been the target also of moral philosophers as diverse in their own views as Bernard Williams, Alasdair MacIntyre, Philippa Foot, Susan Wolf, Claudia Card, her book is of interest as much for its attempt to articulate an alternative to the Kantian justice perspective as for its implicit raising of the question of male bias in Western moral theory, especially liberal-democratic theory. For whether the supposed blind spots of that outlook are due to male bias, or to nonparental bias, or to early traumas of powerlessness or to early resignation to 'detachment' from others, we need first to be persuaded that they *are* blind spots before we will have any interest in their cause and cure. Is justice blind to important social values, or at least only one-eyed? What is it that comes into view from the 'care perspective' that is not seen from the 'justice perspective'?

Gilligan's position here is mostly easily described by contrasting it with that of Kohlberg, against which she developed it. Kohlberg, influenced by Piaget and the Kantian philosophical tradition as developed by John Rawls, developed a theory about typical moral development which saw it to progress from a pre-conventional level, where what is seen to matter is pleasing or not offending parental authority-figures, through a conventional level in which the child tries to fit in with a group, such as a school community, and conform to its standards and rules, to a post-conventional critical level, in which such conventional rules are subjected to tests, and where those tests are of a Utilitarian, or, eventually, a Kantian sort—namely ones that require respect for each person's individual rational will, or autonomy, and conformity to any implicit social contract such wills are deemed to have made, or to any hypothetical ones they would make if thinking clearly. What was found when Kohlberg's questionnaires (mostly by verbal response to verbally sketched moral dilemmas) were applied to female as well as male subjects, Gilligan reports, is that the girls and women not only scored generally lower than the boys and men, but tended to *revert* to the lower stage of the conventional level even after briefly (usually in adolescence) attaining the postconventional level. Piaget's finding that girls were deficient in 'the legal sense' was confirmed.

These results led Gilligan to wonder if there might not be a quite different pattern of development to be discerned, at least in female subjects. She therefore conducted interviews designed to elicit not just how far advanced the subjects were towards an appreciation of the nature and importance of Kantian autonomy, but also to find out what the subjects themselves saw as progress or lack of it, what conceptions of moral maturity they came to possess by the time they were adults. She found that although the Kohlberg version of moral maturity as respect for fellow persons, and for their rights as equals (rights including that of free association), did seem shared by many young men, the women tended to speak in a different voice about morality itself and about moral maturity. To quote Gilligan, 'Since the reality of interconnexion is experienced by women as given rather than freely contracted, they arrive at an understanding of life that reflects the limits of autonomy and control. As a result, women's development delineates the path not only to a less violent life but also to a maturity realized by interdependence and taking care' (D.V., 172). She writes that there is evidence that 'women perceive and construe social reality differently from men, and that these differences center around experiences of attachment and separation . . . because women's sense of integrity appears to be intertwined with an ethics of care, so that to see themselves as women is to see themselves in a relationship of connexion, the major changes in women's lives would seem to involve changes in the understanding and activities of care' (D.V., 171). She contrasts this progressive understanding of care, from merely pleasing others to helping and nurturing, with the sort of progression that is involved in Kohlberg's stages, a progression in the understanding, not of mutual care, but of mutual *respect,* where this has its Kantian overtones of distance, even of some fear for the respected, and where personal autonomy and *in*dependence, rather than more satisfactory interdependence, are the paramount values.

This contrast, one cannot but feel, is one which Gilligan might have used the Marxist language of alienation to make. For the main complaint about the Kantian version of a society with its first virtue justice, constructed as respect for equal rights to formal goods such as having contracts kept, due process, equal opportunity including opportunity to participate in political activities leading to policy and law-making, to basic liberties of speech, free association and assembly, religious worship, is that none of these goods do much to ensure that the people who have and mutually respect such rights will have any other relationships to one another than the minimal relationship needed to keep such a 'civil society' going. They may well be lonely, driven to suicide, apathetic about their work and about participation in political processes, find their lives meaningless and have no wish to leave offspring to face the same meaningless existence. Their rights, and respect for rights, are quite compatible with very great misery, and misery whose causes are not just individual misfortunes and psychic sickness, but social and moral impoverishment.

What Gilligan's older male subjects complain of is precisely this sort of alienation from some dimly glimpsed better possibility for human beings, some richer sort of network of relationships. As one of Gilligan's male subjects put it, 'People have real emotional needs to be attached to something, and equality does not give you attachment. Equality fractures society and places on every person the burden of standing on his own two feet' (D.V., 167). It is not just the difficulty of self-reliance which is complained of, but its socially 'fracturing' effect. Whereas the younger men, in their college years, had seen morality as a matter of reciprocal non-interference, this old man begins to see it as reciprocal attachment. 'Morality is . . . essential . . . for creating the kind of environment, interaction between people, that is a prerequisite to the fulfillment of individual goals. If you want other people not to interfere with your pursuit of whatever you are into, you have to play the game,' says the spokesman for traditional liberalism (D.V., 98). But if what one is 'into' is interconnexion, interdependence rather than an individual autonomy that may involve 'detachment,' such a version of morality will come to seem inadequate. And Gilligan stresses that the interconnexion that her mature women subjects, and some men, wanted to sustain was not merely freely chosen interconnexion, nor interconnexion between equals, but also the sort of interconnexion that can obtain between a child and her unchosen mother and father, or between a child and her unchosen older and younger siblings, or indeed between most workers and their unchosen fellow workers, or most citizens and their unchosen fellow citizens.

A model of a decent community different from the liberal one is involved in the version of moral maturity that Gilligan voices. It has in many ways more in common with the older religion-linked versions of morality and a good society than with the modern Western liberal idea. That perhaps is why some find it so dangerous and retrograde. Yet it seems clear that it also has much in common with what we call Hegelian versions of moral maturity and of social health and malaise, both with Marxist versions and with so-called right-Hegelian views.

Let me try to summarize the main differences, as I see them, between on the one hand Gilligan's version of moral maturity and the sort of social structures that would encourage, express and protect it, and on the other the orthodoxy she sees herself to be challenging. I shall from now on be giving my own interpretation of the significance of her challenges, not merely reporting them. The most obvious point is the challenge to the individualism of the Western tradition, to the fairly entrenched belief in the possibility and desirability of each person pursuing his own good in his own way, constrained only by a minimal formal common good, namely a working legal apparatus that enforces contracts and protects individuals from undue interference by others. Gilligan reminds us that noninterference can, especially for the relatively powerless, such as the very young, amount to neglect, and even between equals can be isolating and alienating. On her less individualist version of individuality, it becomes defined by responses to dependence and to patterns of interconnexion, both chosen and unchosen. It is not something a person *has,* and which she then chooses relationships to suit, but something that develops out of a series of dependencies and interdependencies, and responses to them. This conception of individuality is not flatly at odds with, say, Rawls' Kantian one, but there is at least a difference of tone of voice between speaking as Rawls does of each of us having our own rational life plan, which a just society's moral traffic rules will allow us to follow, and which may or may not include close association with other persons, and speaking as Gilligan does of a satisfactory life as involving 'progress of affiliative relationship' (D.V., 170) where 'the concept of identity expands to include the experience of interconnexion' (D.V., 173). Rawls can allow that progress to Gilligan-style moral maturity may be *a* rational life plan, but not a moral constraint on every life-pattern. The trouble is that it will not do just to say 'let this version of morality be an optional extra. Let us agree on the essential minimum, that is on justice and rights, and let whoever wants to go further and cultivate this more demanding ideal of responsibility and care.' For, first, it cannot be satisfactorily cultivated without closer cooperation from others than respect for rights and justice will ensure, and second, the encouragement of some to cultivate it while others do not could easily lead to exploitation of those who do. It obviously *has* suited some in most societies well enough that others take on the responsibilities of care (for the sick, the helpless, the young) leaving them free to pursue their own less altruistic goods. Volunteer forces of those who accept an ethic of care, operating within a society where the power is exercised and the institutions designed, redesigned, or maintained by those who accept a less communal ethic of minimally constrained self-advancement, will not be the solution. The liberal individualists may be able to 'tolerate' the more communally minded, if they keep the liberals' rules, but it is not so clear that the more communally minded can be content with just those rules, nor be content to be tolerated and possibly exploited.

For the moral tradition which developed the concept of rights, autonomy and justice is the same tradition that provided 'justifications' of the oppression of those whom the primary right-holders depended on to do the sort of work they themselves preferred not to do. The domestic work was left to women and slaves, and the liberal morality for right-holders was surreptitiously supplemented by a different set of demands made on domestic workers. As long as women could be got to assume responsibility for the care of home and children, and to train their children to continue the sexist system, the liberal morality could continue to be the official morality, by turning its eyes away from the contribution made by those it excluded. The long unnoticed moral proletariat were the domestic workers, mostly female. Rights have usually been for the privileged. Talking about laws, and the rights those laws recognize and protect, does not in itself ensure that the group of legislators and rights-holders will not be restricted to some elite. Bills of rights have usually been proclamations of the rights of some in-group, barons, landowners, males, whites, non-foreigners. The 'justice perspective,' and the legal sense that goes with it, are shadowed by their patriarchal past. What did Kant, the great prophet of autonomy, say in his moral theory about women? He said they were incapable of legislation, not fit to vote, that they needed the guidance of more 'rational' males.[2] Autonomy was not for them, only for first-class, really rational persons. It is ironic that Gilligan's original findings in a way confirm Kant's views—it seems that autonomy really may not be for women. Many of them reject that ideal (D.V., 48), and have been found not as good at making rules as are men. But where Kant concludes—'so much the worse for women,' we can conclude—'so much the worse for the male fixation on the special skill of drafting legislation, for the bureaucratic mentality of rule worship, and for the male exaggeration of the importance of independence over mutual interdependence.'

It is however also true that the moral theories that made the concept of a person's rights central were not just the instruments for excluding some persons, but also the instruments used by those who demanded that more and more persons be included in the favored group. Abolitionists, reformers, women, used the language of rights to assert their claims to inclusion in the group of full members of a community. The tradition of liberal moral theory has in fact developed so as to include the women it had for so long excluded, to include the poor as well as rich, blacks and whites, and so on. Women like Mary Wollstonecraft used the male moral theories to good purpose. So we should not be wholly ungrateful for those male moral theories, for all their objectionable earlier content. They were undoubtedly patriarchal, but they also contained the seeds of the challenge, or antidote, to this patriarchal poison.

But when we transcend the values of the Kantians, we should not forget the facts of history—that those values were the values of the oppressors of women. The Christian church, whose version of the moral law Aquinas codified, in his very legalistic moral theory, still insists on the maleness of the God it worships, and jealously reserves for males all the most powerful positions in its hierarchy. Its patriarchical prejudice is open and avowed. In the secular moral theories of men, the sexist patriarchal prejudice is today often less open, not as blatant as it is in Aquinas, in the later natural law tradition, and in Kant and Hegel, but is often still there. No moral theorist today would say that women are unfit to vote, to make laws, or to rule a nation without powerful male advisors (as most queens had), but the old doctrines die hard. In one of the best male theories we have, John Rawls's theory, a key role is played by the idea of the 'head of a household.' It is heads of households who are to deliberate behind a 'veil of ignorance' of historical details, and of details of their own special situation, to arrive at the 'just' constitution for a society. Now of course Rawls does not think or say that these 'heads' are fathers rather than mothers. But if we have really given up the age-old myth of women needing, as Grotius put it, to be under the 'eye' of a more 'rational' male protector and master, then how do families come to have any one 'head,' except by the death or desertion of one parent? They will either be two-headed, or headless. Traces of the old patriarchal poison still remain in even the best contemporary moral theorizing. Few may actually say that women's place is in the home, but there is much muttering, when unemployment figures rise, about how the relatively recent flood of women into the work force complicates the problem, as if it would be a good thing if women just went back home whenever unemployment rises, to leave the available jobs for the men. We still do not really have a wide acceptance of the equal rights of women to employment outside the home. Nor do we have wide acceptance of the equal duty of men to perform those domestic tasks which in no way depend on special female anatomy, namely cooking, cleaning, and the care of weaned children.

All sorts of stories (maybe true stories), about children's need for one 'primary' parent, who must be the mother if the mother breast-feeds the child, shore up the unequal division of domestic responsibility between mothers and fathers, wives and husbands. If we are really to transvalue the values of our patriarchal past, we need to rethink all of those assumptions, really test those psychological theories. And how will men ever develop an understanding of the 'ethics of care' if they continue to be shielded or kept from that experience of caring for a dependent child, which complements the experience we all have had of being cared for as dependent children? These experiences form the natural background for the development of moral maturity as Gilligan's women saw it.

Exploitation aside, why would women, once liberated, not be content to have their version of morality merely tolerated? Why should they not see themselves as voluntarily, for their own reasons, taking on *more* than the liberal rules demand, while having no quarrel with the content of those rules themselves, nor with their remaining the only ones that are expected to be generally obeyed? To see why, we need to move on to three more differences between the Kantian liberals (usually contractarians) and their critics. These concern the relative weight put on relationships between equals, and the relative weight put on freedom of choice, and on the authority of intellect over emotions. It is a typical feature of the dominant moral theories and traditions, since Kant, or perhaps since Hobbes, that relationships between equals or those who are deemed equal in some important sense, have been the relations that morality is concerned primarily to regulate. Relationships between those who are clearly unequal in power, such as parents and children, earlier and later generations in relation to one another, states and citizens, doctors and patients, the well and the ill, large states and small states, have had to be shunted to the bottom of the agenda, and then dealt with by some sort of 'promotion' of the weaker so that an appearance of virtual equality is achieved. Citizens collectively become equal to states, children are treated as adults-to-be, the ill and dying are treated as continuers of their earlier more potent selves, so that their 'rights' could be seen as the rights of equals. This pretence of an equality that is in fact absent may often lead to desirable protection of the weaker, or more dependent. But it somewhat masks the question of what our moral relationships *are* to those who are our superiors or our inferiors in power. A more realistic acceptance of the fact that we begin as helpless children, that at almost every point of our lives we deal with both the more and the less helpless, that equality of power and interdependency, between two persons or groups, is rare and hard to recognize when it does occur, might lead us to a more direct approach to questions concerning the design of institutions structuring these relationships between unequals (families, schools, hospitals, armies) and of the morality of our dealings with the more and the less powerful. One reason why those who agree with the Gilligan version of what morality is about will not want to agree that the liberals' rules are a good minimal set, the only ones we need pressure *everyone* to obey, is that these rules do little to protect the young or the dying or the starving or any of the relatively powerless against neglect, or to ensure an education that will form persons to be *capable* of conforming to an ethics of care and responsibility. Put baldly, and in a way Gilligan certainly has not put it, the liberal morality, if unsupplemented, may *unfit* people to be anything other than what its justifying theories suppose them to be, ones who have no interest in each others' interests. Yet some must take an interest in the next generation's interests. Women's traditional work, of caring for the less powerful, especially for the young, is obviously socially vital. One cannot regard any version of morality that does not ensure that it gets well done as an adequate 'minimal morality,' any more than we could so regard one that left any concern for more distant future generations an optional extra. A moral theory, it can plausibly be claimed, cannot regard concern for new and future persons as an optional charity left for those with a taste for it. If the morality the theory endorses is to sustain itself, it must provide for its own continuers, not just take out a loan on a carefully encouraged maternal instinct or on the enthusiasm of a self-selected group of environmentalists, who make it their business or hobby to be concerned with what we are doing to mother earth.

The recognition of the importance for all parties of relations between those who are and cannot but be unequal, both of these relations in themselves and for their effect on personality formation and so on other relationships, goes along with a recognition of the plain fact that not all morally important relationships can or should be freely chosen. So far I have discussed three reasons women have not to be content to pursue their own values within the framework of the liberal morality. The first was its dubious record. The second was its inattention to relations of inequality or its pretence of equality. The third reason is its exaggeration of the scope of choice, or its inattention to unchosen relations. Showing up the partial myth of equality among actual members of a community, and of the undesirability of trying to pretend that we are treating all of them as equals, tends to go along with an exposure of the companion myth that moral obligations arise from freely *chosen* associations between such equals. Vulnerable future generations do not choose their dependence on earlier generations. The unequal infant does not choose its place in a family or nation, nor is it treated as free to do as it likes until some association is freely entered into. Nor do its parents always choose their parental role, or freely assume their parental responsibilities any more than we choose our power to affect the conditions in which later generations will live. Gilligan's attention to the version of morality and moral maturity found in women, many of whom had faced a choice of whether or not to have an abortion, and who had at some point become mothers, is attention to the perceived inadequacy of the language of rights to help in such choices or to guide them in their parental role. It would not be much of an exaggeration to call the Gilligan 'different voice' the voice of the potential parents. The emphasis on care goes with a recognition of the often unchosen nature of the responsibilities of those who give care, both of children who care for their aged or infirm parents, and of parents who care for the children they in fact have. Contract soon ceases to seem the paradigm source of moral obligation once we attend to parental responsibility, and justice as a virtue of social institutions will come to seem at best only first equal with the virtue, whatever its name, that ensures that each new generation is made appropriately welcome and prepared for their adult lives.

This all constitutes a belated reminder to Western moral theorists of a fact they have always known, that as Adam Ferguson, and David Hume before him emphasized, we are born into families, and the first society we belong to, one that fits or misfits us for later ones, is the small society of parents (or some sort of child-attendants) and children, exhibiting as it may both relationships of near equality and of inequality in power. This simple reminder, with the fairly considerable implications it can have for the plausibility of contractarian moral theory, is at the same time a reminder of the role of human emotions as much as human reason and will in moral development as it actually comes about. The fourth feature of the Gilligan challenge to liberal orthodoxy is a challenge to its typical *rationalism*, or intellectualism, to its assumption that we need not worry what passions persons have, as long as their rational wills can control them. This Kantian picture of a controlling reason dictating to possibly unruly passions also tends to seem less useful when we are led to consider what sort of person we need to fill the role of parent, or indeed want in any close relationship. It might be important for father figures to have rational control over their violent urges to beat to death the children whose screams enrage them, but more than control of such nasty passions seems needed in the mother or primary parent, or parent-substitute, by most psychological theories. They need to love their children, not just to control their irritation. So the emphasis in Kantian theories on rational control of emotions, rather than on cultivating desirable forms of emotion, is challenged by Gilligan, along with the challenge to the assumption of the centrality of autonomy, or relations between equals, and of freely chosen relations.

The same set of challenges to 'orthodox' liberal oral theory has come not just from Gilligan and other women, who are reminding other moral theorists of the role of the family as a social institution and as an influence on the other relationships people want to or are capable of sustaining, but also, as I noted at the start, from an otherwise fairly diverse group of men, ranging from those influenced by both Hegelian and Christian traditions (MacIntyre) to all varieties of other backgrounds. From this group I want to draw attention to the work of one philosopher in particular, namely Laurence Thomas, the author of a fairly remarkable article[3] in which he finds sexism to be a more intractable social evil than racism. . . . Thomas makes a strong case for the importance of supplementing a concern for justice and respect for rights with an emphasis on equally needed virtues, and on virtues seen as appropriate *emotional* as well as rational capacities. Like Gilligan (and unlike MacIntyre) Thomas gives a lot of attention to the childhood beginnings of moral and social capacities, to the role of parental love in making that possible, and to the emotional as well as the cognitive development we have reason to think both possible and desirable in human persons.

It is clear, I think, that the best moral theory has to be a cooperative product of women and men, has to harmonize justice and care. The morality it theorizes about is after all for all persons, for men and for women, and will need their combined insights. As Gilligan said (D.V., 174), what we need now is a 'marriage' of the old male and the newly articulated female insights. If she is right about the special moral aptitudes of women, it will most likely be the women who propose the marriage, since they are the ones with moral natural empathy, with the better diplomatic skills, the ones more likely to shoulder responsibility and take moral initiative, and the ones who find it easiest to empathize and care about how the other party feels. Then, once there is this union of male and female moral wisdom, we maybe can teach each other the moral skills each gender currently lacks, so that the gender difference in moral outlook that Gilligan found will slowly become less marked.

NOTES

1. John Rawls, *A Theory of Justice* (Harvard University Press)

2. Immanuel Kant, *Metaphysics of Morals*, sec. 46

3. Laurence Thomas, 'Sexism and Racism: Some Conceptual Differences,' *Ethics* 90 (1980), 239–50; republished in *Philosophy, Sex and Language*, Vetterling-Braggin, ed. (Totowa, NJ: Littlefield Adams 1980)

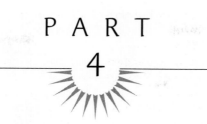

PART
4

Ethical Issues

CHAPTER 8

Abortion

If somehow you had unobstructed access for a single day to all the public and private dramas provoked by the issue of abortion, you might see scenes like this: a forty-year-old mother of five agonizing over whether she should terminate her pregnancy (which is both unexpected and unwanted); antiabortion activists shouting "Thou shall not kill!" at a woman hurrying inside a clinic that performs abortions; a frightened sixteen-year-old rape victim having an abortion against her family's wishes; a Catholic bishop pointing out on the eleven o'clock news that abortion in any form is murder; the head of an abortion rights organization declaring in a CNN interview that antiabortion activists are violent and dangerous; a politician getting elected solely because he favors a constitutional amendment to ban virtually all abortions; two women who have been friends for years disagreeing bitterly about whether a fetus has a right to life; and state legislators angrily debating a bill requiring any woman seeking an abortion to watch a fifteen-minute video titled "The Tragedy of Abortion."

Such scenes are emblematic of the abortion issue in that they are intensely emotional and usually accompanied by uncritical or dogmatic thinking. Passions surge because abortion touches on some of our deepest values and most basic beliefs. When we grapple with the issue of abortion, we must consider whose rights (the mother's or the unborn's) carry the most moral weight, what the meaning of *human being* or *person* is, when—if ever—the unborn achieves personhood, how having an abortion affects the health and mind of the

mother, how much importance to assign to our most fundamental moral principles, and much more. For many women, the abortion controversy is *personal*, involving judgments about their own bodies, their own health and happiness, and their own inner turmoil provoked by life-and-death decisions. Uncritical acceptance of particular moral perspectives on abortion seems to be the norm for people on all sides of the debate. Often discussion of the issue is reduced to shouting; informed reflection, to knee-jerk conclusions; and reasoned argument, to cases built on assumptions never questioned.

In this chapter, we try to do better, relying heavily on critical reasoning and striving for a more objective approach. We begin with a review of the (nonmoral) facts of abortion—biological, medical, psychological, semantic, and legal. Then we consider how the moral theories discussed in previous chapters can be applied to this issue. Finally, we examine a range of common arguments in the debate, from liberal to conservative as well as some intermediate positions.

ISSUE FILE: BACKGROUND

Abortion (also called *induced abortion*) is the deliberate termination of a pregnancy by surgical or medical (with drugs) means. The unintentional termination of a pregnancy (due to a medical disorder or injury) is known as a *spontaneous abortion,* or *miscarriage.* An abortion performed to protect the life or health of the mother is referred to as a **therapeutic abortion.** Therapeutic abortions are usually not thought to be morally problematic. (The Roman Catholic stance, however, is that induced abortion is always wrong, though the unintended death of the fetus during an attempt to save the mother's life is morally permissible.) But induced abortions are intensely controversial and are the focus of the ongoing moral debate.

Throughout our discussion of abortion in this chapter, we will use the word *fetus* to refer to the unborn during its entire development from conception to birth. But technically the term indicates a particular phase of this development. Development begins at **conception,** or fertilization, when a sperm cell enters an ovum and the two merge into a single cell called a *zygote*. The zygote contains a complete set of forty-six chromosomes, half of them from the mother, half from the father—all the genetic information needed to make a unique human individual. Over the next few days the zygote inches down the fallopian tube toward the uterus, expanding as cells divide. In three to five days it reaches the uterus, where it grows in a tiny orb of cells called a *blastocyst*. By day ten the blastocyst fully implants itself in the lining of the uterus, and from implantation until the eighth week after fertilization it is known technically as an *embryo*. In the embryonic phase, most major organs form (though the brain and spinal cord will keep developing during pregnancy), and the embryo will grow to just over an inch long. At about the third week the embryo first acquires a human shape; by the eighth, doctors can detect brain activity. By the end of the eighth week until birth (approximately week forty), the embryo is known in medical terminology as a *fetus*.

In the abortion debate, certain other aspects of fetal development are thought by some to be of special significance. For example, usually at about sixteen to twenty weeks, the mother can feel the fetus moving, an event known as **quickening.**

Abortion in the United States: Facts and Figures

- Nearly half of all pregnancies are unintended (more than 3 million per year).

- About 40 percent of unintended pregnancies end in abortions.

- In 2011, 1,058,500 women had abortions.

- 21 percent of all pregnancies are terminated by abortion.

- In 2011, the abortion rate (number of abortions per 1,000 women of reproductive age in a given year) dropped to 16.9. (The rate in 2008 was 19.4.)

- Overall, the abortion rate has been declining since 1980.

- The risk of death associated with abortion rises with the length of pregnancy: 1 death per 1 million abortions at or before 8 weeks; 1 per 29,000 abortions at 16 to 20 weeks.

- Over half of abortions are obtained by women in their 20s; 18 percent are obtained teenagers; 0.4 percent are obtained by girls younger than 15.

- 45 percent of abortions are obtained by never-married women who are not cohabiting; 61 percent occur in women who have at least one child.

- 36 percent of women having abortions are non-Hispanic white; 30 percent are black non-Hispanic; and 25 percent are Hispanic.

- 37 percent of women having abortions are Protestants; 28 percent are Catholic.*

*Derived from "Fact Sheet" and "National Reproductive Health Profile," data compiled and developed by the Alan Guttmacher Institute, July 2014, www.guttmacher.org (28 October 2014).

At about twenty-three or twenty-four weeks, the fetus may be able to live outside the uterus, a state referred to as **viability.**

Abortion methods vary depending largely on the stage of a woman's pregnancy. Within the first seven weeks or so, drugs can be used to induce an abortion. A combination of mifepristone (RU-486) and prostaglandins (hormonelike agents that provoke uterine contractions) can force the embryo out of the uterus and through the vagina. This approach, sometimes called a medical abortion, has an extremely high success rate.

With a method known as *menstrual aspiration* (or *manual vacuum aspiration*), an abortion can be performed in the first three weeks. In this procedure, a physician expands the opening of the uterus (the cervix) and uses a syringe to draw out the embryo from the uterus wall. Up until twelve weeks of pregnancy (a period when most abortions are performed), a method called *suction curettage* (or *dilation and suction curettage*) is often used. A physician widens the cervix, then inserts a thin, flexible tube through it and into the uterus itself. A vacuum device attached to the other end of the tube then provides suction to empty the uterus. A method often used after twelve weeks is *dilation and evacuation*. After the cervix is opened up, forceps and suction are used to extract the fetus. A nonsurgical technique used in some late abortions involves inducing the contractions of labor so the fetus is expelled from the uterus. To force the contractions, physicians often use drugs as well as *saline injection,* the substitution of saltwater for amniotic fluid in the uterus.

Like any medical procedure, abortion poses some risk of complications. Its risks, however, are relatively low. Fewer than 1 percent of women who have an abortion suffer from a major complication. The risk of death for women who have an abortion at eight weeks or earlier is one death per one million abortions. The risk for all abortions is about 0.6 deaths per 100,000 abortions. By comparison, the risk of death related to childbirth is much higher than that—about twelve times higher.[1] The health risks linked to abortion are directly related to the timing of the procedure. The earlier in the pregnancy an abortion is performed, the lower the risk.

When we try to evaluate arguments in the abortion debate, we must distinguish between the moral question (Is abortion right?) and the legal one (What should the law allow?). Our main concern is the former, not the latter. But to be fully informed about the issue, we should understand, at least in general terms, what the law does allow. In 1973, in the landmark case of *Roe v. Wade*, the United States Supreme Court ruled that a woman has a constitutional, but not unlimited, right to obtain an abortion in a range of circumstances. According to the Court, in the first three months of pregnancy (the first trimester), the woman's right is unrestricted. The decision to have an abortion is up to the woman in consultation with her physician. After the first trimester, a state may regulate (but not ban) abortion to protect the health of the mother. After viability, however, a state may regulate and even forbid abortions in the interests of "the potentiality of human life," except when abortion is necessary to preserve the health or life of the woman.[2]

In *Roe* the Court maintained that a woman's right to an abortion is based on a fundamental right of personal privacy and that this right, derived from several constitutional amendments, applies to numerous situations involving reproduction, families, and children. The Court also pointed out that the word *person* as used in the Constitution "does not include the unborn" and that "the unborn have never been recognized in the law as persons in the whole sense."[3]

[1]"An Overview of Abortion in the United States," developed by Physicians for Reproductive Choice and Health and the Alan Guttmacher Institute, May 2006, www.guttmacher.org (15 November 2011).
[2]*Roe v. Wade*, 410 U.S. 113, 164–65 (1973).
[3]*Roe*, 158, 162.

Majority Opinion in *Roe v. Wade*

Seven justices concurred with the opinion in *Roe v. Wade*, including Justice Harry Blackmun, who wrote it. Here is an excerpt:

> This right of privacy, whether it be founded in the Fourteenth Amendment's concept of personal liberty and restrictions upon state action, as we feel it is, or, as the District Court determined, in the Ninth Amendment's reservation of rights to the people, is broad enough to encompass a woman's decision whether or not to terminate her pregnancy. . . .

> [A]ppellant and some *amici* argue that the woman's right is absolute and that she is entitled to terminate her pregnancy at whatever time, in whatever way, and for whatever reason she alone chooses. With this we do not agree. Appellant's arguments that Texas either has no valid interest at all in regulating the abortion decision, or no interest strong enough to support any limitation upon the woman's sole determination, are unpersuasive. The Court's decisions recognizing a right of privacy also acknowledge that some state regulation in areas protected by that right is appropriate. As noted above, a State may properly assert important interests in safeguarding health, in maintaining medical standards, and in protecting potential life. At some point in pregnancy, these respective interests become sufficiently compelling to sustain regulation of the factors that govern the abortion decision. The privacy right involved, therefore, cannot be said to be absolute. . . .

> We, therefore, conclude that the right of personal privacy includes the abortion decision, but that this right is not unqualified and must be considered against important state interests in regulation. . . .

> [This] decision leaves the State free to place increasing restrictions on abortion as the period of pregnancy lengthens, so long as those restrictions are tailored to the recognized state interests. The decision vindicates the right of the physician to administer medical treatment according to his professional judgment up to the points where important state interests provide compelling justifications for intervention. Up to those points, the abortion decision in all its aspects is inherently, and primarily, a medical decision, and basic responsibility for it must rest with the physician. If an individual practitioner abuses the privilege of exercising proper medical judgment, the usual remedies, judicial and intra-professional, are available.*

*Roe v. Wade, 410 U.S. 113, 153–54, 165–66 (1973).

Over the next thirty years the Court handed down other abortion decisions that clarified or supplemented *Roe*. Among other things, the justices prohibited or constrained the use of Medicaid (a government entitlement program) to subsidize abortions; forbade the use of public employees and facilities to perform abortions (except to save the life of the mother); declared that a woman seeking an abortion does not have to notify her husband of her intent; affirmed that states may not impose restrictions that present an "undue burden," or excessive impediment, to women seeking abortions; and held that states may require a girl under eighteen to obtain either the informed consent of a parent or a court order before getting an abortion.

MORAL THEORIES

How would a utilitarian judge the moral permissibility of abortion? How would a Kantian theorist or a natural law theorist evaluate it? Let us take utilitarianism first. An act-utilitarian would say that an abortion is morally right if it results in the greatest overall happiness, everyone considered. To argue for abortion, she might point to all the unhappiness that could be caused by the mother's remaining pregnant against her wishes: the mother's impaired mental and physical health (and possible death), her loss of personal freedom and future opportunities, financial strain on the mother as well as on her family, the anguish of being pregnant as a result of rape or incest, the agony of bringing a seriously impaired baby to term only to see it die later, and the stress that all these social and financial problems would have on a child after birth. The philosopher Mary Anne Warren cites a possible consequentialist argument that says when women do not have the option of abortion, unhappiness can be created on a *global* scale:

> In the long run, access to abortion is essential for the health and survival not just of individual women and families, but also that of the larger social and biological systems on which all our lives depend. Given the inadequacy of present methods of contraception and the lack of universal access to contraception, the avoidance of rapid population growth generally requires some use of abortion. Unless population growth rates are reduced in those impoverished societies where they remain high, malnutrition and starvation will become even more widespread than at present.[4]

An act-utilitarian, of course, could also argue against abortion on exactly the same grounds— the overall happiness (or unhappiness) brought about by particular actions. She could contend, for example, that *not* having an abortion would produce more net happiness than having one because having one would cause the mother tremendous psychological pain, because the happiness brought into the world with the birth of the child would be considerable, and because the social stigma of having an abortion would be extremely painful for both the mother and her family.

A rule-utilitarian could also view abortion as either morally right or wrong depending on the rule being followed and how much net happiness results from adhering to it. He could argue on various grounds that generally following a rule such as "Abortion is not morally permissible except to save the mother's life" would maximize happiness. Or he could claim that generally following this rule instead would maximize happiness: "Abortion is morally permissible for any reason during the first trimester and always in cases of rape, incest, fetal impairment, and serious threats to the mother's health or life."

A premise (often unstated) in many arguments about abortion is that the fetus is (or is not) a **person**—an entity with full moral rights. In general, utilitarian arguments about abortion do not depend heavily, if at all, on whether the fetus is regarded as a person. Whether the fetus is a person is not likely to dramatically affect the hedonic calculus. The main issue is not personhood but utility. For the Kantian theorist, however, the moral status of the fetus is likely to matter much more. (Whether Kant himself thought the fetus a person is an open question.) If the Kantian maintains that the fetus is a person—that is, an end in itself, a thing of intrinsic value and dignity—then he would insist that it has all the rights and is due all the respect that any other person has. This would mean that the unborn should not be regarded as just another quantity in a utilitarian calculation of consequences. Like any adult human, the fetus has rights, and these rights cannot be overridden merely for utility's sake. Only for the most compelling moral reasons can these rights be set aside. A Kantian might say that one such reason is self-defense: killing a person in self-defense is permissible. He might therefore argue that if the mother's life is being threatened by the fetus she carries (if being pregnant is somehow life-threatening), therapeutic abortion is permissible, just as killing someone who is trying to kill you is permissible. In this view, abortion would seem to be only rarely justified.

[4]Mary Anne Warren, "Abortion," in *A Companion to Ethics*, ed. Peter Singer, corr. ed. (Cambridge, MA: Blackwell, 1993), 304.

On the other hand, if the Kantian does not regard the fetus as a person, he may believe that abortion is often justified to protect the rights and dignity of the mother, who *is* a person. In other words, the fetus—like any other nonperson—can be used as a means to an end, whereas the mother must be treated as an end in herself.

Traditional natural law theorists would view abortion very differently for two reasons. First, to them, there is no question about the moral status of the fetus: it is a person with full moral rights. Second, the theory is very clear about the treatment of innocent persons: it is always morally wrong to directly kill the innocent. So the direct, intentional killing of a fetus through abortion is never permissible. According to the doctrine of double effect, killing an innocent person for the purpose of achieving some greater good is immoral. But indirectly, unintentionally killing an innocent person while trying to do good may be permissible.

Abortion and the Scriptures

Do the Jewish or Christian scriptures forbid abortion? Many people believe that they do, but the philosopher James Rachels argues that they do not:

> It is difficult to derive a prohibition of abortion from either the Jewish or the Christian Scriptures. The Bible does not speak plainly on the matter. There are certain passages, however, that are often quoted by conservatives because they seem to suggest that fetuses have full human status. One of the most frequently cited passages is from the first chapter of Jeremiah, in which God is quoted as saying: "Before I formed you in the womb I knew you, and before you were born I consecrated you." These words are presented as though they were God's endorsement of the conservative position: They are taken to mean that the unborn, as well as the born, are "consecrated" to God.
>
> In context, however, these words obviously mean something quite different. Suppose we read the whole passage in which they occur:
>
>> Now the word of the Lord came to me saying, "Before I formed you in the womb I knew you, and before you were born I consecrated you; I appointed you a prophet to the nations." Then I said, "Ah, Lord God! Behold, I do not know how to speak, for I am only a youth." But the Lord said to me, "Do not say, 'I am only a youth' for to all to whom I send you you shall go, and whatever I command you you shall speak. Be not afraid of them, for I am with you to deliver you," says the Lord.
>
> Neither abortion, the sanctity of fetal life, nor anything else of the kind is being discussed in this passage. Instead, Jeremiah is asserting his authority as a prophet. He is saying, in effect, "God authorized me to speak for him; even though I resisted, he commanded me to speak." But Jeremiah puts the point more poetically; he has God saying that God had intended him to be a prophet even before Jeremiah was born. . . .
>
> The scriptural passage that comes closest to making a specific judgment about the moral status of fetuses occurs in the 21st chapter of Exodus. This chapter is part of a detailed description of the law of the ancient Israelites. Here the penalty for murder is said to be death; however, it is also said that if a pregnant woman is caused to have a miscarriage, the penalty is only a fine, to be paid to her husband. Murder was not a category that included fetuses. The Law of Israel apparently regarded fetuses as something less than full human beings.*

*James Rachels, *The Elements of Moral Philosophy*, 4th Ed. pp. 59–60. Copyright © 2003 McGraw Hill Education. Reprinted by permission.

> ### QUICK REVIEW
>
> **abortion**—The deliberate termination of a pregnancy by surgical or medical (with drugs) means.
>
> **therapeutic abortion**—An abortion performed to protect the life or health of the mother.
>
> **conception**—The merging of a sperm cell and an ovum into a single cell; also called fertilization.
>
> **quickening**—The point in fetal development when the mother can feel the fetus moving (it occurs at about sixteen to twenty weeks).
>
> **viability**—The stage of fetal development at which the fetus is able to survive outside the uterus.
>
> **person**—A being thought to have full moral rights.

Therefore, intentionally killing a fetus through abortion, even to save the mother's life, is wrong. But trying to, say, cure a pregnant woman's cancer by performing a hysterectomy on her or giving her chemotherapy—treatment that has the unintended side effect of aborting the fetus—may be morally acceptable. In this view, very few abortions are morally acceptable.

MORAL ARGUMENTS

Arguments for and against abortion are plentiful and diverse, their quality ranging from good to bad, and their conclusions varying from conservative ("pro-life") to liberal ("pro-choice") with several moderate positions in between. We can sum up the central issue of the debate like this: *When, if ever, is abortion morally permissible?* Recall that in ethics the proper reply to such a question is to provide good reasons for a particular position. The usual fireworks that accompany the abortion debate—strident denunciations of the other side, appeals to emotion and pity, extremist rhetoric, exaggerated claims, political posturing, and the like—are not

appropriate, not germane, and not helpful. So here we try to cut through all that and examine a few of the main arguments offered for a range of views.

The conservative position is that abortion is never, or almost never, morally permissible. Typically the "almost never" refers to situations in which abortion may be permissible to save the life of the mother. (Generally, both the liberal and conservative hold that abortion may be permissible to save the mother's life, usually on the grounds that the mother has a right of self-defense. But as mentioned earlier, the Roman Catholic position is that in any case the death of the fetus must be unintended.)

Like many arguments about abortion, the conservative case is built on a proposition about the moral status of the fetus. For most conservatives, the fetus is a person (a human being, as some would say) with full moral rights, the same rights that any adult human has, and these rights emerge at the moment of conception. Of course, the moral right at the heart of it all is the right to life. Taking the life of a fetal person is just as immoral as killing an innocent adult human.

Here is one version of the conservative argument:

1. The unborn is obviously a human life.
2. It is wrong to take a human life.
3. Abortion is the taking of a human life.
4. Therefore, abortion is wrong.

To evaluate this argument (or *any* argument), we must determine (1) whether the conclusion follows from the premises; and (2) whether the premises are true. A cursory glance at this argument might suggest that the conclusion does follow from the premises and that the premises are true. But we must be careful. This argument commits the fallacy of equivocation. The term *human life* is assigned two different meanings in the premises, rendering the argument invalid. In Premise 1, "human life" means something like "biologically human"—an entity with human DNA, an entity that is from the human species. But in Premises 2 and 3, the term means "person"—a being entitled to full moral rights. If "human life" is used in different senses in the premises, then the argument is not valid (the conclusion does not follow from the premises)—even if the premises, using their respective meanings of the term, are true. As it stands, Premise 1 is unmistakably true: a fetus born of human parents with human DNA is certainly biologically human. And in its present form, Premise 2 is also true: the killing of a person is indeed wrong (except perhaps to save a life). Still, the argument fails and does not provide us with good reasons to accept the conclusion.

Yet there are conservative arguments that do not equivocate. Consider this one:

1. The unborn is an innocent person from conception.

2. It is wrong to kill an innocent person.

3. Abortion is the killing of an innocent person.

4. Therefore, abortion is wrong.

This argument is valid. The only significant difference between it and the previous one is Premise 1, which asserts that the unborn is a being with full moral rights from the very moment of fertilization. If Premise 1 is true, then the argument is sound—the premises are true and the conclusion follows from them.

But *is* the premise true? The conservative insists that it is and can argue for it in this fashion. Birth is generally thought to be the point at which the fetus is most clearly (and legally) a person. The development of the unborn from conception to birth, however, is one continuous process, with no obvious points along the way that might signal a transition into personhood. Moreover, whatever essential properties a born human has that make it a person seem to be present at the moment of conception. Therefore, since no unambiguous point of personhood can be located in this process, the most reasonable option is to identify personhood with conception.

CRITICAL THOUGHT: Late-Term Abortions

Late-term abortion (what some opponents of abortion call "partial-birth abortion") is a controversial procedure known technically as *intact dilation and extraction*. It is a rare operation usually performed after the first trimester because the pregnancy endangers the mother's life, the fetus is seriously deformed or defective, or the mother is mentally impaired, homeless, addicted to drugs, or otherwise unprepared or unwilling to care for an infant. Late-term abortion has been hotly debated in society and frequently adjudicated in the courts.

Some late-term abortions are performed after the fetus becomes viable. Do such procedures then involve, as some have alleged, the killing of babies? Should all late-term abortions be outlawed? Why or why not? Are they different from earlier abortions in morally relevant respects? Why or why not?

Opponents of this argument contend that it is fallacious. We may not be able to pinpoint a precise moment when day becomes night, they say, but that does not mean that day *is* night. Likewise, we may not be able to determine the precise point in the continuous process of human development when a zygote becomes a full-fledged person. But that does not mean that a zygote is a person.

The conservative, however, can propose a more nuanced reason for supposing that conception marks the beginning of personhood:

One evidence of the nonarbitrary character of the line drawn [at conception] is the difference of probabilities on either side of it. If a spermatozoon is destroyed, one destroys a being which had a chance of far less than 1 in 200 million of developing into a reasoning being, possessed of the genetic code, a heart and other organs, and capable of pain. If a fetus is destroyed, one destroys a being already possessed of the genetic code, organs and sensitivity to pain, and one which had an 80 percent chance of developing further into a baby outside the womb who, in time, would reason.

The positive argument for conception as the decision moment of humanization is that at conception the new being receives the genetic code. It is this genetic information which determines his characteristics, which is the biological carrier of the possibility of human wisdom, which makes him a self-evolving being. A being with a human genetic code is man.[5]

Others who oppose abortion argue that although the fetus may not be a person, it has the *potential* to become a person and is therefore entitled to the same rights as full-fledged persons. But critics reject this view:

> This argument is implausible, since in no other case do we treat the potential to achieve some status entailing certain rights as itself entailing those same rights. For instance, every child born in the United States is a potential voter, but no-one under the age of 18 has the right to vote in that country. If a fetus is a potential person, then so is an unfertilized human ovum, together with enough viable spermatozoa to achieve fertilization; yet few would seriously suggest that *these* living human entities should have full and equal moral status.[6]

The liberal position is that abortion is always (or almost always) permissible. Like the conservative's argument, the liberal's is based on a particular view of the moral status of the fetus. But in opposition to the conservative view, the liberal asserts that the fetus is not a person, not a being with full moral rights. Abortion therefore is morally permissible because the fetus does not possess a right to life (unlike the mother, who has a full complement of rights). Generally, for the liberal, the event that makes the unborn a person is not conception but birth.

Here is a version of a common liberal argument:

1. The unborn is not a person until birth (and thus does not have a right to life).

2. It is wrong to kill an innocent person.

3. Abortion before birth would not be the killing of an innocent person.

4. If abortion before birth is not the killing of an innocent person, it is permissible.

5. Therefore, abortion before birth is permissible.

Notice that this argument and the conservative one have a common premise: it is wrong to kill an innocent person. Thus the liberal and the conservative agree on the immorality of murder. Their disagreement is not over this fundamental moral principle, but over the nature of persons and who does or does not qualify as such an entity. Premise 1, then, is the crux of the liberal's argument (just as Premise 1 is the heart of the conservative's argument). How might the liberal defend this premise?

The obvious approach is to plausibly explain what a person is and then show that the fetus does not qualify as one. The most influential argument along these lines is that of Mary Anne Warren. "What characteristics entitle an entity to be considered a person?" she asks. What criteria, for example, would we use to decide whether alien beings encountered on an unknown planet deserve to be treated morally or treated as, say, a source of food? How would we tell whether the creatures are persons? Warren says that the characteristics most important to our idea of personhood are (1) consciousness, (2) the ability to reason, (3) self-motivated activity, (4) the capacity to communicate, and (5) the presence of self-concepts and self-awareness. Any being that has all of these traits we would surely regard as a person. Even a being that has only some of these traits would probably qualify as a person. More to the point, Warren says, we must admit that any being that has none of these traits is unquestionably *not* a person. And since a fetus lacks all these, we have to conclude that it too is not a person.

[5]John T. Noonan Jr., "An Almost Absolute Value in History," in *The Morality of Abortion: Legal and Historical Perspectives,* ed. Noonan (Cambridge, MA: Harvard University Press, 1970), 56–57.
[6]Warren, 312.

These considerations suggest that being genetically human is not the same thing as being a person in the moral sense, the sense of having full moral rights. As Warren notes,

> Now if [these five traits] are indeed the primary criteria of personhood, then it is clear that genetic humanity is neither necessary nor sufficient for establishing that an entity is a person. Some human beings are not people [persons], and there may well be people who are not human beings. A man or woman whose consciousness has been permanently obliterated but who remains alive is a human being which is no longer a person; defective human beings, with no appreciable mental capacity, are not and presumably never will be people; and a fetus is a human being which is not yet a person, and which therefore cannot coherently be said to have full moral rights. Citizens of the next century should be prepared to recognize highly advanced, self-aware robots or computers, should such be developed, and intelligent inhabitants of other worlds, should such be found, as people in the fullest sense, and to respect their moral rights.[7]

Against the liberal's argument, the conservative can lodge the following objections. First, he can point out that if Warren's view of personhood is correct, then a fetus is not a person—but neither is a newborn. After all, it is doubtful that a newborn (or perhaps even an older baby) can meet Warren's criteria for personhood. If a newborn is not a person, then killing it—the crime of infanticide—would seem to be permissible. But we tend to think that infanticide is obviously wrong.

To this criticism the liberal may say that though a newborn is not a person, it still has value—either because it is a potential person or because it is valued by others. The liberal might even argue that though a baby is not a person, infanticide should never be permitted because it is a gruesome act

that cheapens life or cultivates a callous attitude toward it.

The conservative can offer a related objection to the liberal's position. The liberal argument implies that the unborn is a person at birth but not a person a day or even an hour *before* birth, that abortion is immoral after birth but permissible an hour before. But since in such a case the physiological and psychological differences between the born and unborn are virtually nil, the liberal's distinction seems both arbitrary and ghastly.

The moderate rejects the claim that abortions are almost never permissible (as conservatives say) as well as the notion that they almost always are (as liberals maintain). In a variety of ways, moderates take intermediate positions between these two ends of the spectrum, asserting that abortion may be justified in more cases than conservatives would allow and fewer than liberals would like.

One moderate approach is to argue that the fetus becomes a person (and acquires full rights) some time after conception and before birth—at viability, quickening, sentience (sensory experience), or other notable milestone. Each of these points, however, is problematic in one way or another. The viability of the fetus (the point when it can survive outside the womb) is largely a function of modern medical know-how. Physicians are getting better at sustaining fetal life outside the womb, gradually pushing viability further back toward conception. But this suggests, implausibly, that personhood depends on medical expertise. Quickening, the first detection of fetal movement by the mother, signifies nothing that can be plausibly linked to personhood. It does not indicate the start of fetal movement—the fetus begins moving in the very first week of life. Sentience refers to consciousness, specifically the capacity to have sense experiences. If being sentient (especially the capacity to feel pleasure and pain) is proof of personhood, then personhood must not arise in the fetus until the second trimester, when neurologi-

---

[7]Mary Anne Warren, "On the Moral and Legal Status of Abortion," *The Monist* 57, no. 4 (1973): 56.

cal pathways are developed enough to make sense experience possible. But why should we regard sentience as a marker for personhood in the first place? Kittens, birds, crabs, and spiders are sentient, but few of us would insist that they are persons with full moral rights.

Some moderate positions can be mapped out without reference to the issue of personhood. The most impressive argument for this sort of view is that of Judith Jarvis Thomson. She contends that even if we grant that the fetus is a person with full moral rights, abortion still may be permissible in certain cases—more cases than the conservative would permit and fewer than the liberal would. The fetus has a right to life but not a right to sustain that life by using the mother's body against her will. To underscore her argument, Thomson asks us to consider this strange scenario:

> You wake up in the morning and find yourself back to back in bed with an unconscious violinist. A famous unconscious violinist. He has been found to have a fatal kidney ailment, and the Society of Music Lovers has canvassed all the available medical records and found that you alone have the right blood type to help. They have therefore kidnapped you, and last night the violinist's circulatory system was plugged into yours, so that your kidneys can be used to extract poisons from his blood as well as your own. The director of the hospital now tells you, "Look, we're sorry the Society of Music Lovers did this to you—we would never have permitted it if we had known. But still, they did it, and the violinist now is plugged into you. To unplug you would be to kill him. But never mind, it's only for nine months. By then he will have recovered from his ailment, and can safely be unplugged from you."[8]

Would you agree to such an arrangement? Would you be morally obligated to do so? The violinist, like all persons, has a right to life. But does this right, in Thomson's phrase, "[outweigh] your

right to decide what happens in and to your body"? Thomson concludes that the unborn's right to life does not entail the right to use the mother's body without her consent; the mother has a right to defend herself against unauthorized exploitation of her body. Abortion then is morally permissible when pregnancy is forced on the mother—that is, in cases of rape, incest, and defective contraception. (Like most people involved in the abortion debate, Thomson also thinks that abortion is morally acceptable to save the life of the mother.)

While laying out her argument, Thomson makes a distinction that further moderates her views. She points out that though women have a right to terminate a pregnancy in some cases, they do not have a right to "secure the death of the unborn child":

> It is easy to confuse these two things in that up to a certain point in the life of the fetus it is not able to survive outside the mother's body; hence removing it from her body guarantees its death. But they are importantly different. I have argued that you are not morally required to spend nine months in bed, sustaining the life of that violinist; but to say this is by no means to say that if, when you unplug yourself, there is a miracle and he survives, you then have a right to turn round and slit his throat. You may detach yourself even if this costs him his life; you have no right to be guaranteed his death, by some other means, if unplugging yourself does not kill him.[9]

Here is a greatly simplified version of Thomson's basic argument:

1. Whether or not the unborn has a right to life, it does not have a right to sustain its life by using the mother's body against her will.

2. The mother has a right to defend herself against the unborn's use of her body against her will (a right to have an abortion).

[8]Judith Jarvis Thomson, "A Defense of Abortion," *Philosophy & Public Affairs* 1, no. 1 (1971): 48–49.

[9]Thomson, 66.

3. The unborn uses the mother's body against her when the pregnancy is the result of rape, incest, or defective contraception.

4. Therefore, abortion is permissible in cases of rape, incest, or defective contraception.

Probably the most common criticism of this argument is that the mother may in fact not have the right to disconnect herself from the fetus if she bears some responsibility for being connected. In the case of Thomson's violinist, the woman was not at all responsible for being connected to him. However, if the woman's own actions somehow precipitated her being attached to the violinist, then she would be responsible for her predicament and thus would have no right to disconnect herself. Likewise, this objection goes, if a woman consents to sexual intercourse and knows that her actions can lead to pregnancy, she bears some responsibility for getting pregnant and therefore has no right to abort the fetus, even though it is using her body to survive. If this view is right, an abortion would seem to be justified only in cases of rape, when the woman is clearly not responsible for her pregnancy.

SUMMARY

Abortion is the deliberate termination of a pregnancy by surgical or medical means. Therapeutic abortions are those performed to protect the life of the mother. An abortion can be performed at any point in the development of the unborn—from conception to birth.

Abortion methods vary depending on how long the woman has been pregnant. Very early abortions can be done with drugs. Other types of abortions are performed by widening the uterus and drawing out the embryo with a syringe (manual vacuum aspiration), by opening the cervix and using a thin suction tube to empty the uterus (suction curettage), by using forceps and suction to extract the fetus (dilation and evacuation), and by using drugs or saline solution to cause contractions to expel the fetus from the uterus.

In 1973, in the famous case *Roe v. Wade*, the United States Supreme Court ruled that a woman has a constitutional, but limited, right to obtain an abortion. According to the Court, in the first trimester, the woman's right is unrestricted. The decision to have an abortion is up to the woman in consultation with her physician. After the first trimester, a state may regulate but not ban abortion to protect the health of the mother. After the fetus reaches viability, a state may regulate and even forbid abortions in the interests of the fetus, except when an abortion is necessary to preserve the health or life of the woman.

Major moral theories offer different perspectives on the issue of abortion. An act-utilitarian would argue that an abortion is morally right (or wrong) depending on its consequences. A rule-utilitarian could also judge abortion to be either morally right or wrong depending on the rule being followed and how much net happiness results from adhering to it. A Kantian theorist is likely to judge the issue according to the moral status of the fetus. If the Kantian believes that the fetus is a person, then she would say that the fetus has full moral rights and that these rights cannot be overridden on utilitarian grounds. If she does not think the fetus a person, she may believe that abortion is sometimes justified to protect the rights and dignity of the mother.

Arguments for and against abortion can be roughly grouped into three major categories—conservative, liberal, and moderate. The conservative position is that abortion is never, or almost never, morally permissible. The conservative case is built on the supposition that the fetus is a person with full moral rights. The liberal position is that abortion is always, or almost always, permissible. The liberal asserts that the fetus is not a person and therefore does not have a right to life. The moderate can take a number of intermediate positions between these two extremes, asserting on various grounds that abortion may be permissible in more situations than would be allowed by the conservative and in fewer situations than would be accepted by the liberal. A moderate position can be formulated by arguing that the unborn is a person some time after conception and before birth—perhaps at viability, quickening, or sentience.

READINGS

A Defense of Abortion

JUDITH JARVIS THOMSON

Most opposition to abortion relies on the premise that the fetus is a human being, a person, from the moment of conception. The premise is argued for, but, as I think, not well. Take, for example, the most common argument. We are asked to notice that the development of a human being from conception through birth into childhood is continuous; then it is said that to draw a line, to choose a point in this development and say "before this point the thing is not a person, after this point it is a person" is to make an arbitrary choice, a choice for which in the nature of things no good reason can be given. It is concluded that the fetus is, or anyway that we had better say it is, a person from the moment of conception. But this conclusion does not follow. Similar things might be said about the development of an acorn into an oak tree, and it does not follow that acorns are oak trees, or that we had better say they are. Arguments of this form are sometimes called "slippery slope arguments"—the phrase is perhaps self-explanatory— and it is dismaying that opponents of abortion rely on them so heavily and uncritically.

I am inclined to agree, however, that the prospects for "drawing a line" in the development of the fetus look dim. I am inclined to think also that we shall probably have to agree that the fetus has already become a human person well before birth. Indeed, it comes as a surprise when one first learns how early in its life it begins to acquire human characteristics. By the tenth week, for example, it already has a face, arms and legs, fingers and toes; it has internal organs, and brain activity is detectable. On the other hand, I think that the premise is false, that the fetus is not a person from the moment of conception. A newly fertilized ovum, a newly implanted clump of cells, is no

Judith Jarvis Thomson, excerpts from "A Defense of Abortion." *Philosophy & Public Affairs* 1(1): 47–66. Copyright © 1971 Blackwell Publishing Ltd. Reproduced with permission of John Wiley & Sons, Inc.

more a person than an acorn is an oak tree. But I shall not discuss any of this. For it seems to me to be of great interest to ask what happens if, for the sake of argument, we allow the premise. How, precisely, are we supposed to get from there to the conclusion that abortion is morally impermissible? Opponents of abortion commonly spend most of their time establishing that the fetus is a person, and hardly any time explaining the step from there to the impermissibility of abortion. Perhaps they think the step too simple and obvious to require much comment. Or perhaps instead they are simply being economical in argument. Many of those who defend abortion rely on the premise that the fetus is not a person, but only a bit of tissue that will become a person at birth; and why pay out more arguments than you have to? Whatever the explanation, I suggest that the step they take is neither easy nor obvious, that it calls for closer examination than it is commonly given, and that when we do give it this closer examination we shall feel inclined to reject it.

I propose, then, that we grant that the fetus is a person from the moment of conception. How does the argument go from here? Something like this, I take it. Every person has a right to life. So the fetus has a right to life. No doubt the mother has a right to decide what shall happen in and to her body; everyone would grant that. But surely a person's right to life is stronger and more stringent than the mother's right to decide what happens in and to her body, and so outweighs it. So the fetus may not be killed; an abortion may not be performed.

It sounds plausible. But now let me ask you to imagine this. You wake up in the morning and find yourself back to back in bed with an unconscious violinist. A famous unconscious violinist. He has been found to have a fatal kidney ailment, and the Society of Music Lovers has canvassed all the available medical records and found that you alone have the right blood type to help. They have therefore kidnapped you, and last night the violinist's circulatory system was plugged into yours, so that your kidneys can be used to extract poisons from his blood as well as your own. The director of the hospital now tells you, "Look, we're sorry the Society of Music Lovers did this to you—we would never have permitted it if we had known. But still, they did it, and the violinist now is plugged into you. To unplug you would be to kill him. But never mind, it's only for nine months. By then he will have recovered from his ailment, and can safely be unplugged from you." Is it morally incumbent on you to accede to this situation? No doubt it would be very nice of you if you did, a great kindness. But do you *have* to accede to it? What if it were not nine months, but nine years? Or longer still? What if the director of the hospital says, "Tough luck, I agree, but you've now got to stay in bed, with the violinist plugged into you, for the rest of your life. Because remember this. All persons have a right to life, and violinists are persons. Granted you have a right to decide what happens in and to your body, but a person's right to life outweighs your right to decide what happens in and to your body. So you cannot ever be unplugged from him." I imagine you would regard this as outrageous, which suggests that something really is wrong with that plausible-sounding argument I mentioned a moment ago.

In this case, of course, you were kidnapped; you didn't volunteer for the operation that plugged the violinist into your kidneys. Can those who oppose abortion on the ground I mentioned make an exception for a pregnancy due to rape? Certainly. They can say that persons have a right to life only if they didn't come into existence because of rape; or they can say that all persons have a right to life, but that some have less of a right to life than others, in particular, that those who came into existence because of rape have less. But these statements have a rather unpleasant sound. Surely the question of whether you have a right to life at all, or how much of it you have, shouldn't turn on the question of whether or not you are the product of a rape. And in fact the people who oppose abortion on the ground I mentioned do not make

this distinction, and hence do not make an exception in case of rape.

Nor do they make an exception for a case in which the mother has to spend the nine months of her pregnancy in bed. They would agree that would be a great pity, and hard on the mother; but all the same, all persons have a right to life, the fetus is a person, and so on. I suspect, in fact, that they would not make an exception for a case in which, miraculously enough, the pregnancy went on for nine years, or even the rest of the mother's life.

Some won't even make an exception for a case in which continuation of the pregnancy is likely to shorten the mother's life; they regard abortion as impermissible even to save the mother's life. Such cases are nowadays very rare, and many opponents of abortion do not accept this extreme view. All the same, it is a good place to begin: a number of points of interest come out in respect to it.

1. Let us call the view that abortion is impermissible even to save the mother's life "the extreme view." I want to suggest first that it does not issue from the argument I mentioned earlier without the addition of some fairly powerful premises. Suppose a woman has become pregnant, and now learns that she has a cardiac condition such that she will die if she carries the baby to term. What may be done for her? The fetus, being a person, has a right to life, but as the mother is a person too, so has she a right to life. Presumably they have an equal right to life. How is it supposed to come out that an abortion may not be performed? If mother and child have an equal right to life, shouldn't we perhaps flip a coin? Or should we add to the mother's right to life her right to decide what happens in and to her body, which everybody seems to be ready to grant—the sum of her rights now outweighing the fetus' right to life?

The most familiar argument here is the following. We are told that performing the abortion would be directly killing[1] the child, whereas doing nothing would not be killing the mother, but only letting her die. Moreover, in killing the child, one would be killing an innocent person, for the child has committed no crime, and is not aiming at his mother's death.

And then there are a variety of ways in which this might be continued. (1) But as directly killing an innocent person is always and absolutely impermissible, an abortion may not be performed. Or, (2) as directly killing an innocent person is murder, and murder is always and absolutely impermissible, an abortion may not be performed. Or, (3) as one's duty to refrain from directly killing an innocent person is more stringent than one's duty to keep a person from dying, an abortion may not be performed. Or, (4) if one's only options are directly killing an innocent person or letting a person die, one must prefer letting the person die, and thus an abortion may not be performed.

Some people seem to have thought that these are not further premises which must be added if the conclusion is to be reached, but that they follow from the very fact that an innocent person has a right to life. But this seems to me to be a mistake, and perhaps the simplest way to show this is to bring out that while we must certainly grant that innocent persons have a right to life, the theses in (1) through (4) are all false. Take (2), for example. If directly killing an innocent person is murder, and thus is impermissible, then the mother's directly killing the innocent person inside her is murder, and thus is impermissible. But it cannot seriously be thought to be murder if the mother performs an abortion on herself to save her life. It cannot seriously be said that she *must* refrain, that she *must* sit passively by and wait for her death. Let us look again at the case of you and the violinist. There you are, in bed with the violinist, and the director of the hospital says to you, "It's all most distressing, and I deeply sympathize, but you see this is putting an additional strain on your kidneys, and you'll be dead within the month. But you *have* to stay where you are all the same. Because unplugging you would be directly killing an innocent violinist, and that's murder, and that's impermissible." If anything in the world is true, it is that you do not commit murder, you do not do what is impermissible, if you reach around to your back and unplug yourself from that violinist to save your life.

The main focus of attention in writings on abortion has been on what a third party may or may not do in answer to a request from a woman for an abortion. This is in a way understandable. Things being as they are, there isn't much a woman can safely do to abort herself. So the question asked is what a third party may do, and what the mother may do, if it is mentioned at all, is deduced, almost as an afterthought, from what it is concluded that third parties may do. But it seems to me that to treat the matter in this way is to refuse to grant to the mother that very status of person which is so firmly insisted on for the fetus. For we cannot simply read off what a person may do from what a third party may do. Suppose you find yourself trapped in a tiny house with a growing child. I mean a very tiny house, and a rapidly growing child—you are already up against the wall of the house and in a few minutes you'll be crushed to death. The child on the other hand won't be crushed to death; if nothing is done to stop him from growing he'll be hurt, but in the end he'll simply burst open the house and walk out a free man. Now I could well understand it if a bystander were to say, "There's nothing we can do for you. We cannot choose between your life and his, we cannot be the ones to decide who is to live, we cannot intervene." But it cannot be concluded that you too can do nothing, that you cannot attack it to save your life. However innocent the child may be, you do not have to wait passively while it crushes you to death. Perhaps a pregnant woman is vaguely felt to have the status of house, to which we don't allow the right of self-defense. But if the woman houses the child, it should be remembered that she is a person who houses it.

I should perhaps stop to say explicitly that I am not claiming that people have a right to do anything whatever to save their lives. I think, rather, that there are drastic limits to the right of self-defense. If someone threatens you with death unless you torture someone else to death, I think you have not the right, even to save your life, to do so. But the case under consideration here is very different. In our case there are only two people involved, one whose life is threatened, and one who threatens it. Both are innocent: the one who is threatened is not threatened because of any fault, the one who threatens does not threaten because of any fault. For this reason we may feel that we bystanders cannot intervene. But the person threatened can.

In sum, a woman surely can defend her life against the threat to it posed by the unborn child, even if doing so involves its death. And this shows not merely that the theses in (1) through (4) are false; it shows also that the extreme view of abortion is false, and so we need not canvass any other possible ways of arriving at it from the argument I mentioned at the outset.

2. The extreme view could of course be weakened to say that while abortion is permissible to save the mother's life, it may not be performed by a third party, but only by the mother herself. But this cannot be right either. For what we have to keep in mind is that the mother and the unborn child are not like two tenants in a small house which has, by an unfortunate mistake, been rented to both: the mother *owns* the house. The fact that she does adds to the offensiveness of deducing that the mother can do nothing from the supposition that third parties can do nothing. But it does more than this: it casts a bright light on the supposition that third parties can do nothing. Certainly it lets us see that a third party who says "I cannot choose between you" is fooling himself if he thinks this is impartiality. If Jones has found and fastened on a certain coat, which he needs to keep him from freezing, but which Smith also needs to keep him from freezing, then it is not impartiality that says "I cannot choose between you" when Smith owns the coat. Women have said again and again "This body is *my* body!" and they have reason to feel angry, reason to feel that it has been like shouting into the wind. Smith, after all, is hardly likely to bless us if we say to him, "Of course it's your coat, anybody would grant that it is. But no one may choose between you and Jones who is to have it."

We should really ask what it is that says "no one may choose" in the face of the fact that the body that houses the child is the mother's body. It may be simply a failure to appreciate this fact. But it may be something more interesting, namely the sense that one has a right to refuse to lay hands on people, even where it would be just and fair to do so, even where justice seems to require that somebody do so. Thus justice might call for somebody to get Smith's coat back from Jones, and yet you have a right to refuse to be the one to lay hands on Jones, a right to refuse to do physical violence to him. This, I think, must be granted. But then what should be said is not "no one may choose," but only "*I* cannot choose," and indeed not even this, but "*I* will not *act*," leaving it open that somebody else can or should, and in particular that anyone in a position of authority, with the job of securing people's rights, both can and should. So this is no difficulty. I have not been arguing that any given third party must accede to the mother's request that he perform an abortion to save her life, but only that he may.

I suppose that in some views of human life the mother's body is only on loan to her, the loan not being one which gives her any prior claim to it. One who held this view might well think it impartiality to say "I cannot choose." But I shall simply ignore this possibility. My own view is that if a human being has any just, prior claim to anything at all, he has a just, prior claim to his own body. And perhaps this needn't be argued for here anyway, since, as I mentioned, the arguments against abortion we are looking at do grant that the woman has a right to decide what happens in and to her body.

But although they do grant it, I have tried to show that they do not take seriously what is done in granting it. I suggest the same thing will reappear even more clearly when we turn away from cases in which the mother's life is at stake, and attend, as I propose we now do, to the vastly more common cases in which a woman wants an abortion for some less weighty reason than preserving her own life.

3. Where the mother's life is not at stake, the argument I mentioned at the outset seems to have a much stronger pull. "Everyone has a right to life, so the unborn person has a right to life." And isn't the child's right to life weightier than anything other than the mother's own right to life, which she might put forward as ground for an abortion?

This argument treats the right to life as if it were unproblematic. It is not, and this seems to me to be precisely the source of the mistake.

For we should now, at long last, ask what it comes to, to have a right to life. In some views having a right to life includes having a right to be given at least the bare minimum one needs for continued life. But suppose that what in fact *is* the bare minimum a man needs for continued life is something he has no right at all to be given? If I am sick unto death, and the only thing that will save my life is the touch of Henry Fonda's cool hand on my fevered brow, then all the same, I have no right to be given the touch of Henry Fonda's cool hand on my fevered brow. It would be frightfully nice of him to fly in from the West Coast to provide it. It would be less nice, though no doubt well meant, if my friends flew out to the West Coast and carried Henry Fonda back with them. But I have no right at all against anybody that he should do this for me. Or again, to return to the story I told earlier, the fact that for continued life that violinist needs the continued use of your kidneys does not establish that he has a right to be given the continued use of your kidneys. He certainly has no right against you that *you* should give him continued use of your kidneys. For nobody has any right to use your kidneys unless you give him such a right; and nobody has the right against you that you shall give him this right—if you do allow him to go on using your kidneys, this is a kindness on your part, and not something he can claim from you as his due. Nor has he any right against anybody else that *they* should give him continued use of your kidneys. Certainly he had no right against the Society of Music Lovers that they should plug him into you in the first place. And if you now start to unplug yourself, having learned that you will otherwise have to spend nine years in bed with him, there is nobody in the world who must try to prevent you, in order to see to it that he is given something he has a right to be given.

Some people are rather stricter about the right to life. In their view, it does not include the right to be given anything, but amounts to, and only to, the right not to be killed by anybody. But here a related difficulty arises. If everybody is to refrain from killing that violinist, then everybody must refrain from doing a great many different sorts of things. Everybody must refrain from slitting his throat, everybody must refrain from shooting him—and everybody must refrain from unplugging you from him. But does he have a right against everybody that they shall refrain from unplugging you from him? To refrain from doing this is to allow him to continue to use your kidneys. It could be argued that he has a right against us that *we* should allow him to continue to use your kidneys. That is, while he had no right against us that we should give him the use of your kidneys, it might be argued that he anyway has a right against us that we shall not now intervene and deprive him of the use of your kidneys. I shall come back to third-party interventions later. But certainly the violinist has no right against you that *you* shall allow him to continue to use your kidneys. As I said, if you do allow him to use them, it is a kindness on your part, and not something you owe him.

The difficulty I point to here is not peculiar to the right to life. It reappears in connection with all the other natural rights; and it is something which an adequate account of rights must deal with. For present purposes it is enough just to draw attention to it. But I would stress that I am not arguing that people do not have a right to life—quite to the contrary, it seems to me that the primary control we must place on the acceptability of an account of rights is that it should turn out in that account to be a truth that all persons have a right to life. I am arguing only that having a right to life does not guarantee having either a right to be given the use of or a right to be allowed continued use of another person's body—even if one needs it for life itself. So the right to life will not serve the opponents of abortion in the very simple and clear way in which they seem to have thought it would.

4. There is another way to bring out the difficulty. In the most ordinary sort of case, to deprive someone of what he has a right to is to treat him unjustly. Suppose a boy and his small brother are jointly given a box of chocolates for Christmas. If the older boy takes the box and refuses to give his brother any of the chocolates, he is unjust to him, for the brother has been given a right to half of them. But suppose that, having learned that otherwise it means nine years in bed with that violinist, you unplug yourself from him. You surely are not being unjust to him, for you gave him no right to use your kidneys, and no one else can have given him any such right. But we have to notice that in unplugging yourself, you are killing

him; and violinists, like everybody else, have a right to life, and thus in the view we were considering just now, the right not to be killed. So where you do what he supposedly has a right you shall not do, but you do not act unjustly to him in doing it.

The emendation which may be made at this point is this: the right to life consists not in the right not to be killed, but rather in the right not to be killed unjustly. This runs a risk of circularity, but never mind: it would enable us to square the fact that the violinist has a right to life with the fact that you do not act unjustly toward him in unplugging yourself, thereby killing him. For if you do not kill him unjustly, you do not violate his right to life, and so it is no wonder you do him no injustice.

But if this emendation is accepted, the gap in the argument against abortion stares us plainly in the face: it is by no means enough to show that the fetus is a person, and to remind us that all persons have a right to life—we need to be shown also that killing the fetus violates its right to life, i.e., that abortion is unjust killing. And is it?

I suppose we may take it as a datum that in a case of pregnancy due to rape the mother has not given the unborn person a right to the use of her body for food and shelter. Indeed, in what pregnancy could it be supposed that the mother has given the unborn person such a right? It is not as if there were unborn persons drifting about the world, to whom a woman who wants a child says "I invite you in."

But it might be argued that there are other ways one can have acquired a right to the use of another person's body than by having been invited to use it by that person. Suppose a woman voluntarily indulges in intercourse, knowing of the chance it will issue in pregnancy, and then she does become pregnant; is she not in part responsible for the presence, in fact the very existence, of the unborn person inside her? No doubt she did not invite it in. But doesn't her partial responsibility for its being there itself give it a right to the use of her body? If so, then her aborting it would be more like the boy's taking away the chocolates, and less like your unplugging yourself from the violinist—doing so would be depriving it of what it does have a right to, and thus would be doing it an injustice.

And then, too, it might be asked whether or not she can kill it even to save her own life: If she voluntarily called it into existence, how can she now kill it, even in self-defense?

The first thing to be said about this is that it is something new. Opponents of abortion have been so concerned to make out the independence of the fetus, in order to establish that it has a right to life, just as its mother does, that they have tended to overlook the possible support they might gain from making out that the fetus is *dependent* on the mother, in order to establish that she has a special kind of responsibility for it, a responsibility that gives it rights against her which are not possessed by any independent person—such as an ailing violinist who is a stranger to her.

On the other hand, this argument would give the unborn person a right to its mother's body only if her pregnancy resulted from a voluntary act, undertaken in full knowledge of the chance a pregnancy might result from it. It would leave out entirely the unborn person whose existence is due to rape. Pending the availability of some further argument, then, we would be left with the conclusion that unborn persons whose existence is due to rape have no right to the use of their mothers' bodies, and thus that aborting them is not depriving them of anything they have a right to and hence is not unjust killing.

And we should also notice that it is not at all plain that this argument really does go even as far as it purports to. For there are cases and cases, and the details make a difference. If the room is stuffy, and I therefore open a window to air it, and a burglar climbs in, it would be absurd to say, "Ah, now he can stay, she's given him a right to the use of her house—for she is partially responsible for his presence there, having voluntarily done what enabled him to get in, in full knowledge that there are such things as burglars, and that burglars burgle." It would be still more absurd to say this if I had had bars installed outside my windows, precisely to prevent burglars from getting in, and a burglar got in only because of a defect in the bars. It remains equally absurd if we imagine it is not a burglar who climbs in, but an innocent person who blunders or falls in. Again, suppose it were like this: people-seeds drift about in the air like pollen, and if you open your windows, one may drift in and take root in your carpets or upholstery. You don't want children, so you fix up your windows with fine mesh screens, the very best you can buy. As can happen, however, and on very, very rare occasions does happen, one of the screens is defective; and a seed drifts in and takes root. Does the person-plant who now develops have a right to the use of your house? Surely not—despite the fact that you voluntarily opened your windows, you knowingly kept carpets and upholstered furniture, and you knew that screens were sometimes defective. Someone may argue that you are responsible for its rooting, that it does have a right to your house, because after all you *could* have lived out your life with bare floors and furniture, or with sealed windows and doors. But this won't do—for by the same token anyone can avoid a pregnancy due to rape by having a hysterectomy, or anyway by never leaving home without a (reliable!) army.

It seems to me that the argument we are looking at can establish at most that there are *some* cases in which the unborn person has a right to the use of its mother's body, and therefore *some* cases in which abortion is unjust killing. There is room for much discussion and argument as to precisely which, if any. But I think we should sidestep this issue and leave it open, for at any rate the argument certainly does not establish that all abortion is unjust killing.

5. There is room for yet another argument here, however. We surely must all grant that there may be cases in which it would be morally indecent to detach a person from your body at the cost of his life. Suppose you learn that what the violinist needs is not nine years of your life, but only one hour: all you need do to save his life is to spend one hour in that bed with him. Suppose also that letting him use your kidneys for that one hour would not affect your health in the slightest. Admittedly you were kidnapped. Admittedly you did not give anyone permission to plug him into you. Nevertheless it seems to me plain you *ought* to allow him to use your kidneys for that hour—it would be indecent to refuse.

Again, suppose pregnancy lasted only an hour, and constituted no threat to life or health. And suppose that a woman becomes pregnant as a result of rape. Admittedly she did not voluntarily do anything

to bring about the existence of a child. Admittedly she did nothing at all which would give the unborn person a right to the use of her body. All the same it might well be said, as in the newly emended violinist story, that she *ought* to allow it to remain for that hour—that it would be indecent in her to refuse.

Now some people are inclined to use the term "right" in such a way that it follows from the fact that you ought to allow a person to use your body for the hour he needs, that he has a right to use your body for the hour he needs, even though he has not been given that right by any person or act. They may say that it follows also that if you refuse, you act unjustly toward him. This use of the term is perhaps so common that it cannot be called wrong; nevertheless it seems to me to be an unfortunate loosening of what we would do better to keep a tight rein on. Suppose that box of chocolates I mentioned earlier had not been given to both boys jointly, but was given only to the older boy. There he sits, stolidly eating his way through the box, his small brother watching enviously. Here we are likely to say "You ought not to be so mean. You ought to give your brother some of those chocolates." My own view is that it just does not follow from the truth of this that the brother has any right to any of the chocolates. If the boy refuses to give his brother any, he is greedy, stingy, callous—but not unjust. I suppose that the people I have in mind will say it does follow that the brother has a right to some of the chocolates, and thus that the boy does act unjustly if he refuses to give his brother any. But the effect of saying this is to obscure what we should keep distinct, namely the difference between the boy's refusal in this case and the boy's refusal in the earlier case, in which the box was given to both boys jointly, and in which the small brother thus had what was from any point of view clear title to half.

A further objection to so using the term "right" that from the fact that A ought to do a thing for B, it follows that B has a right against A that A do it for him, is that it is going to make the question of whether or not a man has a right to a thing turn on how easy it is to provide him with it; and this seems not merely unfortunate, but morally unacceptable. Take the case of Henry Fonda again. I said earlier that I had no right to the touch of his cool hand on my fevered brow, even though I needed it to save my life. I said it would be frightfully nice of him to fly in from the West Coast to provide me with it, but that I had no right against him that he should do so. But suppose he isn't on the West Coast. Suppose he has only to walk across the room, place a hand briefly on my brow—and lo, my life is saved. Then surely he ought to do it, it would be indecent to refuse. Is it to be said "Ah, well, it follows that in this case she has a right to the touch of his hand on her brow, and so it would be an injustice in him to refuse"? So that I have a right to it when it is easy for him to provide it, though no right when it's hard? It's rather a shocking idea that anyone's rights should fade away and disappear as it gets harder and harder to accord them to him.

So my own view is that even though you ought to let the violinist use your kidneys for the one hour he needs, we should not conclude that he has a right to do so—we should say that if you refuse, you are, like the boy who owns all the chocolates and will give none away, self-centered and callous, indecent in fact, but not unjust. And similarly, that even supposing a case in which a woman pregnant due to rape ought to allow the unborn person to use her body for the hour he needs, we should not conclude that he has a right to do so; we should conclude that she is self-centered, callous, indecent, but not unjust, if she refuses. The complaints are no less grave; they are just different. However, there is no need to insist on this point. If anyone does wish to deduce "he has a right" from "you ought," then all the same he must surely grant that there are cases in which it is not morally required of you that you allow that violinist to use your kidneys, and in which he does not have a right to use them, and in which you do not do him an injustice if you refuse. And so also for mother and unborn child. Except in such cases as the unborn person has a right to demand it—and we were leaving open the possibility that there may be such cases—nobody is morally *required* to make large sacrifices, of health, of all other interests and concerns, of all other duties and commitments, for nine years, or even for nine months, in order to keep another person alive.

6. We have in fact to distinguish between two kinds of Samaritan: the Good Samaritan and what we might call the Minimally Decent Samaritan. The story of the Good Samaritan, you will remember, goes like this:

> A certain man went down from Jerusalem to Jericho, and fell among thieves, which stripped him of his raiment, and wounded him, and departed, leaving him half dead.
>
> And by chance there came down a certain priest that way; and when he saw him, he passed by on the other side.
>
> And likewise a Levite, when he was at the place, came and looked on him, and passed by on the other side.
>
> But a certain Samaritan, as he journeyed, came where he was; and when he saw him he had compassion on him.
>
> And went to him, and bound up his wounds, pouring in oil and wine, and set him on his own beast, and brought him to an inn, and took care of him.
>
> And on the morrow, when he departed, he took out two pence, and gave them to the host, and said unto him, "Take care of him; and whatsoever thou spendest more, when I come again, I will repay thee."
>
> (Luke 10:30–35)

The Good Samaritan went out of his way, at some cost to himself, to help one in need of it. We are not told what the options were, that is, whether or not the priest and the Levite could have helped by doing less than the Good Samaritan did, but assuming they could have, then the fact they did nothing at all shows they were not even Minimally Decent Samaritans, not because they were not Samaritans, but because they were not even minimally decent.

These things are a matter of degree, of course, but there is a difference, and it comes out perhaps most clearly in the story of Kitty Genovese, who, as you will remember, was murdered while thirty-eight people watched or listened, and did nothing at all to help her. A Good Samaritan would have rushed out to give direct assistance against the murderer. Or perhaps we had better allow that it would have been a Splendid Samaritan who did this, on the ground that it would have involved a risk of death for himself. But the thirty-eight not only did not do this, they did not even trouble to pick up a phone to call the police. Minimally

Decent Samaritanism would call for doing at least that, and their not having done it was monstrous.

After telling the story of the Good Samaritan, Jesus said "Go, and do thou likewise." Perhaps he meant that we are morally required to act as the Good Samaritan did. Perhaps he was urging people to do more than is morally required of them. At all events it seems plain that it was not morally required of any of the thirty-eight that he rush out to give direct assistance at the risk of his own life, and that it is not morally required of anyone that he give long stretches of his life—nine years or nine months—to sustaining the life of a person who has no special right (we were leaving open the possibility of this) to demand it.

Indeed, with one rather striking class of exceptions, no one in any country in the world is *legally* required to do anywhere near as much as this for anyone else. The class of exceptions is obvious. My main concern here is not the state of the law in respect to abortion, but it is worth drawing attention to the fact that in no state in this country is any man compelled by law to be even a Minimally Decent Samaritan to any person; there is no law under which charges could be brought against the thirty-eight who stood by while Kitty Genovese died. By contrast, in most states in this country women are compelled by law to be not merely Minimally Decent Samaritans, but Good Samaritans to unborn persons inside them. This doesn't by itself settle anything one way or the other, because it may well be argued that there should be laws in this country—as there are in many European countries—compelling at least Minimally Decent Samaritanism. But it does show that there is a gross injustice in the existing state of the law. And it shows also that the groups currently working against liberalization of abortion laws, in fact working toward having it declared unconstitutional for a state to permit abortion, had better start working for the adoption of Good Samaritan laws generally, or earn the charge that they are acting in bad faith.

I should think, myself, that Minimally Decent Samaritan laws would be one thing, Good Samaritan laws quite another, and in fact highly improper. But we are not here concerned with the law. What we should ask is not whether anybody should be compelled by law to be a Good Samaritan, but whether we must accede to a situation in which somebody is being compelled—by nature, perhaps—to be a Good Samaritan. We have, in other words, to look now at third-party interventions. I have been arguing that no person is morally required to make large sacrifices to sustain the life of another who has no right to demand them, and this even where the sacrifices do not include life itself; we are not morally required to be Good Samaritans or anyway Very Good Samaritans to one another. But what if a man cannot extricate himself from such a situation? What if he appeals to us to extricate him? It seems to me plain that there are cases in which we can, cases in which a Good Samaritan would extricate him. There you are, you were kidnapped, and nine years in bed with that violinist lie ahead of you. You have your own life to lead. You are sorry, but you simply cannot see giving up so much of your life to the sustaining of his. You cannot extricate yourself, and ask us to do so. I should have thought that—in light of his having no right to the use of your body—it was obvious that we do not have to accede to your being forced to give up so much. We can do what you ask. There is no injustice to the violinist in our doing so.

7. Following the lead of the opponents of abortion, I have throughout been speaking of the fetus merely as a person, and what I have been asking is whether or not the argument we began with, which proceeds only from the fetus' being a person, really does establish its conclusion. I have argued that it does not.

But of course there are arguments and arguments, and it may be said that I have simply fastened on the wrong one. It may be said that what is important is not merely the fact that the fetus is a person, but that it is a person for whom the woman has a special kind of responsibility issuing from the fact that she is its mother. And it might be argued that all my analogies are therefore irrelevant—for you do not have that special kind of responsibility for that violinist, Henry Fonda does not have that special kind of responsibility for me. And our attention might be drawn to the fact that men and women both *are* compelled by law to provide support for their children.

I have in effect dealt (briefly) with this argument in section 4 above; but a (still briefer) recapitulation now may be in order. Surely we do not have any such "special responsibility" for a person unless we have assumed it, explicitly or implicitly. If a set of parents do not try to prevent pregnancy, do not obtain an abortion, and then at the time of birth of the child do not put it out for adoption, but rather take it home with them, then they have assumed responsibility for it, they have given it rights, and they cannot *now* withdraw support from it at the cost of its life because they now find it difficult to go on providing for it. But if they have taken all reasonable precautions against having a child, they do not simply by virtue of their biological relationship to the child who comes into existence have a special responsibility for it. They may wish to assume responsibility for it, or they may not wish to. And I am suggesting that if assuming responsibility for it would require large sacrifices, then they may refuse. A Good Samaritan would not refuse—or anyway, a Splendid Samaritan, if the sacrifices that had to be made were enormous. But then so would a Good Samaritan assume responsibility for that violinist; so would Henry Fonda, if he is a Good Samaritan, fly in from the West Coast and assume responsibility for me.

8. My argument will be found unsatisfactory on two counts by many of those who want to regard abortion as morally permissible. First, while I do argue that abortion is not impermissible, I do not argue that it is always permissible. There may well be cases in which carrying the child to term requires only Minimally Decent Samaritanism of the mother, and this is a standard we must not fall below. I am inclined to think it a merit of my account precisely that it does *not* give a general yes or a general no. It allows for and supports our sense that, for example, a sick and desperately frightened fourteen-year-old schoolgirl, pregnant due to rape, may *of course* choose abortion, and that any law which rules this out is an insane law. And it also allows for and supports our sense that in other cases resort to abortion is even positively indecent. It would be indecent in the woman to request an abortion, and indecent in a doctor to perform it, if she is in her seventh month, and wants the abortion just to avoid the nuisance of postponing a trip abroad.

The very fact that the arguments I have been drawing attention to treat all cases of abortion, or even all cases of abortion in which the mother's life is not at stake, as morally on a par ought to have made them suspect at the outset.

Secondly, while I am arguing for the permissibility of abortion in some cases, I am not arguing for the right to secure the death of the unborn child. It is easy to confuse these two things in that up to a certain point in the life of the fetus it is not able to survive outside the mother's body; hence removing it from her body guarantees its death. But they are importantly different. I have argued that you are not morally required to spend nine months in bed, sustaining the life of that violinist; but to say this is by no means to say that if, when you unplug yourself, there is a miracle and he survives, you then have a right to turn round and slit his throat. You may detach yourself even if this costs him his life; you have no right to be guaranteed his death, by some other means, if unplugging yourself does not kill him. There are some people who will feel dissatisfied by this feature of my argument. A woman may be utterly devastated by the thought of a child, a bit of herself, put out for adoption and never seen or heard of again. She may therefore want not merely that the child be detached from her, but more, that it die. Some opponents of abortion are inclined to regard this as beneath contempt—thereby showing insensitivity to what is surely a powerful source of despair. All the same, I agree that the desire for the child's death is not one which anybody may gratify, should it turn out to be possible to detach the child alive.

At this place, however, it should be remembered that we have only been pretending throughout that the fetus is a human being from the moment of conception. A very early abortion is surely not the killing of a person, and so is not dealt with by anything I have said here.

NOTE

1. The term "direct" in the arguments I refer to is a technical one. Roughly, what is meant by "direct killing" is either killing as an end in itself, or killing as a means to some end, for example, the end of saving someone else's life.

On the Moral and Legal Status of Abortion

Mary Anne Warren

We will be concerned with both the moral status of abortion, which for our purposes we may define as the act which a woman performs in voluntarily terminating, or allowing another person to terminate, her pregnancy, and the legal status which is appropriate for this act. I will argue that, while it is not possible to produce a satisfactory defense of a woman's right to obtain an abortion without showing that a fetus is not a human being, in the morally relevant sense of that term, we ought not to conclude that the difficulties involved in determining whether or not a fetus is human make it impossible to produce any satisfactory solution to the problem of the moral status of abortion. For it is possible to show that, on the basis of intuitions which we may expect even the opponents of abortion to share, a fetus is not a person, and hence not the sort of entity to which it is proper to ascribe full moral rights.

Of course, while some philosophers would deny the possibility of any such proof, others will deny that there is any need for it, since the moral permissibility of abortion appears to them to be too obvious to require proof. But the inadequacy of this attitude should be evident from the fact that both the friends and the foes of abortion consider their position to be morally self-evident. Because proabortionists have never adequately come to grips with the conceptual issues surrounding abortion, most if not all, of the arguments which they advance in opposition to laws restricting access to abortion fail to refute or even weaken the traditional antiabortion argument, i.e., that a fetus is a human being, and therefore abortion is murder.

These arguments are typically of one of two sorts. Either they point to the terrible side effects of the restrictive laws, e.g., the deaths due to illegal abor-

tions, and the fact that it is poor women who suffer the most as a result of these laws, or else they state that to deny a woman access to abortion is to deprive her of her right to control her own body. Unfortunately, however, the fact that restricting access to abortion has tragic side effects does not, in itself, show that the restrictions are unjustified, since murder is wrong regardless of the consequences of prohibiting it; and the appeal to the right to control one's body, which is generally construed as a property right, is at best a rather feeble argument for the permissibility of abortion. Mere ownership does not give me the right to kill innocent people whom I find on my property, and indeed I am apt to be held responsible if such people injure themselves while on my property. It is equally unclear that I have any moral right to expel an innocent person from my property when I know that doing so will result in his death.

Furthermore, it is probably inappropriate to describe a woman's body as her property, since it seems natural to hold that a person is something distinct from her property, but not from her body. Even those who would object to the identification of a person with his body, or with the conjunction of his body and his mind, must admit that it would be very odd to describe, say, breaking a leg, as damaging one's property, and much more appropriate to describe it as injuring one*self*. Thus it is probably a mistake to argue that the right to obtain an abortion is in any way derived from the right to own and regulate property.

But however we wish to construe the right to abortion, we cannot hope to convince those who consider abortion a form of murder of the existence of any such right unless we are able to produce a clear and convincing refutation of the traditional antiabortion argument, and this has not, to my knowledge, been done. With respect to the two most vital issues which that argument involves, i.e., the humanity of the fetus and its implication for the moral status of abortion, confusion has prevailed on both sides of the dispute.

Mary Anne Warren, excerpts from "On the Moral and Legal Status of Abortion" in *The Monist* Volume 57, pp. 43–61. Copyright © *The Monist: An International Quarterly Journal of General Philosophical Inquiry*, The Hegeler Institute, Peru, IL. Reprinted by permission.

Thus, both proabortionists and antiabortionists have tended to abstract the question of whether abortion is wrong to that of whether it is wrong to destroy a fetus, just as though the rights of another person were not necessarily involved. This mistaken abstraction has led to the almost universal assumption that if a fetus is a human being, with a right to life, then it follows immediately that abortion is wrong (except perhaps when necessary to save the woman's life), and that it ought to be prohibited. It has also been generally assumed that unless the question about the status of the fetus is answered, the moral status of abortion cannot possibly be determined.

* * *

Judith Thomson is . . . the only writer I am aware of who has seriously questioned this assumption; she has argued that, even if we grant the antiabortionist his claim that a fetus is a human being, with the same right to life as any other human being, we can still demonstrate that, in at least some and perhaps most cases, a woman is under no moral obligation to complete an unwanted pregnancy.[1] Her argument is worth examining, since if it holds up it may enable us to establish the moral permissibility of abortion without becoming involved in problems about what entitles an entity to be considered human, and accorded full moral rights. To be able to do this would be a great gain in the power and simplicity of the proabortion position, since, although I will argue that these problems can be solved at least as decisively as can any other moral problem, we should certainly be pleased to be able to avoid having to solve them as part of the justification of abortion.

On the other hand, even if Thomson's argument does not hold up, her insight, i.e., that it requires *argument* to show that if fetuses are human then abortion is properly classified as murder, is an extremely valuable one. The assumption she attacks is particularly invidious, for it amounts to the decision that it is appropriate, in deciding the moral status of abortion, to leave the rights of the pregnant woman out of consideration entirely, except possibly when her life is threatened. Obviously, this will not do; determining what moral rights, if any, a fetus possesses is only the first step in determining the moral status of abor-

tion. Step two, which is at least equally essential, is finding a just solution to the conflict between whatever rights the fetus may have, and the rights of the woman who is unwillingly pregnant. While the historical error has been to pay far too little attention to the second step, Ms. Thomson's suggestion is that if we look at the second step first we may find that a woman has a right to obtain an abortion *regardless* of what rights the fetus has.

Our own inquiry will also have two stages. In Section I, we will consider whether or not it is possible to establish that abortion is morally permissible even on the assumption that a fetus is an entity with a full-fledged right to life. I will argue that in fact this cannot be established, at least not with the conclusiveness which is essential to our hopes of convincing those who are skeptical about the morality of abortion, and that we therefore cannot avoid dealing with the question of whether or not a fetus really does have the same right to life as a (more fully developed) human being.

In Section II, I will propose an answer to this question, namely, that a fetus cannot be considered a member of the moral community, the set of beings with full and equal moral rights, for the simple reason that it is not a person, and that it is personhood, and not genetic humanity, . . . which is the basis for membership in this community. I will argue that a fetus, whatever its stage of development, satisfies none of the basic criteria of personhood, and is not even enough *like* a person to be accorded even some of the same rights on the basis of this resemblance. Nor, as we will see, is a fetus's *potential* personhood a threat to the morality of abortion, since, whatever the rights of potential people may be, they are invariably overridden in any conflict with the moral rights of actual people.

I

We turn now to Professor Thomson's case for the claim that even if a fetus has full moral rights, abortion is still morally permissible, at least sometimes, and for some reasons other than to save the woman's life. Her argument is based upon a clever, but I think faulty, analogy. She asks us to picture ourselves waking up one day, in bed with a famous violinist. Imagine that you have been kidnapped, and your bloodstream hooked up to that of the violinist, who happens to have an ailment which will certainly kill him unless he is permitted to share your kidneys for a period of nine months. No one else can save him, since you alone have the right type of blood. He will be unconscious all that time, and you will have to stay in bed with him, but after the nine months are over he may be unplugged, completely cured, that is provided that you have cooperated.

Now then, she continues, what are your obligations in this situation? The antiabortionist, if he is consistent, will have to say that you are obligated to stay in bed with the violinist: for all people have a right to life, and violinists are people, and therefore it would be murder for you to disconnect yourself from him and let him die [p. 174]. But this is outrageous, and so there must be something wrong with the same argument when it is applied to abortion. It would certainly be commendable of you to agree to save the violinist, but it is absurd to suggest that your refusal to do so would be murder. His right to life does not obligate you to do whatever is required to keep him alive; nor does it justify anyone else in forcing you to do so. A law which required you to stay in bed with the violinist would clearly be an unjust law, since it is no proper function of the law to force unwilling people to make huge sacrifices for the sake of other people toward whom they have no such prior obligation.

Thomson concludes that, if this analogy is an apt one, then we can grant the antiabortionist his claim that a fetus is a human being, and still hold that it is at least sometimes the case that a pregnant woman has the right to refuse to be a Good Samaritan towards the fetus, i.e., to obtain an abortion. For there is a great gap between the claim that *x* has a right to life, and the claim that *y* is obligated to do whatever is necessary to keep *x* alive, let alone that he ought to be forced to do so. It is *y*'s duty to keep *x* alive only if he has somehow contracted a *special* obligation to do so; and a woman who is unwillingly pregnant, e.g., who was raped, has done nothing which obligates her to make the enormous sacrifice which is necessary to preserve the conceptus.

This argument is initially quite plausible, and in the extreme case of pregnancy due to rape it is probably conclusive. Difficulties arise, however, when we try to specify more exactly the range of cases in which abortion is clearly justifiable even on the assumption that the fetus is human. Professor Thomson considers it a virtue of her argument that it does not enable us to conclude that abortion is *always* permissible. It would, she says, be "indecent" for a woman in her seventh month to obtain an abortion just to avoid having to postpone a trip to Europe. On the other hand, her argument enables us to see that "a sick and desperately frightened schoolgirl pregnant due to rape may *of course* choose abortion, and that any law which rules this out is an insane law" [p. 183]. So far, so good; but what are we to say about the woman who becomes pregnant not through rape but as a result of her own carelessness, or because of contraceptive failure, or who gets pregnant intentionally and then changes her mind about wanting a child? With respect to such cases, the violinist analogy is of much less use to the defender of the woman's right to obtain an abortion.

Indeed, the choice of a pregnancy due to rape, as an example of a case in which abortion is permissible even if a fetus is considered a human being, is extremely significant; for it is only in the case of pregnancy due to rape that the woman's situation is adequately analogous to the violinist case for our intuitions about the latter to transfer convincingly. The crucial difference between a pregnancy due to rape and the *normal* case of an unwanted pregnancy is that in the normal case, we cannot claim that the woman is in no way responsible for her predicament; she could have remained chaste, or taken her pills more faithfully, or abstained on dangerous days, and so on. If, on the other hand, you are kidnapped by strangers, and hooked up to a strange violinist, then you are free of any shred of responsibility for the situation, on the basis of which it could be argued that you are obligated to keep the violinist alive. Only when her pregnancy is due to rape is a woman clearly just as nonresponsible.[2]

Consequently, there is room for the antiabortionist to argue that in the normal case of unwanted pregnancy a woman has, by her own actions, assumed responsibility for the fetus. For if *x* behaves in a way which he could have avoided, and which he knows involves, let us say, a 1 percent chance of bringing into existence a human being, with a right to life, and does so knowing that if this should happen then that human being will perish unless *x* does certain things to keep him alive, then it is by no means clear that when it does happen *x* is free of any obligation to what he knew in advance would be required to keep that human being alive.

The plausibility of such an argument is enough to show that the Thomson analogy can provide a clear and persuasive defense of a woman's right to obtain an abortion only with respect to those cases in which the woman is in no way responsible for her pregnancy, e.g., where it is due to rape. In all other cases, we would almost certainly conclude that it was necessary to look carefully at the particular circumstances in order to determine the extent of the woman's responsibility, and hence the extent of her obligation. This is an extremely unsatisfactory outcome, from the viewpoint of the opponents of restrictive abortion laws, most of whom are convinced that a woman has a right to obtain an abortion regardless of how and why she got pregnant.

Of course a supporter of the violinist analogy might point out that it is absurd to suggest that forgetting her pill one day might be sufficient to obligate a woman to complete an unwanted pregnancy. And indeed it *is* absurd to suggest this. As we will see, the moral right to obtain an abortion is not in the least dependent upon the extent to which the woman is responsible for her pregnancy. But unfortunately, once we allow the assumption that a fetus has full moral rights, we cannot avoid taking this absurd suggestion seriously. Perhaps we can make this point more clear by altering the violinist story just enough to make it more analogous to a normal unwanted pregnancy and less to a pregnancy due to rape, and then seeing whether it is still obvious that you are not obligated to stay in bed with the fellow.

Suppose, then, that violinists are peculiarly prone to the sort of illness the only cure for which is the use of someone else's bloodstream for nine months, and that because of this there has been formed a society of music lovers who agree that whenever a violinist is stricken they will draw lots and the loser will, by some means, be made the one and only person capable of saving him. Now then, would you be obligated to cooperate in curing the violinist if you had voluntarily joined this society, knowing the possible consequences, and then your name had been drawn and you had been kidnapped? Admittedly, you did not promise ahead of time that you would, but you did deliberately place yourself in a position in which it might happen that a human life would be lost if you did not. Surely this is at least a prima facie reason for supposing that you have an obligation to stay in bed with the violinist. Suppose that you had gotten your name drawn deliberately; surely *that* would be quite a strong reason for thinking that you had such an obligation.

It might be suggested that there is one important disanalogy between the modified violinist case and the case of an unwanted pregnancy, which makes the woman's responsibility significantly less, namely, the fact that the fetus *comes into existence* as the result of the woman's actions. This fact might give her a right to refuse to keep it alive, whereas she would not have had this right had it existed previously, independently, and then as a result of her actions become dependent upon her for its survival.

My own intuition, however, is that *x* has no more right to bring into existence, either deliberately or as a foreseeable result of actions he could have avoided, a being with full moral rights (*y*), and then refuse to do what he knew beforehand would be required to keep that being alive, then he has to enter into an agreement with an existing person, whereby he may be called upon to save that person's life, and then refuse to do so when so called upon. Thus, *x*'s responsibility for *y*'s existence does not seem to lessen his obligation to keep *y* alive, if he is also responsible for *y*'s being in a situation in which only he can save him.

Whether or not this intuition is entirely correct, it brings us back once again to the conclusion that once we allow the assumption that a fetus has full moral rights it becomes an extremely complex and difficult question whether and when abortion is justifiable. Thus the Thomson analogy cannot help us produce a clear and persuasive proof of the moral permissibility of abortion. Nor will the opponents of the restrictive laws thank us for anything less; for their conviction (for the most part) is that abortion is obviously *not* a morally serious and extremely unfortunate, even though sometimes justified act, comparable to killing in self-defense or to letting the violinist die, but rather is closer to being a morally neutral act, like cutting one's hair.

The basis of this conviction, I believe, is the realization that a fetus is not a person, and thus does not have a full-fledged right to life. Perhaps the reason why this claim has been so inadequately defended is that it seems self-evident to those who accept it. And so it is, insofar as it follows from what I take to be perfectly obvious claims about the nature of personhood, and about the proper grounds for ascribing moral rights, claims which ought, indeed, to be obvious to both the friends and foes of abortion. Nevertheless, it is worth examining these claims, and showing how they demonstrate the moral innocuousness of abortion, since this apparently has not been adequately done before.

II

The question which we must answer in order to produce a satisfactory solution to the problem of the moral status of abortion is this: How are we to define the moral community, the set of beings with full and equal moral rights, such that we can decide whether a human fetus is a member of this community or not? What sort of entity, exactly, has the inalienable rights to life, liberty, and the pursuit of happiness? . . . What reason is there for identifying the moral community with the set of all human beings, in whatever way we have chosen to define that term?

1. On the Definition of 'Human'

One reason why this vital . . . question is so frequently overlooked in the debate over the moral status of abortion is that the term 'human' has two distinct, but not often distinguished, senses. This fact results in a slide of meaning, which serves to conceal the fallaciousness of the traditional argument that since (1) it is wrong to kill innocent human beings, and (2) fetuses are innocent human beings, then (3) it is wrong to kill fetuses. For if 'human' is used in the same sense in both (1) and (2) then, whichever of the two senses is meant, one of these premises is question-begging. And if it is used in two different senses then of course the conclusion doesn't follow.

Thus, (1) is a self-evident moral truth,[3] and avoids begging the question about abortion, only if 'human being' is used to mean something like "a full-fledged member of the moral community." (It may or may not also be meant to refer exclusively to members of the species *Homo sapiens*.) We may call this the *moral* sense of 'human'. It is not to be confused with what we will call the *genetic* sense, i.e., the sense in which *any* member of the species is a human being, and no member of any other species could be. If (1) is acceptable only if the moral sense is intended, (2) is non-question-begging only if what is intended is the genetic sense.

In "Deciding Who is Human," [John] Noonan argues for the classification of fetuses with human beings by pointing to the presence of the full genetic code, and the potential capacity for rational thought.[4] It is clear that what he needs to show, for his version of the traditional argument to be valid, is that fetuses are human in the moral sense, the sense in which it is analytically true that all human beings have full moral rights. But, in the absence of any argument showing that whatever is genetically human is also morally human, and he gives none, nothing more than genetic humanity can be demonstrated by the presence of the human genetic code. And, as we will see, the *potential* capacity for rational thought can at most show that an entity has the potential for *becoming* human in the moral sense.

2. Defining the Moral Community

Can it be established that genetic humanity is sufficient for moral humanity? I think that there are very good reasons for not defining the moral community in this way. I would like to suggest an alternative way of defining the moral community, which I will argue for only to the extent of explaining why it is, or should be, self-evident. The suggestion is simply that the moral community consists of all and only *people*, rather than all and only human beings;[5] and probably the best way of demonstrating its self-evidence is by considering the concept of personhood, to see what sorts of entity are and are not persons, and what the decision that a being is or is not a person implies about its moral rights.

What characteristics entitle an entity to be considered a person? This is obviously not the place to attempt a complete analysis of the concept of personhood, but we do not need such a fully adequate analysis just to determine whether and why a fetus is or isn't a person. All we need is a rough and approximate list of the most basic criteria of personhood, and some idea of which, or how many, of these an entity must satisfy in order to properly be considered a person.

In searching for such criteria, it is useful to look beyond the set of people with whom we are acquainted, and ask how we would decide whether a totally alien being was a person or not. (For we have no right to assume that genetic humanity is necessary for personhood.) Imagine a space traveler who lands on an unknown planet and encounters a race of beings utterly unlike any he has ever seen or heard of. If he wants to be sure of behaving morally toward these beings, he has to somehow decide whether they are people, and hence have full moral rights, or whether they are the sort of thing which he need not feel guilty about treating as, for example, a source of food.

How should he go about making this decision? If he has some anthropological background, he might look for such things as religion, art, and the manufacturing of tools, weapons, or shelters, since these factors have been used to distinguish our human from our prehuman ancestors, in what seems to be closer to the moral than the genetic sense of 'human'. And no doubt he would be right to consider the presence of such factors as good evidence that the alien beings were people, and morally human. It would, however, be overly anthropocentric of him to take the absence of these things as adequate evidence that they were not, since we can imagine people who have progressed beyond, or evolved without ever developing, these cultural characteristics.

I suggest that the traits which are most central to the concept of personhood, or humanity in the moral sense, are, very roughly, the following:

(1) consciousness (of objects and events external and/ or internal to the being), and in particular the capacity to feel pain;
(2) reasoning (the *developed* capacity to solve new and relatively complex problems);
(3) self-motivated activity (activity which is relatively independent of either genetic or direct external control);
(4) the capacity to communicate, by whatever means, messages of an indefinite variety of types, that is, not just with an indefinite number of possible contents, but on indefinitely many possible topics;
(5) the presence of self-concepts, and self-awareness, either individual or racial, or both.

Admittedly, there are apt to be a great many problems involved in formulating precise definitions of these criteria, let alone in developing universally valid behavioral criteria for deciding when they apply. But I will assume that both we and our explorer know approximately what (1)–(5) mean, and that he is also able to determine whether or not they apply. How, then should he use his findings to decide whether or not the alien beings are people? We needn't suppose that an entity must have *all* of these attributes to be properly considered a person; (1) and (2) alone may well be sufficient for personhood, and quite probably (1)–(3) are sufficient. Neither do we need to insist that any one of these criteria is *necessary* for personhood, although once again (1) and (2) look like fairly good candidates for necessary conditions, as does (3), if 'activity' is construed so as to include the activity of reasoning.

All we need to claim, to demonstrate that a fetus is not a person, is that any being which satisfies *none* of (1)–(5) is certainly not a person. I consider this claim to be so obvious that I think anyone who denied it, and claimed that a being which satisfied none of (1)–(5) was a person all the same, would thereby demonstrate that he had no notion at all of what a person is—perhaps because he had confused the concept of a person with that of genetic humanity. If the opponents of abortion were to deny the appropriateness of these five criteria, I do not know what further arguments would convince them. We would probably have to admit that our conceptual schemes were indeed irreconcilably different, and that our dispute could not be settled objectively.

I do not expect this to happen, however, since I think that the concept of a person is one which is very nearly universal (to people), and that it is common to both proabortionists and antiabortionists, even though neither group has fully realized the relevance of this concept to the resolution of their dispute. Furthermore, I think that on reflection even the antiabortionists ought to agree not only that (1)–(5) are central to the concept of personhood, but also that it is a part of this concept that all and only people have full moral rights. The concept of a person is in part a moral concept; once we have admitted that *x* is a person we have recognized, even if we have not agreed to respect, *x*'s right to be treated as a member of the moral community. It is true that the claim that *x* is a *human being* is more commonly voiced as part of an appeal to treat *x* decently than is the claim that *x* is a person, but this is either because 'human being' is here used in the sense which implies personhood, or because the genetic and moral senses of 'human' have been confused.

Now if (1)–(5) are indeed the primary criteria of personhood, then it is clear that genetic humanity is neither necessary nor sufficient for establishing that an entity is a person. Some human beings are not people, and there may well be people who are not human beings. A man or woman whose consciousness has been permanently obliterated but who remains alive is a human being which is no longer a person; defective human beings, with no appreciable mental capacity, are not and presumably never will be people; and a fetus is a human being which is not yet a person, and which therefore cannot coherently be said to have full moral rights. Citizens of the next century should be prepared to recognize highly advanced, self-aware robots or computers, should such be developed, and intelligent inhabitants of other worlds, should such

be found, as people in the fullest sense, and to respect their moral rights. But to ascribe full moral rights to an entity which is not a person is as absurd as to ascribe moral obligations and responsibilities to such an entity.

3. Fetal Development and the Right to Life

Two problems arise in the application of these suggestions for the definition of the moral community to the determination of the precise moral status of a human fetus. Given that the paradigm example of a person is a normal adult human being, then (1) How like this paradigm, in particular how far advanced since conception, does a human being need to be before it begins to have a right to life by virtue, not of being fully a person as of yet, but of being *like* a person? and (2) To what extent, if any, does the fact that a fetus has the *potential* for becoming a person endow it with some of the same rights? Each of these questions requires some comment.

In answering the first question, we need not attempt a detailed consideration of the moral rights of organisms which are not developed enough, aware enough, intelligent enough, etc., to be considered people, but which resemble people in some respects. It does seem reasonable to suggest that the more like a person, in the relevant respects, a being is, the stronger is the case for regarding it as having a right to life, and indeed the stronger its right to life is. Thus we ought to take seriously the suggestion that, insofar as "the human individual develops biologically in a continuous fashion . . . the rights of a human person might develop in the same way."[6] But we must keep in mind that the attributes which are relevant in determining whether or not an entity is enough like a person to be regarded as having some of the same moral rights are no different from those which are relevant to determining whether or not it is fully a person—i.e., are no different from (1)–(5)—and that being genetically human, or having recognizably human facial and other physical features, or detectable brain activity, or the capacity to survive outside the uterus, are simply not among these relevant attributes.

Thus it is clear that even though a seven- or eight-month fetus has features which make it apt to arouse in us almost the same powerful protective instinct as is commonly aroused by a small infant, nevertheless it is not significantly more personlike than is a very small embryo. It is *somewhat* more personlike; it can apparently feel and respond to pain, and it may even have a rudimentary form of consciousness, insofar as its brain is quite active. Nevertheless, it seems safe to say that it is not fully conscious, in the way that an infant of a few months is, and that it cannot reason, or communicate messages of indefinitely many sorts, does not engage in self-motivated activity, and has no self-awareness. Thus, in the *relevant* respects, a fetus, even a fully developed one, is considerably less personlike than is the average mature mammal, indeed the average fish. And I think that a rational person must conclude that if the right to life of a fetus is to be based upon its resemblance to a person, then it cannot be said to have any more right to life than, let us say, a newborn guppy (which also seems to be capable of feeling pain), and that a right of that magnitude could never override a woman's right to obtain an abortion, at any stage of her pregnancy.

There may, of course, be other arguments in favor of placing legal limits upon the stage of pregnancy in which an abortion may be performed. Given the relative safety of the new techniques of artificially inducing labor during the third trimester, the danger to the woman's life or health is no longer such an argument. Neither is the fact that people tend to respond to the thought of abortion in the later stages of pregnancy with emotional repulsion, since mere emotional responses cannot take the place of moral reasoning in determining what ought to be permitted. Nor, finally, is the frequently heard argument that legalizing abortion, especially late in the pregnancy, may erode the level of respect for human life, leading, perhaps, to an increase in unjustified euthanasia and other crimes. For this threat, if it is a threat, can be better met by educating people to the kinds of moral distinctions which we are making here than by limiting access to abortion (which limitation may, in its disregard for the rights of women, be just as damaging to the level of respect for human rights).

Thus, since the fact that even a fully developed fetus is not personlike enough to have any significant right to life on the basis of its personlikeness shows that no legal restrictions upon the stage of pregnancy in which an abortion may be performed can be justified on the grounds that we should protect the rights of the older fetus; and since there is no other apparent justification for such restrictions, we may conclude that they are entirely unjustified. Whether or not it would be *indecent* (whatever that means) for a woman in her seventh month to obtain an abortion just to avoid having to postpone a trip to Europe, it would not, in itself, be *immoral,* and therefore it ought to be permitted.

4. Potential Personhood and the Right to Life

We have seen that a fetus does not resemble a person in any way which can support the claim that it has even some of the same rights. But what about its *potential*, the fact that if nurtured and allowed to develop naturally it will very probably become a person? Doesn't that alone give it at least some right to life? It is hard to deny that the fact that an entity is a potential person is a strong prima facie reason for not destroying it; but we need not conclude from this that a potential person has a right to life, by virtue of that potential. It may be that our feeling that it is better, other things being equal, not to destroy a potential person is better explained by the fact that potential people are still (felt to be) an invaluable resource, not to be lightly squandered. Surely, if every speck of dust were a potential person, we would be much less apt to conclude that every potential person has a right to become actual.

Still, we do not need to insist that a potential person has no right to life whatever. There may well be something immoral, and not just imprudent, about wantonly destroying potential people, when doing so isn't necessary to protect anyone's rights. But even if a potential person does have some prima facie right to life, such a right could not possibly outweigh the right of a woman to obtain an abortion, since the rights of any actual person invariably outweigh those of any potential person, whenever the two conflict. Since this may not be immediately obvious in the case of a human fetus, let us look at another case.

Suppose that our space explorer falls into the hands of an alien culture, whose scientists decide to create a few hundred thousand or more human beings, by breaking his body into its component cells, and using these to create fully developed human beings, with, of course, his genetic code. We may imagine that each of these newly created men will have all of the original man's abilities, skills, knowledge, and so on, and also have an individual self-concept, in short that each of them will be a bona fide (though hardly unique) person. Imagine that the whole project will take only seconds, and that its chances of success are extremely high, and that our explorer knows all of this, and also knows that these people will be treated fairly. I maintain that in such a situation he would have every right to escape if he could, and thus to deprive all of these potential people of their potential lives; for his right to life outweighs all of theirs together, in spite of the fact that they are all genetically human, all innocent, and all have a very high probability of becoming people very soon, if only he refrains from acting.

Indeed, I think he would have a right to escape even if it were not his life which the alien scientists planned to take, but only a year of his freedom, or, indeed, only a day. Nor would he be obligated to stay if he had gotten captured (thus bringing all these people-potentials into existence) because of his own carelessness, or even if he had done so deliberately, knowing the consequences. Regardless of how he got captured, he is not morally obligated to remain in captivity for *any* period of time for the sake of permitting any number of potential people to come into actuality, so great is the margin by which one actual person's right to liberty outweighs whatever right to life even a hundred thousand potential people have. And it seems reasonable to conclude that the rights of a woman will outweigh by a similar margin whatever right to life a fetus may have by virtue of its potential personhood.

Thus, neither a fetus's resemblance to a person, nor its potential for becoming a person provides any

basis whatever for the claim that it has any significant right to life. Consequently, a woman's right to protect her health, happiness, freedom, and even her life,[7] by terminating an unwanted pregnancy, will always override whatever right to life it may be appropriate to ascribe to a fetus, even a fully developed one. And thus, in the absence of any overwhelming social need for every possible child, the laws which restrict the right to obtain an abortion, or limit the period of pregnancy during which an abortion may be performed, are a wholly unjustified violation of a woman's most basic moral and constitutional rights.

NOTES

1. Judith Thomson, "A Defense of Abortion," *Philosophy & Public Affairs* 1, no. 1 (Fall 1971): 47–66.

2. We may safely ignore the fact that she might have avoided getting raped, e.g., by carrying a gun, since by similar means you might likewise have avoided getting kidnapped, and in neither case does the victim's failure to take all possible precautions against a highly unlikely event (as opposed to reasonable precautions against a rather likely event) mean that he is morally responsible for what happens.

3. Of course, the principle that it is (always) wrong to kill innocent human beings is in need of many other modifications, e.g., that it may be permissible to do so to save a greater number of other innocent human beings, but we may safely ignore these complications here.

4. John Noonan, "Deciding Who Is Human," *Natural Law Forum* 13 (1968): 135.

5. From here on, we will use 'human' to mean genetically human, since the moral sense seems closely connected to, and perhaps derived from, the assumption that genetic humanity is sufficient for membership in the moral community.

6. Thomas L. Hayes, "A Biological View," *Commonweal* 85 (March 17, 1967): 677–78; quoted by Daniel Callahan, in *Abortion: Law, Choice, and Morality* (New York: Macmillan, 1970).

7. That is, insofar as the death rate, for the woman, is higher for childbirth than for early abortion.

Why Abortion Is Immoral

Don Marquis

The view that abortion is, with rare exceptions, seriously immoral has received little support in the recent philosophical literature. No doubt most philosophers affiliated with secular institutions of higher education believe that the anti-abortion position is either a symptom of irrational religious dogma or a conclusion generated by seriously confused philosophical argument. The purpose of this essay is to undermine this general belief. This essay sets out an argument that purports to show, as well as any argument in ethics can show, that abortion is, except possibly in rare cases, seriously immoral, that it is in the same moral category as killing an innocent adult human being.

The argument is based on a major assumption. Many of the most insightful and careful writers on the ethics of abortion . . . believe that whether or not abortion is morally permissible stands or falls on whether or not a fetus is the sort of being whose life it is seriously wrong to end. The argument of this essay will assume, but not argue, that they are correct.

Also, this essay will neglect issues of great importance to a complete ethics of abortion. Some anti-abortionists will allow that certain abortions, such as abortion before implantation or abortion when the life of a woman is threatened by a pregnancy or abortion after rape, may be morally permissible. This essay will not explore the casuistry of these hard cases. The purpose of this essay is to develop a general argument for the claim that the overwhelming majority of deliberate abortions are seriously immoral.

I.

A sketch of standard anti-abortion and pro-choice arguments exhibits how these arguments possess certain symmetries that explain why partisans of those positions are so convinced of the correctness of their own positions, why they are not successful in convincing their opponents, and why, to others, this issue seems to be unresolvable. An analysis of the nature of this standoff suggests a strategy for surmounting it.

Consider the way a typical anti-abortionist argues. She will argue or assert that life is present from the moment of conception or that fetuses look like babies or that fetuses possess a characteristic such as a genetic code that is both necessary and sufficient for being human. Anti-abortionists seem to believe that (1) the truth of all of these claims is quite obvious, and (2) establishing any of these claims is sufficient to show that abortion is morally akin to murder.

A standard pro-choice strategy exhibits similarities. The pro-choicer will argue or assert that fetuses are not persons or that fetuses are not rational agents or that fetuses are not social beings. Pro-choicers seem to believe that (1) the truth of any of these claims is quite obvious, and (2) establishing any of these claims is sufficient to show that an abortion is not a wrongful killing.

In fact, both the pro-choice and the anti-abortion claims do seem to be true, although the "it looks like a baby" claim is more difficult to establish the earlier the pregnancy. We seem to have a standoff. How can it be resolved?

As everyone who has taken a bit of logic knows, if any of these arguments concerning abortion is a good argument, it requires not only some claim characterizing fetuses, but also some general moral principle that ties a characteristic of fetuses to having or not having the right to life or to some other moral characteristic that will generate the obligation or the lack of obligation not to end the life of a fetus. Accordingly, the arguments of the anti-abortionist and the pro-choicer need a bit of filling in to be regarded as adequate.

Note what each partisan will say. The anti-abortionist will claim that her position is supported by such generally accepted moral principles as "It is always prima facie seriously wrong to take a human life" or "It is always prima facie seriously wrong to end

Don Marquis, "Why Abortion Is Immoral," *The Journal of Philosophy* LXXXVI, 4 (April 1989): 183–202. Reprinted by permission of the publisher and the author.

the life of a baby." Since these are generally accepted moral principles, her position is certainly not obviously wrong. The pro-choicer will claim that her position is supported by such plausible moral principles as "Being a person is what gives an individual intrinsic moral worth" or "It is only seriously prima facie wrong to take the life of a member of the human community." Since these are generally accepted moral principles, the pro-choice position is certainly not obviously wrong. Unfortunately, we have again arrived at a standoff.

Now, how might one deal with this standoff? The standard approach is to try to show how the moral principles of one's opponent lose their plausibility under analysis. It is easy to see how this is possible. On the one hand, the anti-abortionist will defend a moral principle concerning the wrongness of killing which tends to be broad in scope in order that even fetuses at an early stage of pregnancy will fall under it. The problem with broad principles is that they often embrace too much. In this particular instance, the principle "It is always prima facie wrong to take a human life" seems to entail that it is wrong to end the existence of a living human cancer-cell culture, on the grounds that the culture is both living and human. Therefore, it seems that the anti-abortionist's favored principle is too broad.

On the other hand, the pro-choicer wants to find a moral principle concerning the wrongness of killing which tends to be narrow in scope in order that fetuses will *not* fall under it. The problem with narrow principles is that they often do not embrace enough. Hence, the needed principles such as "It is prima facie seriously wrong to kill only persons" or "It is prima facie wrong to kill only rational agents" do not explain why it is wrong to kill infants or young children or the severely retarded or even perhaps the severely mentally ill. Therefore, we seem again to have a standoff. The anti-abortionist charges, not unreasonably, that pro-choice principles concerning killing are too narrow to be acceptable; the pro-choicer charges, not unreasonably, that anti-abortionist principles concerning killing are too broad to be acceptable.

Attempts by both sides to patch up the difficulties in their positions run into further difficulties. The anti-abortionist will try to remove the problem in her position by reformulating her principle concerning killing in terms of human beings. Now we end up with: "It is always prima facie seriously wrong to end the life of a human being." This principle has the advantage of avoiding the problem of the human cancer-cell culture counterexample. But this advantage is purchased at a high price. For although it is clear that a fetus is both human and alive, it is not at all clear that a fetus is a human *being*. There is at least something to be said for the view that something becomes a human being only after a process of development, and that therefore first trimester fetuses and perhaps all fetuses are not yet human beings. Hence, the anti-abortionist, by this move, has merely exchanged one problem for another.

The pro-choicer fares no better. She may attempt to find reasons why killing infants, young children, and the severely retarded is wrong which are independent of her major principle that is supposed to explain the wrongness of taking human life, but which will not also make abortion immoral. This is no easy task. Appeals to social utility will seem satisfactory only to those who resolve not to think of the enormous difficulties with a utilitarian account of the wrongness of killing and the significant social costs of preserving the lives of the unproductive. A pro-choice strategy that extends the definition of 'person' to infants or even to young children seems just as arbitrary as an anti-abortion strategy that extends the definition of 'human being' to fetuses. Again, we find symmetries in the two positions and we arrive at a standoff.

There are even further problems that reflect symmetries in the two positions. In addition to counterexample problems, or the arbitrary application problems that can be exchanged for them, the standard anti-abortionist principle "It is prima facie seriously wrong to kill a human being," or one of its variants, can be objected to on the grounds of ambiguity. If 'human being' is taken to be a *biological* category, then the anti-abortionist is left with the problem of explaining why a merely biological category should make a moral difference. Why, it is asked, is it any more reasonable to base a moral conclusion on the number of chromosomes in one's cells than on the color of one's skin? If 'human being', on the other hand, is taken to be a *moral* category, then the claim that a fetus is a human being cannot be taken to be a premise in the anti-abortion argument, for it is precisely what needs to be established. Hence, either the anti-abortionist's main category is a morally irrelevant, merely biological category, or it is of no use to the anti-abortionist in establishing (noncircularly, of course) that abortion is wrong.

Although this problem with the anti-abortionist position is often noticed, it is less often noticed that the pro-choice position suffers from an analogous problem. The principle "Only persons have the right to life" also suffers from an ambiguity. The term 'person' is typically defined in terms of psychological characteristics, although there will certainly be disagreement concerning which characteristics are most important. Supposing that this matter can be settled, the pro-choicer is left with the problem of explaining why *psychological* characteristics should make a *moral* difference. If the pro-choicer should attempt to deal with this problem by claiming that an explanation is not necessary, that in fact we do treat such a cluster of psychological properties as having moral significance, the sharp-witted anti-abortionist should have a ready response. We do treat being both living and human as having moral significance. If it is legitimate for the pro-choicer to demand that the anti-abortionist provide an explanation of the connection between the biological character of being a human being and the wrongness of being killed (even though people accept this connection), then it is legitimate for the anti-abortionist to demand that the pro-choicer provide an explanation of the connection between psychological criteria for being a person and the wrongness of being killed (even though that connection is accepted).

[Joel] Feinberg has attempted to meet this objection (he calls psychological personhood "commonsense personhood"):

The characteristics that confer commonsense personhood are not arbitrary bases for rights and duties, such as race, sex or species membership; rather they are traits that make sense out of rights and duties and without which those moral attributes would have no point or function. It is because people are conscious; have a sense of their personal identities; have plans, goals, and projects; experience emotions; are liable to pains, anxieties, and frustrations; can reason and bargain, and so on—it is because of these attributes that people have values and interests, desires and expectations of their own, including a stake in their own futures, and a personal well-being of a sort we cannot ascribe to unconscious or nonrational beings. Because of their developed capacities they can assume duties and responsibilities and can have and make claims on one another. Only because of their sense of self, their life plans, their value hierarchies, and their stakes in their own futures can they be ascribed fundamental rights. There is nothing arbitrary about these linkages.[1]

The plausible aspects of this attempt should not be taken to obscure its implausible features. There is a great deal to be said for the view that being a psychological person under some description is a necessary condition for having duties. One cannot have a duty unless one is capable of behaving morally, and a being's capability of behaving morally will require having a certain psychology. It is far from obvious, however, that having rights entails consciousness or rationality, as Feinberg suggests. We speak of the rights of the severely retarded or the severely mentally ill, yet some of these persons are not rational. We speak of the rights of the temporarily unconscious. The New Jersey Supreme Court based their decision in the Quinlan case on Karen Ann Quinlan's right to privacy, and she was known to be permanently unconscious at that time. Hence, Feinberg's claim that having rights entails being conscious is, on its face, obviously false.

Of course, it might not make sense to attribute rights to a being that would never in its natural history have certain psychological traits. This modest connection between psychological personhood and moral personhood will create a place for Karen Ann Quinlan and the temporarily unconscious. But then it makes a place for fetuses also. Hence, it does not serve Feinberg's pro-choice purposes. Accordingly, it seems that the pro-choicer will have as much difficulty bridging the gap between psychological personhood and personhood in the moral sense as the anti-abortionist has bridging the gap between being a biological human being and being a human being in the moral sense.

Furthermore, the pro-choicer cannot any more escape her problem by making person a purely moral category than the anti-abortionist could escape by the analogous move. For if person is a moral category, then the pro-choicer is left without the recourses for establishing (noncircularly, of course) the claim that a fetus is not a person, which is an essential premise in her argument. Again, we have both a symmetry and a standoff between pro-choice and antiabortion views.

Passions in the abortion debate run high. There are both plausibilities and difficulties with the standard positions. Accordingly, it is hardly surprising that partisans of either side embrace with fervor the moral generalizations that support the conclusions they preanalytically favor, and reject with disdain the moral generalizations of their opponents as being subject to inescapable difficulties. It is easy to believe that the counterexamples to one's own moral principles are merely temporary difficulties that will dissolve in the wake of further philosophical research, and that the counterexamples to the principles of one's opponents are as straightforward as the contradiction between A and O propositions in traditional logic. This might suggest to an impartial observer (if there are any) that the abortion issue is unresolvable.

There is a way out of this apparent dialectical quandary. The moral generalizations of both sides are not quite correct. The generalizations hold for the most part, for the usual cases. This suggests that they are all *accidental* generalizations, that the moral claims made by those on both sides of the dispute do not touch on the *essence* of the matter.

This use of the distinction between essence and accident is not meant to invoke obscure metaphysical categories. Rather, it is intended to reflect the rather atheoretical nature of the abortion discussion. If the generalization a partisan in the abortion dispute adopts were derived from the reason why ending the life of a human being is wrong, then there could not be exceptions to that generalization unless some special case obtains in which there are even more powerful countervailing reasons. Such generalizations would not be merely accidental generalizations; they would point to, or be based upon, the essence of the wrongness of killing, what it is that makes killing wrong. All this suggests that a necessary condition of resolving the abortion controversy is a more theoretical account of the wrongness of killing. After all, if we merely believe, but do not understand, why killing adult human beings such as ourselves is wrong, how could we conceivably show that abortion is either immoral or permissible?

II.

In order to develop such an account, we can start from the following unproblematic assumption concerning our own case: it is wrong to kill *us*. Why is it wrong? Some answers can be easily eliminated. It might be said that what makes killing us wrong is that a killing brutalizes the one who kills. But the brutalization consists of being inured to the performance of an act that is hideously immoral; hence, the brutalization does not explain the immorality. It might be said that what makes killing us wrong is the great loss others would experience due to our absence. Although such hubris is understandable, such an explanation does not account for the wrongness of killing hermits, or those whose lives are relatively independent and whose friends find it easy to make new friends.

A more obvious answer is better. What primarily makes killing wrong is neither its effect on the murderer nor its effect on the victim's friends and relatives, but its effect on the victim. The loss of one's life is one of the greatest losses one can suffer. The loss of one's life deprives one of all the experiences, activities, projects, and enjoyments that would otherwise have constituted one's future. Therefore, killing someone is wrong, primarily because the killing inflicts (one of) the greatest possible losses on the victim. To describe this as the loss of life can be misleading, however. The change in my biological state does not by itself make killing me wrong. The effect of the loss of my biological life is the loss to me of all those activities, projects, experiences, and enjoyments which would otherwise have constituted my future personal life. These activities, projects, experiences, and enjoyments are either valuable for their own sakes or are means to something else that is valuable for its own sake. Some parts of my future are not valued by me now, but will come to be valued by me as I grow older and as my values and capacities change. When I am killed, I am deprived both of what I now value which would have been part of my future personal life, but also what I would come to value. Therefore, when I die, I am deprived of all of the value of my future. Inflicting this loss on me is ultimately what makes killing me wrong. This being the case, it would seem that what makes killing *any* adult human being prima facie seriously wrong is the loss of his or her future.

How should this rudimentary theory of the wrongness of killing be evaluated? It cannot be faulted for deriving an 'ought' from an 'is', for it does not. The analysis assumes that killing me (or you, reader) is prima facie seriously wrong. The point of the analysis is to establish which natural property ultimately explains the wrongness of the killing, given that it is wrong. A natural property will ultimately explain the wrongness of killing, only if (1) the explanation fits with our intuitions about the matter and (2) there is no other natural property that provides the basis for a better explanation of the wrongness of killing. This analysis rests on the intuition that what makes killing a particular human or animal wrong is what it does to that particular human or animal. What makes killing wrong is some natural effect or other of the killing. Some would deny this. For instance, a divine-command theorist in ethics would deny it. Surely this denial is, however, one of those features of divine-command theory which renders it so implausible.

The claim that what makes killing wrong is the loss of the victim's future is directly supported by two considerations. In the first place, this theory explains why we regard killing as one of the worst of crimes. Killing is especially wrong, because it deprives the victim of more than perhaps any other crime. In the second place, people with AIDS or cancer who know they are dying believe, of course, that dying is a very bad thing for them. They believe that the loss of a future to them that they would otherwise have experienced is what makes their premature death a very bad thing for them. A better theory of the wrongness

of killing would require a different natural property associated with killing which better fits with the attitudes of the dying. What could it be?

The view that what makes killing wrong is the loss to the victim of the value of the victim's future gains additional support when some of its implications are examined. In the first place, it is incompatible with the view that it is wrong to kill only beings who are biologically human. It is possible that there exists a different species from another planet whose members have a future like ours. Since having a future like that is what makes killing someone wrong, this theory entails that it would be wrong to kill members of such a species. Hence, this theory is opposed to the claim that only life that is biologically human has great moral worth, a claim which many anti-abortionists have seemed to adopt. This opposition, which this theory has in common with personhood theories, seems to be a merit of the theory.

In the second place, the claim that the loss of one's future is the wrong-making feature of one's being killed entails the possibility that the futures of some actual nonhuman mammals on our own planet are sufficiently like ours that it is seriously wrong to kill them also. Whether some animals do have the same right to life as human beings depends on adding to the account of the wrongness of killing some additional account of just what it is about my future or the futures of other adult human beings which makes it wrong to kill us. No such additional account will be offered in this essay. Undoubtedly, the provision of such an account would be a very difficult matter. Undoubtedly, any such account would be quite controversial. Hence, it surely should not reflect badly on this sketch of an elementary theory of the wrongness of killing that it is indeterminate with respect to some very difficult issues regarding animal rights.

In the third place, the claim that the loss of one's future is the wrong-making feature of one's being killed does not entail, as sanctity of human life theories do, that active euthanasia is wrong. Persons who are severely and incurably ill, who face a future of pain and despair, and who wish to die will not have suffered a loss if they are killed. It is, strictly speaking, the value of a human's future which makes killing wrong in this theory. This being so, killing does not necessarily wrong some persons who are sick and dying. Of course, there may be other reasons for a prohibition of active euthanasia, but that is another matter. Sanctity-of-human-life theories seem to hold that active euthanasia is seriously wrong even in an individual case where there seems to be good reason for it independently of public policy considerations. This consequence is most implausible, and it is a plus for the claim that the loss of a future of value is what makes killing wrong that it does not share this consequence.

In the fourth place, the account of the wrongness of killing defended in this essay does straightforwardly entail that it is prima facie seriously wrong to kill children and infants, for we do presume that they have futures of value. Since we do believe that it is wrong to kill defenseless little babies, it is important that a theory of the wrongness of killing easily account for this. Personhood theories of the wrongness of killing, on the other hand, cannot straightforwardly account for the wrongness of killing infants and young children. Hence, such theories must add special ad hoc accounts of the wrongness of killing the young. The plausibility of such ad hoc theories seems to be a function of how desperately one wants such theories to work. The claim that the primary wrong-making feature of a killing is the loss to the victim of the value of its future accounts for the wrongness of killing young children and infants directly; it makes the wrongness of such acts as obvious as we actually think it is. This is a further merit of this theory. Accordingly, it seems that this value of a future-like-ours theory of the wrongness of killing shares strengths of both sanctity-of-life and personhood accounts while avoiding weaknesses of both. In addition, it meshes with a central intuition concerning what makes killing wrong.

The claim that the primary wrong-making feature of a killing is the loss to the victim of the value of its future has obvious consequences for the ethics of abortion. The future of a standard fetus includes a set of experiences, projects, activities, and such which are identical with the futures of adult human beings and are identical with the futures of young children. Since the reason that is sufficient to explain why it is wrong to kill human beings after the time of birth is a reason that also applies to fetuses, it follows that abortion is prima facie seriously morally wrong.

This argument does not rely on the invalid inference that, since it is wrong to kill persons, it is wrong to kill potential persons also. The category that is morally central to this analysis is the category of having a valuable future like ours; it is not the category of personhood. The argument to the conclusion that abortion is prima facie seriously morally wrong proceeded independently of the notion of person or potential person or any equivalent. Someone may wish to start with this analysis in terms of the value of a human future, conclude that abortion is, except perhaps in rare circumstances, seriously morally wrong, infer that fetuses have the right to life, and then call fetuses "persons" as a result of their having the right to life. Clearly, in this case, the category of person is being used to state the *conclusion* of the analysis rather than to generate the *argument* of the analysis.

The structure of this anti-abortion argument can be both illuminated and defended by comparing it to what appears to be the best argument for the wrongness of the wanton infliction of pain on animals. This latter argument is based on the assumption that it is prima facie wrong to inflict pain on me (or you, reader). What is the natural property associated with the infliction of pain which makes such infliction wrong? The obvious answer seems to be that the infliction of pain causes suffering and that suffering is a misfortune. The suffering caused by the infliction of pain is what makes the wanton infliction of pain on me wrong. The wanton infliction of pain on other adult humans causes suffering. The wanton infliction of pain on animals causes suffering. Since causing suffering is what makes the wanton infliction of pain wrong and since the wanton infliction of pain on animals causes suffering, it follows that the wanton infliction of pain on animals is wrong.

This argument for the wrongness of the wanton infliction of pain on animals shares a number of structural features with the argument for the serious prima facie wrongness of abortion. Both arguments start with an obvious assumption concerning what it is wrong to do to me (or you, reader). Both then look for the characteristic or the consequence of the wrong action which makes the action wrong. Both recognize that the wrong-making feature of these immoral actions is a property of actions sometimes directed at individuals other than postnatal human beings. If the structure of the argument for the wrongness of the wanton infliction of pain on animals is sound, then the structure of the argument for the prima facie serious wrongness of abortion is also sound, for the structure of the two arguments is the same. The structure common to both is the key to the explanation of how the wrongness of abortion can be demonstrated without recourse to the category of person. In neither argument is that category crucial.

This defense of an argument for the wrongness of abortion in terms of a structurally similar argument for the wrongness of the wanton infliction of pain on animals succeeds only if the account regarding animals is the correct account. Is it? In the first place, it seems plausible. In the second place, its major competition is Kant's account. Kant believed that we do not have direct duties to animals at all, because they are not persons. Hence, Kant had to explain and justify the wrongness of inflicting pain on animals on the grounds that "he who is hard in his dealings with animals becomes hard also in his dealing with men."[2] The problem with Kant's account is that there seems to be no reason for accepting this latter claim unless Kant's account is rejected. If the alternative to Kant's account is accepted, then it is easy to understand why someone who is indifferent to inflicting pain on animals is also indifferent to inflicting pain on humans, for one is indifferent to what makes inflicting pain wrong in both cases. But, if Kant's account is accepted, there is no intelligible reason why one who is hard in his dealings with animals (or crabgrass or stones) should also be hard in his dealings with men. After all, men are persons: animals are no more persons than crabgrass or stones. Persons are Kant's crucial moral category. Why, in short, should a Kantian accept the basic claim in Kant's argument?

Hence, Kant's argument for the wrongness of inflicting pain on animals rests on a claim that, in a world of Kantian moral agents, is demonstrably false. Therefore, the alternative analysis, being more plausi-

ble anyway, should be accepted. Since this alternative analysis has the same structure as the anti-abortion argument being defended here, we have further support for the argument for the immorality of abortion being defended in this essay.

Of course, this value of a future-like-ours argument, if sound, shows only that abortion is prima facie wrong, not that it is wrong in any and all circumstances. Since the loss of the future to a standard fetus, if killed, is, however, at least as great a loss as the loss of the future to a standard adult human being who is killed, abortion, like ordinary killing, could be justified only by the most compelling reasons. The loss of one's life is almost the greatest misfortune that can happen to one. Presumably abortion could be justified in some circumstances, only if the loss consequent on failing to abort would be at least as great. Accordingly, morally permissible abortions will be rare indeed unless, perhaps, they occur so early in pregnancy that a fetus is not yet definitely an individual. Hence, this argument should be taken as showing that abortion is presumptively very seriously wrong, where the presumption is very strong—as strong as the presumption that killing another adult human being is wrong.

III.

How complete an account of the wrongness of killing does the value of a future-like-our account have to be in order that the wrongness of abortion is a consequence? This account does not have to be an account of the necessary conditions for the wrongness of killing. Some persons in nursing homes may lack valuable human futures, yet it may be wrong to kill them for other reasons. Furthermore, this account does not obviously have to be the sole reason killing is wrong where the victim did have a valuable future. This analysis claims only that, for any killing where the victim did have a valuable future like ours, having that future by itself is sufficient to create the strong presumption that the killing is seriously wrong.

One way to overturn the value of a future-like-ours argument would be to find some account of the wrongness of killing which is at least as intelligible and which has different implications for the ethics of abortion.

Two rival accounts possess at least some degree of plausibility. One account is based on the obvious fact that people value the experience of living and wish for that valuable experience to continue. Therefore, it might be said, what makes killing wrong is the discontinuation of that experience for the victim. Let us call this the *discontinuation account*. Another rival account is based upon the obvious fact that people strongly desire to continue to live. This suggests that what makes killing us so wrong is that it interferes with the fulfillment of a strong and fundamental desire, the fulfillment of which is necessary for the fulfillment of any other desires we might have. Let us call this the *desire account*.

Consider first the desire account as a rival account of the ethics of killing which would provide the basis for rejecting the anti-abortion position. Such an account will have to be stronger than the value of a future-like-ours account of the wrongness of abortion if it is to do the job expected of it. To entail the wrongness of abortion, the value of a future-like-ours account has only to provide a sufficient, but not a necessary, condition for the wrongness of killing. The desire account, on the other hand, must provide us also with a necessary condition for the wrongness of killing in order to generate a pro-choice conclusion on abortion. The reason for this is that presumably the argument from the desire account moves from the claim that what makes killing wrong is interference with a very strong desire to the claim that abortion is not wrong because the fetus lacks a strong desire to live. Obviously, this inference fails if someone's having the desire to live is not a necessary condition of its being wrong to kill that individual.

One problem with the desire account is that we do regard it as seriously wrong to kill persons who have little desire to live or who have no desires to live or, indeed, have a desire not to live. We believe it is seriously wrong to kill the unconscious, the sleeping, those who are tired of life, and those who are suicidal. The value-of-a-human-future account renders standard morality intelligible in these cases; these cases appear to be incompatible with the desire account.

The desire account is subject to a deeper difficulty. We desire life, because we value the goods of this life. The goodness of life is not secondary to our desire for

it. If this were not so, the pain of one's own premature death could be done away with merely by an appropriate alteration in the configuration of one's desires. This is absurd. Hence, it would seem that it is the loss of the goods of one's future, not the interference with the fulfillment of a strong desire to live, which accounts ultimately for the wrongness of killing.

It is worth noting that, if the desire account is modified so that it does not provide a necessary, but only a sufficient, condition for the wrongness of killing, the desire account is compatible with the value of a future-like-ours account. The combined accounts will yield an anti-abortion ethic. This suggests that one can retain what is intuitively plausible about the desire account without a challenge to the basic argument of this paper.

It is also worth that, if future desires have moral force in a modified desire account of the wrongness of killing, one can find support for an anti-abortion ethic even in the absence of a value of a future-like-ours account. If one decides that a morally relevant property, the possession of which is sufficient to make it wrong to kill some individual, is the desire at some future time to live—one might decide to justify one's refusal to kill suicidal teenagers on these grounds, for example—then, since typical fetuses will have the desire in the future to live, it is wrong to kill typical fetuses. Accordingly, it does not seem that a desire account of the wrongness of killing can provide a justification of a pro-choice ethic of abortion which is nearly as adequate as the value of a human-future justification of an anti-abortion ethic.

The discontinuation account looks more promising as an account of the wrongness of killing. It seems just as intelligible as the value of a future-like-ours account, but it does not justify an anti-abortion position. Obviously, if it is the continuation of one's activities, experiences, and projects, the loss of which makes killing wrong, then it is not wrong to kill fetuses for that reason, for fetuses do not have experiences, activities, and projects to be continued or discontinued. Accordingly, the discontinuation account does not have the anti-abortion consequences that the value of a future-like-ours account has. Yet, it seems as intelligible as the value of a future-like-ours account, for when we think of what would be wrong with our being killed, it does seem as if it is the discontinuation of what makes our lives worthwhile which makes killing us wrong.

Is the discontinuation account just as good an account as the value of a future-like-ours account? The discontinuation account will not be adequate at all, if it does not refer to the *value* of the experience that may be discontinued. One does not want the discontinuation account to make it wrong to kill a patient who begs for death and who is in severe pain that cannot be relieved short of killing. (I leave open the question of whether it is wrong for other reasons.) Accordingly, the discontinuation account must be more than a bare discontinuation account. It must make some reference to the positive value of the patient's experiences. But, by the same token, the value of a future-like-ours account cannot be a bare future account either. Just having a future surely does not itself rule out killing the above patient. This account must make some reference to the value of the patient's future experiences and projects also. Hence, both accounts involve the value of experiences, projects, and activities. So far we still have symmetry between the accounts.

The symmetry fades, however, when we focus on the time period of the value of the experiences, etc., which has moral consequences. Although both accounts leave open the possibility that the patient in our example may be killed, this possibility is left open only in virtue of the utterly bleak future for the patient. It makes no difference whether the patient's immediate past contains intolerable pain, or consists in being in a coma (which we can imagine is a situation of indifference), or consists in a life of value. If the patient's future is a future of value, we want our account to make it wrong to kill the patient. If the patient's future is intolerable, whatever his or her immediate past, we want our account to allow killing the patient. Obviously, then, it is the value of that patient's future which is doing the work in rendering the morality of killing the patient intelligible.

This being the case, it seems clear that whether one has immediate past experiences or not does not work in the explanation of what makes killing wrong. The addition the discontinuation account makes to the

value of a human future account is otiose. Its addition to the value-of-a-future account plays no role at all in rendering intelligible the wrongness of killing. Therefore, it can be discarded with the discontinuation account of which it is a part.

IV.

The analysis of the previous section suggests that alternative general accounts of the wrongness of killing are either inadequate or unsuccessful in getting around the anti-abortion consequences of the value of a future-like-ours argument. A different strategy for avoiding these anti-abortion consequences involves limiting the scope of the value of a future argument. More precisely, the strategy involves arguing that fetuses lack a property that is essential for the value-of-a-future argument (or for any anti-abortion argument) to apply to them.

One move of this sort is based upon the claim that a necessary condition of one's future being valuable is that one values it. Value implies a valuer. Given this one might argue that, since fetuses cannot value their futures, their futures are not valuable to them. Hence, it does not seriously wrong them deliberately to end their lives.

This move fails, however, because of some ambiguities. Let us assume that something cannot be of value unless it is valued by someone. This does not entail that my life is of no value unless it is valued by me. I may think, in a period of despair, that my future is of no worth whatsoever, but I may be wrong because others rightly see value—even great value—in it. Furthermore, my future can be valuable to me even if I do not value it. This is the case when a young person attempts suicide, but is rescued and goes on to significant human achievements. Such young people's futures are ultimately valuable to them, even though such futures do not seem to be valuable to them at the moment of attempted suicide. A fetus's future can be valuable to it in the same way. Accordingly, this attempt to limit the anti-abortion argument fails.

Another similar attempt to reject the anti-abortion position is based on [Michael] Tooley's claim that an entity cannot possess the right to life unless it has the capacity to desire its continued existence. It follows that, since fetuses lack the conceptual capacity to desire to continue to live, they lack the right to life. Accordingly, Tooley concludes that abortion cannot be seriously prima facie wrong.[3]

What could be the evidence for Tooley's basic claim? Tooley once argued that individuals have a prima facie right to what they desire and that the lack of the capacity to desire something undercuts the basis of one's right to it.[4] This argument plainly will not succeed in the context of the analysis of this essay, however, since the point here is to establish the fetus's right to life on other grounds. Tooley's argument assumes that the right to life cannot be established in general on some basis other than the desire for life. This position was considered and rejected in the preceding section of this paper.

One might attempt to defend Tooley's basic claim on the grounds that, because a fetus cannot apprehend continued life as a benefit, its continued life cannot be a benefit or cannot be something it has a right to or cannot be something that is in its interest. This might be defended in terms of the general proposition that, if an individual is literally incapable of caring about or taking an interest in some X, then one does not have a right to X or X is not a benefit or X is not something that is in one's interest.

Each member of this family of claims seems to be open to objections. As John C. Stevens[5] has pointed out, one may have a right to be treated with a certain medical procedure (because of a health insurance policy one has purchased), even though one cannot conceive of the nature of the procedure. And, as Tooley himself has pointed out, persons who have been indoctrinated, or drugged, or rendered temporarily unconscious may be literally incapable of caring about or taking an interest in something that is in their interest or is something to which they have a right, or is something that benefits them. Hence, the Tooley claim that would restrict the scope of the value of a future-like-ours argument is undermined by counterexamples.

Finally, Paul Bassen[6] has argued that, even though the prospects of an embryo might seem to be a basis for the wrongness of abortion, an embryo cannot be a

victim and therefore cannot be wronged. An embryo cannot be a victim, he says, because it lacks sentience. His central argument for this seems to be that, even though plants and the permanently unconscious are alive, they clearly cannot be victims. What is the explanation of this? Bassen claims that the explanation is that their lives consist of mere metabolism and mere metabolism is not enough to ground victimizability. Mentation is required.

The problem with this attempt to establish the absence of victimizability is that both plants and the permanently unconscious clearly lack what Bassen calls "prospects" or what I have called "a future life like ours." Hence, it is surely open to one to argue that the real reason we believe plants and the permanently unconscious cannot be victims is that killing them cannot deprive them of a future life like ours; the real reason is not their absence of present mentation.

Bassen recognizes that his view is subject to this difficulty, and he recognizes that the case of children seems to support this difficulty, for "much of what we do for children is based on prospects." He argues, however, that, in the case of children and in other such cases, "potentially comes into play only where victimizability has been secured on other grounds" (p. 333).

Bassen's defense of his view is patently question-begging, since what is adequate to secure victimizability is exactly what is at issue. His examples do not support his own view against the thesis of this essay. Of course, embryos can be victims: when their lives are deliberately terminated, they are deprived of their futures of value, their prospects. This makes them victims, for it directly wrongs them.

The seeming plausibility of Bassen's view stems from the fact that paradigmatic cases of imagining someone as a victim involve empathy, and empathy requires mentation of the victim. The victims of flood, famine, rape, or child abuse are all persons with whom we can empathize. That empathy seems to be part of seeing them as victims.

In spite of the strength of these examples, the attractive intuition that a situation in which there is victimization requires the possibility of empathy is subject to counterexamples. Consider a case that Bassen himself offers: "Posthumous obliteration of an author's work constitutes a misfortune for him only if he had wished his work to endure" (p. 318). The conditions Bassen wishes to impose upon the possibility of being victiminized here seem far too strong. Perhaps this author, due to his unrealistic standards of excellence and his low self-esteem, regarded his work as unworthy of survival, even though it possessed genuine literary merit. Destruction of such work would surely victimize its author. In such a case, empathy with the victim concerning the loss is clearly impossible.

Of course, Bassen does not make the possibility of empathy a necessary condition of victimizability; he requires only mentation. Hence, on Bassen's actual view, this author, as I have described him, can be a victim. The problem is that the basic intuition that renders Bassen's view plausible is missing in the author's case. In order to attempt to avoid counterexamples, Bassen has made his thesis too weak to be supported by the intuitions that suggested it.

Even so, the mentation requirement on victimizability is still subject to counterexamples. Suppose a severe accident renders me totally unconscious for a month, after which I recover. Surely killing me while I am unconscious victimizes me, even though I am incapable of mentation during that time. It follows that Bassen's thesis fails. Apparently, attempts to restrict the value of a future-like-ours argument so that fetuses do not fall within its scope do not succeed.

V.

In this essay, it has been argued that the correct ethic of the wrongness of killing can be extended to fetal life and used to show that there is a strong presumption that any abortion is morally impermissible. If the ethic of killing adopted here entails, however, that contraception is also seriously immoral, then there would appear to be a difficulty with the analysis of this assay.

But this analysis does not entail that contraception is wrong. Of course, contraception prevents the actualization of a possible future of value. Hence, it follows from the claim that futures of value should be maximized that contraception is prima facie immoral. This obligation to maximize does not exist, however; furthermore, nothing in the ethics of killing in this paper entails that it does. The ethics of killing in this essay would entail that contraception is wrong only if something were denied a human future of value by contraception. Nothing at all is denied such a future by contraception, however.

Candidates for a subject of harm by contraception fall into four categories: (1) some sperm or other, (2) some ovum or other, (3) a sperm and an ovum separately, and (4) a sperm and an ovum together. Assigning the harm to some sperm is utterly arbitrary, for no reason can be given for making a sperm the subject of harm rather than an ovum. Assigning the harm to some ovum is utterly arbitrary, for no reason can be given for making an ovum the subject of harm rather than a sperm. One might attempt to avoid these problems by insisting that contraception deprives both the sperm and the ovum separately of a valuable future like ours. On this alternative, too many futures are lost. Contraception was supposed to be wrong, because it deprived us of one future of value, not two. One might attempt to avoid this problem by holding that contraception deprives the combination of sperm and ovum of a valuable future like ours. But here the definite article misleads. At the time of contraception, there are hundreds of millions of sperm, one (released) ovum and millions of possible combinations of all of these. There is no actual combination at all. Is the subject of the loss to be a merely possible combination? Which one? This alternative does not yield an actual subject of harm either. Accordingly, the immorality of contraception is not entailed by the loss of a future-like-ours argument simply because there is no nonarbitrarily identifiable subject of the loss in the case of contraception.

VI.

The purpose of this essay has been to set out an argument for the serious presumptive wrongness of abortion subject to the assumption that the moral permissibility of abortion stands or falls on the moral status of the fetus. Since a fetus possesses a property, the possession of which in adult human beings is sufficient to make killing an adult human being wrong, abortion is wrong. This way of dealing with the problem of abortion seems superior to other approaches to the ethics of abortion, because it rests on an ethics of killing which is close to self-evident, because the crucial morally relevant property clearly applies to fetuses, and because the argument avoids the usual equivocations of 'human life', 'human being', or 'person'. The argument rests neither on religious claims nor on Papal dogma. It is not subject to the objection of "speciesism." Its soundness is compatible with the moral permissibility of euthanasia and contraception. It deals with our intuitions concerning young children.

Finally, this analysis can be viewed as resolving a standard problem—indeed, *the* standard problem—concerning the ethics of abortion. Clearly, it is wrong to kill adult human beings. Clearly, it is not wrong to end the life of some arbitrarily chosen single human cell. Fetuses seem to be like arbitrarily chosen human cells in some respects and like adult humans in other respects. The problem of the ethics of abortion is the problem of determining the fetal property that settles this moral controversy. The thesis of this essay is that the problem of the ethics of abortion, so understood, is solvable.

NOTES

1. Joel Feinberg, "Abortion," in *Matters of Life and Death: New Introductory Essays in Moral Philosophy*, ed. Tom Regan (New York: Random House, 1986), p. 270.

2. "Duties to Animals and Spirits," in *Lectures on Ethics*, trans. Loius Infeld (New York: Harper, 1963), p. 239.

3. Michael Tooley, *Abortion and Infanticide* (New York: Oxford, 1984), pp. 46–47.

4. Tooley, *Abortion and Infanticide*, pp. 44–45.

5. "Must the Bearer of a Right Have the Concept of That to Which He Has a Right?" *Ethics* 95, no. 1 (1984): 68–74.

6. "Present Sakes and Future Prospects: The Status of Early Abortion," *Philosophy and Public Affairs* 11, no. 4 (1982): 314–37.

Virtue Theory and Abortion

ROSALIND HURSTHOUSE

* * *

As everyone knows, the morality of abortion is commonly discussed in relation to just two considerations: first, and predominantly, the status of the fetus and whether or not it is the sort of thing that may or may not be innocuously or justifiably killed; and second, and less predominantly (when, that is, the discussion concerns the *morality* of abortion rather than the question of permissible legislation in a just society), women's rights. If one thinks within this familiar framework, one may well be puzzled about what virtue theory, as such, could contribute. Some people assume the discussion will be conducted solely in terms of what the virtuous agent would or would not do * * *. Others assume that only justice, or at most justice and charity, will be applied to the issue, generating a discussion very similar to Judith Jarvis Thomson's.[1]

Rosalind Hursthouse, excerpts from "Virtue Theory and Abortion." *Philosophy and Public Affairs* 20(3): 233–44. Copyright © 1991 Blackwell Publishing Ltd. Reproduced with permission of John Wiley & Sons, Inc.

Now if this is the way the virtue theorist's discussion of abortion is imagined to be, no wonder people think little of it. It seems obvious in advance that in any such discussion there must be either a great deal of extremely tendentious application of the virtue terms *just*, *charitable*, and so on or a lot of rhetorical appeal to "this is what only the virtuous agent knows." But these are caricatures; they fail to appreciate the way in which virtue theory quite transforms the discussion of abortion by dismissing the two familiar dominating considerations as, in a way, fundamentally irrelevant. In what way or ways, I hope to make both clear and plausible.

Let us first consider women's rights. Let me emphasize again that we are discussing the *morality* of abortion, not the rights and wrongs of laws prohibiting or permitting it. If we suppose that women do have a moral right to do as they choose with their own bodies, or, more particularly, to terminate their pregnancies, then it may well follow that a *law* forbidding abortion would be unjust. Indeed, even if they have no such right, such a law might be, as things stand at the moment, unjust, or impractical, or inhumane: on this issue I have nothing to say in this article. But, putting all questions about the justice or injustice of laws to one side, and supposing only that women have such a moral right, *nothing* follows from this supposition about the morality of abortion, according to virtue theory, once it is noted (quite generally, not with particular reference to abortion) that in exercising a moral right I can do something cruel, or callous, or selfish, light-minded, self-righteous, stupid, inconsiderate, disloyal, dishonest—that is, act viciously.[2] Love and friendship do not survive their parties' constantly insisting on their rights, nor do people live well when they think that getting what they have a right to is of preeminent importance; they harm others, and they harm themselves. So whether women have a moral right to terminate their pregnancies is irrelevant within virtue theory, for it is irrelevant to the question "In having an abortion in these circumstances, would the agent be acting virtuously or viciously or neither?"

What about the consideration of the status of the fetus—what can virtue theory say about that? One might say that this issue is not in the province of *any* moral theory; it is a metaphysical question, and an extremely difficult one at that. Must virtue theory then wait upon metaphysics to come up with the answer?

At first sight it might seem so. For virtue is said to involve knowledge, and part of this knowledge consists in having the *right* attitude to things. "Right" here does not just mean "morally right" or "proper" or "nice" in the modern sense; it means "accurate, true." One cannot have the right or correct attitude to something if the attitude is based on or involves false beliefs. And this suggests that if the status of the fetus is relevant to the rightness or wrongness of abortion, its status must be known, as a truth, to the fully wise and virtuous person.

But the sort of wisdom that the fully virtuous person has is not supposed to be recondite; it does not call for fancy philosophical sophistication, and it does not depend upon, let alone wait upon, the discoveries of academic philosophers.[3] And this entails the following, rather startling, conclusion: that the status of the fetus—that issue over which so much ink has been spilt—is, according to virtue theory, simply not

relevant to the rightness or wrongness of abortion (within, that is, a secular morality).

Or rather, since that is clearly too radical a conclusion, it is in a sense relevant, but only in the sense that the familiar biological facts are relevant. By "the familiar biological facts" I mean the facts that most human societies are and have been familiar with—that, standardly (but not invariably), pregnancy occurs as the result of sexual intercourse, that it lasts about nine months, during which time the fetus grows and develops, that standardly it terminates in the birth of a living baby, and that this is how we all come to be.

It might be thought that this distinction—between the familiar biological facts and the status of the fetus—is a distinction without a difference. But this is not so. To attach relevance to the status of the fetus, in the sense in which virtue theory claims it is not relevant, is to be gripped by the conviction that we must go beyond the familiar biological facts, deriving some sort of conclusion from them, such as that the fetus has rights, or is not a person, or something similar. It is also to believe that this exhausts the relevance of the familiar biological facts, that all they are relevant to is the status of the fetus and whether or not it is the sort of thing that may or may not be killed.

These convictions, I suspect, are rooted in the desire to solve the problem of abortion by getting it to fall under some general rule such as "You ought not to kill anything with the right to life but may kill anything else." But they have resulted in what should surely strike any nonphilosopher as a most bizarre aspect of nearly all the current philosophical literature on abortion, namely, that, far from treating abortion as a unique moral problem, markedly unlike any other, nearly everything written on the status of the fetus and its bearing on the abortion issue would be consistent with the human reproductive facts (to say nothing of family life) being totally different from what they are. Imagine that you are an alien extraterrestrial anthropologist who does not know that the human race is roughly 50 percent female and 50 percent male, or that our only (natural) form of reproduction involves heterosexual intercourse, viviparous birth, and the female's (and only the female's) being pregnant for nine months, or that females are capable of childbearing from late childhood to late middle age, or that childbearing is painful, dangerous, and emotionally charged—do you think you would pick up these facts from the hundreds of articles written on the status of the fetus? I am quite sure you would not. And that, I think, shows that the current philosophical literature on abortion has got badly out of touch with reality.

Now if we are using virtue theory, our first question is not "What do the familiar biological facts show—what can be derived from them about the status of the fetus?" but "How do these facts figure in the practical reasoning, actions and passions, thoughts and reactions, of the virtuous and the nonvirtuous? What is the mark of having the right attitude to these facts and what manifests having the wrong attitude to them?" This immediately makes essentially relevant not only all the facts about human reproduction I mentioned above, but a whole range of facts about our emotions in relation to them as well. I mean such facts as that human parents, both male and female, tend to care passionately about their offspring, and that family relationships are among the deepest and strongest in our lives—and, significantly, among the longest-lasting.

These facts make it obvious that pregnancy is not just one among many other physical conditions; and hence that anyone who genuinely believes that an abortion is comparable to a haircut or an appendectomy is mistaken.[4] The fact that the premature termination of a pregnancy is, in some sense, the cutting off of a new human life, and thereby, like the procreation of a new human life, connects with all our thoughts about human life and death, parenthood, and family relationships, must make it a serious matter. To disregard this fact about it, to think of abortion as nothing but the killing of something that does not matter, or as nothing but the exercise of some right or rights one has, or as the incidental means to some desirable state of affairs, is to do something callous and light-minded, the sort of thing that no virtuous and wise person would do. It is to have the wrong attitude not only to fetuses, but more generally to human life and death, parenthood, and family relationships.

Although I say that the facts make this obvious, I know that this is one of my tendentious points. In partial support of it I note that even the most dedi-cated proponents of the view that deliberate abortion is just like an appendectomy or haircut rarely hold the same view of spontaneous abortion, that is, miscarriage. It is not so tendentious of me to claim that to react to people's grief over miscarriage by saying, or even thinking, "What a fuss about nothing!" would be callous and light-minded, whereas to try to laugh someone out of grief over an appendectomy scar or a botched haircut would not be. It is hard to give this point due prominence within act-centered theories, for the inconsistency is an inconsistency in attitude about the seriousness of loss of life, not in beliefs about which acts are right or wrong. Moreover, an act-centered theorist may say, "Well, there is nothing wrong with *thinking* 'What a fuss about nothing!' as long as you do not say it and hurt the person who is grieving. And besides, we cannot be held responsible for our thoughts, only for the intentional actions they give rise to." But the character traits that virtue theory emphasizes are not simply dispositions to intentional actions, but a seamless disposition to certain actions and passions, thoughts and reactions.

To say that the cutting off of a human life is always a matter of some seriousness, at any stage, is not to deny the relevance of gradual fetal development. Notwithstanding the well-worn point that clear boundary lines cannot be drawn, our emotions and attitudes regarding the fetus do change as it develops, and again when it is born, and indeed further as the baby grows. Abortion for shallow reasons in the later stages is much more shocking than abortion for the same reasons in the early stages in a way that matches the fact that deep grief over miscarriage in the later stages is more appropriate than it is over miscarriage in the earlier stages (when, that is, the grief is solely about the loss of *this* child, not about, as might be the case, the loss of one's only hope of having a child or of having one's husband's child). Imagine (or recall) a woman who already has children; she had not intended to have more, but finds herself unexpectedly pregnant. Though contrary to her plans, the pregnancy, once established as a fact, is welcomed—and then she loses the embryo almost immediately. If this were bemoaned as a tragedy, it would, I think, be a misapplication of the concept of what is tragic. But it may still properly be mourned as a loss. The grief is expressed in such terms as "I shall always wonder how she or he would have turned out" or "When I look at the others, I shall think, 'How different their lives would have been if this other one had been part of them.'" It would, I take it, be callous and light-minded to say, or think, "Well, she has already *got* four children; what's the problem?"; it would be neither, nor arrogantly intrusive in the case of a close friend, to try to correct prolonged mourning by saying, "I know it's sad, but it's not a tragedy; rejoice in the ones you have." The application of *tragic* becomes more appropriate as the fetus grows, for the mere fact that one has lived with it for longer, conscious of its existence, makes a difference. To shrug off an early abortion is understandable just because it is very hard to be fully conscious of the fetus's existence in the early stages and hence hard to appreciate that an early abortion is the destruction of life. It is particularly hard for the young and inexperienced to appreciate this, because appreciation of it usually comes only with experience.

I do not mean "with the experience of having an abortion" (though that may be part of it) but, quite generally, "with the experience of life." Many women who have borne children contrast their later pregnancies with their first successful one, saying that in the later ones they were conscious of a new life growing in them from very early on. And, more generally, as one reaches the age at which the next generation is coming up close behind one, the counterfactuals "If I, or she, had had an abortion, Alice, or Bob, would not have been born" acquire a significant application, which casts a new light on the conditionals "If I or Alice have an abortion then some Caroline or Bill will not be born."

The fact that pregnancy is not just one among many physical conditions does not mean that one can never regard it in that light without manifesting a vice. When women are in very poor physical health, or worn out from childbearing, or forced to do very physically demanding jobs, then they cannot be described as self-indulgent, callous, irresponsible, or light-minded if they seek abortions mainly with a view to avoiding pregnancy as the physical condition that it is. To go through with a pregnancy when one is utterly exhausted, or when one's job consists of crawling along tunnels hauling coal, as many women in the nineteenth century were obliged to do, is perhaps heroic, but people who do not achieve heroism are not necessarily vicious. That they can view the pregnancy only as eight months of misery, followed by hours if not days of agony and exhaustion, and abortion only as the blessed escape from this prospect, is entirely understandable and does not manifest any lack of serious respect for human life or a shallow attitude or motherhood. What it does show is that something is terribly amiss in the conditions of their lives, which make it so hard to recognize pregnancy and childbearing as the good that they can be.

* * *

The foregoing discussion, insofar as it emphasizes the right attitude to human life and death, parallels to a certain extent those standard discussions of abortion that concentrate on it solely as an issue of killing. But it does not, as those discussions do, gloss over the fact, emphasized by those who discuss the morality of abortion in terms of women's rights, that abortion, wildly unlike any other form of killing, is the termination of a pregnancy, which is a condition of a woman's body and results in *her* having a child if it is not aborted. This fact is given due recognition not by appeal to women's rights but by emphasizing the relevance of the familiar biological and psychological facts and their connection with having the right attitude to parenthood and family relationships. But it may well be thought that failing to bring in women's rights still leaves some important aspects of the problem of abortion untouched.

Speaking in terms of women's rights, people sometimes say things like, "Well, it's her life you're talking about too, you know; she's got a right to her own life, her own happiness." And the discussion stops there. But in the context of virtue theory, given that we are particularly concerned with what constitutes a good human life, with what true happiness or *eudaimonia* is, this is no place to stop. We go on to ask, "And is this life of hers a good one? Is she living well?"

If we are to go on to talk about good human lives, in the context of abortion, we have to bring in our thoughts about the value of love and family life, and our proper emotional development through a natural life cycle. The familiar facts support the view that parenthood in general, and motherhood and childbearing in particular, are intrinsically worthwhile, are among the things that can be correctly thought to be partially constitutive of a flourishing human life. If this is right, then a woman who opts for not being a mother (at all, or again, or now) by opting for abortion may thereby be manifesting a flawed grasp of what her life should be, and be about—a grasp that is childish, or grossly materialistic, or shortsighted, or shallow.

I said "*may* thereby": this *need* not be so. Consider, for instance, a woman who has already had several children and fears that to have another will seriously affect her capacity to be a good mother to the ones she has—she does not show a lack of appreciation of the intrinsic value of being a parent by opting for abortion. Nor does a woman who has been a good mother and is approaching the age at which she may be looking forward to bring a good grandmother. Nor does a woman who discovers that her pregnancy may well kill her, and opts for abortion and adoption. Nor, necessarily, does a woman who has decided to lead a life centered around some other worthwhile activity or activities with which motherhood would compete.

People who are childless by choice are sometimes described as "irresponsible," or "selfish," or "refusing to grow up," or "not knowing what life is about." But one can hold that having children is intrinsically worthwhile without endorsing this, for we are, after all, in the happy position of there being more worthwhile things to do than can be fitted into one lifetime. Parenthood, and motherhood in particular, even if granted to be intrinsically worthwhile, undoubtedly take up a lot of one's adult life, leaving no room for some other worthwhile pursuits. But some women who choose abortion rather than have their first child, and some men who encourage their partners to choose abortion, are not avoiding parenthood for the sake of other worthwhile pursuits, but for the worthless one of "having a good time," or for the pursuit of some false vision of the ideals of freedom or self-realization. And some others who say "I am not ready for parenthood yet" are making some sort of mistake about the extent to which one can manipulate the circumstances of one's life so as to make it fulfill some dream that one has. Perhaps one's dream is to have two perfect children, a girl and a boy, within a perfect marriage, in financially secure circumstances,

with an interesting job of one's own. But to care too much about that dream, to demand of life that it give it to one and act accordingly, may be both greedy and foolish, and is to run the risk of missing out on happiness entirely. Not only may fate make the dream impossible, or destroy it, but one's own attachment to it may make it impossible. Good marriages, and the most promising children, can be destroyed by just one adult's excessive demand for perfection.

Once again, this is not to deny that girls may quite properly say "I am not ready for motherhood yet," especially in our society, and, far from manifesting irresponsibility or light-mindedness, show an appropriate modesty or humility, or a fearfulness that does not amount to cowardice. However, even when the decision to have an abortion is the right decision—one that does not itself fall under a vice-related term and thereby one that the perfectly virtuous could recommend—it does not follow that there is no sense in which having the abortion is wrong, or guilt inappropriate. For, by virtue of the fact that a human life has been cut short, some evil has probably been brought about,[5] and that circumstances make the decision to bring about some evil the right decision will be a ground for guilt if getting into those circumstances in the first place itself manifested a flaw in character.

What "gets one into those circumstances" in the case of abortion is, except in the case of rape, one's sexual activity and one's choices, or the lack of them, about one's sexual partner and about contraception. The virtuous woman (which here of course does not mean simply "chaste woman" but "woman with the virtues") has such character traits as strength, independence, resoluteness, decisiveness, self-confidence, responsibility, serious-mindedness, and self-determination—and no one, I think, could deny that many women become pregnant in circumstances in which they cannot welcome or cannot face the thought of having *this* child precisely because they lack one or some of these character traits. So even in the cases where the decision to have an abortion is the right one, it can still be the reflection of a moral failing—not because the decision itself is weak or cowardly or irresolute or irresponsible or light-minded, but because lack of the requisite opposite of these failings landed one in the circumstances in the first place. Hence the common universalized claim that guilt and remorse are never appropriate emotions about an abortion is denied. They may be appropriate, and appropriately inculcated, even when the decision was the right one.

Another motivation for bringing women's rights into the discussion may be to attempt to correct the implication, carried by the killing-centered approach, that insofar as abortion is wrong, it is a wrong that only women do, or at least (given the preponderance of male doctors) that only women instigate. I do not myself believe that we can thus escape the fact that nature bears harder on women than it does on men, but virtue theory can certainly correct many of the injustices that the emphasis on women's rights is rightly concerned about. With very little amendment, everything that has been said above applies to boys and men too. Although the abortion decision is, in a natural sense, the woman's decision, proper to her, boys and men are often party to it, for well or ill, and even when they are not, they are bound to have been party to the circumstances that brought it up. No less than girls and women, boys and men can, in their actions, manifest self-centeredness, callousness, and light-mindedness about life and parenthood in relation to abortion. They can be self-centered or courageous about the possibility of disability in their offspring; they need to reflect on their sexual activity and their choices, or the lack of them, about their sexual partner and contraception; they need to grow up and take responsibility for their own actions and life in relation to fatherhood. If it is true, as I maintain, that insofar as motherhood is intrinsically worthwhile, being a mother is an important purpose in women's lives, being a father (rather than a mere generator) is an important purpose in men's lives as well, and it is adolescent of men to turn a blind eye to this and pretend that they have many more important things to do.

* * *

NOTES

1. Judith Jarvis Thomson, "A Defense of Abortion," *Philosophy & Public Affairs* 1, no. 1 (Fall 1971): 47–66. One could indeed regard this article as proto-virtue theory (no doubt to the surprise of the author) if the concepts of callousness and kindness were allowed more weight.

2. One possible qualification: if one ties the concept of justice very closely to rights, then if women do have a moral right to terminate their pregnancies it *may* follow that in doing so they do not act unjustly. (Cf. Thomson, "A Defense of Abortion.") But it is debatable whether even that much follows.

3. This is an assumption of virtue theory, and I do not attempt to defend it here. An adequate discussion of it would require a separate article, since, although most moral philosophers would be chary of claiming that intellectual sophistication is a necessary condition of moral wisdom or virtue, most of us, from Plato onward, tend to write as if this were so. Sorting out which claims about moral knowledge are committed to this kind of elitism and which can, albeit with difficulty, be reconciled with the idea that moral knowledge can be acquired by anyone who really wants it would be a major task.

4. Mary Anne Warren, in "On the Moral and Legal Status of Abortion," *Monist* 57 (1973), sec. 1, says of the opponents of restrictive laws governing abortion that "their conviction (for the most part) is that abortion is not a *morally* serious and extremely unfortunate, even though sometimes justified, act, comparable to killing in self-defense or to letting the violinist die, but rather is closer to being a *morally neutral* act, like cutting one's hair" (italics mine). I would like to think that no one *genuinely* believes this. But certainly in discussion, particularly when arguing against restrictive laws or the suggestion that remorse over abortion might be appropriate, I have found that some people *say* they believe it (and often cite Warren's article, albeit inaccurately, despite its age). Those who allow that it is morally serious, and far from morally neutral, have to argue against restrictive laws, or the appropriateness of remorse, on a very different ground from that laid down by the premise "The fetus is just part of the woman's body (and she has a right to determine what happens to her body and should not feel guilty about anything she does to it)."

5. I say "some evil has probably been brought about" on the ground that (human) life is (usually) a good and hence (human) death usually an evil. The exceptions would be (*a*) where death is actually a good or a benefit, because the baby that would come to be if the life were not cut short would be better off dead than alive, and (*b*) where death, though not a good, is not an evil either, because the life that would be led (e.g., in a state of permanent coma) would not be a good.

CASES FOR ANALYSIS

1. Aborting Daughters

Daily Mail Online—Thousands of female foetuses have been killed due to gender-based abortion within some ethnic groups, the latest data reveals.

Official figures suggest as many as 4,700 females have disappeared from the latest national census records of England and Wales, raising fears that it indicates the illegal practice of sex-selection abortion has become prevalent in the UK.

Campaigners have reacted with concern to the research, calling for action to stop doctors carrying out these abortions and warning the practice 'will damage society'.

In many cultures sons are deemed to be more desirable than daughters for religious or economic reasons, meaning couples seek to terminate pregnancies if they find out the child will be female. . . .

The practice is illegal in many other countries, including those where the practice is widespread. In parts of India and China there are now as many as 120 or 140 boys for every 100 girls despite a ban on gender-based abortion.*

Do you think sex-selection abortions are morally permissible? What reasons can you provide to back up your view? Some Chinese parents could argue that such abortions are acceptable on utilitarian grounds: Aborting female fetuses prevents economic harm to the family. Is this a good moral argument? Why or why not?

*Emily Davies, "Thousands of Girls Are Aborted Due to Gender," DailyMail.com, 14 January 2014, http://www.dailymail.co.uk/news/article-2539648/Thousands-girls-aborted-gender-Study-finds-couples-cultures-sons-deemed-desirable-terminating-female-pregnancies.html

2. Parental Notification

USA Today—Sabrina Holmquist trained as a physician in low-income neighborhoods in the Bronx, N.Y. She says she often saw pregnant teenagers in desperate health and family crises, including some girls who had been abused at home. That, Holmquist says, led her to believe that doctors sometimes should be able to perform abortions on minors without informing a parent.

But in Texas, Linda W. Flower, who practiced obstetrics for two decades, disagrees. She says that in the vast majority of cases in which a teenage girl seeks an abortion, a parent's guidance is helpful and needed. Flower says she knows of young women who have regretted having abortions.

The doctors' views reflect the dueling arguments in the first abortion case to come before the Supreme Court in five years: a New Hampshire dispute that tests whether a state may bar physicians from performing an abortion on a girl younger than 18 unless one of her parents has been notified at least 48 hours in advance—even in instances in which the girl faces a health emergency.

The case, to be heard by the court Wednesday, is the first abortion dispute before the justices since 2000, when they voted 5–4 to strike down Nebraska's ban on a procedure that critics call "partial birth" abortion because the ban lacked an exception for cases in which the woman's health was at risk. The new dispute tests whether such a health exception should be required in parental-involvement mandates, which have been passed in various forms by 43 states.[†]

Which doctor do you think is right about parental notification? Under what circumstances, if any, do you think it morally permissible for an under-eighteen girl to have an abortion without notifying a parent or guardian? when the girl's life is at stake? when she is a victim of sexual abuse, including incest? Would it be reasonable to require parental notification in *all* cases without exception?

[†]Joan Biskupic, "High Court Case May Signal Shift on Abortion" From USA Today, February 7, 2006. © 2006 USA Today. All rights reserved. Used by permission and protected by the Copyright Laws of the United States. The printing, copying, redistribution, or retransmission of this Content without express written permission is prohibited. www.usatoday.com.

---

3. No Abortion to Avert Health Risks

Medical News Today—The European Court of Human Rights on Tuesday began considering the appeal of a Polish woman who says that in 2000 she was denied an abortion despite warnings from physicians that she could become blind if she continued the pregnancy, the *Scotsman* reports (Neighbour, *Scotsman,* 2/8). Alicja Tysiac—who has three children—alleges that Poland's abortion law violated her rights under Article 8 and Article 14 of the European Convention for the Protection of Human Rights and Fundamental Freedoms, which guarantee "respect for privacy and family life" and "prohibition of discrimination," respectively. Polish law allows abortion only if a woman has been raped, if there is danger to the life of the woman or if the fetus will have birth defects, according to the *Jurist* (Onikepe, *Jurist,* 2/8). The European Court could rule that Tysiac's rights were violated but cannot mandate that Poland change its abortion laws (*Reuters,* 2/7).[‡]

Should Alicja Tysiac have been permitted an abortion even though her life was not at risk? Why or why not? How serious must pregnancy-related health problems be before a risk-lowering abortion is permissible (if ever)? When such health dangers are involved, why should—or should not—a woman be allowed to decide for herself about whether to have an abortion?

[‡]Kaiser Daily Health Policy Report, "European Court of Human Rights Considers Appeal of Polish Woman," published in *Medical News Today*, February 10, 2006. Copyright © 2005 The Henry J. Kaiser Family Foundation. Reprinted with permission.

CHAPTER 9

Altering Genes and Cloning Humans

Like atoms, genes are minute, invisible, unnoticed, and seemingly inconsequential to our lives. But science has found that atoms (and their subatomic particles) are anything but inconsequential. Hiroshima, nuclear power plants, and radiological medicine have proved that. Likewise, genes are the most powerful force we know in shaping the physical features of human life (as well as having a substantial influence on behavioral and psychological factors). From the early decades of genetic research, genes have been helping us understand biological life; now our better understanding of genes is allowing us to *change* biological life—a profound and disturbing prospect.

Scientists have peered into the human genome and learned how to identify, at least in some cases, the genetic anomalies responsible for diseases. (A **genome** is an organism's complete set of DNA.) They have devised tests to ascertain genetic defects in a particular person, defects that forewarn her of serious disorders that may—or certainly will—appear later in life. Even more astonishing, researchers are working on ways to reach into a human being's bank of 20,000 to 25,000 genes and alter or replace some to ease or eradicate diseases. Moreover the genetic fantasy of parents selecting the hair color, musical ability, and intelligence of their unborn child is not entirely fantasy any more: it's technologically possible though not yet actual. Someday soon scientists may be able to affect not just an individual's genes, but also the genome of the entire human race. With this power, scientists could alter the genes in germ-line cells (egg and sperm cells) and thus—for better or

worse—change succeeding generations in the same way. And all the while the ultimate genetic technology—cloning—is being quietly investigated; sheep and monkeys and rabbits are being cloned; and the prospect of cloning a human, though not yet feasible, is on the far horizon.

These advances have provoked moral problems at every step. Most of the questions come down to this: Is it morally permissible to use these amazing technologies? Or, as many who condemn them on religious grounds would say, Should we play God?

ISSUE FILE: BACKGROUND

Cells constitute the bodies of every living thing—humans, apes, dogs, ants, tulips, redwoods, and all the rest. But they are far from being just building blocks, for they contain the machinery of life, the biological mechanisms that produce new cells to specification, repair existing cells, and see to it that physical traits are inherited from parent to child indefinitely. Cell mechanisms know what to do because instructions are chemically encoded into each cell's pool of DNA (deoxyribonucleic acid). This DNA is the same in virtually every cell, providing a detailed plan for constructing and operating an entire organism of massive complexity.

The molecular structure of DNA is the double helix, a twisted ladder with many rungs. Each rung consists of a pair of chemical bases, referred to as a base pair. All the rungs are formed by pairing just four bases in various combinations, and all the instructions to the cell are given by the varying sequence of these base pairs along the length of the twisted ladder, the strand of DNA. So just as a computer program's instructions consist merely of zeros and ones, so DNA instructions to the cell—the genetic code—are made up of just four "letters." The DNA in a human being comprises about 3 billion base pairs, and all of these are crammed into nearly every cell.

A cell would find it difficult to make sense of all these base pairs if they were strung together in one long strand. Fortunately the strand is broken into discrete sections, snippets of genetic code, each of which can provide coherent directions to the cell. These sections are **genes,** the workhorses of cell construction and maintenance and the basic conveyors of inheritance. They are further grouped into forty-six larger compartments, actually forty-six molecules, called **chromosomes,** and these are organized into twenty-three pairs of chromosomes residing in the nucleus of the cell.

Many diseases and conditions in humans (and other creatures) arise because of genetic errors: genes may be defective (due to an inheritable mutation or environmental damage) or missing entirely. Until recently, there was no hope of correcting such problems at the genetic level, but now scientists can try to do just that through **gene therapy** (or *genetic modification*). Gene therapy is an experimental technique for directly changing a person's genes to prevent or treat disease. Researchers try to effect these changes by replacing a mutated gene with a normal one, supplying a gene that is missing, or inactivating (turning off) a malfunctioning gene. The hope (not yet realized) is that gene therapy can cure or treat a host of maladies, including heart disease, cancer, immune disorders, and fatal illnesses such as Huntington's disease and Tay-Sachs.

In the most common kind of gene therapy, a normal copy of a gene is introduced into cells that lack a properly functioning version of the gene. But a gene usually cannot be injected directly into cells and still function correctly. Instead it must be shut-tled into the cell's nucleus by a specially designed carrier molecule, or vector, often a modified virus. Viruses have a knack for inserting their own genes into cells, so scientists render viruses harmless and then use their insertion ability to deliver the designated gene into cells. Once the normal gene is in its proper place in the cell, it can start up the manufacturing of proteins to perform cell functions.

Much of the moral controversy surrounding gene therapy hinges on a distinction between two kinds of this technique—somatic cell and germ-line cell. Somatic cells are body cells (like skin, brain, and muscle cells), and gene therapy involving these cells aims to rectify an existing genetic problem. Only the patients getting the treatment are affected; there is no chance that the alterations to genes will be inherited by the patients' offspring. Germ-line cells are egg and sperm cells, and gene therapy designed to repair the genes in these types of cells can affect future generations. If an egg cell is genetically altered, for example, the alteration can appear in the genome of the offspring born from that egg—and the genetic change can in turn be passed on to that offspring's offspring, a cycle can recur indefinitely.

At the current stage of genetic research, scientists have concerns about the safety and effectiveness of all forms of gene therapy, but they are especially worried (and fascinated) by germ-line therapy. The latter is not technically possible yet, and many believe that any premature attempts to use it could have dire consequences, such as birth defects and fatal diseases. Recently scientists issued warnings about a form of germ-line therapy called "gene editing," a technique actually tried by at least one research team. The attempt failed, and leading researchers denounced the experiment for the damage it could do to cells and for its potential to permanently alter DNA and pass the changes to future generations. It's likely that some form of germ-line therapy will eventually be refined, but even a feasible form of it provokes moral concerns. Is it permissible to tinker with the human genome in this way? Is it playing God to meddle in the random processes of nature? Since there is a chance that germ-line therapy will introduce catastrophic errors into the human genome, isn't it wrong to use it? Theoretically, germ-line therapy can make "designer" babies possible, but isn't this the *manufacturing* of children? How could that be morally permissible? For many researchers, these appeals cannot outweigh the gleaming though remote possibility that germ-line therapy offers—the permanent eradication of particular genetic diseases from the human race.

The moral questions asked most often about somatic cell gene therapy have to do with the consequences of using it—whether the good to be gained outweighs the risks. Although many gene therapy studies have been done, and hundreds are in progress, the research is still preliminary. (The U.S. Food and Drug Administration has yet to approve any gene therapy products.) Some research has shown promising results, but a few early experiments harmed patients. Most scientists, however, probably expect that safe and effective treatments will be devised eventually. At that point, the consequentialist moral question will be easier to answer.

Philosophers have also offered nonconsequentialist arguments both for and against gene therapy. Some hold that if through gene therapy scientists can prevent or cure diseases in patients now, or prevent disorders in future generations, they have a moral duty to do so. Many also appeal to the right of self-determination, or autonomy: If would-be parents have a right to decide for themselves whether to reproduce or not, they surely must also have a right to decide whether to use germ-line therapy to avert disorders in their children. Those who oppose the use of this technology argue that changing the human genome is contrary to the natural order of things and therefore should not be attempted. Or they maintain that the principle of respect for human life is violated when germ-line therapy alters or destroys embryos.

Another important distinction has become the starting point for several other moral debates. There is a difference, many contend, between (1) *genetic repair and prevention* and (2) ***genetic enhancement.***

When scientists use gene therapy or any other kind of genetic intervention to correct genetic defects, they are involved in the former. But if they use genetic intervention to make people *better than normal*—to maximize human traits and capabilities—they are doing the latter. To alter a normal person's genome to increase her intelligence or to make her taller is to practice genetic enhancement. Genetic repair and prevention includes several technologies besides gene therapy—for example, genetic testing, selective abortion (destroying embryos that are defective), and prenatal screening. Genetic enhancement can also be achieved in several ways. It has been used in animal breeding and agriculture for centuries, and in modern pharmaceutical production for decades. (Genetically enhanced microorganisms are now being put to work producing insulin, human growth hormone, and many other therapeutic substances.) When genetic enhancement involves direct intervention in an organism's genome, it is called **genetic engineering.** And the most profound and controversial type of genetic engineering in humans involves germ-line modifications.

Some insist that we may have a moral obligation to use gene therapy to cure a person's cancer or to prevent her from getting cancer in the first place, but we have no duty to use genetic engineering to give her superhuman strength or a two-hundred-year life span. Why not? A common answer is that genetic engineering disrupts the natural, optimum state of humans, the genetic design given to us by God or evolution. Playing with the human genome risks disaster. Some argue that genetic engineering can be literally dehumanizing, that it turns humans into nonhumans, gene by gene. Others worry that genetically enhanced people would have an unfair advantage in competing for social status, jobs, wealth, even survival. The main concern is that such drastic inequality would lead to extreme social injustice, especially if only the rich could afford enhancement.

The most radical and controversial form of genetic manipulation is cloning. **Cloning** is the

Gene Therapy: Some Recent Developments

Severe Combined Immune Deficiency (ADA-SCID). ADA-SCID is more commonly known as bubble boy disease. Those who suffer from SCID are born with impaired immune systems, and are unable to withstand common infections and contagions outside their sterilized bubbles. Bone marrow transplants are used to treat SCID, but not all patients can find matching donors. An alternative treatment for those whose SCID is caused by a lack of ADA (adenosine deaminase) protein is the insertion of the ADA enzyme into the bone marrow, which causes significant improvement, but is expensive and requires life-long application. A more permanent solution to SCID is gene therapy, which has been tested on 30 SCID patients so far, most of whom have not needed further treatment. Recent clinical trials have shown that treating patients with a small amount of busulfan, a chemotherapy drug, before grafting the ADA-corrected stem cells to the bone marrow has increased the success rate of gene therapy in SCID. Most patients can now expect gene-corrected lymphocytes to occupy 1–10% of their blood thanks to gene therapy.

Chronic Granulomatus Disorder (CGD). CGD is a genetic immunodeficiency disease which affects the body's ability to protect itself against bacterial and fungal infections, some of which can prove to be fatal. Seventy percent of CGD sufferers have a defective gp91phox gene, which is located on the X chromosome, and so affects males. Clinical trials have shown that when hematopoietic stem cells combined with functional gp91phox were introduced to CGD patients, the patients made full recoveries and were able to fight off serious infections. However, two patients developed bone marrow abnormalities

as a result of treatment, so researchers are currently working with new gene transfer vectors to improve the safety of gp91phox gene therapy.

Other genetic disorders. Treatments for many genetic disorders, such as congenital blindness, muscular dystrophy, lysosomal storage disease, and others, are currently being tested in clinical trials. The results of all the methods have been encouraging, and clinical research continues.

Neurodegenerative Diseases. Those who suffer from neurodegenerative diseases, such as Parkinson's and Huntington's Disease, may one day be able to benefit from gene therapy treatments. Clinical trials on animals have already shown positive results, and human patients will soon be able to take part.

Other acquired diseases. Gene therapy has also been used to treat viral infections, such as the flu, HIV, and hepatitis, as well as heart disease and diabetes. There are several methods being used so far: T-cell–based approaches, cell therapy, stem cell–based approaches, genetic vaccines, and genetic vectors. All methods have been shown to be affective in human/animal trials.

Based on American Society of Gene and Cell Therapy, "Gene Therapy for Genetic Disorders," 2000–2011, http://www.asgct.org/about_gene_therapy/diseases.php (28 October 2014); American Society of Gene and Cell Therapy, "Immunodeficiency Diseases," 2000–2015, http://www.asgct.org/general-public/educational-resources/gene-therapy-and-cell-therapy-for-diseases/immunodeficiency-diseases (16 March 2015); American Society of Gene and Cell Therapy, "Infectious Diseases," 2000–2015, http://www.asgct.org/general-public/educational-resources/gene-therapy-and-cell-therapy-for-diseases/infectious-diseases (16 March 2015).

production of a genetically identical copy of an existing biological entity (a cell, DNA molecule, animal, or human) through an asexual process. The resulting copy is a clone, and the original material is the clone's progenitor. Without much

public attention, researchers have used simple forms of cloning for years to duplicate plant strains and human and animal cells. But in the past fifteen years, public concern about cloning has spread because science showed that more sophisticated sorts of cloning might be possible: the cloning of whole animals or humans.

Scientists are concerned with three types of cloning, only two of which provoke ethical debate. The uncontroversial kind (and the most widely used in science) is known as *DNA cloning*. It involves the copying of particular genes for study. *Therapeutic cloning* duplicates human embryos for use in research aimed at the treatment of disease. From the embryonic clones, researchers harvest stem cells, which have the unique talent of generating almost any kind of specialized human cell (for example, bone cells, muscle cells, and nerve cells). Scientists hope to use stem cells to treat cancer, heart disease, diabetes, Parkinson's, and many other disorders by replacing defective specialized cells. Most of the ethical concerns about therapeutic cloning crop up because the harvesting of stem cells destroys the embryo, a result that many believe shows disrespect for human life.

By far, the most provocative and morally problematic type of cloning is **reproductive cloning,** the genetic duplication of a fully developed adult animal or human. In 1997, reproductive cloning became big news around the world when Scottish researchers cloned the first mammal from a cell taken from an adult animal. The result was Dolly, a lamb cloned from the cell of a six-year-old sheep. Since then, many other animals have been cloned, including cows, goats, horses, cats, deer, dogs, and rabbits.

The method used to clone mammals is known as somatic cell nuclear transfer (SCNT). First, the nucleus of an egg cell is removed. (The nucleus contains most of an organism's DNA.) Then it is replaced with the nucleus of a body (somatic) cell extracted from the living adult animal to be cloned. Electricity or chemicals are used to jump-start the growth of this new cell to the embryo stage, and the cloned embryo is transferred to the uterus of an adult animal, which gives birth to the clone in the normal way.

This simple description of SCNT glosses over the difficulties of using it to produce healthy clones. For one thing, the technique is extremely inefficient. Most clone embryos never make it to healthy adulthood. Dolly survived to maturity, for example, but 276 other clone embryos used in the experiment did not. Clones are also often plagued by serious health problems—abnormalities in vital organs, weakened immune system, premature aging, and other disorders. Many clones die early and, sometimes, mysteriously. Dolly died at age six, six years short of the usual lifespan for sheep.

The public outcry over cloning humans is out of proportion to the actual feasibility of accomplishing such a feat. To date, no humans have been cloned, despite some bogus claims to the contrary, and no successful cloning is likely for years or even decades. Policymakers, researchers, and physicians generally advise against the cloning of humans. They believe the technique is risky, even dangerous, with a good chance of birth defects and other physiological problems. Until they know a great deal more about cloning, they are likely to oppose any attempts to clone humans.

Although many worries about human cloning seem justified in light of available scientific evidence, some concerns are the result of misunderstandings. The silliest confusion is inspired by Hollywood: the belief that clones are like photocopies of their progenitors, full-blown replicas produced in a few hours or days. But of course a clone begins as an embryo and develops as any other embryo does, taking years to acquire its adult characteristics and being years in age behind its DNA donor.

Another mistake is thinking that human clones are artificial, alien entities that have to be produced in a laboratory. But there are natural clones; they're called twins. Identical twins are true clones, possessing almost identical DNA. This is why some argue that if there are moral objections to the very existence of clones, the objections would seem to apply to the existence of twins as well.

Perhaps the most common misapprehension is that an adult human clone would be an exact copy of its adult human donor. That is, the clone would eventually look like and be like the person who donated his or her DNA. This notion yields the fantasy (also inspired by Hollywood) that if we want several more Einsteins, Gandhis, or Platos, all we have to do is clone the original person. But this assumes that genes determine all of a person's physical and behavioral traits, a doctrine known as genetic determinism. This view, however, is false. DNA is not the only factor that determines a person's characteristics. Many environmental factors (such as nutrition and life experiences) also play a role and may interact in unexpected ways with genes. A cat and its clone, for example, may have completely different coloring, and a clone of Gandhi would likely not be like Gandhi despite having the same genetic makeup.

But even if human cloning were feasible, why would anyone want to do it? For many, cloning would be their only chance of having children who are genetically related to them. Through cloning, a couple might have such a child even if they had no eggs or sperm of their own. They might also turn to cloning to avoid transmitting genetic defects to their offspring. Or suppose parents have only one child and she dies. They might find some comfort in cloning her from one of her cells. Or imagine that a child will die unless he gets a kidney transplant. To save him and to ensure that his immune system does not reject a new kidney, parents might clone him so his clone could eventually supply a compatible kidney.

MORAL THEORIES

Even though genetic technologies are relatively new, major moral theories that have been around for hundreds of years still apply to them.

On these issues, many ethicists and policymakers appeal to consequentialist theories. A utilitarian, for example, would approve of gene therapy if its use would result in greater benefits than risks, everyone considered. But right now whether gene

therapy actually does produce more good than bad is still an open question. In genetic research there have been some minor successes and a few alarming failures. Until human genetics and the effects of gene therapy are better understood, utilitarians are not likely to endorse this technology. This cautious view would apply to somatic cell methods but would pertain with even greater force to germ-line cell therapy.

Utilitarians would likely approve of genetic enhancement if it yields greater overall happiness. After all, the point of this method is to improve on existing capabilities and traits. But some philosophers argue that genetic enhancement, if widely available, could do more harm than good. For one thing, they say, social discontent could arise if genetically enhanced people seem to have an unfair social advantage over the non-enhanced.

Currently neither utilitarians nor deontologists are likely to give blanket approval to human reproductive cloning. The unknowns are many, and the risks are great. (The risks include genetic defects and early death.) But if cloning's technical problems and safety issues were worked out so that the risks were minimal, utilitarians might judge human cloning to be morally permissible, even obligatory. The possible benefits would be substantial: infertile parents could have a genetically related child, the risk of transmitting genetic abnormalities could be erased, and perfectly compatible organ transplants could be possible.

As you might expect, natural law theory rejects many types of genetic intervention. The Roman Catholic version of the theory could give its blessing to somatic-cell gene therapy because the purpose is the treatment or prevention of disease. But genetic enhancement through either somatic-cell or germ-line intervention would be viewed as contrary to nature and therefore immoral. Human reproductive cloning would also be condemned as unnatural because it breaks the connection between procreation and the sexual act. And therapeutic cloning would be out of the question because it

CRITICAL THOUGHT: Longer Life Through Gene Therapy?

In a multitude of ways, scientists are working to conquer aging, to achieve what has been described as "Methuselah-like life spans." One avenue of research (in very preliminary stages) involves the use of gene therapy. Here is an example:

> Cynthia Kenyon of the University of California, San Francisco, found that partially disabling a single gene, called daf-2, doubled the life of tiny worms called Caenorhabditis elegans. Altering the daf-16 gene and other cells added to the effect, allowing the worms to survive in a healthy state six times longer than their normal life span. In human terms, they would be the equivalent of healthy, active 500-year-olds.
>
> Experiments with animals are not always applicable to humans, of course, but humans do have the same sort of genetic pathways that Dr. Kenyon manipulated.[†]

Suppose gene therapy can extend a person's life to over 150 years. Would this be a good thing? Would such a longer life enhance our happiness—or bring misery in the form of accumulated disease and dysfunction? Would increasing the human lifespan be "contrary to nature" and therefore immoral? Would longer life destroy any incentive we might have to meet personal objectives or improve ourselves morally?

[†]Sonia Arrison, "Living to 100 and Beyond," *Wall Street Journal*, 27 August 2011, http://online.wsj.com/article/SB10001424053111904875404576528841080315246, adapted from Sonia Arrison, *100 Plus: How the Coming Age of Longevity Will Change Everything*, 2011 (27 August 2011).

entails the destruction of embryos, which constitutes a lack of respect for human life.

Depending on how personhood and respect for persons are interpreted, a Kantian could either welcome or condemn genetic manipulations. On one hand, she could argue that genetic enhancement improves human life but neither respects nor disrespects personhood. The same could be said for genetic therapy. Reproductive cloning could be viewed as a way to bring persons into the world to be respected and cared for. On the other hand, a Kantian could also see genetic enhancement and reproductive cloning as ways to treat children as a means to an end, as products manufactured to satisfy the desires of others.

MORAL ARGUMENTS

The easiest way to argue for or against genetic interventions is to appeal to their risks or benefits.

Just about everyone agrees that if these techniques are inherently dangerous, they should not be used on humans. Most also recognize that right now their use is risky business. But scientists think that with enough research, our understanding of genetic manipulations will improve and so will their safety and effectiveness. If so, risk-benefit arguments against genetic technologies will eventually lose much of their force, and such arguments in their favor will be strengthened.

Many of the moral arguments, however, rely heavily on widely accepted moral principles. Perhaps the strongest argument for using gene therapy and genetic enhancement appeals to the principle of beneficence, the notion that we are morally obligated to do good to others and to refrain from doing them harm. The argument goes something like this: If through somatic-cell gene therapy we are able to prevent or cure diseases, shouldn't we do so? If through germ-line genetic therapy we can prevent the suffering of future persons, aren't we obligated to do so? If we have an obligation to help people using ordinary means (conventional medical care), don't we also have a duty to help them using extraordinary means (genetic interventions)?

Proponents of both therapy and enhancement also appeal to the principle of autonomy, the idea that persons have a right of self-determination. In genetic debates, an autonomy argument might go this way: The principle of autonomy requires that we have reproductive freedom—the right to produce children or not to produce them. But if we have this right, then surely we also have the right to decide whether our children suffer or don't suffer from a disease or disability, or whether they have above-average intelligence or superior athletic ability. And if we have this right, then we have a right to use any safe and effective genetic technology to ensure that our children are blessed with these things. A counterargument is that the principle of autonomy is not absolute: there are limits to our right of self-determination, and genetic interventions (especially germ-line changes) go too far.

Many arguments center on whether there is a morally significant difference between therapy and enhancement. Eventually we may be able to wield gene therapy (both somatic-cell and germ-line) to treat or prevent many disorders—that is, to restore or ensure normal functions. This is what conventional medicine tries to do, so most people would probably think that a genetic approach that aimed at normalcy would also be morally acceptable. Not so with genetic enhancement. Some believe that this method of improving or extending normal functions is wrong because it amounts to "playing God"—a charge that they also level against gene therapy. They contend that through either an act of divine creation or the impersonal machinations of evolution, we humans have been given a particular package of genes that is just right for us. To toy with our genetic inheritance is to tilt against God or nature and to invite disaster,

divine or natural. These critics, however, maintain that treatment or prevention through gene therapy is permissible because its aim is merely to repair what God or nature has given us.

Many philosophers reject the distinction between curing dysfunction and boosting function, arguing that there is no morally significant difference between the two. One way of putting this argument is to propose a hypothetical situation. Suppose a gene could be inserted into humans to both repair damage done by environmental pollutants and dramatically increase the likelihood of an abnormally long healthy life. Wouldn't it be permissible—and perhaps even obligatory—to insert the gene to reduce human suffering? Wouldn't the repair and enhancement be morally equivalent actions? Wouldn't the enhancement be more than merely permissible, just as the introduction of immune-enhancing penicillin was?[1]

To some opponents of enhancement, the most promising argument against it is an appeal to the principle of justice. The gist is that enhancement is unjust because it would give enhanced people an unfair advantage over the unenhanced. Only the well-off could afford genetic enhancement, so the less fortunate would go without it. And those who are enhanced, this argument says, would acquire traits and capacities (such as super intelligence and extraordinary beauty) that would give them an enormous edge over the unenhanced in any competition for society's goods. Thus the use of genetic enhancement would lead to an abhorrent form of social inequality, and that is unjust.

Many arguments for and against human cloning echo those for and against gene therapy and enhancement. For example: Human reproductive cloning should never be done because it's

---

[1]An example from John Harris, "Is Gene Therapy a Form of Eugenics?" in *Bioethics: Anthology*, ed. Helga Kuhse and Peter Singer (Oxford: Blackwell Publishers, 1999), 165–170.

dom to act according to our own lights. By definition, every clone is forced to begin her life after her progenitor has already matured to adulthood. So she grows up watching her genetic duplicate, believing that the life she wants to live has already been lived by her twin. She thinks she has no open future because she sees in her genetic mirror image how her future will unfold. Her sense of personal freedom evaporates as she comes to believe that the direction of her life is already preordained.

Critics of this line assert that a clone might think her future is already determined—but she also might believe that it is not. There is no reason to assume that she *must* believe the former and not the latter. Moreover they insist that her merely *believing* that her future is predestined does not undermine her rights. If her future is in fact open and shaped by her own free choices, then her being led to believe that it is closed does not violate her right to an open future. In any case, genetic determinism is false; a clone is unlikely to be just like her progenitor.

playing God, because it's a violation of the principle of justice, or because cloning would essentially be the manufacture of children, a practice that would undermine respect for persons. Proponents maintain that cloning is permissible because it is in keeping with the principles of autonomy (reproductive liberty) and beneficence, and because cloning could be of enormous benefit to infertile couples.

A few opponents of cloning claim that the practice is immoral because it would infringe on an important moral right—the "right to ignorance" or a "right to an open future." The key premise in this argument is that we all have a right to personal liberty, to the freedom to live our lives according to our own choices and plans and not to be forced into a particular path. But, the argument goes, cloning would severely constrain our free-

SUMMARY

Cells constitute the bodies of all living things, and cell mechanisms know what to do because instructions are encoded into each cell's DNA. DNA is divided into discrete sections called genes; genes are further grouped into forty-six molecules called chromosomes.

Many diseases and conditions arise because of genetic errors, and scientists are learning how to correct them through gene therapy, or gene modification. Much of the controversy surrounding gene therapy depends on a distinction between two kinds of the treatment—somatic cell and germ-line cell. Somatic cell therapy affects only the persons being treated and is usually thought to be morally permissible. Germ-line methods can effect changes that are passed on to future generations, and this approach is controversial. Moral questions about somatic cell therapy concern its risks and benefits; the application of the principles of beneficence, autonomy, and respect for human life; and appeals to what is or is not natural.

Genetic *repair* is widely believed to be permissible, but genetic *enhancement* is not. Some argue that we may have a duty to cure or prevent diseases but not to enhance traits and capacities so people are *better than normal*. Many object to enhancement on the grounds that it thwarts the genetic design given to us by God or evolution, that it can be dehumanizing, and that it leads to social inequality and injustice.

Reproductive cloning is the genetic duplication of a fully developed adult animal or human. No humans have been cloned yet, and scientists think human cloning is currently too risky to attempt. Arguments for and against human cloning echo those for and against gene therapy and enhancement. A few opponents of cloning claim that the practice is impermissible because it would infringe on an important moral right—the "right to ignorance" or a "right to an open future." But others doubt that there is such a right, or they try to show that human cloning violates no rights at all.

READINGS

Genetic Enhancement

WALTER GLANNON

Gene therapy must be distinguished from genetic enhancement. The first is an intervention aimed at treating disease and restoring physical and mental functions and capacities to an adequate baseline. The second is an intervention aimed at improving functions and capacities that already are adequate. Genetic enhancement augments functions and capacities "that without intervention would be considered entirely normal."[1] Its goal is to "amplify 'normal' genes in order to make them better."[2] In chapter 1, I cited Norman Daniels's definitions of health and disease as well as what the notion of just health care entailed. This involved maintaining or restoring mental and physical functions at or to normal levels, which was necessary to ensure fair equality of opportunity for all citizens. Insofar as this aim defines the goal of medicine, genetic enhancement falls outside this goal. Furthermore, insofar as this type of intervention is not

part of the goal of medicine and has no place in a just health care system, there are no medical or moral reasons for genetically enhancing normal human functions and capacities.

Some have argued that it is mistaken to think that a clear line of demarcation can be drawn between treatment and enhancement, since certain forms of enhancement are employed to prevent disease. Leroy Walters and Julie Gage Palmer refer to the immune system as an example to make this point:

In current medical practice, the best example of a widely accepted health-related physical enhancement is immunization against infectious disease.

With immunizations against diseases like polio and hepatitis B, what we are saying is in effect, "The immune system that we inherited from our parents may not be adequate to ward off certain viruses if we are exposed to them." Therefore, we will enhance the capabilities of our immune system by priming it to fight against these viruses.

From the current practice of immunizations against particular diseases, it would seem to be only a small step to try to enhance the general function of the immune system by genetic means. . . . In our view, the genetic enhancement of the immune system would be morally justifiable if this kind of enhancement assisted in preventing disease and did not cause offsetting harms to the people treated by the technique.[3]

Nevertheless, because the goal of the technique would be to prevent disease, it would not, strictly speaking, be enhancement, at least not in terms of the definitions given at the outset of this section. Genetically intervening in the immune system as described by Walters and Palmer is a means of maintaining it in proper working order so that it will be better able to ward off pathogens posing a threat to the organism as a whole. Thus, it is misleading to call this intervention "enhancement." When we consider what is normal human functioning, we refer to the whole human organism consisting of immune, endocrine, nervous, cardiovascular, and other systems, not to these systems understood as isolated parts. The normal functioning in question here pertains to the ability of the immune system to protect the organism from infectious agents and thus ensure its survival. Any preventive genetic intervention in this system would be designed to maintain the normal functions of the organism, not to restore them or raise them above the norm. It would be neither therapy nor enhancement but instead a form of maintenance. Therefore, the alleged ambiguity surrounding what Walters and Palmer call "enhancing" the immune system does not impugn the distinction between treatment and enhancement.

If enhancement could make adequately functioning bodily systems function even better, then presumably there would be no limit to the extent to which bodily functions can be enhanced. Yet, beyond a certain point, heightened immune sensitivity to infectious agents can lead to an overly aggressive response, resulting in autoimmune disease that can damage healthy cells, tissues, and organs. In fact, there would be a limit to the beneficial effects of genetic intervention in the immune system, a limit beyond which the equilibrium between humoral and cellular response mechanisms would be disturbed.[4] If any intervention ensured that the equilibrium of the immune system was maintained in proper working order, then it would be inappropriate to consider it as a form of enhancement.

To further support the treatment-enhancement distinction, consider a nongenetic intervention, the use of a bisphosphonate such as alendronate sodium. Its purpose is to prevent postmenopausal women from developing osteoporosis, or to rebuild bone in women or men who already have osteoporosis. Some might claim that, because it can increase bone density, it is a form of enhancement. But its more general purpose is to prevent bone fractures and thus maintain proper bone function so that one can have normal mobility and avoid the morbidity resulting from fractures. In terms of the functioning of the entire organism, therefore, it would be more accurate to consider the use of bisphosphonates as prevention, treatment, or maintenance rather than enhancement.

Some might raise a different question. Suppose that the parents of a child much shorter than the norm for his age persuaded a physician to give him growth hormone injections in order to increase his height. Suppose further that the child's shortness was not due to an iatrogenic cause, such as radiation to treat a brain tumor. Would this be treatment or enhancement? The question that should be asked regarding this issue is not whether the child's height is normal for his age group. Rather, the question should be whether his condition implies something less than normal physical functioning, such that he would have fewer opportunities for achievement and a decent minimum level of well-being over his lifetime. Diminutive stature alone does not necessarily imply that one's functioning is or will be so limited as to restrict one's opportunities for achievement. Of course, being short might limit one's opportunities if one wanted to become a professional basketball player. But most of us are quite flexible when it comes to formulating and carrying out life plans. Robert Reich, the treasury secretary in President Clinton's first administration, is just one example of how one can achieve very much in life despite diminutive stature. If a child's stature significantly limited his functioning and opportunities, then growth-hormone injections should be considered therapeutic treatment. If his stature were not so limiting, then the injections should be considered enhancement.

Admittedly, there is gray area near the baseline of adequate functioning where it may be difficult to distinguish between treatment and enhancement. Accordingly, we should construe the baseline loosely or thickly enough to allow for some minor deviation above or below what would be considered normal functioning. An intervention for a condition near the baseline that would raise one's functioning clearly above the critical level should be considered an enhancement. An intervention for a condition making one's functioning fall clearly below the baseline, with the aim of raising one's functioning to the critical level, should be considered a treatment. For example, an athlete with a hemoglobin level slightly below the norm for people his age and mildly anemic may want to raise that level significantly in order to be more competitive in his sport. To the extent that his actual hemoglobin level does not interfere with his ordinary physical functioning, an intervention to significantly raise that level would be an instance of enhancement. In contrast, for a child who has severe thalassemia and severe anemia, with the risk of bone abnormalities and heart failure, an intervention to correct the disorder would be an instance of treatment.

The main moral concern about genetic enhancement of physical and mental traits is that it would give some people an unfair advantage over others with respect to competitive goods like beauty, sociability, and intelligence. Unlike the cognitively disabled individual considered earlier, we can assume that their mental states would not be so different and that they would retain their identity. Enhancement would be unfair because only those who could afford the technology would have access to it, and many people are financially worse off than others through no fault of their own. Insofar as the possession of these goods gives some people an advantage over others in careers, income, and social status, the competitive nature of these goods suggests that there would be no limit to the benefits that improvements to physical and mental capacities would yield to those fortunate enough to avail themselves of the technology. This is altogether different from the example of immune-system enhancement. There would be no diminishing marginal value in the degree of competitive advantage that one could have over others for the social goods in question and presumably no limit to the value of enhancing the physical and mental capacities that would give one this advantage. Not having access to the technology that could manipulate genetic traits in such a way as to enhance these capacities would put one at a competitive disadvantage relative to others who would have access to it.

Advancing an argument similar to the one used by those who reject the treatment-enhancement distinction, one might hold that competitive goods collapse the categorical distinction between correcting deficient capacities and improving normal ones. This is because competitive goods are continuous, coming in degrees, and therefore the capacities that enable one to achieve these goods cannot be thought of as either normal or deficient.[5] Nevertheless, to the extent that any form of genetic intervention is motivated by the medical and moral aim to enable people to have adequate mental and physical functioning and fair equality of opportunity for a decent minimum level of well-being, the goods in question are not *competitive* but *basic*. In other words, the aim of any medical intervention by genetic means is to make people better off than they were before by raising or restoring them to an absolute baseline of normal physical and mental functioning, not to make them comparatively better off than others. Competitive goods above the baseline may be continuous; but the basic goods that enable someone to reach or remain at the baseline are not. Given that these two types of goods are distinct, and that they result from the distinct aims and practices of enhancement and treatment, we can affirm that enhancement and treatment can and should be treated separately. We can uphold the claim that the purpose of any genetic intervention should be to treat people's abnormal functions and restore them to a normal level, not to enhance those functions that already are normal.

As I have mentioned, genetic enhancement that gave some people an advantage over others in possessing competitive goods would entail considerable unfairness. A likely scenario would be one in which parents paid to use expensive genetic technology to raise the cognitive ability or improve the physical beauty of their children. This would give them an advantage over other children with whom they would compete for education, careers, and income. Children of parents who could not afford to pay for the technology would be at a comparative disadvantage. Even if the goods in question fell above the normal functional baseline, one still could maintain that such an advantage would be unfair. It would depend on people's ability to pay, and inequalities in income are unfair to the extent that they result from some factors beyond people's control.

* * *

Yet, suppose that we could manipulate certain genes to enhance our noncompetitive virtuous traits, such as altruism, generosity, and compassion.[6] Surely, these would contribute to a stable, well-ordered society and preserve the principle of fair equality of opportunity. Nothing in this program would be incompatible with the goal of medicine as the prevention and treatment of disease. But it would threaten the individual autonomy essential to us as moral agents who can be candidates for praise and blame, punishment and reward. What confers moral worth on our actions, and indeed on ourselves as agents, is our capacity to cultivate certain dispositions leading to actions. This cultivation involves the exercise of practical reason and a process of critical self-reflection, whereby we modify, eliminate, or reinforce dispositions and thereby come to identify with them as our own. Autonomy consists precisely in this process of reflection and identification. It is the capacity for reflective self-control that enables us to take responsibility for our mental states and the actions that issue from them. Given the importance of autonomy, it would be preferable to have fewer virtuous dispositions that we can identify with as our own than to have more virtuous dispositions implanted in us through genetic enhancement. These would threaten to undermine our moral agency because they would derive from an external source.[7] Even if our genes could be manipulated in such a way that our behavior always conformed to an algorithm

for the morally correct course of action in every situation, it is unlikely that we would want it. Most of us would rather make autonomous choices that turned out not to lead to the best courses of action. This is because of the intrinsic importance of autonomy and the moral growth and maturity that come with making our own choices under uncertainty. The dispositions with which we come to identify, imperfect as they may be, are what make us autonomous and responsible moral agents. Enhancing these mental states through artificial means external to our own exercise of practical reason and our own process of identification would undermine our autonomy by making them alien to us.

In sum, there are four reasons why genetic enhancement would be morally objectionable. First, it would give an unfair advantage to some people over others because some would be able to pay for expensive enhancement procedures while others would not. Second, if we tried to remedy the first problem by making genetic enhancement universally accessible, then it would be collectively self-defeating. Although much competitive unfairness at the individual level would be canceled out at the collective level, there would be the unacceptable social cost of some people suffering from adverse cognitive or emotional effects of the enhancement. Third, inequalities resulting from enhancements above the baseline of normal physical and mental functioning could threaten to undermine the conviction in the fundamental importance of equality as one of the bases of self-respect, and in turn social solidarity and stability. Fourth, enhancement of noncompetitive dispositions would threaten to undermine the autonomy and moral agency essential to us as persons.

NOTES

1. Jon Gordon, "Genetic Enhancement in Humans," *Science* 283 (March 26, 1999): 2023–2024.

2. Eric Juengst, "Can Enhancement Be Distinguished from Prevention in Genetic Medicine?" *Journal of Medicine and Philosophy* 22 (1997): 125–142, and "What Does Enhancement Mean?" in Erik Parens, ed., *Enhancing Human Traits: Ethical and Social Implications* (Washington, DC: Georgetown

University Press, 1998): 27–47, at 27. Also, Dan Brock, "Enhancements of Human Function: Some Distinctions for Policymakers," Ibid., 48–69.

3. *The Ethics of Human Gene Therapy*, 110. Instead of distinguishing between treatments and enhancements, Walters and Palmer distinguish between health-related and non-health-related enhancements. But I do not find this distinction to be very helpful.

4. Brock points this out in "Enhancements of Human Function," 59. Marc Lappe makes a more compelling case for the same point in *The Tao of Immunology*.

5. Kavka develops and defends the idea that competitive goods are continuous in "Upside Risks," 164–165.

6. Walters and Palmer present this thought-experiment in *The Ethics of Human Gene Therapy*, 123–128. As they note, Jonathan Glover introduced this idea in *What Sort of People Should There Be?* (Harmondsworth: Penguin, 1984).

7. Drawing on the work of Lionel Trilling and Charles Taylor, Carl Elliott discusses cognitive and affective enhancements that undermine what he calls the "ethics of authenticity" in "The Tyranny of Happiness: Ethics and Cosmetic Psychopharmacology," in Parens, *Enhancing Human Traits*, 177–188. Also relevant to this issue is Harry Frankfurt, "Identification and Externality," in Frankfurt, *The Importance of What We Care About* (New York: Cambridge University Press, 1989): 58–68.

Is Gene Therapy a Form of Eugenics?

JOHN HARRIS

Eugenic A. *adj*. Pertaining or adapted to the production of fine offspring. B. *sh*. in *pl*. The science which treats of this. (*The Shorter Oxford English Dictionary* Third Edition 1965).

It has now become a serious necessity to better the breed of the human race. The average citizen is too base for the everyday work of modern civilization. Civilised man has become possessed of vaster powers than in old times for good or ill but has made no corresponding advance in wits and goodness to enable him to conduct his conduct rightly. (*Sir Francis Galton*)

If, as I believe, gene therapy is in principle ethically sound except for its possible connection with eugenics then there are two obvious ways of giving a simple and straightforward answer to a question such as this. The first is to say "yes it is, and so what?" The second is to say "no it isn't so we shouldn't worry." If we accept the first of the above definitions we might well be inclined to give the first of our two answers. If on the other hand, we accept the sort of gloss that Ruth Chadwick gives on Galton's account, "those who are genetically weak should simply be discouraged from

John Harris, "Is Gene Therapy a Form of Eugenics" from *Bioethics* 7(2/3): 178–187. Copyright © Basil Blackwell Ltd., 1993. Reproduced with permission of John Wiley & Sons, Inc.

reproducing," either by incentives or compulsory measures, we get a somewhat different flavour, and one which might incline a decent person who favours gene therapy towards the second answer.

The nub of the problem turns on how we are to understand the objective of producing "fine children." Does "fine" mean "as fine as children normally are," or does it mean "as fine as a child can be"? Sorting out the ethics of the connection between gene therapy and eugenics seems to involve the resolution of two morally significant issues. The first is whether or not there is a relevant moral distinction between attempts to remove or repair dysfunction on the one hand and measures designed to enhance function on the other, such that it would be coherent to be in favour of curing dysfunction but against enhancing function? The second involves the question of whether gene therapy as a technique involves something specially morally problematic.

THE MORAL CONTINUUM

Is it morally wrong to wish and hope for a fine baby girl or boy? Is it wrong to wish and hope that one's child will not be born disabled? I assume that my feeling that such hopes and wishes are not wrong is shared by every sane decent person. Now consider whether it would be wrong to wish and hope for the reverse? What would we think of someone who hoped and wished that their child would be born with disability? Again I need not spell out the answer to these questions.

But now let's bridge the gap between thought and action, between hopes and wishes and their fulfilment. What would we think of someone who, hoping and wishing for a fine healthy child, declined to take the steps necessary to secure this outcome when such steps were open to them?

Again I assume that unless those steps could be shown to be morally unacceptable our conclusions would be the same.

Consider the normal practice at I.V.F. clinics where a woman who has had say, five eggs fertilised *in vitro*, wishes to use some of these embryos to become pregnant. Normal practice would be to insert two embryos or at most three. If pre-implantation screening had revealed two of the embryos to possess disabilities of one sort or another, would it be right to implant the two embryos with disability rather than the others? Would it be right to choose the implantation embryos randomly? Could it be defensible for a doctor to override the wishes of the mother and implant the disabled embryos rather than the healthy ones—would we applaud her for so doing?[1]

The answer that I expect to all these rhetorical questions will be obvious. It depends however on accepting that disability is somehow disabling and therefore undesirable. If it were not, there would be no motive to try to cure or obviate disability in health care more generally. If we believe that medical science should try to cure disability where possible, and that parents would be wrong to withhold from their disabled children cures as they become available, then we will be likely to agree on our answers to the rhetorical questions posed.

WHAT IS DISABILITY?

It is notoriously hard to give a satisfactory definition of disability although I believe we all know pretty clearly what we mean by it. A disability is surely a physical or mental condition we have a strong rational preference not to be in, it is, more importantly, a condition which is in some sense a 'harmed condition'.[2] I have in mind the sort of condition in which if a patient presented with it unconscious in the casualty department of a hospital and the condition could be easily and immediately reversed, but not reversed unless the doctor acts without delay, a doctor would be negligent were she not to attempt reversal. Or, one which, if a pregnant mother knew that it affected her fetus and knew also she could remove the condition by simple dietary adjustment, then to fail to do so would be to knowingly harm her child.[3]

To make clearer what's at issue here let's imagine that as a result of industrial effluent someone had contracted a condition that she felt had disabled or harmed her in some sense. How might she convince a court say, that she had suffered disability or injury?

The answer is obvious but necessarily vague. Whatever it would be plausible to say in answer to such a question is what I mean (and what is clearly meant) by disability and injury. It is not possible to stipulate exhaustively what would strike us as plausible here, but we know what injury is and we know what disability or incapacity is. If the condition in question was one which set premature limits on their lifespan—made their life shorter than it would be with treatment, or was one which rendered her specially vulnerable to infection, more vulnerable than others, we would surely recognise that she had been harmed and perhaps to some extent disabled. At the very least such events would be plausible candidates for the description "injuries" or "disabilities."

Against a background in which many people are standardly protected from birth or before against pollution hazards and infections and have their healthy life expectancy extended, it would surely be plausible to claim that failure to protect in this way constituted an injury and left them disabled. Because of their vulnerability to infection and to environmental pollutants there would be places it was unsafe for them to go and people with whom they could not freely consort. These restrictions on liberty are surely at least *prima facie* disabling as is the increased relative vulnerability.

These points are crucial because it is sometimes said that while we have an obligation to cure disease—to restore normal functioning—we do not have an obligation to enhance or improve upon a normal healthy life, that enhancing function is permissive but could not be regarded as obligatory. But, what constitutes a normal healthy life, is determined in part by technological and medical and other advances (hygiene, sanitation etc.) It is normal now for example to be protected against tetanus, the continued provision of such protection is not merely permissive. If the AIDS pandemic continues unabated and the only prospect, or the best prospect, for stemming it's [sic] advance is the use of gene therapy to insert genes coding for antibodies to AIDS, I cannot think that it would be coherent to regard making available such therapy as permissive rather than mandatory.[4]

If this seems still too like normal therapy to be convincing, suppose genes coding for repair enzymes which would not only repair radiation damage or damage by other environmental pollutants but would also prolong healthy life expectancy could be inserted into humans. Again, would it be permissible to let people continue suffering such damage when they could be protected against it? Would it in short be O.K. to let them suffer?

It is not normal for the human organism to be self-repairing in this way, this must be eugenic if anything is. But if available, its use would surely, like penicillin before it, be more than merely permissive.

Of course, there will be unclarity at the margins but at least this conception of disability captures and emphasises the central notion that a disability is disabling in some sense, that it is a harm to those who suffer, it, and that to knowingly disable another individual or leave them disabled when we could remove the disability is to harm that individual.[5]

This is not an exhaustive definition of disability but it is a way of thinking about it which avoids certain obvious pitfalls. First it does not define disability in terms of any conception or normalcy. Secondly it does not depend on *post hoc* ratification by the subject of the condition—it is not a prediction about how the subject of the condition will feel. This is important because we need an account of disability

we can use for the potentially self-conscious; gametes, embryos, fetuses and neonates and for the temporarily unconscious, which does not wait upon subsequent ratification by the person concerned.

With this account in mind we can extract the sting from at least one dimension of the charge that attempts to produce fine healthy children might be wrongful. Two related sorts of wrongfulness are often alleged here. One comes from some people and groups of people with disability or from their advocates. The second comes from those who are inclined to label such measures as attempts at eugenic control.

It is often said by those with disability or by their supporters[6] that abortion for disability, or failure to keep disabled infants alive as long as possible, or even positive infanticide for disabled neonates, constitutes discrimination against the disabled as a group, that it is tantamount to devaluing them as persons, to devaluing them in some existential sense. Alison Davis identifies this view with utilitarianism and comments further that "(i)t would also justify using me as a donor bank for someone more physically perfect (I am confined to a wheelchair due to spina bifida) and, depending on our view of relative worth, it would justify using any of us as a donor if someone of the status of Einstein or Beethoven, or even Bob Geldof, needed one of our organs to survive."[7] This is a possible version of utilitarianism of course, but not I believe one espoused by anyone today. On the view assumed here and which I have defended in detail elsewhere,[8] all persons share the same moral status whether disabled or not. To decide not to keep a disabled neonate alive no more constitutes an attack on the disabled than does curing disability. To set the badly broken legs of an unconscious casualty who cannot consent does not constitute an attack on those confined to wheelchairs. To prefer to remove disability where we can is not to prefer non-disabled individuals as persons. To reiterate, if a pregnant mother can take steps to cure a disability affecting her fetus she should certainly do so, for to fail to do so is to deliberately handicap her child. She is not saying that she prefers those without disability as persons when she says she would prefer not to have a disabled child.

The same is analogously true of charges of eugenics in related circumstances. The wrong of practising eugenics is that it involves the assumption that "those who are genetically weak should be discouraged from reproducing" or are less morally important than other persons and that compulsory measures to prevent them reproducing might be defensible.

It is not that the genetically weak should be discouraged from reproducing but that everyone should be discouraged from reproducing children who will be significantly harmed by their genetic constitution.[9]

Indeed, gene therapy offers the prospect of enabling the genetically weak to reproduce and give birth to the genetically strong. It is to this prospect and to possible objections to it that we must now turn.

In so far as gene therapy might be used to delete specific genetic disorders in individuals or repair damage that had occurred genetically or in any other way it seems straightforwardly analogous to any other sort of therapy and to fail to use it would be deliberately to harm those individuals whom its use would protect.

It might thus, as we have just noted, enable individuals with genetic defects to be sure of having healthy rather than harmed children and thus liberate them from the terrible dilemma of whether or not to risk having children with genetic defects.

Suppose now that it becomes possible to use gene therapy to introduce into the human genome genes coding for antibodies to major infections like AIDS, Hepatitis B, Malaria and others, or coding for repair enzymes which could correct the most frequently occurring defects caused by radiation damage, or which could retard the ageing process and so lead to greater healthy longevity, or which might remove predispositions to heart disease, or which would destroy carcinogens or maybe permit human beings to tolerate other environmental pollutants?[10]

I have called individuals who might have these protections built into their germ line a "new breed."[11] It might be possible to use somatic cell therapy to make the same changes. I am not here interested in the alleged moral differences between germ line and somatic line therapy, though elsewhere I have argued strongly that there is no morally relevant difference.[12]

The question we must address is whether it would be wrong to fail to protect individuals in ways like these which would effectively enhance their function rather than cure dysfunction, which would constitute improvements in human individuals or indeed to the human genome, rather than simple (though complex in another sense and sophisticated) repairs? I am assuming of course that the technique is tried, tested and safe.

To answer this question we need to know whether to fail to protect individuals whom we could protect in this way would constitute a harm to them.[13] The answer seems to be clearly that it would. If the gene therapy could enhance prospects for healthy longevity then just as today, someone who had a life expectancy of fifty years rather than one of seventy would be regarded as at a substantial disadvantage, so having one of only seventy when others were able to enjoy ninety or so would be analogously disadvantageous. However even if we concentrate on increased resistance, or reduced susceptibility, to disease there would still be palpable harms involved. True, to be vulnerable is not necessarily to suffer the harm to which one is vulnerable, although even this may constitute some degree of psychological damage. However the right analogy seems here to be drawn from aviation.

Suppose aircraft manufacturers could easily build in safety features which would render an aircraft immune to, or at least much less susceptible to, a wide range of aviation hazards. If they failed to do so we would regard them as culpable whether or not a particular aircraft did in fact succumb to any of these hazards in the course of its life. They would in short be like a parent who failed to protect her children from dangerous diseases via immunization or our imagined parent who fails to protect through gene therapy.

I hope enough has been said to make clear that where gene therapy will affect improvements to human beings or to human nature that provide protections from harm or the protection of life itself in the form of increases in life expectancy ('death postponing' is after all just 'life saving' redescribed) then call it what you will, eugenics or not, we ought to be in favour of it. There is in short no moral difference between attempts to cure dysfunction and attempts to enhance function where the enhancement protects life or health.

WHAT SORTS OF ENHANCEMENT PROTECT HEALTH?

I have drawn a distinction between attempts to protect life and health and other uses of gene therapy. I have done so mostly for the sake of brevity and to avoid the more contentious area of so-called cosmetic or frivolous uses of gene therapy. Equally and for analogous reasons I have here failed to distinguish between gene therapy on the germ line and gene therapy on the somatic line. I avoid contention here not out of distaste for combat but simply because to deploy the arguments necessary to defend cosmetic uses of gene therapy would take up more space than I have available now. Elsewhere I have deployed these arguments.[14] However, the distinction between preservation of life and health or normal medical uses and other uses of gene therapy is difficult to draw and it is worth here just illustrating this difficulty.

The British Governments' [sic] "Committee on the Ethics of Gene Therapy" in its report to Parliament attempted to draw this distinction. The report, known by the surname of its chairman as *The Clothier Report* suggested "in the current state of knowledge it would not be acceptable to attempt to change traits not associated with disease."[15] This was an attempt to rule out so called cosmetic uses of gene therapy which would include attempts to manipulate intelligence.[16]

Imagine two groups of mentally handicapped or educationally impaired children. In one the disability is traceable to a specific disease state or injury, in the other it has no obvious cause. Suppose now that gene therapy offered the chance of improving the intelligence of children generally and those in both these groups in particular. Those who think that using gene therapy to improve intelligence is wrong because it is not a dimension of health care would have to think that neither group of children should be helped and those, like Clothier, who are marginally more enlightened would have to think that it might be ethical to help children in the first group but not those in the second.[17]

I must now turn to the question of whether or not gene therapy as a technique is specially morally problematic.

WHAT'S WRONG WITH GENE THERAPY?

Gene therapy may of course be scientifically problematic in a number of ways and in so far as these might make the procedure unsafe we would have some reason to be suspicious of it. However these problems are ethically uninteresting and I shall continue to assume that gene therapy is tried and tested from a scientific perspective. What else might be wrong with it?

One other ethical problem for gene therapy has been suggested and it deserves the small space left. Ruth Chadwick has given massive importance to the avoidance of doubt over ones [sic] genetic origins. Chadwick suggests that someone:

> who discovers that her parents had an extra gene or genes added . . . may suffer from what today in the 'problem pages' is called an 'identity crisis' . . . Part of this may be an uncertainty about her genetic history. We have stressed the importance of this knowledge, and pointed out that when one does not know where 50 per cent of one's genes come from, it can cause unhappiness.[18]

Chadwick then asks whether this problem can be avoided if only a small amount of genetic make-up is involved. Her answer is equivocal but on balance she seems to feel that "we must be cautious about producing a situation where children feel they do not really belong anywhere, because their genetic history is confused."[19] This sounds mild enough until we examine the cash value of phrases like "can cause unhappiness" or "be cautious" as Chadwick uses them.

In discussing the alleged unhappiness caused by ignorance of 50 per cent of one's genetic origin, Chadwick argued strongly that such unhappiness was so serious that "it seems wise to restrict artificial reproduction to methods that do not involve donation of genetic material. This rules out AID, egg donation, embryo donation and partial surrogacy."[20]

In elevating doubt about one's genetic origin to a cause of unhappiness so poignant that it would be better that a child who might experience it had never been born, Chadwick ignores entirely the (in fact false) truism that while motherhood is a fact paternity is always merely a hypothesis. It is a wise child indeed that knows her father and since such doubt might reasonably cloud the lives of a high proportion of the population of the world, we have reason to be sceptical that its effects are so terrible that people should be prevented from reproducing except where such doubt can be ruled out.

The effect of Chadwick's conclusion is to deny gay couples and single people the possibility of reproducing. Chadwick denies this suggesting "they are not being denied the opportunity to have children. If they are prepared to take the necessary steps ('the primitive sign of wanting is trying to get') their desire to beget can be satisfied." What are we to make of this? It seems almost self-consciously mischievous. In the first place gay couples and single women resorting to what must, *ex hypothesi*, be distasteful sex with third parties merely for procreational purposes, are unlikely to preserve the identity of their sexual partners for the benefit of their offspring's alleged future peace of mind. If this is right then doubt over genetic origin will not be removed. Since Chadwick is explicitly addressing public policy issues she should in consistency advocate legislation against such a course of action rather than recommend it.

But surely, if we are to comtemplate legislating against practices which give rise to doubt about genetic origins we would need hard evidence not only that such practices harm the resulting children but that the harm is of such high order that not only would it have been better that such children had never been born but also better that those who want such children should suffer the unhappiness consequent on a denial of their chance to have children using donated genetic material?

Where such harm is not only unavoidable but is an inherent part of sexual reproduction and must affect to some degree or other a high percentage of all births, it is surely at best unkind to use the fear of it as an excuse for discriminating against already perse-cuted minorities in the provision of reproductive services.

Where, as in the case of gene therapy, such donated[21] material also protects life and health or improves the human condition we have an added reason to welcome it.

NOTES

1. The argument here follows that of my paper "Should We Attempt to Eradicate Disability" to be published in the Proceedings of the Fifteenth International Wittgenstein Symposium.

2. See my discussion of the difference between harming and wronging in my *Wonderwoman & Superman: The Ethics of Human Biotechnology*, Oxford, 1992, Chapter 4.

3. This goes for relatively minor conditions like the loss of a finger or deafness and also for disfiguring conditions right through to major disability like paraplegia.

4. In this sense the definition of disability is like that of "poverty."

5. See my more detailed account of the relationship between harming and wronging in my *Wonderwoman & Superman*, Oxford University Press, Oxford 1992, Chapter 4.

6. Who should of course include us all.

7. Davis 1988, p. 150.

8. See my *The Value of Life*, Routledge, London 1985 & 1990 Ch. 1 and my "Not all babies should be kept alive as long as possible" in Raanan Gillon and Anne Lloyd, eds., *Principles of Health Care Ethics*, John Wiley & Sons, Chichester, in press, publication 1993.

9. I use the term "weak" here to echo Chadwick's use of the term. I take "genetically weak" to refer to those possessing a debilitating genetic condition or those who will inevitably pass on such a condition. All of us almost certainly carry some genetic abnormalities and are not thereby rendered "weak."

10. Here I borrow freely from my *Wonderwoman & Superman: The Ethics of Human Biotechnology*, Oxford University Press, 1992, Chapter 9, where I discuss all these issues in greater depth than is possible here.

11. Ibid.

12. Ibid., Chapter 8.

13. For an elaboration on the importance of this distinction, see my discussion of 'the wrong of wrongful life' in *Wonderwoman & Superman*, Chapter 4.

14. Ibid., Chapter 7.

15. *Report of the Committee on the Ethics of Gene Therapy*, presented to Parliament by Command of Her Majesty, January 1992. London HMSO para. 4.22.

16. In fact intelligence is unlikely to prove responsive to such manipulation because of its multifactorial nature.

17. There would be analogous problems about attempts to block the use of gene therapy to change things like physical stature and height since it might be used in the treatment of achondroplasia or other forms of dwarfism.

18. Ruth Chadwick, *Ethics, Reproduction and Genetic Control*, Routledge, London, 1987, page 126.

19. Ibid., page 127.

20. Ibid., page 39.

21. I use the term 'donated' here but I do not mean to rule out commerce in such genetic material. See my *Wonderwoman & Superman*, Chapter 6.

The Wisdom of Repugnance

Leon R. Kass

Our habit of delighting in news of scientific and technological breakthroughs has been sorely challenged by the birth announcement of a sheep named Dolly. Though Dolly shares with previous sheep the "softest clothing, woolly, bright," William Blake's question, "Little Lamb, who made thee?" has for her a radically different answer: Dolly was, quite literally, made. She is the work not of nature or nature's God but of man, an Englishman, Ian Wilmut, and his fellow scientists. What is more, Dolly came into being not only asexually—ironically, just like "He [who] calls Himself a Lamb"—but also as the genetically identical copy (and the perfect incarnation of the form or blueprint) of a mature ewe, of whom she is a clone. This long-awaited yet not quite expected success in cloning a mammal raised immediately the prospect—and the specter—of cloning human beings: "I a child and Thou a lamb," despite our differences, have always been equal candidates for creative making, only now, by means of cloning, we may both spring from the hand of man playing at being God.

After an initial flurry of expert comment and public consternation, with opinion polls showing overwhelming opposition to cloning human beings, President Clinton ordered a ban on all federal support for human cloning research (even though none was being supported) and charged the National Bioethics Advisory Commission to report in ninety days on the ethics of human cloning research. The commission (an eighteen-member panel, evenly balanced between scientists and nonscientists, appointed by the president and reporting to the National Science and Technology Council) invited testimony from scientists, religious thinkers, and bioethicists, as well as from the general public. In its report, issued in June 1997, the commission concluded that attempting to clone a human being was "at this time . . . morally unacceptable," recommended continuing the president's moratorium on the use of federal funds to support cloning of humans, and called for federal legislation to prohibit anyone from attempting (during the next three to five years) to create a child through cloning.

Even before the commission reported, Congress was poised to act. Bills to prohibit the use of federal funds for human cloning research have been introduced in the House of Representatives and the Senate; and another bill, in the House, would make it

Leon R. Kass, "The Wisdom of Repugnance," by Leon R. Kass. AEI Press, pp. 3–59. Reprinted by permission of the author.

illegal "for any person to use a human somatic cell for the process of producing a human clone." A fateful decision is at hand. To clone or not to clone a human being is no longer an academic question.

TAKING CLONING SERIOUSLY, THEN AND NOW

Cloning first came to public attention roughly thirty years ago, following the successful asexual production, in England, of a clutch of tadpole clones by the technique of nuclear transplantation. The individual largely responsible for bringing the prospect and promise of human cloning to public notice was Joshua Lederberg, a Nobel laureate geneticist and a man of large vision. In 1966 Lederberg wrote a remarkable article in the *American Naturalist* detailing the eugenic advantages of human cloning and other forms of genetic engineering, and the following year he devoted a column in the *Washington Post*, where he wrote regularly on science and society, to the prospect of human cloning. He suggested that cloning could help us overcome the unpredictable variety that still rules human reproduction and would allow us to benefit from perpetuating superior genetic endowments. Those writings sparked a small public debate in which I became a participant. At the time a young researcher in molecular biology at the National Institutes of Health, I wrote a reply to the *Post*, arguing against Lederberg's amoral treatment of that morally weighty subject and insisting on the urgency of confronting a series of questions and objections, culminating in the suggestion that "the programmed reproduction of man will, in fact, dehumanize him."

Much has happened in the intervening years. It has become harder, not easier, to discern the true meaning of human cloning. We have in some sense been softened up to the idea—through movies, cartoons, jokes, and intermittent commentary in the mass media, some serious, most lighthearted. We have become accustomed to new practices in human reproduction: not just in vitro fertilization, but also embryo manipulation, embryo donation, and surrogate pregnancy. Animal biotechnology has yielded transgenic animals and a burgeoning science of genetic engineering, easily and soon to be transferable to humans.

Even more important, changes in the broader culture make it now vastly more difficult to express a common and respectful understanding of sexuality, procreation, nascent life, family, and the meaning of motherhood, fatherhood, and the links between the generations. Twenty-five years ago, abortion was still largely illegal and thought to be immoral, the sexual revolution (made possible by the extramarital use of the pill) was still in its infancy, and few had yet heard about the reproductive rights of single women, homosexual men, and lesbians. (Never mind shameless memoirs about one's own incest!) Then one could argue, without embarrassment, that the new technologies of human reproduction—babies without sex—and their confounding of normal kin relations—who is the mother: the egg donor, the surrogate who carries and delivers, or the one who rears?—would "undermine the justification and support that biological parenthood gives to the monogamous marriage." Today, defenders of stable, monogamous marriage risk charges of giving offense to those adults who are living in "new family forms" or to those children who, even without the benefit of assisted reproduction, have acquired either three or four parents or one or none at all. Today, one must even apologize for voicing opinions that twenty-five years ago were nearly universally regarded as the core of our culture's wisdom on those matters. In a world whose once-given natural boundaries are blurred by technological change and whose moral boundaries are seemingly up for grabs, it is much more difficult to make persuasive the still compelling case against cloning human beings. As Raskolnikov put it, "Man gets used to everything—the beast!"

Indeed, perhaps the most depressing feature of the discussions that immediately followed the news about Dolly was their ironical tone, their genial cynicism, their moral fatigue: "An Udder Way of Making Lambs" (*Nature*), "Who Will Cash in on Breakthrough in Cloning?" (*Wall Street Journal*), "Is Cloning Baaaaaaaad?" (*Chicago Tribune*). Gone from the scene are the wise and courageous voices of

Theodosius Dobzhansky (genetics), Hans Jonas (philosophy), and Paul Ramsey (theology), who, only twenty-five years ago, all made powerful moral arguments against ever cloning a human being. We are now too sophisticated for such argumentation; we would not be caught in public with a strong moral stance, never mind an absolutist one. We are all, or almost all, postmodernists now.

Cloning turns out to be the perfect embodiment of the ruling opinions of our new age. Thanks to the sexual revolution, we are able to deny in practice, and increasingly in thought, the inherent procreative teleology of sexuality itself. But, if sex has no intrinsic connection to generating babies, babies need have no necessary connection to sex. Thanks to feminism and the gay rights movement, we are increasingly encouraged to treat the natural heterosexual difference and its preeminence as a matter of "cultural construction." But if male and female are not normatively complementary and generatively significant, babies need not come from male and female complementarity. Thanks to the prominence and the acceptability of divorce and out-of-wedlock births, stable, monogamous marriage as the ideal home for procreation is no longer the agreed-upon cultural norm. For that new dispensation, the clone is the ideal emblem: the ultimate "single-parent child."

Thanks to our belief that all children should be *wanted* children (the more high-minded principle we use to justify contraception and abortion), sooner or later only those children who fulfill our wants will be fully acceptable. Through cloning, we can work our wants and wills on the very identity of our children, exercising control as never before. Thanks to modern notions of individualism and the rate of cultural change, we see ourselves not as linked to ancestors and defined by traditions, but as projects for our own self-creation, not only as self-made men but also man-made selves; and self-cloning is simply an extension of such rootless and narcissistic self–re-creation.

Unwilling to acknowledge our debt to the past and unwilling to embrace the uncertainties and the limitations of the future, we have a false relation to both: cloning personifies our desire fully to control the future, while being subject to no controls ourselves. Enchanted and enslaved by the glamour of technology, we have lost our awe and wonder before the deep mysteries of nature and of life. We cheerfully take our own beginnings in our hands and, like the last man, we blink.

Part of the blame for our complacency lies, sadly, with the field of bioethics itself, and its claim to expertise in these moral matters. Bioethics was founded by people who understood that the new biology touched and threatened the deepest matters of our humanity: bodily integrity, identity and individuality, lineage and kinship, freedom and self-command, eros and aspiration, and the relations and strivings of body and soul. With its capture by analytic philosophy, however, and its inevitable routinization and professionalization, the field has by and large come to content itself with analyzing moral arguments, reacting to new technological developments, and taking on emerging issues of public policy, all performed with a naïve faith that the evils we fear can all be avoided by compassion, regulation, and a respect for autonomy. Bioethics has made some major contributions in the protection of human subjects and in other areas where personal freedom is threatened; but its practitioners, with few exceptions, have turned the big human questions into pretty thin gruel.

One reason for that is that the piecemeal formation of public policy tends to grind down large questions of morals into small questions of procedure. Many of the country's leading bioethicists have served on national commissions or state task forces and advisory boards, where, understandably, they have found utilitarianism to be the only ethical vocabulary acceptable to all participants in discussing issues of law, regulation, and public policy. As many of those commissions have been either officially under the aegis of the National Institutes of Health or the Health and Human Services Department, or otherwise dominated by powerful voices for scientific progress, the ethicists have for the most part been content, after some "values clarification" and wringing of hands, to pronounce their blessings upon the inevitable. Indeed, it is the bioethicists, not the scientists, who are now the most articulate defenders of human cloning: the two witnesses testifying before the National Bioethics Advisory Commission in favor of cloning human beings were bioethicists, eager to rebut what they regard as the irrational concerns of those of us in opposition. We have come to expect from the "experts" an accommodationist ethic that will rubber-stamp all biomedical innovation, in the mistaken belief that all other goods must bow down to the gods of better health and scientific advance. Regrettably, as we shall see near the end of this essay, the report of the present commission, though better than its predecessors, is finally not an exception.

If we are to correct our moral myopia, we must first of all persuade ourselves not to be complacent about what is at issue here. Human cloning, though it is in some respects continuous with previous reproductive technologies, also represents something radically new, in itself and in its easily foreseeable consequences. The stakes are very high indeed. I exaggerate, but in the direction of the truth, when I insist that we are faced with having to decide nothing less than whether human procreation is going to remain human, whether children are going to be made rather than begotten, whether it is a good thing, humanly speaking, to say yes in principle to the road that leads (at best) to the dehumanized rationality of *Brave New World*. This is not business as usual, to be fretted about for a while but finally to be given our seal of approval. We must rise to the occasion and make our judgments as if the future of our humanity hangs in the balance. For so it does.

THE STATE OF THE ART

If we should not underestimate the significance of human cloning, neither should we exaggerate its imminence or misunderstand just what is involved. The procedure is conceptually simple. The nucleus of a mature but unfertilized egg is removed and replaced with a nucleus obtained from a specialized cell of an adult (or fetal) organism (in Dolly's case, the donor nucleus came from mammary gland epithelium).

Since almost all the hereditary material of a cell is contained within its nucleus, the renucleated egg and the individual into which that egg develops are genetically identical to the organism that was the source of the transferred nucleus. An unlimited number of genetically identical individuals—clones—could be produced by nuclear transfer. In principle, any person, male or female, newborn or adult, could be cloned, and in any quantity. With laboratory cultivation and storage of tissues, cells outliving their sources make it possible even to clone the dead.

The technical stumbling block, overcome by Wilmut and his colleagues, was to find a means of reprogramming the state of the DNA in the donor cells, reversing its differentiated expression and restoring its full totipotency, so that it could again direct the entire process of producing a mature organism. Now that the problem has been solved, we should expect a rush to develop cloning for other animals, especially livestock, to propagate in perpetuity the champion meat or milk producers. Though exactly how soon someone will succeed in cloning a human being is anybody's guess, Wilmut's technique, almost certainly applicable to humans, makes *attempting* the feat an imminent possibility.

Yet some cautions are in order and some possible misconceptions need correcting. For a start, cloning is not Xeroxing. As has been reassuringly reiterated, the clone of Mel Gibson, though his genetic double, would enter the world hairless, toothless, and peeing in his diapers, just like any other human infant. Moreover, the success rate, at least at first, will probably not be very high: the British transferred 277 adult nuclei into enucleated sheep eggs and implanted twenty-nine clonal embryos, but they achieved the birth of only one live lamb clone. For that reason, among others, it is unlikely that, at least for now, the practice would be very popular, and there is no immediate worry of mass-scale production of multicopies. The need of repeated surgery to obtain eggs and, more crucially, of numerous borrowed wombs for implantation will surely limit use, as will the expense; besides, almost everyone who is able will doubtless prefer nature's sexier way of conceiving.

Still, for the tens of thousands of people already sustaining over 200 assisted-reproduction clinics in the United States and already availing themselves of in vitro fertilization, intracytoplasmic sperm injection, and other techniques of assisted reproduction, cloning would be an option with virtually no added fuss (especially when the success rate improves). Should commercial interests develop in "nucleus-banking," as they have in sperm-banking; should famous athletes or other celebrities decide to market their DNA the way they now market their autographs and just about everything else; should techniques of embryo and germline genetic testing and manipulation arrive as anticipated, increasing the use of laboratory assistance to obtain "better" babies—should all this come to pass, then cloning, if it is permitted, could become more than a marginal practice simply on the basis of free reproductive choice, even without any social encouragement to upgrade the gene pool or to replicate superior types. Moreover, if laboratory research on human cloning proceeds, even without any intention to produce cloned humans, the existence of cloned human embryos in the laboratory, created to begin with only for research purposes, would surely pave the way for later baby-making implantations.

In anticipation of human cloning, apologists and proponents have already made clear possible uses of the perfected technology, ranging from the sentimental and compassionate to the grandiose. They include: providing a child for an infertile couple; "replacing" a beloved spouse or child who is dying or has died; avoiding the risk of genetic disease; permitting reproduction for homosexual men and lesbians who want nothing sexual to do with the opposite sex; securing a genetically identical source of organs or tissues perfectly suitable for transplantation; getting a child with a genotype of one's own choosing, not excluding oneself; replicating individuals of great genius, talent, or beauty—having a child who really could "be like Mike"; and creating large sets of genetically identical humans suitable for research on, for instance, the question of nature versus nurture, or for special missions in peace and war (not excluding espionage), in which using identical humans would

be an advantage. Most people who envision the cloning of human beings, of course, want none of those scenarios. That they cannot say why is not surprising. What is surprising, and welcome, is that, in our cynical age, they are saying anything at all.

THE WISDOM OF REPUGNANCE

Offensive, grotesque, revolting, repugnant, and *repulsive*—those are the words most commonly heard regarding the prospect of human cloning. Such reactions come both from the man or woman in the street and from the intellectuals, from believers and atheists, from humanists and scientists. Even Dolly's creator has said he "would find it offensive" to clone a human being.

People are repelled by many aspects of human cloning. They recoil from the prospect of mass production of human beings, with large clones of look-alikes, compromised in their individuality; the idea of father-son or mother-daughter twins; the bizarre prospects of a woman's giving birth to and rearing a genetic copy of herself, her spouse, or even her deceased father or mother; the grotesqueness of conceiving a child as an exact replacement for another who has died; the utilitarian creation of embryonic genetic duplicates of oneself, to be frozen away or created when necessary, in case of need for homologous tissues or organs for transplantation; the narcissism of those who would clone themselves and the arrogance of others who think they know who deserves to be cloned or which genotype any child-to-be should be thrilled to receive; the Frankensteinian hubris to create human life and increasingly to control its destiny; man playing God. Almost no one finds any of the suggested reasons for human cloning compelling; almost everyone anticipates its possible misuses and abuses. Moreover, many people feel oppressed by the sense that there is probably nothing we can do to prevent it from happening. That makes the prospect all the more revolting.

Revulsion is not an argument; and some of yesterday's repugnances are today calmly accepted—though, one must add, not always for the better. In crucial cases, however, repugnance is the emotional expression of deep wisdom, beyond reason's power fully to articulate it. Can anyone really give an argument fully adequate to the horror which is father-daughter incest (even with consent), or having sex with animals, or mutilating a corpse, or eating human flesh, or raping or murdering another human being? Would anybody's failure to give full rational justification for his revulsion at those practices make that revulsion ethically suspect? Not at all. On the contrary, we are suspicious of those who think that they can rationalize away our horror, say, by trying to explain the enormity of incest with arguments only about the genetic risks of inbreeding.

The repugnance at human cloning belongs in that category. We are repelled by the prospect of cloning human beings not because of the strangeness or novelty of the undertaking, but because we intuit and feel, immediately and without argument, the violation of things that we rightfully hold dear. Repugnance, here as elsewhere, revolts against the excesses of human willfulness, warning us not to transgress what is unspeakably profound. Indeed, in this age in which everything is held to be permissible so long as it is freely done, in which our given human nature no longer commands respect, in which our bodies are regarded as mere instruments of our autonomous rational wills, repugnance may be the only voice left that speaks up to defend the central core of our humanity. Shallow are the souls that have forgotten how to shudder.

The goods protected by repugnance are generally overlooked by our customary ways of approaching all new biomedical technologies. The way we evaluate cloning ethically will in fact be shaped by how we characterize it descriptively, by the context into which we place it, and by the perspective from which we view it. The first task for ethics is proper description. And here is where our failure begins.

Typically, cloning is discussed in one or more of three familiar contexts, which one might call the technological, the liberal, and the meliorist. Under the first, cloning will be seen as an extension of existing techniques for assisting reproduction and determining the genetic makeup of children. Like them, cloning is to be regarded as a neutral technique, with no inherent meaning or goodness, but subject to multiple uses, some good, some bad. The morality of cloning thus depends absolutely on the goodness or badness of the motives and intentions of the cloners. As one bioethicist defender of cloning puts it, "The ethics must be judged [only] by the way the parents nurture and rear their resulting child and whether they bestow the same love and affection on a child brought into existence by a technique of assisted reproduction as they would on a child born in the usual way."

The liberal (or libertarian or liberationist) perspective sets cloning in the context of rights, freedoms, and personal empowerment. Cloning is just a new option for exercising an individual's right to reproduce or to have the kind of child that he wants. Alternatively, cloning enhances our liberation (especially women's liberation) from the confines of nature, the vagaries of chance, or the necessity for sexual mating. Indeed, it liberates women from the need for men altogether, for the process requires only eggs, nuclei, and (for the time being) uteri—plus, of course, a healthy dose of our (allegedly "masculine") manipulative science that likes to do all those things to mother nature and nature's mothers. For those who hold this outlook, the only moral restraints on cloning are adequately informed consent and the avoidance of bodily harm. If no one is cloned without her consent, and if the clonant is not physically damaged, then the liberal conditions for licit, hence moral, conduct are met. Worries that go beyond violating the will or maiming the body are dismissed as "symbolic"—which is to say, unreal.

The meliorist perspective embraces valetudinarians and also eugenicists. The latter were formerly more vocal in those discussions, but they are now generally happy to see their goals advanced under the less threatening banners of freedom and technological growth. These people see in cloning a new prospect for improving human beings—minimally, by ensuring the perpetuation of healthy individuals by avoiding the risks of genetic disease inherent in the lottery of sex, and maximally, by producing "optimum babies," preserving outstanding genetic material, and (with the help of soon-to-come techniques for precise genetic engineering) enhancing inborn human capacities on many fronts. Here the morality of cloning as a means is justified solely by the excellence of the end, that is, by the outstanding traits of individuals cloned—beauty, or brawn, or brains.

These three approaches, all quintessentially American and all perfectly fine in their places, are sorely wanting as approaches to human procreation. It is, to say the least, grossly distorting to view the wondrous mysteries of birth, renewal, and individuality, and the deep meaning of parent-child relations, largely through the lens of our reductive science and its potent technologies. Similarly, considering reproduction (and the intimate relations of family life!) primarily under the political-legal, adversarial, and individualistic notion of rights can only undermine the private yet fundamentally social, cooperative, and duty-laden character of child-bearing, child-rearing, and their bond to the covenant of marriage. Seeking to escape entirely from nature (to satisfy a natural desire or a natural right to reproduce!) is self-contradictory in theory and self-alienating in practice. For we are erotic beings only because we are embodied beings and not merely intellects and wills unfortunately imprisoned in our bodies. And, though health and fitness are clearly great goods, there is something deeply disquieting in looking on our prospective children as artful products perfectible by genetic engineering, increasingly held to our willfully imposed designs, specifications, and margins of tolerable error.

The technical, liberal, and meliorist approaches all ignore the deeper anthropological, social, and, indeed, ontological meanings of bringing forth a new life. To this more fitting and profound point of view cloning shows itself to be a major violation of our given nature as embodied, gendered, and engendering beings—and of the social relations built on this natural ground. Once this perspective is recognized, the ethical judgment on cloning can no longer be reduced to a matter of motives and intentions, rights and freedoms, benefits and harms, or even means and ends. It must be regarded primarily as a matter of meaning: Is cloning a fulfillment of human begetting and belonging? Or is cloning rather, as I contend, their pollution and perversion? To pollution and perversion the fitting response can only be horror and revulsion; and conversely, generalized horror and revulsion are prima facie evidence of foulness and violation. The burden of moral argument must fall entirely on those who want to declare the widespread repugnances of humankind to be mere timidity or superstition.

Yet repugnance need not stand naked before the bar of reason. The wisdom of our horror at human cloning can be partially articulated, even if this is finally one of those instances about which the heart has its reasons that reason cannot entirely know.

THE PROFUNDITY OF SEX

To see cloning in its proper context, we must begin not, as I did before, with laboratory technique, but with the anthropology—natural and social—of sexual reproduction.

Sexual reproduction—by which I mean the generation of new life from (exactly) two complementary elements, one female, one male, (usually) through coitus—is established (if that is the right term) not by human decision, culture, or tradition, but by nature; it is the natural way of all mammalian reproduction. By nature, each child has two complementary biological progenitors. Each child thus stems from and unites exactly two lineages. In natural generation, moreover, the precise genetic constitution of the resulting offspring is determined by a combination of nature and chance, not by human design: each human child shares the common natural human species genotype, each child is genetically (equally) kin to each (both) parent(s), yet each child is also genetically unique.

Those biological truths about our origins foretell deep truths about our identity and about our human condition altogether. Every one of us is at once equally human, equally enmeshed in a particular familial nexus of origin, and equally individuated in our trajectory from birth to death—and, if all goes well, equally capable (despite our mortality) of participating, with a complementary other, in the very same renewal of such human possibility through procreation. Though less momentous than our common humanity, our genetic individuality is not humanly trivial. It shows itself forth in our distinctive appearance through which we are everywhere recognized; it is revealed in our "signature" marks of fingerprints and our self-recognizing immune system; it symbolizes and foreshadows exactly the unique, never-to-be-repeated character of each human life.

Human societies virtually everywhere have structured child-rearing responsibilities and systems of identity and relationship on the bases of those deep natural facts of begetting. The mysterious yet ubiquitous "love of one's own" is everywhere culturally exploited, to make sure that children are not just produced but well cared for and to create for everyone clear ties of meaning, belonging, and obligation. But it is wrong to treat such naturally rooted social practices as mere cultural constructs (like left- or right-driving, or like burying or cremating the dead) that we can alter with little human cost. What would kinship be without its clear natural grounding? And what would identity be without kinship? We must resist those who have begun to refer to sexual reproduction as the "traditional method of reproduction," who would have us regard as merely traditional, and by implication arbitrary, what is in truth not only natural but most certainly profound.

Asexual reproduction, which produces "single-parent" offspring, is a radical departure from the natural human way, confounding all normal understandings of father, mother, sibling, and grandparent and all moral relations tied thereto. It becomes even more of a radical departure when the resulting offspring is a clone derived not from an embryo, but from a mature adult to whom the clone would be an identical twin; and when the process occurs not by natural accident (as in natural twinning), but by deliberate human design and manipulation; and when the child's (or children's) genetic constitution is preselected by the parent(s) (or scientists). Accordingly, as we shall see, cloning is vulnerable to three kinds of concerns and objections, related to these three points: cloning threatens confusion of identity and individuality, even in

small-scale cloning; cloning represents a giant step (though not the first one) toward transforming procreation into manufacture, that is, toward the increasing depersonalization of the process of generation and, increasingly, toward the "production" of human children as artifacts, products of human will and design (what others have called the problem of "commodification" of new life); and cloning—like other forms of eugenic engineering of the next generation—represents a form of despotism of the cloners over the cloned, and thus (even in benevolent cases) represents a blatant violation of the inner meaning of parent-child relations, of what it means to have a child, of what it means to say yes to our own demise and "replacement."

Before turning to those specific ethical objections, let me test my claim of the profundity of the natural way by taking up a challenge recently posed by a friend. What if the given natural human way of reproduction were asexual, and we now had to deal with a new technological innovation—artificially induced sexual dimorphism and the fusing of complementary gametes—whose inventors argued that sexual reproduction promised all sorts of advantages, including hybrid vigor and the creation of greatly increased individuality? Would one then be forced to defend natural asexuality because it was natural? Could one claim that it carried deep human meaning?

The response to that challenge broaches the ontological meaning of sexual reproduction. For it is impossible, I submit, for there to have been human life—or even higher forms of animal life—in the absence of sexuality and sexual reproduction. We find asexual reproduction only in the lowest forms of life: bacteria, algae, fungi, some lower invertebrates. Sexuality brings with it a new and enriched relationship to the world. Only sexual animals can seek and find complementary others with whom to pursue a goal that transcends their own existence. For a sexual being, the world is no longer an indifferent and largely homogeneous *otherness*, in part edible, in part dangerous. It also contains some very special and related and complementary beings, of the same kind but of opposite sex, toward whom one reaches out with special interest and intensity. In higher birds and mammals, the outward gaze keeps a lookout not only for food and predators, but also for prospective mates; the beholding of the many-splendored world is suffused with desire for union—the animal antecedent of human eros and the germ of sociality. Not by accident is the human animal both the sexiest animal—whose females do not go into heat but are receptive throughout the estrous cycle and whose males must therefore have greater sexual appetite and energy to reproduce successfully—and also the most aspiring, the most social, the most open, and the most intelligent animal.

The soul-elevating power of sexuality is, at bottom, rooted in its strange connection to mortality, which it simultaneously accepts and tries to overcome. Asexual reproduction may be seen as a continuation of the activity of self-preservation. When one organism buds or divides to become two, the original being is (doubly) preserved, and nothing dies. Sexuality, by contrast, means perishability and serves replacement; the two that come together to generate one soon will die. Sexual desire, in human beings as in animals, thus serves an end that is partly hidden from, and finally at odds with, the self-serving individual. Whether we know it or not, when we are sexually active we are voting with our genitalia for our own demise. The salmon swimming upstream to spawn and die tell the universal story: sex is bound up with death, to which it holds a partial answer in procreation.

The salmon and the other animals evince that truth blindly. Only the human being can understand what it means. As we learn so powerfully from the story of the Garden of Eden, our humanization is coincident with sexual self-consciousness, with the recognition of our sexual nakedness and all that it implies: shame at our needy incompleteness, unruly self-division, and finitude; awe before the eternal; hope in the self-transcending possibilities of children and a relationship to the divine. In the sexually self-conscious animal, sexual desire can become eros, lust can become love. Sexual desire humanly regarded is thus sublimated into erotic longing for wholeness, completion, and immortality, which drives us knowingly into the embrace and its generative fruit—as well as into all the higher human possibilities of deed, speech, and song.

Through children, a good common to both husband and wife, male and female achieve some genuine unification (beyond the mere sexual "union," which fails to do so). The two become one through sharing generous (not needy) love for that third being as good. Flesh of their flesh, the child is the parents' own commingled being externalized and given a separate and persisting existence. Unification is enhanced also by their commingled work of rearing. Providing an opening to the future beyond the grave, carrying not only our seed but also our names, our ways, and our hopes that they will surpass us in goodness and happiness, children are a testament to the possibility of transcendence. Gender duality and sexual desire, which first draws our love upward and outside of ourselves, finally provide for the partial overcoming of the confinement and limitation of perishable embodiment altogether.

Human procreation, in sum, is not simply an activity of our rational wills. It is a more complete activity precisely because it engages us bodily, erotically, and spiritually as well as rationally. There is wisdom in the mystery of nature that has joined the pleasure of sex, the inarticulate longing for union, the communication of the loving embrace, and the deep-seated and only partly articulate desire for children in the very activity by which we continue the chain of human existence and participate in the renewal of human possibility. Whether or not we know it, the severing of procreation from sex, love, and intimacy is inherently dehumanizing, no matter how good the product.

We are now ready for the more specific objections to cloning.

THE PERVERSITIES OF CLONING

First, an important if formal objection: any attempt to clone a human being would constitute an unethical experiment upon the resulting child-to-be. As the animal experiments (frog and sheep) indicate, there are grave risks of mishaps and deformities. Moreover, because of what cloning means, one cannot presume a future cloned child's consent to be a clone, even a healthy one. Thus, ethically speaking, we cannot even get to know whether or not human cloning is feasible.

I understand, of course, the philosophical difficulty of trying to compare a life with defects against nonexistence. Several bioethicists, proud of their philosophical cleverness, use that conundrum to embarrass claims that one can injure a child in its conception, precisely because it is only thanks to that complained-of conception that the child is alive to complain. But common sense tells us that we have no reason to fear such philosophisms. For we surely know that people can harm and even maim children in the very act of conceiving them, say, by paternal transmission of the AIDS virus, maternal transmission of heroin dependence, or, arguably, even by bringing them into being as bastards or with no capacity or willingness to look after them properly. And we believe that to do that intentionally, or even negligently, is inexcusable and clearly unethical.

The objection about the impossibility of presuming consent may even go beyond the obvious and sufficient point that a clonant, were he subsequently to be asked, could rightly resent having been made a clone. At issue are not just benefits and harms, but doubts about the very independence needed to give proper (even retroactive) consent, that is, not just the capacity to choose but the disposition and ability to choose freely and well. It is not at all clear to what extent a clone will fully be a moral agent. For, as we shall see, in the very fact of cloning, and especially of rearing him *as a clone*, his makers subvert the cloned child's independence, beginning with that aspect that comes from knowing that one was an unbidden surprise, a gift, to the world, rather than the designed result of someone's artful project.

Cloning creates serious issues of identity and individuality. The cloned person may experience concerns about his distinctive identity not only because he will be in genotype and appearance iden-tical to another human being, but, in this case, because he may also be twin to the person who is his "father" or "mother"—if one can still call them that. What would be the psychic burdens of being the "child" or "parent" of your twin? The cloned individual, moreover, will be saddled with a genotype that has already lived. He will not be fully a surprise to the world. People are likely always to compare his performances in life with that of his alter ego. True, his nurture and his circumstance in life will be different; genotype is not exactly destiny. Still, one must also expect parental and other efforts to shape that new life after the original—or at least to view the child with the original version always firmly in mind. Why else did they clone from the star basketball player, mathematician, and beauty queen—or even dear old dad—in the first place?

Since the birth of Dolly, there has been a fair amount of doublespeak on the matter of genetic identity. Experts have rushed in to reassure the public that the clone would in no way be the same person or have any confusions about his identity: as previously noted, they are pleased to point out that the clone of Mel Gibson would not be Mel Gibson. Fair enough. But one is shortchanging the truth by emphasizing the additional importance of the intrauterine environment, rearing, and social setting: genotype obviously matters plenty. That, after all, is the only reason to clone, whether human beings or sheep. The odds that clones of Wilt Chamberlain will play in the NBA are, I submit, infinitely greater than they are for clones of Robert Reich.

Curiously, this conclusion is supported, inadvertently, by the one ethical sticking point insisted on by friends of cloning: no cloning without the donor's consent. Though an orthodox liberal objection, it is in fact quite puzzling when it comes from people (such as Ruth Macklin) who also insist that genotype is not identity or individuality and who deny that a child could reasonably complain about being made a genetic copy. If the clone of Mel Gibson would not be Mel Gibson, why should Mel Gibson have grounds to object that someone had been made his clone? We already allow researchers to use blood and tissue samples for research purposes of no benefit to their sources: my falling hair, my expectorations, my urine, and even my biopsied tissues are "not me" and not mine. Courts have held that the profit gained from uses to which scientists put my discarded tissues do not legally belong to me. Why, then, no cloning without consent—including, I assume, no cloning from the body of someone who just died? What harm is done the donor, if genotype is "not me"? Truth to tell, the only powerful justification for objecting is that genotype really does have something to do with identity, and everybody knows it. If not, on what basis could Michael Jordan object that someone cloned "him," say, from cells taken from a "lost" scraped-off piece of his skin? The insistence on donor consent unwittingly reveals the problem of identity in all cloning.

Genetic distinctiveness not only symbolizes the uniqueness of each human life and the independence of its parents that each human child rightfully attains. It can also be an important support for living a worthy and dignified life. Such arguments apply with great force to any large-scale replication of human individuals. But they are sufficient, in my view, to rebut even the first attempts to clone a human being. One must never forget that these are human beings upon whom our eugenic or merely playful fantasies are to be enacted.

Troubled psychic identity (distinctiveness), based on all-too-evident genetic identity (sameness), will be made much worse by the utter confusion of social identity and kinship ties. For, as already noted, cloning radically confounds lineage and social relations, for "offspring" as for "parents." As bioethicist James Nelson has pointed out, a female child cloned from her "mother" might develop a desire for a relationship to her "father" and might understandably seek out the father of her "mother," who is after all also her biological twin sister. Would "grandpa," who thought his paternal duties concluded, be pleased to discover that the clonant looked to him for paternal attention and support?

Social identity and social ties of relationship and responsibility are widely connected to, and supported by, biological kinship. Social taboos on incest (and adultery) everywhere serve to keep clear who is related to whom (and especially which child belongs to which parents), as well as to avoid confounding the social identity of parent-and-child (or brother-and-sister) with the social identity of lovers, spouses, and coparents. True, social identity is altered by adoption (but as a matter of the best interest of already living children: we do not deliberately produce children for adoption). True, artificial insemination and in vitro fertilization with donor sperm, or whole embryo donation, are in some way forms of "prenatal adoption"—a not altogether unproblematic practice. Even here, though, there is in each case (as in all sexual reproduction) a known male source of sperm and a known single female source of egg—a genetic father and a genetic mother—should anyone care to know (as adopted children often do) who is genetically related to whom.

In the case of cloning, however, there is but one "parent." The usually sad situation of the "single-parent child" is here deliberately planned, and with a vengeance. In the case of self-cloning, the "offspring" is, in addition, one's twin; and so the dreaded result of incest—to be parent to one's sibling—is here brought about deliberately, albeit without any act of coitus. Moreover, all other relationships will be confounded. What will *father, grandfather, aunt, cousin,* and *sister* mean? Who will bear what ties and what burdens? What sort of social identity will someone have with one whole side—"father's" or "mother's"—necessarily excluded? It is no answer to say that our society, with its high incidence of divorce, remarriage, adoption, extramarital child-bearing, and the rest, already confounds lineage and confuses kinship and responsibility for children (and everyone else), unless one also wants to argue that this is, for children, a preferable state of affairs.

Human cloning would also represent a giant step toward turning begetting into making, procreation into manufacture (literally, something "handmade"), a process already begun with in vitro fertilization and genetic testing of embryos. With cloning, not only is the process in hand, but the total genetic blueprint of the cloned individual is selected and determined by the human artisans. To be sure, subsequent development will take place according to natural processes; and the resulting children will still be recognizably human. But we here would be taking a major step into making man himself simply another one of the man-made things. Human nature becomes merely the last part of nature to succumb to the technological project, which turns all of nature into raw material at human disposal, to be homogenized by our rationalized technique according to the subjective prejudices of the day.

How does begetting differ from making? In natural procreation, human beings come together, complementarily male and female, to give existence to another being who is formed, exactly as we were, *by what we are:* living, hence perishable, hence aspiringly erotic, human beings. In clonal reproduction, by contrast, and in the more advanced forms of manufacture to which it leads, we give existence to a being not by what we are but by what we intend and design. As with any product of our making, no matter how excellent, the artificer stands above it, not as an equal but as a superior, transcending it by his will and creative prowess. Scientists who clone animals make it perfectly clear that they are engaged in instrumental making; the animals are, from the start, designed as means to serve rational human purposes. In human cloning scientists and prospective "parents" would be adopting the same technocratic mentality to human children: human children would be their artifacts.

Such an arrangement is profoundly dehumanizing, no matter how good the product. Mass-scale cloning of the same individual makes the point vividly; but the violation of human equality, freedom, and dignity is present even in a single planned clone. And procreation dehumanized into manufacture is further degraded by commodification, a virtually inescapable result of allowing baby-making to proceed under the banner of commerce. Genetic and reproductive biotechnology companies are already growth industries, but they will go into commercial orbit once the Human Genome Project nears comple-

tion. Supply will create enormous demand. Even before the capacity for human cloning arrives, established companies will have invested in the harvesting of eggs from ovaries obtained at autopsy or through ovarian surgery, practiced embryonic genetic alteration, and initiated the stockpiling of prospective donor tissues. Through the rental of surrogate-womb services and through the buying and selling of tissues and embryos, priced according to the merit of the donor, the commodification of nascent human life will be unstoppable.

Finally, and perhaps most important, the practice of human cloning by nuclear transfer—like other anticipated forms of genetic engineering of the next generation—would enshrine and aggravate a profound and mischievous misunderstanding of the meaning of having children and of the parent-child relationship. When a couple now chooses to procreate, the partners are saying yes to the emergence of new life in its novelty, saying yes not only to having a child but also, tacitly, to having whatever child the child turns out to be. In accepting our finitude and opening ourselves to our replacement, we are tacitly confessing the limits of our control. In this ubiquitous way of nature, embracing the future by procreating means precisely that we are relinquishing our grip, in the very activity of taking up our own share in what we hope will be the immortality of human life and the human species. This means that our children are not *our* children: they are not our property, not our possessions. Neither are they supposed to live our lives for us, or anyone else's life but their own. To be sure, we seek to guide them on their way, imparting to them not just life but nurturing, love, and a way of life; to be sure, they bear our hopes that they will live fine and flourishing lives, enabling us in small measure to transcend our own limitations. Still, their genetic distinctiveness and independence are the natural foreshadowing of the deep truth that they have their own and never-before-enacted life to live. They are sprung from a past, but they take an uncharted course into the future.

Much harm is already done by parents who try to live vicariously through their children. Children are sometimes compelled to fulfill the broken dreams of unhappy parents; John Doe, Jr., or John Doe III is under the burden of having to live up to his forebear's name. Still, if most parents have hopes for their children, cloning parents will have expectations. In cloning, such overbearing parents take at the start a decisive step that contradicts the entire meaning of the open and forward-looking nature of parent-child relations. The child is given a genotype that has already lived, with full expectation that the blueprint of a past life ought to be controlling of the life that is to come. Cloning is inherently despotic, for it seeks to make one's children (or someone else's children) after one's own image (or an image of one's choosing) and their future according to one's will. In some cases the despotism may be mild and benevolent. In other cases it will be mischievous and downright tyrannical. But despotism—the control of another through one's will—it inevitably will be.

MEETING SOME OBJECTIONS

The defenders of cloning, of course, are not wittingly friends of despotism. Indeed, they regard themselves mainly as friends of freedom: the freedom of individuals to reproduce, the freedom of scientists and inventors to discover and devise and to foster "progress" in genetic knowledge and technique. They want large-scale cloning only for animals, but they wish to preserve cloning as a human option for exercising our "right to reproduce"—our right to have children, and children with "desirable genes." As law professor John Robertson points out, under our "right to reproduce" we already practice early forms of unnatural, artificial, and extramarital reproduction, and we already practice early forms of eugenic choice. For that reason, he argues, cloning is no big deal.

We have here a perfect example of the logic of the slippery slope, and the slippery way in which it already works in that area. Only a few years ago, slippery-slope arguments were advanced to oppose artificial insemination and in vitro fertilization using unrelated sperm donors. Principles used to justify those practices, it was said, will be used to justify more artificial and more eugenic practices, including cloning. Not so,

the defenders retorted, since we can make the necessary distinctions. And now, without even a gesture at making the necessary distinctions, the continuity of practice is held by itself to be justificatory.

The principle of reproductive freedom as currently enunciated by the proponents of cloning logically embraces the ethical acceptability of sliding down the entire rest of the slope—to producing children ectogenetically from sperm to term (should it become feasible) and to producing children whose entire genetic makeup will be the product of parental eugenic planning and choice. If reproductive freedom means the right to have a child of one's own choosing, by whatever means, it knows and accepts no limits.

But, far from being legitimated by a "right to reproduce," the emergence of techniques of assisted reproduction and genetic engineering should compel us to reconsider the meaning and limits of such a putative right. In truth, a "right to reproduce" has always been a peculiar and problematic notion. Rights generally belong to individuals, but this is a right that (before cloning) no one can exercise alone. Does the right then inhere only in couples? Only in married couples? Is it a (woman's) right to carry or deliver or a right (of one or more parents) to nurture and rear? Is it a right to have your own biological child? Is it a right only to attempt reproduction or a right also to succeed? Is it a right to acquire the baby of one's choice?

The assertion of a negative "right to reproduce" certainly makes sense when it claims protection against state interference with procreative liberty, say, through a program of compulsory sterilization. But surely it cannot be the basis of a tort claim against nature, to be made good by technology, should free efforts at natural procreation fail. Some insist that the right to reproduce embraces also the right against state interference with the free use of all technological means to obtain a child. Yet such a position cannot be sustained: for reasons having to do with the means employed, any community may rightfully prohibit surrogate pregnancy, polygamy, or the sale of babies to infertile couples without violating anyone's basic human "right to reproduce." When the exercise of a previously innocuous freedom now involves or impinges on troublesome practices that the original freedom never was intended to reach, the general presumption of liberty needs to be reconsidered.

We do indeed already practice negative eugenic selection, through genetic screening and prenatal diagnosis. Yet our practices are governed by a norm of health. We seek to prevent the birth of children who suffer from known (serious) genetic diseases. When and if gene therapy becomes possible, such diseases could then be treated, in utero or even before implantation. I have no ethical objection in principle to such a practice (though I have some practical worries), precisely because it serves the medical goal of healing existing individuals. But therapy, to be therapy, implies not only an existing "patient." It also implies a norm of health. In this respect, even germline gene "therapy," though practiced not on a human being but on egg and sperm, is less radical than cloning, which is in no way therapeutic. But once one blurs the distinction between health promotion and genetic enhancement, between so-called negative and positive eugenics, one opens the door to all future eugenic designs. "To make sure that a child will be healthy and have good chances in life": that is Robertson's principle, and, owing to its latter clause, it is an utterly elastic principle, with no boundaries. Being over eight feet tall will likely produce some very good chances in life, and so will having the looks of Marilyn Monroe, and so will a genius-level intelligence.

Proponents want us to believe that there are legitimate uses of cloning that can be distinguished from illegitimate uses, but by their own principles no such limits can be found. (Nor could any such limits be enforced in practice.) Reproductive freedom, as they understand it, is governed solely by the subjective wishes of the parents-to-be (plus the avoidance of bodily harm to the child). The sentimentally appealing case of the childless married couple is, on those grounds, indistinguishable from the case of an individual (married or not) who would like to clone someone famous or talented, living or dead. Further, the principle here endorsed justifies not only cloning but, indeed, all future artificial attempts to create (manufacture) "perfect" babies.

A concrete example will show how, in practice no less than in principle, the so-called innocent case will merge with, or even turn into, the more troubling ones. In practice, the eager parent-to-be will necessarily be subject to the tyranny of expertise. Consider an infertile married couple, she lacking eggs or he lacking sperm, that wants a child of their (genetic) own and proposes to clone either husband or wife. The scientist-physician (who is also co-owner of the cloning company) points out the likely difficulties: A cloned child is not really their (genetic) child, but the child of only *one* of them; that imbalance may produce strains on the marriage; the child might suffer identity confusion; there is a risk of perpetuating the cause of sterility. The scientist-physician also points out the advantages of choosing a donor nucleus. Far better than a child of their own would be a child of their own choosing. Touting his own expertise in selecting healthy and talented donors, the doctor presents the couple with his latest catalog containing the pictures, the health records, and the accomplishments of his stable of cloning donors, samples of whose tissues are in his deep freeze. Why not, dearly beloved, a more perfect baby?

The "perfect baby," of course, is the project not of the infertility doctors, but of the eugenic scientists and their supporters. For them, the paramount right is not the so-called right to reproduce but what biologist Bentley Glass called, a quarter of a century ago, "the right of every child to be born with a sound physical and mental constitution, based on a sound genotype . . . the inalienable right to a sound heritage." But to secure that right and to achieve the requisite quality control over new human life, human conception and gestation will need to be brought fully into the bright light of the laboratory, beneath which the child-to-be can be fertilized, nourished, pruned, weeded, watched, inspected, prodded, pinched, cajoled, injected, tested, rated, graded, approved, stamped, wrapped, sealed, and delivered. There is no other way to produce the perfect baby.

Yet we are urged by proponents of cloning to forget about the science fiction scenarios of laboratory manufacture and multiple-copied clones and to focus only on the homely cases of infertile couples exercising their reproductive rights. But why, if the single cases are so innocent, should multiplying their performance be so off-putting? (Similarly, why do others object to people's making money from that practice if the practice itself is perfectly acceptable?) When we follow the sound ethical principle of universalizing our choice—would it be right if everyone cloned a Wilt Chamberlain (with his consent, of course)? would it be right if everyone decided to practice asexual reproduction?—we discover what is wrong with such seemingly innocent cases. The so-called science fiction cases make vivid the meaning of what looks to us, mistakenly, to be benign.

Though I recognize certain continuities between cloning and, say, in vitro fertilization, I believe that cloning differs in essential and important ways. Yet those who disagree should be reminded that the "continuity" argument cuts both ways. Sometimes we establish bad precedents and discover that they were bad only when we follow their inexorable logic to places we never meant to go. Can the defenders of cloning show us today how, on their principles, we shall be able to see producing babies ("perfect babies") entirely in the laboratory or exercising full control over their genotypes (including so-called enhancement) as ethically different, in any essential way, from present forms of assisted reproduction? Or are they willing to admit, despite their attachment to the principle of continuity, that the complete obliteration of "mother" or "father," the complete depersonalization of procreation, the complete manufacture of human beings, and the complete genetic control of one generation over the next would be ethically problematic and essentially different from current forms of assisted reproduction? If so, where and how will they draw the line, and why? I draw it at cloning, for all the reasons given.

BAN THE CLONING OF HUMANS

What, then, should we do? We should declare that human cloning is unethical in itself and dangerous in its likely consequences. In so doing, we shall have the backing of the overwhelming majority of our fellow Americans, of the human race, and (I believe) of most practicing scientists. Next, we should do all that we can to prevent the cloning of human beings. We should do that by means of an international legal ban if possible and by a unilateral national ban at a minimum. Scientists may secretly undertake to violate such a law, but they will be deterred by not being able to stand up proudly to claim the credit for their technological bravado and success. Such a ban on clonal baby-making, moreover, will not harm the progress of basic genetic science and technology. On the contrary, it will reassure the public that scientists are happy to proceed without violating the deep ethical norms and intuitions of the human community.

That still leaves the vexed question about laboratory research using early embryonic human clones, specially created only for such research purposes, with no intention to implant them into a uterus. There is no question that such research holds great promise for gaining fundamental knowledge about normal (and abnormal) differentiation and for developing tissue lines for transplantation that might be used, say, in treating leukemia or in repairing brain or spinal cord injuries—to mention just a few of the conceivable benefits. Still, unrestricted clonal embryo research will surely make the production of living human clones much more likely. Once the genies put the cloned embryos into the bottles, who can strictly control where they go, especially in the absence of legal prohibitions against implanting them to produce a child?

I appreciate the potentially great gains in scientific knowledge and medical treatment available from embryo research, especially with cloned embryos. At the same time, I have serious reservations about creating human embryos for the sole purpose of experimentation. There is something deeply repugnant and fundamentally transgressive about such a utilitarian treatment of prospective human life. Such total, shameless exploitation is worse, in my opinion, than the "mere" destruction of nascent life. But I see no added objections, as a matter of principle, to creating and using *cloned* early embryos for research purposes, beyond the objections that I might raise to doing so with embryos produced sexually.

And yet, as a matter of policy and prudence, any opponent of the manufacture of cloned humans must, I think, in the end oppose also the creating of cloned human embryos. Frozen embryonic clones (belonging to whom?) can be shuttled around without detection. Commercial ventures in human cloning will be developed without adequate oversight. To build a fence around the law, prudence dictates that one oppose—for that reason alone—all production of cloned human embryos, even for research purposes. We should allow all cloning research on animals to go forward, but the only defensible barrier we can erect against the slippery slide, I suspect, is to insist on the inviolable distinction between animal and human cloning.

Some readers and certainly most scientists will not accept such prudent restraints, since they desire the benefits of research. They will prefer, even in fear and trembling, to allow human embryo cloning research to go forward.

Very well. Let us test them. If the scientists want to be taken seriously on ethical grounds, they must at the very least agree that embryonic research may proceed if and only if it is preceded by an absolute and effective ban on all attempts to implant into a uterus a cloned human embryo (cloned from an adult) to produce a living child. Absolutely no permission for the former without the latter.

The National Bioethics Advisory Commission's recommendations regarding these matters were a step in the right direction, but a step made limpingly and without adequate support. To its credit, the commission has indeed called for federal legislation to prevent anyone from attempting to create a child through cloning. That was, frankly, more than I expected. But the *moral basis* for the commission's opposition to cloning is, sadly, much less than expected and needed, and the ban it urges is to be only temporary. Trying to clone a human being, says the commission, is "morally unacceptable" "*at this time*" because the technique has not been perfected to the point of safe usage. In other words, once it becomes readily feasible to clone a human being, with little risk of bodily harm to the resulting child, the commission has offered not one agreed-upon reason to object. Indeed, anticipating such improvements in technique, the commission insists that "it is

critical" that any legislative ban on baby-making through cloning "should include a sunset clause to ensure that Congress will review the issue after a specified time period (three to five years) to decide whether the prohibition continues to be needed." Although it identifies other ethical concerns (beyond the issue of safety), that blue-ribbon ethics commission takes no stand on any of them! It says only that those issues "require much more widespread and careful public deliberation *before this technology may be used*"—not to decide *whether* the technology *should* be used. Relativistically, the commission wants to ensure only that such ethical and social issues be regularly reviewed "in light of public understandings at that time." This is hardly the sort of opposition to cloning that could be made the basis of any lasting prohibition.

Almost as worrisome, the report is silent on the vexed question of creating cloned human embryos for use in research. Silence is, of course, not an endorsement, but neither is it opposition. Given the currently existing ban on the use of federal funds for any research that involves creating human embryos for experimentation, the commission may have preferred to avoid needless controversy by addressing that issue. Besides, those commissioners (no doubt a big majority) who favor proceeding with cloned embryo research have in fact gained their goal precisely by silence: both the moratorium on federal funding and the legislative ban called for by the commission are confined *solely* to attempts to *create a child* through cloning. The commission knows well how vigorously and rapidly embryo research is progressing in the private sector, and the commission surely understands that its silence on the subject—along with Congress's—means that the creation of human embryonic clones will proceed and perhaps is already proceeding in private or commercial laboratories. Indeed, the report expects and tacitly welcomes such human embryo research: for by what other means shall we arrive at the expected improvements in human cloning technology that would require the recommended periodic reconsideration of any legislative ban?

In the end, the report of the commission turns out to be a moral and (despite its best efforts) a practical failure. Morally, this ethics commission has waffled on the main ethical question by refusing to declare the production of human clones unethical (or ethical). Practically, the moratorium and ban on baby-making that it calls for, while welcome as temporary restraints, have not been given the justification needed to provide a solid and lasting protection against the production of cloned human beings. To the contrary, the commission's weak ethical stance may be said to undermine even its limited call for restraint. Do we really need a federal law solely to protect unborn babies from bodily harm?

Opponents of cloning need therefore to be vigilant. They should press for legislation to *permanently* prohibit baby-making through cloning, and they should take steps to make such a prohibition effective.

The proposal for such a legislative ban is without American precedent, at least in technological matters, though the British and others have banned cloning of human beings, and we ourselves ban incest, polygamy, and other forms of "reproductive freedom." Needless to say, working out the details of such a ban, especially a global one, would be tricky, what with the need to develop appropriate sanctions for violators. Perhaps such a ban will prove ineffective; perhaps it will eventually be shown to have been a mistake. But it would at least place the burden of practical proof where it belongs: on the proponents of this horror, requiring them to show very clearly what great social or medical good can be had only by the cloning of human beings.

We Americans have lived by, and prospered under, a rosy optimism about scientific and technological progress. The technological imperative—if it can be done, it must be done—has probably served us well, though we should admit that there is no accurate method for weighing benefits and harms. Even when, as in the cases of environmental pollution, urban decay, or the lingering deaths that are the unintended byproducts of medical success, we recognize the unwel-come outcomes of technological advance, we remain confident in our ability to fix all the "bad" consequences—usually by means of still newer and better technologies. How successful we can continue to be in such post hoc repairing is at least an open question. But there is very good reason for shifting the paradigm around, at least regarding those technological interventions into the human body and mind that will surely effect fundamental (and likely irreversible) changes in human nature, basic human relationships, and what it means to be a human being. Here we surely should not be willing to risk everything in the naïve hope that, should things go wrong, we can later set them right.

The president's call for a moratorium on human cloning has given us an important opportunity. In a truly unprecedented way, we can strike a blow for the human control of the technological project, for wisdom, prudence, and human dignity. The prospect of human cloning, so repulsive to contemplate, is the occasion for deciding whether we shall be slaves of unregulated progress, and ultimately its artifacts, or whether we shall remain free human beings who guide our technique toward the enhancement of human dignity. If we are to seize the occasion, we must, as the late Paul Ramsey wrote,

raise the ethical questions with a serious and not a frivolous conscience. A man of frivolous conscience announces that there are ethical quandaries ahead that we must urgently consider before the future catches up with us. By this he often means that we need to devise a new ethics that will provide the rationalization for doing in the future what men are bound to do because of new actions and interventions science will have made possible. In contrast a man of serious conscience means to say in raising urgent ethical questions that there may be some things that men should never do. The good things that men do can be made complete only by the things they refuse to do.

Cloning Human Beings: An Assessment of the Ethical Issues Pro and Con

Dan W. Brock

The world of science and the public at large were both shocked and fascinated by the announcement in the journal *Nature* by Ian Wilmut and his colleagues that they had successfully cloned a sheep from a single cell of an adult sheep (Wilmut, 1997). But many were troubled or apparently even horrified at the prospect that cloning of adult humans by the same process might be possible as well. The response of most scientific and political leaders to the prospect of human cloning, indeed of Dr. Wilmut as well, was of immediate and strong condemnation.

A few more cautious voices were heard both suggesting some possible benefits from the use of human cloning in limited circumstances and questioning its too quick prohibition, but they were a clear minority. A striking feature of these early responses was that their strength and intensity seemed far to outrun the arguments and reasons offered in support of them—they seemed often to be "gut level" emotional reactions rather than considered reflections on the issues. Such reactions should not be simply dismissed, both because they may point us to important considerations otherwise missed and not easily articulated, and because they often have a major impact on public policy. But the formation of public policy should not ignore the moral reasons and arguments that bear on the practice of human cloning—these must be articulated in order to understand and inform people's more immediate emotional responses. This essay is an effort to articulate, and to evaluate critically, the main moral considerations and arguments for and against human cloning. Though many people's religious beliefs inform their views on human cloning, and it is often difficult to separate religious from sec-

ular positions, I shall restrict myself to arguments and reasons that can be given a clear secular formulation.

On each side of the issue there are two distinct kinds of moral arguments brought forward. On the one hand, some opponents claim that human cloning would violate fundamental moral or human rights, while some proponents argue that its prohibition would violate such rights. While moral and even human rights need not be understood as absolute, they do place moral restrictions on permissible actions that an appeal to a mere balance of benefits over harms cannot justify overriding; for example, the rights of human subjects in research must be respected even if the result is that some potentially beneficial research is more difficult or cannot be done. On the other hand, both opponents and proponents also cite the likely harms and benefits, both to individuals and to society, of the practice. I shall begin with the arguments in support of permitting human cloning, although with no implication that it is the stronger or weaker position.

MORAL ARGUMENTS IN SUPPORT OF HUMAN CLONING

Is There a Moral Right to Use Human Cloning?

What moral right might protect at least some access to the use of human cloning? A commitment to individual liberty, such as defended by J. S. Mill, requires that individuals be left free to use human cloning if they so choose and if their doing so does not cause significant harms to others, but liberty is too broad in scope to be an uncontroversial moral right (Mill, 1859; Rhodes, 1995). Human cloning is a means of reproduction (in the most literal sense) and so the most plausible moral right at stake in its use is a right to reproductive freedom or procreative liberty (Robertson, 1994a; Brock, 1994), understood to include both the choice not to reproduce, for example, by means of contraception or abortion, and also the right to reproduce.

The right to reproductive freedom is properly understood to include the right to use various assisted reproductive technologies (ARTs), such as in vitro fertilization (IVF), oocyte donation, and so forth. The reproductive right relevant to human cloning is a negative right, that is, a right to use ARTs without interference by the government or others when made available by a willing provider. The choice of an assisted means of reproduction should be protected by reproductive freedom even when it is not the only means for individuals to reproduce, just as the choice among different means of preventing conception is protected by reproductive freedom. However, the case for permitting the use of a particular means of reproduction is strongest when it is necessary for particular individuals to be able to procreate at all, or to do so without great burdens or harms to themselves or others. In some cases human cloning could be the only means for individuals to procreate while retaining a biological tie to their child, but in other cases different means of procreating might also be possible.

It could be argued that human cloning is not covered by the right to reproductive freedom because whereas current ARTs and practices covered by that right are remedies for inabilities to reproduce sexually, human cloning is an entirely new means of reproduction; indeed, its critics see it as more a means of manufacturing humans than of reproduction. Human cloning is a different means of reproduction than sexual reproduction, but it is a means that can serve individuals' interest in reproducing. If it is not protected by the moral right to reproductive freedom, I believe that must be not because it is a new means of reproducing, but instead because it has other objectionable or harmful features; I shall evaluate these other ethical objections to it later.

When individuals have alternative means of procreating, human cloning typically would be chosen because it replicates a particular individual's genome. The reproductive interest in question then is not simply reproduction itself, but a more specific interest in choosing what kind of children to have. The right to reproductive freedom is usually understood to cover at least some choice about the kind of children one will have. Some individuals choose reproductive partners in the hope of producing offspring with desirable traits. Genetic testing of fetuses or preimplantation

embryos for genetic disease or abnormality is done to avoid having a child with those diseases or abnormalities. Respect for individual self-determination, which is one of the grounds of a moral right to reproductive freedom, includes respecting individuals' choices about whether to have a child with a condition that will place severe burdens on them, and cause severe burdens to the child itself.

The less a reproductive choice is primarily the determination of one's own life, but primarily the determination of the nature of another, as in the case of human cloning, the more moral weight the interests of that other person, that is the cloned child, should have in decisions that determine its nature (Annas, 1994). But even then parents are typically accorded substantial, but not unlimited, discretion in shaping the persons their children will become, for example, through education and other childrearing decisions. Even if not part of reproductive freedom, the right to raise one's children as one sees fit, within limits mostly determined by the interests of the children, is also a right to determine within limits what kinds of persons one's children will become. This right includes not just preventing certain diseases or harms to children, but selecting and shaping desirable features and traits in one's children. The use of human cloning is one way to exercise that right.

Public policy and the law now permit prospective parents to conceive, or to carry a conception to term, when there is a significant risk or even certainty that the child will suffer from a serious genetic disease. Even when others think the risk or certainty of genetic disease makes it morally wrong to conceive, or to carry a fetus to term, the parents' right to reproductive freedom permits them to do so. Most possible harms to a cloned child are less serious than the genetic harms with which parents can now permit their offspring to be conceived or born.

I conclude that there is good reason to accept that a right to reproductive freedom presumptively includes both a right to select the means of reproduction, as well as a right to determine what kind of children to have, by use of human cloning. However, the specific reproductive interest of determining what kind of children to have is less weighty than are other reproductive interests and choices whose impact falls more directly and exclusively on the parents rather than the child. Even if a moral right to reproductive freedom protects the use of human cloning, that does not settle the moral issue about human cloning, since there may be other moral rights in conflict with this right, or serious enough harms from human cloning to override the right to use it; this right can be thought of as establishing a serious moral presumption supporting access to human cloning.

What Individual or Social Benefits Might Human Cloning Produce?

Largely Individual Benefits

The literature on human cloning by nuclear transfer or by embryo splitting contains a few examples of circumstances in which individuals might have good reasons to want to use human cloning. However, human cloning seems not to be the unique answer to any great or pressing human need and its benefits appear to be limited at most. What are the principal possible benefits of human cloning that might give individuals good reasons to want to use it?

1. *Human cloning would be a new means to relieve the infertility some persons now experience.* Human cloning would allow women who have no ova or men who have no sperm to produce an offspring that is biologically related to them (Eisenberg, 1976; Robertson, 1994b, 1997; LaBar, 1984). Embryos might also be cloned, by either nuclear transfer or embryo splitting, in order to increase the number of embryos for implantation and improve the chances of successful conception (NABER, 1994). The benefits from human cloning to relieve infertility are greater the more persons there are who cannot overcome their infertility by any other means acceptable to them. I do not know of data on this point, but the numbers who would use cloning for this reason are probably not large.

The large number of children throughout the world possibly available for adoption represents an alternative solution to infertility only if we are prepared to discount as illegitimate the strong desire of many persons, fertile and infertile, for the experience of pregnancy and for having and raising a child biologically related to them. While not important to all

infertile (or fertile) individuals, it is important to many and is respected and met through other forms of assisted reproduction that maintain a biological connection when that is possible; that desire does not become illegitimate simply because human cloning would be the best or only means of overcoming an individual's infertility.

2. *Human cloning would enable couples in which one party risks transmitting a serious hereditary disease to an offspring to reproduce without doing so* (Robertson, 1994b). By using donor sperm or egg donation, such hereditary risks can generally be avoided now without the use of human cloning. These procedures may be unacceptable to some couples, however, or at least considered less desirable than human cloning because they introduce a third party's genes into their reproduction instead of giving their offspring only the genes of one of them. Thus, in some cases human cloning could be a reasonable means of preventing genetically transmitted harms to offspring. Here too, we do not know how many persons would want to use human cloning instead of other means of avoiding the risk of genetic transmission of a disease or of accepting the risk of transmitting the disease, but the numbers again are probably not large.

3. *Human cloning to make a later twin would enable a person to obtain needed organs or tissues for transplantation* (Robertson, 1994b, 1997; Kahn, 1989; Harris, 1992). Human cloning would solve the problem of finding a transplant donor whose organ or tissue is an acceptable match and would eliminate, or drastically reduce, the risk of transplant rejection by the host. The availability of human cloning for this purpose would amount to a form of insurance to enable treatment of certain kinds of medical conditions. Of course, sometimes the medical need would be too urgent to permit waiting for the cloning, gestation, and development that is necessary before tissues or organs can be obtained for transplantation. In other cases, taking an organ also needed by the later twin, such as a heart or a liver, would be impermissible because it would violate the later twin's rights.

Such a practice can be criticized on the ground that it treats the later twin not as a person valued and loved for his or her own sake, as an end in itself in Kantian terms, but simply as a means for benefiting another. This criticism assumes, however, that only this one motive defines the reproduction and the relation of the person to his or her later twin. The well-known case some years ago in California of the Ayalas, who conceived in the hopes of obtaining a source for a bone marrow transplant for their teenage daughter suffering from leukemia, illustrates the mistake in this assumption. They argued that whether or not the child they conceived turned out to be a possible donor for their daughter, they would value and love the child for itself, and treat it as they would treat any other member of their family. That one reason they wanted it, as a possible means to saving their daughter's life, did not preclude their also loving and valuing it for its own sake; in Kantian terms, it was treated as a possible means to saving their daughter, but not *solely as a means*, which is what the Kantian view proscribes.

Indeed, when people have children, whether by sexual means or with the aid of ARTs, their motives and reasons for doing so are typically many and complex, and include reasons less laudable than obtaining lifesaving medical treatment, such as having someone who needs them, enabling them to live on their own, qualifying for government benefit programs, and so forth. While these are not admirable motives for having children and may not bode well for the child's upbringing and future, public policy does not assess prospective parents' motives and reasons for procreating as a condition of their doing so.

4. *Human cloning would enable individuals to clone someone who had special meaning to them, such as a child who had died* (Robertson, 1994b). There is no denying that if human cloning were available, some individuals would want to use it for this purpose, but their desire usually would be based on a deep confusion. Cloning such a child would not replace the child the parents had loved and lost, but would only create a different child with the same genes. The child they loved and lost was a unique individual who had been shaped by his or her environment and choices, not just his or her genes, and more importantly who had experienced a particular relationship with them. Even if the later cloned child could not only have the same genes but also be subjected to the same environment, which of course is impossible, it would remain a different child than the one they had loved and lost because it would share a different history with them (Thomas, 1974). Cloning the lost child might help the parents accept and move on from their loss, but another already existing sibling or a new child that was not a clone might do this equally well; indeed, it might do so better since the appearance of the cloned later twin would be a constant reminder of the child they had lost. Nevertheless, if human cloning enabled some individuals to clone a person who had special meaning to them and doing so gave them deep satisfaction, that would be a benefit to them even if their reasons for wanting to do so, and the satisfaction they in turn received, were based on a confusion.

Largely Social Benefits

5. *Human cloning would enable the duplication of individuals of great talent, genius, character, or other exemplary qualities.* Unlike the first four reasons for human cloning which appeal to benefits to specific individuals, this reason looks to benefits to the broader society from being able to replicate extraordinary individuals—a Mozart, Einstein, Gandhi, or Schweitzer (Lederberg, 1966; McKinnell, 1979). Much of the appeal of this reason, like much support and opposition to human cloning, rests largely on a confused and false assumption of genetic determinism, that is, that one's genes fully determine what one will become, do, and accomplish. What made Mozart, Einstein, Gandhi, and Schweitzer the extraordinary individuals they were was the confluence of their particular genetic endowments with the environments in which they were raised and lived and the particular historical moments they in different ways seized. Cloning them would produce individuals with the same genetic inheritances (nuclear transfer does not even produce 100 percent genetic identity, although for the sake of exploring the moral issues I have followed the common assumption that it does), but it is not possible to replicate their environments or the historical contexts in which they lived and their greatness flourished. We do not know the degree or specific respects in which any individual's greatness

depended on "nature" or "nurture," but we do know that it always depends on an interaction of them both. Cloning could not even replicate individuals' extraordinary capabilities, much less their accomplishments, because these too are the product of their inherited genes and their environments, not of their genes alone.

None of this is to deny that Mozart's and Einstein's extraordinary musical and intellectual capabilities, nor even Gandhi's and Schweitzer's extraordinary moral greatness, were produced in part by their unique genetic inheritances. Cloning them might well produce individuals with exceptional capacities, but we simply do not know how close their clones would be in capacities or accomplishments to the great individuals from whom they were cloned. Even so, the hope for exceptional, even if less and different, accomplishment from cloning such extraordinary individuals might be a reasonable ground for doing so.

Worries here about abuse, however, surface quickly. Whose standards of greatness would be used to select individuals to be cloned? Who would control use of human cloning technology for the benefit of society or mankind at large? Particular groups, segments of society, or governments might use the technology for their own benefit, under the cover of benefiting society or even mankind at large.

6. *Human cloning and research on human cloning might make possible important advances in scientific knowledge, for example, about human development* (Walters, 1982; Smith, 1983). While important potential advances in scientific or medical knowledge from human cloning or human cloning research have frequently been cited, there are at least three reasons for caution about such claims. First, there is always considerable uncertainty about the nature and importance of the new scientific or medical knowledge to which a dramatic new technology like human cloning will lead; the road to new knowledge is never mapped in advance and takes many unexpected turns. Second, we do not know what new knowledge from human cloning or human cloning research could also be gained by other means that do not have the problematic moral features to which its opponents object. Third, what human cloning research

would be compatible with ethical and legal requirements for the use of human subjects in research is complex, controversial, and largely unexplored. Creating human clones solely for the purpose of research would be to use them solely for the benefit of others without their consent, and so unethical. But if and when human cloning was established to be safe and effective, then new scientific knowledge might be obtained from its use for legitimate, nonresearch reasons.

Although there is considerable uncertainty concerning most of human cloning's possible individual and social benefits that I have discussed, and although no doubt it could have other benefits or uses that we cannot yet envisage, I believe it is reasonable to conclude at this time that human cloning does not seem to promise great benefits or uniquely to meet great human needs. Nevertheless, despite these limited benefits, a moral case can be made that freedom to use human cloning is protected by the important moral right to reproductive freedom. I shall turn now to what moral rights might be violated, or harms produced, by research on or use of human cloning.

MORAL ARGUMENTS AGAINST HUMAN CLONING

Would the Use of Human Cloning Violate Important Moral Rights?

Many of the immediate condemnations of any possible human cloning following Wilmut's cloning of Dolly claimed that it would violate moral or human rights, but it was usually not specified precisely, or often even at all, what rights would be violated (WHO, 1997). I shall consider two possible candidates for such a right: a right to have a unique identity and a right to ignorance about one's future or to an open future. Claims that cloning denies individuals a unique identity are common, but I shall argue that even if there is a right to a unique identity, it could not be violated by human cloning. The right to ignorance or to an open future has only been explicitly defended, to my knowledge, by two commentators, and in the context of human cloning, only by Hans Jonas; it supports a more promising, but in my view ultimately unsuccessful, argument that human cloning would violate an important moral or human right.

Is there a moral or human right to a unique identity, and if so would it be violated by human cloning? For human cloning to violate a right to a unique identity, the relevant sense of identity would have to be genetic identity, that is, a right to a unique unrepeated genome. This would be violated by human cloning, but is there any such right? It might be thought that cases of identical twins show there is no such right because no one claims that the moral or human rights of the twins have been violated. However, this consideration is not conclusive (Kass, 1985; NABER, 1994). Only human actions can violate others' rights; outcomes that would constitute a rights violation if deliberately caused by human action are not a rights violation if a result of natural causes. If Arthur deliberately strikes Barry on the head so hard as to cause his death, he violates Barry's right not to be killed; if lightning strikes Cheryl, causing her death, her right not to be killed has not been violated. Thus, the case of twins does not show that there could not be a right to a unique genetic identity.

What is the sense of identity that might plausibly be what each person has a right to have uniquely, that constitutes the special uniqueness of each individual (Macklin 1994; Chadwick 1982)? Even with the same genes, homozygous twins are numerically distinct and not identical, so what is intended must be the various properties and characteristics that make each individual qualitatively unique and different from others. Does having the same genome as another person undermine that unique qualitative identity? Only on the crudest genetic determinism, according to which an individual's genes completely and decisively determine everything else about the individual, all his or her other nongenetic features and properties, together with the entire history or biography that constitutes his or her life. But there is no reason whatever to believe that kind of genetic determinism. Even with the same genes, differences in genetically identical twins' psychological and personal characteristics develop over time together with differences in their life histories, personal relationships, and life choices; sharing an identical genome does not prevent twins from developing distinct and unique personal identities of their own.

We need not pursue whether there is a moral or human right to a unique identity—no such right is found among typical accounts and enumerations of moral or human rights—because even if there is such a right, sharing a genome with another individual as a result of human cloning would not violate it. The idea of the uniqueness, or unique identity, of each person historically predates the development of modern genetics. A unique genome thus could not be the ground of this long-standing belief in the unique human identity of each person.

I turn now to whether human cloning would violate what Hans Jonas called a right to ignorance, or what Joel Feinberg called a right to an open future (Jonas, 1974; Feinberg, 1980). Jonas argued that human cloning in which there is a substantial time gap between the beginning of the lives of the earlier and later twin is fundamentally different from the simultaneous beginning of the lives of homozygous twins that occur in nature. Although contemporaneous twins begin their lives with the same genetic inheritance, they do so at the same time, and so in ignorance of what the other who shares the same genome will by his or her choices make of his or her life.

A later twin created by human cloning, Jonas argues, knows, or at least believes she knows, too much about herself. For there is already in the world another person, her earlier twin, who from the same genetic starting point has made the life choices that are still in the later twin's future. It will seem that her life has already been lived and played out by another, that her fate is already determined; she will lose the sense of human possibility in freely and spontaneously creating her own future and authentic self. It is tyrannical, Jonas claims, for the earlier twin to try to determine another's fate in this way.

Jonas's objection can be interpreted so as not to assume either a false genetic determinism, or a belief in it. A later twin might grant that he is not determined to follow in his earlier twin's footsteps, but nevertheless the earlier twin's life might always haunt him, standing as an undue influence on his life, and shaping it in ways to which others' lives are not vulnerable. But the force of the objection still seems to rest on the false assumption that having the same genome as his earlier twin unduly restricts his freedom to create a different life and self than the earlier twin's. Moreover, a family environment also importantly shapes children's development, but there is no force to the claim of a younger sibling that the existence of an older sibling raised in that same family is an undue influence on the younger sibling's freedom to make his own life for himself in that environment. Indeed, the younger twin or sibling might gain the benefit of being able to learn from the older twin's or sibling's mistakes.

A closely related argument can be derived from what Joel Feinberg has called a child's right to an open future. This requires that others raising a child not so close off the future possibilities that the child would otherwise have as to eliminate a reasonable range of opportunities for the child autonomously to construct his or her own life. One way this right might be violated is to create a later twin who will believe her future has already been set for her by the choices made and the life lived by her earlier twin.

The central difficulty in these appeals to a right either to ignorance or to an open future is that the right is not violated merely because the later twin is likely to *believe* that his future is already determined, when that belief is clearly false and supported only by the crudest genetic determinism. If we know the later twin will falsely believe that his open future has been taken from him as a result of being cloned, even though in reality it has not, then we know that cloning will cause the twin psychological distress, but not that it will violate his right. Jonas's right to ignorance, and Feinberg's right of a child to an open future, are not violated by human cloning, though they do point to psychological harms that a later twin may be likely to experience and that I will take up later.

Neither a moral or human right to a unique identity, nor one to ignorance and an open future, would be violated by human cloning. There may be other moral or human rights that human cloning would violate, but I do not know what they might be. I turn now to consideration of the harms that human cloning might produce.

What Individual or Social Harms Might Human Cloning Produce?

There are many possible individual or social harms that have been posited by one or another commentator and I shall only try to cover the more plausible and significant of them.

Largely Individual Harms

1. *Human cloning would produce psychological distress and harm in the later twin.* No doubt knowing the path in life taken by one's earlier twin might often have several bad psychological effects (Callahan, 1993; LaBar, 1984; Macklin, 1994; McCormick, 1993; Studdard, 1978; Rainer, 1978; Verhey, 1994). The later twin might feel, even if mistakenly, that her fate has already been substantially laid out, and so have difficulty freely and spontaneously taking responsibility for and making her own fate and life. The later twin's experience or sense of autonomy and freedom might be substantially diminished, even if in actual fact they are diminished much less than it seems to her. She might have a diminished sense of her own uniqueness and individuality, even if once again these are in fact diminished little or not at all by having an earlier twin with the same genome. If the later twin is the clone of a particularly exemplary individual, perhaps with some special capabilities and accomplishments, she might experience excessive pressure to reach the very high standards of ability and accomplishment of the earlier twin (Rainer, 1978). These various psychological effects might take a heavy toll on the later twin and be serious burdens to her.

While psychological harms of these kinds from human cloning are certainly possible, and perhaps even likely in some cases, they remain at this point only speculative since we have no experience with human cloning and the creation of earlier and later twins. Nevertheless, if experience with human cloning confirmed that serious and unavoidable psychological harms typically occurred to the later twin, that would be a serious moral reason to avoid the practice. Intuitively at least, psychological burdens and harms seem more likely and more serious for a person who is only one of many identical later twins cloned from one original source, so that the clone might run into another identical twin around every street corner. This prospect could be a good reason to place sharp limits on the number of twins that could be cloned from any one source.

One argument has been used by several commentators to undermine the apparent significance of potential psychological harms to a later twin (Chadwick, 1982; Robertson, 1994b, 1997; Macklin, 1994). The point derives from a general problem, called the nonidentity problem, posed by the philosopher Derek Parfit, although not originally directed to human cloning (Parfit, 1984). Here is the argument. Even if all these psychological burdens from human cloning could not be avoided for any later twin, they are not harms to the twin, and so not reasons not to clone the twin. That is because the only way for the twin to avoid the harms is never to be cloned, and so never to exist at all. But these psychological burdens, hard though they might be, are not so bad as to make the twin's life, all things considered, not worth living. So the later twin is not harmed by being given a life even with these psychological burdens, since the alternative of never existing at all is arguably worse—he or she never has a worthwhile life—but certainly not better for the twin. And if the later twin is not harmed by having been created with these unavoidable burdens, then how could he or she be wronged by having been created with them? And if the later twin is not wronged, then why is any wrong being done by human cloning? This argument has considerable potential import, for if it is sound it will undermine the apparent moral importance of any bad consequence of human cloning to the later twin that is not so serious as to make the twin's life, all things considered, not worth living.

I defended elsewhere the position regarding the general case of genetically transmitted handicaps, that if one could have a *different* child without comparable burdens (for the case of cloning, by using a different method of reproduction which did not result in a later twin), there is as strong a moral reason to do

so as there would be not to cause similar burdens to an already existing child (Brock, 1995). Choosing to create the later twin with serious psychological burdens instead of a different person who would be free of them, without weighty overriding reasons for choosing the former, would be morally irresponsible or wrong, even if doing so does not harm or wrong the later twin who could only exist with the burdens. These issues are too detailed and complex to pursue here and the nonidentity problem remains controversial and not fully resolved, but at the least, the argument for disregarding the psychological burdens to the later twin because he or she could not exist without them is controversial, and in my view mistaken. Such psychological harms, as I shall continue to call them, are speculative, but they should not be disregarded because of the nonidentity problem.

2. *Human cloning procedures would carry unacceptable risks to the clone.* There is no doubt that attempts to clone a human being at the present time would carry unacceptable risks to the clone. Further research on the procedure with animals, as well as research to establish its safety and effectiveness for humans, is clearly necessary before it would be ethical to use the procedure on humans. One risk to the clone is the failure to implant, grow, and develop successfully, but this would involve the embryo's death or destruction long before most people or the law consider it to be a person with moral or legal protections of its life.

Other risks to the clone are that the procedure in some way goes wrong, or unanticipated harms come to the clone; for example, Harold Varmus, director of the National Institutes of Health, raised the concern that a cell many years old from which a person is cloned could have accumulated genetic mutations during its years in another adult that could give the resulting clone a predisposition to cancer or other diseases of aging (Weiss, 1997). Risks to an ovum donor (if any), a nucleus donor, and a woman who receives the embryo for implantation would likely be ethically acceptable with the informed consent of the involved parties.

I believe it is too soon to say whether unavoidable risks to the clone would make human cloning forever unethical. At a minimum, further research is needed to better define the potential risks to humans. But we should not insist on a standard that requires risks to be lower than those we accept in sexual reproduction, or in other forms of ART.

Largely Social Harms

3. *Human cloning would lessen the worth of individuals and diminish respect for human life.* Unelaborated claims to this effect were common in the media after the announcement of the cloning of Dolly. Ruth Macklin explored and criticized the claim that human cloning would diminish the value we place on, and our respect for, human life because it would lead to persons being viewed as replaceable (Macklin, 1994). As I have argued concerning a right to a unique identity, only on a confused and indefensible notion of human identity is a person's identity determined solely by his or her genes, and so no individual could be fully replaced by a later clone possessing the same genes. Ordinary people recognize this clearly. For example, parents of a child dying of a fatal disease would find it insensitive and ludicrous to be told they should not grieve for their coming loss because it is possible to replace him by cloning him; it is *their child who is dying* whom they love and value, and that child and his importance to them is not replaceable by a cloned later twin. Even if they would also come to love and value a later twin as much as they now love and value their child who is dying, that would be to love and value that *different child* for its own sake, not as a replacement for the child they lost. Our relations of love and friendship are with distinct, historically situated individuals with whom over time we have shared experiences and our lives, and whose loss to us can never be replaced.

A different version of this worry is that human cloning would result in persons' worth or value seeming diminished because we would come to see persons as able to be manufactured or "hand-made." This demystification of the creation of human life would reduce our appreciation and awe of human life and of its natural creation. It would be a mistake, however, to conclude that a person created by human cloning is of less value or is less worthy of respect than one created by sexual reproduction. At least outside of some religious contexts, it is the nature of a being, not how it is created, that is the source of its value and makes it worthy of respect. For many people, gaining a scientific understanding of the truly extraordinary complexity of human reproduction and development increases, instead of decreases, their awe of the process and its product.

A more subtle route by which the value we place on each individual human life might be diminished could come from the use of human cloning with the aim of creating a child with a particular genome, either the genome of another individual especially meaningful to those doing the cloning or an individual with exceptional talents, abilities, and accomplishments. The child then comes to be objectified, valued only as an object and for its genome, or at least for its genome's expected phenotypic expression, and no longer recognized as having the intrinsic equal moral value of all persons, simply as persons. For the moral value and respect due all persons to come to be seen as resting only on the instrumental value of individuals and of their particular qualities to others would be to fundamentally change the moral status properly accorded to persons. Individuals would lose their moral standing as full and equal members of the moral community, replaced by the different instrumental value each has to others.

Such a change in the equal moral value and worth accorded to persons should be avoided at all costs, but it is far from clear that such a change would result from permitting human cloning. Parents, for example, are quite capable of distinguishing their children's intrinsic value, just as individual persons, from their instrumental value based on their particular qualities or properties. The equal moral value and respect due all persons simply as persons is not incompatible with the different instrumental value of different individuals; Einstein and an untalented physics graduate student have vastly different value as scientists, but share and are entitled to equal moral value and respect as persons. It is a confused mistake to conflate these two kinds of value and respect. If making a large number of clones from one original person would be more likely to foster it, that would be a further reason to limit the number of clones that could be made from one individual.

* * *

4. *Human cloning might be used by commercial interests for financial gain.* Both opponents and proponents of human cloning agree that cloned embryos should not be able to be bought and sold. In a science fiction frame of mind, one can imagine commercial interests offering genetically certified and guaranteed embryos for sale, perhaps offering a catalogue of different embryos cloned from individuals with a variety of talents, capacities, and other desirable properties. This would be a fundamental violation of the equal moral respect and dignity owed to all persons, treating them instead as objects to be differentially valued, bought, and sold in the marketplace. Even if embryos are not yet persons at the time they would be purchased or sold, they would be being valued, bought, and sold for the persons they will become. The moral consensus against any commercial market in embryos, cloned or otherwise, should be enforced by law whatever the public policy ultimately is on human cloning.

5. *Human cloning might be used by governments or other groups for immoral and exploitative purposes.* In *Brave New World*, Aldous Huxley imagined cloning individuals who have been engineered with limited abilities and conditioned to do, and to be happy doing, the menial work that society needed done (Huxley, 1932). Selection and control in the creation of people was exercised not in the interests of the persons created, but in the interests of the society and at the expense of the persons created; nor did it serve individuals' interests in reproduction and parenting. Any use of human cloning for such purposes would exploit the clones solely as means for the benefit of others, and would violate the equal moral respect and dignity they are owed as full moral persons. If human cloning is permitted to go forward, it should be with regulations that would clearly prohibit such immoral exploitation.

Fiction contains even more disturbing or bizarre uses of human cloning, such as Mengele's creation of many clones of Hitler in Ira Levin's *The Boys from*

Brazil (Levin, 1976), Woody Allen's science fiction cinematic spoof *Sleeper* in which a dictator's only remaining part, his nose, must be destroyed to keep it from being cloned, and the contemporary science fiction film *Blade Runner*. These nightmare scenarios may be quite improbable, but their impact should not be underestimated on public concern with technologies like human cloning. Regulation of human cloning must assure the public that even such far-fetched abuses will not take place.

CONCLUSION

Human cloning has until now received little serious and careful ethical attention because it was typically dismissed as science fiction, and it stirs deep, but difficult to articulate, uneasiness and even revulsion in many people. Any ethical assessment of human cloning at this point must be tentative and provisional. Fortunately, the science and technology of human cloning are not yet in hand, and so a public and professional debate is possible without the need for a hasty, precipitate policy response.

The ethical pros and cons of human cloning, as I see them at this time, are sufficiently balanced and uncertain that there is not an ethically decisive case either for or against permitting it or doing it. Access to human cloning can plausibly be brought within a moral right to reproductive freedom, but its potential legitimate uses appear few and do not promise substantial benefits. It is not a central component of the moral right to reproductive freedom and it does not uniquely serve any major or pressing individual or social needs. On the other hand, contrary to the pronouncements of many of its opponents, human cloning seems not to be a violation of moral or human rights. But it does risk some significant individual or social harms, although most are based on common public confusions about genetic determinism, human identity, and the effects of human cloning. Because most potential harms feared from human cloning remain speculative, they seem insufficient to warrant at this time a complete legal prohibition of either research on or later use of human cloning, if and when its safety and efficacy are established. Legitimate moral concerns about the use and effects of human cloning, however, underline the need for careful public oversight of research on its development, together with a wider public and professional debate and review before cloning is used on human beings.

REFERENCES

Annas, G. J. (1994). "Regulatory Models for Human Embryo Cloning: The Free Market, Professional Guidelines, and Government Restrictions." *Kennedy Institute of Ethics Journal* 4, 3:235–249.

Brock, D. W. (1994). "Reproductive Freedom: Its Nature, Bases and Limits," in *Health Care Ethics: Critical Issues for Health Professionals*, eds. D. Thomasma and J. Monagle. Gaithersburg, MD: Aspen Publishers.

Brock, D. W. (1995). "The Non-Identity Problem and Genetic Harm." *Bioethics* 9:269–275.

Callahan, D. (1993). "Perspective on Cloning: A Threat to Individual Uniqueness." *Los Angeles Times*, November 12, 1993:B7.

Chadwick, R. F. (1982). "Cloning." *Philosophy* 57:201–209.

Eisenberg, L. (1976). "The Outcome as Cause: Predestination and Human Cloning." *The Journal of Medicine and Philosophy* 1:318–331.

Feinberg, J. (1980). "The Child's Right to an Open Future," in *Whose Child? Children's Rights, Parental Authority, and State Power*, eds. W. Aiken and H. LaFollette. Totowa, NJ: Rowman and Littlefield.

Harris, J. (1992). *Wonderwoman and Superman: The Ethics of Biotechnology*. Oxford: Oxford University Press.

Huxley, A. (1932). *Brave New World*. London: Chalto and Winders.

Jonas, H. (1974). *Philosophical Essays: From Ancient Creed to Technological Man*. Englewood Cliffs, NJ: Prentice-Hall.

Kahn, C. (1989). "Can We Achieve Immortality?" *Free Inquiry* 9:14–18.

Kass, L. (1985). *Toward a More Natural Science*. New York: The Free Press.

LaBar, M. (1984). "The Pros and Cons of Human Cloning." *Thought* 57:318–333.

Lederberg, J. (1966). "Experimental Genetics and Human Evolution." *The American Naturalist* 100:519–531.

Levin, I. (1976). *The Boys from Brazil*. New York: Random House.

Macklin, R. (1994). "Splitting Embryos on the Slippery Slope: Ethics and Public Policy." *Kennedy Institute of Ethics Journal* 4:209–226.

McCormick, R. (1993). "Should We Clone Humans?" *Christian Century* 110:1148–1149.

McKinnell, R. (1979). *Cloning: A Biologist Reports*. Minneapolis: University of Minnesota Press.

Mill, J. S. (1859). *On Liberty*. Indianapolis, IN: Bobbs-Merrill Publishing.

NABER (National Advisory Board on Ethics in Reproduction) (1994). "Report on Human Cloning Through Embryo Splitting: An Amber Light." *Kennedy Institute of Ethics Journal* 4:251–282.

Parfit, D. (1984). *Reasons and Persons*. Oxford: Oxford University Press.

Rainer, J. D. (1978). "Commentary." *Man and Medicine: The Journal of Values and Ethics in Health Care* 3:115–117.

Rhodes, R. (1995). "Clones, Harms, and Rights." *Cambridge Quarterly of Healthcare Ethics* 4:285–290.

Robertson, J. A. (1994a). *Children of Choice: Freedom and the New Reproductive Technologies*. Princeton, NJ: Princeton University Press.

Robertson, J. A. (1994b). "The Question of Human Cloning." *Hastings Center Report* 24:6–14.

Robertson, J. A. (1997). "A Ban on Cloning and Cloning Research is Unjustified." Testimony Presented to the National Bioethics Advisory Commission, March 1997.

Smith, G. P. (1983). "Intimations of Immortality: Clones, Cyrons and the Law." *University of New South Wales Law Journal* 6:119–137.

Studdard, A. (1978). "The Lone Clone." *Man and Medicine: The Journal of Values and Ethics in Health Care* 3:109–114.

Thomas, L. (1974). "Notes of a Biology Watcher: On Cloning a Human Being." *New England Journal of Medicine* 291:1296–1297.

Verhey, A. D. (1994). "Cloning: Revisiting an Old Debate." *Kennedy Institute of Ethics Journal* 4:227–234.

Walters, W. A. W. (1982). "Cloning, Ectogenesis, and Hybrids: Things to Come?" in *Test-Tube Babies*, eds. W. A. W. Walters and P. Singer. Melbourne: Oxford University Press.

Weiss, R. (1997). "Cloning Suddenly Has Government's Attention." *International Herald Tribune*, March 7, 1997.

WHO (World Health Organization Press Office). (March 11, 1997). "WHO Director General Condemns Human Cloning." World Health Organization, Geneva, Switzerland.

Wilmut, I., et al. (1997). "Viable Offspring Derived from Fetal and Adult Mammalian Cells." *Nature* 385:810–813.

CASES FOR ANALYSIS

1. Gene Therapy and "Bubble Boy" Disease

Children suffering from the notorious "Bubble Boy" disease, or severe combined immunodeficiency, may now place their hopes in gene therapy, researchers say.

According to an article on *WebMD*, 16 children with the rare genetic disease, SCID, received gene therapy for nine years. Out of those 16, 14 showed remarkable improvement and are on their way to becoming fully functional members of their communities.

> "These children, who would have died very young without treatment, are participating in life as fully as their brothers and sisters," researcher H. Bobby Gaspar, MD, PhD, tells *WebMD*. "Most of them are going to school, playing ball, and going to parties.". . .
>
> For most of the children, gene therapy was a success. But one boy who had the X1 form of SCID developed treatment-related leukemia. The complication was not unexpected, Gaspar says, because four children with the X1 from [*sic*] of SCID in a French study had developed leukemia after getting the gene therapy.*

Was it morally permissible for these researchers to use gene therapy even though they knew that some children might get leukemia after treatment? Should the treatment be used only if there are no risks involved? What if gene therapy was the only possible treatment for the genetic disease, and most children died within two years of being diagnosed? How would these facts change your assessment of the morality of using gene therapy?

*Based on Salynn Boyles, "Gene Therapy Works for 'Bubble Boy' Disease," WebMD Health News, 24 August 2011, http://www.webmd.com/children/news/20110824/gene-therapy-effective-for-bubble-boy-disease (8 September 2011).

2. Building Athletes with Gene Doping

It is no secret that in the quest for better sports performance, some athletes and trainers have used performance-enhancing drugs, a prohibited practice known as *doping*. Doping usually has involved the use of drugs such as steroids and growth hormones. But now it is taking a new form called *gene doping*—gene therapy to boost athletic ability. According to the World Anti-Doping Agency (WADA), gene therapy and gene doping are both in experimental phases, but that could change in the next few years.

Play True—In gene doping, an athlete would not be suffering from any disease. Instead, normal genes would be injected into the body to increase the function of a normal cell.

Scientists . . . have experimented with genes that produce insulin-growth factor 1 (IGF-1), which helps muscles grow and repair themselves. The genes, carried into the body by a harmless virus, produce more IGF-1 than the body would normally produce, stimulating muscle growth.

[Theodore Friedmann, director of the Gene Therapy Program at the University of California San Diego and chair of WADA's gene doping panel] envisions a scenario in which some athletes with injuries in a particular part of the body could use IGF-1 to speed healing and repair of the damaged muscles. Others might use gene doping to strengthen, for instance, a weakened knee or other damaged joint or injured tissue, which would give them a significant advantage on the playing field.[†]

Is gene doping unethical? If the use of performance-enhancing drugs is unethical, should gene doping also be considered unethical? Would the widespread practice of gene doping be morally permissible? How would it change the way we normally view exceptional athletic performance? Would the availability of genetic enhancement techniques divide society into two unequal classes of rich enhanced people and less well off unenhanced people? Should scientific research into genetic enhancement be banned? Why or why not?

[†] World Anti-Doping Agency, "Gene Doping," *Play True*, issue 1, 2005, 2–6.

---

3. Mixing Human and Animal Genes

On June 9th, 2011, Argentina's National Institute of Agribusiness announced the birth of the first ever transgenic (with mixed genes) cow. This historic calf, named Rosita ISA, contains both human and Jersey Cow DNA.

Rosita ISA was born on April 6 weighing in at a staggering 45 kilos, or 99 pounds. Due to her large size, nearly twice that of a nontransgenic Jersey cow, she was born via Ceasarian section.

According to the researchers, when Rosita reaches maturity, her human DNA will allow her to produce milk with the same proteins and similar nutrients to a human mother's.

At a press conference, researcher Adrian Mutto stated that the aim in creating Rosita was to increase "the nutritional value of the cow's milk [with] two human genes, the protein lactoferrin, which provides infants with anti-bacterial and anti-viral protection, and lysozyme, which is also an anti-bacterial agent."[‡]

The era of animal-human hybrids is upon us. Scientists are learning how to blend human and animal DNA to produce creatures that are neither entirely human nor entirely animal. Presumably, in the future, the new creatures will be somehow enhanced by the intermingling of DNA. Should such research be allowed? Should scientists be permitted to produce transgenic cows or any other kind of blended organisms? Is it morally permissible to tinker with human or animal genomes in this way? Why or why not? Suppose a human is genetically engineered to have a significant number of genes derived from animals. Would this being be alienated from the human race? Would it have full moral rights?

‡ Based on *Discovery News*, "Cloned Cows to Produce Human-Like Milk," 10 June 2011, http://news.discovery.com/tech/cloned-cows-produce-human-like-milk-110610.htm (10 June 2011).

CHAPTER 10

Euthanasia and Physician-Assisted Suicide

For fifteen years, Terri Schiavo existed between life and death in that shadow land called a persistent vegetative state, a place where she was wakeful but without awareness or any purposeful behavior. Severe brain damage had left her there, with virtually no chance of recovery. And all the while, a storm of caustic debate swirled around her, reaching its greatest strength in the last few days before her death on March 31, 2005. In 1990 her heart had stopped briefly because of a chemical imbalance, leaving her brain-damaged and in a twilight state, kept alive by a feeding tube. She had left no living will, no written record of her wishes should she become indefinitely incapacitated. Her husband, Michael Schiavo, insisted that Terri had told him once that she would prefer death to being kept alive with machines. Her parents rejected his claim and demanded that Terri be kept alive, holding out hope that with proper care she might recover.

The battle between Michael Schiavo and Terri's parents raged on in the courts for years. Again and again, state and federal courts sided with the husband, while the U.S. Supreme Court repeatedly refused to hear the case. In the final days before Terri died, President George W. Bush, the U.S. Congress, the governor of Florida (where she lived), and Florida legislators weighed in on the controversy, supporting Terri's parents.

Finally, a judge allowed the feeding tube to be removed, and Terri Schiavo, age forty-one, died thirteen days later. The parents called the removal "judicial homicide." A Vatican official called it "an attack against God."[1]

So it goes with all public debates on the moral permissibility of euthanasia. Passions rise, claims and counterclaims collide, and stakes are high. In the balance are issues of life and death, science and religion, murder and mercy. The tragic end of Terri Schiavo is only the most dramatic (and dramatized) case in a series of tragic ends that turned into widely publicized moral battlegrounds. (See the box "The Death of Karen Ann Quinlan.") The moral questions it incited are typical of such cases: Was removing Terri Schiavo's feeding tube really a case of murder? Or was it a morally permissible act allowing her to die with dignity and escape her bleak condition? What if instead of stopping the tube feeding, her doctors had never started it because they deemed her situation hopeless? Would *that* have been murder—or a permissible act of mercy? Or suppose that soon after Schiavo collapsed, her doctors had decided to give her a lethal injection? Would such an act have been morally wrong? What if Schiavo had left a living will that clearly specified that she did *not* want to be kept alive by any means if she fell into a persistent vegetative state? Would withdrawing the feeding tube or giving her a lethal injection then have been morally acceptable?

---

[1]Larry Copeland and Laura Parker, "Terri Schiavo's Case Doesn't End with Her Passing," *USA Today*, 31 March 2005, www.usatoday.com/news/nation/2005-03-31-schiavo_x.htm (13 January 2012).

The Death of Karen Ann Quinlan

Like nothing else before it, the case of Karen Ann Quinlan focused the world's attention on the medical truths, the legal complexities, and the moral problems of euthanasia. She was just twenty-one years old when she sustained acute brain damage after imbibing alcohol along with a tranquilizer. She was left in a persistent vegetative state, kept alive by a feeding tube and a respirator, a machine that maintained her breathing mechanically. After several months, members of her family came to accept that her recovery was hopeless and sought permission from the courts to unplug the respirator to allow her to die. Finally in 1976 the New Jersey Supreme Court granted their request. But to everyone's surprise, she continued to breathe without the respirator until 1985, ten years after she slipped into the vegetative state. She died on June 11.[*]

[*]See "Famous Cases: Karen Ann Quinlan," *CBC News Online*, 22 March 2005, http://www.cbc.ca/news2 /background/schiavo/vegetative_state.html (20 January 2015); Barran H. Lerner, "Planning for the Long Goodbye," *New York Times*, 18 June 2004.

Of course, in every instance of euthanasia there are plenty of nonmoral questions too—primarily legal, judicial, medical, scientific, and political. (In the Schiavo case, for example, the moral questions arose side by side with what most informed observers saw as the *real* issue: who, if anyone, had the legal right to decide for Schiavo what was to become of her?) But these nonmoral concerns are intertwined with the moral concerns. Our task here is to apply moral reasoning to try to unravel the knot.

ISSUE FILE: BACKGROUND

Euthanasia is directly or indirectly bringing about the death of another person for that person's sake.[2] It is thought to provide a benefit or a good for the person by ending a life deemed no longer worth living—a situation that typically arises when someone has an incurable or terminal disease that causes great suffering or when someone experiences an irreversible loss of consciousness (as in the Schiavo case). This notion of dying as a kind of blessing is preserved in the Greek roots of *euthanasia*, which literally means "easy death." Euthanasia makes sense to many people because they believe that a quick and painless death would be preferable to a slow and painful dying (such as the kind that some terminal cancer patients endure) or a long, vegetative sleep without a chance for a meaningful life.

As you might expect, the moral permissibility of euthanasia depends heavily on the consent of the patient (the person whose death is being considered). Moral philosophers therefore distinguish between euthanasia that is voluntary, nonvoluntary, and involuntary. In **voluntary euthanasia,** the patient requests or agrees to the act. She may make the request in person or leave instructions to be followed in case she becomes incapacitated. Such instructions are usually in the form of an **advance directive** (for example, a living will), a legal document allowing physicians to withhold or withdraw treatments if a patient becomes terminally ill and unable to express her wishes. For any voluntary euthanasia request to be valid, the patient at the time of the request must be competent—that is, capable of making an informed, rational choice. In **nonvoluntary euthanasia,** others besides the patient (family or physicians, for example) choose euthanasia for her because she is not competent (due to illness or injury) and has left no instructions regarding her end-of-life preferences.

[2]I owe the notion of a good death "for the sake" of the person dying to Philippa Foot (in "Euthanasia," *Philosophy & Public Affairs* 6, no. 2, [1977]: 85–112); and to Helga Kuhse (in "Euthanasia," in *A Companion to Ethics*, ed. Peter Singer, corr. ed. [Oxford: Blackwell, 1993], 294–302).

Euthanasia performed on infants and small children is, of course, nonvoluntary. In **involuntary euthanasia,** the act is carried out against the wishes of the patient and is therefore illegal and widely regarded as immoral.

People also draw a distinction between active and passive euthanasia. **Active euthanasia** is taking a direct action to kill someone, to carry out a "mercy killing." A doctor who gives a patient a lethal injection is performing active euthanasia, and so is a man who suffocates his dying brother to spare him from an unbearably painful passing. **Passive euthanasia** is allowing someone to die by *not* doing something—by withholding or withdrawing measures necessary for sustaining life. A doctor, then, would be performing passive euthanasia if she removed a patient's respirator, did not administer antibiotics to halt a life-threatening infection, or withdrew hydration and nutrition (fluids and nutrients).

Many believe that this active-passive distinction is essential to understanding the moral permissibility of euthanasia. It allows them to maintain that whereas active euthanasia is always wrong, in some cases passive euthanasia may be permissible. This view is widespread among physicians and fits with the popular notion that killing people is morally worse than letting them die. Others, however, argue that there is no moral difference between killing and letting die: in both active and passive euthanasia the patient's death is caused, and they are therefore morally equivalent.

Taking into account the categories of *voluntary, nonvoluntary, active,* and *passive* (and disregarding *involuntary*), we can identify four kinds of euthanasia: (1) *active voluntary* (mercy killing at the patient's request), (2) *active nonvoluntary* (mercy killing without the patient's consent or request), (3) *passive voluntary* (letting the patient die at her request), and (4) *passive nonvoluntary* (letting the patient die without his consent or request). Generally, the law forbids active euthanasia (either voluntary or nonvoluntary), and the medical profession is officially

opposed to it (though the views of individual physicians vary). Passive voluntary euthanasia is legal; by law, competent patients have the right to refuse any kind of medical treatment. Passive nonvoluntary euthanasia may be legal provided that someone (a family member, for example) can be designated to make decisions on behalf of the patient.

Related to, but distinct from, active voluntary euthanasia is **physician-assisted suicide**—the killing of a person by the person's own hand with the help of a physician. Like active voluntary euthanasia, physician-assisted suicide is requested by the patient, and the intended outcome is the patient's death for the relief of pain and suffering. But the agent who ultimately causes the death in active voluntary euthanasia is the physician, whereas the ultimate causal agent in physician-assisted suicide is the patient. In the former, the physician is primarily responsible for the killing; in the latter, the patient is. In most cases, the physician provides help by prescribing a lethal dose of drugs, which the patient then administers to himself.

In the United States, physician-assisted suicide is legal in only four states—Oregon, Washington, Montana, and Vermont. New Mexico may become the fifth if a state judge's ruling is allowed to stand. U.S. Supreme Court rulings allow each state to decide for itself whether to legalize assisted suicide. The official position of the American Medical Association (AMA), the main professional group for American physicians, is that "Physician-assisted suicide is fundamentally incompatible with the physician's role as healer, would be difficult or impossible to control, and would pose serious societal risks.[3]

A factor that can complicate all the foregoing issues is the concept of death itself. One problem is that thanks to modern medical technology,

[3]Issued June 1994 based on the reports "*Decisions Near the End of Life,*" adopted June 1991, and "*Physician-Assisted Suicide,*" adopted December 1993 (*JAMA.* 1992;267(16): 2229–2233); updated June 1996.

Landmark Court Rulings

In the past three decades, U.S. courts have several times weighed in on the controversial issues of euthanasia and physician-assisted suicide. The following are some of the more far-reaching rulings:

- **1976** The New Jersey Supreme Court ruled that a life-sustaining respirator could be legally disconnected from Karen Ann Quinlan, a young woman who had lapsed into a persistent vegetative state. After it was removed, she remained comatose and lived for another ten years, finally dying in June 1985.

- **1990** The U.S. Supreme Court (in *Cruzan v. Director, Missouri Department of Health*) ruled that a feeding tube could be removed from Nancy Cruzan, a woman in a persistent vegetative state due to an automobile accident, if "clear and convincing evidence" shows that she would have approved of the withdrawal. The ruling recognized the legitimacy of living wills, surrogates to act for incapacitated individuals, and a qualified "right to die."

- **1997** The U.S. Supreme Court (in *Washington v. Glucksberg*) ruled that a Washington State prohibition of physician-assisted suicide did not violate the due process clause of the Fourteenth Amendment.

- **1997** The U.S. Supreme Court (in *Vacco v. Quill*) ruled that a New York State prohibition of physician-assisted suicide did not violate the equal protection clause of the Fourteenth Amendment. The Court acknowledged a crucial distinction between withdrawing life-sustaining treatment and assisted suicide. People may refuse life-sustaining treatment, but assisted suicide is prohibited.

- **2006** In a 6–3 decision in *Gonzales v. Oregon*, the U.S. Supreme Court ruled that the U.S. attorney general is not authorized to ban controlled substances used in physician-assisted suicide. The decision had the effect of upholding Oregon's Death with Dignity Act.

- **2009** In a 4–3 decision in *Baxter v. State of Montana*, the Montana Supreme Court ruled that physician-assisted suicide is not "against public policy." The decision applied only to Montana. The court also ruled that doctors who help terminally ill patients commit suicide cannot be prosecuted under Montana state law.

determining when a person is dead is not so straightforward as it once seemed. Death has become more difficult to define. Years ago the prevailing notion was that a person is dead when his breathing and blood flow stop (no respiration and no heartbeat). But nowadays machines can keep an individual's heart and lungs functioning long after the brain permanently and completely shuts down. Thus we can have an individual whose organs are mechanically operated while he is in a coma or persistent vegetative state—*for years*. By the traditional definition of death, such an individual would still be alive, but many people would insist that he is no longer there: he is dead. So the conventional notion of death seems to be inadequate.

Why does correctly defining death matter at all? Say an individual is in the kind of state just described. If we judge him to be dead and thus no longer a person, then perhaps it would be morally permissible to disconnect him from the machines, or administer a fatal drug overdose, or remove his feeding tube, or even harvest his organs for transplant into another person. Or would it? If we deem him alive and still a person, perhaps we are not justified in doing *any* of the above. Maybe taking any one of these actions is to commit murder. Depending on the concept of death accepted by the legal system, killing him or allowing him to die could have serious legal consequences.

To overcome the drawbacks of the traditional definition of death, alternative definitions have

QUICK REVIEW

euthanasia—Directly or indirectly bringing about the death of another person for that person's sake.

voluntary euthanasia—Euthanasia performed on a person with his or her permission.

advance directive—A legal document allowing physicians to withhold or withdraw treatments if a patient becomes terminally ill and unable to express his or her wishes.

nonvoluntary euthanasia—Euthanasia performed on a person who is not competent to decide the issue and has left no instructions regarding end-of-life preferences. In such cases, family or physicians usually make the decision.

involuntary euthanasia—Euthanasia performed on a person against his or her wishes.

active euthanasia—Euthanasia performed by taking a direct action to cause someone's death; "mercy killing."

passive euthanasia—Euthanasia performed by withholding or withdrawing measures necessary for sustaining life.

physician-assisted suicide—The killing of a person by that person's own hand with the help of a physician.

been suggested. According to the *whole-brain* definition of death, an individual is dead when all brain functions (including those performed in the brain stem) permanently stop. It has become the primary standard in both medicine and the law for determining death. Critics of the whole-brain standard, though, have pointed out that it is based on a faulty assumption: that the brain is the control center for all physiological functions. Yet some functions (such as respiration) are partially independent of brain activity. In addition, by the whole-brain standard, individuals in an irreversible persistent

vegetative state (who have some detectable brain activity) are thought to be alive—a result that some regard as counterintuitive or puzzling.

The *higher brain* definition of death says that an individual is dead when higher brain functions—those that give rise to consciousness—permanently stop. Some have maintained that because consciousness is necessary for personhood, an individual whose higher brain functions have disappeared is no longer a person and is therefore rightly considered dead. By the higher-brain standard, individuals in a persistent vegetative state (who continue to breathe and have a heartbeat) but whose higher brain functions have ceased are thought to be dead—also a result that some people find counterintuitive.

MORAL THEORIES

Utilitarianism, Kant's ethics, and natural law theory lead to divergent conclusions on the issue of euthanasia. An act-utilitarian would certainly try to take into account how much overall happiness various possible actions could bring about, everyone considered. But she could make this calculation in different ways. The basic approach would be to consider the patient's suffering (as well as that of others involved, such as family members) and the likely success of any treatments and try to determine how much overall happiness would be generated by different actions, including bringing about the patient's death. If the patient's situation is hopeless and his suffering great, an act-utilitarian could decide that the greatest net happiness would result from killing the patient or letting him die. The patient's consent to euthanasia may or may not be a primary concern, depending on how consent would affect overall happiness. On the other hand, the act-utilitarian might say that euthanasia is contrary to the goal of maximizing happiness because killing a person rules out any possibility of his experiencing happiness in the future. Happiness does not occur in a vacuum; it exists only when persons experience it. So eliminating a person eliminates potential happiness.

Some people—even those who are not thoroughgoing utilitarians—argue against euthanasia on what amounts to rule-utilitarian grounds or something close to it. They contend that regardless of the moral permissibility of euthanasia in specific cases, a general rule (that is, a social policy or law) permitting some types of euthanasia would cause more harm than good. They offer slippery-slope arguments such as the following: Passing a law (making a rule) permitting active voluntary euthanasia would inevitably lead to abuses such as more frequent use of nonvoluntary euthanasia and unnecessary killing; therefore, no such law should be passed. Similarly, some argue that a general rule allowing physician-assisted suicide would destroy the "moral center" of the medical profession; if physicians are allowed to kill patients, they will violate their pledge to protect life and to heal, causing patients to distrust them. Of course, it is also possible to argue *for* euthanasia on rule-utilitarian grounds. (Whether such arguments are sound is another matter.) A rule-utilitarian could devise a rule that he thinks would result in a maximization of happiness for everyone if the rule were consistently followed.

Like the utilitarian, the Kantian theorist could also take several different positions on euthanasia, consistent with Kantian principles. She could argue that euthanasia is never permissible because it would entail treating persons as mere disposable things. Kant underscores this view in his discussion of suicide. He maintains that "suicide is in no circumstances permissible" because it robs individuals of their personhood, which is the very foundation of all moral values. Furthermore, it treats persons as if they had no more value than a beast. As Kant puts it, "But the rule of morality does not admit of [suicide] under any condition because it degrades human nature below the level of animal nature and so destroys it."[4] This stern prohibition against suicide may or may not

apply equally well to euthanasia—depending on whether those considered for euthanasia are to be regarded as persons. Certainly those who are competent (coherent and rational) are persons and therefore should not be killed or allowed to die. But what would Kant say about individuals who have slipped from waking life into a coma or a vegetative state? Are they still persons with full moral rights? If they are persons, then performing euthanasia on them would be immoral. If they are not persons, then euthanasia might be morally acceptable. In fact, a Kantian might argue that performing euthanasia on individuals in comas or vegetative states may be morally permissible precisely because persons have intrinsic worth and dignity. The bioethicist Ronald Munson explains this view well:

> It may be more in keeping with our freedom and dignity for us to instruct others either to put us to death or to take no steps to keep us alive should we ever be in such a state. Voluntary euthanasia may be compatible with (if not required by) Kant's ethics.
>
> By a similar line of reasoning, it may be that nonvoluntary euthanasia might be seen as a duty that we have to others. We might argue that by putting to death a comatose and hopeless person we are recognizing the dignity that person possessed in his or her previous state.[5]

According to the dominant reading of natural law theory, euthanasia is wrong in almost every instance. It is wrong because we have a moral duty to preserve life. So intentionally performing any kind of euthanasia, active or passive, is impermissible. The doctrine of double effect, however, allows one exception to this rule. Recall that this doctrine makes a distinction between (1) performing a good action that happens to have a bad effect and (2) performing a bad action to achieve a good effect. The former may be permissible, but the latter is not. In the case of euthanasia, the doctrine implies that giving a pain-racked patient a large dose of morphine

---

[4]Immanuel Kant, "Suicide," in *Lectures on Ethics,* trans. Louis Infield (New York: Harper & Row, 1963), 147–54.

[5]Ronald Munson, *Intervention and Reflection: Basic Issues in Medical Ethics,* ed. Munson, 7th ed. (Belmont, CA: Wadsworth, 2004), 696–97.

Dr. Jack Kevorkian was known as a champion of the right-to-die movement, having helped many incurably ill people commit suicide. He was also known as "Dr. Death," the physician who helped desperate people kill themselves. After many unsuccessful tries, prosecutors finally won a conviction against him for murder: in 1999, he was sentenced to ten to twenty-five years in prison. The *New York Times* reported that the sentence was handed down "despite emotional courtroom pleas on his behalf from the widow and brother of the terminally ill man he was convicted of killing."*

Do you agree with the verdict in this case? Why or why not? If you do not agree, would your opinion change if you knew that many of Dr. Kevorkian's suicide patients were not mentally competent at the time of their deaths (because of depression), as some people allege? If so, why? If you were terminally ill and in horrendous pain with no hope of relief, might you think it morally permissible to use the services of someone like Dr. Kevorkian? If not, why not?

* Dirk Johnson, "Kevorkian Sentenced to 10 to 25 Years in Prison," *New York Times,* 14 April 1999.

sive euthanasia (both voluntary and nonvoluntary) is legal, provided certain conditions are met, and both forms of it are widely believed to be morally acceptable. So let us confine our evaluation here to moral arguments for and against *active voluntary euthanasia* (mercy killing at the patient's request). The question these arguments address then is straightforward: *Is active voluntary euthanasia morally permissible?*

As we proceed, we must keep an important distinction in mind: moral permissibility is not the same thing as legal permissibility. Whether euthanasia is morally acceptable is a separate issue from whether it should be legalized. It is possible that we could be justified in believing both that euthanasia is morally permissible *and* that it should not be legalized—or vice versa. We might plausibly argue that in some cases, performing active voluntary euthanasia is the right thing to do but that legalizing it would have terrible consequences. Legalization could, say, lead doctors to practice active *nonvoluntary* euthanasia or encourage them to care less about preserving life or cause patients to fear or mistrust doctors. To mix up these two kinds of issues—moral and legal—is to invite confusion.

We begin by examining arguments *for* active voluntary euthanasia. The strongest of these are built on two fundamental moral principles: persons have (1) a right of self-determination and (2) an obligation to help someone in serious distress or peril (if they are in a position to help without great risk to themselves). Principle (1) refers to the patient's right of self-determination, and principle (2) to other persons who might be able to benefit her. Principle (1) assumes that persons have autonomy—the capacity, as Kant would have it, to use reason to guide their own actions and make their own decisions. It asserts that persons have the right to exercise this power to direct their lives as they see fit (with the proviso that their actions not violate the rights of others). Many who appeal to this principle argue that if it applies to how persons live, then it surely applies to how they die,

to end her life (a practice known as *terminal sedation*) is never morally acceptable. But giving her a large dose of morphine with the intention of easing her pain—an act that has the side effect of expediting her death—is permissible. The hastening of the patient's death is permissible because even though it was foreseen, it was not intended. In the doctrine of double effect, intention makes all the difference.

MORAL ARGUMENTS

Most plausible euthanasia arguments are about *active* euthanasia (mercy killing, as opposed to letting the patient die). As suggested earlier, pas-

because their dying is part of their life. This is how the bioethicist Dan W. Brock explains the importance of this end-of-life self-determination:

> Most people are very concerned about the nature of the last stage of their lives. This reflects not just a fear of experiencing substantial suffering when dying, but also a desire to retain dignity and control during this last period of life. Death is today increasingly preceded by a long period of significant physical and mental decline, due in part to the technological interventions of modern medicine. Many people adjust to these disabilities and find meaning and value in new activities and ways. Others find the impairments and burdens in the last stage of their lives at some point sufficiently great to make life no longer worth living. For many patients near death, maintaining the quality of one's life, avoiding great suffering, maintaining one's dignity, and insuring that others remember us as we wish them to become of paramount importance and outweigh merely extending one's life. But there is no single, objectively correct answer for everyone as to when, if at all, one's life becomes all things considered a burden and unwanted. If self-determination is a fundamental value, then the great variability among people on this question makes it especially important that individuals control the manner, circumstances, and timing of their dying and death.[6]

Principle (2) is a duty of beneficence (a duty to benefit others). Applied to euthanasia, it says that if we are in a position to ease the agony of another, and we can do so without excessive cost to ourselves, we should try to render aid. This tenet applies to persons generally, but it carries extra weight for people with a special relationship with the suffering person, such as family members, close friends, and doctors. Physicians have an explicit obligation to try to relieve the misery of their patients—especially dying patients who often must endure horrific pain and suffering. Many advocates of euthanasia contend that if a competent dying patient is in agony and asks to be put

out of her misery (active voluntary euthanasia), rejecting her plea for mercy would be both cruel and wicked. They also insist that merely withholding treatment from her to hasten her death (passive euthanasia) would only prolong her suffering.

Here is one way to incorporate both principles (1) and (2) into a single argument for active voluntary euthanasia:

1. Competent persons have a right of self-determination (as long as exercising this right does not violate others' rights).

2. The right of self-determination includes the right of competent persons to decide the manner of their dying and to choose active (voluntary) euthanasia.

3. We have an obligation to help others in serious distress or peril (if we are in a position to help without great risk to themselves).

4. This duty of beneficence includes the duty, under appropriate conditions, to ease the pain and suffering of competent dying persons by performing active (voluntary) euthanasia.

5. Therefore, active voluntary euthanasia for competent dying persons is permissible.

The central idea behind this argument is that if competent dying persons have a right to choose active euthanasia, and if the duty of beneficence includes performing active voluntary euthanasia, then active voluntary euthanasia is morally permissible. But does the conclusion follow from the premises, and are the premises true? The answer to the first part of this question is yes. The answer to the second part is more complicated. Look at Premises 1 and 3; they articulate the two basic moral principles we began with. These principles qualify as considered moral judgments and are accepted by virtually all parties to the euthanasia debate. We have good reason, then, to say that Premises 1 and 3 are true.

Premises 2 and 4, however, are controversial. Critics of Premise 2 would say that we do indeed have a right of self-determination but that this right

---

[6]Dan W. Brock, "Voluntary Active Euthanasia," *Hastings Center Report* 22, no. 2 (March/April 1992): 11.

Public Opinion and Euthanasia

Many opinion polls have shown that most people favor some form of euthanasia or physician assistance in dying. A 2014 Gallup poll of 1,028 adults aged eighteen and over echoed these findings. The wording of the survey question, however, matters greatly:

- 69 percent of Americans approve of doctor-assisted suicide when the question is asked like this:

  Wording A: "When a person has a disease that cannot be cured, do you think doctors should be allowed by law to end the patient's life by some painless means if the patient and his or her family request it?"

- But only 58 percent of Americans support doctor-assisted suicide when the question is asked like this:

  Wording B: "When a person has a disease that cannot be cured and is living in severe pain, do you think doctors should or should not be allowed by law to assist the patient to commit suicide if the patient requests it?"

  The conclusion of the pollsters regarding this difference is that "Americans are less likely to support euthanasia when the question emphasizes that the doctor would "assist the patient to commit suicide" than when the question does not mention the word suicide."*

*Gallup, Poll "Seven in 10 Americans Back Euthanasia 18 June 2014," http://www.gallup.com/poll/171704/seven-americans-back-euthanasia.aspx.

---

does not include the right to opt for active voluntary euthanasia. The reason is that active euthanasia is killing, and killing is always wrong. We may have all sorts of rights, but killing is still killing.

This reply, though, is based on a superficial understanding of prohibitions against killing.

Some kinds of killing are considered by most people to be morally permissible—for example, killing in self-defense and killing in war. These are regarded as justified killings; unjustified killings are known as *murder*. So even though all killing may be regrettable, not all killing is immoral. Active euthanasia may in fact be a form of acceptable killing.

The opponent of active euthanasia can make a stronger reply along the same lines. He can say that the problem with active euthanasia is not that it is a type of killing but that it is a type of *unwarranted* killing. A dying patient in the grip of unimaginable pain, for example, does not have to be killed to escape her agony. Modern medicine is better than ever at alleviating pain—even very intense pain. Spinal blocks, drug combinations, new ways to deliver powerful analgesics (drugs that ease pain)—these options and others can offer dying patients unprecedented levels of pain relief. So euthanasia is uncalled for. If this claim is correct, then opponents can argue that contrary to Premise 4, active euthanasia will actually harm patients by cutting their lives short unnecessarily and thus depriving them of the benefits that may accrue in their remaining days—benefits such as profoundly meaningful moments spent with their families, the chance to come to terms with their dying, and even the possibility of a newfound cure for their disease.[7] Proponents of active euthanasia, however, charge that this upbeat view of pain management is not accurate. They point to several unpleasant facts: though it is *possible* to manage even severe pain well, too often pain is not well managed (for a variety of reasons, including the reluctance of health care workers to administer large doses of pain-relieving drugs); the side effects of the best pain medications (especially when used long term) often add to the suffering of the patient;

[7] I owe this point to Thomas F. Wall, *Thinking Critically about Moral Problems* (Belmont, CA: Wadsworth, 2003), 176.

and many dying patients endure not physical pain but psychological suffering that is unbearable and untreatable by any medication.

Proponents can put forth another kind of argument for active voluntary euthanasia, this one based on the moral significance of killing (active euthanasia) and letting die (passive euthanasia). As we saw earlier, active euthanasia is taking a direct action to kill someone, while passive euthanasia is allowing someone to die by withholding or withdrawing measures necessary for sustaining life. Passive euthanasia is legal (competent patients have the right to refuse treatment) and widely believed to be morally permissible. Active euthanasia is generally illegal, and debate continues over its moral permissibility. Opponents of active euthanasia generally think that there is a profound *moral* difference between killing and letting die: killing is far worse than letting die; in fact, killing is morally wrong while letting die is permissible. But proponents of active voluntary euthanasia assert that the two are morally equivalent. Using this alleged moral equivalence, proponents can construct an argument like this:

1. Passive euthanasia is morally permissible.

2. If passive euthanasia is morally equivalent to active euthanasia, active euthanasia is also morally permissible.

3. Passive euthanasia is morally equivalent to active euthanasia.

4. Therefore, active (voluntary) euthanasia is morally permissible.

The conclusion follows from the premises, and Premises 1 and 2 are uncontroversial. The crux of the matter is Premise 3. What reasons are there for thinking that it is true? Here is an argument for Premise 3 in the form of a classic thought experiment. Suppose Smith will inherit a fortune if his six-year-old cousin dies. So he decides to take matters into his own hands. He slips into the bathroom while his little cousin is taking a bath and drowns him. He makes the whole thing look like an accident and leaves undetected. Now consider Jones, who also will inherit a fortune if his six-year-old cousin dies. He too decides to kill the child, and he too slips into the bathroom while the boy is bathing. But before Jones has a chance to commit the deed, the boy slips in the tub, gets knocked unconscious, and will surely drown unless Jones rescues him. Jones is happy to do nothing and lets the boy drown on his own—a simple "accident." Now which man behaves better morally? If there is a significant moral difference between killing and letting die, we would want to say that Jones's actions are less blameworthy than Smith's. But this distinction doesn't seem correct. The motives and aims of both men are the same.[8]

The line taken here is that if the difference between killing and letting die really is important morally, then we would judge one man's action (either Smith's or Jones's) to be more blameworthy than that of the other. But our judgment is the same for both, so there must be no moral difference.

Some reject this argument and insist that there is in fact a moral difference between killing and letting die but that the distinction is often obscured in thought experiments like the Smith-Jones story. One critic claims, for example, that in this scenario the two men are equally reprehensible and the two actions appear to be morally equivalent simply because both men *were prepared to kill*. Remove this common factor, and the moral difference between killing and letting die will be apparent.[9]

Some of the strongest arguments *against* active voluntary euthanasia take a slippery-slope approach. The gist of most of them is that lifting a

[8]James Rachels, "Active and Passive Euthanasia," *New England Journal of Medicine* 292, no. 2 (9 January 1975): 79.

[9]Winston Nesbitt, "Is Killing No Worse Than Letting Die?" *Journal of Applied Philosophy* 12, no. 1 (1995): 101–5.

moral or legal prohibition against this kind of mercy killing will dilute respect for life and encourage a slow slide from active voluntary euthanasia to active *nonvoluntary* euthanasia and then perhaps to *involuntary* euthanasia. This argument is therefore consequentialist: active voluntary euthanasia is wrong because it leads to bad consequences. (The argument is also sometimes lodged against legalizing this form of euthanasia.) Here is how one bioethicist describes the descent down the slope:

> A person apparently hopelessly ill may be allowed to take his own life. Then he may be permitted to deputize others to do it for him should he no longer be able to act. The judgment of others then becomes the ruling factor. Already at this point euthanasia is not personal and voluntary, for others are acting "on behalf of" the patient as they see fit. This may well incline them to act on behalf of other patients who have not authorized them to exercise their judgment. It is only a short step, then, from voluntary euthanasia (self-inflicted or authorized), to directed euthanasia administered to a patient who has given no authorization, to involuntary euthanasia conducted as part of a social policy.[10]

We can formulate a version of the argument thus:

1. If the general acceptance or approval of active voluntary euthanasia leads to widespread abuses (unjustified killing), then the practice is morally wrong.

2. The general acceptance or approval of active voluntary euthanasia will lead to widespread abuses (unjustified killing).

3. Therefore, active voluntary euthanasia is morally wrong.

This is a valid argument, an instance of *modus ponens*, so we need to focus only on the truth or fal-

sity of the premises. Probably most people who have thought carefully about this kind of argument accept Premise 1 or a variation of it. Premise 2 is the sticking point. Because of a lack of solid evidence on the subject, the social consequences of a general acceptance of active euthanasia are difficult to ascertain. For example, to prove their case, some opponents of euthanasia cite reports on the Dutch experience with physician-assisted suicide. Proponents point to the same reports to undermine that case. The difficulty is that the research is not robust enough to lend unequivocal support to one side or the other. It therefore does not show that Premise 2 is true. Many of the arguments for Premise 2 are arguments by analogy or inferences based on observations concerning human behavior. Generally, these too are weak and conjectural.

Those who are skeptical of Premise 2 often simply point out that no good reasons have been provided to support it. At best, they say, arguments for Premise 2 show only that dreadful consequences from widespread use of active euthanasia are possible. As one skeptic puts it,

> Now it cannot be denied that it is *possible* that permitting euthanasia could have these fateful consequences, but that cannot be enough to warrant prohibiting it if it is otherwise justified. A similar *possible* slippery slope worry could have been raised to securing competent patients' rights to decide about life support, but recent history shows such a worry would have been unfounded.[11]

SUMMARY

Euthanasia is directly or indirectly bringing about the death of another person for that person's sake. Its moral status depends in large measure on the consent of the patient. In voluntary euthanasia, the patient agrees to the act. In nonvoluntary euthanasia, others besides the patient decide on euthanasia because he or she is incompetent and has left no statement about

[10]J. Gay-Williams, "The Wrongfulness of Euthanasia," in *Intervention and Reflection: Basic Issues in Medical Ethics*, [selected by] Ronald Munson, 7th ed. (Belmont, CA: Wadsworth, 2004), 710–11.

[11]Brock, 20.

end-of-life preferences. In involuntary euthanasia, the act is performed against the patient's wishes. Active euthanasia is taking direct action to kill someone (administering a lethal injection, for example); passive euthanasia is allowing the patient to die by withholding or withdrawing life-sustaining measures.

The traditional notion of death as the cessation of breathing and heartbeat has been revised in light of new developments in medical technology. According to the whole-brain view of death, the individual is dead when all brain functions permanently stop. The higher-brain view of death says that an individual is dead when higher brain functions permanently stop.

An act-utilitarian might see euthanasia as morally permissible because it results in the greatest happiness for all concerned. She could also consistently say that euthanasia is contrary to the goal of maximizing happiness because killing an individual rules out any possibility of that person's future happiness. A rule-utilitarian might say that a general rule permitting some kinds of euthanasia would do more harm than good—or that such a rule would maximize happiness in the long run. A Kantian theorist could consistently reject euthanasia because it entails treating persons as disposable things. Or he could consistently maintain that individuals in comas or persistent vegetative states are no longer persons, and therefore euthanasia is morally acceptable.

Arguments in favor of active voluntary euthanasia are often based on a right of self-determination and a duty to help others in distress. Some arguments for euthanasia, however, depend on the alleged equivalence between active and passive euthanasia. Some of the strongest arguments against euthanasia are of the slippery-slope type: active voluntary euthanasia is wrong because it leads to bad consequences, such as an increased risk of unjustified killings.

READINGS

Active and Passive Euthanasia

JAMES RACHELS

The distinction between active and passive euthanasia is thought to be crucial for medical ethics. The idea is that it is permissible, at least in some cases, to withhold treatment and allow a patient to die, but it is never permissible to take any direct action designed to kill the patient. This doctrine seems to be accepted by most doctors, and it is endorsed in a statement adopted by the House of Delegates of the American Medical Association on December 4, 1973:

> The intentional termination of the life of one human being by another—mercy killing—is contrary

James Rachels, excerpts from "Active and Passive Euthanasia," from *The New England Journal of Medicine*, Vol. 292, No. 2, pp. 78–80. Copyright © 1975 Massachusetts Medical Society. Reprinted with permission from Massachusetts Medical Society.

to that for which the medical profession stands and is contrary to the policy of the American Medical Association.

> The cessation of the employment of extraordinary means to prolong the life of the body when there is irrefutable evidence that biological death is imminent is the decision of the patient and/or his immediate family. The advice and judgment of the physician should be freely available to the patient and/or his immediate family.

However, a strong case can be made against this doctrine. In what follows I will set out some of the relevant arguments, and urge doctors to reconsider their views on this matter.

To begin with a familiar type of situation, a patient who is dying of incurable cancer of the throat is in terrible pain, which can no longer be satisfactorily alleviated. He is certain to die within a few days, even if present treatment is continued, but he does not want to go on living for those days since the pain is unbearable. So he asks the doctor for an end to it, and his family joins in the request.

Suppose the doctor agrees to withhold treatment, as the conventional doctrine says he may. The justification for his doing so is that the patient is in terrible agony, and since he is going to die anyway, it would be wrong to prolong his suffering needlessly. But now notice this. If one simply withholds treatment, it may take the patient longer to die, and so he may suffer more than he would if more direct action were taken and a lethal injection given. This fact provides strong reason for thinking that, once the initial decision not to prolong his agony has been made, active euthanasia is actually preferable to passive euthanasia, rather than the reverse. To say otherwise is to endorse the option that leads to more suffering rather than less, and is contrary to the humanitarian impulse that prompts the decision not to prolong his life in the first place.

Part of my point is that the process of being "allowed to die" can be relatively slow and painful, whereas being given a lethal injection is relatively quick and painless. Let me give a different sort of example. In the United States about one in 600 babies is born with [Down] syndrome. Most of these babies are otherwise healthy—that is, with only the usual pediatric care, they will proceed to an otherwise normal infancy. Some, however, are born with congenital defects such as intestinal obstructions that require operations if they are to live. Sometimes, the parents and the doctor will decide not to operate, and let the infant die. Anthony Shaw describes what happens then:

> . . . When surgery is denied [the doctor] must try to keep the infant from suffering while natural forces sap the baby's life away. As a surgeon whose natural inclination is to use the scalpel to fight off death, standing by and watching a salvageable baby die is the most emotionally exhausting experience I know. It is easy at a conference, in a theoretical discussion, to decide that such infants should be allowed to die. It is altogether different to stand by in the nursery and watch as dehydration and infection wither a tiny being over hours

and days. This is a terrible ordeal for me and the hospital staff—much more so than for the parents who never set foot in the nursery.[1]

I can understand why some people are opposed to all euthanasia, and insist that such infants must be allowed to live. I think I can also understand why other people favor destroying these babies quickly and painlessly. But why should anyone favor letting "dehydration and infection wither a tiny being over hours and days"? The doctrine that says that a baby may be allowed to dehydrate and wither, but may not be given an injection that would end its life without suffering, seems so patently cruel as to require no further refutation. The strong language is not intended to offend, but only to put the point in the clearest possible way.

My second argument is that the conventional doctrine leads to decisions concerning life and death made on irrelevant grounds.

Consider again the case of the infants with [Down] syndrome who need operations for congenital defects unrelated to the syndrome to live. Sometimes, there is no operation, and the baby dies, but when there is no such defect, the baby lives on. Now, an operation such as that to remove an intestinal obstruction is not prohibitively difficult. The reason why such operations are not performed in these cases is, clearly, that the child has [Down] syndrome and the parents and doctor judge that because of that fact it is better for the child to die.

But notice that this situation is absurd, no matter what view one takes of the lives and potentials of such babies. If the life of such an infant is worth preserving, what does it matter if it needs a simple operation? Or, if one thinks it better that such a baby should not live on what difference does it make that it happens to have an unobstructed intestinal tract? In either case, the matter of life and death is being decided on irrelevant grounds. It is the [Down] syndrome, and not the intestines, that is the issue. The matter should be decided, if at all, on that basis, and not be allowed to depend on the essentially irrelevant question of whether the intestinal tract is blocked.

What makes this situation possible, of course, is the idea that when there is an intestinal blockage, one can "let the baby die," but when there is no such defect there is nothing that can be done, for one must not "kill" it. The fact that this idea leads to such results as deciding life or death on irrelevant grounds is another good reason why the doctrine should be rejected.

One reason why so many people think that there is an important moral difference between active and passive euthanasia is that they think killing someone is morally worse than letting someone die. But is it? Is killing, in itself, worse than letting die? To investigate this issue, two cases may be considered that are exactly alike except that one involves killing whereas the other involves letting someone die. Then, it can be asked whether this difference makes any difference to the moral assessments. It is important that the cases be exactly alike, except for this one difference, since otherwise one cannot be confident that it is this difference and not some other that accounts for any variation in the assessments of the two cases. So, let us consider this pair of cases:

In the first, Smith stands to gain a large inheritance if anything should happen to his six-year-old cousin. One evening while the child is taking his bath, Smith sneaks into the bathroom and drowns the child, and then arranges things so that it will look like an accident.

In the second, Jones also stands to gain if anything should happen to his six-year-old cousin. Like Smith, Jones sneaks in planning to drown the child in his bath. However, just as he enters the bathroom Jones sees the child slip and hit his head, and fall face down in the water. Jones is delighted; he stands by, ready to push the child's head back under if it is necessary, but it is not necessary. With only a little thrashing about, the child drowns all by himself, "accidentally," as Jones watches and does nothing.

Now Smith killed the child, whereas Jones "merely" let the child die. That is the only difference between them. Did either man behave better, from a moral point of view? If the difference between killing and letting die were in itself a morally important matter, one should say that Jones's behavior was less reprehensible than Smith's. But does one really want to say

that? I think not. In the first place, both men acted from the same motive, personal gain, and both had exactly the same end in view when they acted. It may be inferred from Smith's conduct that he is a bad man, although that judgment may be withdrawn or modified if certain further facts are learned about him—for example, that he is mentally deranged. But would not the very same thing be inferred about Jones from his conduct? And would not the same further considerations also be relevant to any modification of this judgment? Moreover, suppose Jones pleaded, in his own defense, "After all, I didn't do anything except just stand there and watch the child drown. I didn't kill him: I only let him die." Again, if letting die were in itself less bad than killing, this defense should have at least some weight. But it does not. Such a "defense" can only be regarded as a grotesque perversion of moral reasoning. Morally speaking, it is no defense at all.

Now, it may be pointed out, quite properly, that the case of euthanasia with which doctors are concerned are not like this at all. They do not involve personal gain or the destruction of normal healthy children. Doctors are concerned only with cases in which the patient's life is of no further use to him, or in which the patient's life has become or will soon become a terrible burden. However, the point is the same in these cases: the bare difference between killing and letting die does not, in itself, make a moral difference. If a doctor lets a patient die, for humane reasons, he is in the same moral position as if he had given the patient a lethal injection for humane reasons. If his decision was wrong—if, for example, the patient's illness was in fact curable—the decision would be equally regrettable no matter which method was used to carry it out. And if the doctor's decision was the right one, the method used is not in itself important.

The AMA policy statement isolates the crucial issue very well: the crucial issue is "the intentional termination of the life of one human being by another." But after identifying this issue, and forbidding "mercy killing," the statement goes on to deny that the cessation of treatment is the intentional termination of a life. This is where the mistake comes in, for what is the cessation of treatment, in these circumstances, if it is not "the intentional termination of the life of one human being by another"? Of course it is exactly that, and if it were not, there would be no point to it.

Many people will find this judgment hard to accept. One reason, I think, is that it is very easy to conflate the question of whether killing is, in itself, worse than letting die, with the very different question of whether most actual cases of killing are more reprehensible than most actual cases of letting die. Most actual cases of killing are clearly terrible (think, for example, of all the murders reported in the newspapers), and one hears of such cases every day. On the other hand, one hardly ever hears of a case of letting die, except for the actions of doctors who are motivated by humanitarian reasons. So one learns to think of killing in a much worse light than of letting die. But this does not mean that there is something about killing that makes it in itself worse than letting die, for it is not the bare difference between killing and letting die that makes the difference in these cases. Rather, the other factors—the murderer's motive of personal gain, for example, contrasted with the doctor's humanitarian motivation—account for different reactions to the different cases.

I have argued that killing is not in itself any worse than letting die: if my contention is right, it follows that active euthanasia is not any worse than passive euthanasia. What arguments can be given on the other side? The most common, I believe, is the following:

"The important difference between active and passive euthanasia is that, in passive euthanasia, the doctor does not do anything to bring about the patient's death. The doctor does nothing, and the patient dies of whatever ills already afflict him. In active euthanasia, however, the doctor does something to bring about the patient's death: he kills him. The doctor who gives the patient with cancer a lethal injection has himself caused his patient's death: whereas if he merely ceases treatment, the cancer is the cause of the death."

A number of points need to be made here. The first is that it is not exactly correct to say that in passive euthanasia the doctor does nothing, for he does do one thing that is very important: he lets the patient die. "Letting someone die" is certainly different, in some respects, from other types of action—mainly in that it is a kind of action that one may perform by way of not performing certain other actions. For example, one may let a patient die by way of not giving medication, just as one may insult someone by way of not shaking his hand. But for any purpose of moral assessment, it is a type of action nonetheless. The decision to let a patient die is subject to moral appraisal in the same way that a decision to kill him would be subject to moral appraisal: it may be assessed as wise or unwise, compassionate or sadistic, right or wrong. If a doctor deliberately let a patient die who was suffering from a routinely curable illness, the doctor would certainly be to blame for what he had done, just as he would be to blame if he had needlessly killed the patient. Charges against him would then be appropriate. If so, it would be no defense at all for him to insist that he didn't "do anything." He would have done something very serious indeed, for he let his patient die.

Fixing the cause of death may be very important from a legal point of view, for it may determine whether criminal charges are brought against the doctor. But I do not think that this notion can be used to show a moral difference between active and passive euthanasia. The reason why it is considered bad to be the cause of someone's death is that death is regarded as a great evil—and so it is. However, if it has been decided that euthanasia—even passive euthanasia—is desirable in a given case, it has also been decided that in this instance death is no greater an evil than the patient's continued existence. And if this is true, the usual reason for not wanting to be the cause of someone's death simply does not apply.

Finally, doctors may think that all of this is only of academic interest—the sort of thing that philosophers may worry about but that has no practical bearing on their own work. After all, doctors must be concerned about the legal consequences of what they do, and active euthanasia is clearly forbidden by the law. But even so, doctors should also be concerned with the fact that the law is forcing upon them a moral doctrine that may well be indefensible, and has a considerable effect on their practices. Of course, most doctors are not now in the position of being coerced in this matter, for they do not regard themselves as merely going along with what the law requires. Rather, in statements such as the AMA policy statement that I have quoted, they are endorsing this doctrine as a central point of medical ethics. In that statement, active euthanasia is condemned not merely as illegal but as "contrary to that for which the medical profession stands," whereas passive euthanasia is approved. However, the preceding considerations suggest that there is really no moral difference between the two, considered in themselves (there may be important moral differences in some cases in their *consequences*, but, as I pointed out, these differences may make active euthanasia, and not passive euthanasia, the morally preferable option). So, whereas doctors may have to discriminate between active and passive euthanasia to satisfy the law, they should not do any more than that. In particular, they should not give the distinction any added authority and weight by writing it into official statements of medical ethics.

NOTE

1. Anthony Shaw, "Doctor, Do We Have a Choice?" *New York Times Magazine,* 30 January 1972, 54.

The Wrongfulness of Euthanasia

J. Gay-Williams

My impression is that euthanasia—the idea, if not the practice—is slowly gaining acceptance within our society. Cynics might attribute this to an increasing tendency to devalue human life, but I do not believe this is the major factor. The acceptance is much more likely to be the result of unthinking sympathy and benevolence. Well-publicized, tragic stories like that of Karen Quinlan elicit from us deep feelings of compassion. We think to ourselves, "She and her family would be better off if she were dead." It is an easy step from this very human response to the view that if someone (and others) would be better off dead, then it might be all right to kill that person. Although I respect the compassion that leads to this conclusion, I believe the conclusion is wrong. I want to show that euthanasia is wrong. It is inherently wrong, but it is also wrong judged from the standpoints of self-interest and of practical effects.

Before presenting my arguments to support this claim, it would be well to define "euthanasia." An essential aspect of euthanasia is that it involves taking a human life, either one's own or that of another. Also, the person whose life is taken must be someone who is believed to be suffering from some disease or injury from which recovery cannot reasonably be expected. Finally, the action must be deliberate and intentional. Thus, euthanasia is intentionally taking the life of a presumably hopeless person. Whether the life is one's own or that of another, the taking of it is still euthanasia.

It is important to be clear about the deliberate and intentional aspect of the killing. If a hopeless person is given an injection of the wrong drug by mistake and this causes his death, this is wrongful killing but not euthanasia. The killing cannot be the result of accident. Furthermore, if the person is given an injection of a drug that is believed to be necessary to treat his disease or better his condition and the person dies as a result, then this is neither wrongful killing nor euthanasia. The intention was to make the patient well, not kill him. Similarly, when a patient's condition is such that it is not reasonable to hope that any medical procedures or treatments will save his life, a failure to implement the procedures or treatments is not euthanasia. If the person dies, this will be as a result of his injuries or disease and not because of his failure to receive treatment.

The failure to continue treatment after it has been realized that the patient has little chance of benefiting from it has been characterized by some as "passive euthanasia." This phrase is misleading and mistaken. In such cases, the person involved is not killed (the first essential aspect of euthanasia), nor is the death of the person intended by the withholding of additional treatment (the third essential aspect of euthanasia). The aim may be to spare the person additional and unjustifiable pain, to save him from the indignities of hopeless manipulations, and to avoid increasing the financial and emotional burden on his family. When I buy a pencil it is so that I can use it to write, not to contribute to an increase in the gross national product. This may be the unintended consequence of my action, but it is not the aim of my action. So it is with failing to continue the treatment of a dying person. I intend his death no more than I intend to reduce the GNP by not using medical supplies. His is an unintended dying, and so-called "passive euthanasia" is not euthanasia at all.

1. THE ARGUMENT FROM NATURE

Every human being has a natural inclination to continue living. Our reflexes and responses fit us to fight attackers, flee wild animals, and dodge out of the way of trucks. In our daily lives we exercise the caution and care necessary to protect ourselves. Our bodies are similarly structured for survival right down to the molecular level. When we are cut, our capillaries seal shut, our blood clots, and fibrogen is produced to start the process of healing the wound. When we are invaded by bacteria, antibodies are produced to fight against the alien organisms, and their remains are swept out of the body by special cells designed for clean-up work.

Euthanasia does violence to this natural goal of survival. It is literally acting against nature because all the processes of nature are bent towards the end of bodily survival. Euthanasia defeats these subtle mechanisms in a way that, in a particular case, disease and injury might not.

It is possible, but not necessary, to make an appeal to revealed religion in this connection. Man as trustee of his body acts against God, its rightful possessor, when he takes his own life. He also violates the commandment to hold life sacred and never to take it without just and compelling cause. But since this appeal will persuade only those who are prepared to accept that religion has access to revealed truths, I shall not employ this line of argument.

It is enough, I believe, to recognize that the organization of the human body and our patterns of behavioral responses make the continuation of life a natural goal. By reason alone, then, we can recognize that euthanasia sets us against our own nature. Furthermore, in doing so, euthanasia does violence to our dignity. Our dignity comes from seeking our ends. When one of our goals is survival, and actions are taken that eliminate that goal, then our natural dignity suffers. Unlike animals, we are conscious through reason of our nature and our ends. Euthanasia involves acting as if this dual nature—inclination towards survival and awareness of this as an end—did not exist. Thus, euthanasia denies our basic human character and requires that we regard ourselves or others as something less than fully human.

2. THE ARGUMENT FROM SELF-INTEREST

The above arguments are, I believe, sufficient to show that euthanasia is inherently wrong. But there are reasons for considering it wrong when judged by standards other than reason. Because death is final and irreversible, euthanasia contains within it the possibility that we will work against our own interest if we practice it or allow it to be practiced on us.

Contemporary medicine has high standards of excellence and a proven record of accomplishment, but it does not possess perfect and complete knowledge. A mistaken diagnosis is possible, and so is a mistaken prognosis. Consequently, we may believe that we are dying of a disease when, as a matter of fact, we may not be. We may think that we have no hope of recovery when, as a matter of fact, our chances are quite good. In such circumstances, if euthanasia were permitted, we would die needlessly. Death is final and the chance of error too great to approve the practice of euthanasia.

Also, there is always the possibility that an experimental procedure or a hitherto untried technique will pull us through. We should at least keep this option open, but euthanasia closes it off. Furthermore, spontaneous remission does occur in many cases. For no apparent reason, a patient simply recovers when those all around him, including his physicians, expected him to die. Euthanasia would just guarantee their expectations and leave no room for the "miraculous" recoveries that frequently occur.

Finally, knowing that we can take our life at any time (or ask another to take it) might well incline us to give up too easily. The will to live is strong in all of us, but it can be weakened by pain and suffering and feelings of hopelessness. If during a bad time we allow ourselves to be killed, we never have a chance to reconsider. Recovery from a serious illness requires that we fight for it, and anything that weakens our determination by suggesting that there is an easy way out is ultimately against our own interest. Also, we may be inclined towards euthanasia because of our concern for others. If we see our sickness and suffering as an emotional and financial burden on our family, we may feel that to leave our life is to make their lives easier. The very presence of the possibility of euthanasia may keep us from surviving when we might.

3. THE ARGUMENT FROM PRACTICAL EFFECTS

Doctors and nurses are, for the most part, totally committed to saving lives. A life lost is, for them, almost a personal failure, an insult to their skills and knowledge. Euthanasia as a practice might well alter this. It could have a corrupting influence so that in any case that is severe doctors and nurses might not try hard enough to save the patient. They might

decide that the patient would simply be "better off dead" and take the steps necessary to make that come about. This attitude could then carry over to their dealings with patients less seriously ill. The result would be an overall decline in the quality of medical care.

Finally, euthanasia as a policy is a slippery slope. A person apparently hopelessly ill may be allowed to take his own life. Then he may be permitted to deputize others to do it for him should he no longer be able to act. The judgment of others then becomes the ruling factor. Already at this point euthanasia is not personal and voluntary, for others are acting "on behalf of" the patient as they see fit. This may well incline them to act on behalf of other patients who have not authorized them to exercise their judgment. It is only a short step, then, from voluntary euthanasia (self-inflicted or authorized), to directed euthanasia administered to a patient who has given no authorization, to involuntary euthanasia conducted as part of a social policy. Recently many psychiatrists and sociologists have argued that we define as "mental illness" those forms of behavior that we disapprove of. This gives us license then to lock up those who display the behavior. The category of the "hopelessly ill" provides the possibility of even worse abuse. Embedded in a social policy, it would give society or its representatives the authority to eliminate all those who might be considered too "ill" to function normally any longer. The dangers of euthanasia are too great to all to run the risk of approving it in any form. The first slippery step may well lead to a serious and harmful fall.

I hope that I have succeeded in showing why the benevolence that inclines us to give approval of euthanasia is misplaced. Euthanasia is inherently wrong because it violates the nature and dignity of human beings. But even those who are not convinced by this must be persuaded that the potential personal and social dangers inherent in euthanasia are sufficient to forbid our approving it either as a personal practice or as a public policy.

Suffering is surely a terrible thing, and we have a clear duty to comfort those in need and to ease their suffering when we can. But suffering is also a natural part of life with values for the individual and for others that we should not overlook. We may legitimately seek for others and for ourselves an easeful death, as Arthur Dyck has pointed out.[1] Euthanasia, however, is not just an easeful death. It is a wrongful death. Euthanasia is not just dying. It is killing.

NOTE

1. Arthur Dyck, "Beneficent Euthanasia and Benemortasia," in *Beneficent Euthanasia,* ed. Marvin Kohl (Buffalo, NY: Prometheus Books, 1975), 177–29.

From *Voluntary Active Euthanasia*

DAN W. BROCK

* * *

THE CENTRAL ETHICAL ARGUMENT FOR VOLUNTARY ACTIVE EUTHANASIA

The central ethical argument for euthanasia is familiar. It is that the very same two fundamental ethical values supporting the consensus on patient's rights to decide about life-sustaining treatment also support the ethical permissibility of euthanasia. These values are individual self-determination or autonomy and individual well-being. By self-determination as it bears on euthanasia, I mean people's interest in making important decisions about their lives for themselves according to their own values or conceptions of a good life, and in being left free to act on those decisions. Self-determination is valuable because it permits people to form and live in accordance with their own conception of a good life, at least within the bounds of justice and consistent with others doing so as well. In exercising self-determination people take responsibility for their lives and for the kinds of persons they become. A central aspect of human dignity lies in people's capacity to direct their lives in this way. The value of exercising self-determination presupposes some minimum of decision making

Dan W. Brock, excerpts from "Voluntary Active Euthanasia" from *Hastings Center Report* 22(2): 10–22. Copyright © 1992 The Hastings Center. Reproduced with permission of John Wiley & Sons, Inc.

capacities or competence, which thus limits the scope of euthanasia supported by self-determination; it cannot justifiably be administered, for example, in cases of serious dementia or treatable clinical depression.

Does the value of individual self-determination extend to the time and manner of one's death? Most people are very concerned about the nature of the last stage of their lives. This reflects not just a fear of experiencing substantial suffering when dying, but also a desire to retain dignity and control during this last period of life. Death is today increasingly preceded by a long period of significant physical and mental decline, due in part to the technological interventions of modern medicine. Many people adjust to these disabilities and find meaning and value in new activities and ways. Others find the impairments and burdens in the last stage of their lives at some point sufficiently great to make life no longer worth living. For many patients near death, maintaining the quality of one's life, avoiding great suffering, maintaining one's dignity, and insuring that others remember us as we wish them to become of paramount importance and outweigh merely extending one's life. But there is no single, objectively correct answer for everyone as to when, if at all, one's life becomes all things considered a burden and unwanted. If self-determination is a fundamental value, then the great variability among people on this question makes it especially important that individuals control the manner, circumstances, and timing of their dying and death.

The other main value that supports euthanasia is individual well-being. It might seem that individual well-being conflicts with a person's self-determination when the person requests euthanasia. Life itself is commonly taken to be a central good for persons, often valued for its own sake, as well as necessary for pursuit of all other goods within a life. But when a competent patient decides to forgo all further life-sustaining treatment then the patient, either explicitly or implicitly, commonly decides that the best life possible for him or her with treatment is of sufficiently poor quality that it is worse than no further life at all. Life is no longer considered a benefit by the patient, but has now become a burden. The same judgment underlies a request for euthanasia: continued life is seen by the patient as no longer a benefit, but now a burden. Especially in the often severely compromised and debilitated states of many critically ill or dying patients, there is no objective standard, but only the competent patient's judgment of whether continued life is no longer a benefit.

Of course, sometimes there are conditions, such as clinical depression, that call into question whether the patient has made a competent choice, either to forgo life-sustaining treatment or to seek euthanasia, and then the patient's choice need not be evidence that continued life is no longer a benefit for him or her. Just as with decisions about treatment, a determination of incompetence can warrant not honoring the patient's choice: in the case of treatment, we then transfer decisional authority to a surrogate, though in the case of voluntary active euthanasia a determination that the patient is incompetent means that choice is not possible.

The value or right of self-determination does not entitle patients to compel physicians to act contrary to their own moral or professional values. Physicians are moral and professional agents whose own self-determination or integrity should be respected as well. If performing euthanasia became legally permissible, but conflicted with a particular physician's reasonable understanding of his or her moral or professional responsibilities, the care of a patient who requested euthanasia should be transferred to another.

Most opponents do not deny that there are some cases in which the values of patient self-determination and well-being support euthanasia. Instead, they commonly offer two kinds of arguments against it that on their view outweigh or override this support. The first kind of argument is that in any individual case where considerations of the patient's self-determination and well-being do support euthanasia, it is nevertheless always ethically wrong or impermissible. The second kind of argument grants that in some individual cases euthanasia may not be ethically wrong, but maintains nonetheless that public and legal policy should never permit it. The first kind of argument focuses on features of any individual case of euthanasia, while the second kind focuses on social or legal policy. In the next section I consider the first kind of argument.

* * *

WOULD THE BAD CONSEQUENCES OF EUTHANASIA OUTWEIGH THE GOOD?

The argument against euthanasia at the policy level is stronger than at the level of individual cases, though even here I believe the case is ultimately unpersuasive, or at best indecisive. The policy level is the place where the main issues lie, however, and where moral considerations that might override arguments in favor of euthanasia will be found, if they are found anywhere. It is important to note two kinds of disagreement about the consequences for public policy of permitting euthanasia. First, there is empirical or factual disagreement about what the consequences would be. This disagreement is greatly exacerbated by the lack of firm data on the issue. Second, since on any reasonable assessment there would be both good and bad consequences, there are moral disagreements about the relative importance of different effects. In addition to these two sources of disagreement, there is also no single, well-specified policy proposal for legalizing euthanasia on which policy assessments can focus. But without such specification, and especially without explicit procedures for protecting against well-intentioned misuse and ill-intentioned abuse, the consequences for policy are largely speculative.

Despite these difficulties, a preliminary account of the main likely good and bad consequences is possible. This should help clarify where better data or more moral analysis and argument are needed, as well as where policy safeguards must be developed.

Potential Good Consequences of Permitting Euthanasia

What are the likely good consequences? First, if euthanasia were permitted it would be possible to respect the self-determination of competent patients who want it, but now cannot get it because of its illegality. We simply do not know how many such patients and people there are. In the Netherlands, with a population of about 14.5 million (in 1987), estimates in a recent study were that about 1,900 cases of voluntary active euthanasia or physician-assisted suicide occur annually. No straightforward extrapolation to the United States is possible for many reasons, among them, that we do not know how many people here who want euthanasia now get it, despite its illegality. Even with better data on the number of persons who want euthanasia but cannot get it, significant moral disagreement would remain about how much weight should be given to any instance of failure to respect a person's self-determination in this way.

One important factor substantially affecting the number of persons who would seek euthanasia is the extent to which an alternative is available. The widespread acceptance in the law, social policy, and medical practice of the right of a competent patient to forgo life-sustaining treatment suggests that the number of competent persons in the United States who would want euthanasia if it were permitted is probably relatively small.

A second good consequence of making euthanasia legally permissible benefits a much larger group. Polls have shown that a majority of the American public believes that people should have a right to obtain euthanasia if they want.[1] No doubt the vast majority of those who support this right to euthanasia will never in fact come to want euthanasia for themselves. Nevertheless, making it legally permissible would reassure many people that if they ever do want euthanasia they would be able to obtain it. This reassurance would supplement the broader control over the process of dying given by the right to decide about life-sustaining treatment. Having fire insurance on one's house benefits all who have it, not just those whose houses actually burn down, by reassuring them that in the unlikely event of their house burning down, they will receive the money needed to rebuild it. Likewise, the legalization of euthanasia can be thought of as a kind of insurance policy against being forced to endure a protracted dying process that one has come to find burdensome and unwanted, especially when there is no life-sustaining treatment to forgo. The strong concern about losing control of their care expressed by many people who face serious illness likely to end in death suggests that they give substantial importance to the legalization of euthanasia as a means of maintaining this control.

A third good consequence of the legalization of euthanasia concerns patients whose dying is filled with severe and unrelievable pain or suffering. When there is a life-sustaining treatment that, if forgone, will lead relatively quickly to death, then doing so can bring an end to these patients' suffering without recourse to euthanasia. For patients receiving no such treatment, however, euthanasia may be the only release from their otherwise prolonged suffering and agony. This argument from mercy has always been the strongest argument for euthanasia in those cases to which it applies.

The importance of relieving pain and suffering is less controversial than is the frequency with which patients are forced to undergo untreatable agony that only euthanasia could relieve. If we focus first on suffering caused by physical pain, it is crucial to distinguish pain that could be adequately relieved with modern methods of pain control, though it in fact is not, from pain that is relievable only by death. For a variety of reasons, including some physicians' fear of hastening the patient's death, as well as the lack of a publicly accessible means for assessing the amount of the patient's pain, many patients suffer pain that could be, but is not, relieved.

Specialists in pain control, as for example the pain of terminally ill cancer patients, argue that there are very few patients whose pain could not be adequately controlled, though sometimes at the cost of so sedating them that they are effectively unable to interact with other people or their environment. Thus, the argument from mercy in cases of physical pain can probably be met in a large majority of cases by providing adequate measures of pain relief. This should be a high priority, whatever our legal policy on euthanasia—the relief of pain and suffering has long been, quite properly, one of the central goals of medicine. Those cases in which pain could be effectively relieved, but in fact is not, should only count significantly in favor of legalizing euthanasia if all reasonable efforts to change pain management techniques have been tried and have failed.

Dying patients often undergo substantial psychological suffering that is not fully or even principally the result of physical pain. The knowledge about how to relieve this suffering is much more limited than in the case of relieving pain, and efforts to do so are probably more often unsuccessful. If the argument from mercy is extended to patients experiencing great and unrelievable psychological suffering, the numbers of patients to which it applies are much greater.

One last good consequence of legalizing euthanasia is that once death has been accepted, it is often more humane to end life quickly and peacefully, when that is what the patient wants. Such a death will often be seen as better than a more prolonged one. People who suffer a sudden and unexpected death, for example by dying quickly or in their sleep from a heart attack or stroke, are often considered lucky to have died in this way. We care about how we die in part because we care about how others remember us, and we hope they will remember us as we were in "good times" with them and not as we might be when disease has robbed us of our dignity as human beings. As with much in the treatment and care of the dying, people's concerns differ in this respect, but for at least some people, euthanasia will be a more humane death than what they have often experienced with other loved ones and might otherwise expect for themselves.

Some opponents of euthanasia challenge how much importance should be given to any of these good consequences of permitting it, or even whether some would be good consequences at all. But more frequently, opponents cite a number of bad consequences that permitting euthanasia would or could produce, and it is to their assessment that I now turn.

Potential Bad Consequences of Permitting Euthanasia

Some of the arguments against permitting euthanasia are aimed specifically against physicians, while others are aimed against anyone being permitted to perform it. I shall first consider one argument of the former sort. Permitting physicians to perform euthanasia, it is said, would be incompatible with their fundamental moral and professional commitment as healers to care for patients and to protect life. Moreover, if euthanasia by physicians became common, patients would come to fear that a medication was intended not to treat or care, but instead to kill, and would thus lose trust in their physicians. This position was forcefully stated in a paper by Willard Gaylin and his colleagues:

> The very soul of medicine is on trial.... This issue touches medicine at its moral center; if this moral center collapses, if physicians become killers or are even licensed to kill, the profession—and, therewith, each physician—will never again be worthy of trust and respect as healer and comforter and protector of life in all its frailty.

These authors go on to make clear that, while they oppose permitting anyone to perform euthanasia, their special concern is with physicians doing so:

> We call on fellow physicians to say that they will not deliberately kill. We must also say to each of our fellow physicians that we will not tolerate killing of patients and that we shall take disciplinary action against doctors who kill. And we must say to the broader community that if it insists on tolerating or legalizing active euthanasia, it will have to find non-physicians to do its killing.[2]

If permitting physicians to kill would undermine the very "moral center" of medicine, then almost certainly physicians should not be permitted to perform euthanasia. But how persuasive is this claim? Patients should not fear, as a consequence of permitting voluntary active euthanasia, that their physicians will substitute a lethal injection for what patients want and believe is part of their care. If active euthanasia is restricted to cases in which it is truly voluntary, then no patient should fear getting it unless she or he has voluntarily requested it. (The fear that we might in time also come to accept nonvoluntary, or even involuntary, active euthanasia is a slippery slope worry I address below.) Patients' trust of their physicians could be increased, not eroded, by knowledge that physicians will provide aid in dying when patients seek it.

. . . In spelling out above what I called the positive argument for voluntary active euthanasia, I suggested that two principal values—respective patients' self-determination and promoting their well-being—underlie the consensus that competent patients, or the surrogates of incompetent patients, are entitled to refuse any life-sustaining treatment and to choose from among available alternative treatments. It is the commitment to these two values in guiding physicians' actions as healers, comforters, and protectors of their patients' lives that should be at the "moral center" of medicine, and these two values support physicians' administering euthanasia when their patients make competent requests for it.

What should not be at that moral center is a commitment to preserving patients' lives as such, without regard to whether those patients want their lives preserved or judge their preservation a benefit to them. . . .

A second bad consequence that some foresee is that permitting euthanasia would weaken society's commitment to provide optimal care for dying patients. We live at a time in which the control of health care costs has become, and is likely to continue to be, the dominant focus of health care policy. If euthanasia is seen as a cheaper alternative to adequate care and treatment, then we might become less scrupulous about providing sometimes costly support and other services to dying patients. Particularly if our society comes to embrace deeper and more explicit rationing of health care, frail, elderly, and dying patients will need to be strong and effective advocates for their own health care and other needs,

although they are hardly in a position to do this. We should do nothing to weaken their ability to obtain adequate care and services.

This second worry is difficult to assess because there is little firm evidence about the likelihood of the feared erosion in the care of dying patients. There are at least two reasons, however, for skepticism about this argument. The first is that the same worry could have been directed at recognizing patients' or surrogates' rights to forgo life-sustaining treatment, yet there is no persuasive evidence that recognizing the right to refuse treatment has caused a serious erosion in the quality of care of dying patients. The second reason for skepticism about this worry is that only a very small proportion of deaths would occur from euthanasia if it were permitted. In the Netherlands, where euthanasia under specified circumstances is permitted by the courts, though not authorized by statute, the best estimate of the proportion of overall deaths that result from it is about 2 percent.[3] Thus, the vast majority of critically ill and dying patients will not request it, and so will still have to be cared for by physicians, families, and others. Permitting euthanasia should not diminish people's commitment and concern to maintain and improve the care of these patients.

A third possible bad consequence of permitting euthanasia (or even a public discourse in which strong support for euthanasia is evident) is to threaten the progress made in securing the rights of patients or their surrogates to decide about and to refuse life-sustaining treatment. This progress has been made against the backdrop of a clear and firm legal prohibition of euthanasia, which has provided a relatively bright line limiting the dominion of others over patients' lives. It has therefore been an important reassurance to concerns about how the authority to take steps ending life might be misused, abused, or wrongly extended.

Many supporters of the right of patients or their surrogates to refuse treatment strongly oppose euthanasia, and if forced to choose might well withdraw their support of the right to refuse treatment rather than accept euthanasia. Public policy in the last fifteen years has generally let life-sustaining treatment decisions be made in health care settings between physicians and patients or their surrogates, and without the involvement of the courts. However, if euthanasia is made legally permissible greater involvement of the courts is likely, which could in turn extend to a greater court involvement in life-sustaining treatment decisions. Most agree, however, that increased involvement of the courts in these decisions would be undesirable, as it would make sound decisionmaking more cumbersome and difficult without sufficient compensating benefits.

As with the second potential bad consequence of permitting euthanasia, this third consideration too is speculative and difficult to assess. The feared erosion of patients' or surrogates' rights to decide about life-sustaining treatment, together with greater court involvement in those decisions, are both possible. However, I believe there is reason to discount this generally worry. The legal rights of competent patients and, to a lesser degree, surrogates of incompetent patients to decide about treatment are very firmly embedded in a long line of informed consent and life-sustaining treatment cases, and are not likely to be eroded by a debate over, or even acceptance of, euthanasia. It will not be accepted without safeguards that reassure the public about abuse, and if that debate shows the need for similar safeguards for some life-sustaining treatment decisions they should be adopted there as well. In neither case are the only possible safeguards greater court involvement, as the recent growth of institutional ethics committees shows.

The fourth potential bad consequence of permitting euthanasia . . . turns on the subtle point that making a new option or choice available to people can sometimes make them worse off, even if once they have the choice they go on to choose what is best for them. Ordinarily, people's continued existence is viewed by them as a given, a fixed condition with which they must cope. Making euthanasia available to people as an option denies them the alternative of staying alive by default. If people are offered the option of euthanasia, their continued existence is now a choice for which they can be held responsible and which they can be asked by others to justify. We care, and are right to care, about being able to justify ourselves to others. To the extent that our society is unsympathetic to justifying a severely dependent or impaired existence, a heavy psychological burden of proof may be placed on patients who think their terminal illness or chronic infirmity is not a sufficient reason for dying. Even if they otherwise view their life as worth living, the opinion of others around them that it is not can threaten their reason for living and make euthanasia a rational choice. Thus the existence of the option becomes a subtle pressure to request it.

This argument correctly identifies the reason why offering some patients the option of euthanasia would not benefit them. [David] Velleman takes it not as a reason for opposing all euthanasia, but for restricting it to circumstances where there are "unmistakable and overpowering reasons for persons to want the option of euthanasia,"[4] and for denying the option in all other cases. But there are at least three reasons why such restriction may not be warranted. First, polls and other evidence support that most Americans believe euthanasia should be permitted (though the recent defeat of the referendum to permit it in the state of Washington raises some doubt about this support). Thus, many more people seem to want the choice than would be made worse off by getting it. Second, if giving people the option of ending their life really makes them worse off, then we should not only prohibit euthanasia, but also take back from people the right they now have to decide about life-sustaining treatment. The feared harmful effect should already have occurred from securing people's right to refuse life-sustaining treatment, yet there is no evidence of any such widespread harm or any broad public desire to rescind that right. Third, since there is a wide range of conditions in which reasonable people can and do disagree about whether they would want continued life, it is not possible to restrict the permissibility of euthanasia as narrowly as Velleman suggests without thereby denying it to most persons who would want it; to permit it only in cases in which virtually everyone would want it would be to deny it to most who would want it.

A fifth potential bad consequence of making euthanasia legally permissible is that it might weaken the general legal prohibition of homicide. This prohibition is so fundamental to civilized society, it is argued, that we should do nothing that erodes it. If most cases of stopping life support are killing, as I have already argued, then the court cases permitting such killing have already in effect weakened this prohibition. However, neither the courts nor most people have seen these cases as killing and so as challenging the prohibition of homicide. The courts have usually grounded patients' or their surrogates' rights to refuse life-sustaining treatment in rights to privacy, liberty, self-determination, or bodily integrity, not in exceptions to homicide laws.

Legal permission for physicians or others to perform euthanasia could not be grounded in patients' rights to decide about medical treatment. Permitting euthanasia would require qualifying, at least in effect, the legal prohibition against homicide, a prohibition that in general does not allow the consent of the victim to justify or excuse the act. Nevertheless, the very same fundamental basis of the right to decide about life-sustaining treatment—respecting a person's self-determination—does support euthanasia as well. Individual self-determination has long been a well-entrenched and fundamental value in the law, and so extending it to euthanasia would not require appeal to novel legal values or principles. That suicide or attempted suicide is no longer a criminal offense in virtually all states indicates an acceptance of individual self-determination in the taking of one's own life analogous to that required for voluntary active euthanasia. The legal prohibition (in most states) of assisting in suicide and the refusal in the law to accept the consent of the victim as a possible justification of homicide are both arguably a result of difficulties in the legal process of establishing the consent of the victim after the fact. If procedures can be designed that clearly establish the voluntariness of the person's request for euthanasia it would under those procedures represent a carefully circumscribed qualification on the legal prohibition of homicide. Nevertheless, some remaining worries about this weakening can be captured in the final potential bad consequence, to which I will now turn.

This final potential bad consequence is the central concern of many opponents of euthanasia and, I believe, is the most serious objection to a legal policy permitting it. According to this "slippery slope" worry, although active euthanasia may be morally permissible in cases in which it is unequivocally voluntary and the patient finds his or her condition unbearable, a legal policy permitting euthanasia would inevitably lead to active euthanasia being performed in many other cases in which it would be morally wrong. To prevent those other wrongful cases of euthanasia we should not permit even morally justified performance of it.

Slippery slope arguments of this form are problematic and difficult to evaluate. From one perspective, they are the last refuge of conservative defenders of the status quo. When all the opponent's objections to the wrongness of euthanasia itself have been met, the opponent then shifts ground and acknowledges both that it is not in itself wrong and that a legal policy which resulted only in its being performed would not be bad. Nevertheless, the opponent maintains, it should still not be permitted because doing so would result in its being performed in other cases in which it is not voluntary and would be wrong. In this argument's most extreme form, permitting euthanasia is the first and fateful step down the slippery slope to Nazism. Once on the slope we will be unable to get off.

Now it cannot be denied that it is *possible* that permitting euthanasia could have these fateful consequences, but that cannot be enough to warrant prohibiting it if it is otherwise justified. A similar *possible* slippery slope worry could have been raised to securing competent patients' rights to decide about life support, but recent history shows such a worry would have been unfounded. It must be relevant how likely it is that we will end with horrendous consequences and an unjustified practice of euthanasia. How *like*, and *widespread* would the abuses and unwarranted extensions of permitting it be? By abuses, I mean the performance of euthanasia that fails to satisfy the conditions required for voluntary active euthanasia, for example, if the patient has been subtly pressured to accept it. By unwarranted extensions of policy, I mean later changes in legal policy to permit not just voluntary euthanasia, but also euthanasia in cases in which, for example, it need not be fully voluntary.

Opponents of voluntary euthanasia on slippery slope grounds have not provided the data or evidence necessary to turn their speculative concerns into well-grounded likelihoods.

It is at least clear, however, that both the character and likelihood of abuses of a legal policy permitting euthanasia depend in significant part on the procedures put in place to protect against them. I will not try to detail fully what such procedures might be, but will just give some examples of what they might include:

1. The patient should be provided with all relevant information about his or her medical condition, current prognosis, available alternative treatments, and the prognosis of each.
2. Procedures should ensure that the patient's request for euthanasia is stable or enduring (a brief waiting period could be required) and fully voluntary (an advocate for the patient might be appointed to ensure this).
3. All reasonable alternatives must have been explored for improving the patient's quality of life and relieving any pain or suffering.
4. A psychiatric evaluation should ensure that the patient's request is not the result of a treatable psychological impairment such as depression.

These examples of procedural safeguards are all designed to ensure that the patient's choice is fully informed, voluntary, and competent, and so a true exercise of self-determination. Other proposals for euthanasia would restrict its permissibility further—for example, to the terminally ill—a restriction that cannot be supported by self-determination. Such additional restrictions might, however, be justified by concern for limiting potential harms from abuse. At the same time, it is important not to impose procedural or substantive safeguards so restrictive as to make euthanasia impermissible or practically infeasible in a wide range of justified cases.

These examples of procedural safeguards make clear that it is possible to substantially reduce, though not to eliminate, the potential for abuse of a policy permitting voluntary active euthanasia. Any legalization of the practice should be accompanied by a well-considered set of procedural safeguards together with an ongoing evaluation of its use. Introducing euthanasia into only a few states could be a form of carefully limited and controlled social experiment that would give us evidence about the benefits and harms of the practice. Even then firm and uncontroversial data may remain elusive, as the continuing controversy over what has taken place in the Netherlands in recent years indicates.[5]

* * *

THE ROLE OF PHYSICIANS

If euthanasia is made legally permissible, should physicians take part in it? Should only physicians be permitted to perform it, as is the case in the Netherlands? In discussing whether euthanasia is incompatible with medicine's commitment to curing, caring for, and comforting patients, I argued that it is not at odds with a proper understanding of the aims of medicine, and so need not undermine patients' trust in their physicians. If that argument is correct, then physicians probably should not be prohibited, either by law or by professional norms, from taking part in a legally permissible practice of euthanasia (nor, of course, should they be compelled to do so if their personal or professional scruples forbid it). Most physicians in the Netherlands appear not to understand euthanasia to be incompatible with their professional commitments.

Sometimes patients who would be able to end their lives on their own nevertheless seek the assistance of physicians. Physician involvement in such cases may have important benefits to patients and others beyond simply assuring the use of effective means. Historically, in the United States suicide has carried a strong negative stigma that many today believe unwarranted. Seeking a physician's assistance, or what can almost seem a physician's blessing, may be a way of trying to remove that stigma and show others that the decision for suicide was made with due seriousness and was justified under the circumstances. The physician's involvement provides a kind of social approval, or more accurately helps counter what would otherwise be unwarranted social disapproval.

There are also at least two reasons for restricting the practice of euthanasia to physicians only. First, physicians would inevitably be involved in some of the important procedural safeguards necessary to a defensible practice, such as seeing to it that the patient is well-informed about his or her condition, prognosis, and possible treatments, and ensuring that all reasonable means have been taken to improve the quality of the patient's life. Second, and probably more important, one necessary protection against abuse of the practice is to limit the persons given authority to perform it, so that they can be held accountable for their exercise of that authority. Physicians, whose training and professional norms give some assurance that they would perform euthanasia responsibly, are an appropriate group of persons to whom the practice may be restricted.

* * *

NOTES

1. P. Painton and E. Taylor, "Love or Let Die," *Time*, 19 March 1990, 62–71; Boston Globe/Harvard University Poll, *Boston Globe*, 3 November 1991.

2. Willard Gaylin, Leon R. Kass, Edmund D. Pellegrino, and Mark Siegler, "Doctors Must Not Kill," *Journal of the American Medical Association* 259 (1988): 2139–40.

3. Paul J. Van der Maas et al., "Euthanasia and Other Medical Decisions Concerning the End of Life," *Lancet* 338 (1991): 669–74.

4. David Velleman commented on an earlier version of the paper delivered at the American Philosophical Association Central Division meetings.

5. Richard Fenigsen, "A Case against Dutch Euthanasia," *Special Supplement, Hastings Center Report* 19, no. 1 (1989): 22–30.

Euthanasia

PHILIPPA FOOT

The widely used *Shorter Oxford English Dictionary* gives three meanings for the word "euthanasia": the first, "a quiet and easy death"; the second, "the means of procuring this"; and the third, "the action of inducing a quiet and easy death." It is a curious fact that no one of the three gives an adequate definition of the word as it is usually understood. For "euthanasia" means much more than a quiet and easy death, or the means of procuring it, or the action of inducing it. The definition species only the manner of the death, and if this were all that was implied a murderer, careful to drug his victim, could claim that his act was an act of euthanasia. We find this ridiculous because we

take it for granted that in euthanasia it is death itself, not just the manner of death, that must be kind to the one who dies.

To see how important it is that "euthanasia" should not be used as the dictionary definition allows it to be used, merely to signify that a death was quiet and easy, one has only to remember that Hitler's "euthanasia" program traded on this ambiguity. Under this program, planned before the War but brought into full operation by a decree of 1 September 1939, some 275,000 people were gassed in centers which were to be a model for those in which Jews were later exterminated. Anyone in a state institution could be sent to the gas chambers if it was considered that he could not be "rehabilitated" for useful work. As Dr. Leo Alexander reports, relying on the testimony of a neuropathologist who received 500 brains from one of the killing centers,

In Germany the exterminations included the mentally defective, psychotics (particularly schizophrenics), epileptics and patients suffering from infirmities of old age and from various organic neurological disorders such as infantile paralysis, Parkinsonism, multiple sclerosis and brain tumors. . . . In truth, all those unable to work and considered nonrehabilitable were killed.[1]

These people were killed because they were "useless" and "a burden on society"; only the manner of their deaths could be thought of as relatively easy and quiet.

Let us insist, then, that when we talk about euthanasia we are talking about a death understood as a good or happy event for the one who dies. This stipulation follows etymology, but is itself not exactly in line with current usage, which would be captured by the condition that the death should *not* be an evil rather than that it *should* be a good. That this is how people talk is shown by the fact that the case of Karen Ann Quinlan and others in a state of permanent coma is often discussed under the heading of "euthanasia." Perhaps it is not too late to object to the use of the word "euthanasia" in this sense. Apart from the break with the Greek origins of the word there are other unfortunate aspects of this extension of the term. For if we say that the death must be supposed to be a good to the subject we can also specify that it shall be for his sake that an act of euthanasia is performed. If we say merely that death shall not be an evil to him, we cannot stipulate that benefiting him shall be the motive where euthanasia is in question. Given the importance of the question, For whose sake are we acting? it is good to have a definition of euthanasia which brings under this heading only cases of opting for death for the sake of the one who dies. Perhaps what is most important is to say either that euthanasia is to be for the good of the subject or at least that death is to be no evil to him, thus refusing to talk Hitler's language. However, in this paper it is the first condition that will be understood, with the additional proviso that by an act of euthanasia we mean one of inducing or otherwise opting for death for the sake of the one who is to die.

A few lesser points need to be cleared up. In the first place it must be said that the word "act" is not to be taken to exclude omission: we shall speak of an act of euthanasia when someone is deliberately allowed to die, for his own good, and not only when positive measures are taken to see that he does. The very general idea we want is that of a choice of action or inaction directed at another man's death and causally effective in the sense that, in conjunction with actual circumstances, it is a sufficient condition of death. Of complications such as overdetermination, it will not be necessary to speak.

A second, and definitely minor, point about the definition of an act of euthanasia concerns the question of fact versus belief. It has already been implied that one who performs an act of euthanasia thinks that death will be merciful for the subject since we have said that it is on account of this thought that the act is done. But is it enough that he acts with this thought, or must things actually be as he thinks them to be? If one man kills another, or allows him to die, thinking that he is in the last stages of a terrible disease, though in fact he could have been cured, is this an act of euthanasia or not? Nothing much seems to hang on our decision about this. The same condition has got to enter into the definition whether as an element in reality or only as an element in the agent's belief. And however we define an act of euthanasia culpability or justifiability will be the same: if a man acts through ignorance his ignorance may be culpable or it may not.[2]

These are relatively easy problems to solve, but one that is dauntingly difficult has been passed over in this discussion of the definition, and must now be faced. It is easy to say, as if this raised no problems, that an act of euthanasia is by definition one aiming at the *good* of the one whose death is in question, and that it is *for his sake* that his death is desired. But how is this to be explained? Presumably we are thinking of some evil already with him or to come on him if he continues to live, and death is thought of as a release from this evil. But this cannot be enough. Most people's lives contain evils such as grief or pain, but we do not therefore think that death would be a blessing to them. On the contrary life is generally supposed to be a good even for someone who is unusually unhappy or frustrated. How is it that one can ever wish for death for the sake of the one who is to die? This difficult question is central to the discussion of euthanasia, and we shall literally not know what we are talking about if we ask whether acts of euthanasia defined as we have defined them are ever morally permissible without first understanding better the reason for saying that life is a good, and the possibility that it is not always so.

If a man should save my life he would be my benefactor. In normal circumstances this is plainly true; but does one always benefit another in saving his life? It seems certain that he does not. Suppose, for instance, that a man were being tortured to death and was given a drug that lengthened his sufferings; this would not be a benefit but the reverse. Or suppose that in a ghetto in Nazi Germany a doctor saved the life of someone threatened by disease, but that the man once cured was transported to an extermination camp; the doctor might wish for the sake of the patient that he had died of the disease. Nor would a longer stretch of life always be a benefit to the person who was given it. Comparing Hitler's camps with those of Stalin, Dmitri Panin observes that in the latter the method of extermination was made worse by agonies that could stretch out over months.

> Death from a bullet would have been bliss compared with what many millions had to endure while dying of hunger. The kind of death to which they were condemned has nothing to equal it in treachery and sadism.[3]

These examples show that to save or prolong a man's life is not always to do him a service: it may be better for him if he dies earlier rather than later. It must therefore be agreed that while life is normally a benefit to the one who has it, this is not always so.

The judgment is often fairly easy to make—that life is or is not a good to someone—but the basis for it is very hard to find. When life is said to be a benefit or a good, on what grounds is the assertion made?

The difficulty is underestimated if it is supposed that the problem arises from the fact that one who is dead has nothing, so that the good someone gets from being alive cannot be compared with the amount he would otherwise have had. For why should this particular comparison be necessary? Surely it would be enough if one could say whether or not someone whose life was prolonged had more good than evil in the extra stretch of time. Such estimates are not always possible, but frequently the year; we say, for example, "He was very happy in those last years," or, "He had little but unhappiness then." If the balance of good and evil determined whether life was a good to someone we would expect to find a correlation in the judgments. In fact, of course, we find nothing of the kind. First, a man who has no doubt that existence is a good to him may have no idea about the balance of happiness and unhappiness in his life, or of any other positive and negative factors that may be suggested. So the supposed criteria are not always operating where the judgment is made. And secondly the application of the criteria gives an answer that is often wrong. Many people have more evil than good in their lives; we do not, however, conclude that we would do these people no service by rescuing them from death.

To get around this last difficulty Thomas Nagel has suggested that experience itself is a good which must be brought in to balance accounts.

> . . . life is worth living even when the bad elements of experience are plentiful, and the good ones too meager to outweigh the bad ones on their own. The additional positive weight is supplied by experience itself, rather than by any of its contents.[4]

This seems implausible because if experience itself is a good it must be so even when what we experience is wholly bad, as in being tortured to death. How should one decide how much to count for this experiencing; and why count anything at all?

Others have tried to solve the problem by arguing that it is a man's desire for life that makes us call life a good: if he wants to live then anyone who prolongs his life does him a benefit. Yet someone may cling to life where we would say confidently that it would be better for him if he died, and he may admit it too. Speaking of those same conditions in which, as he said, a bullet would have been merciful, Panin writes,

> I should like to pass on my observations concerning the absence of suicides under the extremely severe conditions of our concentration camps. The more that life became desperate, the more a prisoner seemed determined to hold onto it.[5]

One might try to explain this by saying that hope was the ground of this wish to survive for further days and months in the camp. But there is nothing unintelligible in the idea that a man might cling to life though he knew those facts about his future which would make any charitable man wish that he might die.

The problem remains, and it is hard to know where to look for a solution. Is there a conceptual connection between *life* and *good?* Because life is not always a good we are apt to reject this idea, and to think that it must be a contingent fact that life is usually a good, as it is a contingent matter that legacies are usually a benefit, if they are. Yet it seems not to be a contingent matter that to save someone's life is ordinarily to benefit him. The problem is to find where the conceptual connection lies.

It may be good tactics to forget for a time that it is euthanasia we are discussing and to see how *life* and *good* are connected in the case of living beings other than men. Even plants have things done to them that are harmful or beneficial, and what does them good must be related in some way to their living and dying. Let us therefore consider plants and animals, and then come back to human beings. At least we shall get away from the temptation to think that the connection between life and benefit must everywhere be a matter of happiness and unhappiness or of pleasure and pain; the idea being absurd in the case of animals and impossible even to formulate for plants.

In case anyone thinks that the concept of the beneficial applies only in a secondary or analogical way to plants, he should be reminded that we speak quite straightforwardly in saying, for instance, that a certain amount of sunlight is beneficial to most plants. What is in question here is the habitat in which plants of particular species flourish, but we can also talk, in a slightly different way, of what does them good, where there is some suggestion of improvement or remedy. What has the beneficial to do with sustaining life? It is tempting to answer, "everything," thinking that a healthy condition just is the one apt to secure survival. In fact, however, what is beneficial to a plant may have to do with reproduction rather than the survival of the individ-

ual member of the species. Nevertheless there is a plain connection between the beneficial and the life-sustaining even for the individual plant; if something makes it better able to survive in conditions normal for that species it is ipso facto good for it. We need go no further, and could go no further, in explaining why a certain environment or treatment is good for a plant than to show how it helps this plant to survive.[6]

This connection between the life-sustaining and the beneficial is reasonably unproblematic, and there is nothing fanciful or zoomorphic in speaking of benefiting or doing good to plants. A connection with its survival can make something beneficial to a plant. But this is not, of course, to say that we count life as a good to a plant. We may save its life by giving it what is beneficial; we do not benefit it by saving its life.

A more ramified concept of benefit is used in speaking of animal life. New things can be said, such as that an animal is better or worse off for something that happened, or that it was a good or bad thing for it that it did happen. And new things count as benefit. In the first place, there is comfort, which often is, but need not be, related to health. When loosening a collar which is too tight for a dog we can say, "That will be better for it." So we see that the words "better for it" have two different meanings which we mark when necessary by a difference of emphasis, saying "better *for* it" when health is involved. And secondly an animal can be benefited by having its life saved. "Could you do anything for it?" can be answered by, "Yes, I managed to save its life." Sometimes we may understand this, just as we would for a plant, to mean that we had checked some disease. But we can also do something for an animal by scaring away its predator. If we do this, it is a good thing for the animal that we did, unless of course it immediately meets a more unpleasant end by some other means. Similarly, on the bad side, an animal may be worse off for our intervention, and this not because it pines or suffers but simply because it gets killed.

The problem that vexes us when we think about euthanasia comes on the scene at this point. For if we can do something for an animal—can benefit it—by relieving its suffering but also by saving its life, where does the greater benefit come when only death will end pain? It seemed that life was a good in its own right; yet pain seemed to be an evil with equal status and could therefore make life not a good after all. Is it only life without pain that is a good when animals are concerned? This does not seem a crazy suggestion when we are thinking of animals, since unlike human beings they do not have suffering as part of their normal life. But it is perhaps the idea of ordinary life that matters here. We would not say that we had done anything for an animal if we had merely kept it alive, either in an unconscious state or in a condition where, though conscious, it was unable to operate in an ordinary way; and the fact is that animals in severe and continuous pain simply do not operate normally. So we do not, on the whole, have the option of doing the animal good by saving its life though the life would be a life of pain. No doubt there are borderline cases, but that is no problem. We are not trying to make new judgments possible, but rather to find the principle of the ones we do make.

When we reach human life the problems seem even more troublesome. For now we must take quite new things into account, such as the subject's own view of his life. It is arguable that this places extra constraints on the solution: might it not be counted as a necessary condition of life's being a good to a man that he should see it as such? Is there not some difficulty about the idea that a benefit might be done to him by the saving or prolonging of his life even though he himself wished for death? Of course he might have a quite mistaken view of his own prospects, but let us ignore this and think only of cases where it is life as he knows it that is in question. Can we think that the prolonging of his life would be a benefit to him even though he would rather have it end than continue? It seems that this cannot be ruled out. That there is no simple incompatibility between life as a good and the wish for death is shown by the possibility that a man should wish himself dead, not for his own sake, but for the sake of someone else. And if we try to amend the thesis to say that life cannot be a good to one who wishes *for his own sake* that he should die, we find the crucial concept slipping

through our fingers. As Bishop Butler pointed out long ago not all ends are either benevolent or self-interested. Does a man wish for death for his own sake in the relevant sense if, for instance, he wishes to revenge himself on another by his death? Or what if he is proud and refuses to stomach dependence or incapacity even though there are many good things left in life for him? The truth seems to be that the wish for death is sometimes compatible with life's being a good and sometimes not, which is possible because the description "wishing for death" is one covering diverse states of mind from that of the determined suicide, pathologically depressed, to that of one who is surprised to find that the thought of a fatal accident is viewed with relief. On the one hand, a man may see his life as a burden but go about his business in a more or less ordinary way; on the other hand, the wish for death may take the form of a rejection of everything that is in life, as it does in severe depression. It seems reasonable to say that life is not a good to one permanently in the latter state, and we must return to this topic later on.

When are we to say that life is a good or a benefit to a man? The dilemma that faces us is this. If we say that life as such is a good we find ourselves refuted by the examples given at the beginning of this discussion. We therefore incline to think that it is as bringing good things that life is a good, where it is a good. But if life is a good only because it is the condition of good things why is it not equally an evil when it brings bad things? And how can it be a good even when it brings more evil than good?

It should be noted that the problem has here been formulated in terms of the balance of good and evil, not that of happiness and unhappiness, and that it is not to be solved by the denial (which may be reasonable enough) that unhappiness is the only evil or happiness the only good. In this paper no view has been expressed about the nature of goods other than life itself. The point is that on any view of the goods and evils that life can contain, it seems that a life with more evil than good could still itself be a good.

It may be useful to review the judgments with which our theory must square. Do we think that life can be a good to one who suffers a lot of pain? Clearly we do. What about severely handicapped people; can life be a good to them? Clearly it can be, for even if someone is almost completely paralyzed, perhaps living in an iron lung, perhaps able to move things only by means of a tube held between his lips, we do not rule him out of order if he says that some benefactor saved his life. Nor is it different with mental handicap. There are many fairly severely handicapped people—such as those with [Down] Syndrome (Mongolism)—for whom a simple affectionate life is possible. What about senility? Does this break the normal connection between life and good? Here we must surely distinguish between forms of senility. Some forms leave a life which we count someone as better off having than not having, so that a doctor who prolonged it would benefit the person concerned. With some kinds of senility this is however no longer true. There are some in geriatric wards who are barely conscious, though they can move a little and swallow food put into their mouths. To prolong such a state, whether in the old or in the very severely mentally handicapped is not to do them a service or confer a benefit. But of course it need not be the reverse: only if there is suffering would one wish for the sake of the patient that he should die.

It seems, therefore, that merely being alive even without suffering is not a good, and that we must make a distinction similar to that which we made when animals were our topic. But how is the line to be drawn in the case of men? What is to count as ordinary human life in the relevant sense? If it were only the very senile or very ill who were to be said not to have this life it might seem right to describe it in terms of *operation*. But it will be hard to find the sense in which the men described by Panin were not operating, given that they dragged themselves out to the forest to work. What is it about the life that the prisoners were living that makes us put it on the other side of the dividing line from that of some severely ill or suffering patients, and from most of the physically or mentally handicapped? It is not that they were in captivity, for life in captivity can certainly be a good. Nor is it merely the unusual nature of their life. In some ways the prisoners were living more as other men do than the patient in an iron lung.

The suggested solution to the problem is, then, that there is a certain conceptual connection between *life* and *good* in the case of human beings as in that of animals and even plants. Here, as there, however, it is not the mere state of being alive that can determine, or itself count as, a good, but rather life coming up to some standard of normality. It was argued that it is as part of ordinary life that the elements of good that a man may have are relevant to the question of whether saving his life counts as benefiting him. Ordinary human lives, even very hard lives, contain a minimum of basic goods, but when these are absent the idea of life is no longer linked to that of good. And since it is in this way that the elements of good contained in a man's life are relevant to the question of whether he is benefited if his life is preserved, there is no reason why it should be the balance of good and evil that counts.

It should be added that evils are relevant in one way when, as in the examples discussed above, they destroy the possibility of ordinary goods, but in a different way when they invade a life from which the goods are already absent for a different reason. So, for instance, the connection between *life* and *good* may be broken because consciousness has sunk to a very low level, as in extreme senility or severe brain damage. In itself this kind of life seems to be neither good nor evil, but if suffering sets in one would hope for a speedy end.

The idea we need seems to be that of life which is ordinary human life in the following respect—that it contains a minimum of basic human goods. What is ordinary in human life—even in very hard lives—is that a man is not driven to work far beyond his capacity; that he has the support of a family or community; that he can more or less satisfy his hunger; that he has hopes for the future; that he can lie down to rest at night. Such things were denied to the men in the Vyatlag camps described by Panin; not even rest at night was allowed them when they were tormented by bed-bugs, by noise and stench, and by routines such as body-searches and bath-parades—arranged for the night time so that work norms would not be reduced. Disease too can so take over a man's life that the normal human goods disappear.

When a patient is so overwhelmed by pain or nausea that he cannot eat with pleasure, if he can eat at all, and is out of the reach of even the most loving voice, he no longer has ordinary human life in the sense in which the words are used here. And we may now pick up a thread from an earlier part of the discussion by remarking that crippling depression can destroy the enjoyment of ordinary goods as effectively as external circumstances can remove them.

This, admittedly inadequate, discussion of the sense in which life is normally a good, and of the reasons why it may not be so in some particular case, completes the account of what euthanasia is here taken to be. An act of euthanasia, whether literally act or rather omission, is attributed to an agent who opts for the death of another because in his case life seems to be an evil rather than a good. The question now to be asked is whether acts of euthanasia are ever justifiable. But there are two topics here rather than one. For it is one thing to say that some acts of euthanasia considered only in themselves and their results are morally unobjectionable, and another to say that it would be all right to legalize them. Perhaps the practice of euthanasia would allow too many abuses, and perhaps there would be too many mistakes. Moreover the practice might have very important and highly undesirable side effects, because it is unlikely that we could change our principles about the treatment of the old and the ill without changing fundamental emotional attitudes and social relations. The topics must, therefore, be treated separately. In the next part of the discussion, nothing will be said about the social consequences and possible abuses of the practice of euthanasia, but only about acts of euthanasia considered in themselves.

What we want to know is whether acts of euthanasia, defined as we have defined them, are ever morally permissible. To be more accurate, we want to know whether it is ever sufficient justification of the choice of death for another that death can be counted a benefit rather than harm, and that this is why the choice is made.

It will be impossible to get a clear view of the area to which this topic belongs without first marking the distinct grounds on which objection may lie when one man ops for the death of another. There are two different virtues whose requirements are, in general, contrary to such actions. An unjustified act of killing, or allowing to die, is contrary to justice or to charity, or to both virtues, and the moral failings are distinct. Justice has to do with what men *owe* each other in the way of noninterference and positive service. When used in this wide sense, which has its history in the doctrine of the cardinal virtues, justice is not especially connected with, for instance, law courts but with the whole area of rights, and duties corresponding to rights. Thus murder is one form of injustice, dishonesty another, and wrongful failure to keep contracts a third; chicanery in a law court or defrauding someone of his inheritance are simply other cases of injustice. Justice as such is not directly linked to the good of another, and may require that something be rendered to him even where it will do him harm, as Hume pointed out when he remarked that a debt must be paid even to a profligate debauchee who "would rather receive harm than benefit from large possessions."[7] Charity, on the other hand, is the virtue which attaches us to the good of others. An act of charity is in question only where something is not demanded by justice, but a lack of charity and of justice can be shown where a man is denied something which he both needs and has a right to; both charity and justice demand that widows and orphans are not defrauded, and the man who cheats them is neither charitable nor just.

It is easy to see that the two grounds of objection to inducing death are distinct. A murder is an act of injustice. A culpable failure to come to the aid of someone whose life is threatened is normally contrary, not to justice, but to charity. But where one man is under contract, explicit or implicit, to come to the aid of another injustice too will be shown. Thus injustice may be involved either in an act or an omission, and the same is true of a lack of charity; charity may demand that someone be aided, but also that an unkind word not be spoken.

The distinction between charity and justice will turn out to be of the first importance when voluntary and nonvoluntary euthanasia are distinguished later on. This is because of the connection between justice and rights, and something should now be said about this. I believe it is true to say that wherever a man acts unjustly he has infringed a right, since justice has to do with whatever a man is owed, and whatever he is owed is his as a matter of right. Something should therefore be said about the different kinds of rights. The distinction commonly made is between having a right in the sense of having a liberty, and having a "claim-right" or "right of recipience." The best way to understand such a distinction seems to be as follows. To say that a man has a right in the sense of liberty is to say that no one can demand that he do not do the thing which he has a right to do. The fact that he has a right to do it consists in the fact that a certain kind of objection does not lie against his doing it. Thus a man has a right in this sense to walk down a public street or park his car in a public parking space. It does not follow that no one else may prevent him from doing so. If for some reason I want a certain man not to park in a certain place I may lawfully park there myself or get my friends to do so, thus preventing him from doing what he has a right (in the sense of a liberty) to do. It is different, however, with a claim-right. This is the kind of right which I have in addition to a liberty when, for example, I have a private parking space; now others have duties in the way of noninterference, as in this case, or of service, as in the case where my claim-right is to goods or services promised to me. Sometimes one of these rights gives other people the duty of securing to me that to which I have a right, but at other times their duty is merely to refrain from interference. If a fall of snow blocks my private parking space there is normally no obligation for anyone else to clear it away. Claim-rights generate duties; sometimes these duties are duties of noninterference; sometimes they are duties of service. If your right gives me the duty not to interfere with you I have "no right" to do it; similarly, if your right gives me the duty to provide something for you I have "no right" to refuse to do it. What *I* lack is the right which is a liberty; I am not "at liberty" to interfere with you or to refuse the service.

Where in this picture does the right to life belong? No doubt people have the right to live in the sense of a liberty, but what is important is the cluster of claim-rights brought together under the title of the right to life. The chief of these is, of course, the right to be free from interferences that threaten life. If other people aim their guns at us or try to pour poison into our drink we can, to put it mildly, demand that they desist. And then there are the services we can claim from doctors, health officers, bodyguards, and firemen; the rights that depend on contract or public arrangement. Perhaps there is no particular point in saying that the duties these people owe us belong to the right to life; we might as well say that all the services owed to anyone by tailors, dressmakers, and couturiers belong to a right called the right to be elegant. But contracts such as those understood in the patient-doctor relationship come in an important way when we are discussing the rights and wrongs of euthanasia, and are therefore mentioned here.

Do people have the right to what they need in order to survive, apart from the right conferred by special contracts into which other people have entered for the supplying of these necessities? Do people in the underdeveloped countries in which starvation is rife have the right to the food they so evidently lack? Joel Feinberg, discussing this question, suggests that they should be said to have "a claim," distinguishing this from a "valid claim," which gives a claim-right.

> The manifesto writers on the other side who seem to identify needs, or at least basic needs, with what they call "human rights," are more properly described, I think, as urging upon the world community the moral principle that *all* basic human needs ought to be recognized as *claims* (in the customary *prima facie* sense) worthy of sympathy and serious consideration right now, even though, in many cases, they cannot yet plausibly be treated as *valid* claims, that is, as grounds of any other people's duties. This way of talking avoids the anomaly of ascribing to all human beings now, even those in pre-industrial societies, such "economic and social rights" as "periodic holidays with pay."[8]

This seems reasonable, though we notice that there are some actual rights to service which are not based on anything like a contract, as for instance the right that children have to support from their parents and parents to support from their children in old age, though both sets of rights are to some extent dependent on existing social arrangements.

Let us now ask how the right to life affects the morality of acts of euthanasia. Are such acts sometimes or always ruled out by the right to life? This is certainly a possibility; for although an act of euthanasia is, by our definition, a matter of opting for death for the good of the one who is to die, there is, as we noted earlier, no direct connection between that to which a man has a right and that which is for his good. It is true that men have the right only to the kind of thing that is, in general, a good: we do not think that people have the right to garbage or polluted air. Nevertheless, a man may have the right to something which he himself would be better off without; where rights exist it is a man's will that counts not his or anyone else's estimate of benefit or harm. So the duties complementary to the right to life—the general duty of noninterference and the duty of service incurred by certain persons—are not affected by the quality of a man's life or by his prospects. Even if it is true that he would be, as we say, "better off dead," so long as he wants to live this does not justify us in killing him and may not justify us in deliberately allowing him to die. All of us have the duty of noninterference, and some of us may have the duty to sustain his life. Suppose, for example, that a retreating army has to leave behind wounded or exhausted soldiers in the wastes of an arid or snowbound land where the only prospect is death by starvation or at the hands of an enemy notoriously cruel. It has often been the practice to accord a merciful bullet to men in such desperate straits. But suppose that one of them demands that he should be left alive? It seems clear that his comrades have no right to kill him, though it is a quite different question as to whether they should give him a life-prolonging drug. The right to life can sometimes give a duty of positive service, but does not do so here. What it does give is the right to be left alone.

Interestingly enough we have arrived by way of a consideration of the right to life at the distinction normally labeled "active" versus "passive" euthanasia, and often thought to be irrelevant to the moral issue. Once it is seen that the right to life is a distinct ground of objection to certain acts of euthanasia, and that this right creates a duty of noninterference more widespread than the duties of care there can be no doubt about the relevance of the distinction between passive and active euthanasia. Where everyone may have the duty to leave someone alone, it may be that no one has the duty to maintain his life, or that only some people do.

Where then do the boundaries of the "active" and "passive" lie? In some ways the words are themselves misleading, because they suggest the difference between act and omission which is not quite what we want. Certainly the act of shooting someone is the kind of thing we were talking about under the heading of "interference," and omitting to give him a drug a case of refusing care. But the act of turning off a respirator should surely be thought of as no different from the decision not to start it; if doctors had decided that a patient should be allowed to die, either course of action might follow, and both should be counted as passive rather than active euthanasia if euthanasia were in question. The point seems to be that interference in a course of treatment is not the same as other interference in a man's life, and particularly if the same body of people are responsible for the treatment and for its discontinuance. In such a case we could speak of the disconnecting of the apparatus as killing the man, or of the hospital as allowing him to die. By and large, it is the act of killing that is ruled out under the heading of noninterference, but not in every case.

Doctors commonly recognize this distinction, and the grounds on which some philosophers have denied it seem untenable. James Rachels, for instance, believes that if the difference between active and passive is relevant anywhere, it should be relevant everywhere, and he has pointed to an example in which it seems to make no difference which is done. If someone saw a child drowning in a bath it would seem just as bad to let it drown as to push its head under water. If "it makes no difference" means that one act would be as iniquitous as the other this is true. It is not that killing is *worse* than allowing to die, but that the two are contrary to distinct virtues, which gives the possibility that in some circumstances one is impermissible and the other permissible. In the circumstances invented by Rachels, both are wicked: it is contrary to justice to push the child's head under the water—something one has no right to do. To leave it to drown is not contrary to justice, but it is a particularly glaring example of lack of charity. Here it makes no practical difference because the requirements of justice and charity coincide; but in the case of the retreating army they did not: charity would have required that the wounded soldier be killed had not justice required that he be left alive.[9] In such a case it makes all the difference whether a man opts for the death of another in a positive action, or whether he allows him to die. An analogy with the right to property will make the point clear. If a man owns something he has the right to it even when its possession does him harm, and we have no right to take it from him. But if one day it should blow away, maybe nothing requires us to get it back for him; we could not deprive him of it, but we may allow it to go. This is not to deny that it will often be an unfriendly act or one based on an arrogant judgment when we refuse to do what he wants. Nevertheless, we would be within our rights, and it might be that no moral objection of any kind would lie against our refusal.

It is important to emphasize that a man's rights may stand between us and the action we would dearly like to take for his sake. They may, of course, also prevent action which we would like to take for the sake of others, as when it might be tempting to kill one man to save several. But it is interesting that the limits of allowable interference, however uncertain, seem stricter in the first case than the second. Perhaps there are no cases in which it would be all right to kill a man against his will *for his own sake* unless they could equally well be described as cases of allowing him to die, as in the example of turning off the respirator. However, there are circumstances, even if these are very rare, in which one man's life would justifiably be sacrificed to save others, and "killing" would be the only description of what was being done. For instance, a vehicle which had gone out of control might be steered from a path on which it would kill more than one man to a path on which it would kill one. But it would not be permissible to steer a vehicle towards someone in order to kill him, against his will, for his own good. An analogy with property rights illustrates the point. One may not destroy a man's property against his will on the grounds that he would be better off without it; there are however circumstances in which it could be destroyed for the sake of others. If his house is liable to fall and kill him that is his affair; it might, however, without injustice be destroyed to stop the spread of a fire.

We see then that the distinction between active and passive, important as it is elsewhere, has a special importance in the area of euthanasia. It should also be clear why James Rachels' other argument, that it is often "more humane" to kill than to allow to die, does not show that the distinction between active and passive euthanasia is morally irrelevant. It might be "more humane" in this sense to deprive a man of the property that brings evils on him, or to refuse to pay what is owed to Hume's profligate debauchee; but if we say this we must admit that an act which is "more humane" than its alternative may be morally objectionable because it infringes rights.

So far we have said very little about the right to service as opposed to the right to noninterference, though it was agreed that both might be brought under the heading of "the right to life." What about the duty to preserve life that may belong to special classes of persons such as bodyguards, firemen, or doctors? Unlike the general public they are not within their rights if they merely refrain from interfering and do not try to sustain life. The subject's claim-rights are two-fold as far as they are concerned and passive as well as active euthanasia may be ruled out here if it is against his will. This is not to say that he has the right to any and every service needed to save or prolong his life; the rights of other people set limits to what may be demanded, both because they have the right not to be interfered with and because they may have a competing right to services. Furthermore one must enquire just what the contract or implicit agreement amounts to in each case. Firemen and bodyguards presumably have a duty which is simply to preserve life, within the limits of justice to others and of reasonableness to themselves. With doctors it may however be different, since their duty relates not only to preserving life but also to the relief of suffering. It is not clear what a doctor's duties are to his patient if life can be prolonged only at the cost of suffering or suffering relieved only by measures that shorten life. George Fletcher has argued that what the doctor is under contract to do depends on what is generally done, because this is what a patient will reasonably expect.[10] This seems right. If procedures are part of normal medical practice then it seems that the patient can demand them however much it may be against his interest to do so. Once again it is not a matter of what is "most humane."

That the patient's right to life may set limits to permissible acts of euthanasia seems undeniable. If he does not want to die no one has the right to practice active euthanasia on him, and passive euthanasia may also be ruled out where he has a right to the services of doctors or others.

Perhaps few will deny what has so far been said about the impermissibility of acts of euthanasia simply because we have so far spoken about the case of one who positively wants to live, and about his rights, whereas those who advocate euthanasia are usually thinking either about those who wish to die or about those whose wishes cannot be ascertained either because they cannot properly be said to have wishes or because, for one reason or another, we are unable to form a reliable estimate of what they are. The question that must now be asked is whether the latter type of case, where euthanasia though not involuntary would again be nonvoluntary, is different from the one discussed so far. Would we have the right to kill someone for his own good so long as we had no idea that he positively wished to live? And what about the life-prolonging duties of doctors in the same circumstances? This is a very difficult problem. On the one hand, it seems ridiculous to suppose that a man's right to life is something which generates duties only where he has signaled that he wants to live; as a borrower does indeed have a duty to return something lent on indefinite loan only if the lender indicates that he wants it back. On the other

hand, it might be argued that there is something illogical about the idea that a right has been infringed if someone incapable of saying whether he wants it or not is deprived of something that is doing him harm rather than good. Yet on the analogy of property we would say that a right has been infringed. Only if someone had earlier told us that in such circumstances he would not want to keep the thing could we think that his right had been waived. Perhaps if we could make confident judgments about what anyone in such circumstances would wish, or what he would have wished beforehand had he considered the matter, we could agree to consider the right to life as "dormant," needing to be asserted if the normal duties were to remain. But as things are we cannot make any such assumption; we simply do not know what most people would want, or would have wanted, us to do unless they tell us. This is certainly the case so far as active measures to end life are concerned. Possibly it is different, or will become different, in the matter of being kept alive, so general is the feeling against using sophisticated procedures on moribund patients, and so much is this dreaded by people who are old or terminally ill. Once again the distinction between active and passive euthanasia has come on the scene, but this time because most people's attitudes to the two are so different. It is just possible that we might presume, in the absence of specific evidence, that someone would not wish, beyond a certain point, to be kept alive; it is certainly not possible to assume that he would wish to be killed.

In the last paragraph we have begun to broach the topic of voluntary euthanasia, and this we must now discuss. What is to be said about the case in which there is no doubt about someone's wish to die: either he has told us beforehand that he would wish it in circumstances such as he is now in, and has shown no sign of a change of mind, or else he tells us now, being in possession of his faculties and of a steady mind. We should surely say that the objections previously urged against acts of euthanasia, which it must be remembered were all on the ground of rights, had disappeared. It does not seem that one would infringe someone's right to life in killing him with his permission and in fact at his request. Why should someone not be able to waive his right to life, or rather, as would be more likely to happen, to cancel some of the duties of noninterference that this right entails? (He is more likely to say that he should be killed by this man at this time in this manner, than to say that anyone may kill him at any time and in any way.) Similarly someone may give permission for the destruction of his property, and request it. The important thing is that he gives a critical permission, and it seems that this is enough to cancel the duty normally associated with the right. If someone gives you permission to destroy his property it can no longer be said that you have no right to do so, and I do not see why it should not be the case with taking a man's life. An objection might be made on the ground that only God has the right to take life, but in this paper religious as opposed to moral arguments are being left aside. Religion apart, there seems to be no case to be made out for an infringement of rights if a man who wishes to die is allowed to die or even killed. But of course it does not follow that there is no moral objection to it. Even with property, which is after all a relatively small matter, one might be wrong to destroy what one had the right to destroy. For, apart from its value to other people, it might be valuable to the man who wanted it destroyed, and charity might require us to hold our hand where justice did not.

Let us review the conclusion of this part of the argument, which has been about euthanasia and the right to life. It has been argued that from this side come stringent restrictions on the acts of euthanasia that could be morally permissible. Active nonvoluntary euthanasia is ruled out by that part of the right to life which creates the duty of noninterference though passive nonvoluntary euthanasia is not ruled out, except where the right to life-preserving action has been created by some special condition such as a contract between a man and his doctor, and it is not always certain just what such a contract involves. Voluntary euthanasia is another matter: as the preceding paragraph suggested, no right is infringed if a man is allowed to die or even killed at his own request.

Turning now to the other objection that normally holds against inducing the death of another, that it is against charity, or benevolence, we must tell a very different story. Charity is the virtue that gives attachment to the good of others, and because life is normally a good, charity normally demands that it should be saved or prolonged. But as we so defined an act of euthanasia that it seeks a man's death for his own sake—for his good—charity will normally speak in favor of it. This is not, of course, to say that charity can require an act of euthanasia which justice forbids, but if an act of euthanasia is not contrary to justice—that is, it does not infringe rights—charity will rather be in its favor than against.

Once more the distinction between nonvoluntary and voluntary euthanasia must be considered. Could it ever be compatible with charity to seek a man's death although he wanted to live, or at least had not let us know that he wanted to die? It has been argued that in such circumstances active euthanasia would infringe his right to life, but passive euthanasia would not do so, unless he had some special right to life-preserving service from the one who allowed him to die. What would charity dictate? Obviously when a man wants to live there is a presumption that he will be benefited if his life is prolonged, and if it is so the question of euthanasia does not arise. But it is, on the other hand, possible that he wants to live where it would be better for him to die: perhaps he does not realize the desperate situation he is in, or perhaps he is afraid of dying. So, in spite of a very proper resistance to refusing to go along with a man's own wishes in the matter of life and death, someone might justifiably refuse to prolong the life even of someone who asked him to prolong it, as in the case of refusing to give the wounded soldier a drug that would keep him alive to meet a terrible end. And it is even more obvious that charity does not always dictate that life should be prolonged where a man's own wishes, hypothetical or actual, are not known.

So much for the relation of charity to nonvoluntary passive euthanasia, which was not, like nonvoluntary active euthanasia, ruled out by the right to life. Let us now ask what charity has to say about voluntary euthanasia both active and passive. It was suggested in the discussion of justice that if of sound mind and steady desire a man might give others the *right* to allow him to die or even to kill him, where otherwise this would be ruled out. But it was pointed out that this would not settle the question of whether the act was morally permissible, and it is this that we must now consider. Could not charity speak against what justice allowed? Indeed it might do so. For while the fact that a man wants to die suggests that his life is wretched, and while his rejection of life may itself tend to take the good out of the things he might have enjoyed, nevertheless his wish to die might here be opposed for his own sake just as it might be if suicide were in question. Perhaps there is hope that his mental condition will improve. Perhaps he is mistaken in thinking his disease incurable. Perhaps he wants to die for the sake of someone else on whom he feels he is a burden, and we are not ready to accept this sacrifice whether for ourselves or others. In such cases, and there will surely be many of them, it could not be for his own sake that we kill him or allow him to die, and therefore euthanasia as defined in this paper would not be in question. But this is not to deny that there could be acts of voluntary euthanasia both passive and active against which neither justice nor charity would speak.

We have now considered the morality of euthanasia both voluntary and nonvoluntary, and active and passive. The conclusion has been that nonvoluntary active euthanasia (roughly, killing a man against his will or without his consent) is never justified; that is to say, that a man's being killed for his own good never justifies the act unless he himself has consented to it. A man's rights are infringed by such an action, and it is therefore contrary to justice. However, all the other combinations, nonvoluntary passive euthanasia, voluntary active euthanasia, and voluntary passive euthanasia are sometimes compatible with both justice and charity. But the strong condition carried in the definition of euthanasia adopted in this paper must not be forgotten; an act of euthanasia as here understood is one whose purpose is to benefit the one who dies.

In the light of this discussion let us look at our present practices. Are they good or are they bad? And what changes might be made, thinking now not only of the morality of particular acts of euthanasia but also of the indirect effects of instituting different practices, of the abuses to which they might be subject and of the changes that might come about if euthanasia became a recognized part of the social scene.

The first thing to notice is that it is wrong to ask whether we should introduce the practice of euthanasia as if it were not something we already had. In fact we do have it. For instance it is common, where the medical prognosis is very bad, for doctors to recommend against measures to prolong life, and particularly where a process of degeneration producing one medical emergency after another has already set in. If these doctors are not certainly within their legal rights this is something that is apt to come as a surprise to them as to the general public. It is also obvious that euthanasia is often practiced where old people are concerned. If someone very old and soon to die is attacked by a disease that makes his life wretched, doctors do not always come in with life-prolonging drugs. Perhaps poor patients are more fortunate in this respect than rich patients, being more often left to die in peace; but it is in any case a well recognized piece of medical practice, which is a form of euthanasia.

No doubt the case of infants with mental or physical defects will be suggested as another example of the practice of euthanasia as we already have it, since such infants are sometimes deliberately allowed to die. That they are deliberately allowed to die is certain; children with severe spina bifida malformations are not always operated on even where it is thought that without the operation they will die; and even in the case of children with [Down] Syndrome who have intestinal obstructions the relatively simple operation that would make it possible to feed them is sometimes not performed.[11] Whether this is euthanasia in our sense or only as the Nazis understood it is another matter. We must ask the crucial question, "Is it for the sake of the child himself that the doctors and parents choose his death?" In some cases the answer may really be yes, and what is more important it may really be true that the kind of life which is a good is not possible or likely for this child, and that there is little but suffering and frustration in store for him.[12] But this must presuppose that the medical prognosis is wretchedly bad, as it maybe for some spina bifida children. With children who are born with [Down] Syndrome it is, however, quite different. Most of these are able to live on for quite a time in a reasonably contented way, remaining like children all their lives but capable of affectionate relationships and able to play games and perform simple tasks. The fact is, of course, that the doctors who recommend against life-saving procedures for handicapped infants are usually thinking not of them but rather of their parents and of other children in the family or of the "burden on society" if the children survive. So it is not for their sake but to avoid trouble to others that they are allowed to die. When brought out into the open this seems unacceptable: at least we do not easily accept the principle that adults who need special care should be counted too burdensome to be kept alive. It must in any case be insisted that if children with [Down] Syndrome are deliberately allowed to die this is not a matter of euthanasia except in Hitler's sense. And for our children, since we scruple to gas them, not even the manner of their death is "quiet and easy"; when not treated for an intestinal obstruction a baby simply starves to death. Perhaps some will take this as an argument for allowing active euthanasia, in which case they will be in the company of an S.S. man stationed in the Warthgenau who sent Eichmann a memorandum telling him that "Jews in the coming winter could no longer be fed" and submitting for his consideration a proposal as to whether "it would not be the most humane solution to kill those Jews who were incapable of work through some quicker means."[13] If we say we are *unable* to look after children with handicaps we are no more telling the truth than was the S.S. man who said that the Jews could not be fed.

Nevertheless if it is ever right to allow deformed children to die because life will be a misery to them, or not to take measures to prolong for a little the life of a newborn baby whose life cannot extend beyond a few months of intense medical intervention, there is a genuine problem about active as opposed to passive euthanasia. There are well-known cases in which the medical staff has looked on wretchedly while an infant died slowly from starvation and dehydration because they did not feel able to give a lethal injection. According to the principles discussed in the earlier part of this paper they would indeed have had no right to give it, since an infant cannot ask that it should be done. The only possible solution—supposing that voluntary active euthanasia were to be legalized—would be to appoint guardians to act on the infant's behalf. In a different climate of opinion this might not be dangerous, but at present, when people so readily assume that the life of a handicapped baby is of no value, one would be loath to support it.

Finally, on the subject of handicapped children, another word should be said about those with severe mental defects. For them too it might sometimes be right to say that one would wish for death for their sake. But not even severe mental handicap automatically brings a child within the scope even of a possible act of euthanasia. If the level of consciousness is low enough it could not be said that life is a good to them, any more than in the case of those suffering from extreme senility. Nevertheless if they do not suffer it will not be an act of euthanasia by which someone opts for their death. Perhaps charity does not demand that strenuous measures are taken to keep people in this state alive, but euthanasia does not come into the matter, any more than it does when someone is, like Karen Ann Quinlan, in a state of permanent coma. Much could be said about this last case. It might even be suggested that in the case of unconsciousness this "life" is not the life to which "the right to life" refers. But that is not our topic here.

What we must consider, even if only briefly, is the possibility that euthanasia, genuine euthanasia, and not contrary to the requirements of justice or charity, should be legalized over a wider area. Here we are up against the really serious problem of abuse. Many people want, and want very badly, to be rid of their elderly relatives and even of their ailing husbands or wives. Would any safeguards ever be able to stop them describing as euthanasia what was really for their own benefit? And would it be possible to prevent the occurrence of acts which were genuinely acts of euthanasia but morally impermissible because infringing the rights of a patient who wished to live?

Perhaps the furthest we should go is to encourage patients to make their own contracts with a doctor by making it known whether they wish him to prolong their life in case of painful terminal illness or of incapacity. A document such as the Living Will seems eminently sensible, and should surely be allowed to give a doctor following the previously expressed wishes of the patient immunity from legal proceedings by relatives.[14] Legalizing active euthanasia is, however, another matter. Apart from the special repugnance doctors feel towards the idea of a lethal injection, it may be of the very greatest importance to keep a psychological barrier up against killing. Moreover it is active euthanasia which is the most liable to abuse. Hitler would not have been able to kill 275,000 people in his "euthanasia" program if he had had to wait for them to need life-saving treatment. But there are other objections to active euthanasia, even voluntary active euthanasia. In the first place it would be hard to devise procedures that would protect people from being persuaded into giving their consent. And secondly the possibility of active voluntary euthanasia might change the social scene in ways that would be very bad. As things are, people do, by and large, expect to be looked after if they are old or ill. This is one of the good things that we have, but we might lose it, and be much worse off without it. It might come to be expected that someone likely to need a lot of looking after should call for the doctor and demand his own death. Something comparable could be good in an extremely poverty-stricken community where the children genuinely suffered from lack of food; but in rich societies such as ours it would surely be a spiritual disaster. Such possibilities should make us very wary of supporting large measures of euthanasia, even where moral principle applied to the individual act does not rule it out.

NOTES

1. Leo Alexander, "Medical Science under Dictatorship," *New England Journal of Medicine*, 14 July 1949, p. 40.

2. For a discussion of culpable and nonculpable ignorance see Thomas Aquinas, *Summa Theologica*, First Part of the Second Part, Question 6, article 8, and Question 19, articles 5 and 6.

3. Dmitri Panin, *The Notebooks of Sologdin* (London, 1976), pp. 66–67.

4. Thomas Nagel, "Death," in James Rachels, ed., *Moral Problems* (New York, 1971), p. 362.

5. Panin, *Sologdin*, p. 85.

6. Yet some detail needs to be filled in to explain why we should not say that a scarecrow is beneficial to the plants it protects. Perhaps what is beneficial must either be a feature of the plant itself, such as protective prickles, or else must work on the plant directly, such as a line of trees which give it shade.

7. David Hume, *Treatise*, Book III, Part II, Section 1.

8. Feinberg, "Human Rights," *Moral Problems in Medicine*, p. 465.

9. It is not, however, that justice and charity conflict. A man does not lack charity because he refrains from an act of injustice which would have been for someone's good.

10. George Fletcher, "Legal Aspects of the Decision not to Prolong Life," *Journal of the American Medical Association* 203, no. 1 (1 Jan. 1968): 119–122. Reprinted in Gorovitz.

11. I have been told this by a pediatrician in a well-known medical center in the United States. It is confirmed by Anthony M. Shaw and Iris A. Shaw, "Dilemma of Informed Consent in Children," *The New England Journal of Medicine* 289, no. 17 (25 Oct. 1973): 885–890. Reprinted in Gorovitz.

12. It must be remembered, however, that many of the social miseries of spina bifida children could be avoided. Professor R.B. Zachary is surely right to insist on this. See, for example, "Ethical and Social Aspects of Spina Bifida," *The Lancet*, 3 Aug. 1968, pp. 274–276. Reprinted in Gorovitz.

13. Quoted by Hannah Arendt, *Eichmann in Jerusalem* (London, 1963), p. 90.

14. Details of this document are to be found in J.A. Behnke and Sissela Bok, eds., *The Dilemmas of Euthanasia* (New York, 1975), and in A.B. Downing, ed., *Euthanasia and the Right to Life: The Case for Voluntary Euthanasia* (London, 1969).

Killing and Allowing to Die

DANIEL CALLAHAN

* * *

If a lessened worry about the consequences of legal euthanasia has been gaining ground, there has been an even more powerful threat to the traditional prohibition against it. No valid distinction, many now argue, can be made between killing and allowing to die, or between an act of commission and one of omission. The standard distinction being challenged rests on the commonplace observation that lives can come to an end as the result of: (a) the direct action of another who becomes the cause of death (as in shooting a person), and (b) the result of impersonal forces where no human agent has acted (death by lightning, or by disease). The purpose of the distinction has been to separate those deaths caused by human action, and those caused by nonhuman events. It is, as a distinction, meant to say something about human beings and their relationship to the world. It is a way of articulating the difference between those actions for which human beings can be held rightly responsible, or blamed, and those of which they are innocent. At issue is the difference between physical causality, the realm of impersonal events, and moral culpability, the realm of human responsibility.

The challenges encompass two points. The first is that people can become equally dead by our omissions as well as our commissions. We can refrain from saving them when it is possible to do so, and they will be just as dead as if we shot them. It is our decision itself that is the reason for their death, not necessarily how we effectuate that decision. That fact establishes the basis of the second point: if we *intend* their death, it can be brought about as well by omitted acts as by those we commit. The crucial moral point is not how they die, but our intention about their death. We can, then, be responsible for the death of another by

intending that they die and accomplish that end by standing aside and allowing them to die.

Despite these criticisms—resting upon ambiguities that can readily be acknowledged—the distinction between killing and allowing to die remains, I contend, perfectly valid. It not only has a logical validity but, no less importantly, a social validity whose place must be central in moral judgments. As a way of putting the distinction into perspective, I want to suggest that it is best understood as expressing three different, though overlapping, perspectives on nature and human action. I will call them the metaphysical, the moral, and the medical perspectives.

Metaphysical. The first and most fundamental premise of the distinction between killing and allowing to die is that there is a sharp difference between the self and the external world. Unlike the childish fantasy that the world is nothing more than a projection of the self, or the neurotic person's fear that he or she is responsible for everything that goes wrong, the distinction is meant to uphold a simple notion: there is a world external to the self that has its own, and independent, causal dynamism. The mistake behind a conflation of killing and allowing to die is to assume that the self has become master of everything within and outside of the self. It is as if the conceit that modern man might ultimately control nature has been internalized: that, if the self might be able to influence nature by its actions, then the self and nature must be one.

Of course that is a fantasy. The fact that we can intervene in nature, and cure or control many diseases, does not erase the difference between the self and the external world. It is as "out there" as ever, even if more under our sway. That sway, however great, is always limited. We can cure disease, but not always the chronic illness that comes with the cure. We can forestall death with modern medicine, but death always wins in the long run because of the innate limitations of the body, inherently and stub-

Daniel Callahan, "Can We Return Death to Disease?" from *Hastings Center Report* 19(1): 4–6. Copyright © 1989 The Hastings Center. Reproduced with permission of John Wiley & Sons, Inc.

bornly beyond final human control. And we can distinguish between a diseased body and an aging body, but in the end if we wait long enough they always become one and the same body. To attempt to deny the distinction between killing and allowing to die is, then, mistakenly to impute more power to human action than it actually has and to accept the conceit that nature has now fallen wholly within the realm of human control. Not so.

Moral. At the center of the distinction between killing and allowing to die is the difference between physical causality and moral culpability. To bring the life of another to an end by an injection kills the other directly; our action is the physical cause of the death. To allow someone to die from a disease we cannot cure (and that we did not cause) is to permit the disease to act as the cause of death. The notion of physical causality in both cases rests on the difference between human agency and the action of external nature. The ambiguity arises precisely because we can be morally culpable for killing someone (if we have no moral right to do so, as we would in self-defense) and no less culpable for allowing someone to die (if we have both the possibility and the obligation of keeping that person alive). Thus there are cases where, morally speaking, it makes no difference whether we killed or allowed to die; we are equally responsible. In those instances, the lines of physical causality and moral culpability happen to cross. Yet the fact that they can cross in some cases in no way shows that they are always, or even usually, one and the same. We can normally find the difference in all but the most obscure cases. We should not, then, use the ambiguity of such cases to do away altogether with the distinction between killing and allowing to die. The ambiguity may obscure, but does not erase, the line between the two.

There is one group of ambiguous cases that is especially troublesome. Even if we grant the ordinary validity between killing and allowing to die, what about those cases that combine (a) an illness that renders a patient unable to carry out an ordinary biological function (to breathe or eat on his own, for example), and (b) our turning off a respirator or removing an artificial feeding tube? On the level of physical causality, have we killed the patient or

allowed him to die? In one sense, it is our action that shortens his life, and yet in another sense his underlying disease brings his life to an end. I believe it reasonable to say that, since his life was being sustained by artificial means (respirator or feeding tube) made necessary because of the fact that he had an incapacitating disease, his disease is the ultimate reality behind his death. But for its reality, there would be no need for artificial sustenance in the first place and no moral issue at all. To lose sight of the paramount reality of the disease is to lose sight of the difference between our selves and the outer world.

I quickly add, and underscore, a moral point: the person who, without good moral reason, turns off a respirator or pulls a feeding tube, can be morally culpable; that the patient has been allowed to die of his underlying condition does not morally excuse him. The moral question is whether we are obliged to continue treating a life that is being artificially sustained. To cease treatment may or may not be morally acceptable; but it should be understood, in either case, that the physical cause of death was the underlying disease.

Medical. An important social purpose of the distinction between killing and allowing to die has been that of protecting the historical role of the physician as one who tries to cure or comfort patients rather than to kill patients. Physicians have been given special knowledge about the body, knowledge that can be used to kill or to cure. They are also given great privileges in making use of that knowledge. It is thus all the more important that physicians' social role and power be, and be seen to be, a limited power. It may be used only to cure or comfort, never to kill. They have not been given, nor should they be given, the power to use their knowledge and skills to bring life to an end. It would open the way for powerful misuse and, no less importantly, represent an intrinsic violation of what it has meant to be a physician.

Yet if it is possible for physicians to misuse their knowledge and power to kill people directly, are they thereby required to use that same knowledge always to keep people alive, always to resist a disease that can itself kill the patient? The traditional answer has been: not necessarily. For the physician's ultimate obligation is to the welfare of the patient, and excessive treatment can be as detrimental to that welfare as inadequate treatment. Put another way, the obligation to resist the lethal power of disease is limited—it ceases when the patient is unwilling to have it resisted, or where the resistance no longer serves the patient's welfare. Behind this moral premise is the recognition that disease (of some kind) ultimately triumphs and that death is both inevitable sooner or later and not, in any case, always the greatest human evil. To demand of the physician that he always struggle against disease, as if it was in his power always to conquer it, would be to fall into the same metaphysical trap mentioned above: that of assuming that no distinction can be drawn between natural and human agency.

A final word. I suggested earlier that the most potent motive for active euthanasia and assisted suicide stems from a dread of the power of medicine. That power then seems to take on a drive of its own regardless of the welfare or wishes of patients. No one can easily say no—not physicians, not patients, not families. My guess is that happens because too many have already come to believe that it is their choice, and their choice alone, which brings about death; and they do not want to exercise that kind of authority. The solution is not to erase the distinction between killing and allowing to die, but to underscore its validity and importance. We can bring disease as a cause of death back into the care of the dying.

CASES FOR ANALYSIS

1. Assisted Suicide or Murder?

One of the more bizarre cases of assisted suicide in recent times came to its conclusion on Monday, when New Yorker Kenneth Minor was convicted of manslaughter after stabbing a Long Island motivational speaker. Minor claimed that the man wished to die, and had paid him to help him do so.

Minor received a sentence of 12 years when he accepted the prosecutors' plea deal and pled guilty to first-degree manslaughter.

However, Minor's lawyer claims, "We will be back again . . . Our hope is the appellate division will once again reverse this case."

Minor's lawyer, Daniel J. Gotlin, hopes to overturn the conviction by bringing the case to an appeals court. Gotlin argues that the verdict should be thrown out based on procedural grounds. Minor's indictment includes murder charges and assisted suicide charges, which Gotlin claims are mutually exclusive.

Minor has been incarcerated for more than five years, and, according to Gotlin, accepted the plea deal because "he wants finality; he wants this to be over." If Minor is unsuccessful in his appeal, he will have to serve five more years before he could be released.

Moments before Minor entered his plea, Justice Laura A. Ward of the State Supreme Court in Manhattan denied Gotlin's request to dismiss the case, stating that a man can be charged for both murder and assisted suicide. However, she did not refute that Minor had a right to appeal her ruling, and said, "Perhaps we will get a definite ruling from the appellate division."

The man who Minor admits to killing, Jeffrey Locker, was found tied up in his car in East Harlem in July 2009. Multiple stab wounds were found on his chest.

Minor claims that Locker, a middle-aged father who had fallen deeply into debt, had hired him to assist in his suicide plans. Minor says he held a knife to a steering wheel while Locker flung himself against it multiple times. Minor's prosecutors found his story incredible and brought a murder charge against him instead of assisted suicide.

In 2011, Minor was tried and convicted of second-degree murder by a jury. The judge gave him 20 years to life in prison, but the verdict was invalidated two years later by an appellate panel. They concluded that the trial judge had given the jury an incorrect definition of assisted suicide.

Minor was given another trial in January. This time, an assisted suicide charge was added to his indictment at the request of Cyrus R. Vance Jr., Manhattan district attorney. A jury could now convict him of a lesser charge.

During Minor's first trial, the defense and the prosecution agreed that Minor had participated in Locker's suicide at the request of the deceased, who wished to make his death look like a murder so that his family could claim life insurance.

However, prosecutors argued that it was a case of murder for hire, not assisted suicide, as Minor was still the cause of Locker's death. According to a medical expert, Minor did not simply hold a knife to a steering wheel, but stabbed Locker as he lay in his car. He then used Locker's credit card to withdraw money from an ATM.*

Suppose Minor killed Locker at Locker's request. Would the killing then be morally permissible? Is there a moral difference between physician-assisted suicide and Locker's murder when both actions are taken at the victim's request? What is the difference, if any, between murder and assisted suicide?

Suppose Locker's motive for asking Minor for aid in dying, and for making the death look like murder, was that Locker's life insurance money would pay for the only medical treatment that could save his daughter's life. How would these facts change your moral judgment about the killing?

*Based on James C. McKinley Jr., "Harlem Man Pleads Guilty to Assisting 2009 Death," *New York Times*, September 2014, http://www.nytimes.com/2014/09/30/nyregion/-harlem-man-pleads-guilty-to-assisting-2009-death.html?_r=0 (23 March 2015).

2. Euthanasia for Newborns

Paris (CNSNews.com)—Four years after becoming the first nation formally to legalize euthanasia, the Netherlands is set to amend its legislation to provide for the euthanasia of newborn babies, under certain circumstances.

In 2001, the Dutch government passed a law allowing doctors to end the life of adult patients at their own request.

The new directive, which will be debated in parliament later this month and most likely approved without a vote, will extend the regulations to incorporate what is known as the Groningen Protocol.

Under these guidelines, parents can give consent for children to be killed, if they are suffering from severe pain and are terminally ill.

"This is dangerous because the question is, what will be the next extension?" said Bert Dorenbos, chairman of Cry for Life, a pro-life organization in the Netherlands.

"It can be very dangerous when our lives are in the hands of political parties or subjective groups," he said.

The Groningen Academic Hospital, where doctors drew up the guidelines, made headlines last year when it admitted publicly that it had carried out euthanasia on terminally ill newborn babies.

The hospital claimed the practice was common elsewhere in the world, including in the U.S.

Government officials said there were 10–15 cases of child euthanasia in the Netherlands every year and doctors were eager for the directive to be adopted so they will not be prosecuted. . . .

The Groningen Protocol lists several criteria for making a decision on ending a child's life. There should be severe pain and suffering and no hope for a cure or relief through medical treatment, and an independent doctor must provide a second opinion. Parents must also give consent.[†] [The law now permits the euthanasia of infants provided that the protocol is followed.]

Provide reasons for your answers to the following questions. Under the circumstances described (severe pain, terminal illness), would child euthanasia ever be morally permissible? Would child euthanasia be permissible if the newborn was not terminal but in an unalterable vegetative state? Would it be permissible if the newborn suffered from a severe birth defect such as Down's syndrome, which causes severe disabilities but does not rule out a worthwhile life?

[†]Excerpt from Eva Cahen, "Next Up in the Netherlands: Euthanasia for Babies," CNSNews.com, October 5, 2005. Reprinted with permission.

---

3. The Suicide of Admiral Nimitz

The name of Chester W. Nimitz is legendary in the annals of naval warfare. In June 1942, Admiral Nimitz commanded the U.S. forces assigned to block a Japanese invasion of Midway.

In the Battle of Midway, Nimitz's fighter-bombers caught the Japanese fleet off guard, as its carrier aircraft were being refueled on deck. His pilots swooped in and sent to the bottom four of the Japanese carriers—*Hiryu*, *Soryu*, *Akagi* and *Kaga*—that had led the attack on Pearl Harbor. Midway broke the back of Japanese naval power and was among the most decisive battles in all of history.

Nimitz's son and namesake, Chester W. Nimitz Jr., would rise to the same rank of admiral and become a hero of the Pacific war—a submarine commander who would sink a Japanese destroyer bearing down on his boat by firing torpedoes directly into its bow.

But Chester W. Nimitz Jr., achieved another kind of fame on Jan. 2. In a suicide pact with his 89-year-old wife, the 86-year-old hero ended his life with an overdose of sleeping pills.

Having lost 30 pounds from a stomach disorder, suffering from congestive heart failure and in constant back pain, the admiral had been determined to dictate the hour of his death. His wife, who suffered from osteoporosis so severe her bones were breaking, had gone blind. She had no desire to live without her husband.

So, as the devoted couple had spent their lives together, they decided to end their lives together. The admiral's final order read: "Our decision was made over a considerable period of time and was not carried out in acute desperation. Nor is it the expression of a mental illness. We have consciously, rationally, deliberately and of our own free will taken measures to end our lives today because of the physical limitations on our quality of life placed upon us by age, failing vision, osteoporosis, back and painful orthopedic problems."

According to *The New York Times* obituary, "The Nimitzes did not believe in any afterlife or God, and embraced no religion. But one of Mr. Nimitz's three surviving sisters, Mary Aquinas, 70, is a Catholic nun. . . . Sister Mary said that she could not condone her brother's decision to end his life, but that she felt sympathetic. 'If you cannot see any value to suffering for yourself or others,' she said, 'Then maybe it does make sense to end your life.'"‡

Provide reasons for your answers: Was Admiral Nimitz justified in his decision to commit suicide? Is suicide morally wrong in all circumstances? Is suicide a matter of personal choice, morally permissible if a person freely opts to end her life for whatever reason?

‡Patrick J. Buchanan, "The Sad Suicide of Admiral Nimitz," *World Net Daily*, January 18, 2002. Reprinted by permission of Creators Syndicate.

CHAPTER 11

Capital Punishment

Few moral issues provoke the kind of fiery emotions and fervent debate that capital punishment does. In some circles, the very mention of the words *death penalty* is enough to set off a cross fire of opinions on the subject—as well as an onslaught of zealotry and moral confusion. At the center of all the commotion is a clash of fundamental moral values, a conflict heightened by the realization that weighing in the balance is, ultimately and tragically, the life or death of a human being.

In this controversy, the **abolitionists** (those who wish to abolish capital punishment) most often appeal to basic moral principles such as "Do not kill," "Honor the sanctity of life," or "Respect human dignity." The **retentionists** (those who wish to retain the death penalty) are likely to appeal to other principles: "Punish the guilty," "Give murderers the punishment they deserve," "A life for a life," or "Deter the ultimate crime (murder) with the ultimate punishment." On the most general and fundamental of these principles—not killing, respecting human dignity, and punishing the guilty—almost all parties to the dispute agree. But retentionists and abolitionists are usually at odds over how these principles should be interpreted.

Retentionists like to remind us of murderers whose crimes are so horrific that the death penalty may seem the only fitting punishment. Thus they bring up such moral monsters as Timothy McVeigh (used a bomb to kill 168 men, women, and children), Ted Bundy (murdered, by his own count, more than 100 women), John Wayne Gacy (raped and murdered 33 boys and men), and Adolf Eichmann (facilitated the murder of millions during the Holocaust). Abolitionists, on the other hand, tell of the horrors that often accompany the death penalty: innocent people who are wrongly convicted and executed, executions that go wrong and cause excruciating pain to those executed, and the suspiciously high percentage of poor and minority people who are executed in the United States. Commonplace in the capital punishment debate, such facts may move us to anger, pity, disgust, or sadness, and they may inform our thinking in important ways. But we should not allow our emotional reaction to them to interfere with the vital task that we begin in this chapter—the careful evaluation of arguments for and against capital punishment.

ISSUE FILE: BACKGROUND

In the legal sense, **punishment** is the deliberate and authorized causing of pain or harm to someone thought to have broken a law. It is a legal sanction imposed by society on offenders for violating society's official norms. The justification for punishment—the reason why society uses it—generally takes one of two forms. As we will see later, many believe that the sole reason we should punish the wrongdoer is because he morally *deserves* punishment. His desert is the only justification required, and meting out punishment to those who deserve it is morally obligatory and a morally good thing. Others believe that the only proper justification is the good consequences for society that the punishment of offenders will bring—most notably, the prevention of future crimes and the maintenance of an orderly society.

Capital punishment is punishment by execution of someone officially judged to have committed a serious, or capital, crime. For thousands of years, this extreme sanction has been used countless times in the Western world for a variety of offenses—rape, murder, horse theft, kidnapping, treason, sodomy, spying, blasphemy, witchcraft, and many others. A wide assortment of execution methods have also been employed, ranging from the ancient and medieval (crucifixion, drawing and quartering, burning alive, impalement, etc.) to the handful of standard techniques of the past two centuries (hanging, firing squad, lethal gas, electrocution, and lethal injection). In twenty-first-century America, most death-penalty states (thirty-two in 2013) reserve capital punishment for the crime of murder, and lethal injection is authorized in all of them. Seventeen states authorize other modes of execution, including lethal gas, hanging, and firing squad.[1]

At the end of 2013, there were 2,979 prisoners on death row in the United States, and in that year nine states carried out 39 executions. In 2013, 56 percent of death row inmates were white, 42 percent were black, and 14 percent were Latino. In the same year, Texas executed sixteen inmates—more by far than any other state. Florida executed seven; Oklahoma six; Ohio three; Alabama one; and all other states three or fewer. By the end of 2013, eighteen states and the District of Columbia had abolished their death penalty statutes: Alaska, Connecticut, Illinois, Hawaii, Iowa, Maine, Maryland, Massachusetts, Michigan, Minnesota, New Jersey, New Mexico, New York, North Dakota, Rhode Island, Vermont, West Virginia, and Wisconsin.[2]

The trend in executions in the United States has varied over the past few decades. The number of executions carried out each year between the mid-1930s and the 1970s gradually declined, from a high of 200 down to 0 in 1976. But from 1977 to 1999, the annual toll ramped up again, from 1 in 1977 to 98 in 1999. Since this high point, another downward trend has set in, with the number of executions in 2004 dropping to 59, and in 2013 to 39.[3] The gradual decrease in executions has coincided with significant public support for the death penalty for convicted murderers. Gallup polls show that between 1994 and 2014, the percentage of American adults in favor of capital punishment for murder has fluctuated annually but always stayed within the 60 to 80 percent range. In the last seven years, however, the range has been 60 to 65 percent. These numbers decreased significantly when people were asked to consider life in prison without parole as an option.[4]

Most other countries have officially abolished the death penalty or simply stopped using it. One hundred forty nations—including Canada, Mexico, and all the western European countries—are in this category. Fifty-eight countries and territo-

---

[1]Death Penalty Information Center, "States With and Without the Death Penalty, 2014," http://www.deathpenaltyinfo.org/states-and-without-death-penalty; "Methods of Execution, 2011," http://www.deathpenaltyinfo.org/methods-execution (29 October 2014); Death Penalty Information Center, "The Death Penalty in 2013: Year End Report," http://deathpenaltyinfo.org/YearEnd2013; Death Row Population Figures from NAACP-LDF "Death Row USA (July 1, 2014)," http://www.deathpenaltyinfo.org/death-row-usa/DRUSAFall2014.pdf; Bureau of Justice Statistics: "Capital Punishment, 2013—Statistical Tables," http://www.bjs.gov/cp13st.pdf.

[2]Bureau of Justice Statistics: "Capital Punishment, 2013—Statistical Tables," http://www.bjs.gov/cp13st.pdf. [3]*Bureau of Justice Statistics Bulletin*, Capital Punishment, 2003 (November 2004), 10; Bureau of Justice Statistics: "Capital Punishment, 2013—Statistical Tables," http://www.bjs.gov/cp13st.pdf.

[4]"Facts about the Death Penalty," Death Penalty Information Center, www.deathpenaltyinfo.org (20 January 2012).

ries, however, continue to employ capital punishment. In 2013, three nations accounted for almost 80 percent of executions: Iran (369), Iraq (169), and Saudi Arabia (79).[5]

The use of capital punishment in the United States has been shaped by several landmark Supreme Court decisions. In 1972, in *Furman v. Georgia*, the Court ruled that capital punishment as it was then being applied in certain states was unconstitutional. The ruling put a halt to executions across the country. Yet the Court declared not that the death penalty itself was unconstitutional, only that its current method of administration was. The majority on the Court thought that the usual administration—which allowed juries to impose the death penalty arbitrarily without any legal guidance—constituted "cruel and unusual punishment," a violation of the Eighth Amendment of the Constitution.

Many states then promptly rewrote their death penalty statutes to try to minimize administrative arbitrariness. A few states passed laws decreeing that the death penalty would be mandatory for particular capital crimes. But in *Woodson v. North Carolina* (1976), the Supreme Court declared mandatory death sentences unconstitutional. Some states instituted sentencing guidelines to provide standards for the judge or jury deliberating about whether to impose the death penalty. In *Gregg v. Georgia* (1976), the Court ruled that such death penalty laws prescribing proper guidelines were constitutional, at least in cases of murder. This ruling in effect reinstated capital punishment in the country, and executions resumed in the following year. Since 1976, few state statutes have allowed the death penalty for anything but homicide cases.

More recently the Court has banned the use of the death penalty for particular kinds of offenders.

[5]Amnesty International, "The Death Penalty in 2013," 2013, http://www.amnesty.org/en/death-penalty/death-sentences-and-executions-in-2013 (29 October 2014).

In *Atkins v. Virginia* (2002), the Court held that the execution of mentally retarded persons is cruel and unusual punishment and is therefore unconstitutional. In *Roper v. Simmons* (2005), the Court held that executing those who were under the age of eighteen when they committed their crimes is also a violation of Eighth Amendment protection against cruel and unusual punishment. Before *Roper*, seven states had no minimum age for execution, and fifteen states had set the minimum at between fourteen and seventeen years old. In *Kennedy v. Louisiana* (2008) the Court ruled a Louisiana statute unconstitutional. The law permitted the death penalty for child rape in cases where the child did not die.

An important tradition in law that bears on capital punishment is the distinction between types of punishable killing: namely, between first-degree murder, second-degree murder, and manslaughter. Statutes vary by jurisdiction, but generally first-degree murder is killing (1) with premeditation; (2) while performing a major crime (felony) such as armed robbery, kidnapping, or rape; or (3) involving particular egregious circumstances such as the deaths of several people or of a child or police officer. Second-degree murder is killing without premeditation but with some degree of intent ("malice aforethought"). Manslaughter is killing without premeditation or intent, as when one person kills another in "the heat of passion" or by driving drunk. Usually, only first-degree murder makes a defendant eligible for the death penalty.

MORAL THEORIES

Both retentionists and abolitionists appeal to consequentialist and nonconsequentialist moral theories. Retentionist arguments are often thoroughly utilitarian, contending that use of capital punishment can create a favorable balance of happiness over unhappiness for society. One common argument is that the death penalty achieves such utility through *prevention*—by preventing the criminal

CRITICAL THOUGHT: Medicated for the Death Penalty

In 2004, 44-year-old Charles Singleton was executed by lethal injection in Arkansas. The event became one of the more infamous executions in the United States because Singleton was insane—except when he took his medication for his schizophrenia. And he was fully medicated for his date with death. According to a CNN account,

> Singleton . . . was rational only when he was on medication. It was that fact, as well as an 18-year-old Supreme Court ruling barring executing the insane, that his attorney, some members of the legal and medical communities and death penalty critics pointed to in opposing Singleton's execution.*

The prosecutor, however, emphasized the fact that Singleton was sane when he committed his crime.*

Do you think it is morally permissible to execute a convicted murderer who was sane at the time of his crime but is now insane? Why or why not? Is it morally permissible to medicate such a person to ensure that he is sane enough for execution? To what moral theory, if any, are you appealing to help you decide?

*Excerpt from Kevin Drew, "Executed Mentally Ill Inmate Heard Voices Until End," *CNN.com,* 6 January 2004, www.cnn.com/2004/LAW/01/06/singleton.death.row/index.html (26 January 2015). © 2004 Cable News Network. Reprinted courtesy of CNN.

---

from striking again. Better than any other form of punishment, the retentionist says, the death penalty protects society from repeat criminals, those violent and dangerous offenders who cannot be reformed. The retentionist claims that life in prison without parole—the usual alternative to the death penalty—is an inadequate substitute. Violent lifers can kill other inmates and prison guards, or they can escape to terrorize society again. By also appealing to utility, the abolitionist may object to this line by insisting that the retentionist produce empirical evidence showing that executing violent criminals does indeed protect society better than the use of life sentences. After all, such premises about deterrence are empirical claims, and empirical claims require supporting evidence.

A related retentionist argument asserts that the death penalty, more than any other form of punishment (including life in prison), can achieve great overall utility through *deterrence*—the dissuading of possible offenders from committing capital crimes. This utilitarian argument is thought by many to be the retentionist's strongest. The utilitarian philosopher John Stuart Mill claims that for a particular kind of would-be criminal, capital punishment is the most effective deterrent of all:

> But the influence of punishment is not to be estimated by its effect on hardened criminals. Those whose habitual way of life keeps them, so to speak, at all times within sight of the gallows, do grow to care less about it; as, to compare good things with bad, an old soldier is not much affected by the chance of dying in battle. I can afford to admit all that is often said about the indifference of the professional criminals to the gallows. Though of that indifference one-third is probably bravado and another third confidence that they shall have the luck to escape, it is quite probable that the remaining third is real. But the efficacy of a punishment which acts principally through the imagination, is chiefly to be measured by the impression it makes on those who are still innocent; by the horror with which it surrounds

the first promptings of guilt; the restraining influence it exercises over the beginning of the thought which, if indulged, would become a temptation; the check which it exerts over the graded declension towards the state—never suddenly attained—in which crime no longer revolts, and punishment no longer terrifies.[6]

Like the prevention appeal, the deterrence argument requires supporting evidence—specifically, evidence showing that the execution of criminals really does deter serious criminal behavior better than lesser punishments such as imprisonment. Abolitionists, however, are quick to question any such evidence. In fact, even many retentionists agree that the relevant scientific studies on the deterrence question are conflicting or otherwise inconclusive.

The central difficulty in conducting these studies is the number of variables that must be controlled to get reliable results. A social scientist, for example, could select two very similar jurisdictions, one with the death penalty and one without, and compare the murder rates in each. Presumably, if capital punishment deters murderers, then the jurisdiction using the death penalty should have a lower murder rate than the no-death penalty jurisdiction. But it is virtually impossible to rule out the influence of extraneous factors on the study results. Besides being influenced by the penal system, murder rates may be affected by many variables—unemployment, cultural conventions, moral beliefs, political climate, media influence, availability of lethal weapons, incidence of illegal drug use, history of violence, income level, and on and on. No two jurisdictions are exactly alike, and many differences (both known and unknown) could contribute to the rise or fall of serious crime rates.

Despite these research problems, many retentionists still consider the case for deterrence strong. They argue that even if science does not yet offer unequivocal support for the death penalty's power to deter capital crimes, common sense does. The philosopher Louis Pojman takes this tack. He contends that it is obvious that most people want to avoid jail and that long sentences will deter most potential criminals better than short ones—and that there are good reasons to believe that the death penalty deters better still. One reason, he says, is that a large proportion of crimes are committed by criminals who weigh the risks and benefits of their criminal activity and become more attracted to particular crimes the milder the punishments are. And there are good indications that the death penalty would exert maximum deterrence in these cases: "The fact that those who are condemned to death do everything in their power to get their sentences postponed or reduced to long-term prison sentences, in the way *lifers* do not, shows that they fear death more than life in prison."[7]

The abolitionist can offer a couple of responses to this argument from common sense. First, even if the death penalty is a more severe punishment than life in prison, it does not follow that the death penalty deters murderers better. The prospect of life in prison may very well deter future murderers just as effectively as the death penalty can. Second, it is possible that the threat of capital punishment motivates potential killers not to avoid killing but to try harder not to get caught.

Recognizing the uncertainties in trying to assess levels of deterrence, some retentionists argue that despite the unknowns, our wisest and most

[6]John Stuart Mill, "Speech in Favor of Capital Punishment," to the English Parliament, 1868, http://ethics.sandiego.edu/books/Mill/Punishment/ (26 January 2015).

[7]Louis P. Pojman, "Why the Death Penalty Is Morally Permissible," in *Debating the Death Penalty: Should America Have Capital Punishment? The Experts on Both Sides Make Their Best Case*, eds. Hugo Adam Bedau and Paul G. Cassell (Oxford: Oxford University Press, 2004), 60–61.

morally responsible move is to bet that capital punishment does deter murderers. The reasoning that leads to this conclusion is essentially a utilitarian calculation. The philosopher Ernest van den Haag was the first to articulate this argument. The choice we are faced with, he says, is either to use the death penalty or not to use it—and we must choose while not knowing for sure whether it is a superior deterrent. If we use the penalty, we risk killing convicted murderers (and saving innocent lives). If we abolish the penalty, we risk bringing about the deaths of innocent victims (and saving the lives of murderers). If we must risk something, he says, it is better to risk the lives of convicted murderers than those of innocent people. Thus, our best bet is to retain the death penalty. "I believe we have no right to risk additional future victims of murder for the sake of sparing convicted murderers," van den Haag asserts, "on the contrary, our moral obligation is to risk the possible ineffectiveness of executions."[8]

A common abolitionist reply to this argument is that the utilitarian calculation is incomplete. The assessment of net happiness, says the abolitionist, fails to take into account the possibility that the death penalty could *encourage* violent crime instead of just deterring it. How? Some argue that violent criminals who know they are likely to get the death penalty may commit murder to avoid being captured. In addition, some abolitionists maintain that capital punishment has a brutalizing effect on society—it makes killing human beings seem more morally and psychologically acceptable. If so, executing people could cause more harm than good and be a very poor bet for society.

On utilitarian grounds, abolitionists can attack capital punishment directly (as opposed to simply

countering retentionist arguments). In perhaps the most common of such approaches, the abolitionist argues that more net happiness is created in society by sentencing murderers to life in prison without parole than by executing them. Life sentences promote the welfare of society by preventing murderers from killing again—and they do so without generating the disadvantages and pain inherent in a system of capital punishment.

Another utilitarian argument against the death penalty is that this form of punishment is simply too costly:

> The death penalty is much more expensive than its closest alternative—life imprisonment with no parole. Capital trials are longer and more expensive at every step than other murder trials. Pre-trial motions, expert witness investigations, jury selection, and the necessity for two trials—one on guilt and one on sentencing—make capital cases extremely costly, even before the appeals process begins. Guilty pleas are almost unheard of when the punishment is death. In addition, many of these trials result in a life sentence rather than the death penalty, so the state pays

QUICK REVIEW

abolitionists—Those who wish to abolish capital punishment.

retentionists—Those who wish to retain the death penalty.

punishment—The deliberate and authorized causing of pain or harm to someone thought to have broken a law.

capital punishment—Punishment by execution of someone officially judged to have committed a serious, or capital, crime.

retributivism—The view that offenders deserve to be punished, or "paid back," for their crimes and to be punished in proportion to the severity of their offenses.

---

[8]Ernest van den Haag, "On Deterrence and the Death Penalty," *Journal of Criminal Law, Criminology, and Police Science* 60, no. 2 (1969).

CRITICAL THOUGHT: Botched Executions

In 2014, several executions by lethal injection went terribly wrong. In at least three executions, instead of dying within ten or fifteen minutes, the prisoners writhed or gasped for much longer, up to nearly two hours in one case. Consider this description of one such procedure:

> On Wednesday afternoon, a prisoner named Joseph Rudolph Wood III suffered what was one of the longest executions in U.S. history. Executioners in Arizona began pumping the lethal drugs into Wood's veins at 1:57 p.m. His death was not pronounced until nearly two hours later at 3:49 p.m. According to Michael Kiefer, a reporter with the *Arizona Republic* who witnessed the execution, Wood gasped 660 times before he died. A witness from the attorney general's office said he was merely snoring, but another attending reporter used what has become, in descriptions of botched

executions, a familiar metaphor, saying Wood looked "like a fish on shore gulping for air."*

Do you think botched executions like these constitute "cruel and unusual punishment" and therefore are prohibited by the Constitution? Are executions morally permissible (or impermissible) regardless of their cruelty? Why or why not? Do you believe botched executions offer good reasons to do away with the death penalty? Or do they merely suggest there should be a ban on lethal injections but not other forms of execution? Why or why not?

*Ben Crair, "2014 Is Already the Worst Year in the History of Lethal Injection," *New Republic*, July 24, 2014, http://www.newrepublic.com/article/118833/2014-botched-executions-worst-year-lethal-injection-history (30 October 2014).

the cost of life imprisonment on top of the expensive trial.[9]

Retentionists often respond to this argument by questioning whether the costs have been calculated accurately and fairly. Perhaps more often, they offer a nonconsequentialist reply: if the death penalty is a just punishment, then the costs involved are irrelevant.

In the death penalty debate, appeals to nonconsequentialist theories are common on both sides of the issue. Abolitionists devise arguments against capital punishment using what they take to be fundamental moral principles regarding the value or dignity of human life. For them, regard-

[9]Richard C. Dieter, "Millions Misspent: What Politicians Don't Say about the High Cost of the Death Penalty," Fall 1994, www.deathpenaltyinfo.org/node /599 (26 January 2015).

less of its social utility, the death penalty is wrong because it violates these principles. For example, they may argue that everyone has a right to life (a basic moral principle), even hardened criminals, and that the death penalty is a violation of this right—therefore, executing criminals is wrong. To this argument, retentionists usually reply along these lines: people do indeed have a right to life, but this right is not absolute. That is, a person's right to life can sometimes be overridden for good reasons. For example, if your life is being threatened, it is morally permissible to kill an attacker in self-defense. So the right to life does not hold in every situation no matter what. It may be morally permissible, then, to sometimes set this right aside.

To make their case, abolitionists often appeal to notions of fairness or justice. One prevalent argument is based on the assertion that our penal system is inherently unjust, sometimes executing innocent people (numerous cases have come to light in which people who had been executed or who were on death row were later found to be innocent). Because the death penalty is irrevocable—that is, there is no way to "undo" an execution or to compensate the executed—the execution of the innocent is an especially egregious miscarriage of justice. Therefore, we should get rid of the death penalty, since abolition is the only way to avoid such tragedies. Retentionists are generally unmoved by this argument, offering counterarguments like this one:

> Miscarriages of justice result in innocent people being sentenced to death and executed, even in criminal-law systems in which greatest care is taken to ensure that it never comes to that. But this does not stem from the intrinsic nature of the institution of capital punishment; it results from deficiencies, limitations, and imperfections of the criminal law procedures in which this punishment is meted out. Errors of justice do not demonstrate the need to do away with capital punishment; they simply make it incumbent on us to do everything possible to improve even further procedures of meting it out.[10]

The main nonconsequentialist argument for the death penalty is based on the theory of punishment known as **retributivism**—the view that offenders deserve to be punished, or "paid back," for their crimes and to be punished in proportion to the severity of their offenses. Retributivism says that offenders should be punished because *they deserve to be punished*. Punishment is a matter of justice, not social utility. If offenders are not punished, justice is not done. Kant, probably the most influential retributivist, declares that there is only one reason to punish someone for his offenses:

> Juridical punishment can never be administered merely as a means for promoting another good

either with regard to the criminal himself or to civil society, but must in all cases be imposed only because the individual on whom it is inflicted has committed a crime.[11]

We can distinguish two kinds of retributivism according to the nature of the penal payback required. Kant accepts retributivism based on the doctrine of *lex talionis*—the idea that the punishment should match the crime in kind, that justice demands "an eye for an eye, a life for a life." He thinks that whatever harm the criminal does to the innocent, that same kind of harm should be done to the criminal. Thus, the only just punishment for a man who wrongfully and deliberately takes someone's life is the taking of *his* life. Other retributivists are uncomfortable with the notion of punishing in kind (should rapists be raped? should torturers be tortured?). They favor *proportional retributivism*, in which punishment reflects the seriousness of the crime but does not necessarily *resemble* the crime. For these retributivists, murder is the worst possible crime and deserves the worst possible punishment—the death of the offender.

Underpinning many retributive views of capital punishment is a Kantian emphasis on respect for persons. Persons have dignity and inherent worth and are ends in themselves. Deliberately killing an innocent person, says the retributivist, is so heinous a crime, such an intolerable evil, that it merits the ultimate punishment—the death of the murderer. So when the killer takes a life, she must forfeit her own. As Kant says,

> Even if a civil society resolved to dissolve itself with the consent of all its members . . . the last murderer lying in prison ought to be executed before the resolution was carried out. This ought to be done in order that every one may realize the desert of his deeds, and that blood-guiltiness may not remain on the people; for otherwise they will all be regarded as

---

[10]Igor Primoratz, *Justifying Legal Punishment* (Atlantic Highlands, NJ: Humanities Press International, 1989), 165.

[11]Immanuel Kant, *The Philosophy of Law*, trans. W. Hastie (Edinburgh: Clark, 1887), 195.

participants in the murder as a public violation of justice.[12]

Perhaps surprisingly, often the retributivist also appeals to the dignity and worth of the murderer. As Kant notes, treating persons with respect means treating them as rational agents who make free choices and are responsible for their actions. To justly punish persons—to give them what they deserve—is to acknowledge their status as responsible agents deserving of respect. He asserts, then, that executing a murderer is not an affront to human dignity but a recognition of it.

A frequent reaction to the retributivist view is that penal retribution is not justice—but revenge. The retributivist replies that this charge is muddled: vengeance refers to making the offender suffer because of one's sense of outrage, grief, or frustration toward her and her crime; retribution involves moral deliberation about an offender's just deserts.

MORAL ARGUMENTS

Is the death penalty a morally permissible form of punishment? As you know by now, many arguments have been put forth on both sides of this issue—too many for any single book to tackle, let alone a single chapter. But we can dissect one of the more widely used (and interesting) examples. Let us begin with a popular argument *against* the death penalty:

1. If the death penalty discriminates against blacks, it is unjust.

2. If the death penalty is unjust, it should be abolished.

3. The death penalty discriminates against blacks.

4. Therefore, the death penalty should be abolished.

This argument is valid, so our evaluation of it should focus on the truth of the premises. Premises 1 and 2 are moral statements; Premise 3 is an empirical statement about the use of the death penalty against African Americans. (Arguments like this are used with equal force when focusing on other minority groups as well as the poor and uneducated; for simplicity's sake we focus on blacks, who make up the largest segment of minority death row inmates.)

Let us examine the empirical claim first: is Premise 3 true? We can give it more precision by recasting it like this: The administration of the death penalty is biased against blacks. Many abolitionists insist that this claim is indeed accurate. They say, for example, that blacks convicted of murder are more likely to be sentenced to death than whites convicted of murder. How is this claim supported? Here is one way:

> [T]he Reverend Jesse Jackson, in his book *Legal Lynching*, argues that "[n]umerous researchers have shown conclusively that African American defendants are far more likely to receive the death penalty than are white defendants charged with the same crime." The support for this claim is said to be the undisputed fact that when compared to their percentage in the overall population African Americans are overrepresented on death row. For example, while 12 percent of the population is African American, about 43 percent of death row inmates are African American, and 38 percent of prisoners executed since 1977 are African American.[13]

But such statistical comparisons can be misleading, say some retentionists:

> The relevant population for comparison is not the general population, but rather the population of murderers. If the death penalty is administered without regard to race, the percentage of African American death row inmates found at the end of the process should not exceed the percentage of African

---

[12]Kant, 198.

[13]Paul G. Cassell, "In Defense of the Death Penalty," in Bedau and Cassell, eds., *Debating the Death Penalty*, 201.

CRITICAL THOUGHT: Different Cases, Same Punishment

Consider the contrasts in the description of two men executed on the same day for a capital crime:

> One is Troy Davis, a black man who was convicted of killing a white off-duty police officer in Savannah, Georgia, in 1989. The other is Lawrence Brewer, a white man who in 1998 participated in the grisly murder of James Byrd Jr., a black man whom Brewer and two other men attacked.*

Davis said to the last that he was innocent, no physical evidence or weapon tied him to the crime, and many witnesses against him at the trial later recanted their testimony. Millions of people, including the pope, pleaded for mercy for Davis. Brewer admitted his crime in which he and two other men chained a black man to a pickup truck and dragged him until his body was torn into pieces. Later in letters he wrote in jail, Brewer

bragged about the murder and touted the thrill it gave him. Few asked for mercy for Brewer.

What do these very different cases suggest about the system of capital punishment in the United States? Despite the contrast between these two men—one despicable and clearly guilty, the other a sympathetic character whose guilt was in doubt—they were both executed by the state. Does this outcome suggest that an injustice was perpetrated? Should the nature of the crime, the character of the accused, or the degree of certainty about guilt affect the penalty for a crime? Based on the information given here, would you say that justice was done?

*Trymaine Lee, "Troy Davis and Lawrence Brewer, a Tale of Two Executions," *Huffington Post*, 21 September 2011, http://www.huffingtonpost.com/2011/09/21/troy-davis-and-lawrence-b_n_974293.html.

American defendants charged with murder at the beginning. The available statistics indicate that is precisely what happens. The Department of Justice found that while African Americans constituted 48 percent of adults charged with homicide, they were only 41 percent of those admitted to prison under sentence of death. In other words, once arrested for murder, blacks are actually less likely to receive a capital sentence than are whites.[14]

Needless to say, Premise 3 (in the form examined here and in several other variations) is controversial. That does not mean, of course, that its truth or falsity is unknowable. New research or conscientious examination of existing research may provide the support that Premise 3 requires. In any event, the support must come in the form

of solid statistical data carefully interpreted. Anecdotal evidence—for example, news stories of apparent unequal treatment of whites and blacks—cannot help us much.

As we did with Premise 3, we can restate Premise 1 to make it more specific: If the administration of the death penalty is biased against blacks, it is unjust. On a straightforward reading, this assertion would seem to be acceptable to both retentionists and abolitionists. Few would deny that applying the death penalty in a discriminatory fashion is unjust, for equals must be treated equally. On this reading, the premise is almost certainly true. But many abolitionists would interpret the statement differently. They would contend that if the administration of the death penalty is biased against blacks, then the death penalty itself is unjust. Some abolitionists accept this view because they believe there is no way to apply the death

[14]Cassell, 201.

penalty fairly; the administration of capital punishment is inherently unjust. Others would say that there is no way to separate the "death penalty itself" from the way it is administered. In the real world, there is only the death-penalty-as-actually-applied, which is inescapably unfair.

A common reply to the abolitionist understanding of Premise 1 is that it misses an important distinction: the unjust administration of a punishment does not entail the injustice of the punishment itself. As one retentionist says,

> [This charge of unfairness] is not an argument, either against the death penalty or against any other form of punishment. It is an argument against unjust and inequitable distribution of penalties. If the trials of wealthy men are less likely to result in convictions than those of poor men, then something must be done to reform the procedure in criminal courts. . . . But the maldistribution of penalties is no argument against any particular form of penalty.[15]

It seems that we cannot decide the truth of Premise 1 without a much more thorough examination of the arguments for and against it, a task beyond the scope of this discussion. So let us move to our revised Premise 2: If the administration of the death penalty is unjust, it should be abolished. As you can see, this premise has the same kind of ambiguity that we see in Premise 1. Again the abolitionist reading is that an unjust application of the death penalty is an indictment against capital punishment itself, so capital punishment should be abolished. Thus the same arguments and counterarguments surrounding Premise 1 also apply here.

At this point, we have not determined whether this abolitionist argument is a good one. But we have gained insight into this part of the capital punishment debate. Look again at the argument in its revised form:

---

[15]B. M. Leiser, *Liberty, Justice and Morals: Contemporary Value Conflicts* (New York: Macmillan, 1973), 225.

1. If the administration of the death penalty is biased against blacks, it is unjust.

2. If the administration of the death penalty is unjust, it should be abolished.

3. The administration of the death penalty is biased against blacks.

4. Therefore, the death penalty should be abolished.

We have seen how difficult it can be to make this argument work. If any one of the premises is false, the conclusion is not supported and the argument fails. (Also, the argument is now valid only on the reading preferred by abolitionists.) But we have also found that the lynchpin of the argument is the abolitionist view that injustice in the system of capital punishment is the same as injustice in lethal punishment itself. If abolitionists can establish this equivalence, the argument is much more likely to succeed. The other links in the chain of reasoning—the injustice of discrimination and the need to abolish unjust punishments—are generally accepted by all parties to the dispute.

We have also learned something about the retentionist position. We have discovered how retentionists can readily agree that the application of the death penalty discriminates against blacks, that this biased treatment is unconscionable and unjust, and that such a discriminatory system should be reformed or abolished—and still consistently believe that it can be morally permissible for the state to put a convicted murderer to death.

SUMMARY

Capital punishment is a form of legal punishment—execution—reserved for someone convicted of committing a capital crime, usually some form of murder. Abolitionists wish to abolish capital punishment; retentionists want to retain it. In several decisions, the U.S. Supreme Court has sanctioned and circumscribed the use of the death penalty. In *Gregg v. Georgia*, the Court ruled that administration of the death penalty—if used according to proper guidelines—is constitutional in cases of murder. Other rulings banned the execution of retarded persons and of those who were under eighteen when they committed their crimes.

Both retentionists and abolitionists appeal to utilitarianism and nonconsequentialist moral theories to make their case. Retentionists often argue that the death penalty maximizes the welfare of society by preventing repeat crimes or deterring future crimes. Retributivists argue on nonconsequentialist grounds that capital punishment is morally permissible because it accords with the demands of justice. Abolitionists, on the other hand, often contend that the death penalty does more harm than good to society and that life in prison without parole results in more net happiness than executions do. Many abolitionists also take the nonconsequentialist route by insisting that the death penalty violates some fundamental moral principles—the right to life, the dignity of human beings, and the injustice of executing the innocent.

READINGS

The Ultimate Punishment: A Defense

Ernest van den Haag

In an average year about 20,000 homicides occur in the United States. Fewer than 300 convicted murderers are sentenced to death. But because no more than thirty murderers have been executed in any recent year, most convicts sentenced to death are likely to die of old age.[1] Nonetheless, the death penalty looms large in discussions: it raises important moral questions independent of the number of executions.[2]

The death penalty is our harshest punishment.[3] It is irrevocable: it ends the existence of those punished, instead of temporarily imprisoning them. Further, although not intended to cause physical pain, execution is the only corporal punishment still applied to adults. These singular characteristics contribute to the perennial, impassioned controversy about capital punishment.

Ernest van den Haag, republished with permission of Harvard Law Review Association, from "The Ultimate Punishment: A Defense," *Harvard Law Review* 99: 1662–69. Copyright © 1986 by Harvard Law Review Association; permission conveyed through Copyright Clearance Center, Inc.

I. DISTRIBUTION

Consideration of the justice, morality, or usefulness, of capital punishment is often conflated with objections to its alleged discriminatory or capricious distribution among the guilty. Wrongly so. If capital punishment is immoral *in se*, no distribution among the guilty could make it moral. If capital punishment is moral, no distribution would make it immoral. Improper distribution cannot affect the quality of what is distributed, be it punishment or rewards. Discriminatory or capricious distribution thus could not justify abolition of the death penalty. Further, maldistribution inheres no more in capital punishment than in any other punishment.

Maldistribution between the guilty and the innocent is, by definition, unjust. But the injustice does not lie in the nature of the punishment. Because of the finality of the death penalty, the most grievous maldistribution occurs when it is imposed upon the innocent. However, the frequent allegations of discrimination and capriciousness refer to maldistribution among the guilty and not to the punishment of the innocent.

Maldistribution of any punishment among those who deserve it is irrelevant to its justice or morality. Even if poor or black convicts guilty of capital offenses suffer capital punishment, and other convicts equally guilty of the same crimes do not, a more equal distribution, however desirable, would merely be more equal. It would not be more just to the convicts under sentence of death.

Punishments are imposed on persons, not on racial or economic groups. Guilt is personal. The only relevant question is: does the person to be executed deserve the punishment? Whether or not others who deserved the same punishment, whatever their economic or racial group, have avoided execution is irrelevant. If they have, the guilt of the executed convicts would not be diminished, nor would their punishment be less deserved. To put the issue starkly, if the death penalty were imposed on guilty blacks, but not on guilty whites, or, if it were imposed by a lottery among the guilty, this irrationally discriminatory or capricious distribution would neither make the penalty unjust, nor cause anyone to be unjustly punished, despite the undue impunity bestowed on others.

Equality, in short, seems morally less important than justice. And justice is independent of distributional inequalities. The ideal of equal justice demands that justice be equally distributed, not that it be replaced by equality. Justice requires that as many of the guilty as possible be punished, regardless of whether others have avoided punishment. To let these others escape the deserved punishment does not do justice to them, or to society. But it is not unjust to those who could not escape.

These moral considerations are not meant to deny that irrational discrimination, or capriciousness, would be inconsistent with constitutional requirements. But I am satisfied that the Supreme Court has in fact provided for adherence to the constitutional requirement of equality as much as is possible. Some inequality is indeed unavoidable as a practical matter in any system.[4] But, *ultra posse nemo obligatur*. (Nobody is bound beyond ability.)

Recent data reveal little direct racial discrimination in the sentencing of those arrested and convicted of murder.[5] The abrogation of death penalty for rape has eliminated a major source of racial discrimination. Concededly, some discrimination based on the race of murder victims may exist; yet, this discrimination affects criminal victimizers in an unexpected way. Murderers of whites are thought more likely to be executed than murderers of blacks. Black victims, then, are less fully vindicated than white ones. However, because most black murderers kill blacks, black murderers are spared the death penalty more often than are white murderers. They fare better than most white murderers.[6] The motivation behind unequal distribution of the death penalty may well have been to discriminate against blacks, but the result has favored them. Maldistribution is thus a straw man for empirical as well as analytical reasons.

II. MISCARRIAGES OF JUSTICE

In a recent survey Professors Hugo Adam Bedau and Michael Radelet found that 7000 persons were executed in the United States between 1900 and 1985 and that 25 were innocent of capital crimes.[7] Among the innocents they list Sacco and Vanzetti as well as Ethel and Julius Rosenberg. Although their data may be questionable, I do not doubt that, over a long enough period, miscarriages of justice will occur even in capital cases.

Despite precautions, nearly all human activities, such as trucking, lighting, or construction, cost the lives of some innocent bystanders. We do not give up these activities, because the advantages, moral or material, outweigh the unintended losses.[8] Analogously, for those who think the death penalty just, miscarriages of justice are offset by the moral benefits and the usefulness of doing justice. For those who think the death penalty unjust even when it does not miscarry, miscarriages can hardly be decisive.

III. DETERRENCE

Despite much recent work, there has been no conclusive statistical demonstration that the death penalty is a better deterrent than are alternative punishments. However, deterrence is less than decisive for either side. Most abolitionists acknowledge that they would continue to favor abolition even if the death penalty were shown to deter more murders than alternatives could deter.[9] Abolitionists appear to value the life of a convicted murderer or, at least, his non-execution, more highly than they value the lives of the innocent victims who might be spared by deterring prospective murderers.

Deterrence is not altogether decisive for me either. I would favor retention of the death penalty as retribution even if it were shown that the threat of execution could not deter prospective murderers not already deterred by the threat of imprisonment.[10] Still, I believe the death penalty, because of its finality, is more feared than imprisonment, and deters some prospective murderers not deterred by the threat of imprisonment. Sparing the lives of even a few prospective victims by deterring their murderers is more important than preserving the lives of convicted murderers because of the possibility, or even the probability, that executing them would not deter others. Whereas the lives of the victims who might be saved are valuable, that of the murderer has only negative value, because of his crime. Surely the criminal law is meant to protect the lives of potential victims in preference to those of actual murderers.

Murder rates are determined by many factors; neither the severity nor the probability of the threatened sanction is always decisive. However, for the long run, I share the view of Sir James Fitzjames Stephen: "Some men, probably, abstain from murder because they fear that if they committed murder they would be hanged. Hundreds of thousands abstain from it because they regard it with horror. One great reason why they regard it with horror is that murderers are hanged."[11] Penal sanctions are useful in the long run for the formation of the internal restraints so necessary to control crime. The severity and finality of the death penalty is appropriate to the seriousness and the finality of murder.[12]

IV. INCIDENTAL ISSUES: COST, RELATIVE SUFFERING, BRUTALIZATION

Many nondecisive issues are associated with capital punishment. Some believe that the monetary cost of appealing a capital sentence is excessive. Yet most comparisons of the cost of life imprisonment with the cost of execution, apart from their dubious relevance, are flawed at least by the implied assumption that life prisoners will generate no judicial costs during their imprisonment. At any rate, the actual monetary costs are trumped by the importance of doing justice.

Others insist that a person sentenced to death suffers more than his victim suffered, and that this (excess) suffering is undue according to the *lex talionis* (rule of retaliation). We cannot know whether the murderer on death row suffers more than his victim suffered; however, unlike the murderer, the victim deserved none of the suffering inflicted. Further, the limitations of the *lex talionis* were meant to restrain private vengeance, not the social retribution that has taken its place. Punishment—regardless of the motivation—is not intended to revenge, offset, or compensate for the victim's suffering, or to be measured by it. Punishment is to vindicate the law and the social order undermined by the crime. This is why a kidnapper's penal confinement is not limited to the period for which he imprisoned his victim; nor is a burglar's confinement meant merely to offset the suffering or the harm he caused his victim; nor is it meant only to offset the advantage he gained.[13]

Another argument heard . . . is that, by killing a murderer, we encourage, endorse, or legitimize unlawful killing. Yet, although all punishments are meant to be unpleasant, it is seldom argued that they legitimize the unlawful imposition of identical unpleasantness. Imprisonment is not thought to legitimize kidnapping; neither are fines thought to legitimize robbery. The difference between murder and execution, or between kidnapping and imprisonment, is that the first is unlawful and undeserved, the second a lawful and deserved punishment for an unlawful act. The physical similarities of the punishment to the crime are irrelevant. The relevant difference is not physical, but social.[14]

V. JUSTICE, EXCESS, DEGRADATION

We threaten punishments in order to deter crime. We impose them not only to make the threats credible but also as retribution (justice) for the crimes that were not deterred. Threats and punishments are necessary to deter and deterrence is a sufficient practical justification for them. Retribution is an independent moral justification. Although penalties can be unwise, repulsive, or inappropriate, and those punished can be pitiable, in a sense the infliction of legal punishment on a guilty person cannot be unjust. By committing the crime, the criminal volunteered to assume the risk of receiving a legal punishment that he could have avoided by not committing the crime. The punishment he suffers is the punishment he voluntarily risked suffering and, therefore, it is no more unjust to him than any other event for which one knowingly volunteers to assume the risk. Thus, the death penalty cannot be unjust to the guilty criminal.[15]

There remain, however, two moral objections. The penalty may be regarded as always excessive as retribution and always morally degrading. To regard the death penalty as always excessive, one must believe that no crime—no matter how heinous—could possibly justify capital punishment. Such a belief can be neither corroborated nor refuted; it is an article of faith.

Alternatively, or concurrently, one may believe that everybody, the murderer no less than the victim, has an imprescriptible (natural?) right to life. The law therefore should not deprive anyone of life. I share Jeremy Bentham's view that any such "natural and imprescriptible rights" are "nonsense upon stilts."[16]

Justice Brennan has insisted that the death penalty is "uncivilized," "inhuman," inconsistent with "human dignity" and with "the sanctity of life," that it "treats members of the human race as nonhumans, as objects to be toyed with and discarded," that it is "uniquely degrading to human dignity" and "by its very nature, [involves] a denial of the executed person's humanity." Justice Brennan does not say why he thinks execution "uncivilized." Hitherto most civilizations have had the death penalty, although it has been discarded in Western Europe, where it is currently unfashionable probably because of its abuse by totalitarian regimes.

By "degrading," Justice Brennan seems to mean that execution degrades the executed convicts. Yet philosophers, such as Immanuel Kant and G. W. F. Hegel, have insisted that, when deserved, execution, far from degrading the executed convict, affirms his humanity by affirming his rationality and his responsibility for his actions. They thought that execution, when deserved, is required for the sake of the convict's dignity. (Does not life imprisonment violate human dignity more than execution, by keeping alive a prisoner deprived of all autonomy?)

Common sense indicates that it cannot be death—our common fate—that is inhuman. Therefore, Justice Brennan must mean that death degrades when it comes not as a natural or accidental event, but as a deliberate social imposition. The murderer learns through his punishment that his fellow men have found him unworthy of living; that because he has murdered, he is being expelled from the community of the living. This degradation is self-inflicted. By murdering, the murderer has so dehumanized himself that he cannot remain among the living. The social recognition of his self-degradation is the punitive essence of execution. To believe, as Justice Brennan appears to, that the degradation is inflicted by the execution reverses the direction of causality.

Execution of those who have committed heinous murders may deter only one murder per year. If it does, it seems quite warranted. It is also the only fitting retribution for murder I can think of.

NOTES

1. Death row as a semipermanent residence is cruel, because convicts are denied the normal amenities of prison life. Thus, unless death row residents are integrated into the prison population, the continuing accumulation of convicts on death row should lead us to accelerate either the rate of executions or the rate of communications. I find little objection to integration.

2. The debate about the insanity defense is important for analogous reasons.

3. Some writers, for example, Cesare Bonesana, Marchese di Beccaria, have thought that life imprisonment is more severe. However, the overwhelming majority of both abolitionists and of convicts under death sentence prefer life imprisonment to execution.

4. The ideal of equality, unlike the ideal of retributive justice (which can be approximated separately in each instance), is clearly unattainable unless all guilty persons are apprehended, and therefore tried, convicted and sentenced by the same court, at the same time. Unequal justice is the best we can do; it is still better than the injustice, equal or unequal, which occurs if, for the sake of equality, we deliberately allow some who could be punished to escape.

5. *See* Bureau of Justice Statistics, U.S. Dep't of Justice, Bulletin No. NJC-98,399, Capital Punishment 1984, at 9 (1985); Johnson, *The Executioner's Bias*, Nat'l Rev., Nov. 15, 1985, at 44.

6. It barely need be said that any discrimination *against* (for example, black murderers of whites) must also be discrimination *for* (for example, black murderers of blacks).

7. Bedau & Radelet, *Miscarriages of Justice in Potentially Capital Cases* (1st draft, Oct. 1985) (on file at Harvard Law School Library).

8. An excessive number of trucking accidents or of miscarriages of justice could offset the benefits gained by trucking or the practice of doing justice. We are, however, far from this situation.

9. For most abolitionists, the discrimination argument, *see supra* pp. 1662–64, is similarly nondecisive: they would favor abolition even if there could be no racial discrimination.

10. If executions were shown to increase the murder rate in the long run, I would favor abolition. Sparing the innocent victims who would be spared by the nonexecution of murderers would be more important to me than the execution, however just, of murderers. But although there is a lively discussion of the subject, no serious evidence exists to support the hypothesis that executions produce a higher murder rate.

11. H. Gross, A Theory of Criminal Justice 489 (1979) (attributing this passage to Sir James Fitzjames Stephen).

12. Weems v. United States, 217 U.S. 349 (1910), suggests that penalties be proportionate to the seriousness of the crime—a common theme of the criminal law. Murder, therefore, demands more than life imprisonment, if, as I believe, it is a more serious crime than other crimes punished by life imprisonment. In modern times, our sensibility requires that the range of punishments be narrower than the range of crimes—but not so narrow as to exclude the death penalty.

13. Thus restitution (a civil liability) cannot satisfy the punitive purpose of penal sanctions, whether the purpose be retributive or deterrent.

14. Some abolitionists challenge: if the death penalty is just and serves as a deterrent, why not televise executions? The answer is simple. The death even of a murderer, however well-deserved, should not serve as public entertainment. It so served in earlier centuries. But in this respect our sensibility has changed for the better, I believe. Further, television unavoidably would trivialize executions, wedged in, as they would be, between game shows, situation comedies and the like. Finally, because televised executions would focus on the physical aspects of the punishment, rather than the nature of the crime and the suffering of the victim, a televised execution would present the murderer as the victim of the state. Far from communicating the moral significance of the execution, television would shift the focus to the pitiable fear of the murderer. We no longer place in cages those sentenced to imprisonment to expose them to public view. Why should we so expose those sentenced to execution?

15. An explicit threat of punitive action is necessary to the justification of any legal punishment: *nulla poena sine lege* (no punishment without [preexisting] law). To be sufficiently justified, the threat must in turn have a rational and legitimate purpose. "Your money or your life" does not qualify; nor does the threat of an unjust law; nor, finally, does a threat that is altogether disproportionate to the importance of its purpose. In short, preannouncement legitimizes the threatened punishment only if the threat is warranted. But this leaves a very wide range of justified threats. Furthermore, the punished person is aware of the penalty for his actions and thus volunteers to take the risk even of an unjust punishment. His victim, however, did not volunteer to risk anything. The question whether any self-inflicted injury—such as a legal punishment—ever can be unjust to a person who knowingly risked it is a matter that requires more analysis than is possible here.

16. The Works of Jeremy Bentham 105 (J. Bowring ed. 1972).

From *Justice, Civilization, and the Death Penalty: Answering van den Haag*

Jeffrey H. Reiman

On the issue of capital punishment, there is as clear a clash of moral intuitions as we are likely to see. Some (now a majority of Americans) feel deeply that justice requires payment in kind and thus that murderers should die; and others (once, but no longer, nearly a majority of Americans) feel deeply that the state ought not be in the business of putting people to death.[1] Arguments for either side that do not do justice to the intuitions of the other are unlikely to persuade anyone not already convinced. And, since, as I shall suggest, there is truth on both sides, such arguments are easily refutable, leaving us with nothing but conflicting intuitions and no guidance from reason in distinguishing the better from the worse. In this context, I shall try to make an argument for the abolition of the death penalty that does justice to the intuitions on both sides. I shall sketch out a conception of retributive justice that accounts for the justice of executing murderers, and then I shall argue that *though the death penalty is a just punishment for murder*, abolition of the death penalty is part of the civilizing mission of modern states.

* * *

[I.] JUST DESERTS AND JUST PUNISHMENTS

In my view, the death penalty is a just punishment for murder because the *lex talionis*, an eye for an eye, and so on, is just, although, as I shall suggest at the end of this section, it can only be rightly applied when its implied preconditions are satisfied. The *lex talionis* is a version of retributivism. Retributivism—as the word itself suggests—is the doctrine that the offender should be *paid back* with suffering he deserves because of the evil he has done, and the *lex talionis* asserts that injury equivalent to that he

imposed is what the offender deserves.[2] But the *lex talionis* is not the only version of retributivism. Another, which I shall call "proportional retributivism," holds that what retribution requires is not equality of injury between crimes and punishments, but "fit" or proportionality, such that the worst crime is punished with the society's worst penalty, and so on, though the society's worst punishment need not duplicate the injury of the worst crime.[3] Later, I shall try to show how a form of proportional retributivism is compatible with acknowledging the justice of the *lex talionis*. Indeed, since I shall defend the justice of the *lex talionis*, I take such compatibility as a necessary condition of the validity of any form of retributivism.

There is nothing self-evident about the justice of the *lex talionis* nor, for that matter, of retributivism. The standard problem confronting those who would justify retributivism is that of overcoming the suspicion that it does no more than sanctify the victim's desire to hurt the offender back. Since serving that desire amounts to hurting the offender simply for the satisfaction that the victim derives from seeing the offender suffer, and since deriving satisfaction from the suffering of others seems primitive, the policy of imposing suffering on the offender for no other purpose than giving satisfaction to his victim seems primitive as well. Consequently, defending retributivism requires showing that the suffering imposed on the wrongdoer has some worthy point beyond the satisfaction of victims. In what follows, I shall try to identify a proposition—which I call the *retributivist principle*—that I take to be the nerve of retributivism. I think this principle accounts for the justice of the *lex talionis* and indicates the point of the suffering demanded by retributivism. Not to do too much of the work of the death penalty advocate, I shall make no extended argument for the principle beyond suggesting the considerations that make it plausible. I shall identify these considerations by drawing, with considerable license, on Hegel and Kant.

I think that we can see the justice of the *lex talionis* by focusing on the striking affinity between it and the *golden rule*. The *golden rule* mandates "Do unto others as you would have others do unto you," while the *lex talionis* counsels "Do unto others as they have done unto you." It would not be too far-fetched to say that the *lex talionis* is the law enforcement arm of the golden rule, at least in the sense that if people were actually treated as they treated others, then everyone would necessarily follow the golden rule because then people could only willingly act toward others as they were willing to have others act toward them. This is not to suggest that the *lex talionis* follows from the golden rule, but rather that the two share a common moral inspiration: the equality of persons. Treating others as you *would* have them treat you means treating others as equal to you, because adopting the golden rule as one's guiding principle implies that one counts the suffering of others to be as great a calamity as one's own suffering, that one counts one's right to impose suffering on others as no greater than their right to impose suffering on one, and so on. This leads to the *lex talionis* by two approaches that start from different points and converge.

I call the first approach "Hegelian" because Hegel held (roughly) that crime upsets the equality between persons and retributive punishment restores that equality by "annulling" the crime.[4] As we have seen, acting according to the golden rule implies treating others as your equals. Conversely, violating the golden rule implies the reverse: Doing to another what you would *not* have that other do to you violates the equality of persons by asserting a right toward the other that the other does not possess toward you. Doing back to you what you did "annuls" your violation by reasserting that the other has the same right toward you that you assert toward him. Punishment according to the *lex talionis* cannot heal the injury that the other has suffered at your hands, rather it rectifies the indignity he has suffered, by restoring him to equality with you.

"Equality of persons" here does not mean equality of concern for their happiness, as it might for a utilitarian. On such a (roughly) utilitarian under-

standing of equality, imposing suffering on the wrongdoer equivalent to the suffering he has imposed would have little point. Rather, equality of concern for people's happiness would lead us to impose as little suffering on the wrongdoer as was compatible with maintaining the happiness of others. This is enough to show that retributivism (at least in this "Hegelian" form) reflects a conception of morality quite different from that envisioned by utilitarianism. Instead of seeing morality as administering doses of happiness to individual recipients, the retributivist envisions morality as maintaining the relations appropriate to equally sovereign individuals. A crime, rather than representing a unit of suffering added to the already considerable suffering in the world, is an assault on the sovereignty of an individual that temporarily places one person (the criminal) in a position of illegitimate sovereignty over another (the victim). The victim (or his representative, the state) then has the right to rectify this loss of standing relative to the criminal by meting out a punishment that reduces the criminal's sovereignty in the degree to which he vaunted it above his victim's. It might be thought that this is a duty, not just a right, but that is surely too much. The victim has the right to forgive the violator without punishment, which suggests that it is by virtue of having the right to punish the violator (rather than the duty), that the victim's equality with the violator is restored.

I call the second approach "Kantian" since Kant held (roughly) that, since reason (like justice) is no respecter of the sheer difference between individuals, when a rational being decides to act in a certain way toward his fellows, he implicitly authorizes similar action by his fellows toward him.[5] A version of the golden rule, then, is a requirement of reason: acting rationally, one always acts as he would have others act toward him. Consequently, to act toward a person as he has acted toward others is to treat him as a rational being, that is, as if his act were the product of a rational decision. From this, it may be concluded that we have a duty to do to offenders what they have done, since this amounts to according them the respect due rational beings.[6] Here too, however, the assertion of a duty to punish seems excessive, since, if this duty arises because doing to people what they have done to others is necessary to accord them the respect due rational beings, then we would have a duty to do to all rational persons *everything*—good, bad, or indifferent—that they do to others. The point rather is that, by his acts, a rational being *authorizes* others to do the same to him, he doesn't *compel* them to. Here too, then, the argument leads to a right, rather than a duty, to exact the *lex talionis*. And this is supported by the fact that we can conclude from Kant's argument that a rational being cannot validly complain of being treated in the way he has treated others, and where there is no valid complaint, there is no injustice, and where there is no injustice, others have acted within their rights.[7] It should be clear that the Kantian argument also rests on the equality of persons, because a rational agent only implicitly authorizes having done to him action similar to what he has done to another, if he and the other are similar in the relevant ways.

The "Hegelian" and "Kantian" approaches arrive at the same destination from opposite sides. The "Hegelian" approach starts from the victim's equality with the criminal, and infers from it the victim's right to do to the criminal what the criminal has done to the victim. The "Kantian" approach starts from the criminal's rationality, and infers from it the criminal's authorization of the victim's right to do to the criminal what the criminal has done to the victim. Taken together, these approaches support the following proposition: The equality and rationality of persons implies that an offender deserves and his victim has the right to impose suffering on the offender equal to that which he imposed on the victim. This is the proposition I call the *retributivist principle*, and I shall assume henceforth that it is true. This principle provides that the *lex talionis* is the criminal's just desert and the victim's (or as his representative, the state's) right. Moreover, the principle also indicates the point of retributive punishment, namely, it affirms the equality and rationality of persons, victims and offenders alike. And the point of this affirmation is, like any moral affirmation, to make a statement, to the criminal, to impress upon him his

equality with his victim (which earns him a like fate) and his rationality (by which his actions are held to authorize his fate), and to the society, so that recognition of the equality and rationality of persons becomes a visible part of our shared moral environment that none can ignore in justifying their actions to one another.

* * *

The truth of the retributivist principle establishes the justice of the *lex talionis*, but, since it establishes this as a right of the victim rather than a duty, it does not settle the question of whether or to what extent the victim or the state should exercise this right and exact the *lex talionis*. This is a separate moral question because strict adherence to the *lex talionis* amounts to allowing criminals, even the most barbaric of them, to dictate our punishing behavior. It seems certain that there are at least some crimes, such as rape or torture, that we ought not try to match. And this is not merely a matter of imposing an alternative punishment that produces an equivalent amount of suffering, as, say, some number of years in prison that might "add up" to the harm caused by a rapist or a torturer. Even if no amount of time in prison would add up to the harm caused by a torturer, it still seems that we ought not torture him even if this were the only way of making him suffer as much as he has made his victim suffer. Or, consider someone who has committed several murders in cold blood. On the *lex talionis*, it would seem that such a criminal might justly be brought to within an inch of death and then revived (or to within a moment of execution and then reprieved) as many times as he has killed (minus one), and then finally executed. But surely this is a degree of cruelty that would be monstrous.

Since the retributivist principle establishes the *lex talionis* as the victim's right, it might seem that the question of how far this right should be exercised is "up to the victim." And indeed, this would be the case in the state of nature. But once, for all the good reasons familiar to readers of John Locke, the state comes into existence, public punishment replaces private, and the victim's right to punish reposes in the state. With this, the decision as to how far to exercise this right goes to the state as well. To be sure, since (at least with respect to retributive punishment) the victim's right is the source of the state's right to punish, the state must exercise its right in ways that are faithful to the victim's right. Later, when I try to spell out the upper and lower limits of just punishment, these may be taken as indicating the range within which the state can punish and remain faithful to the victim's right.

I suspect that it will be widely agreed that the state ought not administer punishments of the sort described above even if required by the letter of the *lex talionis*, and thus, even granting the justice of *lex talionis*, there are occasions on which it is morally appropriate to diverge from its requirements. We must, of course, distinguish such morally based divergence from that which is based on practicality. Like any moral principle, the *lex talionis* is subject to "ought implies can." It will usually be impossible to do to an offender exactly what he has done—for example, his offense will normally have had an element of surprise that is not possible for a judicially imposed punishment, but this fact can hardly free him from having to bear the suffering he has imposed on another. Thus, for reasons of practicality, the *lex talionis* must necessarily be qualified to call for doing to the offender *as nearly as possible* what he has done to his victim. When, however, we refrain from raping rapists or torturing torturers, we do so for reasons of morality, not of practicality. And, given the justice of the *lex talionis*, these moral reasons cannot amount to claiming that it would be *unjust* to rape rapists or torture torturers. Rather the claim must be that, even though it would be just to rape rapists and torture torturers, other moral considerations weigh against doing so.

* * *

This way of understanding just punishment enables us to formulate proportional retributivism so that it is compatible with acknowledging the justice of the *lex talionis:* If we take the *lex talionis* as spelling out the offender's just deserts, and if other moral considerations require us to refrain from matching the injury caused by the offender while still allowing us to punish justly, then surely we impose just punish-

ment if we impose the closest morally acceptable approximation to the *lex talionis*. Proportional retributivism, then, in requiring that the worst crime be punished by the society's worst punishment and so on, could be understood as translating the offender's just desert into its nearest equivalent in the society's table of morally acceptable punishments. Then the two versions of retributivism (*lex talionis* and proportional) are related in that the first states what just punishment would be if nothing but the offender's just desert mattered, and the second locates just punishment at the meeting point of the offender's just deserts and the society's moral scruples. And since this second version only modifies the requirements of the *lex talionis* in light of other moral considerations, it is compatible with believing that the *lex talionis* spells out the offender's just deserts, much in the way that modifying the obligations of promisers in light of other moral considerations is compatible with believing in the binding nature of promises.

* * *

[II.] CIVILIZATION, PAIN, AND JUSTICE

As I have already suggested, from the fact that something is justly deserved, it does not automatically follow that it should be done, since there may be other moral reasons for not doing it such that, all told, the weight of moral reasons swings the balance against proceeding. The same argument that I have given for the justice of the death penalty for murderers proves the justice of beating assaulters, raping rapists, and torturing torturers. Nonetheless, I believe, and suspect that most would agree, that it would not be right for us to beat assaulters, rape rapists, or torture torturers, *even though it were their just deserts*—and even if this were the only way to make them suffer as much as they had made their victims suffer. Calling for the abolition of the death penalty, though it be just, then, amounts to urging that as a society we place execution in the same category of sanction as beating, raping, and torturing, and treat it as something it would also not be right for us to do to offenders, *even if it were their just deserts*.

To argue for placing execution in this category, I must show what would be gained therefrom; and to show that, I shall indicate what we gain from placing torture in this category and argue that a similar gain is to be had from doing the same with execution. I select torture because I think the reasons for placing it in this category are, due to the extremity of torture, most easily seen—but what I say here applies with appropriate modification to other severe physical punishments, such as beating and raping. First, and most evidently, placing torture in this category broadcasts the message that we as a society judge torturing so horrible a thing to do to a person that we refuse to do it even when it is deserved. Note that such a judgment does not commit us to an absolute prohibition on torturing. No matter how horrible we judge something to be, we may still be justified in doing it if it is necessary to prevent something even worse. Leaving this aside for the moment, what is gained by broadcasting the public judgment that torture is too horrible to inflict even if deserved?

I think the answer to this lies in what we understand as civilization. In *The Genealogy of Morals*, Nietzsche says that in early times "pain did not hurt as much as it does today."[8] The truth in this puzzling remark is that progress in civilization is characterized by a lower tolerance for one's own pain and that suffered by others. And this is appropriate, since, via growth in knowledge, civilization brings increased power to prevent or reduce pain and, via growth in the ability to communicate and interact with more and more people, civilization extends the circle of people with whom we empathize. If civilization is characterized by lower tolerance for our own pain and that of others, then publicly refusing to do horrible things to our fellows both signals the level of our civilization *and, by our example, continues the work of civilizing*. And this gesture is all the more powerful if we refuse to do horrible things to those who deserve them. I contend then that the more things we are able to include in this category, the more civilized we are and the more civi*lizing*. Thus we gain from including torture in this category, and if execution is especially horrible, we gain still more by including it.

* * *

Thus far, by analogy with torture, I have argued that execution should be avoided because of how horrible it is to the one executed. But there are reasons of another sort that follow from the analogy with torture. Torture is to be avoided not only because of what it says about *what* we are willing to do to our fellows, but also because of what it says about *us* who are willing to do it. To torture someone is an awful spectacle not only because of the intensity of pain imposed, but because of what is required to be able to impose such pain on one's fellows. The tortured body cringes, using its full exertion to escape the pain imposed upon it—it literally begs for relief with its muscles as it does with its cries. To torture someone is to demonstrate a capacity to resist this begging, and that in turn demonstrates a kind of hardheartedness that a society ought not parade.

And this is true not only of torture, but of all severe corporal punishment. Indeed, I think this constitutes part of the answer to the puzzling question of why we refrain from punishments like whipping, even when the alternative (some months in jail versus some lashes) seems more costly to the offender. Imprisonment is painful to be sure, but it is a reflective pain, one that comes with comparing what is to what might have been, and that can be temporarily ignored by thinking about other things. But physical pain has an urgency that holds body and mind in a fierce grip. Of physical pain, as Orwell's Winston Smith recognized, "you could only wish one thing: that it should stop."[9] Refraining from torture in particular and corporal punishment in general, we both refuse to put a fellow human being in this grip *and* refuse to show our ability to resist this wish. The death penalty is the last corporal punishment used officially in the modern world. And it is corporal not only because administered via the body, but because the pain of foreseen, humanly administered death strikes us with the urgency that characterizes intense physical pain, causing grown men to cry, faint, and lose control of their bodily functions. There is something to be gained by refusing to endorse the hardness of heart necessary to impose such a fate.

By placing execution alongside torture in the category of things we will not do to our fellow human beings even when they deserve them, we broadcast the message that totally subjugating a person to the power of others *and* confronting him with the advent of his own humanly administered demise is too horrible to be done by civilized human beings to their fellows even when they have earned it: too horrible to do, and too horrible to be capable of doing. And I contend that broadcasting this message loud and clear would in the long run contribute to the general detestation of murder and be, to the extent to which it worked itself into the hearts and minds of the populace, a deterrent. In short, refusing to execute murderers though they deserve it both reflects and continues the taming of the human species that we call civilization. Thus, I take it that the abolition of the death penalty, though it is a just punishment for murder, is part of the civilizing mission of modern states.

* * *

NOTES

1. Asked, in a 1981 Gallup Poll, "Are you in favor of the death penalty for persons convicted of murder?" 66.25% were in favor, 25% were opposed, and 8.75% had no opinion. Asked the same question in 1966, 47.5% were opposed, 41.25% were in favor, and 11.25% had no opinion (Timothy J. Flanagan, David J. van Alstyne, and Michael R. Gottfredson, eds., *Sourcebook of Criminal Justice Statistics—1981*, U.S. Department of Justice, Bureau of Justice Statistics [Washington, D.C.: U.S. Government Printing Office, 1982], p. 209).

2. I shall speak throughout of retribution as paying back for "harm caused," but this is shorthand for "harm intentionally attempted or caused"; likewise when I speak of the death penalty as punishment for murder, I have in mind premeditated, first-degree murder. Note also that the harm caused by an offender, for which he is to be paid back, is not necessarily limited to the harm done to his immediate victim. It may include as well the suffering of the victim's relatives or the fear produced in the general populace, and the like. For simplicity's sake, however, I shall continue to speak as if the harm for which retributivism would have us pay the offender back is the harm (intentionally attempted or done) to his immediate victim. Also, retribution is not to be confused with *restitution*. Restitution involves restoring the *status quo ante*, the condition prior to the offense. Since it was in this condition that the criminal's offense was committed, it is this condition that constitutes the baseline against which

retribution is exacted. Thus retribution involves imposing a loss on the offender measured from the status quo ante. For example, returning a thief's loot to his victim so that thief and victim now own what they did before the offense is *restitution*. Taking enough from the thief so that what he is left with is less than what he had before the offense is *retribution*, since this is just what he did to his victim.

3. "The most extreme form of retributivism is the law of retaliation: 'an eye for an eye'" (Stanley I. Benn, "Punishment," *The Encyclopedia of Philosophy* 7, ed. Paul Edwards [New York: Macmillan, 1967], p. 32). Hugo Bedau writes: "retributive justice need not be thought to consist of *lex talionis*. One may reject that principle as too crude and still embrace the retributive principle that the severity of punishments should be graded according to the gravity of the offense" (Hugo Bedau, "Capital Punishment," in *Matters of Life and Death*, ed. Tom Regan [New York: Random House, 1980], p. 177).

4. Hegel writes that "The sole positive existence which the injury [i.e., the crime] possesses is that it is the particular will of the criminal [i.e., it is the criminal's intention that distinguishes criminal injury from, say, injury due to an accident]. Hence to injure (or penalize) this particular will as a will determinately existent is to annul the crime, which otherwise would have been held valid, and to restore the right" (G. W. F. Hegel, *The Philosophy of Right*, trans. by T. M. Knox [Oxford: Clarendon Press, 1962; originally published in German in 1821], p. 69, see also p. 331n). I take this to mean that the right is a certain equality of sovereignty between the wills of individuals, crime disrupts that equality by placing one will above others, and punishment restores the equality by annulling the illegitimate ascendance. On these grounds, as I shall suggest below, the desire for revenge (strictly limited to the desire "to even the score") is more respectable than philosophers have generally allowed. And so Hegel writes that "The annulling of crime in this sphere where right is immediate [i.e., the condition prior to conscious morality] is principally revenge, which is just in its content in so far as it is retributive" (ibid., p. 73).

5. Kant writes that "any undeserved evil that you inflict on someone else among the people is one that you do to yourself. If you vilify him, you vilify yourself; if you steal from him, you steal from yourself; if you kill him, you kill yourself." Since Kant holds that "If what happens to someone is also willed by him, it cannot be a punishment," he takes pains to distance himself from the view that the offender *wills* his punishment. "The chief error contained in this sophistry," Kant writes, "consists in the confusion of the

criminal's [that is, the murderer's] own judgment (which one must necessarily attribute to his reason) that he must forfeit his life with a resolution of the will to take his own life" (Immanuel Kant, *The Metaphysical Elements of Justice, Part I of The Metaphysics of Morals*, trans. by J. Ladd [Indianapolis: Bobbs-Merrill, 1965; originally published in 1797], pp. 101, 105–106). I have tried to capture this notion of attributing a judgment to the offender rather than a resolution of his will with the term 'authorizes.'

6. "Even if a civil society were to dissolve itself by common agreement of all its members . . . , the last murderer remaining in prison must first be executed, so that everyone will duly receive what his actions are worth" (Kant, ibid., p. 102).

7. "It may also be pointed out that no one has ever heard of anyone condemned to death on account of murder who complained that he was getting too much [punishment] and therefore was being treated unjustly; everyone would laugh in his face if he were to make such a statement" (Kant, *Metaphysical Elements of Justice*, p. 104; see also p. 133).

8. Friedrich Nietzsche, *The Birth of Tragedy and The Genealogy of Morals*, trans. Francis Golffing (New York: Doubleday, 1956), pp. 199–200.

9. George Orwell, *1984* (New York: New American Library, 1983; originally published in 1949), p. 197.

Against the Death Penalty: The Minimal Invasion Argument

HUGO ADAM BEDAU

Abolitionists attacking the death penalty typically employ a wide variety of moral arguments. The value of human life, respect for human life—these norms play a decisive role for some. Others object on the ground that the state has no right to kill any of its prisoners. Some oppose it because they regard it as an affront to human dignity. Many others object on the ground that the death penalty violates the offender's right to life. Some will insist that it is the unfair administration of the death penalty, and the impossibility of making it fair, that warrants abolishing it. Still others insist that the risk of executing the innocent outweighs whatever alleged benefits the death penalty provides, or that, all things considered, a policy of selective death sentences has less overall social utility—in particular, it squanders scarce resources—than does a policy of no death sentencing. Or (to borrow language from the Supreme Court) "evolving standards of decency" condemn the death penalty today, even if they did not a century ago. Some oppose the death penalty not so much for what it does to the offender as for what it reveals about *us* in tolerating, not to say advocating, such killings. These and perhaps other moral concerns can be connected in various ways; they show that there is much to think about from the moral point of view in evaluating and criticizing the death penalty.

This occasion does not present the opportunity to develop an adequate review and critique of all the arguments implied by these varied moral norms. For that reason I propose to present and discuss only one argument—the one I now think is the best argument against the death penalty. Its lineage can be traced back to the little book by Cesare Beccaria, *An Essay on Crimes and Punishments* (1764), the tract usually credited with inspiring the abolition movement during the period of the Enlightenment in Europe and a version of which reappears in the recent papal encyclical, *Evangelium Vitae*. The argument rests on a fundamental principle that neither Beccaria nor the Pope explicitly formulated: Given a compelling state interest in some goal or purpose, the government in a constitutional democracy built on the principle of equal freedom and human rights for all must use the least restrictive means sufficient to achieve that goal or purpose. More expansively, the principle (a near-neighbor to what students of constitutional law would recognize as the principle of "substantive due process") holds that if individual privacy, liberty, and autonomy (or other fundamental values) are to be invaded and deliberately violated, it must be because the end to be achieved is of undeniable importance to society, and no less severe interference will suffice. For convenience of reference, let us henceforth call this the Minimal Invasion argument against the death penalty and the principle that generates it the Minimal Invasion principle.

The Minimal Invasion argument is unlike most arguments against the death penalty in two important respects. First, it does not rely on such familiar values as the right to life, values that either are not widely shared or are widely shared but at the cost of excessive vagueness. Second, the argument (with the exception of the debate over deterrence) does not hinge on establishing the usual faults that plague this form of punishment as actually administered. Thus, this argument sidesteps worries about the risk of executing the innocent, the arbitrariness of death sentencing and executions, and demonstrable effects of racial bias (especially in the South), the evident vulnerability of the poor, the unavoidable economic costs that exceed those of imprisonment. Opponents of the death penalty are often challenged to declare where they would stand were these flaws to be corrected. Despite the current interest in reforming our several systems of capital punishment, it is doubtful whether all or even most of the reforms so far proposed will be adopted. In any case, the Minimal Invasion argument does not depend on such contingencies. While it is a far cry from a philosopher's a priori argument, it comes close to sharing with such arguments immunity to a wide variety of factual considerations.

If an argument against the death penalty is to be constructed around the Minimal Invasion principle, at least three further propositions must be accepted. First, punishment for crime must be judged to be a legitimate practice in society under a constitution such as ours. Second, the death penalty by its very nature must be judged to be more severe, invasive, and irremediable than the alternative of some form of long-term imprisonment. Third, the death penalty must be judged not to play a necessary role in securing public safety either by way of general deterrence or specific incapacitation. If these three propositions are true, as I think they are, then in conjunction with the principle with which we began they lead to the conclusion that we ought to abolish the death penalty for all crimes and all offenders. Restating this argument in semi-formal style, this is what we get:

The principle. Invasions by the government of an individual's privacy, liberty, and autonomy (or other fundamental value) are justified only if no less invasive practice is sufficient to achieve an important social goal.

1. Punishment is justified only if it is necessary as a means to some socially valid end.
2. The death penalty is more severe—more invasive—than long-term imprisonment.
3. Long-term imprisonment is sufficient as an invasion of individual liberty, privacy, and autonomy (and other fundamental values) to achieve valid social goals.
4. Society ought to abolish any lawful practice that imposes more violation of individual liberty, privacy, or autonomy (or other fundamental value) when it is known that a less invasive practice is available and is sufficient.

The conclusion. Society ought to abolish the death penalty.

There's the argument. What can be said on behalf of the truth of each of its premises? Consider first the Minimal Invasion principle (and its corollary, step [4]). How much defense does it require? Surely it is clear that only extreme socialists, fascists, theocrats, or other totalitarians who for various reasons want to extend state power and intervention into the lives of citizens as far as possible will quarrel with this principle. Liberals and conservatives alike, who accept the basic tenets of constitutional democracy and believe in human rights, should readily embrace it. The only issue calling for further discussion among these supporters is whether this principle might ever conflict with other principles worthier of respect in certain cases, so that it must yield to them. What might such an incompatible but superior principle be? What sort of case might arise where such a conflict occurs? A fuller account of the rationale behind this principle would require us to connect it with more fundamental principles of social justice, a topic that cannot be pursued here. As for the three other steps in the argument, each warrants a closer look.

The first premise. Affirming the legitimacy of a system of punishment poses no problem for supporters of the death penalty nor for any but a few of its opponents. No one disputes that public security—protection against criminal victimization—is a salient value and that intervention by government into the behavior of its citizens to achieve that goal is warranted. But pursuit of such a goal is subject to constraints. Not every imaginable weapon to fight crime is morally permissible. Principles of various sorts (e.g., due process of law) restrict the tactics of intervention. These constraints to the side, as things stand, society needs recourse to punitive methods as a necessary condition of public safety.

This is not, however, because punishment is an end in itself; it is because we know of no less invasive responses to individual behavior sufficient as a means to achieve the purpose. If we did, then it would be difficult and perhaps impossible to defend punishment as a morally permissible practice. After all, punishment by its very nature involves deliberately inflicting deprivations and hardships on persons that, if inflicted by private citizens, would be crimes. So punishment needs to be justified, and the only justification available is that it is a necessary means to a fundamental social goal. For present purposes, then, we can say that there is little dispute over the truth of the first proposition.

The second premise. Few will deny the greater brutality and violence of the death penalty when compared to imprisonment. From time to time one hears a friend of the death penalty—and even on occasion some of its enemies—claiming that life in prison is a much more severe punishment than death. Beccaria and his English admirer, Jeremy Bentham (1748–1832), both pioneering abolitionists, believed that life in prison involved more suffering than a few moments on the gallows. I think it is sufficient by way of a reply to point out that those in the best position to know behave in a manner that suggests otherwise.

Few death row prisoners try to commit suicide and fewer succeed. Few death row prisoners insist that all appeals on their behalf be dropped. Few convicted murderers sentenced to life in prison declare years later that they wish they had been sentenced instead to death and executed. Few if any death row prisoners refuse clemency if it is offered to them. No doubt prison life can be made unbearable and hideous; no doubt death row can be managed by the authorities in an inhumane fashion. But none of this is necessary. No doubt not all life-term prisoners find ways to make their imprisonment something more than an inhumane endurance test. So it should hardly come as a surprise that the vast majority of friends of the death penalty as well as its opponents believe that death is worse than imprisonment. This is why its opponents want to abolish it—and its supporters want to keep it. So we can accept the second proposition without further ado.

The third premise. The third proposition affirms that whatever the legitimate purposes of punishment are, imprisonment serves them as well as or better than the death penalty. This proposition rests on a variety of kinds of empirical evidence, ranging from statistical research on deterrence, the behavior in prison and on parole of convicted murderers not sentenced to death and executed, and above all on the experience of jurisdictions such as Michigan that have gone without the death penalty for decades.

Here is what the record shows: There is no evidence that prison officials, guards, or visitors in prisons where there is no death penalty are more at risk than are their counterparts in the death penalty states. There is no evidence that residents of abolition jurisdictions are at greater risk of murderous victimization than are residents in the death penalty jurisdictions. (The District of Columbia in recent years has had a very high homicide rate and is an abolition jurisdiction; but there is no research that connects the one fact with the other. Most other abolition jurisdictions have a noticeably lower homicide rate than do neighboring death penalty jurisdictions.) To be sure, some convicted murderers commit another murder while in prison or after release—the U.S. Bureau of Justice Statistics reports that 9 percent of those currently on death row had a previous homicide conviction.[1] But not all of these recidivist murderers were guilty in their first homicide of a death-eligible murder. For these murderers, their second homicide could not have been prevented by inflicting the death penalty on them for the first homicide, since their first homicide was not death-eligible. Furthermore, there is no way to predict in advance which convicted murderers are likely to recidivate: the predictions of future dangerousness are plagued with false positives. If we could make accurate and reliable predictions of which prisoners would be dangerous in the future, these offenders could be kept under confinement, just as a typhoid carrier may be quarantined as a public health menace. The only way to prevent such recidivism would be to execute *every* convicted murderer—a policy that is politically unavailable and morally indefensible. Today's defenders of the death penalty must accept a pick-and-choose system of death sentences and executions, with all the adverse effects—as they see it—that such a system has on prevention and retribution.

It is also true that opponents of the death penalty who want to rest their case on the argument under discussion would be vulnerable to evidence—if there were any—showing that the death penalty is a better deterrent than imprisonment. Were there such evidence, opponents would have to rely on some other argument. (I have not claimed that the Minimal Invasion argument is the only argument for abolition, I claim only that I find it the most persuasive.)[2] But since there is so little reason to suppose that the death penalty is ever a marginally superior deterrent over imprisonment, or that such superiority (if any) can be detected by the currently available methods of social science, this "what-if" counterargument can be put to the side and disregarded. (Below, I return to the issue of deterrence.)

With worries about prevention, deterrence, and incapacitation behind us (for the moment), what might we reasonably expect to be the public response in quarters where the death penalty currently has wide support? Is there reason to believe that if the death penalty were abolished, the police would take to administering curbstone justice and the public would revolt? Would the clamor of surviving family members of murder victims force the authorities to restore the death penalty? Would outspoken abolitionists become targets for violent rage, as have some doctors in abortion clinics? Nothing of the sort has happened in any current abolition jurisdiction. However, given the utter lack of political leadership on all aspects of the death penalty in states in the Deep South, where the death penalty has been so conspicuously used, I must admit to some uneasiness over what might happen if Texas were told—say, by a Supreme Court ruling—that it could no longer use the death penalty. The heirs of those who plastered the South in the 1950s with billboards shouting "Impeach Earl Warren" would rise to the occasion and denounce whatever political leadership brought about abolition. Fundamentalist Christians, Mormons, and others who have persuaded themselves that the Bible decrees the death penalty for murder pose a somewhat different problem. How members of these religious groups—clergy and laity, concentrated in (but by no means confined to) the Bible Belt across the South—would behave is far from obvious.

The upshot is that the third premise in the argument under discussion is reasonably supported by the available facts; and that suffices to prove the conclusion.

* * *

Nevertheless, many friends of the death penalty will not be persuaded by my argument. They will advance at least two objections, one empirical and the other conceptual and normative. First, they will insist on the superiority of the death penalty as a deterrent. Second, they will object that my argument simply ignores a crucial conceptual element and normative principle that, when properly taken into account, leads to a different conclusion.

* * *

. . . The question that defenders of the death penalty need to answer is not "Does the death penalty deter?" Common sense assures us that punishments generally serve to deter some persons from some crimes on some occasions. There is no reason to think that the death penalty is an exception. As for measuring how much it deters, as econometricians try to do, that is a side issue. Answering the question above would be dispositive only if opponents of the death penalty favored *no* punishment for capital crimes. But of course they don't favor no punishment (with the exception, perhaps, of some pacificists). The question that death penalty advocates need to answer is this: "Does the death penalty deter *as well as or better than* imprisonment?" To date, no one has even tried to determine the extent to which imprisonment is a deterrent to murder. For all we know, it is as good a deterrent as death, or even better. For all we know, the alleged deterrent effect detected by econometric methods is owing to increases in the use of long-term imprisonment concurrent with executions. Defenders of the death penalty who want to rest their case in whole or in part on the alleged deterrent effect of the death penalty at best refute those abolitionists who think (erroneously) that the death penalty never deters. They leave untouched those abolitionists who think there is no evidence that the death penalty is marginally a better deterrent than executions.

But for the sake of the argument, let us suppose that the death penalty as currently employed does have a marginally superior deterrent effect. Such an effect is of little use in defending the death penalty because the supposed benefit is obtained at an unacceptable cost. The cost comes in the many ways our death penalty system is dysfunctional. The latest study by James S. Liebman and his associates documents this conclusion in alarming detail. Perhaps their most disturbing finding was that the more a jurisdiction uses the death penalty, the greater the likelihood that it will make mistakes—notably, the mistake of convicting the innocent or the mistake of sentencing to death offenders whose crimes should not have made them death-eligible. Everyone agrees that the deterrent effect of a penalty is a function of the frequency with which it is employed; Liebman's research shows that the more courts strive for a deterrent effect by increasing the frequency of death sentences, the more likely they are to err in their judgments and sentences.[3] We have no right to secure a benefit for some (innocents protected by superior marginal deterrence), *knowing* that we do so by methods that impose injustice on others—defendants who may not be guilty (or not guilty of first-degree murder) and whose guilt is determined by violations of due process and equal protection of the law.

Today, would-be defenders of the death penalty no longer rely, as they once did, mainly on the claim of superior deterrence. And that is just as well. Quite apart from the difficulties just discussed in defending the death penalty on grounds of deterrence, those who rely on the principle that severe punishments are justified by their superior deterrent and incapacitative effects are implicitly invited to go further. If death deters more than imprisonment, then death preceded by torture presumably deters more than death alone. If so, on what ground is the defender of the death penalty able to resist embracing torture as well as death? Surely, all sides agree that morality and politics require that there be some upper bound to the permissible severity of punishments no matter what their deterrent effect might be. The dispute is not over whether there is such a limit, but where to place that limit and why. The Minimal Invasion argument provides a reasonable solution to that problem. Preferring the death penalty because of its allegedly superior deterrent effects does not.

* * *

NOTES

1. U.S. Department of Justice, Bureau of Justice Statistics, "Capital Punishment 1998," Washington, D.C., 1999, p. 10.

2. A strong candidate for an argument equally as concise as but otherwise very different from mine is the "knockdown argument" offered by Stephen Nathanson, *An Eye for an Eye*, 2nd ed. (Lanham, Md.: Rowman and Littlefield, 2001), p. 175. Here it is, addressed to a death penalty supporter: "You accept justice and respect for human life as fundamental values; the death penalty is inconsistent with these values; therefore, based on your own values, you ought to reject the death penalty."

3. James S. Liebman et al., *Why There Is So Much Error in Capital Cases, and What Can Be Done about It* (New York: Columbia Law School, February 2002).

In Defense of the Death Penalty

LOUIS P. POJMAN

THE RETRIBUTIVIST ARGUMENT FOR THE DEATH PENALTY

Let me say a word about the notion of *desert*. Part of justice, going back to Plato, Aristotle, Kant, the Biblical tradition, and virtually every major religion, holds that people ought to get what they deserve. Those who work hard for worthy goals deserve reward; those who do not make the effort deserve nothing; and those who purposefully do evil deserve punishment. The virtuous deserve to flourish to the degree of their virtue, and the vicious deserve to suffer to the degree of their vice. "Whatsoever a man soweth, that shall he reap," is an ancient adage perhaps as old as its metaphysical counterpart of eternal judgment (Jewish/Christian tradition) or karma (Hindu/Buddhist tradition)—that what one does in this life will be part of one's essential constitution in the next life. This notion presumes the notion of responsibility, that people are accountable for their actions and should be rewarded and punished accordingly. Even Karl Marx objected to applying the principle "From each

Louis Pojman, "The Death Penalty" from *Life and Death*, 2E. © 2000 Wadsworth, a part of Cengage Learning, Inc. Reproduced by permission. www.cengage.com/permissions.

according to his ability, to each according to his need," to people who did not work, who did not deserve to be helped.[1] Only in contemporary liberalism, such as Rawls's theory of justice as fairness, has the notion of natural desert been seriously undermined. But Rawls is wrong here. Although we may not deserve our initial endowments or capacities, we do deserve what we make with them. Our effort and contribution are worthy of moral assessment, and as agents we can be held accountable for our effort and contributions. That is, without the concept of desert, responsibility has no validity, and without the notion of responsibility, neither morality nor law has a footing.

Suppose, as most of us do, that each person has a right to life. That right, however, is not absolute, but conditional (otherwise we could not kill even in self-defense). Like our right to property and liberty, it can be overridden for weighty moral reasons. When an offender threatens or attempts to kill an innocent person, the offender deserves a punishment appropriate to the severity of the crime. When an offender with malice aforethought takes the life of an innocent person, he or she forfeits his or her own life. But the main idea in the retributivist theory is that not only is the death penalty permissible for the murderer, it is also deserved. The guilty deserve punishment, and that punishment should be proportional to the severity of their crime. A complete retributivist like Kant *** holds that all and only those who are guilty should be so punished. The moderate retributivist holds that only the guilty should be so punished—but not necessarily all of the guilty. Mitigating circumstances, the external costs of punishment, the possibility of reform, and so forth may prescribe lesser degrees of punishment than are deserved. Hell itself may be a just desert for Hitler, but morality doesn't require that we torture him. The moderate retributivist holds that giving people what they deserve (positive and negative) is a *prima facie* duty, not an absolute, nonoverridable one.

Some have objected that the death penalty is itself murder. To quote eighteenth-century abolitionist Cesare di Beccaria, "Putting the criminal to death only compounds evil. If killing is an evil, then the State actually doubles the evil by executing the murderer. The State violates the criminal's right to life. It carries out *legalized murder*. The death penalty cannot be useful because of the example of barbarity it gives to men. . . . it seems to me absurd that the laws which punish homicide should themselves commit it." But there is a difference. The murderer volunteered for his crime. The victim didn't volunteer for his fate. The murderer had reason to believe that he would be justly and severely punished for his crime, so he has no reason to complain when the state executes him. The murderer violated the victim's right to life, thereby forfeiting his own *prima facie* right to life. The Fifth and Fourteenth Amendments of our Bill of Rights state that no one should be deprived of life, liberty, or property without due process of the law, implying that so long as due process of the law has been observed, condemning a murderer to death is both legally and morally justified.

Society may rank punishments corresponding roughly to the gravity of the crime. That is, it draws up two lists. The first list consists of a list of crimes, from the most to the least serious. The second is a list of punishments that it considers acceptable, from the most severe to the least severe. So long as there is a rough correspondence between the two lists, a society is permitted to consult its own sense of justice in linking the various punishments with each crime in question. The death penalty, it seems, is at the head of the list of severe punishments, linked retributively with the worst crimes. Whether torture is also permitted for a torturer, mutilation for a rapist, and so forth, may be debated. Strictly speaking I have no argument against the appropriate use of torture, though I think it is not necessary. It seems to me that death is a sufficient punishment for the most heinous crimes, but it's not part of my thesis to sort out these matters. Where to put the limit of harm to be imposed on the murderer is partly a cultural matter, as the history of legal punishment indicates.[2] Our notion of what is or is not "humane," connected with repulsion against torture and corporal punishment in general, is largely a cultural matter. It has to do with how we have been socialized. Torture shocks our sensibilities, but not those of our ancestors, and not necessarily our moral principles. Although I am a moral objectivist, holding that moral truth exists, part of morality is relative to culture, to the sensibilities of the majority of its members.

One objection to the retributivist argument is that although a criminal may deserve the death penalty, the justification of the State's execution of the criminal is another matter. It needs a separate justification. The correct response is that justice consists of giving people what they deserve. As Locke noted, in the state of nature we would each have the right and duty to punish the offender, but in organized society, we surrender that right and duty to the State. We may override justice because of mitigating circumstances, but insofar as the State has duty to dispense justice, it is justified in executing those who commit murder.

THE UTILITARIAN ARGUMENT

The utilitarian argument for capital punishment is that it deters would-be offenders from committing first-degree murder. If the death penalty deters, we have an auxiliary argument for its use. This argument may supplement (but not replace) the retributivist argument. Isaac Ehrlich's study, to my knowledge the most thorough study to date, takes into account the complex sociological data and concludes that over the period 1933–1969, "an additional execution per year. . . . may have resulted on the average in seven or eight fewer murders."[3] Ehrlich's findings have been challenged by many opponents with the result that the issue is left in doubt. It seems an enormous undertaking to prove either that the death penalty deters or that it does not deter. The statistical evidence is inconclusive—which is different from saying that it is "zero," as abolitionists sometimes claim.

Commonsense reasons exist for believing that the death penalty deters some would-be murderers from murdering. Richard Herrnstein and James Q. Wilson have argued in *Crime and Human Nature* that a great deal of crime is committed in a cost-benefit scheme, wherein the criminal engages in some form of risk assessment as to his or her chances of getting caught and punished in some manner. If a would-be criminal estimates the punishment to be mild, the crime will become inversely attractive, and vice versa. If a potential murderer judges that he may be punished by imprisonment or death, he will be more deterred than if he judges that he will be punished only by imprisonment. Doesn't the fact that those condemned to death do everything in their power to postpone it, and to get their sentences reduced to long-term prison sentences, show that the death penalty is feared as an evil to be avoided? The potential criminal need not go through deliberate cost-benefit analysis. The association of murder with the death penalty may have embedded in the subconscious mind of potential criminals a powerful deterrence. Perhaps the abolition of the death penalty from the 1960s until the late 1970s, and the fact that it is only recently being carried out with any regularity, have eroded the association, accounting for the increased murder rate from 1980 until 1993. The fact that the death penalty is beginning to be carried out may partially account for the decrease of homicides in recent years.

Former Prosecuting Attorney for the State of Florida, Richard Gernstein, has set forth the commonsense case for deterrence. First of all, the death penalty certainly deters the murderer from committing any further murders, including those he or she might commit within the prison in which he is confined. Second, statistics cannot tell us how many potential criminals have refrained from taking another's life through fear of the death penalty. As Hyman Barshay puts it:

> The death penalty is a warning, just like a lighthouse throwing its beams out to sea. We hear about shipwrecks, but we do not hear about the ships the lighthouse guides safely on their way. We do not have proof of the number of ships it saves, but we do not tear the lighthouse down.

Some of the commonsense evidence is anecdotal, as reported by British member of parliament Arthur Lewis, who was converted from being an abolitionist to a retentionist:

> One reason that has stuck in my mind, and which has proved to me beyond question, is that there was once a professional burglar in my constituency who consistently boasted of the fact that the had spent about one-third of his life in prison. . . . he said to me, "I am a professional burglar. Before we go out on a job we plan it down to every detail. Before we go into the boozer to have a drink we say, 'Don't forget, no shooters'—shooters being guns." He adds, "We did our job and didn't have shooters because at that time there was capital punishment. Our wives, girlfriends and our mums said, 'Whatever you do, do not carry a shooter because if you are caught you might be topped.' If you do away with capital punishment they will all be carrying shooters."

It's difficult to know how widespread this kind of reasoning is. My own experience, growing up in a neighborhood where some of my acquaintances were criminals, corroborates this testimony. These criminals admitted being constrained in their behavior by the possibility of the death penalty. No doubt some crimes are committed in the heat of passion or by the temporarily insane, but not all crime fits that mold. Perhaps rational risk assessment, which involves the cost-benefit analysis of crime, is mainly confined to certain classes of potential and professional criminals, including burglars and kidnappers. It probably applies to people who are tempted to kill their enemies. We simply don't know how much capital punishment deters, but this sort of commonsense, anecdotal evidence cannot be dismissed as worthless. Common sense tells us that people will be deterred by greater punishments such as death than by lesser ones such as imprisonment.

I have been arguing that we do have some statistical and commonsense evidence that the death penalty deters would-be killers. Even if you are skeptical about that evidence, another argument, based on the *possibility* that it deters, is available to us. This is the argument set forth by Ernest van den Haag, which he calls the "Best Bet argument."[4] Van den Haag argues that even though we don't know for certain whether the death penalty deters or prevents other murders, we should bet that it does. Indeed, due to our ignorance, any social policy we take is a gamble. Not to choose capital punishment for first-degree murder is as much a bet that capital punishment doesn't deter as choosing the policy is a bet that it does. There is a significant difference in the betting, however: to bet *against* capital punishment is to bet against the innocent and for the murderer; while to bet *for* it is to bet against the murderer and for the innocent.[5]

The point is this: we are accountable for what we let happen as well as for what we actually do. If I fail to bring up my children properly and they are a menace to society, I am to some extent responsible for their bad behavior. I could have caused it to be somewhat better. If I have good evidence that a bomb will blow up the building in which you are working and I fail to notify you (assuming that I can), I am partly responsible for your death, if and when the bomb explodes. To refrain purposefully from a lesser evil that we know will allow a greater evil to occur, is to be at least partially responsible for the greater evil.

This responsibility for our omissions underlies van den Haag's argument, to which we now return. Suppose that we choose a policy of capital punishment for capital crimes. In this case we are betting that the death of some murderers will be more than compensated for by the lives of some innocents who will not be murdered (by either these murderers or others). If we're right, we have saved the lives of the innocent. If we're wrong, unfortunately, we've sacrificed the lives of some murderers. Suppose we choose not to have a social policy of capital punishment. If capital punishment doesn't work as a deterrent, we've come out ahead, but if it does, we've missed an opportunity to save innocent lives. If we value the saving of innocent lives more highly than the loss of the guilty, betting on a policy of capital punishment turns out to be rational. The reasoning goes like this: Let "CP" stand for Capital Punishment:

The Wager

CP works	CP doesn't work
We bet on CP	
a. We win: some murderers die and some innocents are saved.	b. We lose: some murderers die for no purpose.
We bet against CP	
c. We lose: murderers live and some innocents die needlessly.	d. We win: murderers live and the lives of others are unaffected.

Suppose that we estimate the utility value of a murderer's life a 5 while the value of an innocent's life is 10. Although we cannot give lives exact numerical values, we can make rough comparative estimates: Mother Teresa's life is greater than Adolf Hitler's, and all things being equal, the life of an innocent person is at least twice the value of a murderer's. (My own sense is that the murderer has forfeited most, if not all, of his worth, but if I had to put a figure on it, that figure would be 1,000 to 1). Given van den Haag's figures, the sums work out this way:

A murderer saved	+5
A murderer executed	−5
An innocent saved	+10
An innocent murdered	−10

Suppose that for each execution only two innocent lives are spared. Then the outcomes read as follows:

1. $-5 + 20 = +15$
2. -5
3. $+5 - 20 = -15$
4. $+5$

If all of the possibilities are roughly equal, we can sum their outcomes as follows:

If we bet on capital punishment, (a) and (b) obtain = +10.

If we bet against capital punishment, (c) and (d) obtain = −10.

So to execute convicted murderers turns out to be a good bet. To abolish the death penalty for convicted murderers would be a bad bet. We unnecessarily put the innocent at risk.

Even if we value the utility of an innocent life only slightly more than that of a murderer, it is still rational to execute convicted murderers. As van den Haag writes, "Though we have no proof of the positive deterrence of the penalty, we also have no proof of zero or negative effectiveness. I believe we have no right to risk additional future victims of murder for the sake of sparing convicted murderers; on the contrary, our moral obligation is to risk the possible ineffectiveness of executions."[6]

THE GOLDEN RULE ARGUMENT

One more argument should be set forth, and that is the Golden Rule argument for the death penalty. The Golden Rule states that we should do unto others as we would have them do unto us if we were in their shoes. Reflect on the evil deeds perpetrated by Nazi war criminals, or by those who blew up the Murrah Federal Building in Oklahoma City on April 19, 1995, killing 168 people, or on any number of heinous murders well known to us. If you had yielded to temptation and blown up the Federal Building, or like Steven Judy had raped and murdered a helpless woman and then drowned her three small children, or if you had kidnapped a young girl, placed her in your trunk and then killed her, what punishment do you think would be fitting for *you*? What would you deserve? Would you want to live? Would not the moral guilt that you would doubtless feel demand the death penalty? And would you not judge that such moral guilt was appropriate and that anyone who did not feel it was morally defective? Would you not agree that you had forfeited your right to life, that you had brought upon yourself the hangman's noose? Would you not agree that you deserved nothing less than death? Should we not apply these sentiments to murderers?

OBJECTIONS TO CAPITAL PUNISHMENT

Let us examine three major objections to capital punishment, as well as the retentionist's responses to those objections.

1. Objection: Capital punishment is a morally unacceptable thirst for revenge. As former British Prime Minister Edward Heath put it,

> The real point which is emphasized to me by many constituents is that even if the death penalty is not a deterrent, murderers deserve to die. This is the question of revenge. Again, this will be a matter of moral judgment for each of us. I do not believe in revenge. If I were to become the victim of terrorists, I would not wish them to be hanged or killed in any other way for revenge. All that would do is deepen the bitterness which already tragically exists in the conflicts we experience in society, particularly in Northern Ireland.[7]

Response: Retributivism is not the same thing as revenge, although the two attitudes are often intermixed in practice. Revenge is a personal response to a perpetrator for an injury. Retribution is an impartial and impersonal response to an offender for an offense done against someone. You cannot desire revenge for the harm of someone to whom you are indifferent. Revenge always involves personal concern for the victim. Retribution is not personal but based on objective factors: the criminal has deliberately harmed an innocent party and so deserves to be punished, whether I wish it or not. I would agree that I, my son, or my daughter deserves to be punished for our crimes, but I don't wish any vengeance on myself, my son, or my daughter.

Furthermore, while revenge often leads us to exact more suffering from the offender than the offense warrant, retribution stipulates that the offender be punished in proportion to the gravity of the offense. In this sense, the *lex talionis* that we find in the Old Testament is actually a progressive rule, where retribution replaces revenge as the mode of punishment. It says that there are limits to what one may do to an offender. Revenge demands a life for an eye or a tooth, but Moses provides a rule that exacts a penalty equal to the harm done by the offender.

2. Objection: Miscarriages of justice occur. Capital punishment is to be rejected because of human fallibility in convicting innocent parties and sentencing them to death. In a survey done in 1985, Hugo Adam Bedau and Michael Radelet found that of the 7,000 persons executed in the United States between 1900 and 1985, 25 were innocent of capital crimes.[8] Although some compensation is available to those unjustly imprisoned, the death sentence is irrevocable. We can't compensate the dead. As John Maxton, a member of the British Parliament, puts it, "If we allow one innocent person to be executed, morally we are committing the same, or, in some ways, a worse crime than the person who committed the murder."[9]

Response: Mr. Maxton is incorrect in saying that mistaken judicial execution is morally the same as or worse than murder. A deliberate intention to kill the innocent occurs in a murder, whereas no such intention occurs in wrongful capital punishment.

Sometimes the objection is framed this way: It is better to let ten criminals go free than to execute one innocent person. If this dictum is a call for safeguards, it is well taken, but somewhere there seems to be a limit on the society's tolerance of capital offenses. Would these abolitionists argue that it is better that 50 or 100 or 1,000 murderers go free than that one innocent person be executed? Society has a right to protect itself from capital offenses even if this means taking a finite chance of executing an innocent person. If the basic activity or process is justified, it is regrettable but morally acceptable that some mistakes are made. Fire trucks occasionally kill innocent pedestrians while racing to fires, but we accept these losses as justified by the greater good of the activity of using fire trucks. We judge the use of automobiles to be acceptable even though such use causes an average of 50,000 traffic fatalities each year. We accept the morality of a defensive war even though it will result in our troops accidentally or mistakenly killing innocent people.

The fact that we can err in applying the death penalty should give us pause and cause us to build an appeals process into the judicial system. Such a process is already in the American and British legal systems. Occasional errors may be made, but as regrettable as this is, it is not a sufficient reason for us to refuse to use the death penalty if, on balance, it serves a just and useful function.

Furthermore, abolitionists are simply misguided in thinking that prison sentences are a satisfactory alternative. It's not clear that we can always or typically compensate innocent parties who waste away in prison. Jacques Barzun has argued that a prison sentence can be worse than death and carries all the problems that the death penalty does regarding the impossibility of compensation:

> In the preface of his useful volume of cases, *Hanged in Error*, Mr. Leslie Hale refers to the tardy recognition of a minor miscarriage of justice—one year in jail: "The prisoner emerged to find that his wife had died and that his children and his aged parents had been removed to the workhouse. By the time a small payment had been assessed as 'compensation' the victim was incurably insane." So far we are as indignant with the law as Mr. Hale. But what comes next? He cites the famous Evans case, in which it is very probable that the wrong man was hanged, and he exclaims: "While such mistakes are possible, should society impose an irrevocable sentence?" Does Mr. Hale really ask us to believe that the sentence passed on the first man, whose wife died and who went insane, was in any sense *revocable*? Would not any man rather be Evans dead than that other wretch "emerging" with his small compensation and his reason for living gone?[10]

The abolitionist is incorrect in arguing that death is different than long-term prison sentences because it is irrevocable. Imprisonment also takes good things away from us that may never be returned. We cannot restore to an inmate the freedom or opportunities he or she lost. Suppose an innocent twenty-five-year-old man is given a life sentence for murder. Thirty years later the mistake is discovered and he is set free. Suppose he equates three years of freedom to every one year of life. That is, he would rather live ten years as a free man than thirty as a prisoner. Given this man's values, the criminal justice system has taken the equivalent of ten years of life from him. If he lives until he is sixty-five, he has, by his estimate, lost ten years, so he may be said to have lived only fifty-five years.[11]

The numbers in this example are arbitrary, but the basic point is sound. Most of us would prefer a short life of high quality to a longer one of low quality. Death prevents all subsequent quality, but imprisonment also irrevocably harms one in diminishing the quality of life of the prisoner.

3. *Objection:* The death penalty is unjust because it discriminates against the poor and minorities, particularly African Americans. Former Supreme Court Justice William Douglas wrote that "a law which reaches that [discriminatory] result in practice has no more sanctity than a law which in terms provides the same."[12] Nathanson argues that "in many cases, whether one is treated justly or not depends not only on what one deserves but on how other people are treated."[13] He offers the example of unequal justice in a plagiarism case. "I tell the students in my class that anyone who plagiarizes will fail the course. Three students plagiarize papers, but I give only one a failing grade. The other two, in describing their motivation, win my sympathy, and I give them passing grades." Arguing that this is patently unjust, he likens this case to the imposition of the death penalty and concludes that it too is unjust.

Response: First of all, it is not true that a law applied in a discriminatory manner is unjust. Unequal justice is no less justice, however uneven its application. The discriminatory application, not the law itself, is unjust. A just law is still just, even if it is not applied consistently. For example, a friend of mine once got two speeding tickets during a 100-mile trip (having borrowed my car). He complained to the police officer who gave him his second ticket that many drivers were driving faster than he was at the time. They had escaped detection, he argued, so it wasn't fair for him to get two tickets on one trip. The officer acknowledged the imperfections of the system but, justifiably, had no qualms about giving him the second ticket. Unequal justice is still justice, however regrettable. So Justice Douglas is wrong in asserting that discriminatory results invalidate the law itself. The discriminatory

practice should be reformed, and in many cases it can be. But imperfect practices in themselves do not entail that the laws engendering these practices are themselves unjust.

With regard to Nathanson's analogy in the plagiarism case, two things should be said against it. First, if the teacher is convinced that the motivational factors are mitigating factors, then he or she may be justified in passing two of the plagiarizing students. Suppose that one student did no work whatsoever, showed no interest (Nathanson's motivation factor) in learning, and exhibited no remorse in cheating, whereas the other two spent long hours seriously studying the material and, upon apprehension, showed genuine remorse for their misdeeds. To be sure, they yielded to temptation at certain—though limited—sections of their long papers, but the vast majority of their papers represented their own diligent work. Suppose also that all three had C averages at this point. The teacher gives the unremorseful, gross plagiarizer an F but relents and gives the other two Ds. Her actions parallel the judge's use of mitigating circumstances and cannot be construed as arbitrary, let alone unjust.

The second problem with Nathanson's analogy is that it would have disastrous consequences for law and benevolent practices alike. If we concluded that we should abolish a rule or practice unless we always treated everyone by exactly the same rules, we would have to abolish, for example, traffic laws and laws against imprisonment for rape, theft, and even murder. Carried to its logical limits, we would also have to refrain from saving drowning victims if a number of people were drowning but only a few of them could be saved. Imperfect justice is the best that we humans can attain. We should reform our practices as much as possible to eradicate unjust discrimination wherever we can, but if we are not allowed to have a law without perfect application, we will be forced to have no laws at all.

Nathanson acknowledges this response but argues that the case of death is different. "Because of its finality and extreme severity of the death penalty, we need to be more scrupulous in applying it as punishment than is necessary with any other punishment."[14]

The retentionist agrees that the death penalty is a severe punishment and that we need to be scrupulous in applying it. The difference between the abolitionist and the retentionist seems to lie in whether we are wise and committed enough as a nation to reform our institutions so that they approximate fairness. Apparently Nathanson is pessimistic here, whereas I have faith in our ability to learn from our mistakes and reform our systems. If we can't reform our legal system, what hope is there for us?

More specifically, the charge that a higher percentage of blacks than whites are executed was once true but is no longer so. Many states have made significant changes in sentencing procedures, with the result that currently whites convicted of first-degree murder are sentenced to death at a higher rate than blacks.[15]

One must be careful in reading too much into these statistics. Although great disparities in statistics should cause us to examine our judicial procedures, they do not in themselves prove injustice. For example, more males than females are convicted of violent crimes (almost 90 percent of those convicted of violent crimes are males—a virtually universal statistic), but this is not strong evidence that the law is unfair, for there are psychological explanations for the disparity in convictions. Males are on average and by nature more aggressive (usually tied to testosterone) than females. Likewise, there may be good explanations for why people of one ethnic group commit more crimes than do those of other groups, explanations that do not impugn the processes of the judicial system.[16]

4. *Objection:* The death penalty is a "cruel and unusual punishment." It constitutes a denial of the wrongdoer's essential dignity as a human being. No matter how bad a person becomes, no matter how terrible one's deed, we must never cease to regard a person as an end in himself or herself, as someone with inherent dignity. Capital punishment violates that dignity. As such, it violates the Constitution of the United States of America, which forbids "cruel and unusual" punishments. Here is how Justice Thurgood Marshall stated it in *Gregg v. Georgia:*

To be sustained under the Eighth Amendment, the death penalty must [comport] with the basic concept of human dignity at the core of the Amendment; the objective in imposing it must be [consistent] with our respect for the dignity of [other] men. Under these standards, the taking of life "because the wrongdoer deserves it" surely must fail, for such a punishment has as its very basis the total denial of the wrongdoer's dignity and worth. The death penalty, unnecessary to promote the goal of deterrence or to further any legitimate notion of retribution, is an excessive penalty forbidden by the Eighth and Fourteenth Amendments.[17]

Similarly, in *Furman v. Georgia* (1972) Justice William Brennan condemned capital punishment because it treats "members of the human race as nonhumans, as objects to be toyed with and discarded," adding that it is "inconsistent with the fundamental premise of the Clause that even the vilest criminal remains a human being possessed of common human dignity."[18]

Response: First of all, Justice Marshall differs with the framers of the Constitution about the meaning of "cruel and unusual" in declaring that the death penalty violates the Eighth Amendment's prohibition against "cruel and unusual" punishments—unless one would accuse the framers of the Constitution of contradicting themselves. The Fifth and Fourteenth Amendments clearly authorize the death penalty.[19] The phrase "cruel and unusual" in the Eighth Amendment seems to mean cruel and *uncustomary or new* punishments, for, as van den Haag notes, "the framers did not want judges to invent *new* cruel punishments, but did not abolish customary ones."[20] However, even if the framers did intend to prohibit the death penalty, I would argue that it is morally justified. The law is not always identical to what is morally correct.

Rather than being a violation of a wrongdoer's dignity, capital punishment may constitute a recognition of human dignity. As noted in the discussion in Kant's view of retribution, the use of capital punishment respects the worth of victims in calling for an equal punishment to be extracted from offenders, and it respects the dignity of the offenders in treating them as free agents who must be respected for their decisions and who must bear the cost of their acts as responsible agents.

Let's look at these two points a bit more closely. The first—that capital punishment respects the worth of the victim—is bluntly articulated by newspaper columnist Mike Royko:

> When I think of the thousands of inhabitants of Death Rows in the hundreds of prisons in this country, I don't react the way the kindly souls do—with revulsion that the state would take these lives. My reaction is: What's taking us so long? Let's get that electrical current flowing. Drop the pellets now!
>
> Whenever I argue this with friends who have opposite views, they say that I don't have enough regard for that most marvelous of miracles—human life.
>
> Just the opposite: It's because I have so much regard for human life that I favor capital punishment. Murder is the most terrible crime there is. Anything less than the death penalty is an insult to the victim and society. It says, in effect, that we don't value the victim's life enough to punish the killer fully.[21]

It is precisely because the victim's life is sacred that the death penalty is sometimes the only fitting punishment for first-degree murder. I am accepting here the idea that there is something "sacred" or "dignified" about human life, although earlier I gave reasons that should cause secularists to doubt this.

Second, it's precisely because murderers are autonomous, free agents that we regard their acts of murder as their own and hold them responsible. Not to hold a murderer responsible for his crime is to treat him as less than autonomous. Just as we praise and reward people in proportion to the merit of their good deeds, so we blame and punish them in proportion to the evil of their bad deeds. If there is evidence that the offender did not act freely, we would mitigate his sentence, but if he acted of his own free will, he bears the responsibility for those actions and deserves to be punished accordingly.

Of course, there are counterresponses to all of the retentionist's responses. Consider the utilitarian matter of cost. The appeals process, which is necessary to our system of justice, is so prolonged and expensive that it might not be worth the costs simply to satisfy

our sense of retribution. Furthermore, most moderate retributivists do not argue that there is an absolute duty to execute first-degree murderers. Even the principle that the guilty should suffer in proportion to the harm they caused is not absolute; it can be overridden by mercy. But such mercy must be judicious, serving the public good.

In the same vein many argue that life imprisonment without parole will accomplish just as much as the death penalty. The retentionist would respond that death is a more fitting punishment for one who kills in cold blood, and utilitarians (deterrentists) would be concerned about the possibility of escape, murders committed by the murderer while incarcerated, and the enormous costs of keeping a prisoner incarcerated for life. Imprisonment without parole, advocated by many abolitionists as an alternative to the death penalty, should be given serious consideration in special cases, such as when there is evidence that the murderer has suitably repented. Even in these cases, however, the desert argument and the Best Bet argument lean toward the death penalty.

No doubt we should work toward the day when capital punishment is no longer necessary: when the murder rate becomes a tiny fraction of what it is today, when a civilized society can safely incarcerate the few violent criminals in its midst, and when moral reform of the criminal is a reality. Perhaps this is why several European nations have abolished capital punishment (e.g., the murder rate in one year in Detroit alone was 732 times that of the nation of Austria). I for one regret the use of the death penalty. I would vote for its abolition in an instant if only one condition were met: that those contemplating murder would set an example for me. Otherwise, it is better that the murderer perish than that innocent victims be cut down by the murderer's knife or bullet.

ENDNOTES

1. Karl Marx, "Critique of the Gotha Program," *Karl Marx: Selected Writings*, ed. B. McLellan (Oxford: Oxford University Press, 1977). For a fuller discussion of desert, see my article "Equality and Desert," *What Do We Deserve*, eds. L. Pojman and O. McLeod (Oxford: Oxford University Press, 1998).

2. Michael Davis has an excellent discussion of "humane punishment" in "Death, Deterrence, and the Method of Common Sense," *Social Theory and Practice* (summer 1981).

3. Isaac Ehrlich, "The Deterrent Effect of Capital Punishment: A Question of Life and Death," *American Economic Review* 65 (June 1975): 397–417.

4. Ernst van den Haag, "On Deterrence and the Death Penalty," *Ethics*, 78 (July 1968).

5. The Best Bet argument rejects the passive–active distinction involved in killing and letting die. Many people think that it is far worse to kill someone than to let him die, even with the same motivation. More generally, they hold that it is worse to *do* something bad than to *allow* something bad to happen. I think people feel this way because they are tacitly supposing different motivational stances. Judith Jarvis Thomson gives the following counterexample to this doctrine: John is a trolley driver who suddenly realizes that his brakes have failed. He is heading for a group of workers on the track before him and will certainly kill them if something isn't done immediately. Fortunately, there is a side track to the right onto which John can turn the trolley. Unfortunately, there is one worker on that track who will be killed if John steers the trolley onto the side track.

   If the passive–active distinction holds, John should do nothing but simply allow the trolley to take its toll of the five men on the track before him, but that seems terrible. Surely by turning quickly and causing the trolley to move onto the side track, John will be saving a total of four lives. It seems morally preferable for John to turn the trolley onto the side track and actively cause the death of one man rather than passively allow the death of five. John is caught in a situation in which he cannot help doing or allowing harm, but he can act so that the lesser of the evils obtains.

6. van den Haag, op. cit.

7. British Parliamentary Debates, 1982, quoted in Sorrell, *Moral Theory*, 43.

8. Hugo Adam Bedau and Michael Radelet, *Miscarriages of Justice in Potential Capital Cases* (1st draft Oct. 1985, on file at Harvard Law School Library), quoted in E. van den Haag, "The Ultimate Punishment: A Defense," *Harvard Law Review*, 99, no. 7 (May 1896): 1664.

9. Ibid., 47.

10. Jacques Barzun, "In Favor of Capital Punishment," *The American Scholar*, 31, no. 2 (spring 1962).

11. I have been influenced by similar arguments by Michael Levin (unpublished manuscript) and Michael Davis, "Is the Death Penalty Irrevocable?" *Social Theory and Practice* 10:2 (summer 1984).

12. Justice William Douglas in *Furman v. Georgia* 408 U.S. 238 (1972).

13. Stephen Nathanson, *An Eye for an Eye?* (Totowa, NJ: Roman & Littlefield, 1987) 62.

14. Ibid., 67.

15. The Department of Justice's *Bureau of Justice Statistics Bulletin* for 1994 reports that between 1977 and 1994, 2,336 (51%) of those arrested for murder were white, 1838 (40%) were black, 316 (7%) were Hispanic. Of the 257 who were executed, 140 (54%) were white, 98 (38%) were black, 17 (7%) were Hispanic, and 2 (1%) were of other races. In 1994, 31 prisoners, 20 white men and 11 black men, were executed, although whites made up only 7,532 (41%) and blacks 9,906 (56%) of those arrested for murder. Of those sentenced to death in 1994, 158 were white men, 133 were black men, 25 were Hispanic men, 2 were Native American men, 2 were white women, and 3 were black women. Of those sentenced, relatively more blacks (72%) than whites (65%) or Hispanics (60%), had prior felony records. Overall, the criminal justice system does not seem to favor white criminals over black, though it does seem to favor rich defendants over poor ones.

16. For instance, according to FBI figures for 1992, the U.S. murder rate was 9.3, far higher than that of France (4.5), Germany (3.9) or Austria (3.9). Of the 23,760 murders committed in the United States that year, 55% of the offenders whose race was known were black and 43% white. Since blacks compose 12.1% of the U.S. population, the murder rate for blacks in 1992 was 45 per 100,000, while that for whites was 4.78— a figure much closer to that for European whites.

17. Justice Thurgood Marshall, *Gregg v. Georgia* (1976).

18. Justice William Brennan, *Furman v. Georgia* (1972).

19. The Fifth Amendment permits depriving people of "life, liberty or property" if the deprivation occurs with "due process of law," and the Fourteenth Amendment applies this provision to the states: "no State shall . . . deprive any person of life, liberty, or property, without due process of law."

20. Ernest van den Haag, "Why Capital Punishment?" *Albany Law Review* 54 (1990).

21. Mike Royko, *Chicago Sun-Times*, September 1983.

CASES FOR ANALYSIS

1. Redemption and Capital Punishment

In 2005, 51-year-old Stanley Tookie Williams, convicted murderer and Crips gang co-founder, was executed by the State of California. His many supporters—including celebrities such as Jamie Foxx and Snoop Dogg—denounced the execution as unjust because while in prison he had sought and found redemption. As one report says,

> The case became the state's highest-profile execution in decades. Hollywood stars and capital punishment foes argued that Williams' sentence should be commuted to life in prison because he had made amends by writing children's books about the dangers of gangs and violence.

Gov. Arnold Schwarzenegger rejected Williams' plea for clemency on the grounds that Williams was not genuinely remorseful about the Crips' killings. Williams was convicted of murdering four people—a 26-year-old store clerk and a couple and their 43-year-old daughter. At the trial, witnesses said he bragged and laughed about the murders.

The Associated Press quoted Williams saying, "There is no part of me that existed then that exists now."*

Suppose Williams was guilty of the murders for which he was convicted, and suppose he had a genuine change of heart and performed many commendable deeds while in prison. Should Williams's sentence then have been commuted to life in prison? Why or why not? Is redemption compatible with justice? If a murderer mends his ways, should this change have an effect on his punishment? Is mercy (giving someone a break) compatible with justice (giving someone what he deserves)?

*"Tookie Williams Is Executed," CBSNews.com, 13 December 2005, http://www.cbsnews.com/news/tookie-williams-is-executed-13-12-2005/ (27 January 2015).

2. Cruel and Unusual Punishment

A new order by the Supreme Court yesterday brought a Florida prisoner's execution to a standstill. The man had already been tied to the gurney and needles had entered his arm, when the news came that death row inmates may now contest lethal injection as a form of capital punishment.

The 48-year-old convict, Clarence E. Hill, was found guilty of murdering a Pensacola police officer in 1982. He will now be given the opportunity to present his case against lethal injection before the Supreme Court. Hill claims that the chemical mixture used in executions would cause him extreme pain and would therefore amount to cruel and unusual punishment, a violation of his civil rights. While capital defense lawyers have been using this claim more and more frequently in recent years, it has not aided many convicts in escaping lethal injection.

The death penalty is legal in 38 states; 37 of those allow lethal injection as a means of execution. Because the chemicals used in Florida are similar to those used in other states, as well as in the U.S. military and federal government, the result of Hill's case could impact death row inmates across the country.

"It certainly could be a mess," states criminal law professor Douglas A. Berman (Ohio State University). Twenty-five inmates are currently scheduled for execution between now and when the Supreme Court is due to make its decision in June.

Hill's case does not directly concern the legality of lethal injection as a form of execution—the Supreme Court will be asked to make a ruling on whether the presence of specific chemicals used in such executions is constitutional. In short, will they cause the prisoner undue suffering and so violate his civil rights?

The idea that such chemicals cause prisoners extreme pain came from a 2005 study published in the medical journal *The Lancet*. The study found that 21 out of 49 prisoners who were executed via lethal injection "may have been conscious and feeling pain."

Hill had attempted to use this study to convince the U.S. Court of Appeals for the 11th Circuit to give him an opportunity to challenge Florida's lethal injection protocol, but was ultimately unsuccessful. Now, with the Supreme Court's new ruling, he will have a chance to argue his case against the current form of lethal injection.

Suppose neither lethal injection nor any other form of execution can be made painless. Would this fact justify the abolition of the death penalty or provide any evidence against it? Why or why not? Does it really matter that executions not constitute cruel and unusual punishment? If so, why?

Based on Charles Lane, "High Court to Hear Lethal-Injection Case," *The Washington Post*, January 26 2006, http://www.washingtonpost.com/wp-dyn/content/article/2006/01/25/AR2006012502018.html (23 March 2015).

---

3. Poor Representation

Delma Banks, Jr. was charged in the 1980 murder of Richard Whitehead of Texas. The only evidence against Banks was the testimony of an informant who in exchange for his testimony received $200 and the dismissal of an arson charge that could have resulted in his [sic] life sentence as a habitual offender. Banks' lawyer did not vigorously cross-examine the informant, nor did he investigate the case. Had he done so, he would have learned of strong evidence that Banks was in another city at the time of the crime. Banks received such poor representation that former FBI director and United States District Court Judge William Sessions weighed in to urge the Supreme Court to temporarily stay his execution. On April 21, 2003 the U.S. Supreme Court accepted Banks' case for review.[‡]

Do you think Banks should have gotten a new trial? Assuming capital punishment is morally permissible, would it ever be right to put someone to death who had not received adequate legal representation? Why or why not? What do you think would constitute adequate legal representation?

Suppose someone who is duly sentenced to die got excellent legal representation except for one minor point—her lawyer dozed off for fifteen seconds during her trial. Should this small lapse be a good enough reason to throw out her conviction and demand a new trial?

‡American Civil Liberties Union, "Inadequate Representation," from ACLU.org, October 8, 2003. Copyright © 2003 American Civil Liberties Union, www.aclu.org/capital-punishment/inadequate-representation. Reprinted by permission of the ACLU.

CHAPTER 12

Drug Use, Harm, and Personal Liberty

Decades ago, the administration of U.S. President Richard M. Nixon called for a national "war on drugs." It soon became a global conflict, and the struggle to stop the production, sale, and use of illicit substances has been raging ever since. Some experts say these efforts have failed miserably to curb America's drug habit; others reject this verdict; and some believe we have no choice but to continue the fight.

But no matter how drug use and its accompanying harms are measured, the conclusion to be drawn is the same: the damage to society's institutions and people's lives has been both pervasive and tragic. The most common legal drugs—alcohol, nicotine, and prescription medication—cause well over a half million deaths a year.[1] As for illicit drugs, the U.S. government estimates that in 2013, about 24.6 million Americans (age twelve and older) were users of illegal drugs. That's 9.4 percent of the total population of this age group. Marijuana was the most common illicit drug used

(19.8 million users), followed by the nonmedical use of prescription drugs (4.5 million), cocaine (1.5 million), hallucinogens (1.3 million), inhalants (496,000), and heroin (289,000).[2] The resulting injury to the heart, liver, kidneys, lungs, mind, and many other systems is well documented, and annual drug-related deaths number in the tens of thousands. The National Institute on Drug Abuse sums up the effects of drug abuse like this:

> Drug-related deaths have more than doubled since the early 1980s. There are more deaths, illnesses, and disabilities from substance abuse than from any other preventable health condition. Today, one in four deaths is attributable to alcohol, tobacco, and illicit drug use.[3]

Some commentators say the war on drugs has caused more misery than the actual use of drugs. Violence has always accompanied drug trafficking by dealers and cartels, and death and injury are unavoidable in efforts to enforce drug laws. Thousands have been killed in drug-related violence,

[1]Centers for Disease Control and Prevention, U.S. Department of Health and Human Services, "Alcohol Use and Your Health," http://www.cdc.gov/alcohol/fact-sheets/alcohol-use.htm (14 February 2015); U.S. Department of Health and Human Services, *The Health Consequences of Smoking—50 Years of Progress: A Report of the Surgeon General, 2014*, http://www.surgeongeneral.gov/library/reports/50-years-of-progress/ (14 February 2015); Centers for Disease Control and Prevention, CDC WONDER (Wide-ranging Online Data for Epidemiologic Research), Compressed Mortality File: Underlying Cause of Death, http://wonder.cdc.gov/mortsql.html (14 February 2015).

[2]Substance Abuse and Mental Health Services Administration, Center for Behavioral Health Statistics and Quality, September 4, 2014, "The NSDUH Report: Substance Use and Mental Health Estimates from the 2013 National Survey on Drug Use and Health: Overview of Findings," available at http://jpo.wrlc.org/bitstream/handle/11204/3782/2013%20Subst%20Use%20and%20Ment%20Hlth%20Ests.SAMHSA.pdf?sequence=1 (15 February 2015).

[3]National Institutes of Health, National Institute of Drug Abuse, "Medical Consequences of Drug Abuse," December 2012, http://www.drugabuse.gov/related-topics/medical-consequences-drug-abuse/mortality (15 February 2015).

including many innocents who had nothing to do with illegal drugs. In 2012, about 1.5 million Americans were arrested for violating drug laws. The great majority of these arrests were for possession; less than 20 percent were for selling or producing drugs.[4]

State and federal prisons have been filled to capacity with people arrested for drug violations, many of them sentenced to long prison terms for possessing small amounts of marijuana. Thousands of lengthy prison terms for breaking drug laws have been handed down because many statutes—often enacted as part of zero-tolerance drug policies—require mandatory minimum sentences. Some states, however, have repealed laws that mandate tough sentences for nonviolent drug offenses, and two-thirds of Americans agree with these changes.[5]

In the United States, attitudes toward drug use and drug law enforcement are changing. Two-thirds of Americans now think the government should pay more attention to treatment for users of hard drugs (cocaine and heroin, for example) than to prosecution of these users. Some states are abandoning mandatory prison sentences for those guilty of nonviolent drug offenses. In 2001, only 47 percent thought such a move was a good idea; in 2014, 63 percent thought that.

The legalization of marijuana is receiving much more support from the public than it did a few years ago. In 2004, 60 percent of Americans were against legalization; 32 percent were for it. In 2014, only 42 percent were against legalization; 54 percent were for legalization.[6]

From whatever perspective we wish to view the issue of drug use and abuse, there are moral questions that demand our attention. These questions fall into two broad categories: (1) the moral permissibility of using drugs; and (2) the morality of legal and social policies that address the use of drugs. Type (1) questions are concerned with personal autonomy, individual liberty, moral and legal rights, harm to oneself, and harm to others. Type (2) questions are about the ethics of drug laws and policies, and the prosecution and punishment of drug users.

ISSUE FILE: BACKGROUND

The term **drug** has been surprisingly difficult to define to everyone's satisfaction. A general definition that can aid our discussions is "a nonfood chemical substance that can affect the functions or makeup of the body." Thus, cocaine and marijuana are drugs, but so are nicotine, alcohol, and caffeine. When doctors, nurses, and medical researchers use the word *drugs*, they mean substances designed to treat or prevent disease. In this category are all prescription drugs and nonfood over-the-counter (OTC) medicines (which do not include vitamins, which are considered food substances). *Drug abuse* and *drug habit* usually refer to the nonmedical, proscribed use of psychotropic (mind-altering) substances. Marijuana, prescription medicines (used nonmedically), alcohol, nicotine, and cocaine are all drugs in this sense.

Several terms prominent in discussions of drugs are important but are often misused and misunderstood. **Drug addiction**, like *drug*, is a term whose definition is debated by experts and nonexperts alike. An authoritative medical manual says that drug addiction is

---

[4]U.S. Department of Justice, Federal Bureau of Investigation, "Crime in the United States 2012: Persons Arrested," FBI Uniform Crime Report, http://www.fbi.gov /about-us/cjis/ucr/crime-in-the-u.s/2012/crime-in-the -u.s.-2012/persons-arrested/persons-arrested (15 February 2015).

[5]Pew Research Center, "America's New Drug Policy Landscape," April 2, 2014, http://www.people-press .org/2014/04/02/americas-new-drug-policy-landscape/ (15 February 2015).

[6]Pew Research Center, "America's New Drug Policy Landscape."

an intense craving for the drug and compulsive, uncontrolled use of the drug despite harm done to the user or other people. People who are addicted spend more and more time obtaining the drug, using the drug, or recovering from its effects. Thus, addiction usually interferes with the ability to work, study, or interact normally with family and friends.[7]

Drug dependence is a condition in which discontinuing the use of a drug is extremely difficult, involving psychological or physical symptoms. In *physical* dependence, discontinuing the drug leads to uncomfortable physical symptoms of withdrawal—symptoms that can be physically painful, even life threatening. In *psychological* dependence, there is both a strong craving (an acute desire to repeat taking the drug) and an unpleasant experience of withdrawal (an intense distress when not taking the drug).

> The intense desire and compulsion to use a drug lead to using it in larger amounts, more frequently, or over a longer period than at first intended. People who are psychologically dependent on a drug give up social and other activities because of drug use. They also continue to use the drug even though they know that the drug is physically harmful or interferes with other aspects of their life, including family and work.[8]

Debates about the morality of producing, selling, or using illicit drugs are often muddied by misunderstandings of the terms *legalization*, *criminalization*, and *decriminalization*. **Legalization** is the making of the production and sale of drugs legal—that is, making their sale and production no longer a punishable crime. Drugs could be legalized by giving the government the exclusive right to regulate and sell them to the public, much

---

[7] *The Merck Manual (Home Edition)*, "Overview of Drug Abuse," January 2009, http://www.merckmanuals.com/home/special_subjects/drug_use_and_abuse/overview_of_drug_abuse.html?qt=%22Overview%20of%20Drug%20Abuse%22&alt=sh (15 February 2015).

[8] *The Merck Manual (Home Edition)*, "Overview of Drug Abuse."

DIVERSE VIEWS IN THE UNITED STATES ON USING MARIJUANA

Should marijuana use be legal?

	Yes %	No %
Total	54	42
White	55	42
Black	60	37
Age 18–29	70	28
Age 50–64	55	43

Should people get jail time for possessing small amounts of marijuana?

	Yes	No
Total	22	76
Age 18–29	18	81
Age 50–64	18	81
Republican	29	69
Democrat	19	79

Pew Research Center, "America's New Drug Policy Landscape," April 2, 2014, http://www.people-press.org/2014/04/02/americas-new-drug-policy-landscape/ (15 February 2015).

---

as states now regulate and sell alcohol. Or they could be legalized by allowing individuals to freely buy and sell them without incurring criminal punishment. **Criminalization** makes the *use* (and possession) of drugs a criminal offense. Under a criminalized system, merely possessing drugs in a specified amount can be punished by fines or prison. **Decriminalization** allows people to use drugs legally, without being liable to criminal prosecution and punishment.

How different states apply these policies can vary. They can criminalize the use of particular drugs or virtually all of them. They can punish the production and sale of drugs while decriminalizing their use. (Even in full decriminalization, drug use under particular circumstances—while driving a car or flying an airplane, for example—would likely remain a crime.) Or they can opt for a strict zero-tolerance policy and outlaw their use, production, and sale.

A much-debated alternative to punishing people for drug offenses is what experts call **harm reduction**. The idea is to concentrate not on decreasing the number of users or the quantity of available drugs in society, but on reducing the harm that arises from drugs and drug laws. Douglas Husak explains this option:

> Many sensible and enlightened commentators propose that the best drug policy is whatever will minimize harm. Their basic insight is that current drug policy initiatives are almost always evaluated by a criterion we should reject: the test of *use-reduction* (or *prevalence-reduction*). In other words, at the present time, no suggestion about how to improve our policy will be accepted unless it offers the potential to reduce the numbers of persons who use drugs. Theorists who favor a standard of harm-reduction point out that the total amount of harm that drugs cause in our society might actually decrease, even though the number of drug users would increase. If the average harm caused per user were reduced, total social harm might go down while the number of users went up.
>
> The most promising harm-reduction programs are needle exchange programs for heroin addicts and medical programs for patients whose symptoms are alleviated by smoking marijuana. Both of these ideas can effectively reduce harm in society.[9]

MORAL THEORIES

Traditional moral theories have interesting implications for drug use. A utilitarian would judge the moral permissibility of using illicit drugs by how well that choice maximizes happiness, everyone considered. So she might reason like this: On the positive side, using drugs (nonmedically or recreationally) could provide the user with pleasure, euphoria, a respite from stress, a break from the mundane, or some other desirable experience. She might then balance these benefits with several alleged negatives (depending on the kind of drug): addiction, dependence, withdrawal, physical disability, psychological impairment, loss of employment, damage done to personal relationships, and harm to other people. On the list of negatives she must also include the legal ramifications of drug use: the possibility of arrest, prosecution, imprisonment, and having a criminal record. She would have to make a judgment about the extent and likelihood of all these legal and nonlegal problems, difficult calculations about which experts disagree. She might finally conclude that the cost of using a particular drug far outweighs the benefits. Or she might assess the evidence differently and decide that the negatives for all concerned are not as bad as some people suggest.

These considerations of course pertain to the morality of personal drug use, but our utilitarian could also make a similar calculation about drug laws and policy generally. For example, based on her assessment of the overall effects of an antidrug law, she might conclude that enforcement of the law causes more unhappiness than the drug itself does, or that using the drug does more harm to more people than the law does.

Kantian ethics is likely to condemn the use of illicit drugs on the grounds that it violates a version of the categorical imperative: never use persons merely as a means to an end but always as an end in themselves. Kant would have us include ourselves in this formula. When we use illicit drugs, he might say, we use ourselves merely as a means to the end of drug-induced pleasure, stress reduction, or altered consciousness. What's more, we impair the very thing that constitutes our personhood—our autonomy, our capacity for reasoned self-determination. Some commentators argue that in full-blown drug addiction, our autonomy is destroyed altogether. In addiction,

[9]Douglas Husak and Peter de Marneffe, *The Legalization of Drugs: For and Against* (Cambridge: Cambridge University Press, 2005), 34–35.

CRITICAL THOUGHT: Does Legalizing Medical Marijuana Encourage Use among Teenagers?

Between 1999 and 2006, ten states legalized medical marijuana: Alaska, California, Colorado, Hawaii, Maine, Montana, Nevada, Oregon, Vermont, and Washington. How did these changes affect recreational marijuana use among teenagers? Existing data show that during this period there was no statistically significant rise in teen marijuana use in any of these states. There was, however, a statistically significant drop in four of the states: Alaska, California, Hawaii, and Montana.*

What do these data suggest about teen marijuana use? Do they show that marijuana use is harmless? Do they prove that medical marijuana should be legalized in every state? What claim about medical marijuana do they disprove?

*Substance Abuse and Mental Health Services Administration (SAMHSA), National Household Surveys on Drug Abuse (NHSDA), 1999–2006; Statistical Assessment Service (STATS).

they say, the addict's freedom to choose is lost, for he is a slave to his chemical master. Others contend, however, that free will is not diminished as much as some critics say, especially if the drug addict freely chooses to use drugs in the first place.

It's hard to see how natural law theory could ever condone hardcore drug use. Recall that in this theory, the morally right action is one that follows the dictates of nature. Whatever people do, they must fulfill their God-given, natural purpose. Lying is immoral, for example, because it goes against human nature, which naturally inclines toward social living where truth contributes to peaceful coexistence. Using mind-altering drugs, however, can lead to addiction, which forces the mind into an unnatural state in which autonomy is weakened and the moral law is obscured.

MORAL ARGUMENTS

Some of the more compelling arguments for and against drug use involve Type (2) questions, those concerning the morality of legal restrictions or bans on the use of drugs. The essential query is, Under what circumstances is the government justified in preventing or stopping people from using

drugs recreationally? The answers, or justifications, are usually derived from three principles: (1) the harm principle; (2) the paternalism principle; or (3) the legal moralism principle. When people try to explain their reasons for advocating a "war on drugs" or any other kind of interference with drug use, they almost always appeal to one or more of these fundamental ideas.

The **harm principle** says that authorities are justified in restricting some people's freedom to prevent harm to others. The government claims for itself the right to arrest, subdue, punish, or quarantine anyone if doing so will prevent harm to the public. Numerous civil laws, crime laws, and judicial rulings rest firmly on the harm principle. The great utilitarian John Stuart Mill articulated this principle best when he said, "the only purpose for which power can be rightfully exercised over any member of a civilized community, against his will, is to prevent harm to others."[10]

Many who are opposed to recreational drug use assert that drug users hurt plenty of people. Users, they say, are more likely to neglect their children, abuse their spouses, cheat their employers by

[10] John Stuart Mill, *On Liberty* (1859).

doing poor work, steal to support their drug habit, and hurt other people through accidents and negligence. In addition, drug users burden society with the costs of drug-law enforcement, drug treatment, legal prosecution, and imprisonment. As James Q. Wilson says, "The notion that abusing drugs such as cocaine is a 'victimless crime' is not only absurd but dangerous."[11]

Proponents of decriminalization counter that the harms of illicit drug use are exaggerated, are based on worst-case scenarios, and lack supporting evidence. Furthermore, they maintain that most of the harms that accompany drug use are not the direct result of drug use but of antidrug laws and policies. Douglas Husak itemizes some of these alleged harms:

> In the first place, prohibition [of drugs and drug use] has always been aimed—or selectively enforced—against minorities. . . . In addition, drug prohibition is destructive of public health. Since the vast majority of illicit drugs taken for recreational purposes are purchased on the street from unlicensed sellers, consumers can have no confidence about what they are buying. . . . Street drugs may contain deadly impurities, and unknown potencies can contribute to deaths from overdose. . . . Truth is among the foremost casualties of our misguided drug policy. The demonization of illicit drugs is so pervasive that frank and honest discourse is all but impossible. . . . There may be no greater threat to the rule of law than corruption and abuse of authority among government officials. Prohibition and the huge amounts of money in the illicit drug trade create irresistible temptations for law-enforcement agents to place themselves above the law. . . . Our punitive drug policies cost exorbitant amounts of money. . . . Most of this money has been wasted. If we stopped punishing drug users, taxpayers would reap enormous savings.[12]

For some who favor decriminalization, trying to judge the issue by some utilitarian standard—that is, by weighing harms and benefits—is entirely wrongheaded. The real issue, they say, is not harms but justice. The decision to punish someone for breaching a law should be decided according to *what is just*. If Jones commits a crime, we don't decide his fate by balancing the good and bad effects of his actions. The utilitarian calculus is useless here. We try instead to determine what a just treatment of him would be, what his rights are, and what he deserves. Underlying this view is the idea that people are rational, autonomous beings whose freedom to choose and act should not be constrained without strong justification.

The **paternalism principle** asserts that authorities are sometimes justified in limiting people's freedom to prevent them from harming themselves. To act paternally is to curtail a person's liberty for her own good, regardless of what her preferences are. A paternalistic drug law would, say, criminalize a drug user's actions to prevent him from doing something that might injure or impair him. One paternalistic argument concludes that people must be protected from freely and knowingly choosing to take addictive drugs that can undermine their autonomy.

Peter de Marneffe takes a paternalistic view. He declares that there is only one good reason for drug prohibition—that some people will be worse off if drugs are legalized. He argues:

> Drug prohibition is justified, in my view, as reducing the independent harms of drug abuse [harms besides those caused by drug-law enforcement]. But it is commonly objected that drug laws "don't work." If so, it is no argument for drug legalization. In this sense laws against murder and theft do not work either, but this does not mean that we should abolish them.[13]

---

[11]James Q. Wilson, "Against the Legalization of Drugs," *Commentary*, February 1990, https://www.commentary magazine.com/article/against-the-legalization-of-drugs/ (15 February 2015).
[12]Husak, *The Legalization of Drugs: For and Against*, 92–95.

[13]De Marneffe, *The Legalization of Drugs: For and Against*, 110.

QUICK REVIEW

drug—A nonfood chemical substance that can affect the functions and makeup of the body.

drug addiction—An intense craving for a drug and compulsive, uncontrolled use of the drug despite harm done to the user or other people.

drug dependence—A condition in which discontinuing the use of a drug is extremely difficult, involving psychological or physical symptoms.

legalization—The process of making the production and sale of drugs legal.

criminalization—Making the use (and possession) of drugs a criminal offense.

decriminalization—Permitting the use of drugs without incurring criminal penalties.

harm reduction—A drug policy aimed at reducing the harm that arises from drugs and drug laws.

harm principle—The view that authorities are justified in restricting some people's freedom to prevent harm to others.

paternalism principle—The view that authorities are sometimes justified in limiting people's freedom to prevent them from harming themselves.

legal moralism—The doctrine that the government is justified in curbing people's freedom in order to force them to obey moral rules.

As you might expect, those who condemn paternalistic drug laws usually base their arguments on the supreme value of autonomy. Whatever the form of such laws, they say, they are still unacceptable assaults on individual liberty, even if they are intended to somehow protect autonomy.

The **legal moralism** principle is the doctrine that the government is justified in curbing people's freedom in order to force them to obey moral rules. For the legal moralist, if an act is immoral, that's reason enough to make it a crime and prosecute those who violate the law. Estimations of harm need not be involved. The principle of course can be applied not just to drug use but to any action thought to breach moral standards. Wilson's attitude toward antidrug laws is decidedly moralistic:

> Even now, when the dangers of drug use are well-understood, many educated people still discuss the drug problem in almost every way except the right way. They talk about the "costs" of drug use and the "socioeconomic factors" that shape that use. They rarely speak plainly—drug use is wrong because it is immoral and it is immoral because it enslaves the mind and destroys the soul.[14]

A common reply to the doctrine of legal moralism is that it conflicts with other commonsense moral beliefs or policies we have. Decriminalization supporters ask why drug use, and not other kinds of behavior, should be outlawed simply because it is deemed immoral. Many actions are thought to be immoral—cheating at golf, plagiarizing, lying to a spouse, breaking a solemn vow, betraying a confidence—but few think these actions should be regarded as crimes and prosecuted as such. Critics of legal moralism say that legal moralists must explain why drug use should be a crime just because it's immoral, but not other presumably immoral acts like betraying a confidence. Why is drug use a crime and not cheating at golf or lying to a spouse? Decriminalization proponents say legal moralists have yet to explain this inconsistency, so the doctrine of legal moralism is an inadequate justification for making drug use illegal.

[14]John Q. Wilson, quoted in *Body Count: Moral Poverty . . . and How to Win America's War on Drugs*, by William J. Bennett, John DiIulio, Jr., and John Walters (New York: Simon & Schuster, 1996), 140–41.

SUMMARY

A *drug* is a nonfood chemical substance that can affect the functions or makeup of the body. *Drug addiction* is "an intense craving for the drug and compulsive, uncontrolled use of the drug despite harm done to the user or other people." *Drug dependence* is a condition in which discontinuing the use of a drug is extremely difficult, involving psychological or physical symptoms. *Drug legalization* refers to making the production and sale of drugs legal—that is, making their sale and production no longer a punishable crime. *Criminalization* makes the use (and possession) of drugs a criminal offense. *Decriminalization* allows people to use drugs legally, to use them without being liable to criminal prosecution and punishment.

A utilitarian would judge the moral permissibility of using illicit drugs by how well that choice maximizes happiness, everyone considered. Kantian ethics is likely to condemn the use of illicit drugs on the grounds that it violates a version of the categorical imperative: never use persons merely as a means to an end but always as an end in themselves. Natural law theorists condemn hardcore drug use on the grounds that mind-altering drugs can lead to addiction, which forces the mind into an unnatural state in which autonomy is weakened and the moral law is obscured.

Arguments against decriminalization are often derived from three principles: (1) the harm principle; (2) the paternalism principle; or (3) the legal moralism principle. When people try to explain their reasons for advocating a "war on drugs" or any other kind of interference with drug use, they almost always appeal to one or more of these fundamental ideas.

READINGS

The Ethics of Addiction

THOMAS SZASZ

Lest we take for granted that we know what drug addiction is, let us begin with some definitions.

According to the World Health Organization's Expert Committee on Drugs Liable to Produce Addiction,

> Drug addiction is a state of periodic or chronic intoxication detrimental to the individual and to society, produced by the repeated consumption of a drug (natural or synthetic). Its characteristics include: (1) an overpowering desire or need (compulsion) to continue taking the drug and to obtain it by any means, (2) a tendency to increase the dosage, and (3) a psychic (psychological) and sometimes physical dependence on the effects of the drug.[1]

Thomas Szasz, "The Ethics of Addiction," from *The Theology of Medicine* (1977). Reprinted with permission from the Estate of Thomas Szasz.

Since this definition hinges on the harm done to the individual and to society by the consumption of the drug, it is clearly an ethical one. Moreover, by not specifying what is "detrimental" or who shall ascertain it and on what grounds, this definition immediately assimilates the problem of addiction with other psychiatric problems in which psychiatrists define the patient's dangerousness to himself and others. Actually, physicians regard as detrimental what people do to themselves but not what they do to people. For example, when college students smoke marijuana, that is detrimental; but when psychiatrists administer psychotropic drugs to involuntary mental patients, that is not detrimental.

The rest of the definition proposed by the World Health Organization is of even more dubious value. It speaks of an "overpowering desire" or "compulsion" to take the drug and of efforts to obtain it "by any means." Here again, we sink into the conceptual and semantic morass of psychiatric jargon. What is an "overpowering desire" if not simply a desire by which we choose to let ourselves be overpowered? And what is a "compulsion" if not simply an unresisted inclination to do something, and keep on doing it, even though someone thinks we should not be doing it?

Next, we come to the effort to obtain the addictive substance "by any means." That suggests that the substance is prohibited, or is very expensive for some other reason, and is hence difficult to obtain for the ordinary person rather than that the person who wants it has an inordinate craving for it. If there were an abundant and inexpensive supply of what the "addict" wants, there would be no reason for him to go to "any means" to obtain it. Does the World Health Organization's definition mean that one can be addicted only to a substance that is illegal or otherwise difficult to obtain? If so—and there is obviously some truth to the view that forbidden fruit tastes sweeter, although it cannot be denied that some things are sweet regardless of how the law treats them—then that surely removes the problem of addiction from the sphere of medicine and psychiatry and puts it squarely into that of morals and law.

The definition of addiction offered in *Webster's Third New International Dictionary of the English Language, Unabridged* exhibits the same difficulties. It defines addiction as "the compulsory uncontrolled use of habit-forming drugs beyond the period of medical need or under conditions harmful to society." This definition imputes lack of self-control to the addict over his taking or not taking a drug, a dubious proposition at best; at the same time, by qualifying an act as an addiction depending on whether or not it harms society, it offers a moral definition of an ostensibly medical condition.

Likewise, the currently popular term *drug abuse* places this behavior squarely in the category of ethics. For it is ethics that deals with the right and wrong uses of man's powers and possessions.

Clearly, drug addiction and drug abuse cannot be defined without specifying the proper and improper uses of certain pharmacologically active agents. The regular administration of morphine by a physician to a patient dying of cancer is the paradigm of the proper use of a narcotic, whereas even its occasional self-administration by a physically healthy person for the purpose of pharmacological pleasure is the paradigm of drug abuse.

I submit that these judgments have nothing whatever to do with medicine, pharmacology, or psychiatry. They are moral judgments. Indeed, our present views on addiction are astonishingly similar to some of our former views on sex. Intercourse in marriage with the aim of procreation used to be the paradigm of the proper use of one's sexual organs, whereas intercourse outside of marriage with the aim of carnal pleasure used to be the paradigm of their improper use. Until recently, masturbation—or self-abuse, as it was called—was professionally declared and popularly accepted as both the cause and the symptom of a variety of illnesses.[2]

To be sure, it is now virtually impossible to cite a contemporary American (or foreign) medical authority to support the concept of self-abuse. Medical opinion now holds that there is simply no such thing, that whether a person masturbates or not is medically irrelevant, and that engaging in the practice or refraining from it is a matter of personal morals or life-style. On the other hand, it is now virtually impossible to cite a contemporary American (or foreign) medical authority to oppose the concept of drug abuse. Medical opinion now holds that drug abuse is a major medical, psychiatric, and public-health problem; that drug addiction is a disease similar to diabetes, requiring prolonged (or lifelong) and carefully supervised medical treatment; and that taking or not taking drugs is primarily, if not solely, a matter of medical concern and responsibility.

Like any social policy, our drug laws may be examined from two entirely different points of view—technical and moral. Our present inclination is either to ignore the moral perspective or to mistake the technical for the moral.

An example of our misplaced overreliance on a technical approach to the so-called drug problem is the professionalized mendacity about the dangerousness of certain types of drugs. Since most of the propagandists against drug abuse seek to justify certain repressive policies by appeals to the alleged dangerousness of various drugs, they often falsify the facts about the true pharmacological properties of the drugs they seek to prohibit. They do so for two reasons: first, because many substances in daily use are just as harmful as the substances they want to prohibit; second, because they realize that dangerousness alone is never a sufficiently persuasive argument to justify the prohibition of any drug, substance, or artifact. Accordingly, the more the "addiction-mongers" ignore the moral dimensions of the problem, the more they must escalate their fraudulent claims about the dangers of drugs.

To be sure, some drugs are more dangerous than others. It is easier to kill oneself with heroin than with aspirin. But it is also easier to kill oneself by jumping off a high building than a low one. In the case of drugs, we regard their potentiality for self-injury as justification for their prohibition; in the case of buildings, we do not.

Furthermore, we systematically blur and confuse the two quite different ways in which narcotics may cause death—by a deliberate act of suicide and by accidental overdosage.

As I have suggested elsewhere, we ought to consider suicide a basic human right. If so, it is absurd to deprive an adult of a drug (or of anything else) because he might use it to kill himself. To do so is to treat everyone the way institutional psychiatrists treat the so-called suicidal mental patient: they not only imprison such a person but take everything away from him—shoelaces, belts, razor blades, eating utensils, and so forth—until the "patient" lies naked on a mattress in a padded cell, lest he kill himself. The result is the most degrading tyrannization in the annals of human history.

Death by accidental overdose is an altogether different matter. But can anyone doubt that this danger now looms so large precisely because the sale of narcotics and many other drugs is illegal? People who buy illicit drugs cannot be sure what drug they are getting or how much of it. Free trade in drugs, with governmental action limited to safeguarding the purity of the product and the veracity of the labeling, would reduce the risk of accidental overdose with "dangerous drugs" to the same levels that prevail, and that we find acceptable, with respect to other chemical agents and physical artifacts that abound in our complex technological society.

Although this essay is not intended as an exposition on the pharmacological properties of narcotics and other mind-affecting drugs, it might be well to say something more about the medical and social dangers they pose. Before proceeding to that task, I want to make clear, however, that in my view, regardless of their dangerousness, all drugs should be legalized (a misleading term I employ reluctantly as a concession to common usage). Although I recognize that some drugs—notably heroin, the amphetamines, and LSD among those now in vogue—may have undesirable personal or social consequences, I favor free trade in drugs for the same reason the Founding Fathers favored free trade in ideas: in an open society, it is none of the government's business what idea a man puts into his mind; likewise, it should be none of the government's business what drug he puts into his body.

It is a fundamental characteristic of human beings that they get used to things: one becomes habituated, or addicted, not only to narcotics, but to cigarettes, cocktails before dinner, orange juice for breakfast, comic strips, sex, and so forth. It is similarly a fundamental characteristic of living organisms that they acquire increasing tolerance to various chemical agents and physical stimuli: the first cigarette may cause nothing but nausea and headache; a year later, smoking three packs a day may be pure joy. Both alcohol and opiates are addictive, then, in the sense that the more regularly they are used, the more the user craves them and the greater his tolerance for them becomes. However, there is no mysterious process of "getting hooked" involved in any of this. It is simply an aspect of the universal biological propensity for learning, which is especially well-developed in man. The opiate habit, like the cigarette habit or the food habit, can be broken—usually without any medical assistance—provided the person wants to break it. Often he doesn't. And why indeed should he if he has nothing better to do with his life? Or as happens to be the case with morphine, if he can live an essentially normal life while under its influence? That, of course, sounds completely unbelievable, or worse—testimony to our "addiction" to half a century of systematic official mendacity about opiates, which we can break only by suffering the intellectual withdrawal symptoms that go with giving up treasured falsehoods.

Actually, opium is much less toxic than alcohol. Moreover, just as it is possible to be an alcoholic and work and be productive, so it is (or rather, it used to be) possible to be an opium addict and work and be productive. Thomas De Quincey and Samuel Taylor Coleridge were both opium takers, and "Kubla Khan," considered one of the most beautiful poems in the English language, was written while Coleridge was under the influence of opium.[3] According to a definitive study by Light and others published by the American Medical Association in 1929, "morphine addiction is not characterized by physical deterioration or impairment of physical fitness. . . . There is no evidence of change in the circulatory, hepatic, renal, or endocrine functions. When it is considered that these subjects had been addicted for at least five years, some of them as long as twenty years, these negative observations are highly significant."[4] In a 1928 study, Lawrence Kolb, an assistant surgeon general of the United States Public Health Service, found that of 119 persons addicted to opiates through medical practice, 90 had good industrial records and only 29 had poor ones. . . .

I am not citing this evidence to recommend the opium habit. The point is that we must, in plain honesty, distinguish between pharmacological effects and personal inclinations. Some people take drugs to cope—to help them function and conform to social expectations. Others take them to cop out—to ritualize their refusal to function and conform to social expectations. Much of the drug abuse we now witness—perhaps nearly all of it—is of the second type. But instead of acknowledging that addicts are unable or unfit or unwilling to work and be normal, we prefer to believe that they act as they do because certain drugs—especially heroin, LSD, and the amphetamines—make them sick. If only we could get them well, so runs this comfortable and comforting view, they would become productive and useful citizens. To believe that is like believing that if an illiterate cigarette smoker would only stop smoking, he would become an Einstein. With a falsehood like that, one can go far. No wonder that politicians and psychiatrists love it.

The idea of free trade in drugs runs counter to another cherished notion of ours—namely, that everyone must work and that idleness is acceptable only under special conditions. In general, the obligation to work is greatest for healthy adult white males. We tolerate idleness on the part of children, women, blacks, the aged, and the sick, and we even accept the responsibility of supporting them. But the new wave of drug abuse affects mainly young adults, often white males who are, in principle at least, capable of working and supporting themselves. But they refuse: they drop out, adopting a life-style in which *not* working, *not* supporting oneself, *not* being useful to others, are positive values. These people challenge some of the most basic values of our society. It is hardly surprising, then, that society wants to retaliate, to strike back. Even though it would be cheaper to support addicts on welfare than to "treat" them, doing so would be legitimizing their life-style. That, "normal" society refuses to do. Instead, the majority acts as if it felt that, so long as it is going to spend its money on addicts, it is going to get something out of it. What society gets out of its war on addiction is what every persecutory movement provides for the persecutors: by defining a minority as evil (or sick), the majority confirms itself as good (or healthy). (If that can be done for the victim's own good, so much the better.) In short, the war on addiction is a part of that vast modern enterprise which I have named the "manufacture of madness." It is indeed a therapeutic enterprise, but with this grotesque twist: its beneficiaries are the therapists, and its victims are the patients.

Most of all perhaps, the idea of free trade in narcotics frightens people because they believe that vast masses of our population would spend their days and nights smoking opium or mainlining heroin instead of working and shouldering their responsibilities as citizens. But that is a bugaboo that does not deserve to be taken seriously. Habits of work and idleness are deep-seated cultural patterns; I doubt that free trade in drugs would convert industrious people from hustlers into hippies at the stroke of a legislative pen.

The other side of the economic coin regarding drugs and drug controls is actually far more important. The government is now spending millions of dollars—the hard-earned wages of hard-working Americans—to support a vast and astronomically expensive bureaucracy whose efforts not only drain our economic resources and damage our civil liberties but create ever more addicts and, indirectly, the crime associated with the traffic in illicit drugs. Although my argument about drug taking is moral and political and does not depend upon showing that free trade in drugs would also have fiscal advantages over our present policies, let me indicate briefly some of the economic aspects of the drug-control problem.

On April 1, 1967, New York State's narcotics addiction-control program, hailed as "the most massive ever tried in the nation," went into effect. "The program, which may cost up to $400 million in three years," reported *The New York Times*, "was hailed by Governor Rockefeller as 'the start of an unending war.'"[5] Three years later, it was conservatively estimated that the number of addicts in the state had tripled or quadrupled. New York State Senator John Hughes reported that the cost of caring for each addict during that time was $12,000 per year (as against $4,000 per year for patients in state mental hospitals).[6] It was a great time, though, for some of the ex-addicts themselves. In New York City's Addiction Services Agency, one ex-addict started at $6,500 a year on November 27, 1967, and was making $16,000 seven months later. Another started at $6,500 on September 12, 1967, and went up to $18,100 by July 1, 1969.[7] The salaries of the medical bureaucrats in charge of the programs are similarly attractive. In short, the detection and rehabilitation of addicts is good business; and so was, in former days, the detection and rehabilitation of witches. We

now know that the spread of witchcraft in the late Middle Ages was due more to the work of witchmongers than to the lure of witchcraft. Is it not possible that, similarly, the spread of addiction in our day is due more to the work of addictmongers than to the lure of narcotics? . . .

Clearly, the argument that marijuana—or heroin, or methadone, or morphine—is prohibited because it is addictive or dangerous cannot be supported by facts. For one thing, there are many drugs—from insulin to penicillin—that are neither addictive nor dangerous but are nevertheless also prohibited—they can be obtained only through a physician's prescription. For another, there are many things—from dynamite to guns—that are much more dangerous than narcotics (especially to others) but are not prohibited. As everyone knows, it is still possible in the United States to walk into a store and walk out with a shotgun. We enjoy that right not because we do not believe that guns are dangerous, but because we believe even more strongly that civil liberties are precious. At the same time, it is not possible in the United States to walk into a store and walk out with a bottle of barbiturates, codeine, or other drugs. We are now deprived of that right because we have come to value medical paternalism more highly than the right to obtain and use drugs without recourse to medical intermediaries.

I submit, therefore, that our so-called drug-abuse problem is an integral part of our present social ethic, which accepts "protections" and repressions justified by appeals to health similar to those that medieval societies accepted when they were justified by appeals to faith.[8] Drug abuse (as we now know it) is one of the inevitable consequences of the medical monopoly over drugs—a monopoly whose value is daily acclaimed by science and law, state and church, the professions and the laity. As the Church formerly regulated man's relations to God, so Medicine now regulates his relations to his body. Deviation from the rules set forth by the Church was then considered to be heresy and was punished by appropriate theological sanctions, called *penance*; deviation from the rules set forth by Medicine is now considered to be drug abuse (or some sort of mental illness) and is punished by appropriate medical sanctions, called *treatment*.

The problem of drug abuse will thus be with us so long as we live under medical tutelage. This is not to say that if all access to drugs were free, some people would not medicate themselves in ways that might upset us or harm them. That of course is precisely what happened when religious practices became free.

What I am suggesting is that although addiction is ostensibly a medical and pharmacological problem, actually it is a moral and political problem. We talk as if we were trying to ascertain which drugs *are* toxic, but we act as if we were trying to decide which drugs *ought to be* prohibited.

We ought to know, however, that there is no necessary connection between facts and values, between what is and what ought to be. Thus, objectively quite harmful acts, objects, or persons may be accepted and tolerated—by minimizing their dangerousness. Conversely, objectively quite harmless acts, objects, or persons may be prohibited and persecuted—by exaggerating their dangerousness. It is always necessary to distinguish—and especially so when dealing with social policy—between description and prescription, fact and rhetoric, truth and falsehood.

To command adherence, social policy must be respected; and to be respected, it must be considered legitimate. In our society, there are two principal methods of legitimizing policy—social tradition and scientific judgment. More than anything else, time is the supreme ethical arbiter. Whatever a social practice might be, if people engage in it generation after generation, then that practice becomes acceptable.

Many opponents of illegal drugs admit that nicotine may be more harmful to health than marijuana; nevertheless, they argue that smoking cigarettes should be legal but smoking marijuana should not be, because the former habit is socially accepted while the latter is not. That is a perfectly reasonable argument. But let us understand it for what it is—a plea for legitimizing old and accepted practices and illegitimizing novel and unaccepted ones. It is a justification that rests on precedence, not on evidence.

The other method of legitimizing policy, increasingly more important in the modern world, is through the authority of science. In matters of health, a vast and increasingly elastic category, physicians thus play important roles as legitimizers and illegitimizers. One result is that, regardless of the pharmacological effects of a drug on the person who takes it, if he obtains it through a physician and uses it under medical supervision, that use is, ipso facto, legitimate and proper; but if he obtains it through nonmedical channels and uses it without medical supervision (and especially if the drug is illegal and the individual uses it solely for the purpose of altering his mental state), then that use is, ipso facto, illegitimate and improper. In short, being medicated by a doctor is drug use, while self-medication (especially with certain classes of drugs) is drug abuse.

That too is a perfectly reasonable arrangement. But let us understand it for what it is—a plea for legitimizing what doctors do, because they do it with good, therapeutic intent; and for illegitimizing what laymen do, because they do it with bad, self-abusive (masturbatory) intent. It is a justification that rests on the principles of professionalism, not of pharmacology. That is why we applaud the systematic medical use of methadone and call it "treatment for heroin addiction," but decry the occasional nonmedical use of marijuana and call it "dangerous drug abuse."

Our present concept of drug abuse thus articulates and symbolizes a fundamental policy of scientific medicine—namely, that a layman should not medicate his own body but should place its medical care under the supervision of a duly accredited physician. Before the Reformation, the practice of true Christianity rested on a similar policy—namely, that a layman should not himself commune with God but should place his spiritual care under the supervision of a duly accredited priest. The self-interests of the Church and of Medicine in such policies are obvious enough. What might be less obvious is the interest of the laity in them: by delegating responsibility for the spiritual and medical welfare of the people to a class of authoritatively accredited specialists, those policies—and the practices they ensure—relieve individuals from assuming the burdens of those responsibilities for themselves. As I see it, our present problems with drug use and drug abuse are just one of the consequences of our pervasive ambivalence about personal autonomy and responsibility. . . .

I propose a medical reformation analogous to the Protestant Reformation—specifically, a "protest" against the systematic mystification of man's relationship to his body and his professionalized separation from it. The immediate aim of the reform would be to remove the physician as intermediary between man and his body and to give the layman direct access to the language and contents of the pharmacopoeia. It is significant that until recently physicians wrote prescriptions in Latin and that medical diagnoses and treatments are still couched in a jargon whose chief aim is to awe and mystify the laity. If man had unencumbered access to his own body and the means of chemically altering it, it would spell the end of Medicine, at least as we now know it. That is why, with faith in Medicine so strong, there is little interest in this kind of medical reform: physicians fear the loss of their privileges; laymen, the loss of their protections.

Our present policies with respect to drug use and drug abuse thus constitute a covert plea for legitimizing certain privileges on the part of physicians and illegitimizing certain practices on the part of everyone else. The upshot is that we act as if we believed that only doctors should be allowed to dispense narcotics, just as we used to believe that only priests should be allowed to dispense holy water.

Finally, since luckily we still do not live in the utopian perfection of one world, our technical approach to the drug problem has led, and will undoubtedly continue to lead, to some curious attempts to combat it. . . .

I believe that just as we regard freedom of speech and religion as fundamental rights, so we should also regard freedom of self-medication as a fundamental right; and that instead of mendaciously opposing or mindlessly promoting illicit drugs, we should, paraphrasing Voltaire, make this maxim our rule: I disapprove of what you take, but I will defend to the death your right to take it!

To be sure, like most rights, the right of self-medication should apply only to adults; and it should not be an unqualified right. Since these are important qualifications, it is necessary to specify their precise range.

John Stuart Mill said (approximately) that a person's right to swing his arm ends where his neighbor's nose begins. Similarly, the limiting condition with respect to self-medication should be the inflicting of actual (as against symbolic) harm on others.

Our present practices with respect to alcohol embody and reflect this individualistic ethic. We have the right to buy, possess, and consume alcoholic beverages. Regardless of how offensive drunkenness might be to a person, he cannot interfere with another person's right to become inebriated so long as that person drinks in the privacy of his own home or at some other appropriate location and so long as he conducts himself in an otherwise law-abiding manner. In short, we have a right to be intoxicated—in private. Public intoxication is considered to be an offense against others and is therefore a violation of the criminal law.

The same principle applies to sexual conduct. Sexual intercourse, especially between husband and wife, is surely a right. But it is a right that must be exercised at home or at some other appropriate location; it is not a right in a public park or on a downtown street. It makes sense that what is a right in one place may become, by virtue of its disruptive or disturbing effect on others, an offense somewhere else.

The right to self-medication should be hedged in by similar limits. Public intoxication, not only with alcohol but with any drug, should be an offense punishable by the criminal law. Furthermore, acts that may injure others—such as driving a car—should, when carried out in a drug-intoxicated state, be punished especially strictly and severely. The habitual use of certain drugs, such as alcohol and opiates, may also harm others indirectly by rendering the subject unmotivated for working and thus unemployed. In a society that supports the unemployed, such a person would, as a consequence of his own conduct, place a burden on the shoulders of his working neighbors. How society might best guard itself against that sort of hazard I cannot discuss here. However, it is obvious that prohibiting the use of habit-forming drugs offers no protection against that risk, but only adds to the tax burdens laid upon the productive members of society.

The right to self-medication must thus entail unqualified responsibility for the effects of one's drug-intoxicated behavior on others. For unless we are willing to hold ourselves responsible for our own behavior and hold others responsible for theirs, the liberty to ingest or inject drugs degenerates into a license to injure others. But here is the catch: we are exceedingly reluctant to hold people responsible for their misbehavior. That is why we prefer diminishing rights to increasing responsibilities. The former requires only the passing of laws, which can then be more or less freely violated or circumvented; whereas the latter requires prosecuting and punishing offenders, which can be accomplished only by just laws justly enforced. The upshot is that we increasingly substitute tender-hearted tyranny for tough-spirited liberty.

Such then would be the situation of adults were we to regard the freedom to take drugs as a fundamental right similar to the freedom to read and to worship. What would be the situation of children? Since many people who are now said to be drug addicts or drug abusers are minors, it is especially important that we think clearly about this aspect of the problem.

I do not believe, and I do not advocate, that children should have a right to ingest, inject, or otherwise use any drug or substance they want. Children do not have the right to drive, drink, vote, marry, or make binding contracts. They acquire those rights at various ages, coming into their full possession at maturity, usually between the ages of eighteen and twenty-one. The right to self-medication should similarly be withheld until maturity. . . .

In short, I suggest that "dangerous" drugs be treated more or less as alcohol and tobacco are treated now. (That does not mean that I believe the state should make their use a source of tax revenue.) Neither the use of narcotics nor their possession should be prohibited, but only their sale to minors. Of course, that would result in the ready availability of all kinds of drugs among minors—though perhaps their availability would be no greater than it is now

but only more visible and hence more easily subject to proper controls. That arrangement would place responsibility for the use of all drugs by children where it belongs: on parents and their children. That is where the major responsibility rests for the use of alcohol and tobacco. It is a tragic symptom of our refusal to take personal liberty and responsibility seriously that there appears to be no public desire to assume a similar stance toward other dangerous drugs. . . .

Sooner or later, we shall have to confront the basic moral dilemma underlying our drug problem: does a person have the right to take a drug—any drug—not because he needs it to cure an illness, but because he wants to take it?

The Declaration of Independence speaks of our inalienable right to "life, liberty, and the pursuit of happiness." How are we to interpret that phrase? By asserting that we ought to be free to pursue happiness by playing golf or watching television but not by drinking alcohol, or smoking marijuana, or ingesting amphetamines?

The Constitution and the Bill of Rights are silent on the subject of drugs. Their silence would seem to imply that the adult citizen has, or ought to have, the right to medicate his own body as he sees fit. Were that not the case, why should there have been a need for a constitutional amendment to outlaw drinking? But if ingesting alcohol was, and is now again, a constitutional right, is ingesting opium, or heroin, or barbiturates, or anything else not also such a right? If it is, then the Harrison Narcotic Act is not only a bad law but unconstitutional as well, because it prescribes in a legislative act what ought to be promulgated in a constitutional amendment.

The nagging questions remain. As American citizens, do we and should we have the right to take narcotics or other drugs? Further, if we take drugs and conduct ourselves as responsible and law-abiding citizens, do we and should we have a right to remain unmolested by the government? Lastly, if we take drugs and break the law, do we and should we have a right to be treated as persons accused of a crime rather than as patients accused of being mentally ill?

These are fundamental questions that are conspicuous by their absence from all contemporary discussions of problems of drug addiction and drug abuse. In this area as in so many others, we have allowed a moral problem to be disguised as a medical question and have then engaged in shadowboxing with metaphorical diseases and medical attempts, ranging from the absurd to the appalling, to combat them.

The result is that instead of debating the use of drugs in moral and political terms, we define our task as the ostensibly narrow technical problem of protecting people from poisoning themselves with substances for whose use they cannot possibly assume responsibility. That, I think, best explains the frightening national consensus against personal responsibility for taking drugs and for one's conduct while under their influence. In 1965, for example, when President Johnson sought a bill imposing tight federal controls over "pep pills" and "goof balls," the bill cleared the House by a unanimous vote, 402 to 0. . . .

Finally, those repeated unanimous votes on far-reaching measures to combat drug abuse are bitter reminders that when the chips are really down, that is, when democratic lawmakers can preserve their intellectual and moral integrity only by going against certain popular myths, they prove to be either mindless or spineless. They prefer running with the herd to courting unpopularity and risking reelection.

After all is said and done—after millions of words are written, thousands of laws are enacted, and countless numbers of people are "treated" for "drug abuse"—it all comes down to whether we accept or reject the ethical principle John Stuart Mill so clearly enunciated in 1859:

> The only purpose for which power can be rightfully exercised over any member of a civilized community, against his will, is to prevent harm to others. His own good, either physical or moral, is not a sufficient warrant. He cannot rightfully be compelled to do or forebear because it will make him happier, because, in the opinions of others, to do so would be wise, or even

right. . . . In the part [of his conduct] which merely concerns himself, his independence is, of right, absolute. Over himself, over his own body and mind, the individual is sovereign.[9]

The basic issue underlying the problem of addiction—and many other problems, such as sexual activity between consenting adults, pornography, contraception, gambling, and suicide—is simple but vexing: in a conflict between the individual and the state, where should the former's autonomy end and the latter's right to intervene begin?

One way out of the dilemma lies through concealment: by disguising the moral and political question as a medical and therapeutic problem, we can, to protect the physical and mental health of patients, exalt the state, oppress the individual, and claim benefits for both.

The other way out of it lies through confrontation: by recognizing the problem for what it is, we can choose to maximize the sphere of action of the state at the expense of the individual or of the individual at the expense of the state. In other words, we can commit ourselves to the view that the state, the representative of many, is more important than the individual and that it therefore has the right, indeed the duty, to regulate the life of the individual in the best interests of the group. Or we can commit ourselves to the view that individual dignity and liberty are the supreme values of life and that the foremost duty of the state is to protect and promote those values.

In short, we must choose between the ethic of collectivism and the ethic of individualism and pay the price of either—or of both.

NOTES

1. Quoted in L. C. Kolb, *Noyes' Modern Clinical Psychiatry*, 7th ed. (Philadelphia: Saunders, 1968), p. 516.

2. See my *The Manufacture of Madness: A Comparative Study of the Inquisition and the Mental Health Movement* (New York: Harper & Row, 1970), pp. 180–206.

3. A. Montagu, "The Long Search for Euphoria," *Reflections* 1 (May–June 1966): 65.

4. A. B. Light et al., *Opium Addiction* (Chicago: American Medical Association, 1929), p. 115; quoted in Alfred R. Lindesmith, *Addiction and Opiates* (Chicago: Aldine, 1968), p. 40.

5. *The New York Times*, April 1, 1967.

6. Editorial, "About Narcotics," *Syracuse Herald-Journal*, March 6, 1969.

7. *The New York Times*, June 29, 1970.

8. See my *Ideology and Insanity: Essays on the Psychiatric Dehumanization of Man* (Garden City, N.Y.: Doubleday, Anchor Press, 1970).

9. J. S. Mill, *On Liberty* (Chicago: Regnery, 1955), p. 13.

The Fallacy of the "Hijacked Brain"

PEG O'CONNOR

Of all the philosophical discussions that surface in contemporary life, the question of free will—mainly, the debate over whether or not we have it—is certainly one of the most persistent.

That might seem odd, as the average person rarely seems to pause to reflect on whether their choices on, say, where they live, whom they marry, or what they eat for dinner, are their own or the inevitable outcome of a deterministic universe. Still, as James Atlas pointed out last month, the spate of "can't help yourself" books would indicate that people are in fact deeply concerned with how much of their lives they can control. Perhaps that's because, upon further reflection, we find that our understanding of free will lurks beneath many essential aspects of our existence.

One particularly interesting variation on this question appears in scientific, academic and therapeutic discussions about addiction. Many times, the question is framed as follows: "Is addiction a disease or a choice?"

The argument runs along these lines: If addiction is a disease, then in some ways it is out of our control and forecloses choices. A disease is a medical condition that develops outside of our control; it is, then, not a matter of choice. In the absence of choice, the addicted person is essentially relieved of responsibility. The addict has been overpowered by her addiction.

The counterargument describes addictive behavior as a choice. People whose use of drugs and alcohol leads to obvious problems but who continue to use them anyway are making choices to do so. Since those choices lead to addiction, blame and responsibility clearly rest on the addict's shoulders. It then becomes more a matter of free will.

Recent scientific studies on the biochemical responses of the brain are currently tipping the scales toward the more deterministic view—of addiction as a disease. The structure of the brain's reward system combined with certain biochemical responses and certain environments, they appear to show, cause people to become addicted.

In such studies, and in reports of them to news media, the term "the hijacked brain" often appears, along with other language that emphasizes the addict's lack of choice in the matter. Sometimes the pleasure-reward system has been "commandeered." Other times it "goes rogue." These expressions are often accompanied by the conclusion that there are "addicted brains."

The word "hijacked" is especially evocative; people often have a visceral reaction to it. I imagine that this is precisely why this term is becoming more commonly used in connection with addiction. But it is important to be aware of the effects of such language on our understanding.

When most people think of a hijacking, they picture a person, sometimes wearing a mask and always wielding some sort of weapon, who takes control of a car, plane or train. The hijacker may not himself drive or pilot the vehicle, but the violence involved leaves no doubt who is in charge. Someone can hijack a vehicle for a variety of reasons, but mostly it boils down to needing to escape or wanting to use the vehicle itself as a weapon in a greater plan. Hijacking is a means to an end; it is always and only oriented to the goals of the hijacker. Innocent victims are ripped from their normal lives by the violent intrusion of the hijacker.

In the "hijacked" view of addiction, the brain is the innocent victim of certain substances—alcohol, cocaine, nicotine or heroin, for example—as well as certain behaviors like eating, gambling or sexual activity. The drugs or the neurochemicals produced by the behaviors overpower and redirect the brain's normal responses, and thus take control of (hijack) it. For addicted people, that martini or cigarette is the weapon-wielding hijacker who is going to compel certain behaviors.

To do this, drugs like alcohol and cocaine and behaviors like gambling light up the brain's pleasure circuitry, often bringing a burst of euphoria. Other studies indicate that people who are addicted have lower dopamine and serotonin levels in their brains, which means that it takes more of a particular substance or behavior for them to experience pleasure or to reach a certain threshold of pleasure. People tend to want to maximize pleasure; we tend to do things that bring more of it. We also tend to chase it when it subsides, trying hard to recreate the same level of pleasure we have experienced in the past. It is not uncommon to hear addicts talking about wanting to experience the euphoria of a first high. Often they never reach it, but keep trying. All of this lends credence to the description of the brain as hijacked.

Analogies and comparisons can be very effective and powerful tools in explanation, especially when the objects compared are not overtly and obviously similar at first glance. A comparison can be especially compelling when one of the objects is familiar or common and is wrested from its usual context. Similarities shared between disparate cases can help to highlight features in each that might otherwise escape notice. But analogies and comparisons always start to break down at some point, often when the differences are seen to be greater than similarities. This, I submit, is the case with understanding addiction as hijacking.

A hijacker comes from outside and takes control by violent means. A hijacker takes a vehicle that is not his; hijacking is always a form of stealing and kidnapping. A hijacker always takes someone else's vehicle; you cannot hijack your own car. That is a type of nonsense or category mistake. Ludwig Wittgenstein offered that money passed from your left hand to your right is not a gift. The practical consequences of this action are not the same as those of a gift. Writing yourself a thank-you note would be absurd.

The analogy of addiction and hijacking involves the same category mistake as the money switched from hand to hand. You can treat yourself poorly, callously or violently. In such cases, we might say the person is engaging in acts of self-abuse and self-harm. Self-abuse can involve acting in ways that you know are not in your self-interest in some larger sense or that are contrary to your desires. This, however, is not hijacking; the practical consequences are quite different.

It might be tempting to claim that in an addiction scenario, the drugs or behaviors are the hijackers. However, those drugs and behaviors need to be done by the person herself (barring cases in which someone is given drugs and may be made chemically dependent). In the usual cases, an individual is the one putting chemicals into her body or engaging in certain behaviors in the hopes of getting high. This simply pushes the question back to whether a person can hijack herself.

There is a kind of intentionality to hijacking that clearly is absent in addiction. No one plans to become an addict. One certainly may plan to drink in reckless or dangerous ways, not with the intention of becoming an addict somewhere down the road. Addiction develops over time and requires repeated and worsening use.

In a hijacking situation, it is very easy to assign blame and responsibility. The villain is easy to identify. So are the victims, people who have had the bad luck to be in the wrong place at the wrong time. Hijacked people are given no choice in the matter.

A little logic is helpful here, since the "choice or disease" question rests on a false dilemma. This fallacy posits that only two options exist. Since there are only two options, they must be mutually exclusive. If we think, however, of addiction as involving both choice *and* disease, our outlook is likely to become more nuanced. For instance, the progression of many medical diseases is affected by the choices that individuals make. A patient who knows he has chronic obstructive pulmonary disease and refuses to wear a respirator or at least a mask while using noxious chemicals is making a choice that exacerbates his condition. A person who knows he meets the D.S.M.-IV criteria for chemical abuse, and that abuse is often the precursor to dependency, and still continues to use drugs, is making a choice, and thus bears responsibility for it.

Linking choice and responsibility is right in many ways, so long as we acknowledge that choice can be constrained in ways other than by force or overt coercion. There is no doubt that the choices of people progressing to addiction are constrained; compulsion and impulsiveness constrain choices. Many addicts will say that they choose to take that first drink or drug and that once they start they cannot stop. A classic binge drinker is a prime example; his choices are constrained with the first drink. He both has and does not have a choice. (That moment before the first drink or drug is what the philosopher Owen Flanagan describes as a "zone of control.") But he still bears some degree of responsibility to others and to himself.

The complexity of each person's experience with addiction should caution us to avoid false quandaries, like the one that requires us to define addiction as either disease or choice, and to adopt more nuanced conceptions. Addicts are neither hijackers nor victims. It is time to retire this analogy.

Against the Legalization of Drugs

JAMES Q. WILSON

In 1972, the President appointed me chairman of the National Advisory Council for Drug Abuse Prevention. Created by Congress, the Council was charged with providing guidance on how best to coordinate the national war on drugs. (Yes, we called it a war then, too.) In those days, the drug we were chiefly concerned with was heroin. When I took office, heroin use had been increasing dramatically. Everybody was worried that this increase would continue. Such phrases as "heroin epidemic" were commonplace.

That same year, the eminent economist Milton Friedman published an essay in *Newsweek* in which he called for legalizing heroin. His argument was on

James Q. Wilson, "Against the Legalization of Drugs." Reprinted from *Commentary*, February 1990, by permission; copyright © 1990 by Commentary, Inc.

two grounds: as a matter of ethics, the government has no right to tell people not to use heroin (or to drink or to commit suicide); as a matter of economics, the prohibition of drug use imposes costs on society that far exceed the benefits. Others, such as the psychoanalyst Thomas Szasz, made the same argument.

We did not take Friedman's advice. (Government commissions rarely do.) I do not recall that we even discussed legalizing heroin, though we did discuss (but did not take action on) legalizing a drug, cocaine, that many people then argued was benign. Our marching orders were to figure out how to win the war on heroin, not to run up the white flag of surrender.

That was 1972. Today, we have the same number of heroin addicts that we had then—half a million, give or take a few thousand. Having that many heroin addicts is no trivial matter; these people deserve our attention. But not having had an increase in that number for over fifteen years is also something that deserves our attention. What happened to the "heroin epidemic" that many people once thought would overwhelm us?

The facts are clear: a more or less stable pool of heroin addicts has been getting older, with relatively few new recruits. In 1976 the average age of heroin users who appeared in hospital emergency rooms was about twenty-seven; ten years later it was thirty-two. More than two-thirds of all heroin users appearing in emergency rooms are now over the age of thirty. Back in the early 1970's, when heroin got onto the national political agenda, the typical heroin addict was much younger, often a teenager. Household surveys show the same thing—the rate of opiate use (which includes heroin) has been flat for the better part of two decades. More fine-grained studies of inner-city neighborhoods confirm this. John Boyle and Ann Brunswick found that the percentage of young blacks in Harlem who used heroin fell from 8 percent in 1970-71 to about 3 percent in 1975-76.

Why did heroin lose its appeal for young people? When the young blacks in Harlem were asked why they stopped, more than half mentioned "trouble with the law" or "high cost" (and high cost is, of course, directly the result of law enforcement). Two-thirds said that heroin hurt their health; nearly all said they had had a bad experience with it. We need not rely, however, simply on what they said. In New York City in 1973-75, the street price of heroin rose dramatically and its purity sharply declined, probably as a result of the heroin shortage caused by the success of the Turkish government in reducing the supply of opium base and of the French government in closing down heroin-processing laboratories located in and around Marseilles. These were short-lived gains for, just as Friedman predicted, alternative sources of supply—mostly in Mexico—quickly emerged. But the three-year heroin shortage interrupted the easy recruitment of new users.

Health and related problems were no doubt part of the reason for the reduced flow of recruits. Over the preceding years, Harlem youth had watched as more and more heroin users died of overdoses, were poisoned by adulterated doses, or acquired hepatitis from dirty needles. The word got around: heroin can kill you. By 1974 new hepatitis cases and drug-overdose deaths had dropped to a fraction of what they had been in 1970.

Alas, treatment did not seem to explain much of the cessation in drug use. Treatment programs can and do help heroin addicts, but treatment did not explain the drop in the number of *new* users (who by definition had never been in treatment) nor even much of the reduction in the number of experienced users.

No one knows how much of the decline to attribute to personal observation as opposed to high prices or reduced supply. But other evidence suggests strongly that price and supply played a large role. In 1972 the National Advisory Council was especially worried by the prospect that U.S. servicemen returning to this country from Vietnam would bring their heroin habits with them. Fortunately, a brilliant study by Lee Robins of Washington University in St. Louis put that fear to rest. She measured drug use of Vietnam veterans shortly after they had returned home. Though many had used heroin regularly while in Southeast Asia, most gave up the habit when back in the United States. The reason: here, heroin was less available and sanctions on its use were more pronounced. Of course, if a veteran had been willing to pay enough—which might have meant traveling to another city and would certainly have meant making an illegal contact with a disreputable dealer in a threatening neighborhood in order to acquire a (possibly) dangerous dose—he could have sustained his drug habit. Most veterans were unwilling to pay this price, and so their drug use declined or disappeared.

RELIVING THE PAST

Suppose we had taken Friedman's advice in 1972. What would have happened? We cannot be entirely certain, but at a minimum we would have placed the young heroin addicts (and, above all, the prospective addicts) in a very different position from the one in which they actually found themselves. Heroin would have been legal. Its price would have been reduced by 95 percent (minus whatever we chose to recover in taxes.) Now that it could be sold by the same people who make aspirin, its quality would have been assured—no poisons, no adulterants. Sterile hypodermic needles would have been readily available at the neighborhood drugstore, probably at the same counter where the heroin was sold. No need to travel to big cities or unfamiliar neighborhoods—heroin could have been purchased anywhere, perhaps by mail order.

There would no longer have been any financial or medical reason to avoid heroin use. Anybody could have afforded it. We might have tried to prevent children from buying it, but as we have learned from our efforts to prevent minors from buying alcohol and tobacco, young people have a way of penetrating markets theoretically reserved for adults. Returning Vietnam veterans would have discovered that Omaha and Raleigh had been converted into the pharmaceutical equivalent of Saigon.

Under these circumstances, can we doubt for a moment that heroin use would have grown exponentially? Or that a vastly larger supply of new users would have been recruited? Professor Friedman is a Nobel Prize-winning economist whose understanding of market forces is profound. What did he think would happen to consumption under his legalized regime? Here are his words: "Legalizing drugs might increase the number of addicts, but it is not clear that it would. Forbidden fruit is attractive, particularly to the young."

Really? I suppose that we should expect no increase in Porsche sales if we cut the price by 95 percent, no increase in whiskey sales if we cut the price by a comparable amount—because young people only want fast cars and strong liquor when they are "forbidden." Perhaps Friedman's uncharacteristic lapse from the obvious implications of price theory can be explained by a misunderstanding of how drug users are recruited. In his 1972 essay he said that "drug addicts are deliberately made by pushers, who give likely prospects their first few doses free." If drugs were legal it would not pay anybody to produce addicts, because everybody would buy from the cheapest source. But as every drug expert knows, pushers do not produce addicts. Friends or acquaintances do. In fact, pushers are usually reluctant to deal with non-users because a non-user could be an undercover cop. Drug use spreads in the same way any fad or fashion spreads: somebody who is already a user urges his friends to try, or simply shows already-eager friends how to do it.

But we need not rely on speculation, however plausible, that lowered prices and more abundant supplies would have increased heroin usage. Great Britain once followed such a policy and with almost exactly those results. Until the mid-1960's, British physicians were allowed to prescribe heroin to certain classes of addicts. (Possessing these drugs without a doctor's prescription remained a criminal offense.) For many years this policy worked well enough because the addict patients were typically middle-class people who had become dependent on opiate painkillers while undergoing hospital treatment. There was no drug culture. The British system worked for many years, not because it prevented drug abuse, but because there was no problem of drug abuse that would test the system.

All that changed in the 1960's. A few unscrupulous doctors began passing out heroin in wholesale amounts. One doctor prescribed almost 600,000 heroin tablets—that is, over thirteen pounds—in just one year. A youthful drug culture emerged with a demand for drugs far different from that of the older addicts. As a result, the British government required doctors to refer users to government-run clinics to receive their heroin.

But the shift to clinics did not curtail the growth in heroin use. Throughout the 1960's the number of addicts increased—the late John Kaplan of Stanford estimated by fivefold—in part as a result of the diversion of heroin from clinic patients to new users on the streets. An addict would bargain with the clinic doctor over how big a dose he would receive. The patient wanted as much as he could get, the doctor wanted to give as little as was needed. The patient had an advantage in this conflict because the doctor could not be certain how much was really needed.

Many patients would use some of their "maintenance" dose and sell the remaining part to friends, thereby recruiting new addicts. As the clinics learned of this, they began to shift their treatment away from heroin and toward methadone, an addictive drug that, when taken orally, does not produce a "high" but will block the withdrawal pains associated with heroin abstinence.

Whether what happened in England in the 1960's was a mini-epidemic or an epidemic depends on whether one looks at numbers or at rates of change. Compared to the United States, the numbers were small. In 1960 there were 68 heroin addicts known to the British government; by 1968 there were 2,000 in treatment and many more who refused treatment. (They would refuse in part because they did not want to get methadone at a clinic if they could get heroin on the street.) Richard Hartnoll estimates that the actual number of addicts in England is five times the number officially registered. At a minimum, the number of British addicts increased by thirtyfold in ten years; the actual increase may have been much larger.

In the early 1980's the numbers began to rise again, and this time nobody doubted that a real epidemic was at hand. The increase was estimated to be 40 percent a year. By 1982 there were thought to be 20,000 heroin users in London alone. Geoffrey Pearson reports that many cities—Glasgow, Liverpool, Manchester, and Sheffield among them—were now experiencing a drug problem that once had been largely confined to London. The problem, again, was supply. The country was being flooded with cheap, high-quality heroin, first from Iran and then from Southeast Asia.

The United States began the 1960's with a much larger number of heroin addicts and probably a bigger at-risk population than was the case in Great Britain. Even though it would be foolhardy to suppose that the British system, if installed here, would have worked the same way or with the same results, it would be equally foolhardy to suppose that a combination of heroin available from leaky clinics and from street dealers who faced only minimal law-enforcement risks would not have produced a much greater increase in heroin use than we actually experienced. My guess is that if we had allowed either doctors or clinics to prescribe heroin, we would have had far worse results than were produced in Britain, if for no other reason than the vastly larger number of addicts with which we began. We would have had to find some way to police thousands (not scores) of physicians and hundreds (not dozens) of clinics. If the British civil service found it difficult to keep heroin in the hands of addicts and out of the hands of recruits when it was dealing with a few hundred people, how well would the American civil service have accomplished the same tasks when dealing with tens of thousands of people?

BACK TO THE FUTURE

Now cocaine, especially in its potent form, crack, is the focus of attention. Now as in 1972 the government is trying to reduce its use. Now as then some people are advocating legalization. Is there any more reason to yield to those arguments today than there was almost two decades ago?

I think not. If we had yielded in 1972 we almost certainly would have had today a permanent population of several million, not several hundred thousand, heroin addicts. If we yield now we will have a far more serious problem with cocaine.

Crack is worse than heroin by almost any measure. Heroin produces a pleasant drowsiness and, if hygienically administered, has only the physical side effects of constipation and sexual impotence. Regular heroin use incapacitates many users, especially poor ones, for any productive work or social responsibility. They will sit nodding on a street corner, helpless but at least harmless. By contrast, regular cocaine use leaves the user neither helpless nor harmless. When smoked (as with crack) or injected, cocaine produces instant, intense, and short-lived euphoria. The experience generates a powerful desire to repeat it. If the drug is readily available, repeat use will occur. Those people who progress to "bingeing" on cocaine become devoted to the drug and its effects to the exclusion of almost all other considerations—job, family, children, sleep, food, even sex. Dr. Frank Gawin at Yale and Dr. Everett Ellinwood at Duke report that a substantial percentage of all high-dose, binge users become uninhibited, impulsive, hyper-sexual, compulsive, irritable, and hyperactive. Their moods vacillate dramatically, leading at times to violence and homicide.

Women are much more likely to use crack than heroin, and if they are pregnant, the effects on their babies are tragic. Douglas Besharov, who has been following the effects of drugs on infants for twenty years, writes that nothing he learned about heroin prepared him for the devastation of cocaine. Cocaine harms the fetus and can lead to physical deformities or neurological damage. Some crack babies have for all practical purposes suffered a disabling stroke while still in the womb. The long-term consequences of this brain damage are lowered cognitive ability and the onset of mood disorders. Besharov estimates that about 30,000 to 50,000 such babies are born every year, about 7,000 in New York City alone. There may be ways to treat such infants, but from everything we now know the treatment will be long, difficult, and expensive. Worse, the mothers who are most likely to produce crack babies are precisely the ones who, because of poverty or temperament, are least able and willing to obtain such treatment. In fact, anecdotal evidence suggests that crack mothers are likely to abuse their infants.

The notion that abusing drugs such as cocaine is a "victimless crime" is not only absurd but dangerous. Even ignoring the fetal drug syndrome, crack-dependent people are, like heroin addicts, individuals who regularly victimize their children by neglect, their spouses by improvidence, their employers by lethargy, and their co-workers by carelessness. Society is not and could never be a collection of autonomous individuals. We all have a stake in ensuring that each of us displays a minimal level of dignity, responsibility, and empathy. We cannot, of course, coerce people into goodness, but we can and should insist that some standards must be met if society itself—on which the very existence of the human personality depends—is to persist. Drawing the line that defines those standards is difficult and contentious, but if crack and heroin use do not fall below it, what does?

The advocates of legalization will respond by suggesting that my picture is overdrawn. Ethan Nadel-mann of Princeton argues that the risk of legalization is less than most people suppose. Over 20 million Americans between the ages of eighteen and twenty-five have tried cocaine (according to a government survey), but only a quarter million use it daily. From this Nadelmann concludes that at most 3 percent of all young people who try cocaine develop a problem with it. The implication is clear: make the drug legal and we only have to worry about 3 percent of our youth.

The implication rests on a logical fallacy and a factual error. The fallacy is this: the percentage of occasional cocaine users who become binge users *when the drug is illegal* (and thus expensive and hard to find) tells us nothing about the percentage who will become dependent when the drug is legal (and thus cheap and abundant). Drs. Gawin and Ellinwood report, in common with several other researchers, that controlled or occasional use of cocaine changes to compulsive and frequent use "when access to the drug increases" or when the user switches from snorting to smoking. More cocaine more potently administered alters, perhaps sharply, the proportion of "controlled" users who become heavy users.

The factual error is this: the federal survey Nadelmann quotes was done in 1985, *before* crack had become common. Thus the probability of becoming dependent on cocaine was derived from the responses of users who snorted the drug. The speed and potency of cocaine's action increases dramatically when it is smoked. We do not yet know how greatly the advent of crack increases the risk of dependency, but all the clinical evidence suggests that the increase is likely to be large.

It is possible that some people will not become heavy users even when the drug is readily available in its most potent form. So far there are no scientific grounds for predicting who will and who will not become dependent. Neither socioeconomic background nor personality traits differentiate between casual and intensive users. Thus, the only way to settle the question of who is correct about the effect of easy availability on drug use, Nadelmann or Gawin and Ellinwood, is to try it and see. But that social experiment is so risky as to be no experiment at all, for if cocaine is legalized and if the rate of its abusive use increases dramatically, there is no way to put the genie back in the bottle, and it is not a kindly genie.

HAVE WE LOST?

Many people who agree that there are risks in legalizing cocaine or heroin still favor it because, they think, we have lost the war on drugs. "Nothing we have done has worked" and the current federal policy is just "more of the same." Whatever the costs of greater drug use, surely they would be less than the costs of our present, failed efforts.

That is exactly what I was told in 1972—and heroin is not quite as bad a drug as cocaine. We did not surrender and we did not lose. We did not win, either. What the nation accomplished then was what most efforts to save people from themselves accomplish: the problem was contained and the number of victims minimized, all at a considerable cost in law enforcement and increased crime. Was the cost worth it? I think so, but others may disagree. What are the lives of would-be addicts worth? I recall some people saying to me then, "Let them kill themselves." I was appalled. Happily, such views did not prevail.

Have we lost today? Not at all. High-rate cocaine use is not commonplace. The National Institute of Drug Abuse (NIDA) reports that less than 5 percent of high-school seniors used cocaine within the last thirty days. Of course this survey misses young people who have dropped out of school and miscounts those who lie on the questionnaire, but even if we inflate the NIDA estimate by some plausible percentage, it is still not much above 5 percent. Medical examiners reported in 1987 that about 1,500 died from cocaine use; hospital emergency rooms reported about 30,000 admissions related to cocaine abuse.

These are not small numbers, but neither are they evidence of a nationwide plague that threatens to engulf us all. Moreover, cities vary greatly in the proportion of people who are involved with cocaine. To get city-level data we need to turn to drug tests carried out on arrested persons, who obviously are more likely to be drug users than the average citizen. The National Institute of Justice, through its Drug Use Forecasting (DUF) project, collects urinalysis data on arrestees in 22 cities. As we have already seen, opiate (chiefly heroin) use has been flat or declining in most of these cities over the last decade. Cocaine use has gone up sharply, but with great variation among cities. New York, Philadelphia, and Washington, D.C., all report that two-thirds or more of their arrestees tested positive for cocaine, but in Portland, San Antonio, and Indianapolis the percentage was one-third or less.

In some neighborhoods, of course, matters have reached crisis proportions. Gangs control the streets, shootings terrorize residents, and drug-dealing occurs in plain view. The police seem barely able to contain matters. But in these neighborhoods—unlike at Palo Alto cocktail parties—the people are not calling for legalization, they are calling for help. And often not much help has come. Many cities are willing to do almost anything about the drug problem except spend more money on it. The federal government cannot change that; only local voters and politicians can. It is not clear that they will.

It took about ten years to contain heroin. We have had experience with crack for only about three or four years. Each year we spend perhaps $11 billion on law enforcement (and some of that goes to deal with marijuana) and perhaps $2 billion on treatment. Large sums, but not sums that should lead anyone to say, "We just can't afford this any more."

The illegality of drugs increases crime, partly because some users turn to crime to pay for their habits, partly because some users are stimulated by certain drugs (such as crack or PCP) to act more violently or ruthlessly than they otherwise would, and partly because criminal organizations seeking to control drug supplies use force to manage their markets. These also are serious costs, but no one knows how much they would be reduced if drugs were legalized. Addicts would no longer steal to pay black-market prices for drugs, a real gain. But some, perhaps a great deal, of that gain would be offset by the great increase in the number of addicts. These people, nodding on heroin or living in the delusion-ridden high of cocaine, would hardly be ideal employees. Many would steal simply to support themselves, since snatch-and-grab, opportunistic crime can be manged [*sic*] even by people unable to hold a regular job or plan an elaborate crime. Those British addicts who get their supplies from government clinics are not models of law-abiding decency. Most are in crime, and though their per-capita rate of criminality may be lower thanks to the cheapness of their drugs, the total volume of crime they produce may be quite large. Of course, society could decide to support all unemployable addicts on welfare, but that would mean that gains from lowered rates of crime would have to be offset by large increases in welfare budgets.

Proponents of legalization claim that the costs of having more addicts around would be largely if not entirely offset by having more money available with which to treat and care for them. The money would come from taxes levied on the sale of heroin and cocaine.

To obtain this fiscal dividend, however, legalization's supporters must first solve an economic dilemma. If they want to raise a lot of money to pay for welfare and treatment, the tax rate on the drugs will have to be quite high. Even if they themselves do not want a high rate, the politicians' love of "sin taxes" would probably guarantee that it would be high anyway. But the higher the tax, the higher the price of the drug, and the higher the price the greater the likelihood that addicts will turn to crime to find the money for it and that criminal organizations will be formed to sell tax-free drugs at below-market rates. If we managed to keep taxes (and thus prices) low, we would get that much less money to pay for welfare and treatment and more people could afford to become addicts. There may be an optimal tax rate for drugs that maximizes revenue while minimizing crime, bootlegging, and the recruitment of new addicts, but our experience with alcohol does not suggest that we know how to find it.

THE BENEFITS OF ILLEGALITY

The advocates of legalization find nothing to be said in favor of the current system except, possibly, that it keeps the number of addicts smaller than it would otherwise be. In fact, the benefits are more substantial than that.

First, treatment. All the talk about providing "treatment on demand" implies that there is a demand for treatment. That is not quite right. There are some drug-dependent people who genuinely want treatment and will remain in it if offered; they should receive it. But there are far more who want only short-term help after a bad crash; once stabilized and bathed, they are back on the street again, hustling. And even many of the addicts who enroll in a program honestly wanting help drop out after a short while when they discover that help takes time and commitment. Drug-dependent people have very short time horizons and a weak capacity for commitment. These two groups—those looking for a quick fix and those unable to stick with a long-term fix—are not easily helped. Even if we increase the number of treatment slots—as we should—we would have to do something to make treatment more effective.

One thing that can often make it more effective is compulsion. Douglas Anglin of UCLA, in common with many other researchers, has found that the longer one stays in a treatment program, the better the chances of a reduction in drug dependency. But he, again like most other researchers, has found that drop-out rates are high. He has also found, however, that patients who enter treatment under legal compulsion stay in the program longer than those not subject to such pressure. His research on the California civil-commitment program, for example, found that heroin users involved with its required drug-testing program had over the long term a lower rate of heroin use than similar addicts who were free of such constraints. If for many addicts compulsion is a useful component of treatment, it is not clear how compulsion could be achieved in a society in which purchasing, possessing, and using the drug were legal. It could be managed, I suppose, but I would not want to have to answer the challenge from the American Civil Liberties Union that it is wrong to compel a person to undergo treatment for consuming a legal commodity.

Next, education. We are now investing substantially in drug-education programs in the schools. Though we do not yet know for certain what will work, there are some promising leads. But I wonder how credible such programs would be if they were aimed at dissuading children from doing something perfectly legal. We could, of course, treat drug education like smoking education: inhaling crack and inhaling tobacco are both legal, but you should not do it because it is bad for you. That tobacco is bad for you is easily shown; the Surgeon General has seen to that. But what do we say about crack? It is pleasurable, but devoting yourself to so much pleasure is not a good idea (though perfectly legal)? Unlike tobacco, cocaine will not give you cancer or emphysema, but it will lead you to neglect your duties to family, job, and neighborhood? Everybody is doing cocaine, but you should not?

Again, it might be possible under a legalized regime to have effective drug-prevention programs, but their effectiveness would depend heavily, I think, on first having decided that cocaine use, like tobacco use, is purely a matter of practical consequences; no fundamental moral significance attaches to either. But if we believe—as I do—that dependency on certain mind-altering drugs *is* a moral issue and that their illegality rests in part on their immorality, then legalizing them undercuts, if it does not eliminate altogether, the moral message.

That message is at the root of the distinction we now make between nicotine and cocaine. Both are highly addictive; both have harmful physical effects. But we treat the two drugs differently, not simply because nicotine is so widely used as to be beyond the reach of effective prohibition, but because its use does not destroy the user's essential humanity. Tobacco shortens one's life, cocaine debases it. Nicotine alters one's habits, cocaine alters one's soul. The heavy use of crack, unlike the heavy use of tobacco, corrodes those natural sentiments of sympathy and duty that constitute our human nature and make possible our social life. To say, as does Nadelmann, that distinguishing morally between tobacco and cocaine is "little more than a transient prejudice" is close to saying that morality itself is but a prejudice.

THE ALCOHOL PROBLEM

Now we have arrived where many arguments about legalizing drugs begin: is there any reason to treat heroin and cocaine differently from the way we treat alcohol?

There is no easy answer to that question because, as with so many human problems, one cannot decide simply on the basis either of moral principles or of individual consequences; one has to temper any policy by a common-sense judgment of what is possible. Alcohol, like heroin, cocaine, PCP, and marijuana, is a drug—that is, a mood-altering substance—and consumed to excess it certainly has harmful consequences: auto accidents, barroom fights, bedroom shootings. It is also, for some people, addictive. We cannot confidently compare the addictive powers of these drugs, but the best evidence suggests that crack and heroin are much more addictive than alcohol.

Many people, Nadelmann included, argue that since the health and financial costs of alcohol abuse are so much higher than those of cocaine or heroin abuse, it is hypocritical folly to devote our efforts to preventing cocaine or drug use. But as Mark Kleiman of Harvard has pointed out, this comparison is quite misleading. What Nadelmann is doing is showing that a *legalized* drug (alcohol) produces greater social harm than *illegal* ones (cocaine and heroin). But of course. Suppose that in the 1920's we had made heroin and cocaine legal and alcohol illegal. Can anyone doubt that Nadelmann would now be writing that it is folly to continue our ban on alcohol because cocaine and heroin are so much more harmful?

And let there be no doubt about it—widespread heroin and cocaine use are associated with all manner of ills. Thomas Bewley found that the mortality rate of British heroin addicts in 1968 was 28 times as high as the death rate of the same age group of nonaddicts, even though in England at the time an addict could obtain free or low-cost heroin and clean needles from British clinics. Perform the following mental experiment: suppose we legalized heroin and cocaine in this country. In what proportion of auto fatalities would the state police report that the driver was nodding off on heroin or recklessly driving on a coke high? In what proportion of spouse-assault and child-abuse cases would the local police report that crack was involved? In what proportion of industrial accidents would safety investigators report that the forklift or drill-press operator was in a drug-induced stupor or frenzy? We do not know exactly what the proportion would be, but anyone who asserts that it would not be much higher than it is now would have to believe that these drugs have little appeal except when they are illegal. And that is nonsense.

An advocate of legalization might concede that social harm—perhaps harm equivalent to that already produced by alcohol—would follow from making cocaine and heroin generally available. But at least, he might add, we would have the problem "out in the open" where it could be treated as a matter of "public health." That is well and good, *if* we knew how to treat—that is, cure—heroin and cocaine abuse. But we do not know how to do it for all the people who would need such help. We are having only limited success in coping with chronic alcoholics. Addictive behavior is immensely difficult to change, and the best methods for changing it—living in drug-free therapeutic communities, becoming faithful members of Alcoholics Anonymous or Narcotics Anonymous—require great personal commitment, a quality that is, alas, in short supply among the very persons—young people, disadvantaged people—who are often most at risk for addiction.

Suppose that today we had, not 15 million alcohol abusers, but half a million. Suppose that we already knew what we have learned from our long experience with the widespread use of alcohol. Would we make whiskey legal? I do not know, but I suspect there would be a lively debate. The Surgeon General would remind us of the risks alcohol poses to pregnant women. The National Highway Traffic Safety Administration would point to the likelihood of more highway fatalities caused by drunk drivers. The Food and Drug Administration might find that there is a nontrivial increase in cancer associated with alcohol consumption. At the same time the police would report great difficulty in keeping illegal whiskey out of our cities, officers being corrupted by bootleggers, and alcohol addicts often resorting to crime to feed their habit. Libertarians, for their part, would argue that every citizen has a right to drink anything he wishes and that drinking is, in any event, a "victimless crime."

However the debate might turn out, the central fact would be that the problem was still, at that point, a small one. The government cannot legislate away the addictive tendencies in all of us, nor can it remove completely even the most dangerous addictive substances. But it can cope with harms when the harms are still manageable.

SCIENCE AND ADDICTION

One advantage of containing a problem while it is still containable is that it buys time for science to learn more about it and perhaps to discover a cure. Almost unnoticed in the current debate over legalizing drugs is that basic science has made rapid strides in identifying the underlying neurological processes involved in some forms of addiction. Stimulants such as cocaine and amphetamines alter the way certain brain cells communicate with one another. That alteration is complex and not entirely understood, but in simplified form it involves modifying the way in which a neurotransmitter called dopamine sends signals from one cell to another.

When dopamine crosses the synapse between two cells, it is in effect carrying a message from the first cell to activate the second one. In certain parts of the brain that message is experienced as pleasure. After the message is delivered, the dopamine returns to the first cell. Cocaine apparently blocks this return, or "reuptake," so that the excited cell and others nearby continue to send pleasure messages. When the exaggerated high produced by cocaine-influenced dopamine finally ends, the brain cells may (in ways that are still a matter of dispute) suffer from an extreme lack of dopamine, thereby making the individual unable to experience any pleasure at all. This would explain why cocaine users often feel so depressed after enjoying the drug. Stimulants may also affect the way in which other neurotransmitters, such as serotonin and noradrenaline, operate.

Whatever the exact mechanism may be, once it is identified it becomes possible to use drugs to block either the effect of cocaine or its tendency to produce dependency. There have already been experiments using desipramine, imipramine, bromocriptine, carbamazepine, and other chemicals. There are some promising results.

Tragically, we spend very little on such research, and the agencies funding it have not in the past occupied very influential or visible posts in the federal bureaucracy. If there is one aspect of the "war on drugs" metaphor that I dislike, it is its tendency to focus attention almost exclusively on the troops in the trenches, whether engaged in enforcement or treatment, and away from the research-and-development efforts back on the home front where the war may ultimately be decided.

I believe that the prospects of scientists in controlling addiction will be strongly influenced by the size and character of the problem they face. If the problem is a few hundred thousand chronic, high-dose users of an illegal product, the chances of making a difference at a reasonable cost will be much greater than if the problem is a few million chronic users of legal substances. Once a drug is legal, not only will its use increase but many of those who then use it will prefer the drug to the treatment: they will want the pleasure, whatever the cost to themselves or their families, and they will resist—probably successfully—any effort to wean them away from experiencing the high that comes from inhaling a legal substance.

IF I AM WRONG . . .

No one can know what our society would be like if we changed the law to make access to cocaine, heroin, and PCP easier. I believe, for reasons given, that the result would be a sharp increase in use, a more widespread degradation of the human personality, and a greater rate of accidents and violence.

I may be wrong. If I am, then we will needlessly have incurred heavy costs in law enforcement and some forms of criminality. But if I am right, and the legalizers prevail anyway, then we will have consigned millions of people, hundreds of thousands of infants, and hundreds of neighborhoods to a life of oblivion and disease. To the lives and families destroyed by alcohol we will have added countless more destroyed by cocaine, heroin, PCP, and whatever else a basement scientist can invent.

Human character is formed by society; indeed, human character is inconceivable without society, and good character is less likely in a bad society. Will we, in the name of an abstract doctrine of radical individualism, and with the false comfort of suspect predictions, decide to take the chance that somehow individual decency can survive amid a more general level of degradation?

I think not. The American people are too wise for that, whatever the academic essayists and cocktail-party pundits may say. But if Americans today are less wise than I suppose, then Americans at some future time will look back on us now and wonder, what kind of people were they that they could have done such a thing?

CASES FOR ANALYSIS

1. Decriminalization in Portugal

On July 1, 2001, Portugal decriminalized every imaginable drug, from marijuana, to cocaine, to heroin. Some thought Lisbon would become a drug tourist haven, others predicted usage rates among youths to surge.

Eleven years later, it turns out they were both wrong.

Over a decade has passed since Portugal changed its philosophy from labeling drug users as criminals to labeling them as people affected by a disease. This time lapse has allowed statistics to develop and in time, has made Portugal an example to follow.

First, some clarification.

Portugal's move to decriminalize does not mean people can carry around, use, and sell drugs free from police interference. That would be legalization. Rather, all drugs are "decriminalized," meaning drug possession, distribution, and use is still illegal. While distribution and trafficking is still a criminal offense, possession and use is moved out of criminal courts and into a special court where each offender's unique situation is judged by legal experts, psychologists, and social workers. Treatment and further action is decided in these courts, where addicts and drug use is treated as a public health service rather than referring it to the justice system (like the US), reports Fox News.

The resulting effect: a drastic reduction in addicts, with Portuguese officials and reports highlighting that this number, at 100,000 before the new policy was enacted, has been **halved in the following 10 years.** Portugal's **drug usage rates are now among the lowest of EU member states,** according to the same report.[*]

Can you logically conclude from Portugal's example that decriminalization would achieve the same results in the United States? Why or why not?

What, if anything, does the success of the Portuguese approach prove?

[*]Sam Blackstone, "Portugal Decriminalized All Drugs Eleven Years Ago and the Results Are Staggering," *Business Insider*, July 17, 2012. Copyrighted 2015. Business Insider, Inc. 114921:0715DS. Reprinted with permission.

---

2. Against Legalization or Decriminalization of Drugs

Position Statement from Drug Watch International: The legalization or decriminalization of drugs would make harmful, psychoactive, and addictive substances affordable, available, convenient, and marketable. It would expand the use of drugs. It would remove the social stigma attached to illicit drug use, and would send a message of tolerance for drug use, especially to youth. . . .

The use of illicit drugs is illegal because of their intoxicating effects on the brain, damaging impact on the body, adverse impact on behavior, and potential for abuse. Their use threatens the health, welfare, and safety of all people, of users and non-users alike.[†]

Explain your answers. Do you agree with this position statement? Is the description of the effects of drug use accurate or exaggerated? Does legalization or decriminalization imply that the government approves of drug use?

[†]Drug Watch International, "Position Statement," August 1, 1994, http://www.drugwatch.org/resources /publications/position-statements-and-resolutions/ (15 February 2015).

3. Is Marijuana Medicine?

The marijuana plant contains several chemicals that may prove useful for treating a range of illnesses or symptoms, leading many people to argue that it should be made legally available for medical purposes. In fact, a growing number of states (20 as of March 2014) have legalized marijuana's use for certain medical conditions.

The term "medical marijuana" is generally used to refer to the whole unprocessed marijuana plant or its crude extracts, which are not recognized or approved as medicine by the U.S. Food and Drug Administration (FDA). But scientific study of the active chemicals in marijuana, called *cannabinoids*, has led to the development of two FDA-approved medications already, and is leading to the development of new pharmaceuticals that harness the therapeutic benefits of cannabinoids while minimizing or eliminating the harmful side effects (including the "high") produced by eating or smoking marijuana leaves.[‡]

Should marijuana be made available to people for medical reasons? It is not legal in most states; should it stay that way, or should all states legalize it? Why or why not? Suppose you think using marijuana for medical or recreational purposes is immoral or harmful to society. Would you change your mind about its use if it were found to be a cure for hard-to-treat cancers? Explain.

[‡]National Institute on Drug Abuse, "DrugFacts: Is Marijuana Medicine?," December 2014, http://www.drugabuse.gov/publications/drugfacts/marijuana-medicine (15 February 2015).

CHAPTER 13

Sexual Morality

Sex has probably always been controversial, a volatile subject that triggers intense emotions, social angst, and legal and religious sanctions. Fortunately, it has also attracted the interest of moral philosophers who have tried to shed light on its ethical uncertainties. The moral issues most often focus on the morality of specific sexual acts and the context of those acts—aspects of sexuality on which people never fail to have strong opinions. Thus many commend or condemn oral sex, anal sex, masturbation, homosexuality, group sex, premarital sex, promiscuous sex, prostitution, contraception, and whatever is labeled "sexual perversion."

Unfortunately, people's positions on these questions usually have more to do with their upbringing, religious tradition, or cultural background than with plausible moral arguments. So let's see what critical thinking can tell us about the ethics of sex and marriage.

ISSUE FILE: BACKGROUND

As suggested above, the central question in the morality of sex is, What kind of sexual behavior is morally permissible, and under what circumstances? People generally give one of three answers: (1) sex is permissible only in a marriage between a man and a woman; (2) sex is permissible between informed, consenting adults; and (3) sex is permissible between informed, consenting adults who are bound by love or commitment.

The first answer is the **conventional view:** sex is morally acceptable only between one man and one woman who are married to each other by

legal authority. Sex involving the unmarried or sex in adulterous relationships is impermissible—that is, premarital sex and extramarital sex are wrong. In a religious strain of the conventional view, some sex acts performed by married partners—acts that are incompatible with procreation—are also prohibited. These include masturbation, oral sex, anal sex, and sex using contraceptives.

The conventional attitude has been championed by Christianity, Judaism, and Islam, and has been vigorously defended in the natural law teachings of the Roman Catholic Church. For a long time it was the dominant view of sexual ethics in the West, but since the 1960s its influence has faded. In a recent public opinion poll, 66 percent of respondents said they believe it morally acceptable for a man and woman to have sex before marriage.[1] And whatever people say they believe about the subject, their actual behavior is a far cry from the conventional standard. Research shows that sex before marriage is almost universal among Americans. By age forty-four, 95 percent have had premarital sexual relations.[2]

The second answer is the **liberal view** (not to be confused with the political outlook with the same name). Directly counter to the conventional stance, it says that as long as basic moral

[1]Gallup Poll, "Marriage," May 8–11, 2014, gallup.com/poll/117328/marriage.aspx (16 February 2015).
[2]Lawrence B. Finer, "Trends in Premarital Sex in the United States, 1954–2003," *Public Health Reports* 122 (January–February 2007), www.publichealthreports.org/issueopen.cfm?articleID=1784 (16 February 2015).

standards are respected (for example, no one is harmed or coerced), any sexual activity engaged in by informed, consenting adults is permissible. Provided that people adhere to the relevant moral principles, all kinds of sexual behavior condemned by the conventionalist would be morally acceptable, including premarital sex, extramarital sex, group sex, masturbation, and homosexuality.

The third answer is the **moderate view,** which says that sex is permissible, whether in marriage or not, if the consenting partners have a serious emotional connection. Moral sex does not require marriage, but it does entail more than just the informed, freely given consent of the people involved. For some, this needed connection is love, affection, or mutual caring; for others it's a commitment to sustaining the relationship. Provided that the necessary

element is present, both premarital and extramarital sex could be permitted, but promiscuous sex would likely be disallowed.

As you would expect, the conventionalist and the liberal take opposing views on the rightness of **homosexuality** (sexual relations between people of the same sex). The conventionalist denounces it as abnormal, unnatural, harmful, or dangerous. It is always and everywhere wrong. The liberal sees no morally relevant difference between heterosexual and homosexual sex. The behavior is morally permissible if it conforms to legitimate moral standards and involves consenting adults.

All these diverse views are related to issues involving the sale and use of pornography. **Pornography** is sexually explicit images or text meant to cause sexual excitement or arousal.

VITAL STATS: Sexual Behavior

- By age 20, 77 percent of adults have had sex, and 75 percent have had premarital sex.

- By age 44, 94 percent of women and 96 percent of men have had premarital sex.

- Among adults aged 25–44, 98 percent of women and 97 percent of men have had vaginal intercourse; 89 percent of women and 90 percent of men have had oral sex with an opposite-sex partner; and 36 percent of women and 44 percent of men have had anal sex with an opposite-sex partner.

- Half or more of women ages 18 to 39 report giving or receiving oral sex in the past 90 days.

- The sexual repertoires of U.S. adults vary dramatically, with more than 40 combinations of sexual activity described at adults' most recent sexual event. Adult men and women rarely engage in just one sex act when they have sex.

- 46 percent of high school students report having sexual intercourse; 14 percent report sexual intercourse with four or more persons.

- Among teenagers and young adults (age 15–21), 11 percent of women and 4 percent of men have reported a same-sex sexual experience.

- On average, men experience first intercourse at 16.9 years; women at 17.4.

Statistic from CBS/*New York Times* Poll, January 11–15, 2009, N = 1,112 adults nationwide, MoE ± 3; The Alan Guttmacher Institute, published and unpublished data, 2002, 2011, www.guttmacher.org (3 May 2012); Lawrence B. Finer, "Trends in Premarital Sex in the United States, 1954–2003," *Public Health Reports*, 122 (January–February 2007), www.publichealthreports.org/issueopen.cfm?articleID =1784 (16 February 2015); National Health Statistics Reports, "Sexual Behavior, Sexual Attraction, and Sexual Identity in the United States (2006-2008)," number 36, 3 March 2011; Centers for Disease Control and Prevention, "Trends in the Prevalence of Sexual Behaviors," National YRBS, 1991–2009; compiled data from The Kinsey Institute.

Many who take a conventional view of sexual morality are likely to favor censorship of pornographic material on the grounds that it encourages the very behavior they oppose—premarital sex, extramarital sex, and unacceptable sexual behavior. They may oppose pornography because they believe it is bad for people and institutions. Personal and institutional immorality, lowering of moral standards, decay of religious values and traditions, the undermining of personal virtue, the debasement and subordination of women, increase in crime and social disorder, psychological damage—these and other ills are said to be the possible results of producing or using pornography. Those who adopt a liberal view of sexual morality are likely to condone the use of pornography (but oppose child pornography and underage exposure to pornography). They may reject claims about the harm that pornography causes, pointing to a lack of supporting evidence for them. Many who argue against censorship may also appeal to a principle of individual liberty. They may hold that the only legitimate reason for limiting liberty is the prevention of harm to others. We are free to think, believe, say, desire, and choose as we see fit—as long as we do not harm our fellow citizens.

MORAL THEORIES

Major moral theories have important implications for the morality of sexual behavior. As we have seen (in Chapter 6), natural law theory holds that right actions are those directed towards the aims revealed in nature. According to the Roman Catholic account of the theory, since procreation is foremost among these aims, actions consistent with it are permissible and actions incompatible with it are forbidden. Sexual intercourse between a man and a woman is the supreme act of procreation, and marriage provides the necessary stable context to nurture the fruits of procreation—children. Thus, only sex between a man and a

woman joined by marriage can be morally legitimate. The Vatican declares:

> Experience teaches us that love must find its safeguard in the stability of marriage, if sexual intercourse is truly to respond to the requirements of its own finality and to those of human dignity. These requirements call for a conjugal contract sanctioned and guaranteed by society—a contract which establishes a state of life of capital importance both for the exclusive union of the man and the woman and for the good of their family and of the human community.[3]

Premarital sex is, therefore, proscribed, as well as contraception and sexual activity not directed at procreation such as oral sex, masturbation, and homosexuality.

Although Immanuel Kant favored a conventional approach to sex and marriage, some thinkers have derived from his theory a liberal view of sexual ethics. Recall Kant's dictum that we must always treat people as ends in themselves, never merely as a means to an end. Thomas Mappes says that to treat someone merely, or solely, as a means is to *use* that person, to treat that person without the respect that she deserves. He defines *using another person* as violating the requirement that interactions with that person be based on her voluntary informed consent. This implies that "using another person (in the morally significant sense) can arise in at least two ways: via *coercion*, which is antithetical to voluntary consent, and via *deception*, which undermines the informed character of voluntary consent."[4]

According to these guidelines, any sexual activity in which one person deceives or coerces another is wrong. But when the principle of

---

[3]Sacred Congregation for the Doctrine of the Faith, "*Persona Humana*: Declaration on Certain Questions Concerning Sexual Ethics" (29 December 1975).
[4]Thomas A. Mappes, "Sexual Morality and the Concept of Using Another Person," in *Social Ethics: Morality and Social Policy,* ed. Thomas A. Mappes and Jane S. Zembaty, 7th ed. (New York: McGraw-Hill, 2007), 171.

voluntary informed consent is respected, a broad range of sexual practices is permissible.

A utilitarian is likely to sanction many kinds of sexual activity on the grounds that they produce the greatest overall happiness or good for all concerned. Sexual behavior that results in the greatest net good (the greatest utility) is morally right regardless of whether it is unconventional, "unnatural," deviant, marital, extramarital, procreative, or recreational.

Maximizing utility in sexual matters, however, requires weighing many possible harms and benefits. Those involved in a sexual relationship may risk sexually transmitted disease, pregnancy, emotional distress (humiliation, disappointment, guilt, etc.), disruptions in family life (as a result of adultery, for example), and social or legal censure. But they may also experience a great deal of sexual pleasure, attain a sense of well-being and psychological satisfaction, and forge strong bonds of affection and mutual caring.

MORAL ARGUMENTS

The key difference between the conventional and the liberal view of sexuality is that the former insists that sexual behavior has a morally significant goal, and the latter assumes that sex has no goal at all. This anyway is the central premise in an argument for sexual liberalism put forth by Alan Goldman. He says that several faulty theories of sexuality are based on the idea that sex's rightful goal is procreation, communication, or the expression of love and that "sex which does not fit one of these models or fulfill one of these functions is in some way deviant or incomplete."[5] The Roman Catholic view, for example, is that homosexuality, masturbation, and oral or anal sex are not aimed at the prescribed goal of procreation and are therefore immoral or perverted. Goldman, however, rejects this goal-directed (or, as he says,

"means-end") analysis of sex. He maintains instead that sex is not a means to some other goal—sex is just "plain sex." Sexual desire, he says, is "desire for contact with another person's body and for the pleasure which such contact produces. . . ."

> The desire for physical contact with another person is a minimal criterion for (normal) sexual desire, but is both necessary and sufficient to qualify normal desire as sexual. Of course, we may want to express other feelings through sexual acts in various contexts; but without the desire for the physical contact in and for itself, or when it is sought for other reasons, activities in which contact is involved are not predominantly sexual. Furthermore, the desire for physical contact in itself, without the wish to express affection or other feelings through it, is sufficient to render sexual the activity of the agent which fulfills it.[6]

Sexual pleasure, he says, is what is most valuable about sex, and pleasure is intrinsically valuable. So sex does not need to be assigned some larger goal or purpose. On this point, Igor Primoratz agrees:

> We have no reason to believe that there is only one morally acceptable aim or purpose of human sexual experience and behavior, whether prescribed by nature or enjoined by society . . . Sex has no special moral significance; it is morally neutral. No act is either morally good or bad, right or wrong, merely in virtue of being a sexual act. . . . Accordingly, there is neither need nor room for a set of moral considerations that apply only to sex and constitute sexual morality in the strict sense of the terms. What does apply to choices, acts, and practices in the field of sex are the same moral rules and principles that apply in nonsexual matters.[7]

Goldman and Primoratz do not affirm that sexual behavior can never be immoral, only that it cannot be immoral merely because it is sexual. If sexual behavior is immoral, it is so because it violates moral principles or rules that apply to any

---

[5]Alan H. Goldman, "Plain Sex," *Philosophy and Public Affairs* 6, no. 3 (Spring 1977): 267–287.

[6]Goldman, 269.
[7]Igor Primoratz, *Ethics and Sex* (London: Routledge, 1999), 173.

VITAL STATS: Sex and Relationships

- More than half the participants in the 2010 national sex survey ages 18–24 indicated that their most recent sexual partner was a casual or dating partner. For all other age groups, the majority of study participants indicated that their most recent sexual partner was a relationship partner.

- Men whose most recent sexual encounter was with a relationship partner reported greater arousal, greater pleasure, fewer problems with erectile function, orgasm, and less pain during the event than men whose last sexual encounter was with a non-relationship partner.

- Sexual dissatisfaction is associated with increased risk of divorce and relationship dissolution.

- A study of married couples found age and marital satisfaction to be the two variables most associated with amount of sex. As couples age, they engage in sex less frequently with half of couples age 65–75 still engaging in sex, but less than one fourth of couples over 75 still sexually active.

- Across all ages couples who reported higher levels of marital satisfaction also reported higher frequencies of sex.

Quoted from a report by The Kinsey Institute (kinsey institute.org) summarizing available data.

---

other kinds of actions. "Our first conclusion regarding morality and sex," Goldman says, "is therefore that no conduct otherwise immoral should be excused because it is sexual conduct, and nothing in sex is immoral unless condemned by rules which apply elsewhere as well."[8]

According to Goldman, the views that posit a proper goal for sex (the means-end analyses) inevitably fall into inconsistency. For example, the sex-as-procreation theory condemns oral-genital sex (because it is not a reproductive function) yet fails to denounce kissing or handholding, which are also sexual but not reproductive.

As you would expect, those who champion conventional sexual morality reject "plain sex" arguments. They hold that sexual encounters have a deeper, more significant meaning than sexual liberals would admit. Sexual experiences are not just physical events; they involve the comingling of persons' spiritual and moral selves. As such, they

express and affirm moral values, and the right kind of sex expresses and affirms the right kind of values (specifically, the conventional values of mutual commitment through marriage). Sex that is devoid of these values is morally deficient or perverse.

One of the more contentious—and divisive—issues in sexual ethics is homosexuality. The most heated arguments concern whether homosexual behavior is immoral, and many of these center around the charge that homosexuality is unnatural or abnormal.

Some people take *unnatural* to mean something like "not commonly done by animals." If homosexual behavior is not found among animals in nature, then it is unnatural and, therefore, morally unacceptable. But biologists and others dispute this contention. For example:

> We know that in species after species, right through the animal kingdom, students of animal behavior report unambiguous evidence of homosexual attachments and behavior—in insects, fish, birds, and lower and higher mammals. . . . Whatever the moral implications of homosexuality and naturalness may

[8]Goldman, 280.

be, it is false that homosexuality is immoral because it does not exist amongst animals.[9]

For many who denounce homosexuality, *unnatural* means "out of the norm," "a deviation from the usual pattern," and this unnaturalness is reason enough to call homosexual behavior immoral. A common counterargument is that it does not follow from an action's statistical abnormality that it is immoral. Many acts are statistically out of the norm—skydiving, composing operas, eating snails—but we do not necessarily think them morally wrong.

While acknowledging the weaknesses of the foregoing definitions, some conventionalists offer more sophisticated abnormality arguments. Consider this line of reasoning:

> This paper defends the view that homosexuality is abnormal and hence undesirable—not because it is immoral or sinful, or because it weakens society or hampers evolutionary development, but for a purely mechanical reason. It is a misuse of bodily parts. Clear empirical sense attaches to the idea of *the use* of such bodily parts as genitals, the idea that they are *for* something, and consequently to the idea of their misuse. I argue on grounds involving natural selection that misuse of bodily parts can with high probability be connected to unhappiness. . . . I . . . draw a seemingly evident corollary from my view that homosexuality is abnormal and likely to lead to unhappiness.[10]

The argument here is that homosexuality is a misuse of a bodily part—specifically, the penis, which is for injecting sperm into the vagina, not for the abnormal functions that gay men prefer. This misuse leads to unhappiness because it frustrates "an innately rewarding desire." Society has an

QUICK REVIEW

conventional view (of sexuality)—The idea that sex is morally acceptable only between a man and a woman who are legally married to each other.

liberal view (of sexuality)—The idea that as long as basic moral standards are respected, any sexual activity engaged in by informed, consenting adults is permissible.

moderate view (of sexuality)—The idea that sex is permissible, whether in marriage or not, if the consenting partners have a serious emotional connection.

homosexuality—Sexual relations between people of the same sex.

pornography—Sexually explicit images or text meant to cause sexual excitement or arousal.

interest in promoting happiness; and since homosexuality makes for unhappiness, society ought to discourage it by not legalizing it.

A typical rejoinder to this argument is that evolutionary adaptations, whatever their form, tell us nothing about how people *ought* to behave. Just because blind accidents of nature have shaped humans in a particular way, that doesn't mean people are obligated to stay as they are. As one philosopher puts it, "Human beings are completely at liberty to dispose of their work, their behavior, and even such things as their anatomy and physiology as they see fit."[11] Contrary to natural law theory, knowing how nature *is* tells us nothing about how we *ought to be*.

[9]Michael Ruse, "Is Homosexuality Bad Sexuality?" in *Homosexuality: A Philosophical Inquiry* (Oxford: Blackwell, 1988), 179–192.

[10]Michael Levin, "Why Homosexuality Is Abnormal," *The Monist* (April 1984).

[11]Timothy F. Murphy, "Homosexuality and Nature: Happiness and the Law at Stake," *Journal of Applied Philosophy* 4, no. 2 (1987).

SUMMARY

The main question in the morality of sex is, What kind of sexual behavior is morally permissible, and under what circumstances? The most common answers are: (1) sex is permissible only in a marriage between a man and a woman (the conventional view); (2) sex is permissible between informed, consenting adults (the liberal view); and (3) sex is permissible between informed, consenting adults who are bound by love or commitment (the moderate view).

Natural law theory offers a conventional account of sexual morality, exemplified by Roman Catholic teachings on the subject. Premarital and extramarital sex are forbidden, as well as contraception, oral and anal sex, masturbation, and homosexuality. A liberal view of sexual ethics can be derived from Kantian theory. It says that any sexual activity in which one person deceives or coerces another is wrong, but when the principle of voluntary informed consent is respected, a broad range of sexual practices is permissible. Utilitarianism is likely to endorse many kinds of sexual activity on the grounds that they maximize utility.

Some philosophers reject the idea that sex's rightful goal is procreation, communication, or the expression of love. This goal-oriented view implies that sex that does not aim at one of these objectives is deviant or incomplete. But for many sexual liberals, sex does not have a lofty goal; it is simply sexual desire for the pleasure that comes from physical contact. Since pleasure is intrinsically valuable, a further goal for sexual acts is not needed.

A common charge against homosexuality is that it is unnatural or abnormal. People rebut these claims by trying to show that they are unfounded or confused, or by arguing that abnormality does not imply immorality.

READINGS

Plain Sex

ALAN H. GOLDMAN

I

* * *

I shall suggest here that sex continues to be misrepresented in recent writings, at least in philosophical writings, and I shall criticize the predominant form of analysis which I term "means-end analysis." Such conceptions attribute a necessary external goal or purpose to sexual activity, whether it be reproduction, the expression of love, simple communication, or interpersonal awareness. They analyze sexual activity as a means to one of these ends, implying that sexual desire is a desire to reproduce, to love or be loved, or to communicate with others. All definitions of this type suggest false views of the relation of sex to perversion and morality by implying that sex which does not fit one of these models or fulfill one of these functions is in some way deviant or incomplete.

The alternative, simpler analysis with which I will begin is that sexual desire is desire for contact with another person's body and for the pleasure which such contact produces; sexual activity is activity which tends to fulfill such desire of the agent. Whereas Aristotle and Butler were correct in holding that pleasure is normally a byproduct rather than a goal of purposeful action, in the case of sex this is not so clear. The desire for another's body is, principally among other things, the desire for the pleasure that physical contact brings. On the other hand, it is not a desire for a

Alan H. Goldman, "Plain Sex" from *Philosophy and Public Affairs* 6(3): 268–75 and 278–87. Copyright © 1977 Blackwell Publishing Ltd. Reproduced with permission of John Wiley & Sons, Inc.

particular sensation detachable from its causal context, a sensation which can be derived in other ways. This definition in terms of the general goal of sexual desire appears preferable to an attempt to more explicitly list or define specific sexual activities, for many activities such as kissing, embracing, massaging, or holding hands may or may not be sexual, depending upon the context and more specifically upon the purposes, needs, or desires into which such activities fit. The generality of the definition also represents a refusal (common in recent psychological texts) to overemphasize orgasm as the goal of sexual desire or genital sex as the only norm of sexual activity (this will be hedged slightly in the discussion of perversion below).

Central to the definition is the fact that the goal of sexual desire and activity is the physical contact itself, rather than something else which this contact might express. By contrast, what I term "means-end analyses" posit ends which I take to be extraneous to plain sex, and they view sex as a means to these ends. Their fault lies not in defining sex in terms of its general goal, but in seeing plain sex as merely a means to other separable ends. I term these "means-end analyses" for convenience, although "means-separable-end analyses," while too cumbersome, might be more fully explanatory. The desire for physical contact with another person is a minimal criterion for (normal) sexual desire, but is both necessary and sufficient to qualify normal desire as sexual. Of course, we may want to express other feelings through sexual acts in various contexts; but without the desire for the physical contact in and for itself, or when it is sought for other reasons, activities in which contact is involved are not predominantly sexual. Furthermore, the desire for physical contact in itself, without the wish to express affection or other feelings through it, is sufficient to render sexual the activity of the agent which fulfills it. Various activities with this goal alone, such as kissing and caressing in certain contexts, qualify as sexual even without the presence of genital symptoms of sexual excitement. The latter are not therefore necessary criteria for sexual activity.

This initial analysis may seem to some either over- or underinclusive. It might seem too broad in leading us to interpret physical contact as sexual desire in activities such as football and other contact sports. In these cases, however, the desire is not for contact with another body per se, it is not directed toward a particular person for that purpose, and it is not the goal of the activity—the goal is winning or exercising or knocking someone down or displaying one's prowess. If the desire is purely for contact with another specific person's body, then to interpret it as sexual does not seem an exaggeration. A slightly more difficult case is that of a baby's desire to be cuddled and our natural response in wanting to cuddle it. In the case of the baby, the desire may be simply for the physical contact, for the pleasure of the caresses. If so, we may characterize this desire, especially in keeping with Freudian theory, as sexual or protosexual. It will differ nevertheless from full-fledged sexual desire in being more amorphous, not directed outward toward another specific person's body. It may also be that what the infant unconsciously desires is not physical contact per se but signs of affection, tenderness, or security, in which case we have further reason for hesitating to characterize its wants as clearly sexual. The intent of our response to the baby is often the showing of affection, not the pure physical contact, so that our definition in terms of action which fulfils sexual desire *on the part of the agent* does not capture such actions, whatever we say of the baby. (If it is intuitive to characterize our response as sexual as well, there is clearly no problem here for my analysis.) The same can be said of signs of affection (or in some cultures polite greeting) among men or women: these certainly need not be homosexual when the intent is only to show friendship, something extrinsic to plain sex although valuable when added to it.

Our definition of sex in terms of the desire for physical contact may appear too narrow in that a person's personality, not merely her or his body, may be sexually attractive to another, and in that looking or conversing in a certain way can be sexual in a given context without bodily contact. Nevertheless, it is not the contents of one's thoughts per se that are sexually appealing, but one's personality as embodied in certain manners of behavior. Furthermore, if a person is sexually attracted by another's personality, he or she will desire not just further conversation, but actual sexual contact. While looking at or conversing with someone can be interpreted as sexual in given contexts it is so when intended as preliminary to, and hence parasitic upon, elemental sexual interest. Voyeurism or viewing a pornographic movie qualifies as a sexual activity, but only as an imaginative substitute for the real thing (otherwise a deviation from the norm as expressed in our definition). The same is true of masturbation as a sexual activity without a partner.

That the initial definition indicates at least an ingredient of sexual desire and activity is too obvious to argue. We all know what sex is, at least in obvious cases, and do not need philosophers to tell us. My preliminary analysis is meant to serve as a contrast to what sex is not, at least, not necessarily. I concentrate upon the physically manifested desire for another's body, and I take as central the immersion in the physical aspect of one's own existence and attention to the physical embodiment of the other. One may derive pleasure in a sex act from expressing certain feelings to one's partner or from awareness of the attitude of one's partner, but sexual desire is essentially desire for physical contact itself: it is a bodily desire for the body of another that dominates our mental life for more or less brief periods. Traditional writings were correct to emphasize the purely physical or animal aspect of sex; they were wrong only in condemning it. This characterization of sex as an intensely pleasurable physical activity and acute physical desire may seem to some to capture only its barest level. But it is worth distinguishing and focusing upon this least common denominator in order to avoid the false views of sexual morality and perversion which emerge from thinking that sex is essentially something else.

II

We may turn then to what sex is not, to the arguments regarding supposed conceptual connections between sex and other activities which it is necessary to conceptually distinguish. The more comprehensible attempt to build an extraneous purpose into the sex act identifies that purpose as reproduction, its primary biological function. While this may be "nature's" purpose, it certainly need not be ours (the analogy

with eating, while sometimes overworked, is pertinent here). While this identification may once have had a rational basis which also grounded the identification of the value and morality of sex with that applicable to reproduction and childrearing, the development of contraception rendered the connection weak. Methods of contraception are by now so familiar and so widely used that it is not necessary to dwell upon the changes wrought by these developments in the concept of sex itself and in a rational sexual ethic dependent upon that concept. In the past, the ever present possibility of children rendered the concepts of sex and sexual morality different from those required at present. There may be good reasons, if the presence and care of both mother and father are beneficial to children, for restricting reproduction to marriage. Insofar as society has a legitimate role in protecting children's interests, it may be justified in giving marriage a legal status, although this question is complicated by the fact (among others) that children born to single mothers deserve no penalties. In any case, the point here is simply that these questions are irrelevant at the present time to those regarding the morality of sex and its potential social regulation. . . .

It is obvious that the desire for sex is not necessarily a desire to reproduce, that the psychological manifestation has become, if it were not always, distinct from its biological roots. There are many parallels, as previously mentioned, with other natural functions. The pleasures of eating and exercising are to a large extent independent of their roles in nourishment or health (as the junk-food industry discovered with a vengeance). Despite the obvious parallel with sex, there is still a tendency for many to think that sex acts which can be reproductive are, if not more moral or less immoral, at least more natural. These categories of morality and "naturalness," or normality, are not to be identified with each other, as will be argued below, and neither is applicable to sex by virtue of its connection to reproduction. The tendency to identify reproduction as the conceptually connected end of sex is most prevalent now in the pronouncements of the Catholic church. There the assumed analysis is clearly tied to a restrictive sexual morality according to which acts become immoral and unnatural when they are not oriented towards reproduction, a morality which has independent roots in the Christian sexual ethic as it derives from Paul. However, the means-end analysis fails to generate a consistent sexual ethic: homosexual and oral-genital sex is condemned while kissing or caressing, acts equally unlikely to lead in themselves to fertilization, even when properly characterized as sexual according to our definition, are not.

III

Before discussing further relations of means-end analyses to false or inconsistent sexual ethics and concepts of perversion, I turn to other examples of these analyses. One common position views sex as essentially an expression of love or affection between the partners. It is generally recognized that there are other types of love besides sexual, but sex itself is taken as an expression of one type, sometimes termed "romantic" love.[1] Various factors again ought to weaken this identification. First, there are other types of love besides that which it is appropriate to express sexually, and "romantic" love itself can be expressed in many other ways. I am not denying that sex can take on heightened value and meaning when it becomes a vehicle for the expression of feelings of love or tenderness, but so can many other usually mundane activities such as getting up early to make breakfast on Sunday, cleaning the house, and so on. Second, sex itself can be used to communicate many other emotions besides love, and, as I will argue below, can communicate nothing in particular and still be good sex.

On a deeper level, an internal tension is bound to result from an identification of sex, which I have described as a physical-psychological desire, with love as a long-term, deep emotional relationship between two individuals. As this type of relationship, love is permanent, at least in intent, and more or less exclusive. A normal person cannot deeply love more than a few individuals even in a lifetime. We may be suspicious that those who attempt or claim to love many love them weakly if at all. Yet, fleeting sexual desire can arise in relation to a variety of other individuals one finds sexually attractive. It may even be, as some

have claimed, that sexual desire in humans naturally seeks variety, while this is obviously false of love. For this reason, monogamous sex, even if justified, almost always represents a sacrifice or the exercise of self-control on the part of the spouses, while monogamous love generally does not. There is no such thing as casual love in the sense in which I intend the term "love." It may occasionally happen that a spouse falls deeply in love with someone else (especially when sex is conceived in terms of love), but this is relatively rare in comparison to passing sexual desires for others; and while the former often indicates a weakness or fault in the marriage relation, the latter does not.

If love is indeed more exclusive in its objects than is sexual desire, this explains why those who view sex as essentially an expression of love would again tend to hold a repressive or restrictive sexual ethic. As in the case of reproduction, there may be good reasons for reserving the total commitment of deep love to the context of marriage and family—the normal personality may not withstand additional divisions of ultimate commitment and allegiance. There is no question that marriage itself is best sustained by a deep relation of love and affection; and even if love is not naturally monogamous, the benefits of family units to children provide additional reason to avoid serious commitments elsewhere which weaken family ties. It can be argued similarly that monogamous sex strengthens families by restricting and at the same time guaranteeing an outlet for sexual desire in marriage. But there is more force to the argument that recognition of a clear distinction between sex and love in society would help avoid disastrous marriages which result from adolescent confusion of the two when sexual desire is mistaken for permanent love, and would weaken damaging jealousies which arise in marriages in relation to passing sexual desires. The love and affection of a sound marriage certainly differs from the adolescent romantic variety, which is often a mere substitute for sex in the context of a repressive sexual ethic.

In fact, the restrictive sexual ethic tied to the means-end analysis in terms of love again has failed to be consistent. At least, it has not been applied consistently, but forms part of the double standard which has curtailed the freedom of women. It is predictable in light of this history that some women would now advocate using sex as another kind of means, as a political weapon or as a way to increase unjustly denied power and freedom. The inconsistency in the sexual ethic typically attached to the sex-love analysis, according to which it has generally been taken with a grain of salt when applied to men, is simply another example of the impossibility of tailoring a plausible moral theory in this area to a conception of sex which builds in conceptually extraneous factors.

I am not suggesting here that sex ought never to be connected with love or that it is not a more significant and valuable activity when it is. Nor am I denying that individuals need love as much as sex and perhaps emotionally need at least one complete relationship which encompasses both. Just as sex can express love and take on heightened significance when it does, so love is often naturally accompanied by an intermittent desire for sex. But again love is accompanied appropriately by desires for other shared activities as well. What makes the desire for sex seem more intimately connected with love is the intimacy which is seen to be a natural feature of mutual sex acts. Like love, sex is held to lay one bare psychologically as well as physically. Sex is unquestionably intimate, but beyond that the psychological toll often attached may be a function of the restrictive sexual ethic itself, rather than a legitimate apology for it. The intimacy involved in love is psychologically consuming in a generally healthy way, while the psychological tolls of sexual relations, often including embarrassment as a correlate of intimacy, are too often the result of artificial sexual ethics and taboos. The intimacy involved in both love and sex is insufficient in any case in light of previous points to render a means-end analysis in these terms appropriate.

*   *   *

V

I have now criticized various types of analysis sharing or suggesting a common means-end form. I have suggested that analyses of this form relate to attempts to limit moral or natural sex to that which fulfills some purpose or function extraneous to basic sexual desire.

The attempts to brand forms of sex outside the idealized models as immoral or perverted fail to achieve consistency with intuitions that they themselves do not directly question. The reproductive model brands oral-genital sex a deviation, but cannot account for kissing or holding hands; the communication account holds voyeurism to be perverted but cannot accommodate sex acts without much conscious thought or seductive nonphysical foreplay; the sex-love model makes most sexual desire seem degrading or base. The first and last condemn extramarital sex on the sound but irrelevant grounds that reproduction and deep commitment are best confined to family contexts. The romanticization of sex and the confusion of sexual desire with love operate in both directions: sex outside the context of romantic love is repressed; once it is repressed, partners become more difficult to find and sex becomes romanticized further, out of proportion to its real value for the individual.

What all these analyses share in addition to a common form is accordance with and perhaps derivation from the Platonic-Christian moral tradition, according to which the animal or purely physical element of humans is the source of immorality, and plain sex in the sense I defined it is an expression of this element, hence in itself to be condemned. All the analyses examined seem to seek a distance from sexual desire itself in attempting to extend it conceptually beyond the physical. The love and communications analyses seek refinement or intellectualization of the desire; plain physical sex becomes vulgar, and too straightforward sexual encounters without an aura of respectable cerebral communicative content are to be avoided. [Robert] Solomon explicitly argues that sex cannot be a "mere" appetite, his argument being that if it were, subway exhibitionism and other vulgar forms would be pleasing.[2] This fails to recognize that sexual desire can be focused or selective at the same time as being physical. Lower animals are not attracted by every other member of their species, either. Rancid food forced down one's throat is not pleasing, but that certainly fails to show that hunger is not a physical appetite. Sexual desire lets us know that we are physical beings and, indeed, animals; this is why traditional Platonic morality is so thorough in its condemnation. Means-end analyses continue to reflect this tradition, sometimes unwittingly. They show that in conceptualizing sex it is still difficult, despite years of so-called revolution in this area, to free ourselves from the lingering suspicion that plain sex as physical desire is an expression of our "lower selves," that yielding to our animal natures is subhuman or vulgar.

VI

Having criticized these analyses for the sexual ethics and concepts of perversion they imply, it remains to contrast my account along these lines. To the question of what morality might be implied by my analysis, the answer is that there are no moral implications whatever. Any analysis of sex which imputes a moral character to sex acts in themselves is wrong for that reason. There is no morality intrinsic to sex, although general moral rules apply to the treatment of others in sex acts as they apply to all human relations. We can speak of a sexual ethic as we can speak of a business ethic, without implying that business in itself is either moral or immoral or that special rules are required to judge business practice which are not derived from rules that apply elsewhere as well. Sex is not in itself a moral category, although like business it invariably places us into relations with others in which moral rules apply. It gives us opportunity to do what is otherwise recognized as wrong, to harm others, deceive them or manipulate them against their wills. Just as the fact that an act is sexual in itself never renders it wrong or adds to its wrongness if it is wrong on other grounds (sexual acts towards minors are wrong on other grounds, as will be argued below), so no wrong act is to be excused because done from a sexual motive. If a "crime of passion" is to be excused, it would have to be on grounds of temporary insanity rather than sexual context (whether insanity does constitute a legitimate excuse for certain actions is too big a topic to argue here). Sexual motives are among others which may become deranged, and the fact that they are sexual has no bearing in itself on the moral character, whether negative or exculpatory, of the actions deriving from them. Whatever might be true of war, it is certainly not the case that all's fair in love or sex.

Our first conclusion regarding morality and sex is therefore that no conduct otherwise immoral should be excused because it is sexual conduct, and nothing in sex is immoral unless condemned by rules which apply elsewhere as well. The last clause requires further clarification. Sexual conduct can be governed by particular rules relating only to sex itself. But these precepts must be implied by general moral rules when these are applied to specific sexual relations or types of conduct. The same is true of rules of fair business, ethical medicine, or courtesy in driving a car. In the latter case, particular acts on the road may be reprehensible, such as tailgating or passing on the right, which seem to bear no resemblance as actions to any outside the context of highway safety. Nevertheless their immorality derives from the fact that they place others in danger, a circumstance which, when avoidable, is to be condemned in any context. This structures of general and specifically applicable rules describes a reasonable sexual ethic as well. To take an extreme case, rape is always a sexual act and it is always immoral. A rule against rape can therefore be considered an obvious part of sexual morality which has no bearing on nonsexual conduct. But the immorality of rape derives from its being an extreme violation of a person's body, of the right not to be humiliated, and of the general moral prohibition against using other persons against their wills, not from the fact that it is a sexual act.

The application elsewhere of general moral rules to sexual conduct is further complicated by the fact that it will be relative to the particular desires and preferences of one's partner (these may be influenced by and hence in some sense include misguided beliefs about sexual morality itself). This means that there will be fewer specific rules in the area of sexual ethics than in other areas of conduct, such as driving cars, where the relativity of preference is irrelevant to the prohibition of objectively dangerous conduct. More reliance will have to be placed upon the general moral rule, which in this area holds simply that the preferences, desires, and interests of one's partner or potential partner ought to be taken into account. This rule is certainly not specifically formulated to govern sexual relations; it is a form of the central principle of morality itself. But when applied to sex, it prohibits certain actions, such as molestation of children, which cannot be categorized as violations of the rule without at the same time being classified as sexual. I believe this last case is the closest we can come to an action which is wrong *because* it is sexual, but even here its wrongness is better characterized as deriving from the detrimental effects such behavior can have on the future emotional and sexual life of the naive victims, and from the fact that such behavior therefore involves manipulation of innocent persons without regard for their interests. Hence, this case also involves violation of a general moral rule which applies elsewhere as well.

Aside from faulty conceptual analyses of sex and the influence of the Platonic moral tradition, there are two more plausible reasons for thinking that there are moral dimensions intrinsic to sex acts per se. The first is that such acts are normally intensely pleasurable. According to a hedonistic, utilitarian moral theory they therefore should be at least prima facie morally right, rather than morally neutral in themselves. To me this seems incorrect and reflects unfavorably on the ethical theory in question. The pleasure intrinsic to sex acts is a good, but not, it seems to me, a good with much positive moral significance. Certainly I can have no duty to pursue such pleasure myself, and while it may be nice to give pleasure of any form to others, there is no ethical requirement to do so, given my right over my own body. The exception relates to the context of sex acts themselves, when one partner derives pleasure from the other and ought to return the favor. This duty to reciprocate takes us out of the domain of hedonistic utilitarianism, however, and into a Kantian moral framework, the central principles of which call for just such reciprocity in human relations. Since independent moral judgments regarding sexual activities constitute one area in which ethical theories are to be tested, these observations indicate here, as I believe others indicate elsewhere, the fertility of the Kantian, as opposed to the utilitarian, principles in reconstructing reasoned moral consciousness.

It may appear from this alternative Kantian viewpoint that sexual acts must be at least prima facie wrong in themselves. This is because they invariably involve at different stages the manipulation of one's partner for one's own pleasure, which might appear to be prohibited on the formulation of Kant's principle which holds that one ought not to treat another as a means to such private ends. A more realistic rendering of this formulation, however, one which recognizes its intended equivalence to the first universalizability principle, admits no such absolute prohibition. Many human relations, most economic transactions for example, involve using other individuals for personal benefit. These relations are immoral only when they are one-sided, when the benefits are not mutual, or when the transactions are not freely and rationally endorsed by all parties. The same holds true of sexual acts. The central principle governing them is the Kantian demand for reciprocity in sexual relations. In order to comply with the second formulation of the categorical imperative, one must recognize the subjectivity of one's partner (not merely by being aroused by her or his desire, as [Thomas] Nagel describes). Even in an act which by its nature "objectifies" the other, one recognizes a partner as a subject with demands and desires by yielding to those desires, by allowing oneself to be a sexual object as well, by giving pleasure or ensuring that the pleasures of the acts are mutual. It is this kind of reciprocity which forms the basis for morality in sex, which distinguished right acts from wrong in this area as in others. (Of course, prior to sex acts one must gauge their effects upon potential partners and take these longer range interests into account.)

VII

I suggested earlier that in addition to generating confusion regarding the rightness or wrongness of sex acts, false conceptual analyses of the means-end form cause confusion about the value of sex to the individual. My account recognizes the satisfaction of desire and the pleasure this brings as the central psychological function of the sex act for the individual. Sex affords us a paradigm of pleasure, but not a cornerstone of value. For most of us it is not only a needed outlet for desire but also the most enjoyable form of recreation we know. Its value is nevertheless easily mistaken by being confused with that of love, when it is taken as essentially an expression of that emotion. Although intense, the pleasures of sex are brief and repetitive rather than cumulative. They give value to the specific acts which generate them, but not the lasting kind of value which enhances one's whole life. The briefness of these pleasures contributes to their intensity (or perhaps their intensity makes them necessarily brief), but it also relegates them to the periphery of most rational plans for the good life.

By contrast, love typically develops over a long term relation; while its pleasures may be less intense and physical, they are of more cumulative value. The importance of love to the individual may well be central in a rational system of value. And it has perhaps an even deeper moral significance relating to the identification with the interests of another person, which broadens one's possible relationships with others as well. Marriage is again important in preserving this relation between adults and children, which seems as important to the adults as it is to the children in broadening concerns which have a tendency to become selfish. Sexual desire, by contrast, is desire for another which is nevertheless essentially self-regarding. Sexual pleasure is certainly a good for the individual, and for many it may be necessary in order for them to function in a reasonably cheerful way. But it bears little relation to those other values just discussed, to which some analyses falsely suggest a conceptual connection.

VIII

While my initial analysis lacks moral implications in itself, as it should, it does suggest by contrast a concept of sexual perversion. Since the concept of perversion is itself a sexual concept, it will always be defined relative to some definition of normal sex; and any conception of the norm will imply a contrary notion of perverse forms. The concept suggested by my account again differs sharply from those implied by the means-end analyses examined above. Perversion does not represent a deviation from the reproductive function (or kissing would be perverted), from a loving relationship (or most sexual desire and many heterosexual acts would be perverted), or from efficiency in communicating (or unsuccessful seduction attempts would be perverted). It is a deviation from a norm, but the norm in question is merely statistical. Of course,

not all sexual acts that are statistically unusual are perverted—a three-hour continuous sexual act would be unusual but not necessarily abnormal in the requisite sense. The abnormality in question must relate to the *form of the desire* itself in order to constitute sexual perversion; for example, desire, not for contact with another, but for merely looking, for harming or being harmed, for contact with items of clothing. This concept of sexual abnormality is that suggested by my definition of normal sex in terms of its typical desire. However not all unusual desires qualify either, only those with the typical physical sexual effects upon the individual who satisfies them. These effects, such as erection in males, were not built into the original definition of sex in terms of sexual desire, for they do not always occur in activities that are properly characterized as sexual, say, kissing for the pleasure of it. But they do seem to bear a closer relation to the definition of activities as perverted. (For those who consider only genital sex sexual, we could build such symptoms into a narrower definition, then speaking of sex in a broad sense as well as "proper" sex.)

Solomon and Nagel disagree with this statistical notion of perversion. For them the concept is evaluative rather than statistical. I do not deny that the term "perverted" is often used evaluatively (and purely emotively for that matter), or that it has a negative connotation for the average speaker. I do deny that we can find a norm, other than that of statistically usual desire, against which all and only activities that properly count as sexual perversions can be contrasted. Perverted sex is simply abnormal sex, and if the norm is not to be an idealized or romanticized extraneous end or purpose, it must express the way human sexual desires usually manifest themselves. Of course not all norms in other areas of discourse need be statistical in this way. Physical health is an example of a relatively clear norm which does not seem to depend upon the numbers of healthy people. But the concept in this case achieves its clarity through the connection of physical health with other clearly desirable physical functions and characteristics, for example, living longer. In the case of sex, that which is statistically abnormal is not necessarily incapacitating in other ways, and yet these abnormal desires with

sexual effects upon their subject do count as perverted to the degree to which their objects deviate
from usual ones. The connotations of the concept of
perversion beyond those connected with abnormality or statistical deviation derive more from the attitudes of those likely to call certain acts perverted than
from specifiable features of the acts themselves. These
connotations add to the concept of abnormality that
of *sub*normality, but there is no norm against which
the latter can be measured intelligibly in accord with
all and only acts intuitively called perverted.

The only proper evaluative norms relating to sex
involve degrees of pleasure in the acts and moral
norms, but neither of these scales coincides with statistical degrees of abnormality, according to which
perversion is to be measured. The three parameters
operate independently (this was implied for the first
two when it was held above that the pleasure of sex is
a good, but not necessarily moral good). Perverted sex
may be more or less enjoyable to particular individuals than normal sex, and more or less moral, depending upon the particular relations involved. Raping a
sheep may be more perverted than raping a woman,
but certainly not more condemnable morally.[3] It is
nevertheless true that the evaluative connotations
attaching to the term "perverted" derive partly from
the fact that most people consider perverted sex highly
immoral. Many such acts are forbidden by long standing taboos, and it is sometimes difficult to distinguish
what is forbidden from what is immoral. Others, such
as sadistic acts, are genuinely immoral, but again not
at all because of their connection with sex or abnormality. The principles which condemn these acts
would condemn them equally if they were common
and nonsexual. It is not true that we properly could
continue to consider acts perverted which were found
to be very common practice across societies. Such acts,
if harmful, might continue to be condemned properly
as immoral, but it was just shown that the immorality
of an act does not vary with its degree of perversion.
If not harmful, common acts previously considered
abnormal might continue to be called perverted for a
time by the moralistic minority; but the term when
applied to such cases would retain only its emotive
negative connotation without consistent logical

criteria for application. It would represent merely
prejudiced moral judgments.

To adequately explain why there is a tendency
to so deeply condemn perverted acts would require a
treatise in psychology beyond the scope of this paper.
Part of the reason undoubtedly relates to the tradition of repressive sexual ethics and false conceptions
of sex; another part to the fact that all abnormality
seems to disturb and fascinate us at the same time. The
former explains why sexual perversion is more abhorrent to many than other forms of abnormality; the
latter indicates why we tend to have an emotive and
evaluative reaction to perversion in the first place. It
may be, as has been suggested according to a Freudian
line,[4] that our uneasiness derives from latent desires
we are loathe to admit, but this thesis takes us into
psychological issues I am not competent to judge.
Whatever the psychological explanation, it suffices
to point out here that the conceptual connection
between perversion and genuine or consistent moral
evaluation is spurious and again suggested by misleading means-end idealizations of the concept of sex.

The position I have taken in this paper against
those concepts is not totally new. Something similar
to it is found in Freud's view of sex, which of course
was genuinely revolutionary, and in the body of writings deriving from Freud to the present time. But in
his revolt against romanticized and repressive conceptions, Freud went too far—from a refusal to view sex as
merely a means to a view of it as the end of all human
behavior, although sometimes an elaborately disguised
end. This pansexualism led to the thesis (among others) that repression was indeed an inevitable and necessary part of social regulation of any form, a strange
consequence of a position that began by opposing
the repressive aspects of the means-end view. Perhaps
the time finally has arrived when we can achieve a
reasonable middle ground in this area, at least in philosophy if not in society.

NOTES

1. Even Bertrand Russell, whose writing in this area was a
model of rationality, at least for its period, tends to make this
identification and to condemn plain sex in the absence of

love: "sex intercourse apart from love has little value, and is to be regarded primarily as experimentation with a view to love." *Marriage and Morals* (New York: Bantam, 1959), p. 87.

2. [Robert] Solomon, "Sex and Perversion," *Philosophy and Sex,* ed. R. Baker and F. Elliston (Buffalo: Prometheus, 1975), p. 285.

3. The example is like one from Sara Ruddick, "Better Sex," *Philosophy and Sex,* p. 96.

4. See Michael Slote, "Inapplicable Concepts and Sexual Perversion," *Philosophy and Sex.*

Sexual Morality

ROGER SCRUTON

* * *

We must now attempt to apply the Aristotelian strategy to the subject-matter of this book, and ask whether there is such a thing as sexual virtue, and, if so, what is it, and how is it acquired? Clearly, sexual desire, which is an interpersonal attitude with the most far-reaching consequences for those who are joined by it, cannot be morally neutral. On the contrary, it is in the experience of sexual desire that we are most vividly conscious of the distinction between virtuous and vicious impulses, and most vividly aware that, in the choice between them, our happiness is at stake.

The Aristotelian strategy enjoins us to ignore the actual conditions of any particular person's life, and to look only at the permanent features of human nature. We know that people feel sexual desire; that they feel erotic love, which may grow from desire; that they may avoid both these feelings, by dissipation or self-restraint. Is there anything to be said about desire, other than that it falls within the general scope of the virtue of temperance, which enjoins us to desire only what reason approves?

The first, and most important, observation to be made is that the capacity for love in general, and for erotic love in particular, is a virtue. In Chapter 8 I tried to show that erotic love involves an element of mutual self-enhancement; it generates a sense of the irre-

Roger Scruton, excerpts from *Sexual Desire: A Moral Philosophy of the Erotic.* Copyright © 1986 by Roger Scruton. Reprinted by permission of Continuum, an imprint of Bloomsbury Publishing Plc and with the permission of Free Press, a Division of Simon & Schuster, Inc.

placeable value, both of the other and of the self, and of the activities which bind them. To receive and to give this love is to achieve something of incomparable value in the process of self-fulfilment. It is to gain the most powerful of all interpersonal *guarantees*; in erotic love the subject becomes conscious of the full reality of his personal existence, not only in his own eyes, but in the eyes of another. Everything that he is and values gains sustenance from his love, and every project receives a meaning beyond the moment. All that exists for us as mere hope and hypothesis—the attachment to life and to the body—achieves under the rule of *erōs* the aspect of a radiant certainty. Unlike the cold glances of approval, admiration and pride, the glance of love sees value precisely in that which is the course of anxiety and doubt: in the merely contingent, merely 'empirical', existence of the flesh, the existence which we did not choose, but to which we are condemned. It is the answer to man's fallen condition—to his *Geworfenheit.*

To receive erotic love, however, a person must be able to give it: or if he cannot, the love of others will be a torment to him, seeking from him that which he cannot provide, and directing against him the fury of a disappointed right. It is therefore unquestionable that we have reason to acquire the capacity for erotic love, and, if this means bending our sexual impulses in a certain direction, that will be the direction of sexual virtue. Indeed, the argument of the last two chapters has implied that the development of the sexual impulse towards love may be impeded: there are sexual habits which are vicious, precisely in neutralising the capacity for love. The first thing that can be said, therefore, is that we all have reason to avoid those habits and to educate our children not to possess them.

Here it may be objected that not every love is happy, that there are many—Anna Karenina, for example, or Phaedra—whose capacity for love was the cause of their downfall. But we must remind ourselves of the Aristotelian strategy. In establishing that courage or wisdom is a virtue, the Aristotelian does not argue that the possession of these virtues is in every particular circumstance bound to be advantageous. A parable of Derek Parfit's, adapted from T. C. Schelling, adequately shows what is a stake: Suppose a man breaks into my house and commands me to open the safe for him, saying that, if I do not comply, he will begin to shoot my children. He has heard me telephone the police, and knows that, if he leaves any of us alive, we will be able to give information sufficient to arrest him if he takes what the safe contains. Clearly it is irrational in these circumstances to open the safe—since that will not protect any of us—and also not to open it, since that would cause the robber to kill my children one by one in order to persuade me of his sincerity. Suppose, however, I possess a drug that causes me to become completely irrational. I swallow the pill, and cry out: 'I love my children, therefore kill them'; the man tortures me and I beg him to continue; and so on. In these changed circumstances, my assailant is powerless to obtain what he wants and can only flee before the police arrive. In other words, in such a case, it is actually in the interests of the subject to be irrational: he has overwhelming circumstantial *reason* to be irrational, just as Anna Karenina had an overwhelming circumstantial *reason* to be without the capacity for love. Clearly, however, it would be absurd, on these grounds, to inculcate a habit of irrationality in our children; indeed no *reason* could be given, in the absence of detailed knowledge of a person's future, for acquiring such a habit. In so far as reasons can be given now, for the cultivation of this or that state of character, they must justify the cultivation of rationality before all else—for how can I flourish according to my nature as a rational agent if I am not at least rational?

In like manner, it is not the particular personal tragedy but the generality of the human condition that determines the basis of sexual morality. Tragedy and loss are the rare but necessary outcomes of a process which we all have reason to undergo. (Indeed, it is part of the point of tragedy that it divorces in our imagination the right and the good from the merely prudential: that it sets the value of life against the value of mere survival.) We wish to know, in advance of any particular experience, which dispositions a person must have if he is successfully to express himself in sexual desire and to be fulfilled in his sexual endeavours. Love is the fulfilment of desire, and therefore love is its *telos*. A life of celibacy may also be fulfilled; but, assuming the general truth that most of us have a powerful, and perhaps overwhelming, urge to make love, it is in our interests to ensure that love—and not some other thing—is made.

Love, I have argued, is prone to jealousy, and the object of jealousy is defined by the thought of the beloved's desire. Because jealousy is one of the greatest of psychical catastrophes, involving the possible ruin of both partners, a morality based in the need for erotic love must forestall and eliminate jealousy. It is in the deepest human interest, therefore, that we form the habit of fidelity. This habit is natural and normal; but it is also easily broken, and the temptation to break it is contained in desire itself—in the element of generality which tempts us always to experiment, to verify, to detach ourselves from that which is too familiar in the interest of excitement and risk. Virtuous desire is faithful; but virtuous desire is also an artefact, made possible by a process of moral education which we do not, in truth, understand in its complexity.

If that observation is correct, a whole section of traditional sexual morality must be upheld. The fulfilment of sexual desire defines the nature of desire: *to telos phuseis estin*. And the nature of desire gives us our standard of normality. There are enormous varieties of human sexual conduct, and of 'common-sense' morality: some societies permit or encourage polygamy, others look with indifference upon pre-marital intercourse, or regard marriage itself as no more than an episode in a relation that pre-exists and perhaps survives it. But no society, and no 'common-sense' morality—not even, it seems, the morality of Samoa—looks with favour upon promiscuity or infidelity, unless influenced by a doctrine of 'emancipation' or 'liberation' which is dependent for its sense upon the very conventions which it defies. Whatever the institutional forms of human sexual union, and whatever the range of permitted partners, sexual desire is itself inherently 'nuptial': it involves concentration upon the embodied existence of the other, leading through tenderness to the 'vow' of erotic love. It is a telling observation that the civilisation which has most tolerated the institution of polygamy—the Islamic—has also, in its erotic literature, produced what are perhaps the intensest and most poignant celebrations of monogamous love, precisely through the attempt to capture, not the institution of marriage, but the human datum of desire.

The nuptiality of desire suggests, in its turn, a natural history of desire: a principle of development which defines the 'normal course' of sexual education. 'Sexual maturity' involves incorporating the sexual impulse into the personality, and so making sexual desire into an expression of the subject himself, even though it is, in the heat of action, a force which also overcomes him. If the Aristotelian approach to these things is as plausible as I think it is, the virtuous habit will also have the character of a 'mean': it will involve the disposition to desire what is desirable, despite the competing impulses of animal lust (in which the intentionality of desire may be demolished) and timorous frigidity (in which the sexual impulse is impeded altogether). Education is directed towards the special kind of temperance which shows itself, sometimes as chastity, sometimes as fidelity, sometimes as passionate desire, according to the 'right judgement' of the subject. In wanting what is judged to be desirable, the virtuous person wants what may also be loved, and what may therefore be obtained without hurt or humiliation.

Virtue is a matter of degree, rarely attained in its completion, but always admired. Because traditional sexual education has pursued sexual virtue, it is worthwhile summarising its most important features, in order to see the power of the idea that underlies and justifies it.

The most important feature of traditional sexual education is summarised in anthropological language as the 'ethic of pollution and taboo'. The child was taught to regard his body as sacred, and as subject to pollution by misperception or misuse. The sense of pollution is by no means a trivial side-effect of the 'bad sexual encounter': it may involve a penetrating disgust, at oneself, one's body and one's situation, such as is experienced by the victim of rape. Those sentiments—which arise from our 'fear of the obscene'—express the tension contained within the experience of embodiment. At any moment we can become 'mere body', the self driven from its incarnation, and its habitation ransacked. The most important root idea of personal morality is that I am *in* my body, not (to borrow Descartes' image) as a pilot in a ship, but as an incarnate self. My body is identical with me, and sexual purity is the precious guarantee of this.

Sexual purity does not forbid desire: it simply ensures the status of desire as an interpersonal feeling. The child who learns 'dirty habits' detaches his sex from himself, sets it outside himself as something curious and alien. His fascinated enslavement to the body is also a withering of desire, a scattering of erotic energy and a loss of union with the other. Sexual purity sustains the *subject* of desire, making him present as a self in the very act which overcomes him.

The extraordinary spiritual significance accorded to sexual 'purity' has, of course, its sociobiological and its psychoanalytical explanations. But what, exactly, is its *meaning*, and have people been right to value it? In Wagner's *Parsifal*, the 'pure fool' is uniquely credited with the power to heal the terrible wound which is the physical sign of Amfortas's sexual 'pollution'. He alone can redeem Kundry, the 'fallen' woman, whose sexual licence is so resistant to her penitent personality, that it must be confined to another world, of which she retains only a dim and horrified consciousness. That other world is a world of pleasure and opportunity, a world of the 'permitted'. It is governed, however, by the impure eunuch Klingsor, whose rule is a kind of slavery. Wagner finds the meaning of Christian redemption in the fool's chastity, which leads him to renounce the rewards of an impure desire for the sake of another's salvation. Parsifal releases Amfortas from the hold of 'magic', from the 'charm' which tempts Szymanowski's King Roger towards a vain apotheosis. Parsifal is the harbinger of peace and freedom, in a world that has been enslaved by the magic of desire.

The haunting symbols of this opera owe their power to feelings that are too deep to be lightly dismissed as aesthetic artefacts. But what is their meaning for people who live unsheltered by religion? The answer is to be found, not in religious, but in sexual, feeling. The purely human redemption which is offered to us in love is dependent, in the last analysis, upon public recognition of the value of chastity, and of the sacrilege involved in a sexual impulse that wanders free from the controlling impulse of respect. The 'pollution' of the prostitute is not that she gives herself for money, but that she gives herself to those whom she hates or despises. This is the 'wound' of unchastity, which cannot be healed in solitude by the one who suffers it, but only by his acceptance into a social order which confines the sexual impulse to the realm of intimate relations. The chaste person sustains the ideal of sexual innocence, by giving honourable form to chastity as a way of life. Through his example, it becomes not foolish but admirable to ignore the promptings of a desire that brings no intimacy or fulfilment. Chastity is not a private policy, followed by one individual alone for the sake of his peace of mind. It has a wider and more generous significance: it attempts to draw others into complicity, and to sustain a social order that confines the sexual impulse to the personal sphere.

Chastity exists in two forms: as a publicly declared and publicly recognised role or policy (the chastity of the monk, priest or nun); or as a private resolution, a recognition of the morality that lies dormant in desire. Thus Hans Sachs, in *Die Meistersinger*, who has the opportunity to fulfil his desire, chooses rather to renounce it, knowing that it will not be reciprocated. Sachs is loved and admired for the irreproachable aloneness which makes him the property of all. He is the buttress of Nuremberg, whose satisfactions are public satisfactions, precisely because his own seed has not been sown. His melancholy and bookish contemplation of the trivialities of progenerative man are in one sense a sigh from the genetic depth: the species

is alive in this sigh, just as the individual dies in it. In another sense, however, his melancholy is the supreme affirmation of the reality of others' joys: the recognition that desire must be silenced, in order that others may thrive in their desire.

The child was traditionally brought up to achieve sexual fulfilment only *through* chastity, which is the condition which surrounds him on his first entering the adult world—the world of commitments and obligations. At the same time, he was encouraged to ponder certain 'ideal objects' of desire. These, presented to him under the aspect of an idealised physical beauty, were never *merely* beautiful, but also endowed with the moral attributes that fitted them for love. This dual inculcation of 'pure' habits and 'ideal' love might seem, on the face of it, to be unworthy of the name of education. Is it not, rather, like the mere *training* of a horse or a dog, which arbitrarily forbids some things and fosters others, without offering the first hint of a reason why? And is it not the distinguishing mark of education that it engages with the rational nature of its recipient, and does not merely mould him indifferently to his own understanding of the process? Why, in short, is this moral education, rather than a transference into the sexual sphere—as Freud would have it—of those same processes of interdiction that train us to defecate, not in our nappies, but in a porcelain pot?

The answer is clear. The cult of innocence is an attempt to generate rational conduct, by incorporating the sexual impulse into the self-activity of the subject. It is an attempt to impede the impulse, until such a time as it may attach itself to the interpersonal project that leads to its fulfilment: the project of union with another person, who is wanted not merely for his body, but for the person who *is* this body. Innocence is the disposition to avoid sexual encounter, except with the person whom one may fully desire. Children who have lost their innocence have acquired the habit of gratification through the body alone, in a state of partial or truncated desire. Their gratification is detached from the conditions of personal fulfilment and wanders from object to object with no settled tendency to attach itself to any, pursued all the while by a sense of the body's obscene dominion. 'Debauching of the innocent' was traditionally regarded as a most serious offence, and one that offered genuine *harm* to the victim. The harm in question was not physical, but moral: the undermining of the process which prepares the child to enter the world of *erōs*. (Thus Nabokov's Lolita, who passes with such rapidity from childish provocativeness to a knowing interest in the sexual act, finds, in the end, a marriage devoid of passion, and dies without knowledge of desire.)

The personal and the sexual can become divorced in many ways. The task of sexual morality is to unite them, to sustain thereby the intentionality of desire, and to prepare the individual for erotic love. Sexual morality is the morality of embodiment: the posture which strives to unite us with our bodies, precisely in those situations when our bodies are foremost in our thoughts. Without such a morality the human world is subject to a dangerous divide, a gulf between self and body, at the verge of which all our attempts at personal union falter and withdraw. Hence the prime focus of sexual morality is not the attitude to others, but the attitude to one's own body and its uses. Its aim is to safeguard the integrity of our embodiment. Only on that condition, it is thought, can we inculcate either innocence in the young or fidelity in the adult. Such habits are, however, only one part of sexual virtue. Traditional morality has combined its praise of them with a condemnation of other things—in particular of the habits of lust and perversion. And it is not hard to find the reason for these condemnations.

Perversion consists precisely in a diverting of the sexual impulse from its interpersonal goal, or towards some act that is intrinsically destructive of personal relations and of the values that we find in them. The 'dissolution' of the flesh, which the Marquis de Sade regarded as so important an element in the sexual aim, is in fact that dissolution of the soul; the perversions described by de Sade are not so much attempts to destroy the flesh of the victim as to rid his flesh of its personal meaning, to wring out, with the blood, the rival perspective. That is true in one way or another of all perversion, which can be simply described as the habit of finding a sexual release that avoids or abolishes the *other*, obliterating his embodiment with the obscene perception of his body. Perversion

is narcissistic, often solipsistic, involving strategies of replacement which are intrinsically destructive of personal feeling. Perversion therefore prepares us for a life without personal fulfilment, in which no human relation achieves foundation in the acceptance of the other, as this acceptance is provided by desire.

Lust may be defined as a genuine sexual desire, from which the goal of erotic love has been excluded, and in which whatever tends towards their goal—tenderness, intimacy, fidelity, dependence—is curtailed or obstructed. There need be nothing perverted in this. Indeed the special case of lust which I have discussed under the title of Don Juanism, in which the project of intimacy is constantly abbreviated by the flight towards another sexual object, provides one of our paradigms of desire. Nevertheless, the traditional condemnation of lust is far from arbitrary, and the associated contrast between lust and love far from a matter of convention. Lust is also a habit, involving the disposition to give way to desire, without regard to any personal relation with the object. (Thus perversions are all forms of lust even though lust is not in itself a perversion.) Naturally, we all feel the promptings of lust, but the rapidity with which sexual acts become sexual habits, and the catastrophic effect of a sexual act which cannot be remembered without shame or humiliation, give us strong reasons to resist them, reasons that Shakespeare captured in these words:

> Th'expence of Spirit in a waste of shame
> Is lust in action, and till action, lust
> Is perjur'd, murdrous, blouddy, full of blame,
> Savage, extreame, rude, cruell, not to trust,
> Injoyd no sooner but dispised straight,
> Past reason hunted, and no sooner had,
> Past reason hated as a swollowed bayt,
> On purpose layd to make the taker mad:
> Mad in pursuit and in possession so,
> Had, having, and in quest to have, extreame,
> A blisse in proofe, and prov'd, a very woe,
> Before a joy proposd, behind, a dreame,
>   All this the world well knowes, yet none knowes well
>   To shun the heaven that leads men to this hell.

In addition to the condemnation of lust and perversion, however, some part of traditional sexual education can be seen as a kind of sustained war against fantasy. It is undeniable that fantasy can play an important part in all our sexual doings, and even the most passionate and faithful lover may, in the act of love, rehearse to himself other scenes of sexual abandon than the one in which he is engaged. Nevertheless, there is truth in the contrast (familiar, in one version, from the writings of Freud) between fantasy and reality, and in the sense that the first is in some way destructive of the second. Fantasy replaces the real, resistant, objective world with a pliant substitute—and that, indeed, is its purpose. Life in the actual world is difficult and embarrassing. Most of all it is difficult and embarrassing in our confrontation with other people, who, by their very existence, make demands that we may be unable or unwilling to meet. It requires a great force, such as the force of sexual desire, to overcome the embarrassment and self-protection that shield us from the most intimate encounters. It is tempting to take refuge in substitutes, which neither embarrass us nor resist the impulse of our spontaneous cravings. The habit grows, in masturbation, of creating a compliant world of desire, in which unreal objects become the focus of real emotions, and the emotions themselves are rendered incompetent to participate in the building of personal relations. The fantasy blocks the passage to reality, which becomes inaccessible to the will.

Even if the fantasy can be overcome so far as to engage in the act of love with another, a peculiar danger remains. The other becomes veiled in substitutes; he is never fully himself in the act of love; it is never clearly *him* that I desire, or *him* that I possess, but always rather a composite object, a universal body, of which he is but one among a potential infinity of instances. Fantasy fills our thoughts with a sense of the obscene, and the orgasm becomes, not the possession of another, but the expenditure of energy on his depersonalised body. Fantasies are private property, which I can dispose according to my will, with no answerability to the other whom I abuse through them. He, indeed, is of no intrinsic interest to me, and serves merely as my opportunity for self-regarding

pleasure. For the fantasist, the ideal partner is indeed the prostitute, who, because she can be purchased, solves at once the moral problem presented by the presence of another at the scene of sexual release.

The connection between fantasy and prostitution is deep and important. The effect of fantasy is to 'commodify' the object of desire, and to replace the law of sexual relationship between people with the law of the market. Sex itself can then be seen as a commodity: something that we pursue and obtain in quantifiable form, and which comes in a variety of packages: in the form of a woman or a man; in the form of a film or a dream; in the form of a fetish or an animal. In so far as the sexual act is seen in this way, it seems morally neutral—or, at best, impersonal. Such criticism as may be offered will concern merely the dangers for the individual and his partner of this or that sexual package: for some bring diseases and discomforts of which others are free. The most harmless and hygienic act of all, on this view, is the act of masturbation, stimulated by whatever works of pornography are necessary to prompt the desire for it in the unimaginative. This justification for pornography has, indeed, recently been offered.

As I have already argued, however, fantasy does not exist comfortably with reality. It has a natural tendency to realise itself: to remake the world in its own image. The harmless wanker with the video-machine can at any moment turn into the desperate rapist with a gun. The 'reality principle' by which the normal sexual act is regulated is a principle of personal encounter, which enjoins us to respect the other person, and to respect, also, the sanctity of his body, as the tangible expression of another self. The world of fantasy obeys no such rule, and is governed by monstrous myths and illusions which are at war with the human world—the illusions, for example, that women wish to be raped, that children have only to be awakened in order to give and receive the intensest sexual pleasure, that violence is not an affront but an affirmation of a natural right. All such myths, nurtured in fantasy, threaten not merely the consciousness of the man who lives by them, but also the moral structure of his surrounding world. They render the world unsafe for self and other, and cause the subject to look on everyone, not as an end in himself, but as a possible means to his private pleasure. In his world, the sexual encounter has been 'fetishised', to use the apt Marxian term, and every other human reality has been poisoned by the sense of the expendability and replaceability of the other.

It is a small step from the preoccupation with sexual virtue, to a condemnation of obscenity and pornography (which is its published form). Obscenity is a direct assault on the sentiment of desire, and therefore on the social order that is based on desire and which has personal love as its goal and fulfilment. There is no doubt that the normal conscience cannot remain neutral towards obscenity, any more than it can remain neutral towards paedophilia and rape (which is not to say that obscenity must also be treated as a *crime*). It is therefore unsurprising that traditional moral education has involved censorship of obscene material, and a severe emphasis on 'purity in thought, word and deed'—an emphasis which is now greeted with irony or ridicule.

Traditional sexual education was, despite its exaggerations and imbecilities, truer to human nature than the libertarian culture which has succeeded it. Through considering its wisdom and its shortcomings, we may understand how to resuscitate an idea of sexual virtue, in accordance with the broad requirements of the Aristotelian argument that I have, in this chapter, been presenting. The ideal of virtue remains one of 'sexual integrity'; of a sexuality that is entirely integrated into the life of personal affection, and in which the self and its responsibility are centrally involved and indissolubly linked to the pleasures and passions of the body.

Traditional sexual morality has therefore been the morality of the body. Libertarian morality, by contrast, has relied almost entirely on a Kantian view of the human subject, as related to his body by no coherent moral tie. Focussing as he does on an idea of purely personal respect, and assigning no distinctive place to the body in our moral endeavour, the Kantian inevitably tends towards permissive morality. No sexual act can be wrong merely by virtue of its physical character, and the ideas of obscenity, pollution and perversion

have no obvious application. His attitude to homosexuality is conveniently summarised in this passage from a Quaker pamphlet:

> We see no reason why the physical nature of the sexual act should be the criterion by which the question whether it is moral should be decided. An act which (for example) expresses true affection between two individuals and gives pleasure to them both, does not seem to us to be sinful by reason *alone* of the fact that it is homosexual. The same criteria seem to apply whether a relationship is heterosexual or homosexual.

Such sentiments are the standard offering of the liberal and utilitarian moralities of our time. However much we may sympathise with their conclusions, it is not possible to accept the shallow reasoning that leads up to them, and which bypasses the great metaphysical conundrum to which all sexual morality is addressed: the conundrum of embodiment. [D. H.] Lawrence asserts that 'sex is *you*', and offers some bad but revealing lines on the subject:

> And don't, with the nasty, prying mind, drag it
>   out from its deeps
> And finger it and force it, and shatter the rhythm
>   it keeps
> When it is left alone, as it stirs and rouses and
>   sleeps.

If anything justifies Lawrence's condemnation of the 'nasty, prying mind', it is the opposite of what he supposes. Sex 'sleeps' in the soul precisely because, and to the extent that, it is buried there by education. If sex is you, it is because you are the product of that education, and not just its victim. It has endowed you with what I have called 'sexual integrity': the ability to be *in* your body, in the very moment of desire.

The reader may be reluctant to follow me in believing that traditional morality is largely justified by the ideal of sexual integrity. But if he accepts the main tenor of my argument, he must surely realise that the ethic of 'liberation', far from promising the release of the self from hostile bondage, in fact heralds the dissipation of the self in loveless fantasy: th'expence of Spirit, in a waste of shame.

Sexual Perversion

THOMAS NAGEL

There is something to be learned about sex from the fact that we possess a concept of sexual perversion. I wish to examine the concept, defending it against the charge of unintelligibility and trying to say exactly what about human sexuality qualifies it to admit of perversions. Let me make some preliminary comments about the problem before embarking on its solution.

Some people do not believe that the notion of sexual perversion makes sense, and even those who do disagree over its application. Nevertheless I think it will be widely conceded that, if the concept is viable at all, it must meet certain general conditions. First, if there are any sexual perversions, they will have to be sexual desires or practices that can be plausibly described as in some sense unnatural, though the explanation of this natural / unnatural distinction is of course the main problem. Second, certain practices will be perversions if anything is, such as shoe fetishism, bestiality, and sadism; other practices, such as unadorned sexual intercourse, will not be; about still others there is controversy. Third, if there are perversions, they will be unnatural sexual *inclinations* rather than merely unnatural practices adopted not from inclination but for other reasons. I realize that this is at variance with the view, maintained by some Roman Catholics, that contraception is a sexual perversion. But although contraception may qualify as a deliberate perversion of the sexual and reproductive functions, it cannot be significantly described as a *sexual* perversion. A sexual perversion must reveal itself in conduct that expresses an unnatural *sexual* preference. And although there might be a form of fetishism focused on the employment of contraceptive devices, that is not the usual explanation for their use.

I wish to declare at the outset my belief that the connection between sex and reproduction has no bearing on sexual perversion. The latter is a concept

of psychological, not physiological interest, and it is a concept that we do not apply to the lower animals, let alone to plants, all of which have reproductive functions that can go astray in various ways. (Think of seedless oranges.) Insofar as we are prepared to regard higher animals as perverted, it is because of their psychological, not their anatomical similarity to humans. Furthermore, we do not regard as a perversion every deviation from the reproductive function of sex in humans: sterility, miscarriage, contraception, abortion.

Another matter that I believe has no bearing on the concept of sexual perversion is social disapprobation or custom. Anyone inclined to think that in each society the perversions are those sexual practices of which the community disapproves, should consider all the societies that have frowned upon adultery and fornication. These have not been regarded as unnatural practices, but have been thought objectionable in other ways. What is regarded as unnatural admittedly varies from culture to culture, but the classification is not a pure expression of disapproval or distaste. In fact it is often regarded as a *ground* for disapproval, and that suggests that the classification has an independent content.

I am going to attempt a psychological account of sexual perversion, which will depend on a specific psychological theory of sexual desire and human sexual interactions. To approach this solution I wish first to consider a contrary position, one which provides a basis for skepticism about the existence of any sexual perversions at all, and perhaps about the very significance of the term. The skeptical argument runs as follows:

"Sexual desire is simply one of the appetites, like hunger and thirst. As such it may have various objects, some more common than others perhaps, but none in any sense 'natural'. An appetite is identified as sexual by means of the organs and erogenous zones in which its satisfaction can be to some extent localized, and the special sensory pleasures which form the core of that satisfaction. This enables us to recognize widely

Thomas Nagel, "Sexual Perversion," *The Journal of Philosophy* LXVI, 1 (January 1969): 5–17. Reprinted with permission of the publisher and the author.

divergent goals, activities, and desires as sexual, since it is conceivable in principle that anything should produce sexual pleasure and that a nondeliberate, sexually charged desire for it should arise (as a result of conditioning, if nothing else). We may fail to empathize with some of these desires, and some of them, like sadism, may be objectionable on extraneous grounds, but once we have observed that they meet the criteria for being sexual, there is nothing more to be said on *that* score. Either they are sexual or they are not: sexuality does not admit of imperfection, or perversion, or any other such qualification—it is not that sort of affection."

This is probably the received radical position. It suggests that the cost of defending a psychological account may be to deny that sexual desire is an appetite. But insofar as that line of defense is plausible, it should make us suspicious of the simple picture of appetites on which the skepticism depends. Perhaps the standard appetites, like hunger, cannot be classed as pure appetites in that sense either, at least in their human versions.

Let us approach the matter by asking whether we can imagine anything that would qualify as a gastronomical perversion. Hunger and eating are importantly like sex in that they serve a biological function and also play a significant role in our inner lives. It is noteworthy that there is little temptation to describe as perverted an appetite for substances that are not nourishing. We should probably not consider someone's appetites as *perverted* if he liked to eat paper, sand, wood, or cotton. Those are merely rather odd and very unhealthy tastes: they lack the psychological complexity that we expect of perversions. (Coprophilia, being already a sexual perversion, may be disregarded.) If on the other hand someone liked to eat cookbooks, or magazines with pictures of food in them, and preferred these to ordinary food—or if when hungry he sought satisfaction by fondling a napkin or ashtray from his favorite restaurant—then the concept of perversion might seem appropriate (in fact it would be natural to describe this as a case of gastronomical fetishism). It would be natural to describe as gastronomically perverted someone who could eat only by having food forced down his throat through a funnel, or only if the meal were a living animal. What helps

in such cases is the peculiarity of the desire itself, rather than the inappropriateness of its object to the biological function that the desire serves. Even an appetite, it would seem, can have perversions if in addition to its biological function it has a significant psychological structure.

In the case of hunger, psychological complexity is provided by the activities that give it expression. Hunger is not merely a disturbing sensation that can be quelled by eating; it is an attitude toward edible portions of the external world, a desire to relate to them in rather special ways. The method of ingestion: chewing, savoring, swallowing, appreciating the texture and smell, all are important components of the relation, as is the passivity and controllability of the food (the only animals we eat live are helpless mollusks). Our relation to food depends also on our size: we do not live upon it or burrow into it like aphids or worms. Some of these features are more central than others, but any adequate phenomenology of eating would have to treat it as a relation to the external world and a way of appropriating bits of that world, with characteristic affection. Displacements or serious restrictions of the desire to eat could then be described as perversions, if they undermined that direct relation between man and food which is the natural expression of hunger. This explains why it is easy to imagine gastronomical fetishism, voyeurism, exhibitionism, or even gastronomical sadism and masochism. Indeed some of these perversions are fairly common.

If we can imagine perversions of an appetite like hunger, it should be possible to make sense of the concept of sexual perversion. I do not wish to imply that sexual desire is an appetite—only that being an appetite is no bar to admitting of perversions. Like hunger, sexual desire has as its characteristic object a certain relation with something in the external world; only in this case it is usually a person rather than an omelet, and the relation is considerably more complicated. This added complication allows scope for correspondingly complicated perversions.

The fact that sexual desire is a feeling about other persons may tempt us to take a pious view of its psychological content. There are those who believe that sexual desire is properly the expression of some other attitude, like love, and that when it occurs by itself it is incomplete and unhealthy—or at any rate subhuman. (The extreme Platonic version of such a view is that sexual practices are all vain attempts to express something they cannot in principle achieve: this makes them all perversions, in a sense.) I do not believe that any such view is correct. Sexual desire is complicated enough without having to be linked to anything else as a condition for phenomenological analysis. It cannot be denied that sex may serve various functions—economic, social, altruistic—but it also has its own content as a relation between persons, and it is only by analyzing that relation that we can understand the conditions of sexual perversion.

I believe it is very important that the object of sexual attraction is a particular individual, who transcends the properties that make him attractive. When different persons are attracted to a single person for different reasons: eyes, hair, figure, laugh, intelligence—we feel that the object of their desire is nevertheless the same, namely that person. There is even an inclination to feel that this is so if the lovers have different sexual aims, if they include both men and women, for example. Different specific attractive characteristics seem to provide enabling conditions for the operation of a single basic feeling, and the different aims all provide expressions of it. We approach the sexual attitude toward the person through the features that we find attractive, but these features are not the objects of that attitude.

This is very different from the case of an omelet. Various people may desire it for different reasons, one for its fluffiness, another for its mushrooms, another for its unique combination of aroma and visual aspect; yet we do not enshrine the transcendental omelet as the true common object of their affections. Instead we might say that several desires have accidentally converged on the same object: any omelet with the crucial characteristics would do as well. It is not similarly true that any person with the same flesh distribution and way of smoking can be substituted as object for a particular sexual desire that has been elicited by those characteristics. It may be that they will arouse attraction whenever they recur, but it will be a new sexual attraction with a new particular object, not merely a

transfer of the old desire to someone else. (I believe this is true even in cases where the new object is unconsciously identified with a former one.)

The importance of this point will emerge when we see how complex a psychological interchange constitutes the natural development of sexual attraction. This would be incomprehensible if its object were not a particular person, but rather a person of a certain *kind*. Attraction is only the beginning, and fulfillment does not consist merely of behavior and contact expressing this attraction, but involves much more.

The best discussion of these matters that I have seen appears in part III of Sartre's *Being and Nothingness*.[1] Since it has influenced my own views, I shall say a few things about it now. Sartre's treatment of sexual desire and of love, hate, sadism, masochism, and further attitudes toward others, depends on a general theory of consciousness and the body which we can neither expound nor assume here. He does not discuss perversion, and this is partly because he regards sexual desire as one form of the perpetual attempt of an embodied consciousness to come to terms with the existence of others, an attempt that is as doomed to fail in this form as it is in any of the others, which include sadism and masochism (if not certain of the more impersonal deviations) as well as several nonsexual attitudes. According to Sartre, all attempts to incorporate the other into my world as another subject, i.e., to apprehend him at once as an object for me and as a subject for whom I am an object, are unstable and doomed to collapse into one or other of the two aspects. Either I reduce him entirely to an object, in which case his subjectivity escapes the possession or appropriation I can extend to that object; or I become merely an object for him, in which case I am no longer in a position to appropriate his subjectivity. Moreover, neither of these aspects is stable; each is continually in danger of giving way to the other. This has the consequence that there can be no such thing as a *successful* sexual relation, since the deep aim of sexual desire cannot in principle be accomplished. It seems likely, therefore, that the view will not permit a basic distinction between successful or complete and unsuccessful or incomplete sex, and therefore cannot admit the concept of perversion.

I do not adopt this aspect of the theory, nor many of its metaphysical underpinnings. What interests me is Sartre's picture of the attempt. He says that the type of possession that is the object of sexual desire is carried out by "a double reciprocal incarnation" and that this is accomplished, typically in the form of a caress, in the following way: "I make myself flesh in order to impel the Other to realize *for-herself* and *for me* her *own* flesh, and my caresses cause my flesh to be born for me in so far as it is for the Other *flesh causing her to be born as flesh*" (391; italics Sartre's). The incarnation in question is described variously as a clogging or troubling of consciousness, which is inundated by the flesh in which it is embodied.

The view I am going to suggest, I hope in less obscure language, is related to this one, but it differs from Sartre's in allowing sexuality to achieve its goal on occasion and thus in providing the concept of perversion with a foothold.

Sexual desire involves a kind of perception, but not merely a single perception of its object, for in the paradigm case of mutual desire there is a complex system of superimposed mutual perceptions—not only perceptions of the sexual object, but perceptions of oneself. Moreover, sexual awareness of another involves considerable self-awareness to begin with—more than is involved in ordinary sensory perception. The experience is felt as an assault on oneself by the view (or touch, or whatever) of the sexual object.

Let us consider a case in which the elements can be separated. For clarity we will restrict ourselves initially to the somewhat artificial case of desire at a distance. Suppose a man and a woman, whom we may call Romeo and Juliet, are at opposite ends of a cocktail lounge, with many mirrors on the walls which permit unobserved observation, and even mutual unobserved observation. Each of them is sipping a martini and studying other people in the mirrors. At some point Romeo notices Juliet. He is moved, somehow, by the softness of her hair and the diffidence with which she sips her martini, and this arouses him sexually. Let us say that *X senses Y* whenever *X* regards *Y* with sexual desire. (*Y* need not be a person, and *X*'s apprehension of *Y* can be visual, tactile, olfactory, etc., or purely imaginary; in the present example we shall concentrate on vision.) So Romeo senses Juliet, rather than merely noticing her. At this stage he is aroused by an unaroused object, so he is more in the sexual grip of his body than she of hers.

Let us suppose, however, that Juliet now senses Romeo in another mirror on the opposite wall, though neither of them yet knows that he is seen by the other (the mirror angles provide three-quarter views). Romeo then begins to notice in Juliet the subtle signs of sexual arousal: heavy-lidded stare, dilating pupils, faint flush, et cetera. This of course renders her much more bodily, and he not only notices but senses this as well. His arousal is nevertheless still solitary. But now, cleverly calculating the line of her stare without actually looking her in the eyes, he realizes that it is directed at him through the mirror on the opposite wall. That is, he notices, and moreover senses, Juliet sensing him. This is definitely a new development, for it gives him a sense of embodiment not only through his own reactions but through the eyes and reactions of another. Moreover, it is separable from the initial sensing of Juliet; for sexual arousal might begin with a person's sensing that he is sensed and being assailed by the perception of the other person's desire rather than merely by the perception of the person.

But there is a further step. Let us suppose that Juliet, who is a little slower than Romeo, now senses that he senses her. This puts Romeo in a position to notice, and be aroused by, her arousal at being sensed by him. He senses that she senses that he senses her. This is still another level of arousal, for he becomes conscious of his sexuality through his awareness of its effect on her and of her awareness that this effect is due to him. Once she takes the same step and senses that he senses her sensing him, it becomes difficult to state, let alone imagine, further iterations, though they may be logically distinct. If both are alone, they will presumably turn to look at each other directly, and the proceedings will continue on another plane. Physical contact and intercourse are perfectly natural extensions of this complicated visual exchange, and mutual touch can involve all the complexities of awareness present in the visual case, but with a far greater range of subtlety and acuteness.

Ordinarily, of course, things happen in a less orderly fashion—sometimes in a great rush—but I believe that some version of this overlapping system of distinct sexual perceptions and interactions is the basic framework of any full-fledged sexual relation and that relations involving only part of the complex are significantly incomplete. The account is only schematic, as it must be to achieve generality. Every real sexual act will be psychologically far more specific and detailed, in ways that depend not only on the physical techniques employed and on anatomical details, but also on countless features of the participants' conceptions of themselves and of each other, which become embodied in the act. (It is a familiar enough fact, for example, that people often take their social roles and the social roles of their partners to bed with them.)

The general schema is important, however, and the proliferation of levels of mutual awareness it involves is an example of a type of complexity that typifies human interactions. Consider aggression, for example. If I am angry with someone, I want to make him feel it, either to produce self-reproach by getting him to see himself through the eyes of my anger, and to dislike what he sees—or else to produce reciprocal anger or fear, by getting him to perceive my anger as a threat or attack. What I want will depend on the details of my anger, but in either case it will involve a desire that the object of that anger be aroused. This accomplishment constitutes the fulfillment of my emotion, through domination of the object's feelings.

Another example of such reflexive mutual recognition is to be found in the phenomenon of meaning, which appears to involve an intention to produce a belief or other effect in another by bringing about his recognition of one's intention to produce that effect. (That result is due to H. P. Grice,[2] whose position I shall not attempt to reproduce in detail.) Sex has a related structure: it involves a desire that one's partner be aroused by the recognition of one's desire that he or she be aroused.

It is not easy to define the basic types of awareness and arousal of which these complexes are composed, and that remains a lacuna in this discussion.

I believe that the object of awareness is the same in one's own case as it is in one's sexual awareness of another, although the two awarenesses will not be the same, the difference being as great as that between feeling angry and experiencing the anger of another. All stages of sexual perception are varieties of identification of a person with his body. What is perceived is one's own or another's *subjection* to or *immersion* in his body, a phenomenon which has been recognized with loathing by St. Paul and St. Augustine, both of whom regarded "the law of sin which is in my members" as a grave threat to the dominion of the holy will.[3] In sexual desire and its expression the blending of involuntary response with deliberate control is extremely important. For Augustine, the revolution launched against him by his body is symbolized by erection and the other involuntary physical components of arousal. Sartre too stresses the fact that the penis is not a prehensile organ. But mere involuntariness characterizes other bodily processes as well. In sexual desire the involuntary responses are combined with submission to spontaneous impulses: not only one's pulse and secretions but one's actions are taken over by the body; ideally, deliberate control is needed only to guide the expression of those impulses. This is to some extent also true of an appetite like hunger, but the takeover there is more localized, less pervasive, less extreme. One's whole body does not become saturated with hunger as it can with desire. But the most characteristic feature of a specifically sexual immersion in the body is its ability to fit into the complex of mutual perceptions that we have described. Hunger leads to spontaneous interactions with food; sexual desire leads to spontaneous interactions with other persons, whose bodies are asserting their sovereignty in the same way, producing involuntary reactions and spontaneous impulses in *them*. These reactions are perceived, and the perception of them is perceived, and that perception is in turn perceived; at each step the domination of the person by his body is reinforced, and the sexual partner becomes more possessible by physical contact, penetration, and envelopment.

Desire is therefore not merely the perception of a preexisting embodiment of the other, but ideally a contribution to his further embodiment which in turn enhances the original subject's sense of himself.

This explains why it is important that the partner be aroused, and not merely aroused, but aroused by the awareness of one's desire. It also explains the sense in which desire has unity and possession as its object: physical possession must eventuate in creation of the sexual object in the image of one's desire, and not merely in the object's recognition of that desire, or in his or her own private arousal. (This may reveal a male bias: I shall say something about that later.)

To return, finally, to the topic of perversion: I believe that various familiar deviations constitute truncated or incomplete versions of the complete configuration, and may therefore be regarded as perversions of the central impulse.

In particular, narcissistic practices and intercourse with animals, infants, and inanimate objects seem to be stuck at some primitive version of the first stage. If the object is not alive, the experience is reduced entirely to an awareness of one's own sexual embodiment. Small children and animals permit awareness of the embodiment of the other, but present obstacles to reciprocity, to the recognition by the sexual object of the subject's desire as the source of his (the object's) sexual self-awareness.

Sadism concentrates on the evocation of passive self-awareness in others, but the sadist's engagement is itself active and requires a retention of deliberate control which impedes awareness of himself as a bodily subject of passion in the required sense. The victim must recognize him as the source of his own sexual passivity, but only as the active source. De Sade claimed that the object of sexual desire was to evoke involuntary responses from one's partner, especially audible ones. The infliction of pain is no doubt the most efficient way to accomplish this, but it requires a certain abrogation of one's own exposed spontaneity. All this, incidentally, helps to explain why it is tempting to regard as sadistic an excessive preoccupation with sexual technique, which does not permit one to abandon the role of agent at any stage of the sexual act. Ideally one should be able to surmount one's technique at some point.

A masochist on the other hand imposes the same disability on his partner as the sadist imposes on himself. The masochist cannot find a satisfactory embodiment as the object of another's sexual desire, but only as the object of his control. He is passive not in relation to his partner's passion but in relation to his non-passive agency. In addition, the subjection to one's body characteristic of pain and physical restraint is of a very different kind from that of sexual excitement: pain causes people to contract rather than dissolve.

Both of these disorders have to do with the second stage, which involves the awareness of oneself as an object of desire. In straightforward sadism and masochism other attentions are substituted for desire as a source of the object's self-awareness. But it is also possible for nothing of that sort to be substituted, as in the case of a masochist who is satisfied with self-inflicted pain or of a sadist who does not insist on playing a role in the suffering that arouses him. Greater difficulties of classification are presented by three other categories of sexual activity: elaborations of the sexual act; intercourse of more than two persons; and homosexuality.

If we apply our model to the various forms that may be taken by two-party heterosexual intercourse, none of them seem clearly to qualify as perversions. Hardly anyone can be found these days to inveigh against oral-genital contact, and the merits of buggery are urged by such respectable figures as D. H. Lawrence and Norman Mailer. There may be something vaguely sadistic about the latter technique (in Mailer's writings it seems to be a method of introducing an element of rape), but it is not obvious that this has to be so. In general, it would appear that any bodily contact between a man and a woman that gives them sexual pleasure is a possible vehicle for the system of multi-level interpersonal awareness that I have claimed is the basic psychological content of sexual interaction. Thus a liberal platitude about sex is upheld.

About multiple combinations, the least that can be said is that they are bound to be complicated. If one considers how difficult it is to carry on two conversations simultaneously, one may appreciate the problems of multiple simultaneous interpersonal perception that can arise in even a small-scale orgy. It may be inevitable that some of the component relations should degenerate into mutual epidermal stimulation by participants otherwise isolated from each other. There may also be a tendency toward voyeurism and exhibitionism, both of which are incomplete relations. The exhibitionist wishes to display his desire without needing to be desired in return; he may even fear the sexual attentions of others. A voyeur, on the other hand, need not require any recognition by his object at all: certainly not a recognition of the voyeur's arousal.

It is not clear whether homosexuality is a perversion if that is measured by the standard of the described configuration, but it seems unlikely. For such a classification would have to depend on the possibility of extracting from the system a distinction between male and female sexuality; and much that has been said so far applies equally to men and women. Moreover, it would have to be maintained that there was a natural tie between the type of sexuality and the sex of the body, and also that two sexualities of the same type could not interact properly.

Certainly there is much support for an aggressive-passive distinction between male and female sexuality. In our culture the male's arousal tends to initiate the perceptual exchange, he usually makes the sexual approach, largely controls the course of the act, and of course penetrates whereas the woman receives. When two men or two women engage in intercourse they cannot both adhere to these sexual roles. The question is how essential the roles are to an adequate sexual relation. One relevant observation is that a good deal of deviation from these roles occurs in heterosexual intercourse. Women can be sexually aggressive and men passive, and temporary reversals of role are not uncommon in heterosexual exchanges of reasonable length. If such conditions are set aside, it may be urged that there is something irreducibly perverted in attraction to a body anatomically like one's own. But alarming as some people in our culture may find such attraction, it remains psychologically unilluminating to class it as perverted. Certainly if homosexuality is a perversion, it is so in a very different sense from that in which shoe-fetishism is a perversion, for some version of the full range of interpersonal perceptions seems perfectly possible between two persons of the same sex.

In any case, even if the proposed model is correct, it remains implausible to describe as perverted every deviation from it. For example, if the partners in heterosexual intercourse indulge in private heterosexual fantasies, that obscures the recognition of the real partner and so, on the theory, constitutes a defective sexual relation. It is not, however, generally regarded as a perversion. Such examples suggest that a simple dichotomy between perverted and unperverted sex is too crude to organize the phenomena adequately.

I should like to close with some remarks about the relation of perversion to good, bad, and morality. The concept of perversion can hardly fail to be evaluative in some sense, for it appears to involve the notion of an ideal or at least adequate sexuality which the perversions in some way fail to achieve. So, if the concept is viable, the judgment that a person or practice or desire is perverted will constitute a sexual evaluation, implying that better sex, or a better specimen of sex, is possible. This in itself is a very weak claim, since the evaluation might be in a dimension that is of little interest to us. (Though, if my account is correct, that will not be true.)

Whether it is a moral evaluation, however, is another question entirely—one whose answer would require more understanding of both morality and perversion than can be deployed here. Moral evaluation of acts and of persons is a rather special and very complicated matter, and by no means all our evaluations of persons and their activities are moral evaluations. We make judgments about people's beauty or health or intelligence which are evaluative without being moral. Assessments of their sexuality may be similar in that respect.

Furthermore, moral issues aside, it is not clear that unperverted sex is necessarily *preferable* to the perversions. It may be that sex which receives the highest marks for perfection *as sex* is less enjoyable than certain perversions; and if enjoyment is considered very important, that might outweigh considerations of sexual perfection in determining rational preference.

That raises the question of the relation between the evaluative content of judgments of perversion and the rather common *general* distinction between good and bad sex. The latter distinction is usually confined to sexual acts, and it would seem, within limits, to cut across the other: even someone who believed, for example, that homosexuality was a perversion could admit a distinction between better and worse homosexual sex, and might even allow that good homosexual sex could be better *sex* than not very good unperverted sex. If this is correct, it supports the position that, if judgments of perversion are viable at all, they represent only one aspect of the possible evaluation of sex, even *qua sex*. Moreover it is not the only important aspect: certainly sexual deficiencies that evidently do not constitute perversions can be the object of great concern.

Finally, even if perverted sex is to that extent not so good as it might be, bad sex is generally better than none at all. This should not be controversial: it seems to hold for other important matters, like food, music, literature, and society. In the end, one must choose from among the available alternatives, whether their availability depends on the environment or on one's own constitution. And the alternatives have to be fairly grim before it becomes rational to opt for nothing.

NOTES

1. Translated by Hazel E. Barnes (New York: Philosophical Library: 1956).

2. "Meaning," *Philosophical Review*, LXVI, 3 (July 1957): 377–388.

3. See Romans, VII, 23; and the *Confessions*, Book 8, v.

Feminists against the First Amendment

WENDY KAMINER

Despite efforts to redevelop it, New York's Forty-second Street retains its underground appeal, especially for consumers of pornography. What city officials call "sex-related uses"—triple-X video (formerly book) stores, peep shows, and topless bars—have declined in number since their heyday in the 1970s, and much of the block between Seventh and Eighth avenues is boarded up, a hostage to development. New sex businesses—yuppie topless bars and downscale lap-dancing joints (don't ask)—are prospering elsewhere in Manhattan. But Peepland (MULTI-VIDEO BOOTHS! NUDE DANCING GIRLS!) still reigns, and Show World, a glitzy sex emporium, still anchors the west end of the block, right around the corner from *The New York Times*.

In the late 1970s I led groups of suburban women on tours through Show World and other Forty-second Street hot spots, exposing them, in the interests of consciousness-raising, to pornography's various genres: Nazi porn, nurse porn, lesbian porn, bondage

porn—none of it terribly imaginative. The women didn't exactly hold hands as they ventured down the street with me, but they did stick close together; traveling en masse, they were not so conspicuous as individuals. With only a little less discomfort than resolve, they dutifully viewed the pornography.

This was in the early days of the feminist anti-porn movement, when legislative strategies against pornography were mere gleams in the eye of the feminist writer Andrea Dworkin, when it seemed possible to raise consciousness about pornography without arousing demands for censorship. That period of innocence did not last long. By 1981 the New Right had mounted a nationwide censorship campaign to purge schools and public libraries of sex education and other secular-humanist forms of "pornography." Sex education was "filth and perversion," Jerry Falwell announced in a fund-raising letter that included, under the label "Adults Only, Sexually Explicit Material," excerpts from a college health text. By the mid-1980s right-wing advocates of traditional family values had co-opted feminist anti-porn protests—or, at least, they'd co-opted feminist rhetoric. The feminist attorney and law professor Catharine

MacKinnon characterized pornography as the active subordination of women, and Phyllis Schlafly wrote, "Pornography really should be defined as the degradation of women. Nearly all porn involves the use of women in subordinate, degrading poses for the sexual, exploitative, and even sadistic and violent pleasures of men." Just like a feminist, Schlafly worried about how pornography might "affect a man who is already prone to violence against women." President Ronald Reagan deplored the link between pornography and violence against women.

PORNOGRAPHY AS SEX DISCRIMINATION

Of course, while feminists blamed patriarchy for pornography, moral majoritarians blamed feminism and other humanist rebellions. The alliance between feminists and the far right was not ideological but political. In 1984 anti-porn legislation devised by Andrea Dworkin and Catharine MacKinnon, defining pornography as a violation of women's civil rights, was introduced in the Indianapolis city council by an anti-ERA activist, passed with the support of the right, and signed into law by the Republican mayor, William Hudnut.

With the introduction of this bill, a new legislative front opened in the war against pornography, alienating civil-libertarian feminists from their more censorious sisters, while appealing to populist concerns about declining moral values. By calling for the censorship of pornography, some radical feminists found their way into the cultural mainstream—and onto the margins of First Amendment law.

The legislation adopted in Indianapolis offered a novel approach to prohibiting pornography which had all the force of a semantic distinction: pornography was not simply speech, Catharine MacKinnon suggested, but active sex discrimination, and was therefore not protected by the First Amendment. (In her 1989 book *Toward a Feminist Theory of the State*, MacKinnon characterized pornography as "a form of forced sex.") Regarding pornography as action, defining it broadly as any verbal or visual sexually explicit material (violent or not) that subordinates women, presuming that the mere existence of pornography

oppresses women, the Indianapolis ordinance gave any woman offended by any arguably pornographic material the right to seek an order prohibiting it, along with damages for the harm it presumably caused. In other words, any woman customer browsing in a bookstore or patrolling one, glancing at a newsstand or a triple-X video store, was a potential plaintiff in a sex-discrimination suit. Given all the literature, films, and videos on the mass market that could be said to subordinate women, this ordinance would have created lots of new business for lawyers—but it did not stand. Within a year of its enactment the Dworkin-MacKinnon law was declared unconstitutional by a federal appeals court, in a decision affirmed by the U.S. Supreme Court.

The feminist anti-porn movement retreated from the legislative arena and passed out of public view in the late 1980s, only to re-emerge with renewed strength on college campuses. College professors following fashions in poststructuralism asserted that legal principles, like those protecting speech, were mere rhetorical power plays: without any objective, universal merit, prevailing legal ideals were simply those privileged by the mostly white male ruling class. The dominant poststructural dogma of the late 1980s denied the First Amendment the transcendent value that the liberal belief in a marketplace of ideas has always awarded it.

MASSACHUSETTS MISCHIEF

This unlikely convergence of First Amendment critiques from multiculturalists, poststructuralists, and advocates of traditional family values, recently combined with high-profile rape and harassment cases and women's abiding concern with sexual violence, buoyed the feminist anti-porn movement. This year [1992] it re-emerged on the national and local scene with renewed legislative clout. The presumption that pornography oppresses women and is a direct cause of sexual violence is the basis for bills introduced in the U.S. Senate and the Massachusetts legislature. Last June the Senate Judiciary Committee passed the Pornography Victims' Compensation Act, which would make producers, distributors, exhibitors, and retailers convicted of disseminating material adjudged obscene liable for damages to victims of crimes who could claim that the material caused their victimization. The Massachusetts legislature held hearings on a much broader anti-porn bill, closely modeled on the Indianapolis ordinance. Disarmingly titled "An Act to Protect the Civil Rights of Women and Children," the Massachusetts bill would not only make purveyors of pornography liable for crimes committed by their customers; it would also allow any woman, whether or not she has been the victim of a crime, to sue the producers, distributors, exhibitors, or retailers of any sexually explicit visual material that subordinates women. (The exclusion of verbal "pornography" from the anti-trafficking provision would protect the likes of Norman Mailer, whom many feminists consider a pornographer, so long as his works are not adapted for the screen.) What this bill envisions is that the First Amendment would protect only that speech considered sexually correct.

The feminist case against pornography is based on the presumption that the link between pornography and sexual violence is clear, simple, and inexorable. The argument is familiar; censorship campaigns always blame unwanted speech for unwanted behavior: Jerry Falwell once claimed that sex education causes teenage pregnancy, just as feminists claim that pornography causes rape. One objection to this assertion is that it gives rapists and batterers an excuse for their crimes, and perhaps even a "pornography made me do it" defense.

The claim that pornography causes rape greatly oversimplifies the problem of sexual violence. We can hardly say that were it not for pornography, there would be no rape or battering. As feminists opposed to anti-porn legislation have pointed out, countries in which commercial pornography is illegal—Saudi Arabia, for example—are hardly safe havens for women.

This is not to deny that there probably is some link between violence in the media and violence in real life, but it is complicated, variable, and difficult to measure. Not all hate speech is an incantation; not all men are held spellbound by pornography. Poststructural feminists who celebrate subjectivism should be among the first to admit that different people respond to the same images differently. All we can confidently claim is that the way women are imagined is likely to have a cumulative effect on the way they're treated, but that does not mean any single image is the clear and simple cause of any single act.

The Dworkin-MacKinnon bill, however, did more than assume that pornography causes sex discrimination and other crimes against women. It said that pornography *is* violence and discrimination: the active subordination of women (and it assumed that we can all agree on what constitutes subordination). MacKinnon and her followers deny that prohibiting pornography is censorship, because they effectively deny that pornography is speech—and that is simply Orwellian. The line between speech and behavior is sometimes blurred: dancing nude down a public street is one way of expressing yourself which may also be a form of disorderly conduct. But if pornography is sex discrimination, then an editorial criticizing the President is treason.

Most feminists concerned about pornography are probably not intent on suppressing political speech, but the legislation they support, like the Massachusetts anti-porn bill, is so broad, and its definition of pornography so subjective, that it would be likely to jeopardize sex educators and artists more than it would hard-core pornographers, who are used to operating outside the law. Feminist legislation makes no exception for "pornography" in which some might find redeeming social value; it could, for example, apply in the case of a woman disfigured by a man who had seen too many paintings by Willem de Kooning. "If a woman is subjected," Catharine MacKinnon writes, "why should it matter that the work has other value?"

With this exclusive focus on prohibiting material that reflects incorrect attitudes toward women, anti-porn feminists don't deny the chilling effect of censorship; they embrace it. Any speech that subordinates women—any pornography—is yelling "Fire!" in a crowded theater, they say, falling back on a legal canard. But that's true only if, just as all crowds are deemed potential mobs, all men are deemed potential abusers whose violent impulses are bound to be sparked by pornography. It needs to be said, by feminists, that efforts to censor pornography reflect a profound disdain for men. Catharine MacKinnon has written that "pornography works as a behavioral conditioner, reinforcer and stimulus, not as idea or advocacy. It is more like saying 'kill' to a trained guard dog—and also the training process itself." That's more a theory of sexuality than of speech: pornography is action because all men are dogs on short leashes.

This bleak view of male sexuality condemns heterosexuality for women as an exercise in wish fulfillment (if only men weren't all dogs) or false consciousness (such as male-identified thinking). True feminism, according to MacKinnon, unlike liberal feminism, "sees sexuality as a social sphere of male power, of which forced sex is paradigmatic." With varying degrees of clarity, MacKinnon and Dworkin suggest that in a context of pervasive, institutionalized inequality, there can be no consensual sex between men and women: we can never honestly distinguish rape from intercourse.

AN ESOTERIC DEBATE

A modified version of this message may well have particular appeal to some college women today, who make up an important constituency for the anti-porn movement. In their late teens and early twenties, these women are still learning to cope with sexuality, in a violent and unquestionably misogynistic world. Feminism on campus tends to focus on issues of sexuality, not of economic equity. Anxiety about date rape is intense, along with anxiety about harassment and hate speech. Understanding and appreciation of the First Amendment is a lot less evident, and concern about employment discrimination seems somewhat remote. It's not hard to understand why: college women, in general, haven't experienced overt repression of opinions and ideas, or many problems in the workplace, but from childhood they've known what it is to fear rape. In the age of AIDS, the fear can be crippling.

Off campus the anti-porn feminist critique of male sexuality and heterosexuality for women has little appeal, but it is not widely known. MacKinnon's theoretical writings are impenetrable to readers who lack familiarity with poststructural jargon and the patience to decode sentences like this: "If objectivity is the epistemological stance of which women's sexual objectification is the social process, its imposition the paradigm of power in the male form, then the state will appear most relentless in imposing the male point of view when it comes closest to achieving its highest formal criterion of distanced aperspectivity." Dworkin is a much more accessible polemicist, but she is also much less visible outside feminist circles. Tailored, with an air of middle-class respectability and the authority of a law professor, MacKinnon looks far less scary to mainstream Americans than her theories about sexuality, which drive the anti-porn movement, might sound.

If anti-pornography crusades on the right reflect grassroots concern about changing sexual mores and the decline of the traditional family, anti-pornography crusades on the feminist left reflect the concerns and perceptions of an educated elite. In the battle for the moral high ground, anti-porn feminists claim to represent the interests of a racially diverse mixture of poor and working-class women who work in the pornography industry—and they probably do represent a few. But many sex-industry workers actively oppose anti-porn legislation (some feminists would say they've been brainwashed by patriarchy or actually coerced), and it's not at all clear that women who are abused in the making of pornography would be helped by forcing it deeper underground; working conditions in an illegal business are virtually impossible to police. It's hard to know how many other alleged victims of pornography feel represented by the anti-porn movement, and I know of no demographic study of the movement's active members.

Leaders of the feminist anti-porn movement, however, do seem more likely to emerge from academia and the professions than from the streets or battered-women's shelters. Debra Robbin, a former director of the New Bedford Women's Center, one of the first shelters in Massachusetts, doesn't believe that "women on the front lines," working with victims of sexual violence, will "put much energy into a fight against pornography." Activists don't have time: "They can barely leave their communities to go to the statehouses to fight for more funding." The poor and working-class women they serve would say, "Yeah, pornography is terrible, but I don't have food on my table." Carolin Ramsey, the executive director of the Massachusetts Coalition of Battered Women Service Groups, says that the pornography debate "doesn't have a lot to do with everyday life for me and the women I'm serving." She explains, "Violence in the home and the streets that directly threatens our lives and our families is more pressing than a movie. Keeping my kids away from drugs is more important than keeping them away from literature."

Ramsey is sympathetic to anti-porn feminists ("there's room in the movement for all of us"), and she believes that "violence in the media contributes to violence in real life." Still, she considers the pornography debate "esoteric" and "intellectual" and feels under no particular pressure from her constituents to take a stand against pornography.

If censoring pornography is the central feminist issue for Catharine MacKinnon, it is a peripheral issue for activists like Robbin and Ramsey. Robbin in particular does not believe that eliminating pornography would appreciably lessen the incidence of sexual abuse. David Adams, a co-founder and the executive director of Emerge, a Boston counseling center for male batterers, believes that only a minority of his clients (perhaps 10 to 20 percent) use hard-core pornography. He estimates that half may have substance-abuse problems, and adds that alcohol seems more directly involved in abuse than pornography. Adams agrees with feminists that pornography is degrading to women but does not support legislation regulating it, because "the legislation couldn't work and would only open the door to censorship."

What might work instead? Emerge conducts programs in Boston and Cambridge public schools on violence, aimed at both victims and perpetrators. "There's a lot of violence in teen relationships," Adams observes. Debra Robbin wishes that women in the anti-porn movement would "channel their energies into funding battered-women's shelters and rape-crisis centers."

Reforming the criminal-justice system is also a priority for many women concerned about sexual violence. Anti-stalking laws could protect many more women than raids on pornographic video stores are ever likely to; so could the efficient processing of cases against men who abuse women.

SENSATIONALISM AS AN ORGANIZING TOOL

Why do some women channel their energies into a fight against pornography? Antiporn legislation has the appeal of a quick fix, as Robbin notes. And, she adds, "there's notoriety to be gained from protesting pornography." The "harder work"—promoting awareness and understanding of sexual violence, changing the way children are socialized, and helping women victims of violence—is less sensationalist and less visible.

Sensationalism, however, is an organizing tool for anti-porn feminists. If questions about the effects of pornography seem intellectual to some women involved in social-service work, the popular campaign against pornography is aggressively anti-intellectual. Although advocates of First Amendment freedoms are stuck with intellectual defenses of the marketplace of ideas, anti-porn feminists whip up support for their cause with pornographic slide shows comprising hard-core pictures of women being tortured, raped, and generally degraded. Many feminists are equally critical of the soft-core porn movies available at local video stores and on cable TV, arguing that the violence in pornography is often covert (and they include mainstream advertising images in their slide shows). But hard-core violence is what works on the crowd. Feminist rhetoric often plays on women's worst fears about men: "Pornography tells us that there but for the grace of God go us." Gail Dines, a sociology professor at Wheelcock College, exclaimed during her recent slide show at Harvard, as she presented photographs of women being brutalized.

Dines's porn show was SRO, its audience some three hundred undergraduates who winced and gasped at the awful slides and cheered when Dines pointed to a pornographic picture of a woman and said, "When I walk down the street, what they know about me is what they know about her!" She warned her mostly female audience that pornographers have "aggressively targeted college men." She seemed preoccupied with masturbation. Part of the problem of pornography, she suggested, is that men use it to masturbate, and "women weren't put on this world to facilitate masturbation." She advised a student concerned about the presence of *Playboy* in the college library that library collections of pornography aren't particularly worrisome, because men are not likely to masturbate in libraries.

In addition to condemnations of male sexuality, Dines offered questionable horror stories about pornography's atrocities, like this: Rape vans are roaming the streets of New York. Women are dragged into the vans and raped on camera; when their attackers sell the rape videos in commercial outlets, the women have no legal recourse.

A story like this is impossible to disprove (how do you prove a negative?), but it should probably not be taken at face value, as many students in Dines's audience seemed to take it. William Daly, the director of New York City's Office of Midtown Enforcement, which is responsible for monitoring the sex industry in New York, has never heard of rape vans; almost anything is possible on Forty-second Street, but he is skeptical that rape vans are a problem. Part of Dines's story, however, is simply untrue: under New York State privacy law, says Nan Hunter, a professor of law at Brooklyn Law School, women could seek damages for the sale of the rape videos, and also an injunction against their distribution.

It would be difficult even to raise questions about the accuracy of the rape-van story, however, in the highly emotional atmosphere of a slide show; you'd be accused of "not believing the women." Just as slides of bloody fetuses pre-empt rational debate about abortion, pornographic slide shows pre-empt argumentative questions and rational consideration of First Amendment freedoms, the probable effect of efforts to censor pornography, and the actual relationship between pornography and violence.

A PORNOGRAPHIC CULTURE?

Does pornography cause violence against women, as some feminists claim? Maybe, in some cases, under some circumstances involving explicitly violent material. Readers interested in the social-science

debate should see both the report of the Attorney General's Commission on Pornography, which found a link between pornography and violence against women, and the feminist writer Marcia Pally's "Sense and Censorship," published by Americans for Constitutional Freedom and the Freedom to Read Foundation. In addition to the equivocal social-science data, however, we have the testimony of women who claim to have been brutalized by male consumers of pornography. Anti-porn feminists generally characterize pornography as a "how to" literature on abusing women, which men are apparently helpless to resist. But evidence of this is mainly anecdotal: At a hearing last March on the anti-porn bill in the Massachusetts legislature, several women told awful, lurid tales of sexual abuse, said to have been inspired by pornography. Like a TV talk show, the Attorney General's commission presented testimony from pornography's alleged victims, which may or may not have been true. It's difficult to cross-examine a sobbing self-proclaimed victim; you either take her testimony at face value or you don't.

Still, many people don't need reliable, empirical evidence about a link between pornography and behavior to believe that one exists. When feminists talk about pornography, after all, they mean a wide range of mainstream media images—Calvin Klein ads, Brian De Palma films, and the endless stream of TV shows about serial rapist stranglers and housewives who moonlight as hookers. How could we not be affected by the routine barrage of images linking sex and violence and lingerie? The more broadly pornography is defined, the more compelling are assertions about its inevitable effect on behavior, but the harder it is to control. How do we isolate the effect of any particular piece of pornography if we live in a pornographic culture?

Narrowly drawn anti-porn legislation, which legislators are most likely to pass and judges most likely to uphold, would not begin to address the larger cultural problem of pornography. Feminists themselves usually claim publicly that they're intent on prohibiting only hard-core pornography, although on its face their legislation applies to a much broader range of material. But if you accept the feminist critique of sexism in the media, hard-core porn plays a relatively minor role in shaping attitudes and behavior. If feminists are right about pornography, it is a broad social problem, not a discrete legal one—that is, pornography is not a problem the law can readily solve, unless perhaps we suspend the First Amendment entirely and give feminists the power to police the mainstream media, the workplace, and the schools.

The likelihood that feminists would not be the ones to police Forty-second Street should anti-porn legislation pass is one reason that many feminists oppose the anti-porn campaign. If society is as sexist as Andrea Dworkin and Catharine MacKinnon claim, it is not about to adopt a feminist agenda when it sets out to censor pornography. The history of anti-porn campaigns in this country is partly a history of campaigns against reproductive choice and changing roles for men and women. The first federal obscenity legislation, known as the Comstock Law, passed in 1873, prohibited the mailing of not only dirty pictures but also contraceptives and information about abortion. Early in this century Margaret Sanger and the sex educator Mary Ware Dennett were prosecuted for obscenity violations. Recently the New Right campaign against socially undesirable literature has focused on sex education in public schools. Anti-porn activists on the right consider feminism and homosexuality (which they link) to be threats to traditional family life (which, in fact, they are). In Canada a landmark Supreme Court ruling this year which adopted a feminist argument against pornography was first used to prohibit distribution of a small lesbian magazine, which a politically correct feminist would be careful to label erotica.

Gay and lesbian groups, as well as advocates of sex education and the usual array of feminist and nonfeminist civil libertarians, actively oppose anti-pornography legislation. Some state chapters of the National Organization for Women—New York, California, and Vermont—have taken strong anti-censorship stands, but at the national level NOW has not taken a position in the pornography debate. Its president, Patricia Ireland, would like to see pornography become socially unacceptable, "like smoking," but is wary of taking legal action against it, partly because she's wary of "giving people like Jesse Helms the power to decide what we read and see." But for major, national feminist organizations, like NOW and the NOW Legal Defense and Education Fund, the pornography debate is a minefield to be carefully avoided. Pornography is probably the most divisive issue feminists have faced since the first advocates of the ERA, in the 1920s, squared off against advocates of protective labor legislation for women. Feminists for and against anti-porn legislation are almost as bitterly divided as pro-choice activists and members of Operation Rescue.

Renewed concern about abortion rights may drain energy from the anti-porn movement. Feminists may awaken to the danger that anti-pornography laws will be used against sex educators and advocates of choice. (The imposition of a gag rule on family-planning clinics may have made some feminists more protective of the First Amendment.) Politicians courting women voters may find that anti-porn legislation alienates more feminists than it pleases. Still, censorship campaigns will always have considerable appeal. Like campaigns to reinstate the death penalty, they promise panaceas for profound social pathologies. They make their case by exploiting the wrenching anecdotal testimony of victims: politicians pushing the death penalty hold press conferences flanked by mothers of murdered children, just as feminists against pornography spotlight raped and battered women.

Rational argument is no match for highly emotional testimony. But it may be wishful thinking to believe that penalizing the production and distribution of hard-core pornography would have much effect on sexual violence. It would probably have little effect even on pornography given the black market. It would, however, complicate campaigns to distribute information about AIDS, let alone condoms, in the public schools. It would distract us from the harder, less popular work of reforming sexual stereotypes and roles, and addressing actual instead of metaphorical instruments of violence. The promise of the anti-porn movement is the promise of a world in which almost no one can buy pornography and almost anyone can buy a gun.

"The Price We Pay?": Pornography and Harm

SUSAN J. BRISON

Defenders of civil liberties have typically held, with J. S. Mill, that governments may justifiably exercise power over individuals, against their will, only to prevent harm to others (Mill, 1978: ch. 1).[1] Until the 1970s, liberals and libertarians assumed that since producers and consumers of pornography clearly didn't harm anyone else, the only reasons their opponents had for regulating pornography were that they considered it harmful to the producers or consumers, that they thought it an offensive nuisance, and that they objected, on moral or religious grounds, to certain private sexual pleasures of others. None of these reasons was taken to provide grounds for regulating pornography, however, since individuals are considered to be the best judges of what is in their own interest (and, in any case, they cannot be harmed by something to which they consent), what is merely offensive may be avoided (with the help of plain brown wrappers and zoning restrictions), and the private sexual activities, of consenting adults anyway, are no one else's, certainly not the state's, business.

In the 1970s, however, the nature of the pornography debate changed as an emerging group of feminists argued that what is wrong with pornography is not that it morally defiles its producers and consumers, nor that it is offensive or sinful, but, rather, that it is a species of hate literature as well as a particularly insidious method of sexist socialization. Susan Brownmiller was one of the first to take this stance in proclaiming that "[p]ornography is the undiluted essence of anti-female propaganda" (1975: 443). On this view, pornography (of the violent degrading variety) harms women by sexualizing misogynistic violence. According to Catharine MacKinnon, "[p]ornography sexualizes rape, battery, sexual harassment, prostitution, and child sexual abuse; it thereby celebrates, promotes, authorizes, and legitimizes them" (1987: 171).

The claim that women are harmed by pornography has changed the nature of the pornography debate, which is, for the most part, no longer a debate between liberals who subscribe to Mill's harm principle and legal moralists who hold that the state can legitimately legislate against so-called "morals offenses" that do not harm any non-consenting adults. Rather, the main academic debates now take place among those who subscribe to Mill's harm principle, but disagree about what its implications are for the legal regulation of pornography. Some theorists hold that violent degrading pornography does not harm anyone and, thus, cannot justifiably be legally regulated, socially stigmatized, or morally condemned. Others maintain that, although it is harmful to women, it cannot justifiably be regulated by either the civil or the criminal law, since that would cause even greater harms and/or violate the legal rights of pornography producers and consumers, but that, nevertheless, private individuals should do what they can (through social pressure, educational campaigns, boycotts, etc.) to put an end to it. Still others claim that such pornography harms women by violating their civil right to be free from sex discrimination and should, for that reason, be addressed by the law (as well as by other means), just as other forms of sex discrimination are. But others argue that restricting such pornography violates the moral right of pornography producers and consumers and, thus, restrictions are morally impermissible. Later in this chapter I will argue that there is no moral right to such pornography.

WHAT IS PORNOGRAPHY?

First, however, I need to articulate what is at issue, but this is hard to do, given various obstacles to describing the material in question accurately. (I have encountered the same problem in writing about sexual violence.) There is too much at stake to be put off writing about issues of urgent import to women because of squeamishness or fear of academic impropriety—but how can one write about this particular issue without reproducing the violent degrading pornography itself? (Recall the labeling of Anita Hill as "a little nutty and a little slutty" because she repeated, in public, the sexually demeaning language that Clarence Thomas had uttered to her in private.) However, if one doesn't write graphically about the content of violent degrading pornography, one risks being viewed as either crazy ("she must be imagining things!") or too prudish to talk frankly about sex. And what tone should one adopt—one of scholarly detachment or of outrage? There is a double bind here, similar to that faced by rape victims on the witness stand. If they appear calm and rational enough for their testimony to be credible, that may be taken as evidence that they cannot have been raped. But if they are emotional and out of control enough to appear traumatized, then their testimony is not considered reliable.

Any critic of violent degrading pornography risks being viewed not only as prudish (especially if the critic is a woman), but also as meddling in others' "private" business, since we tend not to see the harm in pornography—harm which is often made invisible and considered unspeakable. But "we" used not to see the harm in depriving women and minorities of their civil rights. And "we" used not to see the harm in distributing postcards depicting and celebrating lynchings. More recently, "we" didn't see the harm in marital or "date" rape, spousal battering, or sexual harassment. Even now, as Richard Delgado and Jean Stefancic point out:

[M]embers of the empowered group may simply announce to the disaffected that they do not see their problem, that they have looked for evidence of harm but cannot find it. Later generations may well marvel, "how could they have been so blind?" But paradigms change slowly. In the meantime, one may describe oneself as a cautious and principled social scientist interested only in the truth. And one's opponent, by a neat reversal, becomes an intolerant zealot willing to trample on the liberties of others without good cause. (1997: 37)

A further problem arises in critically analyzing violent degrading pornography, deriving from precisely those harmful aspects of it being critiqued,

which is that descriptions of it and quotations from it can themselves be degrading, or even retraumatizing, especially for women who have been victimized by sexual violence. But one thing that is clear is that feminist critics of such pornography are *not* criticizing it on the grounds that it is erotic, or sexually arousing, or that it constitutes "obscenity," defined by the Court as "works which, taken as a whole, appeal to the prurient interest in sex, which portray sexual conduct in a patently offensive way, and which, taken as a whole, do not have serious literary, artistic, political or scientific value" (*Miller v. California*, 1973: 24). Those who work on this issue—and have familiarized themselves with the real world of the pornography industry—know all too well that pornography is not merely offensive. In contrast, here is how some of them define "pornography":

[T]he graphic sexually explicit subordination of women through pictures or words that also includes women dehumanized as sexual objects, things, or commodities; enjoying pain or humiliation or rape; being tied up, cut up, mutilated, bruised, or physically hurt; in postures of sexual submission, servility or display; reduced to body parts, penetrated by objects or animals, or presented in scenarios of degradation, injury, torture; shown as filthy or inferior; bleeding, bruised, or hurt in a context that makes these conditions sexual. (MacKinnon, 1987: 176)[2]

I define "pornography," for the purposes of this chapter, as violent degrading misogynistic hate speech (where "speech" includes words, pictures, films, etc.). I will argue that, if pornography unjustly harms women (as there is reason to suppose it does), then there is no moral right to produce, sell, or consume it. (I will not here be arguing for or against its legal restriction and no position on that issue is dictated by my argument against the alleged moral right.)

PORNOGRAPHY AND HARM

I cannot hope to portray adequately the harms inflicted on girls and women in the production of pornography (for the reasons given above), but there is plenty of research documenting them. One of the most powerful forms of evidence for such harms is the first-person testimony of "participants" in pornography. * * * A not uncommon scenario in which a girl becomes trapped in the pornography industry is described by Evelina Giobbe in her testimony to the US Attorney-General's Commission on Pornography. After running away from home at age 13 and being raped her first night on the streets, Giobbe was befriended by a man who seemed initially kind and concerned, but who, after taking nude photographs of her, sold her to a pimp who raped and battered her, threatening her life and those of her family until she "agreed" to work as a prostitute for him. Her "customers" knew she was an adolescent and sexually inexperienced. "So," she testified, "they showed me pornography to teach me and ignored my tears and they positioned my body like the women in the pictures, and used me." She tried on many occasions to escape, but, as a teenager with no resources, cut off from friends and family, who believed she was a criminal, she was an easy mark for her pimp: "He would drag me down streets, out of restaurants, even into taxis, all the while beating me while I protested, crying and begging passers-by for help. No one wanted to get involved" (quoted in Russell, 1993: 38). She was later sold to another pimp who "was a pornographer and the most brutal of all." According to her testimony, he recruited other girls and women into pornography by advertising for models:

When a woman answered his ad, he'd offer to put her portfolio together for free, be her agent, and make her a "star." He'd then use magazines like *Playboy* to convince her to pose for "soft-core" porn. He'd then engage her in a love affair and smooth talk her into prostitution. "Just long enough," he would say, "to get enough money to finance your career as a model." If sweet talk didn't work, violence and blackmail did. She became one of us. (Quoted in Russell, 1993: 39)

Giobbe escaped the pornography industry by chance, after "destroy[ing] herself with heroin" and becoming "no longer usable." She considers herself one of the lucky ones—"a rare survivor" (quoted in Russell, 1993: 39–40). And this was *before* the AIDS epidemic.

More recently, according to an article in the *Sunday New York Times Magazine*, pornography—of an increasingly violent sort—has played an important role in the global sex trafficking of girls and women who, lured by promises of employment (for example, as nannies or waitresses), end up trapped in foreign countries, with no money, no (legal) papers, no family or friends, and no ability to speak the local language. Immigrations and Customs Enforcement (ICE) agents at the Cyber Crimes Center in Fairfax, Virginia are "tracking a clear spike in the demand for harder-core pornography on the Internet. 'We've become desensitized by the soft stuff; now we need a harder and harder hit', says ICE Special Agent Perry Woo." With ICE agents, the author of the article looked up a website purporting to offer sex slaves for sale: "There were streams of Web pages of thumbnail images of young girls of every ethnicity in obvious distress, bound, gagged, contorted. The agents in the room pointed out probable injuries from torture" (Landesman, 2004: 72). "'With new Internet technology', Woo said, 'pornography is becoming more pervasive. With Web cams we're seeing more live molestation of children'" (Landesman, 2004: 74).

It is not enough to say that the participants in pornography consent, *even* in the case of adult women who apparently do, given the road many have been led (or dragged) down, since childhood in some cases, to get to that point. Genuine autonomous consent requires the ability to evaluate critically and to choose from a range of significant and worthwhile options. Even if all the participants genuinely consented to their use in the pornography industry, however, we would need to consider how pornography influences how *other* non-consenting women are viewed and treated. Compare the (thankfully imaginary) scenario in which some blacks consented to act servile or even to play the part of slaves—who are humiliated, beaten, and whipped for the pleasure of their masters. Suppose a *lot* of whites got off on this and some people got a lot of money from tapping into (and pumping up) the desire for such films. And suppose the widespread consumption of such entertainment—a multibillion-dollar industry, in fact—influenced how whites generally viewed and treated blacks, making it harder than it would otherwise be for blacks to overcome a brutal and ongoing legacy of hate and oppression. It is unimaginable that we would tolerate such "entertainment" simply because some people got off on it.

To give another analogy, the fact that scabs will work for less money (in worse conditions) than strikers harms the strikers. It makes it harder for the strikers to work under fair conditions. Sure, the scabs benefit; however, that's not the point. The point is that the strikers suffer. Suppose there were "slave auction" clubs where some blacks allowed themselves to be brutalized and degraded for the pleasure of their white customers. Suppose the black "performers" determined that, given the options, it was in their best interest to make money in this way. Their financial gain—imagine that they are highly paid—more than compensates for the social harm to them as individuals of being subjected to a slightly increased risk (resulting from the prevalence of such clubs) of being degraded and brutalized outside their workplace. Some of them even enjoy the work, having a level of ironic detachment that enables them to view their customers as pathetic or contemptible. Some, who don't actually enjoy their work, don't suffer distress, since they manage to dissociate during it. Others are distressed by it, but they have determined that the financial benefit outweighs the psychic and physical pain. For those blacks who did not work in the clubs, however, there would be nothing that compensated for their slightly increased risk of being degraded and brutalized as a result of it. They would be better off if the clubs did not exist. The work done by the blacks in the clubs would make it harder for other blacks to live their lives free of fear.

The harms caused by pornography to non-participants in its production—often called "indirect" or "diffuse" harms, which makes them sound less real and less serious than they actually are—include (1) harms to those who have pornography forced on them, (2) increased or reinforced discrimination against—and sexual abuse of—girls and women, (3) harms to boys and men whose attitudes toward women and whose sexual desires are influenced by pornography, and (4) harms to those who have already been victimized by sexual violence. The first three categories of harm have been amply documented. * * * That the proliferation of pornography leads to attitudinal changes in men, which, in turn, led to harmful behavior, should not be surprising, especially given the high rates of exposure to pornography of pre-teen and teenage boys. On the contrary, as Frederick Schauer, Frank Stanton Professor of the First Amendment at the John F. Kennedy School of Government at Harvard University, testified at the Pornography Civil Rights hearing in Boston, Massachusetts on March 16, 1992:

I find it a constant source of astonishment that a society that so easily and correctly accepts the possibility that a cute drawing of a camel can have such an effect on the number of people who take up smoking, has such difficulty accepting the proposition that endorsing images of rape or other forms of sexual violence can have an effect on the number of people who take up rape. (cited in MacKinnon and Dworkin, 1997: 396)

One might object, though, that pornography is merely a symptom (of a misogynistic, patriarchal society), not a cause. Even if this were the case, however, that would not mean that we should not be concerned about it. The fact that there are so few female legislators in the US at the federal level (and that it's still inconceivable that a woman could be elected president) is a symptom, not a cause, of patriarchy. But this does not mean that we should not do anything about the political status quo. In any case, pornography is more than a mere symptom: it fosters and perpetuates the sexist attitudes that are essential for its enjoyment, even if it does not create them.

It should be noted here that the fact that the *point* of pornography (from the standpoint of the producers) is to make money by giving pleasure does not mean that it cannot also be harmfully degrading. On the contrary, it is pleasurable (and profitable) *precisely because* it is degrading to others. And it is reasonable to expect a spill-over effect in the public domain, since its enjoyment requires the adoption of certain attitudes. Compare the case of pornography with that of sexist humor. Until quite recently, it used to be maintained that women who were offended by sexist jokes were simply humorless. After all, it was held, one can laugh at a sexist joke (because it's funny) and not *be* a sexist. Now it is widely acknowledged that such jokes are funny only if one holds certain sexist beliefs: in other words, the humor is contingent upon the beliefs.[3] With regard to pornographic depictions, it would be difficult to argue that the degradation and subordination of women they involve are merely incidental to their ability to arouse. The arousal is dependent on the depiction of degradation, just as, in sexist humor, the humor is dependent on the sexism. I stress this in order to deflect the objection that the *point* of pornography is to give pleasure, not to defame or degrade women.

It might be argued that one could laugh at sexist jokes and enjoy sexist pornography *in private* without this having any effect on one's ability to view women as equals *in public* and to treat them accordingly. But are we really so good at keeping our private and public attitudes distinct? Suppose it became known that a white public official—say, a judge—privately relished racist humor, collected racist paraphernalia, and showed old racist films at home for the entertainment of his close friends and family. Although one might not want there to be laws against such reprehensible behavior (for their enforcement would require gross invasions of privacy), one would presumably consider such *private* behavior to compromise the integrity of the judge's public position. (Were this judge's pastime to be made public during his confirmation hearings for a set on the Supreme Court, for example, it would presumably defeat his nomination.)

It is easier for us, now, to see the harm in the dehumanization of blacks and Jews in racist and anti-Semitic propaganda. We are well aware that the Nazis' campaign to exterminate the Jews utilized anti-Semitic propaganda which portrayed Jews as disgusting, disease-ridden vermin. In addition, "Nazis made Jews do things that would further associate them with the disgusting," making them scrub latrines to which they were then denied access (Nussbaum, 2001, p. 348). This in turn made them appear less than human. As Primo Levi observed in *The Drowned and the Saved*:

The SS escorts did not hide their amusement at the sight of men and women squatting wherever they could, on the platforms and in the middle of the tracks, and the German passengers openly expressed their disgust: people like this deserve their fate, just look how they behave. These are not *Menschen*, human beings, but animals, it's as clear as day. (Quoted in Nussbaum, 2001: 348)

It is harder for us to see the same process of dehumanization at work when girls and women are rou-

tinely portrayed as being worthy of degradation, torture, and even death. But empirical studies have shown that exposure to such portrayals increases the likelihood that people will take actual sexual violence less seriously—and even consider it to be justified in some cases (see Lederer and Delgado, 1995: 61–112; MacKinnon and Dworkin, 1993: 46–60; Russell, 1993: 113–213).

There is another connection between the dehumanization of girls and women in pornography and their brutalization in rape, battering, forced prostitution, and sexual murder, which is that, in a society where women are victimized in these ways at an alarming rate, it shows a callous disregard for the actual victims to have depictions of sexual violence bought and sold as entertainment. For a short while, after 9/11, we empathized so much with the victims of the terrorist attacks that films of similarly horrifying attacks were withdrawn because they were no longer considered entertaining. But victims of sexual violence are given so little respect that many of us see nothing wrong with being entertained by depictions of what they have had to endure.

If we take seriously the harm of pornography, then we want to know what to do about it. Should the government intervene by regulating it? The standard debate over pornography has framed it as a free speech issue. The drafters of an anti-pornography ordinance adopted by the city of Indianapolis argued that pornography constitutes a violation of the civil rights of women. In response to those who asserted that the First Amendment protected pornography, they argued that pornography violated the First Amendment rights of women (by "silencing" them—depriving them of credibility and making "no" appear to mean "yes" in rape scenarios) as well as their Fourteenth Amendment rights to equal protection. In his opinion in *American Booksellers Association v. Hudnut*, which ruled unconstitutional the Indianapolis anti-pornography ordinance, Judge Frank Easterbrook acknowledged that pornography harms women in very significant and concrete ways:

Depictions of subordination tend to perpetuate subordination. The subordinate status of women in turn leads to affront and lower pay at work, insult and injury at home, battery and rape on the streets. In the language of the legislature, "[p]ornography is central in creating and maintaining sex as a basis of discrimination. Pornography is a systematic practice of exploitation and subordination based on sex which differentially harms women. The bigotry and contempt it produces, with the acts of aggression it fosters, harm women's opportunities for equality and rights [of all kinds]." Indianapolis Code §16-1(a) (2). "Yet this simply demonstrates the power of pornography as speech" (*American Booksellers Association, Inc.* v. *Hudnut*, 1985: 329).[4]

Easterbrook seems to take the harms of pornography seriously, but he then goes on to talk about its "unhappy effects" which he considers to be the result of "mental intermediation." He assumes that speech has no (or merely negligible) effects that are not under the conscious control of the audience, although this assumption is undermined not only by the widely acknowledged power of advertising, but also by recent work in cognitive neuroscience on the prevalence of unconscious imitation in human beings.[5] It might be argued, though, that, if we consider the producers of pornography to be even partially responsible for the violence perpetrated by some of its consumers, then we must consider the perpetrators *not* to be responsible or to be less than fully responsible for their crimes. But this does not follow. Even if the perpetrators are considered to be 100 percent responsible, some responsibility can still be attributed to the pornographers. (In fact, two or more people can each be 100 percent responsible for the same crime, as in the case of multiple snipers who simultaneously fire many shots, fatally wounding their victim.)

The courts have, for now, decided that even if serious harm to women results from it, pornography is, qua speech, protected (except for that material which also meets the legal definition of obscenity). That is, there is, currently, a *legal* right to it, falling under the right to free speech. But *should* there be?

A MORAL RIGHT TO PORNOGRAPHY?

Of course we value freedom of speech. But how should we value it? What should we do when speech

is genuinely harmful? Traditionally, in the US, the right to free speech is held to be of such high importance that it trumps just about everything else. For example, in the *Hudnut* case, discussed above, it was acknowledged that the pornography producers' and consumers' right to free speech was in conflict with women's right to equal protection, but it was asserted (without argumentation) that the free speech right had priority. Acceptance of this claim without requiring a defense of it, however, amounts to adopting a kind of free speech fundamentalism. To see how untenable such a view is, suppose that uttering the words "you're dead" caused everyone within earshot (but the speaker) to fall down dead. Would anyone seriously say that such speech deserved protection? Granted, the harms of pornography are less obvious and less severe, but there is sufficient evidence for them for it to be reasonable to require an argument for why the legal right to it should take priority over others' legal rights not to be subjected to such harms.

If we reject free speech fundamentalism, the question of whether pornography should be legally restricted becomes much more complicated. My aim here is not to articulate or defend a position on this question, but I do want to stress that whatever view we take on it should be informed by an understanding of the harms of pornography—the price some people pay so that other people may get off on it.

In . . . "The Right to Get Turned On: Pornography, Autonomy, Equality," Andrew Altman shifts the debate over pornography in a promising way by arguing that there is a *moral* right to (even violent misogynistic) pornography, falling not under a right to free speech, but, rather, under a right to sexual autonomy (which also covers the right to use contraceptives and the right to homosexual sex).[6] On this view, which Altman dubs "liberal sexual morality," whatever harm results from pornography is just the price we pay for the right to sexual autonomy. Sexuality is an important, arguably central, aspect of a flourishing human life. Sexual expression is one of the primary ways we define ourselves and our relations to others, and a healthy society should value and celebrate it. But what does it add to these claims to say that we have a moral *right* to sexual autonomy? And, if we do have such a right, does it include a right to produce, distribute, and consume pornography (defined, as above, as violent degrading misogynistic hate speech)?

Although philosophers disagree about the nature of rights (and, indeed, even about whether such things exist at all), most hold that to say that someone, X, has a moral right to do something, y, means that others are under a duty not to interfere with X's doing y. (Of course, X's right is limited by others' rights, as expressed by the saying "your right to swing your arm ends at my face.") But beyond this, there is little agreement. Some hold that rights are natural, inalienable, and God-given. Others hold that rights-talk is just short-hand for talk about those interests that are especially important to us (for example, because protecting them tends to increase our welfare). Some hold that we have positive rights, just by virtue of being human, such that other people are under an obligation to provide us with whatever we need to exercise those rights. (If there is a positive right to education, for example, then society has an obligation to provide free public education for all.) Others hold that we have only negative rights (unless individuals *grant* us positive rights by, for example, making promises to assist us), which require only that other people do not interfere with our exercising those rights. (The right to privacy, if taken to be simply a right to be left alone, is an example of a negative right.)

On any account, the concept of a right is diffuse. To say that X has a moral right to do y does not, by itself, say very much, unless we specify what others are required to do (or to refrain from doing) in order not to violate that right. There is a wide range of different responses to X's doing y, given that X has a right to do y—from complete acceptance (or perhaps even positive support) to something just short of physical restraint or intervention. Where is the alleged right to pornography located on this spectrum of moral assessment?

Altman considers the right to pornography and the right to sexual orientation to have the same foundation in a right to sexual autonomy. What should our (society's) attitude be toward the exercising of that right? Should we tolerate it, that is, have no laws against it, while allowing private individuals to lobby against it or to try to dissuade people from it? Or

should we actively embrace it? Assimilating the right to pornography to the right to sexual orientation muddies the waters here. Presumably, according to liberal sexual morality, the right to sexual orientation requires more than mere tolerance. It requires society's complete acceptance (and, I would argue, positive support, given that prejudice and violence against gays and lesbians persist in our society). It is wrong to hold that gays and lesbians have "bad characters" or to try to get them to "reform."

The right to pornography, however, does not lie on the same end of the spectrum, since Altman claims that getting off on pornography is a sign of a bad character. Some feminists and liberals who defend a legal right to pornography hold at the same time that all sorts of private pressure—protests, boycotts, educational campaigns—should be brought to bear on the pornographers. Altman's position is that there is not just a legal right, but also a *moral* right to pornography, even if there is something bad about exercising it. There are persuasive reasons for holding that we have legal rights to do some things that are morally wrong, in cases in which enforcement would be impossible or would involve gross violations of privacy. But Altman seems to hold that we have a *moral* right to do some things that are morally wrong. What does this mean? It cannot mean that people have a right to do things that are wrong in that they harm others. It might mean that people have the right to do things that other people consider wrong (but that are not harmful to others)—that is, people have the right to do harmless things that other people morally disapprove of. However, if the behavior, e.g. engaging in homosexual sex, is not unjustly harming others, then liberals who subscribe to Mill's harm principle have no grounds for considering it to be wrong.

So where should the right to pornography be located on the spectrum of moral assessment? There is no one answer to this question. We need to look at particular cases. Suppose I have a 21-year-old son—leaving aside the question of whether minors have a right to pornography—who is a heavy consumer of pornography (of the kind I've been talking about). What does his (alleged) right to pornography entail? Given my opposition to pornography, presumably I would not be under an obligation positively to support his pornography habit by buying it for him. But would I have to pretend that I'm not aware of it? Would I be under a duty not to try to dissuade him from viewing pornography? Would his sister be under a duty not to throw the magazines out when she saw them in common areas of the house? Would it be wrong for his buddies to try to talk him out of it? Would his teachers have a duty to refrain from arguing against it? Would it be wrong for his neighbors to boycott the local convenience store that sold it? Would his girlfriend (or boyfriend) who became convinced it was ruining their relationship be under a moral duty not to rip it out of his hands? If the answer to each of the above questions is "no," which I think it is, then it's not clear what, if anything, his right entitles him to.[7] What is clear is that, if a right to pornography exists, it is quite unlike a right to engage in homosexual sex or to use contraceptives, and is located at the opposite end of the spectrum of moral assessment.

Perhaps there is, nevertheless, something special about sexual arousal ("getting turned on") that gives it special moral status. But Altman has not said what makes sexual arousal different (in a morally significant way) from other forms of arousal—for example, that of racial animus. It makes sense to say that there is a right to be turned on—not a special right, but, rather, one falling under a general right to liberty, but this general right to liberty is delimited by the harm principle. There is no general right to have pleasurable feelings (of any sort, sexual or otherwise) that override others' rights not to be harmed. There is no moral right to achieve a feeling of comfort by unjustly discriminating against homosexuals on the grounds that associating with them makes you uncomfortable. Likewise, there is no moral right to achieve a feeling of superiority (no matter how pleasurable such a feeling might be) by discriminating against those of a different race. And it doesn't matter how central to one's self-definition the feeling in question might be. For parents, the satisfaction of ensuring the good upbringing and education of their children is of paramount importance, and yet this degree of importance does not give racist parents the right to racially segregated housing or schools.

It might be argued that sexual arousal is special in that it is a bodily pleasure and, thus, more natural,

possibly even immutable. Even if this were so, it would not follow that one has a right to achieve it by any means necessary. To take an example of another kind of "bodily" pleasure, suppose that there are gustatory pleasures that can be achieved only in immoral ways— for example, by eating live monkey brains (which some people used to do), or organs or flesh "donated" by (or purchased from) living human beings, or food that has been stolen from the people on the verge of starvation. That there is a (general) right to enjoy eating what one chooses to eat—it would be (in general) wrong, for example, for me to force you to eat, or not to eat, something—does not mean that one has a right to eat whatever gives one pleasure.

But it is not the case that what people find sexually arousing is a simple biological fact about them, a given, something immutable. People can be conditioned to be aroused by any number of things. In one study, for example, men were conditioned to be aroused by a picture of a woman's boot (Russell, 1993: 129). Emotions, especially ones with strong physiological components, such as sexual arousal, *feel* natural. They don't seem to be socially constructed, because we don't (at the time) consciously choose them: they just *are*. But emotions are, at least to some extent, learned reactions to things. There are gender differences in emotional reactions; for example, men tend to get angry in some situations in which women tend to feel not angry, but hurt. But this does not mean that such differences are *natural*.

Given the wide variety of sexual fantasies and fetishes we know about, it's conceivable that just about *anything* could be a turn on for someone— looking at photos of dead, naked bodies piled in mass graves in Nazi death camps, for example, or looking at photos of lynched black men. According to liberal sexual morality, the only reason for supposing that there might not be a moral right to make a profit from and get off on such "pornography" would be that the photographed people are posthumously harmed by it (given that they did not consent to their images being used in this way). But suppose they had consented. Or suppose, more plausibly, that the images were computer-generated—completely realistic-looking, but not images *of* actual individuals. Liberal sexual morality would have to allow (some) people to make money by others' getting turned on by these images. Not only that, but, given that sexual desires are malleable, the pornographer also has a right to make money by acculturating others to be turned on by such images. (In other words, the pornographer has a right to turn the world into a place where people get turned on by such images.) And, if our attitude toward this is grounded in the right to sexual autonomy, it should be similar to our attitude toward homosexuality: we shouldn't merely tolerate it, we should come to accept and support it.

While conceding that there are limits to the right to sexual autonomy—it is constrained by the harm principle—Altman assumes (as most liberals do) that one cannot be harmed by something to which one consents. I argued earlier that the way many models get lured into the pornography industry should make us at least question the extent to which they are consenting to what is being done to them. But suppose they do consent. Does that mean that we must tolerate the production and use of whatever pornography results? Unfortunately, one doesn't have to construct a thought experiment to test our intuitions about this. According to *The New York Times*, Armin Meiwes, "[a] German computer technician who killed and ate a willing victim he found through the Internet" was recently convicted of manslaughter. His "victim," Bernd-Jürgen Brandes, had "responded to an Internet posting by Mr Meiwes seeking someone willing to be 'slaughtered'." "'Both were looking for the ultimate kick'," the judge said. It was "an evening of sexual role-playing and violence, much of it videotaped by Mr Meiwes," enough to convince the court that the "victim" had consented (Landler, 2004: A3). Does the right to sexual autonomy include the rights to produce, sell, and get turned on by the videotape of this "slaughter"—a real-life instance of a snuff film? If we cannot *prove* that there is a causal connection between the film and harm to others, the answer, according to liberal sexual morality, is "yes."

Altman claims that "even if a causal connection between violent pornography and sexual violence were clearly established, it would still be insufficient to conclude that, in contemporary society, the production, distribution and viewing of violent pornog-raphy lay beyond the limits of an adult's right to sexual autonomy" because *other* media—he cites "slasher films"—arguably "cause at least some amount of violence against women, sexual and otherwise. However, it is unreasonable to deny that adults have a right to produce, distribute, and view such movies" (2005: 229). Why, if one has established that, say, "slasher films" are harmful, we must hold that adults have a right to them is not explained. But even if we agree that adults have the right to produce/consume non-pornographic media even if it is as harmful as pornography, it does not follow that adults have the right to produce/consume pornography. To assume that it does would be like arguing against prohibiting driving while talking on cell phones on the grounds that this is not the *only* thing (or even the main thing) contributing to automobile accidents.

Altman accepts that "it is reasonable to hold that the existence of . . . pornography makes it more difficult for women to live their lives as the sexual equals of men—i.e., more difficult relative to a society which was ruled by a liberal sexual morality and had fewer women, or none at all, who were willing to engage in humiliating conduct as part of the production of pornographic materials" (Altman, 2005: 233), but he notes that women are better off in a society with liberal sexual morality than in a society with traditional sexual morality (for example, Saudi Arabia). I agree, but surely these are not the only two possibilities. I would advocate the alternative of a progressive sexual morality. What might that look like? We don't even know. Even our most deep-seated assumptions about sexuality may turn out to be mistaken. We used to view rape as being motivated purely by lust and battering as a way of showing spousal love. Some of us still do. Gradually, however, we are breaking the link between sexuality and violence. Perhaps some day we'll have reached the point where sexual violence is no longer arousing, where it makes no sense to talk of killing and being killed as the "ultimate" sexual "kick."

According to liberal sexual morality, the harms of pornography are the price we pay for having the right to sexual autonomy in other areas—e.g. the right to have sex (including homosexual sex) outside of marriage and the right to use contraceptives. But this view (of the right to sexual autonomy as an all-or-nothing package) is formed in response to legal moralism, and makes sense only if one considers all these rights to be rights to do harmless things that some people nevertheless morally condemn. In such cases, proponents of liberal sexual morality say: "If you don't like it, don't look at it (or hear about it or think about it)." This is a satisfactory response only if the behavior in question isn't harming anyone. But as our views about what constitutes harm have changed, our views of what is our business have also changed. Just as we no longer look the other way in response to marital or "date" rape, domestic violence, and sexual harassment, we should no longer accept pornography's harms as the price we pay for sexual autonomy.

NOTES

* * *

1. Mill considered his harm principle to apply equally to governmental regulation and to "the moral coercion of public opinion." The harm principle states that " . . . the only purpose for which power can be rightfully exercised over any member of a civilized community, against his will, is to prevent harm to others" (1978: 9). Mill does not specify what counts as harm. Following Joel Feinberg (1984), I consider it to be a wrongful setback to one's significant interests.

2. This is the definition used in the anti-pornography ordinance drafted by Andrea Dworkin and Catharine MacKinnon, passed by the city of Indianapolis, but ruled unconstitutional by the courts.

3. For a persuasive argument to that effect, see de Sousa (1987). In comparing sexist fantasies with sexist and racist humor, one might reply, however, that we have less control over, and thus are less responsible for, our fantasies than our jokes. This seems right, to the extent that we can refrain from laughing at or telling certain jokes (even though we might not be able to resist finding them funny). But the same distinction applies to fantasies. We do not always choose the fantasies that occur to us, but we can choose whether or not to cultivate them (voluntarily return to them repeatedly, make or view films about them, etc.). Even in the case of dreams, over which we, at the time, anyway, have no control, a white male liberal would be alarmed if he often

had pleasurable dreams of watching blacks getting lynched. This would presumably prompt some probing of his unconscious attitudes about blacks.

4. This view can't consistently be held, however, by liberals and feminists who support laws against sex or race discrimination and segregation in schools, workplace, and even private clubs. One doesn't hear the argument that if segregation harms minorities' opportunities for equal rights this simply demonstrates the power of freedom of association, which is also protected by the First Amendment.

5. The recent research discussed in Hurley (2004) suggests that the imitation of others' behavior, including others' violent acts, is not a consciously mediated process, under the autonomous control of the viewers/imitators.

6. Since some theorists ground the right to free speech in a right to autonomy, however, there may not be such a sharp distinction between these two approaches. See Brison (1998).

7. I also mean for the above thought experiment to illustrate the fact that the nature of the duty one has with respect to the holder of the alleged moral right to pornography depends on one's relationship to the right-holder. Presumably a neighbor would be under a duty not to snatch pornography out of the right-holder's hands. But if someone *else*, the right-holder's lover, say, is under no such duty, then it's not clear what the right amounts to.

REFERENCES

Altman, Andrew (2005). "The right to get turned on: pornography, autonomy, equality." In Andrew I. Cohen and Christopher Heath Wellman (eds.), *Contemporary Debates in Applied Ethics* (pp. 223–35). Oxford: Blackwell, 2005.

American Booksellers Association, Inc. v. *Hudnut* (1985). 771 F.2d 323.

Attorney General's Commission on Pornography (1986). *Final Report.* Washington, DC: US Department of Justice.

Brison, Susan J. (1998). "The autonomy defense of free speech." *Ethics*, 108: 312–39.

Brownmiller, Susan (1975). *Against Our Will: Men, Women and Rape.* New York: Bantam Books.

Delgado, Richard and Jean Stefancic (1997). *Must We Defend Nazis? Hate Speech, Pornography, and the New First Amendment.* New York: New York University Press.

de Sousa, Ronald (1987). "When is it wrong to laugh?" In *The Rationality of Emotion* (pp. 275–99). Cambridge, MA: MIT Press.

Feinberg, Joel (1984). *The Moral Limits of the Criminal Law*, vol. 1: *Harm to Others*. New York: Oxford University Press.

Hurley, Susan L. (2004). "Imitation, media violence, and freedom of speech." *Philosophical Studies*, 17/1–2 (January): 165–218.

Itzen, Catherine (ed.) (1992). *Pornography: Women, Violence and Civil Liberties*. New York: Oxford University Press.

Landesman, Peter (2004). "The girls next door." *Sunday New York Times Magazine* (January 25): 30–9, 66–74.

Landler, Mark (2004). "German court convicts Internet cannibal of manslaughter." *New York Times* (January 31): A3.

Lederer, Laura (ed.) (1980). *Take Back the Night: Women on Pornography*. New York: William Morrow and Co., Inc.

Lederer, Laura J. and Richard Delgado (eds.) (1995). *The Price We Pay: The Case Against Racist Speech, Hate Propaganda, and Pornography*. New York: Hill and Wang.

MacKinnon, Catharine A. (1987). *Feminism Unmodified: Discourses on Life and Law*. Cambridge, MA: Harvard University Press.

MacKinnon, Catharine A. (1993). *Only Words*. Cambridge, MA: Harvard University Press.

MacKinnon, Catharine A. and Andrea Dworkin (eds.) (1997). *In Harms' Way: The Pornography Civil Rights Hearings*. Cambridge, MA: Harvard University Press.

Mill, John Stuart (1978). *On Liberty*. Indianapolis, IN: Hackett Publishing Co. (Originally published 1859).

Miller v. California (1973). 413 US 15.

Nussbaum, Martha (2001). *Upheavals of Thought*. Cambridge: Cambridge University Press.

Russell, Diana E. H. (ed.) (1993). *Making Violence Sexy: Feminist Views on Pornography*. Buckingham: Open University Press.

CASES FOR ANALYSIS

1. Avoiding Morality in Sex Lessons

London (*The Sunday Times*)—Parents should avoid trying to convince their teenage children of the difference between right and wrong when talking to them about sex, a new government leaflet is to advise.

Instead, any discussion of values should be kept "light" to encourage teenagers to form their own views, according to the brochure, which one critic has called "amoral."

"Talking to Your Teenager About Sex and Relationships" will be distributed in pharmacies from next month as part of an initiative led by Beverley Hughes, the children's minister.

The leaflet comes in the wake of the case of Alfie Patten, the 13-year-old boy from East Sussex who fathered a child with a 15-year-old girl and sparked a debate about how to cut rates of teenage parenthood.

It advises: "Discussing your values with your teenagers will help them to form their own. Remember, though, that trying to convince them of what's right and wrong may discourage them from being open."*

Should parents keep issues of right and wrong out of discussions about sex with their children? Should parents convey the idea that right and wrong has nothing to do with sex? Why or why not? In school sex education, should discussions of ethics be forbidden? Is ethics irrelevant to contemporary sexual behavior?

*Jack Grimston, "Parents Told: Avoid Morality in Sex Lessons," *Times Online*, February 22, 2009. Reprinted by permission of NI Syndication.

2. Premarital Abstinence Pledges

(*Washington Post*)—Teenagers who pledge to remain virgins until marriage are just as likely to have premarital sex as those who do not promise abstinence and are significantly less likely to use condoms and other forms of birth control when they do, according to a study released today.

The new analysis of data from a large federal survey found that more than half of youths became sexually active before marriage regardless of whether they had taken a "virginity pledge," but that the percentage who took precautions against pregnancy or sexually transmitted diseases was 10 points lower for pledgers than for non-pledgers.

"Taking a pledge doesn't seem to make any difference at all in any sexual behavior," said Janet E. Rosenbaum of the Johns Hopkins Bloomberg School of Public Health, whose report appears in the January issue of the journal *Pediatrics*. "But it does seem to make a difference in condom use and other forms of birth control that is quite striking."

The study is the latest in a series that have raised questions about programs that focus on encouraging abstinence until marriage, including those that specifically ask students to publicly declare their intention to remain virgins. The new analysis, however, goes beyond earlier analyses by focusing on teens who had similar values about sex and other issues before they took a virginity pledge.[†]

Give reasons for your answers. Suppose, as this report suggests, abstinence pledges are ineffective and can reduce condom use and increase the risk of teen pregnancy. Would it be immoral to promote the pledges among teens? Should the effectiveness of the pledges in reducing teen pregnancy or STDs have any bearing on the morality of promoting the pledges? Is premarital sex among teens morally wrong regardless of its physical and social risks?

3. Pornography and Rape

Here is part of the abstract of a scientific study published in the *International Journal of Law and Psychiatry* in 1991:

> We have looked at the empirical evidence of the well-known feminist dictum: "pornography is the theory—rape is the practice" (Morgan, 1980). While earlier research, notably that generated by the U.S. Commission on Obscenity and Pornography (1970), had found no evidence of a causal link between pornography and rape, a new generation of behavioral scientists have, for more than a decade, made considerable effort to prove such a connection, especially as far as "aggressive pornography" is concerned. The first part of the article examines and discusses the findings of this new research. A number of laboratory experiments have been

conducted, much akin to the types of experiments developed by researchers of the effects of nonsexual media violence. As in the latter, a certain degree of increased "aggressiveness" has been found under certain circumstances, but to extrapolate from such laboratory effects to the commission of rape in real life is dubious. Studies of rapists' and nonrapists' immediate sexual reactions to presentations of pornography showed generally greater arousal to non-violent scenes, and no difference can be found in this regard between convicted rapists, nonsexual criminals and noncriminal males. In the second part of the paper an attempt was made to study the necessary precondition for a substantial causal relationship between the availability of pornography, including aggressive pornography, and rape—namely, that obviously increased availability of such material was followed by an increase in cases of reported rape. The development of rape and attempted rape during the period 1964–1984 was studied in four countries: the U.S.A., Denmark, Sweden and West Germany. In all four countries there is clear and undisputed evidence that during this period the availability of various forms of pictorial pornography including violent/dominant varieties (in the form of picture magazines, and films/videos used at home or shown in arcades or cinemas) has developed from extreme scarcity to relative abundance. If (violent) pornography causes rape, this exceptional development in the availability of (violent) pornography should definitely somehow influence the rape statistics. Since, however, the rape figures could not simply be expected to remain steady during the period in question (when it is well known that most other crimes increased considerably), the development of rape rates was compared with that of non-sexual violent offences and nonviolent sexual offences (in so far as available statistics permitted). The results showed that in none of the countries did rape increase more than nonsexual violent crimes. This finding in itself would seem sufficient to discard the hypothesis that pornography causes rape.[‡]

Does this study prove conclusively that access to pornography does not cause rape? Why or why not? Suppose exposure to pornography does indeed lead to rape (increases its incidence). Would this fact justify the banning of all pornographic materials? How would you balance this harm (increased risk of rape) with freedom of expression? To which one would you give more weight?

But say pornography is harmless. Would you still want to see it banned? If so, on what grounds?

Suppose pornography was actually helpful to people (enhancing sexuality, improving relationships, decreasing divorce rates, etc.). Would you still want it censored? Why or why not?

[‡]Berl Kutchinsky, excerpt reprinted from *International Journal of Law and Psychiatry*, Vol. 14, Nos. 1–2, "Pornography and Rape: Theory and Practice? Evidence from Crime Data in Four Countries Where Pornography Is Easily Available," pp. 47–64, Copyright © 1991 Pergamon Press plc, with permission from Elsevier.

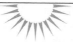

CHAPTER 14

Same-Sex Marriage

On June 26, 2015, the Supreme Court ruled in a 5 to 4 decision that the U.S. Constitution establishes a right to same-sex marriage. But the issue has been and will continue to be the subject of debate. For twenty years or so, it has been provoking consternation and fury in the legislatures, the courts, the church, and the media. Many—probably most—of the debates have been useless to anyone who wants to arrive at well-supported opinions on the subject. Appeals to plausible argument and evidence have generally been few and feeble. But the moral philosopher's approach to the issue should be more helpful. Try to view same-sex marriage in this clearer light and see if your opinions become better focused and better supported.

ISSUE FILE: BACKGROUND

Same-sex marriage refers to the marriage, in the full legal sense, of gay and lesbian couples. This is the meaning of the term in common usage and the starting point for the verbal fights surrounding the issue. For most people—both those for and against same-sex marriage—the central question is whether homosexuals should be permitted to enter into legally sanctioned marriage, with all its civic and social benefits, just as heterosexual couples can. The benefits include property rights, social status, inheritance rights, health and life insurance, adoption, hospital visitation rights, tax breaks, and pension rights. Legal arrangements for same-sex couples that had fallen short of the marriage standard (such as civil unions and domestic partnerships) were less controversial. They granted some official legitimacy to same-sex relationships without giving them the full marriage rights that heterosexuals have. People on both sides of the gay marriage issue favored or opposed these legal options, but the main battles were fought over marriage proper.

Before the final Supreme Court ruling, a minority of states had no place for same-sex marriage, but thirty-seven allowed gay and lesbian couples to marry. In February 2015, a court ruling compelled Alabama to allow same-sex marriages. In 2014 Alaska permitted gay marriage after the U. S. Supreme Court refrained from overruling a lower court's decision to strike down the state's gay-marriage ban. Other states seemed likely to follow suit. States allowing same-sex marriage include New York, Iowa, Massachusetts, Vermont, New Hampshire, Connecticut, and Idaho, in addition to Washington, D. C.

In 1996 Congress passed (and President Bill Clinton signed) the **Defense of Marriage Act**, which forbade the federal government to recognize same-sex marriages. It denied benefits to gay and lesbian marriages and allowed states to discount such marriages recognized by other states. Later a federal judge struck down the law, and in 2013 the Supreme Court did the same.

Public attitudes toward same-sex marriage have also been shifting. In 2003, 37 percent of adults believed the marriage of gay and lesbian couples should be legal; 55 percent believed it should be illegal. In 2014 the situation had almost reversed: 55 percent thought it should be legal while 42 percent thought it should not.

Religion is as divided on same-sex marriage as the general public is. Many Protestant churches are trying to figure out how they should feel about the issue. Some mainline denominations (such as the United Church of Christ) have formally endorsed same-sex marriage, and some (such as the Episcopal Church) have opened positions in the clergy to gay and lesbian members. The Catholic Church, the Southern Baptist Convention, and other evangelical Christians strongly and publicly oppose same-sex marriages. Conservative Judaism is split on the question; most Orthodox rabbis are against same-sex marriage, but Reform Judaism has no objection to rabbis officiating at gay and lesbian ceremonies. Islam condemns homosexuality and considers same-sex marriages to be violations of Islamic law or principles.

Arguments against same-sex marriage concentrate on four themes: (1) Same-sex marriage is contrary to custom, tradition, or nature; (2) it's a distortion of the true meaning or essence of marriage; (3) it's wrong because homosexuality is wrong; and (4) the consequences of allowing same-sex marriage would be dangerous or harmful. Opponents of same-sex marriage offer several variations on these kinds of arguments.

Proponents generally argue their case on two grounds: (1) Permitting same-sex marriage is a matter of justice, which demands equal treatment and equal opportunity for all; and (2) allowing it would be beneficial both to homosexuals and society as a whole. This is how one philosopher summarizes variations on reason 1:

> Marriage provides benefits which are denied to same-sex couples on the basis of their orientation; if the function of marriage is the legal recognition of loving, or "voluntary intimate," relationships, the exclusion of same-sex relationships appears arbitrary and unjustly discriminatory. Same-sex relationships are relevantly similar to heterosexual relationships recognized as marriages, yet the state denies gays and lesbians access to the benefits of marriage, hence treating them unequally.[1]

[1]Elizabeth Brake, "Marriage and Domestic Partnerships," *Stanford Encyclopedia of Philosophy,* 2009, http://plato.stanford.edu/entries/marriage/#SamSexMar (14 August 2011).

And this is how Andrew Sullivan elaborates on reason 2:

> Like straight marriage, [same-sex marriage] would foster social cohesion, emotional security, and economic prudence. Since there's no reason gays should not be allowed to adopt or be foster parents, it could also help nurture children . . . A law institutionalizing gay marriage would merely reinforce a healthy social trend. It would also, in the wake of AIDS, qualify as a genuine public health measure. . . . [Gay marriage] provides role models for young gay people, who after the exhilaration of coming out, can easily lapse into short-term relationships and insecurity with no tangible goal in sight. My own guess is that most gays would embrace such a goal with as much (if not more) commitment as straights. Even in our society as it is, many lesbian relationships are virtual textbook cases of monogamous commitment. Legal gay marriage could also help bridge the gulf often found between gays and their parents.[2]

MORAL THEORIES

Natural law theory generally condemns same-sex marriage, just as it condemns homosexuality. The Roman Catholic version rejects the former for the same reason it does the latter: the practice is contrary to the divinely mandated aim of procreation. The church is crystal clear on this:

> There are absolutely no grounds for considering homosexual unions to be in any way similar or even remotely analogous to God's plan for marriage and family. Marriage is holy, while homosexual acts go against the natural moral law. Homosexual acts "close the sexual act to the gift of life." They do not proceed from a genuine affective and sexual complementarity. Under no circumstances can they be approved.[3]

[2]Andrew Sullivan, "Here Comes the Groom: A (Conservative) Case for Gay Marriage," in *Beyond Queer*, Bruce Bawer, ed. (New York: Free Press, 1996), 252–258.
[3]The Vatican, Congregation for The Doctrine of The Faith, "Considerations Regarding Proposals to Give Legal Recognition to Unions Between Homosexual Persons," June 2003, http://www.vatican.va/roman_curia/congregations/cfaith/documents/rc_con_cfaith_doc_2003073_homosexual-unions_en.html (18 February 2015).

OPINION POLLS: Same-Sex Marriage

"Do you think it should be legal or illegal for same-sex couples to marry?"

Legal	Not Legal	Unsure/No Answer
56%	37%	7%

CBS News/New York Times Poll. Sept. 12–15, 2014, N = 1,009 adults nationwide.

"Do you think marriages of same-sex couples should or should not be recognized by the law as valid, with the same rights as traditional marriages?"

Should	Should Not	Unsure
55%	42%	3%

Gallup Poll. May 8–11, 2014, N = 1,028 adults nationwide.

"Suppose that on Election Day you could vote on key issues as well as candidates. Would you vote for or against a federal law that would make same-sex marriages legal in all 50 states?"

Vote for	Vote against	Unsure
52%	43%	4%

Gallup Poll. July 10–14, 2013. N = 1,055 adults nationwide. Margin of error ± 4.

Kant would not have liked the notion of same-sex marriage, but it's possible to harness some of his insights to support this practice. Recall that at the core of Kant's moral theory is the principle of respect for persons, which requires that they not be treated merely as a means to an end and that their rights be given the highest priority. To violate people's right to equal treatment and equal opportunity is to treat them merely as a means—to regard them as less than persons with full moral rights. Proponents of same-sex marriage argue that outlawing the practice denies gays and lesbians the equal treatment and opportunity they are due.

In the debates over same-sex marriage, both proponents and opponents have argued in a consequentialist vein. Andrew Sullivan takes this tack in the previous quotation. But Maggie Gallagher, among others, thinks same-sex marriage would bring disaster to the family:

> Same-sex marriage would enshrine in law a public judgment that the desire of adults for families of choice outweighs the need of children for mothers and fathers. It would give sanction and approval to the creation of a motherless or fatherless family as a deliberately chosen "good." It would mean the law was neutral as to whether children had mothers and fathers. Motherless and fatherless families would be deemed just fine.[4]

William Bennett also warns of the dire consequences of legalizing same-sex unions:

> Consider: the legal union of same-sex couples would shatter the conventional definition of marriage, change the rules which govern behavior, endorse practices which are completely antithetical to the tenets of all the world's major religions, send conflicting signals about marriage and sexuality, particularly to the young, and obscure marriage's enormously consequential function—procreation and child-rearing.[5]

[4]Maggie Gallagher, "What Marriage Is For: Children Need Mothers and Fathers," *Weekly Standard* 8, no. 45 (4–11 August 2003): 22–25.

[5]William Bennett, "Leave Marriage Alone," *Newsweek* 3 June 1996.

VITAL STATS: Gays, Lesbians, and Same-Sex Couples

- **3.5%** Approximate percentage of Americans who identify as lesbian, gay, or bisexual (Gallup Poll, 2012).

- **646,464** Number of same-sex households in the United States (Census Bureau, 2010).

- **20** Number of countries worldwide where same-sex marriage has been approved in all or part of the entire country: Argentina, Belgium, Brazil, Canada, Denmark, Finland, France, Iceland, Ireland, Luxembourg, the Netherlands, New Zealand, Norway, Portugal, South Africa, Spain, Sweden, the United Kingdom (England, Scotland, Wales), the United States, and Uruguay (Freedom to Marry, Inc., 2015).

MORAL ARGUMENTS

To many, homosexuality challenges ideas about gender and biology, but same-sex marriage threatens one of the fundamental pillars of society itself—the institution of marriage. So both those who favor and those who oppose same-sex marriage realize that the stakes are high and that a great deal depends on the answer to the central moral question, Should same-sex marriages be permitted?

The traditional answer is, of course, no. One argument for this position appeals to the benefits to society of preserving long-standing customs and traditions. The idea is that because these structures have evolved and endured in human societies, they embody a collective wisdom that must be preserved. However arbitrary or unjust they may seem, they work, and we are stuck with them. If we tamper with them, we risk wrecking their complex internal workings and destroying whole systems. The tradition of marriage is one such intricate structure, now solidly established as an institution joining male and female only.

Jonathan Rauch calls this the Hayekian view, which "argues strongly against gay marriage." It asserts that

> once you say that marriage need not be male-female, soon marriage will stop being anything at all. You can't mess with the formula without causing unfore-

seen consequences, possibly including the implosion of marriage itself.[6]

But this position has serious problems, Rauch says:

> In its extreme form, it implies that no social reforms should ever be undertaken. Indeed, no laws should be passed, because they interfere with the natural evolution of social mores. How could Hayekians abolish slavery?[7]

Other arguments against same-sex marriage appeal to the essence or real meaning of marriage. The idea is that the true purpose and meaning of marriage is procreation and child-rearing. Heterosexual couples can procreate and fulfill marriage's purpose; homosexual couples cannot. Same-sex marriage, therefore, amounts to a degradation of true marriage, a desertion from its essential meaning. Maggie Gallagher takes this view:

> Marriage is the fundamental, cross-cultural institution for bridging the male-female divide so that children have loving, committed mothers and fathers. . . . Privately, religiously, emotionally, individually, marriage may have many meanings. But this is the core

---

[6]Jonathan Rauch, "For Better or Worse? The Case for Gay (and Straight) Marriage," *The New Republic* (6 May 1996): 18–23.
[7]Rauch, "For Better or Worse?"

of its public, shared meaning: Marriage is the place where having children is not only tolerated but welcomed and encouraged, because it gives children mothers and fathers. . . . The problem with endorsing gay marriage is not that it would allow a handful of people to choose alternative family forms, but that it would require society at large to gut marriage of its central presumptions about family in order to accommodate a few adults' desires.[8]

Critics of this reasoning reply that the traditional notion of marriage preferred by Gallagher and others is too narrow. Procreation is just one of several aims of marriage. This is how Rauch makes the point:

> For the record, I would be the last to deny that children are one central reason for the privileged status of marriage. When men and women get together, children are a likely outcome; and, as we are learning in ever more unpleasant ways, when children grow up without two parents, trouble ensues. Children are not a trivial reason for marriage; they just cannot be the only reason.
>
> What are the others? It seems to me that the two strongest candidates are these: domesticating men and providing reliable caregivers. Both purposes are critical to the functioning of a humane and stable society, and both are much better served by marriage—that is, by one-to-one lifelong commitment—than by any other institution.[9]

These other purposes, Rauch says, can be realized through both same-sex and heterosexual marriage, so there is no reason to bar homosexual couples from this important social practice.

Some argue for the same conclusion another way. They doubt that procreation is the essential function of marriage because our civil marriage laws do not require procreation or fertility to be a necessary part of marriage. People who are infertile or who cannot or will not consummate their marriage may legally marry as easily as anyone else.

[8]Gallagher, "What Marriage Is For."
[9]Rauch, "For Better or Worse?"

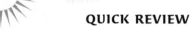

QUICK REVIEW

same-sex marriage—Marriage, in the full legal sense, of gay and lesbian couples.

Defense of Marriage Act—A law passed by Congress in 1996 forbidding the federal government to recognize same-sex marriages, effectively denying federal benefits to gay and lesbian marriages.

SUMMARY

Same-sex marriage is marriage—in the full legal sense—of gay and lesbian couples. The central moral question is, Should same-sex couples be permitted to enter into marriage of this kind?

Arguments against same-sex marriage concentrate on four themes: (1) Same-sex marriage is contrary to custom, tradition, or nature; (2) it's a distortion of the true meaning or essence of marriage; (3) it's wrong because homosexuality is wrong; and (4) the consequences of allowing same-sex marriage would be dangerous or harmful. Proponents generally argue that (1) permitting same-sex marriage is a matter of justice, which demands equal treatment and equal opportunity for all, or (2) allowing it would be beneficial both to homosexuals and society as a whole.

The Roman Catholic account of natural law theory condemns same-sex marriage, just as it condemns homosexuality. Kant's theory may sanction same-sex marriages on the grounds that allowing the practice entails respect for persons. Consequentialism can be interpreted to support or reject same-sex marriage, depending on how the consequences are reckoned.

Some appeal to tradition to argue against same-sex marriage. Others argue against it by insisting that it is an abandonment of the true meaning of marriage. Marriage is for procreation and child-rearing, but same-sex couples cannot procreate. The main counterargument is that marriage has several purposes beyond procreation, and same-sex couples can participate in these as well as heterosexual couples can.

On Gay Rights

RICHARD D. MOHR

I. WHO ARE GAYS ANYWAY?

A recent Gallup poll found that only one in five Americans reports having a gay acquaintance. This finding is extraordinary given the number of practicing homosexuals in America. Alfred Kinsey's 1948 study of the sex lives of 5000 white males shocked the nation: 37 percent had at least one homosexual experience to orgasm in their adult lives; an additional 13 percent had homosexual fantasies to orgasm; 4 percent were exclusively homosexual in their practices; another 5 percent had virtually no heterosexual experience, and nearly 20 percent had at least as many homosexual as heterosexual experiences. With only slight variations, these figures held across all social categories: region, religion, political belief, class, income, occupation, and education.

Two out of five men one passes on the street have had orgasmic sex with men. Every second family in the country has a member who is essentially homosexual, and many more people regularly have homosexual experiences. Who are homosexuals? They are your friends, your minister, your teacher, your bankteller, your doctor, your mailcarrier, your secretary, your congressional representative, your sibling, parent, and spouse. They are everywhere, virtually all ordinary, virtually all unknown.

What follows? First, the country is profoundly ignorant of the actual experience of gay people. Second, social attitudes and practices that are harmful to gays have a much greater overall negative impact on society than is usually realized. Third, most gay people live in hiding—in the closet—making the "coming out" experience the central fixture of gay consciousness and invisibility the chief social characteristic of gays.

II. IGNORANCE, STEREOTYPE, AND MORALITY

Society's ignorance of gay people is, however, not limited to individuals' lack of personal acquaintance with gays. Stigma against gay people is so strong that even discussions of homosexuality are taboo. This taboo is particularly strong in academe, where it is reinforced by the added fear of the teacher as molester. So even within the hearth of reason irrational forces have held virtually unchallenged and largely unchallengeable sway. The usual sort of clarifying research that might be done on a stigmatized minority has with gays only just begun—haltingly—in history, literature, sociology, and the sciences.

Yet ignorance about gays has not stopped people from having strong opinions about them. The void which ignorance leaves has been filled with stereotypes. Society holds chiefly two groups of antigay stereotypes; the two are an oddly contradictory lot. One set of stereotypes revolves around alleged mistakes in an individual's gender identity: lesbians are women that want to be, or at least look and act like, men—bulldykes, diesel dykes; while gay men are those who want to be, or at least look and act like, women—queens, fairies, limp-wrists, nellies. Gays are "queer," which, remember, means at root not merely weird but chiefly counterfeit—"he's as queer as a three dollar bill." These stereotypes of mismatched or fraudulent genders provide the materials through which gays and lesbians become the butts of ethnic-like jokes. These stereotypes and jokes, though derisive, basically view gays and lesbians as ridiculous.

Another set of stereotypes revolves around gays as a pervasive, sinister, conspiratorial, and corruptive threat. The core stereotype here is the gay person as child molester and, more generally, as sex-crazed maniac. These stereotypes carry with them fears of the very destruction of family and civilization itself. Now, that which is essentially ridiculous can hardly have such a staggering effect. Something must be afoot in this incoherent amalgam.

Sense can be made of this incoherence if the nature of stereotypes is clarified. Stereotypes are not *simply* false generalizations from a skewed sample of cases examined. Admittedly, false generalizing plays a part in most stereotypes a society holds. If, for instance, one takes as one's sample homosexuals who are in psychiatric hospitals or prisons, as was done in nearly all early investigations, not surprisingly one will probably find homosexuals to be of a crazed and criminal cast. Such false generalizations, though, simply confirm beliefs already held on independent grounds, ones that likely led the investigator to the prison and psychiatric ward to begin with. Evelyn Hooker, who in the mid-fifties carried out the first rigorous studies to use nonclinical gays, found that psychiatrists, when presented with results of standard psychological diagnostic tests—but with indications of sexual orientation omitted—were able to do no better than if they had guessed randomly in their attempts to distinguish gay files from nongay ones, even though the psychiatrists believed gays to be crazy and supposed themselves to be experts in detecting craziness. These studies provided a foundation embarrassment to the psychiatric establishment, the financial well-being of which was substantially enhanced by 'curing' allegedly insane gays. Eventually the studies contributed to the American Psychiatric Association's dropping homosexuality from its registry of mental illnesses in 1973. Nevertheless, the stereotype of gays as sick continues apace in the mind of America.

False generalizations *help maintain* stereotypes; they do not *form* them. As the history of Hooker's discoveries shows, stereotypes have a life beyond facts. Their origin lies in a culture's ideology—the general system of beliefs by which it lives—and they are sustained across generations by diverse cultural transmissions, hardly any of which, including slang and jokes, even purport to have a scientific basis. Stereotypes, then, are not the products of bad science, but are social constructions that perform central functions in maintaining society's conception of itself.

On this understanding, it is easy to see that the antigay stereotypes surrounding gender identification are chiefly means of reinforcing still powerful gender roles in society. If, as this stereotype presumes (and condemns), one is free to choose one's social roles independently of gender, many guiding social divisions, both domestic and commercial, might be threatened. The socially gender-linked distinctions would blur between breadwinner and homemaker, protector and protected, boss and secretary, doctor and nurse, priest and nun, hero and whore, saint and siren, lord and helpmate, and God and his world. The accusations "fag" and "dyke" (which recent philology has indeed shown to be rooted in slang referring to gender-bending, especially cross-dressing) exist in significant part to keep women in their place and to prevent men from breaking ranks and ceding away theirs.

The stereotypes of gays as child molesters, sex-crazed maniacs, and civilization destroyers function to displace (socially irresolvable) problems from their actual source to a foreign (and so, it is thought, manageable) one. Thus, the stereotype of child molester functions to give the family unit a false sheen of absolute innocence. It keeps the unit from being examined too closely for incest, child abuse, wife-battering, and the terrorism of constant threats. The stereotype teaches that the problems of the family are not internal to it, but external.

Because this stereotype has this central social function, it could not be dislodged even by empirical studies, paralleling Hooker's efforts, that showed heterosexuals to be child molesters to a far greater extent than the actual occurrence of heterosexuals in the general population. But one need not even be aware of such debunking empirical studies in order to see the same cultural forces at work in the social belief that gays are molesters as in its belief that they are crazy. For one can see them now in society's and the media's treatment of current reports of violence, especially domestic violence. When a mother kills her child or a father rapes his daughter—regular Section B fare even in major urbane papers—this is never taken by reporters, columnists, or pundits as evidence that there is something wrong with heterosexuality or with traditional families. These issues are not even raised.

But when a homosexual child molestation is reported it is taken as confirming evidence of the way homosexuals are. One never hears of heterosexual murders, but one regularly reads of "homosexual" ones. Compare the social treatment of Richard Speck's sexually motivated mass murder in 1966 of Chicago nurses with that of John Wayne Gacy's serial murders of Chicago youths. Gacy was in the culture's mind taken as symbolic of gay men in general. To prevent the possibility that The Family was viewed as anything but an innocent victim in this affair, the mainstream press knowingly failed to mention that most of Gacy's adolescent victims were homeless hustlers, even though this was made obvious at his trial. That knowledge would be too much for the six o'clock news and for cherished beliefs.

The stereotype of gays as sex-crazed maniacs functions socially to keep individuals' sexuality contained. For this stereotype makes it look as though the problem of how to address one's considerable sexual drives can and should be answered with repression, for it gives the impression that the cyclone of dangerous psychic forces is *out there* where the fags are, not within one's own breast. With the decline of the stereotype of the black man as raping pillaging marauder (found in such works as *Birth of a Nation, Gone with the Wind,* and *Soul on Ice*), the stereotype of gay men as sex-crazed maniacs has become more aggravated. The stereotype of the sex-crazed threat seems one that society desperately needs to have somewhere in its sexual cosmology.

For the repressed homosexual, this stereotype has an especially powerful allure—by hating it consciously, he subconsciously appears to save himself from himself, at least as long as the ruse does not exhaust the considerable psychic energies required to maintain it, or until, like ultraconservative Congressman Robert E. Bauman (R-Md.) and Jon C. Hinson (R-Miss.), he is caught importuning hustlers or gentlemen in washrooms. If, as Freud and some of his followers thought, everyone feels an urge for sex partners of both genders, then the fear of gays works to show us that we have not "met the enemy and he is us."

By directly invoking sex acts, this second set of stereotypes is the more severe and serious of the two—one never hears child-molester jokes. These stereotypes are aimed chiefly against men, as in turn stereotypically the more sexed of the genders. They are particularly divisive for they create a very strong division between those conceived as "us" and those conceived as "them." This divide is not so strong in the case of the stereotype of gay men as effeminate. For women (and so the woman-like) after all do have their place. Nonstrident, nonuppity useful ones can even be part of "us," indeed, belong, like "our children," to "us." Thus, in many cultures with overweening gender-identified social roles (like prisons, truckstops, the armed forces, Latin America, and the Islamic world) only passive partners in male couplings are derided as homosexual.

Because "the facts" largely do not matter when it comes to the generation and maintenance of stereotypes, the effects of scientific and academic research and of enlightenment generally will be, at best, slight and gradual in the changing fortunes of gays. If this account of stereotypes holds, society has been profoundly immoral. For its treatment of gays is a grand scale rationalization and moral sleight-of-hand. The problem is not that society's usual standards of evidence and procedure in coming to judgments of social policy have been misapplied to gays, rather when it comes to gays, the standards themselves have simply been ruled out of court and disregarded in favor of mechanisms that encourage unexamined fear and hatred.

III. ARE GAYS DISCRIMINATED AGAINST? DOES IT MATTER?

Partly because lots of people suppose they do not know a gay person and partly through their willful ignorance of society's workings, people are largely unaware of the many ways in which gays are subject to discrimination in consequence of widespread fear and hatred. Contributing to this social ignorance of discrimination is the difficulty for gay people, as an invisible minority, even to complain of discrimination. For if one is gay, to register a complaint would suddenly target one as a stigmatized person, and so, in the absence of any protections against discrimination, would in turn invite additional discrimination.

Further, many people, especially those who are persistently downtrodden and so lack a firm sense of self to begin with, tend either to blame themselves for their troubles or to view their troubles as a matter of bad luck or as the result of an innocent mistake by others—as anything but an injustice indicating something wrong with society. Alfred Dreyfus went to his grave believing his imprisonment for treason and his degradation from the French military, in which he was the highest ranking Jewish officer, had all just been a sort of clerical error, merely requiring recomputation, rather than what it was—lightning striking a promontory from out of a storm of national bigotry. The recognition of injustice requires doing something to rectify wrong; the recognition of systematic injustices requires doing something about the system, and most people, especially the already beleaguered, simply are not up to the former, let alone the latter.

For a number of reasons, then, discrimination against gays, like rape, goes seriously underreported. What do they experience? First, gays are subject to violence and harassment based simply on their perceived status rather than because of any actions they have performed. A recent extensive study by the National Gay and Lesbian Task Force found that over 90 percent of gays and lesbians had been victimized in some form on the basis of their sexual orientation. Greater than one in five gay men and nearly one in ten lesbians had been punched, hit, or kicked; a quarter of all gays had had objects thrown at them; a third had been chased; a third had been sexually harassed and 14 percent had been spit on—all just for being perceived to be gay.

The most extreme form of antigay violence is queerbashing—where groups of young men target another man who they suppose is gay and beat and kick him unconscious and sometimes to death amid a torrent of taunts and slurs. Such seemingly random but in reality socially encouraged violence has the same social origin and function as lynchings of blacks—to keep a whole stigmatized group in line. As with lynchings of the recent past, the police and courts have routinely averted their eyes, giving their implicit approval to the practice.

Few such cases with gay victims reach the courts. Those that do are marked by inequitable procedures and results. Frequently judges will describe queerbashers as "just All-American Boys." In 1984, a District of Columbia judge handed suspended sentences to queerbashers whose victim had been stalked, beaten, stripped at knife point, slashed, kicked, threatened with castration, and pissed on, because the judge thought the bashers were good boys at heart—after all they went to a religious prep school.

In the summer of 1984, three teenagers hurled a gay man to his death from a bridge in Bangor, Maine. Though the youths could have been tried as adults and normally would have been, given the extreme violence of their crime, they were tried rather as children and will be back on the streets again automatically when they turn twenty-one.

Further, police and juries simply discount testimony from gays. They typically construe assaults on and murders of gays as "justified" self-defense—the killer need only claim his act was a panicked response to a sexual overture. Alternatively, when guilt seems patent, juries will accept highly implausible insanity or other "diminished capacity" defenses. In 1981 a former New York City Transit Authority policeman, later claiming he was just doing the work of God, machine-gunned down nine people, killing two, in two Greenwich Village gay bars. His jury found him innocent due to mental illness. The best known example of a successful "diminished capacity" defense is Dan White's voluntary manslaughter conviction for the 1978 assassination of openly gay San Francisco city councilman Harvey Milk—Hostess Twinkies, his lawyer successfully argued, made him do it.

These inequitable procedures and results collectively show that the life and liberty of gays, like those of blacks, simply count for less than the life and liberty of members of the dominant culture.

The equitable role of law is the heart of an orderly society. The collapse of the rule of law for gays shows that society is willing to perpetrate the worst possible injustices against them. Conceptually there is a difference only in degree between the collapse of the rule of law and systematic extermination of members of a population simply for having some group status independent of any act an individual has performed. In the Nazi concentration camps, gays were forced to wear pink triangles as identifying badges, just as Jews were forced to wear yellow stars. In remembrance of that collapse of the rule of law, the pink triangle has become the chief symbol of the gay rights movement.

Gays have been widely subject to discrimination in employment—the very means by which one puts bread on one's table and one of the chief means by which a person identifies himself to himself and achieves individual dignity. Governments are leading offenders here. They do a lot of discriminating themselves. They require that others, like government contractors, do it, and they set precedents and establish models favoring discrimination in the private sector. The federal government explicitly discriminates against gays in the armed forces, the CIA, the FBI, the National Security Agency, and the state department. The federal government refuses to give security clearances to gays and so forces the country's considerable private-sector military and aerospace contractors to fire known gay employees. State and local governments regularly fire gay teachers, police and fire personnel, social workers, and anyone who has contact with the public. Further, states through licensing laws officially bar gays from a vast array of occupations and professions—everything from doctors, lawyers, accountants, and nurses to hairdressers, morticians, and used car dealers. The American Civil Liberties Union's handbook *The Rights of Gay People* (1975) lists 307 such prohibited occupations.

Gays are subject to discrimination in a wide variety of other ways, including private-sector employment, public accommodations, housing, immigration and naturalization, insurance of all types, custody and adoption, and zoning regulations that bar "singles" or "non-related" couples. All of these discriminations affect central components of a meaningful life; some even reach to the means by which life itself is sustained. In half the states, where gay sex is illegal, the central role of sex to meaningful life is officially denied to gays.

All these sorts of discriminations also affect the ability of people to have significant intimate relations. It is difficult for people to live together as couples without having their sexual orientation perceived in the public realm and so becoming targets for discrimination. Illegality, discrimination, and the absorption by gays of society's hatred of them—all interact to impede or block altogether the ability of gays and lesbians to create and maintain significant personal relations with loved ones. So every facet of life is affected by discrimination. Only the most compelling reasons could justify it.

IV. BUT AREN'T THEY IMMORAL?

Many people think society's treatment of gays is justified because gays are extremely immoral. To evaluate this claim, different senses of "moral" must be distinguished. Sometimes by "morality" is meant the overall beliefs affecting behavior in a society—its current mores, norms, and customs. On this understanding, gays certainly are not moral: lots of people hate them and social customs are designed to register widespread disapproval of gays. The problem here is that this sense of morality is merely a *descriptive* one. On this understanding of what morality is, *every* society has a morality—even Nazi society, which had racism and mob rule as central features of its popular "morality." What is needed in order to use the notion of morality to praise or condemn behavior is a sense of morality that is *prescriptive* or *normative*—what is needed is a sense of morality whereby, for instance, the descriptive morality of the Nazis is found wanting.

Moral thinking that carries a prescriptive or normative force has certain basic ground rules to which all people consent when attention is drawn to them. First, normative moral beliefs are not merely expressions of feelings. Rather we—normatively moral agents—both expect and are expected to be able to give reasons or justifications for them. We suspect that beliefs, especially strongly held ones, for which no reasons or justifications can be tendered, are mere expressions of phobias and neuroses. Second, moral thinking must be consistent and fair—we must recognize that our specific moral beliefs commit us to general moral principles in light of which we must be willing to treat relevantly similar cases similarly. Third, we must avoid prejudice and rationalization: we must be willing to apply to ourselves the same rules and standards of evidence and argument that we apply to others. And we must avoid being so peculiar and particular in the scope of our principles that we stand accused of being whimsical and arbitrary in picking them.

Even from this sketch of minimum requirements of a critical or normative morality, it should be clear that something's being descriptively moral or immoral is nowhere near enough to make it normatively moral or immoral. For one of our principles itself is that simply a lot of people's saying something is good, even over eons, does not make it so. Our rejection of the long history of socially approved and state-enforced slavery is a good example of this principle at work. Slavery would be wrong even if nearly everyone liked it. So consistency and fairness requires that the culture abandon the belief that gays are immoral simply because most people dislike or disapprove of gays or gay acts, or even because gay sex acts are illegal.

Further, recent historical and anthropological research has shown that opinion about gays has been by no means universally negative. Historically, it has varied widely even within the larger part of the Christian era and even within the Church itself. There are even societies—current ones—where homosexuality is not only tolerated but even a universal and compulsory part of social maturation. Society holds its current descriptive morality of gays not because it has to, but because it chooses to. Within the last thirty years, American society has undergone a grand turnabout from deeply ingrained, near total condemnation to near total acceptance on two emotionally charged "moral" or "family" issues: adult contraception and divorce. America could do the same with homosexuality if it thought to.

If popular opinion and custom are not enough to ground moral condemnation of homosexuality, perhaps religion can. Such argument proceeds along two lines. One claims that the condemnation is a direct revelation of God, usually through the Bible; the other claims to be able to detect condemnation in God's plan as manifested in nature.

One of the more remarkable discoveries of recent gay research is that the Bible may not be as univocal in its condemnation of homosexuality as has been usually believed. Christ never mentions homosexuality. Recent interpreters of the Old Testament have pointed out that the story of Lot at Sodom is probably intended to condemn inhospitality rather than homosexuality. Further, some of the Old Testament condemnations of homosexuality seem simply to be ways of tarring those of the Israelites' opponents who happen to accept homosexual practices when the Israelites themselves did not. If so, the condemnation is merely a quirk of history and rhetoric rather than a moral precept. All of this is hotly contested, and the debate continues.

What does seem clear, though, is that those who regularly cite the Bible to condemn an activity like homosexuality do so by reading it selectively. Do ministers who cite what they take to be condemnations of homosexuality in Leviticus maintain in their lives all the hygienic and dietary laws of Leviticus? If they cite the story of Lot at Sodom to condemn homosexuality, do they also cite the story of Lot in the Cave to praise incestuous rape? If not, they may be hypocrites (against whom Christ frequently riles) [sic], but more importantly they violate the normatively moral notions of consistency and fairness—unless of course they can cite some higher principle which generates exceptions to the (now) lower level principle: obey the Bible. But what could that be? It seems then not that the Bible is being used to ground condemnations of homosexuality as much as society's dislike of homosexuality is being used to interpret the Bible.

Even if a consistent portrait of condemnation could be gleaned from the Bible, what social significance should it be given? One of the guiding principles of society, enshrined in the Constitution as a check against the government, is that decisions affecting social policy are not made on religious grounds. If the real ground of the alleged immorality invoked by governments to discriminate against gays is religious, then one of the major commitments of our nation is violated. But this principle is widely accepted as holding even beyond government. Usually one does not pick one's friends and acquaintances according to their religious beliefs or their accidental conformity to one's own religious tenets. And this is so because in America people deeply believe that one's religious life is a private matter. Indeed, one has to have built up a relationship of friendly trust with another for the question of religious beliefs even to be broached. No one (other than someone who is despicable on other grounds) points out with pride one's membership in a club that excludes Jews or Catholics—even where the exclusion is legal. People recognize that holding others accountable for religious beliefs is properly a source of shame, even if they go ahead and do it anyway. In respecting religious privacy, then, one does not hold others accountable to the beliefs one holds *solely* on religious grounds. Those who invoke religious sentiments for their attitudes toward gays, then, need to examine whether their religious beliefs are here not really a disguise for some animus for which they have no reasons.

V. BUT AREN'T THEY UNNATURAL?

The most noteworthy feature of the accusation of something being unnatural (where a moral rather than an advertising point is being made) is that the plaint is being made so infrequently. One used to hear the charge leveled against abortion, but it has dropped from public discourse as anti-abortionists have come to lay their chips on the hope that people in general will come to view abortion as murder. Incest used to be considered unnatural but discourse now usually assimilates it to the moral machinery of rape and violated trust. The charge comes up now in ordinary discourse only against homosexuality. This social pattern suggests that the charge is highly idiosyncratic and has little, if any, explanatory force. It fails to put homosexuality in a class with anything else so that one can learn by comparison with clear cases of the class just what exactly it is that is allegedly wrong with it. Nor is homosexuality even a paradigm case for a class of unnatural acts. In popular morality, the charge that homosexuality is immoral because unnatural appeals to a principle so narrow as to be arbitrary.

What the charge of unnaturalness lacks in moral content is compensated for by the emotional thrust with which it is delivered. In ordinary discourse, when the accusation of unnaturalness is applied to homosexuality, it is usually delivered with venom of forethought. It carries a high emotional charge, usually

expressing disgust and evincing queasiness. Probably it has no content other than its expression of emotional aversion. For people get equally disgusted and queasy at all sorts of things that are perfectly natural—to be expected in nature apart from artifice—and that could hardly be fit subjects for moral condemnation. Two examples from current American culture are some people's responses to mothers suckling in public and to women who do not shave body hair. When people have strong emotional reactions, as they do in these cases, without being able to give good reasons for the reactions, one thinks of them not as operating morally and certainly not as grounding a morality for others, but rather as being obsessed and manic. So the feelings of disgust that some people have to gays will hardly ground a charge of immorality. People fling the term "unnatural" against gays in the same breath and with the same force as calling gays "sick" and "gross," and when they do this, they give every appearance of being neurotically fearful, while at the same time violating the moral principle that one needs justifying reasons for moral beliefs.

When "nature" is taken in *technical* rather than ordinary usages, it looks like the notion also will not ground a charge of homosexual immorality. When unnatural means "by artifice" or "made by man," one need only point out that virtually everything that is good about life is unnatural in this sense, that one feature that distinguished people from most other animals is people's ability to make over the world to meet their needs and desires, and that people's well-being depends upon these departures from nature. On this understanding of the natural and people's nature, homosexuality is perfectly unobjectionable.

Another technical sense of natural is that something is natural, and so good, if it fulfills some function in nature. Homosexuality in this view is unnatural because it allegedly violates the function of genitals, which is to produce babies. One problem with this view is that lots of bodily parts have lots of functions and just because some one activity can be fulfilled by only one organ (say, the mouth for eating) this activity does not condemn other functions of the organ to immorality (say, the mouth for talking, licking stamps, blowing bubbles, or having sex). So the possible use of the genitals to produce children does not, without more, condemn the use of the genitals for other purposes, say, achieving ecstasy and intimacy.

The functional view of nature will provide a morally condemnatory sense to the unnatural only if a thing which might have many uses has but one proper function to the exclusion of all other possible functions. But whether this is so cannot be established simply by looking at the thing. For what is seen is all its possible functions: "it's a stamp-licker," "no, its a talker," "no, it's a bubble-blower," "no, it's a sex organ." It was thought that the notion of function might ground moral authority, but instead it turns out that moral authority is needed to define proper function.

Some people try to fill in this moral authority by appeal to the "design" or "order" of an organ, saying, for instance, that the genitals are designed for the purpose of procreation. But these people intellectually cheat if they fail to make explicit *who* the designer and orderer is. If it is God, the discussion is back to square one—they are holding others accountable for religious beliefs.

Further, ordinary moral attitudes about child-rearing will not provide the needed supplement which in conjunction with the natural-function view of bodily parts would produce a positive obligation to use the genitals for procreation. Society's attitude toward a childless couple is that of pity, not censure—even if the couple could have children. The pity may be an unsympathetic one—that is, not registering a course one would choose *for oneself*—but this does not make it a course one would *require* of others. The couple who discovers they cannot have children are viewed not as having thereby had a debt canceled, but rather as having to forgo some of the richness of life, just as a quadriplegic is not viewed as absolved from some moral obligation to hop, skip, and jump, but is viewed as missing some of the richness of life. Consistency requires, then, that, at most, gays who do not or cannot have children are to be pitied rather than condemned. What *is* immoral is the willful preventing of people from achieving the richness of life. Immorality in this regard lies with those social customs, regulations, and statutes that prevent lesbians and gay men from establishing blood or adoptive families, not with gays themselves.

Sometimes people attempt to establish authority for a moral obligation to use certain bodily parts in only one way simply by claiming that moral laws are natural laws and vice versa. On this account, inanimate objects and plants are good in that they follow natural laws by necessity, animals by instinct, and persons by a rational will. People are special in that they must first discover the laws that govern the species. Now, even if one believes the view—dubious in the post-Newtonian, post-Darwinian world—that natural laws in the usual sense ($e = mc^2$, for instance) have some moral content, it is not at all clear how one is to discover the laws in nature that apply to people.

If, on the one hand, one looks to people themselves for a model—and looks hard enough—one finds amazing variety, including homosexual behavior as a social ideal (upper-class fifty-century B.C. Athenians) and even as socially mandatory (Melanesia today). When one looks to people, one is simply unable to strip away the layers of social custom, history, and taboo in order to see what's really there to any degree more specific than that people are the creatures which make over their world and are capable of abstract thought.

Most people, though, do not even try to see *what's there* but instead simply and by default end up projecting the peculiarities of their culture into the universe as cosmic principles. Anthropology has shown that each and every society—however much it may differ from the next—thinks that its own central norms are dictated by and conform with nature writ large. That this is so should raise doubts that neutral principles are to be found in man's nature that will condemn homosexuality. Man may very well be, as Hannah Arendt claimed, the creature whose nature it is to have no nature. It is by virtue of this human condition that people can be creative and make moral progress.

On the other hand, if for models one looks to nature apart from people, the possibilities are staggering. There are fish that change gender over their lifetimes: should people "follow nature" and be operative transsexuals? Orangutans, genetically our next of kin, live completely solitary lives without social organization of any kind: ought people to "follow nature" and be hermits? There are many species where only two

members per generation reproduce: shall we be bees? The search in nature for people's purpose, far from finding sure models for action, is likely to leave people morally rudderless.

What Marriage Is For: Children Need Mothers and Fathers
Maggie Gallagher

Gay marriage is no longer a theoretical issue. Canada has it. Massachusetts is expected to get it any day. The Goodridge decision there could set off a legal, political, and cultural battle in the courts of 50 states and in the U.S. Congress. Every politician, every judge, every citizen has to decide: Does same-sex marriage matter? If so, how and why?

The timing could not be worse. Marriage is in crisis, as everyone knows: High rates of divorce and illegitimacy have eroded marriage norms and created millions of fatherless children, whole neighborhoods where lifelong marriage is no longer customary, driving up poverty, crime, teen pregnancy, welfare dependency, drug abuse, and mental and physical health problems. And yet, amid the broader negative trends, recent signs point to a modest but significant recovery.

Divorce rates appear to have declined a little from historic highs; illegitimacy rates, after doubling every decade from 1960 to 1990, appear to have leveled off, albeit at a high level (33 percent of American births are to unmarried women); teen pregnancy and sexual activity are down; the proportion of homemaking mothers is up; marital fertility appears to be on the rise. Research suggests that married adults are more committed to marital permanence than they were twenty years ago. A new generation of children of divorce appears on the brink of making a commitment to life-

long marriage. In 1977, 55 percent of American teenagers thought a divorce should be harder to get; in 2001, 75 percent did.

A new marriage movement—a distinctively American phenomenon—has been born. The scholarly consensus on the importance of marriage has broadened and deepened; it is now the conventional wisdom among child welfare organizations. As a Child Trends research brief summed up: "Research clearly demonstrates that family structure matters for children, and the family structure that helps children the most is a family headed by two biological parents in a low-conflict marriage. Children in single-parent families, children born to unmarried mothers, and children in stepfamilies or cohabiting relationships face higher risks of poor outcomes. . . . There is thus value for children in promoting strong, stable marriages between biological parents."

What will court-imposed gay marriage do to this incipient recovery of marriage? For, even as support for marriage in general has been rising, the gay marriage debate has proceeded on a separate track. Now the time has come to decide: Will unisex marriage help or hurt marriage as a social institution?

Why should it do either, some may ask? How can Bill and Bob's marriage hurt Mary and Joe? In an exchange with me in the just-released book "Marriage and Same Sex Unions: A Debate," Evan Wolfson, chief legal strategist for same-sex marriage in the Hawaii case, Baer v. Lewin, argues that there is "enough marriage to share." What counts, he says, "is not family

Maggie Gallagher, "What Marriage Is For: Children Need Mothers and Fathers," from *The Weekly Standard*, August 4, 2003, Vol. 8, Issue 45, 22–25. Reprinted with permission from the Weekly Standard.

structure, but the quality of dedication, commitment, self-sacrifice, and love in the household."

Family structure does not count. Then what is marriage for? Why have laws about it? Why care whether people get married or stay married? Do children need mothers and fathers, or will any sort of family do? When the sexual desires of adults clash with the interests of children, which carries more weight, socially and legally?

These are the questions that same-sex marriage raises. Our answers will affect not only gay and lesbian families, but marriage as a whole.

In ordering gay marriage on June 10, 2003, the highest court in Ontario, Canada, explicitly endorsed a brand new vision of marriage along the lines Wolfson suggests: "Marriage is, without dispute, one of the most significant forms of personal relationships. . . . Through the institution of marriage, individuals can publicly express their love and commitment to each other. Through this institution, society publicly recognizes expressions of love and commitment between individuals, granting them respect and legitimacy as a couple."

The Ontario court views marriage as a kind of Good Housekeeping Seal of Approval that government stamps on certain registered intimacies because, well, for no particular reason the court can articulate except that society likes to recognize expressions of love and commitment. In this view, endorsement of gay marriage is a no-brainer, for nothing really important rides on whether anyone gets married or stays married. Marriage is merely individual expressive conduct, and there is no obvious reason why some individuals' expression of gay love should hurt other individuals' expressions of non-gay love.

There is, however, a different view—indeed, a view that is radically opposed to this: Marriage is the fundamental, cross-cultural institution for bridging the male-female divide so that children have loving, committed mothers and fathers. Marriage is inherently normative: It is about holding out a certain kind of relationship as a social ideal, especially when there are children involved. Marriage is not simply an artifact of law; neither is it a mere delivery mechanism for a set of legal benefits that might as well be shared more broadly. The laws of marriage do not create marriage, but in societies ruled by law they help trace the boundaries and sustain the public meanings of marriage.

In other words, while individuals freely choose to enter marriage, society upholds the marriage option, formalizes its definition, and surrounds it with norms and reinforcements, so we can raise boys and girls who aspire to become the kind of men and women who can make successful marriages. Without this shared, public aspect, perpetuated generation after generation, marriage becomes what its critics say it is: a mere contract, a vessel with no particular content, one of a menu of sexual lifestyles, of no fundamental importance to anyone outside a given relationship.

The marriage idea is that children need mothers and fathers, that societies need babies, and that adults have an obligation to shape their sexual behavior so as to give their children stable families in which to grow up.

Which view of marriage is true? We have seen what has happened in our communities where marriage norms have failed. What has happened is not a flowering of libertarian freedom, but a breakdown of social and civic order that can reach frightening proportions. When law and culture retreat from sustaining the marriage idea, individuals cannot create marriage on their own.

In a complex society governed by positive law, social institutions require both social and legal support. To use an analogy, the government does not create private property. But to make a market system a reality requires the assistance of law as well as culture. People have to be raised to respect the property of others, and to value the traits of entrepreneurship, and to be law-abiding generally. The law cannot allow individuals to define for themselves what private property (or law-abiding conduct) means. The boundaries of certain institutions (such as the corporation) also need to be defined legally, and the definitions become socially shared knowledge. We need a shared system of meaning, publicly enforced, if market-based economies are to do their magic and individuals are to maximize their opportunities.

Successful social institutions generally function without people's having to think very much about how they work. But when a social institution is contested—as marriage is today—it becomes critically important to think and speak clearly about its public meanings.

Again, what is marriage for? Marriage is a virtually universal human institution. In all the wildly rich and various cultures flung throughout the ecosphere, in society after society, whether tribal or complex, and however bizarre, human beings have created systems of publicly approved sexual union between men and women that entail well-defined responsibilities of mothers and fathers. Not all these marriage systems look like our own, which is rooted in a fusion of Greek, Roman, Jewish, and Christian culture. Yet everywhere, in isolated mountain valleys, parched deserts, jungle thickets, and broad plains, people have come up with some version of this thing called marriage. Why?

Because sex between men and women makes babies, that's why. Even today, in our technologically advanced contraceptive culture, half of all pregnancies are unintended: Sex between men and women still makes babies. Most men and woman are powerfully drawn to perform a sexual act that can and does generate life. Marriage is our attempt to reconcile and harmonize the erotic, social, sexual, and financial needs of men and women with the needs of their partner and their children.

How to reconcile the needs of children with the sexual desires of adults? Every society has to face that question, and some resolve it in ways that inflict horrendous cruelty on children born outside marriage. Some cultures decide these children don't matter: Men can have all the sex they want, and any children they create outside of marriage will be throwaway kids; marriage is for citizens—slaves and peasants need not apply. You can see a version of this elitist vision of marriage emerging in America under cover of acceptance of family diversity. Marriage will continue to exist as the social advantage of elite communities. The poor and the working class? Who cares whether their kids have dads? We can always import people from abroad to fill our need for disciplined, educated workers.

Our better tradition, and the only one consistent with democratic principles, is to hold up a single ideal for all parents, which is ultimately based on our deep cultural commitment to the equal dignity and social worth of all children. All kids need and deserve a married mom and dad. All parents are supposed to at least try to behave in ways that will give their own children this important protection. Privately, religiously, emotionally, individually, marriage may have many meanings. But this is the core of its public, shared meaning: Marriage is the place where having children is not only tolerated but welcomed and encouraged, because it gives children mothers and fathers.

Of course, many couples fail to live up to this ideal. Many of the things men and women have to do to sustain their own marriages, and a culture of marriage, are hard. Few people will do them consistently if the larger culture does not affirm the critical importance of marriage as a social institution. Why stick out a frustrating relationship, turn down a tempting new love, abstain from sex outside marriage, or even take pains not to conceive children out of wedlock if family structure does not matter? If marriage is not a shared norm, and if successful marriage is not socially valued, do not expect it to survive as the generally accepted context for raising children. If marriage is just a way of publicly celebrating private love, then there is no need to encourage couples to stick it out for the sake of the children. If family structure does not matter, why have marriage laws at all? Do adults, or do they not, have a basic obligation to control their desires so that children can have mothers and fathers?

The problem with endorsing gay marriage is not that it would allow a handful of people to choose alternative family forms, but that it would require society at large to gut marriage of its central presumptions about family in order to accommodate a few adults' desires.

The debate over same-sex marriage, then, is not some sideline discussion. It is the marriage debate. Either we win—or we lose the central meaning of marriage. The great threat unisex marriage poses to marriage as a social institution is not some distant or nearby slippery slope, it is an abyss at our feet. If we cannot explain why unisex marriage is, in itself, a disaster, we have already lost the marriage ideal.

Same-sex marriage would enshrine in law a public judgment that the desire of adults for families of choice outweighs the need of children for mothers and fathers. It would give sanction and approval to the creation of a motherless or fatherless family as a deliberately chosen "good." It would mean the law was neutral as to whether children had mothers and fathers. Motherless and fatherless families would be deemed just fine.

Same-sex marriage advocates are startlingly clear on this point. Marriage law, they repeatedly claim, has nothing to do with babies or procreation or getting mothers and fathers for children. In forcing the state legislature to create civil unions for gay couples, the high court of Vermont explicitly ruled that marriage in the state of Vermont has nothing to do with procreation. Evan Wolfson made the same point in "Marriage and Same Sex Unions": "[I]sn't having the law pretend that there is only one family model that works (let alone exists) a lie?" He goes on to say that in law, "marriage is not just about procreation—indeed is not necessarily about procreation at all."

Wolfson is right that in the course of the sexual revolution the Supreme Court struck down many legal features designed to reinforce the connection of marriage to babies. The animus of elites (including legal elites) against the marriage idea is not brand new. It stretches back at least thirty years. That is part of the problem we face, part of the reason 40 percent of our children are growing up without their fathers.

It is also true, as gay-marriage advocates note, that we impose no fertility tests for marriage: Infertile and older couples marry, and not every fertile couple chooses procreation. But every marriage between a man and a woman is capable of giving any child they create or adopt a mother and a father. Every marriage between a man and a woman discourages either from creating fatherless children outside the marriage vow. In this sense, either older married couples nor childless husbands and wives publicly challenge or dilute the core meaning of marriage. Even when a man marries an older woman and they do not adopt, this marriage helps protect children. How? His marriage means, if he keeps his vows, that he will not produce out-of-wedlock children.

Does marriage discriminate against gays and lesbians? Formally speaking, no. There are no sexual-orientation tests for marriage; many gays and lesbians do choose to marry members of the opposite sex, and some of these unions succeed. Our laws do not require a person to marry the individual to whom he or she is most erotically attracted, so long as he or she is willing to promise sexual fidelity, mutual caretaking, and shared parenting of any children of the marriage.

But marriage is unsuited to the wants and desires of many gays and lesbians, precisely because it is designed to bridge the male-female divide and sustain the idea that children need mothers and fathers. To make a marriage, what you need is a husband and a wife. Redefining marriage so that it suits gays and lesbians would require fundamentally changing our legal, public, and social conception of what marriage is in ways that threaten its core public purposes.

Some who criticize the refusal to embrace gay marriage liken it to the outlawing of interracial marriage, but the analogy is woefully false. The Supreme Court overturned anti-miscegenation laws because they frustrated the core purpose of marriage in order to sustain a racist legal order. Marriage laws, by contrast, were not invented to express animus toward homosexuals or anyone else. Their purpose is not negative, but positive: They uphold an institution that developed, over thousands of years, in thousands of cultures, to help direct the erotic desires of men and women into a relatively narrow but indispensably fruitful channel. We need men and women to marry and make babies for our society to survive. We have no similar public stake in any other family form—in the union of same-sex couples or the singleness of single moms.

Meanwhile, cui bono? To meet the desires of whom would we put our most basic social institution at risk? No good research on the marriage intentions of homosexual people exists. For what it's worth, the Census Bureau reports that 0.5 percent of households now consist of same-sex partners. To get a proxy for how many gay couples would avail themselves of the health insurance benefits marriage can provide, I asked the top 10 companies listed on the Human Rights Campaign's website as providing same-sex insurance benefits how many of their employees use this option. Only one company, General Motors, released its data. Out of 1.3 million employees, 166 claimed benefits for a same-sex partner, one one-hundredth of one percent.

People who argue for creating gay marriage do so in the name of high ideals: justice, compassion, fairness. Their sincerity is not in question. Nevertheless, to take the already troubled institution most responsible for the protection of children and throw out its most basic presumption in order to further adult interests in sexual freedom would not be high-minded. It would be morally callous and socially irresponsible.

If we cannot stand and defend this ground, then face it: The marriage debate is over. Dan Quayle was wrong. We lost.

Here Comes the Groom: A (Conservative) Case for Gay Marriage

ANDREW SULLIVAN

Last month in New York, a court ruled that a gay lover had the right to stay in his deceased partner's rent-control apartment because the lover qualified as a member of the deceased's family. The ruling deftly annoyed almost everybody. Conservatives saw judicial activism in favor of gay rent control: three reasons to be appalled. Chastened liberals (such as the *New York Times* editorial page), while endorsing the recognition of gay relationships, also worried about the abuse of already stretched entitlements that the ruling threatened. What neither side quite contemplated is that they both might be right, and that the way to tackle the issue of unconventional relationships in conventional society is to try something both more radical and more conservative than putting courts in the business of deciding what is and is not a family. That alternative is the legalization of civil gay marriage.

The New York rent-control case did not go anywhere near that far, which is the problem. The rent-control regulations merely stipulated that a "family" member had the right to remain in the apartment. The judge ruled that to all intents and purposes a gay lover is part of his lover's family, inasmuch as a "family" merely means an interwoven social life, emotional commitment, and some level of financial interdependence.

It's a principle now well established around the country. Several cities have "domestic partnership" laws, which allow relationships that do not fit into the category of heterosexual marriage to be registered with the city and qualify for benefits that up till now have been reserved for straight married couples. San Francisco, Berkeley, Madison, and Los Angeles all have legislation, as does the politically correct Washington, D.C., suburb, Takoma Park. In these cities, a variety of interpersonal arrangements qualify for health insurance, bereavement leave, insurance, annuity and pension rights, housing rights (such as rent-control apartments), adoption and inheritance rights. Eventually, according to gay lobby groups, the aim is to include federal income tax and veterans' benefits as well. A recent case even involved the right to use a family member's accumulated frequent-flier points. Gays are not the only beneficiaries; heterosexual "live-togethers" also qualify.

There's an argument, of course, that the current legal advantages extended to married people unfairly discriminate against people who've shaped their lives in less conventional arrangements. But it doesn't take a genius to see that enshrining in the law a vague principle like "domestic partnership" is an invitation to qualify at little personal cost for a vast array of entitlements otherwise kept crudely under control.

To be sure, potential DPs have to prove financial interdependence, shared living arrangements, and a commitment to mutual caring. But they don't need to have a sexual relationship or even closely mirror old-style marriage. In principle, an elderly woman and her live-in nurse could qualify. A couple of uneuphemistically confirmed bachelors could be DPs. So could two close college students, a pair of seminarians, or a couple of frat buddies. Left as it is, the concept of domestic partnership could open a Pandora's box of litigation and subjective judicial decision-making about who qualifies. You either are or are not married; it's not a complex question. Whether you are in a "domestic partnership" is not so clear.

More important, the concept of domestic partnership chips away at the prestige of traditional relationships and undermines the priority we give them. This priority is not necessarily a product of heterosexism. Consider heterosexual couples. Society has good reason to extend legal advantages to heterosexuals who choose the formal sanction of marriage over simply living together. They make a deeper commitment to one another and to society; in exchange, society extends certain benefits to them. Marriage provides an anchor, if an arbitrary and weak one, in the chaos of sex and relationships to which we are all prone. It provides a mechanism for emotional stability, economic security, and the healthy rearing of the next generation. We rig the law in its favor not because we disparage all forms of relationship other than the nuclear family, but because we recognize that not to promote marriage would be to ask too much of human virtue. In the context of the weakened family's effect upon the poor, it might also invite social disintegration. One of the worst products of the New Right's "family values" campaign is that its extremism and hatred of diversity has disguised this more measured and more convincing case for the importance of the marital bond.

The concept of domestic partnership ignores these concerns, indeed directly attacks them. This is a pity, since one of its most important objectives—providing some civil recognition for gay relationships—is a noble cause and one completely compatible with the defense of the family. But the way to go about it is not to undermine straight marriage; it is to legalize old-style marriage for gays.

The gay movement has ducked this issue primarily out of fear of division. Much of the gay leadership clings to notions of gay life as essentially outsider, anti-bourgeois, radical. Marriage, for them, is co-optation into straight society. For the Stonewall generation, it is hard to see how this vision of conflict will ever fundamentally change. But for many other gays—my guess, a majority—while they don't deny the importance of rebellion 20 years ago and are grateful for what was done, there's now the sense of a new opportunity. A need to rebel has quietly ceded to a desire to belong. To be gay and to be bourgeois no longer seems such an absurd proposition. Certainly since AIDS, to be gay and to be responsible has become a necessity.

Gay marriage squares several circles at the heart of the domestic partnership debate. Unlike domestic partnership, it allows for recognition of gay relationships, while casting no aspersions on traditional marriage. It merely asks that gays be allowed to join in. Unlike domestic partnership, it doesn't open up avenues for heterosexuals to get benefits without the responsibilities of marriage, or a nightmare of definitional litigation. And unlike domestic partnership, it harnesses to an already established social convention the yearnings for stability and acceptance among a fast-maturing gay community.

Gay marriage also places more responsibilities upon gays; it says for the first time that gay relationships are not better or worse than straight relationships, and that the same is expected of them. And it's clear and dignified. There's a legal benefit to a clear, common symbol of commitment. There's also a personal benefit. One of the ironies of domestic partnership is that it's not only more complicated than marriage, it's more demanding, requiring an elaborate statement of intent to qualify. It amounts to a substantial invasion of privacy. Why, after all, should gays be required to prove commitment before they get married in a way we would never dream of asking of straights?

Legalizing gay marriage would offer homosexuals the same deal society now offers heterosexuals: general social approval and specific legal advantages in exchange for a deeper and harder-to-extract-yourself-from commitment to another human being. Like straight marriage, it would foster social cohesion, emotional security, and economic prudence. Since there's no reason gays should not be allowed to adopt or be foster parents, it could also help nurture children. And its introduction would not be some sort of radical break with social custom. As it has become more acceptable for gay people to acknowledge their loves publicly, more and more have committed themselves to one another for life in full view of their families and their friends. A law institutionalizing gay marriage would merely reinforce a healthy social trend. It would also, in the wake of AIDS, qualify as a genuine public health measure. Those conservatives who deplore promiscuity among some homosexuals should be among the first to support it. Burke could have written a powerful case for it.

The argument that gay marriage would subtly undermine the unique legitimacy of straight marriage is based upon a fallacy. For heterosexuals, straight marriage would remain the most significant—and only legal social bond. Gay marriage could only delegitimize straight marriage if it were a real alternative to it, and this is clearly not true. To put it bluntly, there's precious little evidence that straights could be persuaded by any law to have sex with—let alone marry—someone of their own sex. The only possible effect of this sort would be to persuade gay men and women who force themselves into heterosexual marriage (often at appalling cost to themselves and their families) to find a focus for their family instincts in a more personally positive environment. But this is clearly a plus, not a minus: gay marriage could both avoid a lot of tortured families and create the possibility for many happier ones. It is not, in short, a denial of family values. It's an extension of them.

Of course, some would claim that any legal recognition of homosexuality is a de facto attack upon heterosexuality. But even the most hardened conservatives recognize that gays are a permanent minority and aren't likely to go away. Since persecution is not an option in a civilized society, why not coax gays into traditional values rather than rail incoherently against them?

There's a less elaborate argument for gay marriage: it's good for gays. It provides role models for young gay people who, after the exhilaration of coming out, can easily lapse into short-term relationships and insecurity with no tangible goal in sight. My own guess is that most gays would embrace such a goal with as much (if not more) commitment as straights. Even in our society as it is, many lesbian relationships are virtual textbook cases of monogamous commitment. Legal gay marriage could also help bridge the gulf often found between gays and their parents. It could bring the essence of gay life—a gay couple—into the heart of the traditional straight family in a way the family can most understand and the gay offspring can most easily acknowledge. It could do as much to heal the gay-straight rift as any amount of gay rights legislation.

If these arguments sound socially conservative, that's no accident. It's one of the richest ironies of our society's blind spot toward gays that essentially conservative social goals should have the appearance of being so radical. But gay marriage is not a radical step. It avoids the mess of domestic partnership; it is humane; it is conservative in the best sense of the word. It's also about relationships. Given that gay relationships will always exist, what possible social goal is advanced by framing the law to encourage those relationships to be unfaithful, undeveloped, and insecure?

CASES FOR ANALYSIS

1. Rabbis and Gay Marriage

The differing views of two Conservative rabbis in New York State exemplify the diverging opinions in Conservative Judaism on same-sex marriage. At a Conservative congregation in Manhattan, Rabbi Allan Schranz refused to officiate at a same-sex wedding, even though he supports the law that authorizes same-sex marriage in New York State. Yet at a Conservative congregation in White Plains, Rabbi Gordon Tucker officiated at a Jewish wedding for two gay men. Such disagreements come at a time when New York and five other states have passed legislation to make same-sex marriages legal.*

Regardless of which stance these two rabbis take on same-sex marriage, on what grounds should they base their views? Tradition? Scripture? Reason? Ancient religious traditions and doctrines often conflict with the ethics of contemporary society. When they do, which perspective should prevail? Why?

*Joseph Berger, "Among Conservative Rabbis, a Wide Disagreement Over Same-Sex Marriage," *New York Times*, 1 August 2001, http://www.nytimes.com/2011/08/02/nyregion/conservative-rabbis-disagree-on-same-sex-marriage .html?pagewanted=all&_r=0 (15 February 2015).

2. Supreme Court Guarantees Right to Same-Sex Marriage

In a truly momentous decision in June, 2015, the Supreme Court ruled that it is unconstitutional to deny same-sex couples the right to marry in the United States, overruling the decisions of many state governments.

Advocates of gay marriage hailed the decision as a huge victory for LGBT rights, but conservatives claim that the Supreme Court has threatened the stability of the country by altering the definition of marriage.

Notably, Justice Antonin Scalia wrote in his dissent that the court's ruling was a "threat to American democracy." Scalia's fellow conservative Justices, John G. Roberts Jr., Clarence Thomas, and Samuel A. Alito Jr., also dissented.

They are not alone in their belief that Friday's decision was unconstitutional, but President Obama has made it clear that he sides with the liberal Justices in this case, citing his belief that when we are treated as equals "we are more free." *

Do you agree with the Supreme Court's ruling? Why or why not? Will a huge increase in same-sex marriages be good or bad for America? What effect, if any, do you think legalizing same-sex marriage will have on heterosexual marriage?

* Based on Robert Barnes, "Supreme Court rules gay couples nationwide have a right to marry," *Washington Post*, 26 June 2015, http://www.washingtonpost.com/politics/gay-marriage-and-other-major-rulings-at-the-supreme -court/2015/06/25/ef75a120-1b6d-11e5-bd7f-4611a60dd8e5_story.html (26 June 2015).

3. Same-Sex Marriage Undermines Public's Morality?

(Syracuse.com/*Syracuse Post-Standard*)—Conservatives and some clergy condemned the New York State Legislature's vote to legalize same-sex marriages as a move that will harm society and denigrate the institution of marriage.

The passage of the bill that will "alter radically and forever humanity's historic understanding of marriage leaves us deeply disappointed and troubled," read a statement from the state's Catholic bishops.

"We worry that both marriage and the family will be undermined by this tragic presumption of government in passing this legislation that attempts to redefine these cornerstones of civilization."

Opponents decried the vote as a blow to public morality.

"I think it represents a low point in the decay of our culture," said Rick Guy, a former city councilman and a Republican candidate last year for Assembly. "The fact that so many legislators were unable to see the unique dignity of marriage between one man and one woman is very discouraging and disheartening." . . .

"It is a troubling indicator of where the values and morals of where our community are going," [Austin Olmsted] said. "Seeing social mores change like that is going to affect future generations."‡

Does the legalization of same-sex marriage undermine public morality, as these critics suggest? If so, how? If not, why not? Isn't the charge that same-sex marriage degrades morality and culture an empirical claim? If so, what evidence, if any, can be used to support or oppose the practice?

‡Glenn Coin, "Passage of Same-Sex Marriage Law Represents a Blow to Public Morality, Opponents Say." *Syracuse Post-Standard*, June 26, 2001. Reprinted by permission of the Syracuse Post-Standard.

CHAPTER 15

Environmental Ethics

For most of its history, Western ethics has focused on the moral values, rights, and obligations of *humans*. The relevant questions have been, What is the good for *humans*? What value should we place on a *human* life or person? What obligations or duties do we have to our fellow *humans*? What moral rights, if any, do *humans* have? In large part, the rest of the planet seems to have been left out of our moral equations. The nonhuman animals, the plants, the waters, the land—these have mattered, if at all, largely because they affect the well-being of humankind.

But the planet is not what it used to be. The world's natural resources are being depleted. Human technology, culture, and avarice are devouring forests and meadows, poisoning water and air, wiping out ecosystems and species—and threatening the interests of the very beings who have wielded so much technological and cultural power. Some predict doom. They say that humans have gone too far and that the world as we know it will end not with a bang or a whimper, but a gasp: a gasp for uncontaminated air, water, or food. But whether the situation is or is not this dire, the profound environmental changes that humans have produced on earth have inspired many to see the proper purview of ethics as encompassing not just humans but the whole natural world. Consequently a new set of ethical questions is demanding our attention: Is the environment valuable in its own right, regardless of its usefulness for people? Do animals or plants have moral rights? Are they somehow intrinsically valuable? If they are intrinsically valuable or worthy of moral con-

sideration, what makes them so? Does a dolphin have more moral value than a rat? or a rat more than a redwood? or an individual mongoose more than its species? What obligations, if any, do humans have to the natural world? Should the interests of people take precedence over the interests or needs of the environment? Is it morally permissible, for example, to halt the construction of a dam that will bring prosperity to thousands of poor people but will also destroy a species of crayfish?

Trying to answer such questions through critical reasoning is the main business of *environmental ethics,* a branch of applied ethics. Let us explore how these questions arise, determine whether traditional moral theories can shed any light on them, and evaluate arguments that are frequently used to address important environmental issues.

ISSUE FILE: BACKGROUND

Environmental issues can emerge from a variety of real-world challenges: endangered species, pollution, wilderness preservation, treatment of animals, ecosystem protection, climate change, waste disposal, global population, resource allocation, energy use, economics, food production, world hunger, social justice, and the welfare of future generations. The problems are often intractable and maddeningly entangled.

As you would expect, serious disputes about environmental issues involve both the nonmoral and the moral—nonmoral facts (often scientific or technical) and moral principles or judgments. More often than not, there is substantial agreement on the former but serious divergence on the latter. All parties may agree, for instance, that building a road through a forest would help a struggling town prosper and that the project would wipe out a rare species of butterfly, but the debate rages over whether prosperity is more valuable than the butterfly.

Moral arguments in environmental ethics depend heavily on notions of *value* and *moral status*. The distinction between *instrumental* and *intrinsic* value is especially important. Recall that something with instrumental (or extrinsic) value is valuable as a means to something else; something with intrinsic value is valuable in itself, for its own sake. For many people, nature possesses instrumental value (some think it has instrumental value *only*). They may therefore believe that a forest has value because of its economic worth, because it provides the raw materials for making houses, furniture, and paper. Or because it helps make the environment livable for humans by cleaning the air as it absorbs carbon dioxide and releases oxygen. Or because it adds to the quality of human life simply by being beautiful, inspiring, or impressive. Or because it provides a home to many animal and plant species that are themselves instrumentally valuable to humans. In all these cases, the value of the forest is measured by its positive effects on human well-being. The forest is good because it is good for human beings. On the other hand, for many other people, nature has intrinsic value—it is valuable regardless of its usefulness to humanity. (Keep in mind that nature or objects in nature can have both instrumental and intrinsic value.) So they might say that the forest should be cherished for what it is, for its own sake, regardless of whether it can contribute to the welfare or happiness of humankind. The forest has intrinsic value because of its aesthetic qualities, its organizational complexity, its status as a living thing, or some other value-granting property. Even without utility, it can have great intrinsic worth.

Many debates in environmental ethics revolve around the concept of **moral status,** or **moral considerability.** Something has moral status if it is a suitable candidate for moral concern or respect in its own right. A being with moral status is of moral importance regardless of whether it is a means to something else, and in our dealings with it we must somehow take this fact into account. Everyone agrees that humans have moral status; many believe that nonhuman animals also have moral status; some insist that *all* living things have moral status (including plants and even one-celled creatures); and a few think that the natural environment generally—mountains, oceans, rivers, and all—has moral status. A fundamental issue in environmental ethics is precisely what sorts of entities have moral status—and why.

Many things can have instrumental or intrinsic value yet have no moral status—that is, they may not deserve our direct moral concern. A bicycle can have instrumental value as a mode of transportation, but it is not the kind of thing that can have moral status. Michelangelo's magnificent sculpture *David* is generally thought to have intrinsic aesthetic value, but few philosophers would think that it has moral status. Some theorists draw such a distinction as follows: "We can have obligations *regarding* a painting, but not *to* a painting. We ought to treat beautiful paintings with respect, but not because we have obligations to the paintings. We ought to respect them because they are beautiful (or because their owners have rights), not because they have rights."[1]

Often the question at issue in environmental debates is not whether something has moral status, but whether it has greater or lesser moral status than something else. Does an ape have the same moral status as a domestic cow? Do animals (human and

---

[1]David Schmidtz and Elizabeth Willott, *Environmental Ethics: What Really Matters, What Really Works,* Introduction (New York: Oxford University Press, 2002), xvii.

nonhuman) deserve the same level of moral concern as plants? Do humans and nonhuman animals have the same moral status? Is a cat as morally important as a cabbage? Does a species have a stronger claim on our moral concern than any individual of a species? As we will soon see, on various grounds many people give priority to one or more species over others, some think all living things equal, and some rank species over individuals.

In light of these considerations, we should not be surprised that a central question in environmental ethics is, What entities have moral status and to what degree do they have it? The answer that has been assumed in the Western world for much of its history is known as **anthropocentrism,** the notion that only humans have moral standing. By anthropocentric (human-centered) lights, the rest of nature has only instrumental value—that is, nonhuman animals, plants, mountains, and streams have value only because they are valuable in some way to humans. An anthropocentrist sees animals, plants, and ecosystems as means to enhance the well-being of humankind, to serve the ends of human beings. This stance, however, does not imply a disregard for the environment. He may be genuinely concerned about the destruction of rain forests, the extinction of species, river and lake pollution, the destruction of wetlands, animal cruelty, and global warming—but only because these calamities might lead to a less livable environment for humans, or their loss of enjoyable aesthetic or spiritual experiences of nature, or their feelings of distress at the thought of animal suffering, or dramatic climate changes that could endanger human lives.

On what grounds should humans be granted this exclusive moral status? The traditional justification has been along Kantian lines: that humans are moral agents or persons—they are capable of making free, rational moral choices.

Another influential answer to our question is what could be called **zoocentrism,** the notion that animals—both human and nonhuman—

have moral status. Advocates for animal rights, notably the philosophers Peter Singer and Tom Regan, take this view, insisting that human and nonhuman animals are equally deserving of moral considerability or respect. Singer contends that moral status is justified for nonhuman animals when they, like humans, possess the psychological property of sentience. Sentient nonhuman animals can experience pain and pleasure, just as humans can; therefore, he says, they are entitled to the same level of moral respect. Some critics, however, object to this kind of animal egalitarianism, affirming that all sentient animals do have moral status but that humans have greater moral considerability than nonhuman animals.

Some theorists want to expand the sphere of moral status to include more than just animals. They hold to **biocentrism,** or life-centered ethics, the view that all living entities have moral status, whether sentient or not. People, cats, trees, weeds, algae, amoebas, germs—all these are worthy of some sort of moral concern simply because they are alive. This moral concern, many biocentrists say, is justified by the teleological nature of living things (*telos* is Greek for "goal"). Living things are goal directed, striving consciously or unconsciously toward some good. They therefore have moral status. But biocentrists differ on how much respect to grant living things. Some assert that all living things have *equal* moral status: exactly the same moral considerability is accorded to human beings, dogs, redwood trees, and amoebas. These biocentrists are therefore **species egalitarians.** Other biocentrists, **species nonegalitarians,** think that not all living beings are created equal—some have more moral worth than others. A nonegalitarian might argue that a human deserves more respect than an elk, an elk more than a rat, and a rat more than a cactus.

In either form, biocentrism implies that in our moral deliberations we cannot ignore how our actions might affect both sentient and nonsentient living beings, as some forms of anthropocentrism

Some Major Environmental Issues

GLOBAL WARMING

The Problem: *Global warming* refers to the increase in the average temperature of the earth, a rise that occurred most dramatically over the twentieth century and has accelerated in the past thirty years. It worries scientists because even a tiny increase in the average temperature could affect climate worldwide. According to a growing scientific consensus, this warming is due largely to the "greenhouse effect" in which radiation from the sun is trapped in the earth's atmosphere by greenhouse gases such as carbon dioxide (CO_2) and CFCs (chlorofluorocarbons), heating up the lower atmosphere and the earth's surface. Scientists also generally agree that human activity in the past fifty years—notably the combustion of fossil fuels (which produces carbon dioxide)—is responsible for most of the buildup of these gases. Climate change due to global warming will have both positive and negative potential effects. The possible negative effects include melting glaciers and an accompanying rise in sea level (which could mean a loss of habitable land, extensive flooding, and displacement of populations), drought in some regions, the expansion of deserts, increased world hunger, changes in regional climates (for example, from dry to wet or cool to warm), and more hurricanes or even superhurricanes.

The Numbers: The earth's surface temperature has increased about 1.4 degrees F in the past century. Scientists predict a warming of 4.7 to 8.6 degrees F by the end of this century. Annually, more than 60 percent of global CO_2 comes from industrialized nations. As of 1996, per capita emissions of carbon in the United States (5.37 thousand tons) are twenty times higher than emissions in India (0.29), and seven times higher than emissions in China (0.76). The United States has 4 percent of the world's population, but emits 23 percent of global greenhouse gases. The European Union nations constitute 3 percent of the world's population but account for 10 percent of global emissions.

The Questions: Should governments take steps to prevent global warming even if such measures would result in some human suffering—such as the loss of jobs and economic harm to businesses or whole industries? How should we weigh the benefits to a future generation against current economic harm to industries?

OZONE DEPLETION

The Problem: In the upper reaches of the earth's atmosphere, there is an airy layer of material known as ozone. The ozone layer absorbs a particularly harmful form of the sun's radiation, a segment of ultraviolet light known as UVB. Scientists have linked UVB to skin cancer and cataracts in humans and have shown that it can damage crops and marine life. A hole in the ozone layer or even its slight thinning in a particular area will allow more UVB to reach the earth's surface, increasing the risk of harm. The amount of ozone in the atmosphere waxes and wanes naturally over time, but scientists have discovered that some commercial products contain chemicals that can deplete the ozone layer faster than it can be replenished. Chlorofluorocarbons (CFCs)—found in refrigerants, aerosol sprays, solvents, and other products—were determined to be the main culprits. CFCs are stable compounds that drift into the ozone layer, undergo a chemical reaction, and destroy ozone. Ozone depletion happens over most of the planet, including North America, Europe, and Asia. Beginning in the 1970s, nations started to ban the use of CFCs, and eventually international agreements made the prohibition against CFCs almost universal. Consequently, the emissions of CFCs and other ozone-depleting substances have been dropping. Scientists say that if all goes well, the ozone layer may restore itself—in fifty years or so. At the same time, NASA reports that in a few years, climate change may do more to deplete the ozone layer than CFCs had done.

The Numbers: For every 1 percent decrease in the ozone layer, rates of skin cancer increase 5 percent.

Ninety percent of ozone exists in the stratosphere, 6 to 30 miles above the earth. It is estimated that without international agreements banning ozone-depleting products, 50 percent of the ozone over the Northern Hemisphere's mid-latitudes would be depleted by the year 2050, resulting in a doubling of the amount of UVB reaching the earth's surface.

The Questions: How should we weigh the saving of lives (by eliminating the risk of skin cancer) against the harm done to people's livelihoods? How much is one life worth? or a thousand lives? What if a single nation was responsible for most of the damage to the ozone layer and refused to be restrained by any international agreements? Should that nation be forced to comply?

FOREST CONSERVATION

The Problem: To a surprising degree, the planet and its inhabitants depend on its forests. From forests, people derive a long list of valuable products—aesthetic wood (for example, mahogany and teak), lumber, firewood, paper, rubber, fruit, nuts, and medicines. For many people, the commercial value of forests is mostly beside the point—forests are valuable for their beauty, their inspirational power, and their educational potential. For tribal hunter-gatherers, forests provide livelihoods, fuel, fiber, and homes. Tropical forests are an especially powerful force for biodiversity, offering habitats for tens of thousands of plant and animal species and enriching the world with potential sources of scientific, genetic, and evolutionary knowledge. At the most basic level, forests nourish life: they use up carbon dioxide and give off oxygen, helping to neutralize the global greenhouse effect in the process. But the world's forests are vanishing, along with many of the species they supported. As a consequence of the timber trade in valuable woods (both illegal and legal), the clearing of forests for agriculture and industry, the felling of trees for firewood, and the building of roads through wooded areas, millions of acres of forests are disappearing each year.

The Numbers: Forests now cover about 30 percent of the earth's land area. Each year more than 56,000 square miles of natural forests are lost. By the year 2050, global wood consumption is expected to increase 50 percent. Americans use 27 percent of the world's commercially harvested wood. Of the world's 1.2 billion people living in dire poverty, 80 to 90 percent depend on forests to make their living.

The Questions: How far should we go in preserving forests? Various industries, millions of impoverished people, and many tribal cultures depend economically on the clearing of forests. Are we justified in causing economic harm to save the world's forests? Are we justified in destroying someone's way of life to achieve that end?

Sources: National Academy of Sciences and the Royal Society, "Climate Change: Evidence and Causes," 2013, http://nas-sites.org/americasclimatechoices/events/a-discussion-on-climate-change-evidence-and-causes/ (21 February 2015); National Academy of Sciences, "Understanding and Responding to Climate Change, 2008, http://www.nrcs.usda.gov/Internet/FSE_DOCUMENTS/stelprdb1048006.pdf (21 February 2015); Committee on the Science of Climate Change, Division of Earth and Life Studies, National Research Council, "Climate Change Science: An Analysis of Some Key Questions, Washington, DC: National Academy Press, 2001, available at http://www.nap.edu/openbook.php?record_id=10139&page=R1 (21 February 2015); U.S. Environmental Protection Administration, Climate Change: Basic Information, http://www.epa.gov/climatechange/basics/ (21 February 2015).

U.S. Environmental Protection Administration, Ozone Layer Protection, http://www.epa.gov/ozone/basicinfo.html (21 February 2015).

United Nations Environment Programme, Backgrounder: Basic Facts and Data on the Science and Politics of Ozone Protection, September 2008, http://ozone.unep.org/Events/ozone_day_2009/press_backgrounder.pdf (21 February 2015); J. Louise Mastrantonio and John K. Francis, "A Student Guide to Tropical Forest Conservation," 1997, http://www.treesearch.fs.fed.us/pubs/2792 (21 February 2015).

might have us do. If we want to build a shopping mall on wetlands, we must consider all the plants and animals that the project would destroy—and judge whether their deaths would outweigh any benefits that the mall would provide to humans and other living things.

In both zoocentrism and biocentrism, the fundamental unit of moral consideration is the *individual*—the individual animal or plant. Only individuals have moral status. This perspective then is *individualistic,* its advocates being called **ecological individualists.** In contrast, some theorists say that the proper focus of moral concern is not the individual but the entire biosphere and its ecosystems, what has been called the "biotic community." This view then is *holistic;* its proponents, **ecological holists.** It implies that in considering our moral obligations to the environment, the good of the whole will always outweigh the good of an individual. An elk, for example, may be killed to preserve a species of plant or to ensure the health of its ecosystem. As one theorist expressed it, "A thing is right when it tends to preserve the integrity, stability, and beauty of the biotic community. It is wrong when it tends otherwise."[2] What properties might confer moral considerability on the biotic community or an ecosystem? A holist might say that such an environmental whole deserves our respect because it is a unity of beautifully integrated parts, or it is a self-regulating system, or its destruction would diminish the world's genetic possibilities.

MORAL THEORIES

On environmental issues, some traditional moral theories have been strongly anthropocentric. Kant's theory is a good example, mandating duties to people because they are ends in themselves but establishing no direct duties to animals. For Kant,

> ### QUICK REVIEW
>
> *moral status (or moral considerability)*—The property of being a suitable candidate for direct moral concern or respect.
>
> *anthropocentrism*—The notion that only humans have moral status.
>
> *zoocentrism*—The notion that both human and nonhuman animals have moral status.
>
> *biocentrism*—The view that all living entities have moral status, whether sentient or not.
>
> *species egalitarian*—One who believes that all living things have equal moral status.
>
> *species nonegalitarian*—One who believes that some living things have higher moral status than others.
>
> *ecological individualist*—One who believes that the fundamental unit of moral consideration in environmental ethics is the individual.
>
> *ecological holist*—One who believes that the fundamental unit of moral consideration in environmental ethics is the biosphere and its ecosystems.

animals have instrumental value only. As he puts it, "Animals . . . are there merely as means to an end. That end is man."[3] Thomas Aquinas, author of the most famous version of natural law theory, also thinks animals are tools to be employed at the discretion of humans. In addition, the Bible has seemed to many to suggest an anthropocentric attitude toward nature, commanding that humans "subdue" the earth and "have dominion over the fish of the sea and over the birds of the air and over every living thing that moves upon the earth" (Genesis 1.28). But traditional theories can also be—and have been—construed in various

---

[2]Aldo Leopold, "The Land Ethic," in *A Sand County Almanac* (Oxford: Oxford University Press, 1981), 237–65.

[3]Immanuel Kant, *Lectures on Ethics,* trans. Louis Infield (New York: Harper and Row, 1963), 239–40.

CRITICAL THOUGHT: Should Pandas Pay the Price?

Some of the most controversial disputes in environmental ethics involve conflicts between concern for endangered species and the economic needs and demands of humans. Here is just one of many recent examples:

> (*China Daily*)—The more than 100 wild giant pandas in Northwest China's Gansu Province are now stepping onto the verge of extinction because of a decline in their ability to reproduce, according to Xinhua reports.
>
> Researchers from the Gansu Baishuijiang Giant Panda Nature Reserve said the giant pandas in the province now live in five separate habitats, making mating among the groups almost impossible.
>
> According to basic principles of genetics and the pandas' reproduction habits, a group of less than 50 giant pandas are predicted to become extinct at some point as a result of a weakening reproductive ability caused by inbreeding.
>
> Wang Hao, a giant panda expert of Peking University, said the fragmentation of wild pandas' habitats had become the biggest threat to the survival of the species.
>
> Wang said that the construction of highways is cutting large panda habitats into smaller and

smaller ones, increasing the risk of degeneration of the species. . . .

> Wang estimated that the annual cost to protect one wild panda exceeds 5 million yuan (US$617,000).*

Which should be given more moral weight—the people or the pandas? What are your reasons for preferring one over the other? If you agree that we should try to save endangered species like the panda, how much should we be willing to pay to do so? Is $617,000 per panda an acceptable price? How about $1 million? Suppose saving one panda would put one thousand people out of a job, forcing scores of families into poverty. Would saving the pandas be worth that cost? Why or why not? What moral principle would you devise to help you answer these questions (and similar questions regarding any endangered species)?

*Guo Nei, reprinted with permission of SydiGate Media Inc. from "Road Construction Segregates Giant Pandas' Habitats in Gansu," *China Daily*, December 5, 2006; permission conveyed through Copyright Clearance Center, Inc.

ways to support nonanthropocentric approaches to environmental ethics.

As we have seen, some theorists adopt a nonconsequentialist or Kantian-like perspective on nature. They reject instrumentalist views in favor of the notion that the environment or its constituents have intrinsic value, just as persons are thought to be intrinsically valuable. Probably the most overtly Kantian theorist is the philosopher Paul Taylor, a biocentrist who argues that "it is the good (well-being, welfare) of individual organisms, considered as entities having inherent worth, that determines our moral relations with the Earth's wild communities of life" and that "[their] well-being, as well as human well-being, is something to be realized *as an*

end in itself."[4] Some zoocentrists also have a Kantian bent. For example, Tom Regan argues that sentient animals, human and nonhuman, possess equal intrinsic worth and therefore have an equal moral right not to be treated as mere things.[5] In this account, just as there are certain things that we should not do to humans regardless of the resulting utilitarian benefits, so there are ways of treating nonhuman animals that are wrong regardless of the advantages to humans. According to Regan, the

[4]Paul W. Taylor, "The Ethics of Respect for Nature," *Environmental Ethics* 3, no. 3 (1981): 198.
[5]Tom Regan, "Animal Rights, Human Wrongs," *Environmental Ethics* 2, no. 2 (Summer 1980): 99–120.

result of applying this outlook to the treatment of animals would be the eradication of factory farming, animal experimentation, and hunting.

Utilitarianism has also been put to use in defense of nonhuman animals. Following the lead of the philosopher Jeremy Bentham, utilitarianism's founder, Peter Singer maintains that in calculating which action will produce the greatest overall satisfaction of interests (for example, an interest in avoiding pain), we must include the interests of all sentient creatures and give their interests equal weight. The pain suffered by a human is no more important than that experienced by a nonhuman animal. This view seems to imply that any factory farming in which animals suffer greatly before being slaughtered is wrong. But it also seems to suggest that if the animals could be raised without such suffering, factory farming may be morally permissible, even if they are killed in the end.

MORAL ARGUMENTS

Serious environmental issues and the arguments that surround them are numerous, varied, and complex, so for the purposes of evaluation let us focus on arguments pertaining to the one question that has concerned us most throughout this chapter: *When, if ever, do environmental entities or beings have moral status?* As we have seen, environmental philosophers and other thinkers have argued for and against different kinds of entities having moral considerability and for and against various justifications for that status. The entities thought to be worthy of such moral concern include human beings exclusively (anthropocentrism), human and nonhuman animals (zoocentrism), living things (biocentrism), and collections or systems of living things such as species or ecosystems (ecological holism). The properties that are supposed to validate their claim to moral worth range across a broad spectrum of possibilities—from

moral agency or sentience to complexity to self-regulation to beauty.

To begin, let us examine a simple argument containing a premise that offers a common answer to our question—the answer that entities in the environment have moral status because they are *natural* (lacking human interference or contrivance).

1. All natural entities have moral status (intrinsic value or rights, for example).

2. Old-growth forests are natural entities.

3. Therefore, old-growth forests have moral status.

We can see right away that this is a valid argument, but—as is so often the case in moral arguments—the moral premise (Premise 1) is not obviously true (though the other premise definitely is). What reasons might someone give to support the statement that objects in nature deserve our respect just because their properties are due solely to natural processes?

One reason that could be put forth is that Premise 1 is supported by our moral intuitions (our considered moral judgments, for example). To test this idea, mull over this thought experiment:

> Imagine that a certain mine requires the destruction of a group of trees on a rocky outcrop and of the outcrop itself. Environmentalists protest that such destruction involves an uncompensated loss of value. The mining company promises to reconstruct the outcrop from synthetic parts and to replace the trees with plastic models. This bit of artificial environment will be indistinguishable, except by laboratory analysis, from what was originally there. It will be exactly as appealing to look at, no animals will be harmed as a consequence, and no ecosystem will be disrupted.[6]

[6]Robert Elliot, "Environmental Ethics," in *A Companion to Ethics*, ed. Peter Singer, corr. ed. (Oxford: Blackwell, 1993), 291.

What, if anything, would be wrong with replacing these natural entities with synthetic ones? A few trees would be destroyed, and thus there is a loss of living things, but let us mentally discount the loss. Would this substitution of nonnatural for natural make a moral difference? Would the mining company be guilty of wrongdoing? If this scenario suggests to us that the property of naturalness does confer some kind of moral standing on objects, then perhaps our moral intuitions do support Premise 1.

The obvious move for a critic is to assert that it is not at all clear whether moral intuitions offer such support. Perhaps we are merely confused, actually worrying not about unnaturalness but about harm to ecosystems or extermination of wildlife.[7]

A defender of Premise 1 could try another tack. She could attempt to take our moral intuitions in a different direction, declaring that just as fake works of art seem to have less value for us than the originals, so synthetic objects in the environment have less intrinsic value than their natural counterparts or originals. We simply do not appreciate replicas of fine sculptures as much as we do the originals, and we do not respect artificial trees as much as we do natural ones. The property of being natural, then, appears to confer some value on objects—and thus some level of moral standing.[8]

A detractor could cast doubt on this line by pointing out that there seem to be instances in which we do in fact value the artificial more than the natural. For example, Niagara Falls on the American side of the border with Canada is undeniably beautiful and majestic, exemplifying the ideal waterfall in its natural state. But oddly enough, the majestic, "natural" state of the falls is largely a product of human ingenuity. Because of natural erosion, the falls deteriorate over time and—without human intervention—would suffer so much damage that it would no longer look much like the falls people have come to expect. Through reconstruction and control of water flow, engineers have saved Niagara Falls, a now largely artificial phenomenon that people would almost certainly prefer over the natural but less impressive version.[9]

Let us now consider a "higher level" sort of argument, one that tries to establish the truth of a particular environmental theory, in this case biocentric egalitarianism. Recall that this doctrine asserts that all living things possess equal moral status—no being is superior to any other in moral considerability. Humans, then, are not entitled to more respect than apes or redwoods or elk. Here is how the philosopher Paul Taylor argues for this position:[10]

1. Humans are members of earth's community of life in exactly the same way that all other living things are members.

2. Human beings and all other living things constitute a dynamic system of interlinked and interdependent parts.

3. Each living thing is a "teleological center of life, pursuing its own good in its own way."

4. Human beings are not superior to other species.

5. Therefore, all living things have equal moral status.

[7]Elliot, 292.
[8]This argument is a vastly oversimplified rendering of Robert Elliot's argument in "Faking Nature," *Inquiry* 25, no. 1 (1982): 81–93.

[9]This example is adapted from Martin H. Krieger, "What's Wrong with Plastic Trees?" *Science* 179 (1973): 446–55.
[10]Taylor, 207.

This argument is complex and deserves far more close analysis than we can provide here. But we can home in on a few interesting elements.

Consider Premise 4. At the outset, note that the argument is not valid: the conclusion does not follow from the first four premises. Taylor acknowledges this fact but suggests that if we accept Premises 1–4, then it would at least be more reasonable than not to accept the conclusion. He says the same thing about Premise 4: if we accept Premises 1–3, it would not be unreasonable to accept the fourth premise. But some argue that Premise 4 does not follow from Premises 1–3. More to the point, it could be argued that even if we accept that humans are part of an interdependent community of life in which all members are teleological centers pursuing their own good, we are not necessarily being unreasonable if we then reject the idea that humans are on a par with all other species. Even if Premises 1–3 are true, we are not obliged to accept Premise 4.

Some philosophers have argued directly against Taylor's conclusion (Statement 5) by drawing out its implications. If all species are morally equal, what would that imply about how we treat various species? One critic gives this answer:

> What seems far more problematic for species egalitarianism is that it seems to suggest that it makes no difference *what* we kill. Vegetarians typically think it worse to kill a cow than to kill a carrot. Are they wrong? Yes they are, according to species egalitarianism. In this respect, species egalitarianism cannot be right. I believe we have reason to respect nature. But we fail to give nature due respect if we say we should have no more respect for a cow than for a potato.[11]

This counterargument is, of course, another appeal to our moral intuitions. We are asked to reflect on whether it would be morally permissible to treat a cow as if it had the same moral status as a potato. If they do deserve the same level of respect, then if we must kill one of them, we should not care which. They are moral equals. But if we think that it does matter which one we kill, we have reason to reject the notion that they are moral equals—and thus deny biocentric egalitarianism.

SUMMARY

Environmental ethics, a branch of applied ethics, explores questions about the value of nature and its constituents, the relationship between the environment and humans, and the moral obligations that humans have toward the environment. Logical arguments in the field rely on several key concepts, including instrumental value, intrinsic value, and moral status or considerability. Something with instrumental value is valuable as a means to something else; something with intrinsic value is valuable in itself. An entity has *moral status* if it is a suitable candidate for moral concern or respect in its own right.

Several positions have been staked out regarding the proper attitude of humans toward nature. Anthropocentrism is the view that only humans have moral standing; zoocentrism, that animals do; and biocentrism, that all living things do. Species egalitarians believe that all living things have equal moral status; species nonegalitarians, that they do not. Ecological individualists think that only individuals have moral status; ecological holists, that only the biosphere and its ecosystems do.

Some theorists have adopted a Kantian-like perspective on the environment. Paul Taylor insists that organisms have inherent worth and should not be treated merely as means to ends. Tom Regan asserts that sentient beings possess equal intrinsic worth and should not be considered mere things. A utilitarian stance is also possible, as Peter Singer has demonstrated in his position on animal rights.

---

[11]David Schmidtz, "Are All Species Equal?" *Journal of Applied Philosophy* 15, no. 1 (1998): 59.

READINGS

People or Penguins

WILLIAM F. BAXTER

I start with the modest proposition that, in dealing with pollution, or indeed with any problem, it is helpful to know what one is attempting to accomplish. Agreement on how and whether to pursue a particular objective, such as pollution control, is not possible unless some more general objective has been identified and stated with reasonable precision. We talk loosely of having clean air and clean water, of preserving our wilderness areas, and so forth. But none of these is a sufficiently general objective: each is more accurately viewed as a means rather than as an end.

With regard to clean air, for example, one may ask, "how clean?" and "what does clean mean?" It is even reasonable to ask, "why have clean air?" Each of these questions is an implicit demand that a more general community goal be stated—a goal sufficiently general in its scope and enjoying sufficiently general assent among the community of actors that such "why" questions no longer seem admissible with respect to that goal.

If, for example, one states as a goal the proposition that "every person should be free to do whatever he wishes in contexts where his actions do not interfere with the interests of other human beings," the speaker is unlikely to be met with a response of "why." The goal may be criticized as uncertain in its implications or difficult to implement, but it is so basic a tenet of our civilization—it reflects a cultural value so broadly shared, at least in the abstract—that the question "why" is seen as impertinent or imponderable or both.

I do not mean to suggest that everyone would agree with the "spheres of freedom" objective just stated. Still less do I mean to suggest that a society could subscribe to four or five such general objectives that would be adequate in their coverage to serve as testing criteria by which all other disagreements might be measured. One difficulty in the attempt to construct such a list is that each new goal added will conflict, in certain applications, with each prior goal listed; and thus each goal serves as a limited qualification on prior goals.

Without any expectation of obtaining unanimous consent to them, let me set forth four goals that I generally use as ultimate testing criteria in attempting to frame solutions to problems of human organization. My position regarding pollution stems from these four criteria. If the criteria appeal to you and any part of what appears hereafter does not, our disagreement will have a helpful focus: which of us is correct, analytically, in supposing that his position on pollution would better serve these general goals. If the criteria do not seem acceptable to you, then it is to be expected that our more particular judgments will differ, and the task will then be yours to identify the basic set of criteria upon which your particular judgments rest.

My criteria are as follows:

1. The spheres of freedom criterion stated above.
2. Waste is a bad thing. The dominant feature of human existence is scarcity—our available resources, our aggregate labors, and our skill in employing both have always been, and will continue for some time to be, inadequate to yield to every man all the tangible and intangible satisfactions he would like to have. Hence, none of those resources, or labors, or skills, should be wasted—that is, employed so as to yield less than they might yield in human satisfactions.
3. Every human being should be regarded as an end rather than as a means to be used for the

betterment of another. Each should be afforded dignity and regarded as having an absolute claim to an evenhanded application of such rules as the community may adopt for its governance.

4. Both the incentive and the opportunity to improve his share of satisfactions should be preserved to every individual. Preservation of incentive is dictated by the "no-waste" criterion and enjoins against the continuous, totally egalitarian redistribution of satisfactions, or wealth; but subject to that constraint, everyone should receive, by continuous redistribution if necessary, some minimal share of aggregate wealth so as to avoid a level of privation from which the opportunity to improve his situation becomes illusory.

The relationship of these highly general goals to the more specific environmental issues at hand may not be readily apparent, and I am not yet ready to demonstrate their pervasive implications. But let me give one indication of their implications. Recently scientists have informed us that use of DDT in food production is causing damage to the penguin population. For the present purposes let us accept that assertion as an indisputable scientific fact. The scientific fact is often asserted as if the correct implication—that we must stop agricultural use of DDT—followed from the mere statement of the fact of penguin damage. But plainly it does not follow if my criteria are employed.

My criteria are oriented to people, not penguins. Damage to penguins, or sugar pines, or geological marvels is, without more, simply irrelevant. One must go further, by my criteria, and say: Penguins are important because people enjoy seeing them walk about rocks; and furthermore, the well-being of people would be less impaired by halting use of DDT than by giving up penguins. In short, my observations about environmental problems will be people-oriented, as are my criteria. I have no interest in preserving penguins for their own sake.

It may be said by way of objection to this position, that it is very selfish of people to act as if each person represented one unit of importance and nothing else was of any importance. It is undeniably

selfish. Nevertheless I think it is the only tenable starting place for analysis for several reasons. First, no other position corresponds to the way most people really think and act—i.e., corresponds to reality.

Second, this attitude does not portend any massive destruction of nonhuman flora and fauna, for people depend on them in many obvious ways, and they will be preserved because and to the degree that humans do depend on them.

Third, what is good for humans is, in many respects, good for penguins and pine trees—clean air for example. So that humans are, in these respects, surrogates for plant and animal life.

Fourth, I do not know how we could administer any other system. Our decisions are either private or collective. Insofar as Mr. Jones is free to act privately, he may give such preferences as he wishes to other forms of life: he may feed birds in winter and do with less himself, and he may even decline to resist an advancing polar bear on the ground that the bear's appetite is more important than those portions of himself that the bear may choose to eat. In short my basic premise does not rule out private altruism to competing life-forms. It does rule out, however, Mr. Jones's inclination to feed Mr. Smith to the bear, however hungry the bear, however despicable Mr. Smith.

Insofar as we act collectively on the other hand, only humans can be afforded an opportunity to participate in the collective decisions. Penguins cannot vote now and are unlikely subjects for the franchise—pine trees more unlikely still. Again each individual is free to cast his vote so as to benefit sugar pines if that is his inclination. But many of the more extreme assertions that one hears from some conservationists amount to tacit assertions that they are specially appointed representatives of sugar pines, and hence that their preferences should be weighted more heavily than the preferences of other humans who do not enjoy equal rapport with "nature." The simplistic assertion that agricultural use of DDT must stop at once because it is harmful to penguins is of that type.

Fifth, if polar bears or pine trees or penguins, like men, are to be regarded as ends rather than means, if they are to count in our calculus of social organization, someone must tell me how much each one counts, and someone must tell me how these life-forms are to be permitted to express their preferences, for I do not know either answer. If the answer is that certain people are to hold their proxies, then I want to know how those proxy-holders are to be selected: self-appointment does not seem workable to me.

Sixth, and by way of summary of all the foregoing, let me point out that the set of environmental issues under discussion—although they raise very complex technical questions of how to achieve any objective—ultimately raise a normative question: what *ought* we to do. Questions of *ought* are unique to the human mind and world—they are meaningless as applied to a nonhuman situation.

I reject the proposition that we *ought* to respect the "balance of nature" or to "preserve the environment" unless the reason for doing so, express or implied, is the benefit of man.

I reject the idea that there is a "right" or "morally correct" state of nature to which we should return. The word "nature" has no normative connotation. Was it "right" or "wrong" for the earth's crust to heave in contortion and create mountains and seas? Was it "right" for the first amphibian to crawl up out of the primordial ooze. Was it "wrong" for plants to reproduce themselves and alter the atmospheric composition in favor of oxygen? For animals to alter the atmosphere in favor of carbon dioxide both by breathing oxygen and eating plants? No answers can be given to these questions because they are meaningless questions.

All this may seem obvious to the point of being tedious, but much of the present controversy over environment and pollution rests on tacit normative assumptions about just such nonnormative phenomena that it is "wrong" to impair penguins with DDT, but not to slaughter cattle for prime rib roasts. That it is wrong to kill stands of sugar pines with industrial fumes, but not to cut sugar pines and build housing for the poor. Every man is entitled to his own preferred definition of Walden Pond, but there is no definition that has any moral superiority over another, except by reference to the selfish needs of the human race.

From the fact that there is no normative definition of the natural state, it follows that there is no

normative definition of clean air or pure water—hence no definition of polluted air—or of pollution—except by reference to the needs of man. The "right" composition of the atmosphere is one which has some dust in it and some lead in it and some hydrogen sulfide in it—just those amounts that attend a sensibly organized society thoughtfully and knowledgeably pursuing the greatest possible satisfaction for its human members.

The first and most fundamental step toward solution of our environmental problems is a clear recognition that our objective is not pure air or water but rather some optimal state of pollution. That step immediately suggests the question: How do we define and attain the level of pollution that will yield the maximum possible amount of human satisfaction?

Low levels of pollution contribute to human satisfaction but so do food and shelter and education and music. To attain ever lower levels of pollution, we must pay the cost of having less of these other things. I contrast that view of the cost of pollution control with the more popular statement that pollution control will "cost" very large numbers of dollars. The popular statement is true in some senses, false in others; sorting out the true and false senses is of some importance. The first step in that sorting process is to achieve a clear understanding of the difference between dollars and resources. Resources are the wealth of our nation; dollars are merely claim checks upon those resources. Resources are of vital importance; dollars are comparatively trivial.

Four categories of resources are sufficient for our purposes: At any given time a nation, or a planet if you prefer, has a stock of labor, of technological skill, of capital goods, and of natural resources (such as mineral deposits, timber, water, land, etc.). These resources can be used in various combinations to yield goods and services of all kinds—in some limited quantity. The quantity will be larger if they are combined efficiently, smaller if combined inefficiently. But in either event the resource stock is limited, the goods and services that they can be made to yield are limited; even the most efficient use of them will yield less than our population, in the aggregate, would like to have.

If one considers building a new dam, it is appropriate to say that it will be costly in the sense that it will require *x* hours of labor, *y* tons of steel and concrete, and *z* amount of capital goods. If these resources are devoted to the dam, then they cannot be used to build hospitals, fishing rods, schools, or electric can openers. That is the meaningful sense in which the dam is costly.

Quite apart from the very important question of how wisely we can combine our resources to produce goods and services, is the very different question of how they get distributed—who gets how many goods? Dollars constitute the claim checks which are distributed among people and which control their share of national output. Dollars are nearly valueless pieces of paper except to the extent that they do represent claim checks to some fraction of the output of goods and services. Viewed as claim checks, all the dollars outstanding during any period of time are worth, in the aggregate, the goods and services that are available to be claimed with them during that period—neither more nor less.

It is far easier to increase the supply of dollars than to increase the production of goods and services—printing dollars is easy. But printing more dollars doesn't help because each dollar then simply becomes a claim to fewer goods, i.e., becomes worth less.

The point is this: many people fall into error upon hearing the statement that the decision to build a dam, or to clean up a river, will cost $X million. It is regrettably easy to say: "It's only money. This is a wealthy country, and we have lots of money." But you cannot build a dam or clean a river with $X million—unless you also have a match, you can't even make a fire. One builds a dam or cleans a river by diverting labor and steel and trucks and factories from making one kind of goods to making another. The cost in dollars is merely a shorthand way of describing the extent of the diversion necessary. If we build a dam for $X million, then we must recognize that we will have $X million less housing and food and medical care and electric can openers as a result.

Similarly, the costs of controlling pollution are best expressed in terms of the other goods we will have to give up to do the job. This is not to say the job should not be done. Badly as we need more housing, more medical care, and more can openers, and more symphony orchestras, we could do with somewhat less of them, in my judgment at least, in exchange for somewhat cleaner air and rivers. But that is the nature of the trade-off, and analysis of the problem is advanced if that unpleasant reality is kept in mind. Once the trade-off relationship is clearly perceived, it is possible to state in a very general way what the optimal level of pollution is. I would state it as follows:

People enjoy watching penguins. They enjoy relatively clean air and smog-free vistas. Their health is improved by relatively clean water and air. Each of these benefits is a type of good or service. As a society we would be well advised to give up one washing machine if the resources that would have gone into that washing machine can yield greater human satisfaction when diverted into pollution control. We should give up one hospital if the resources thereby freed would yield more human satisfaction when devoted to elimination of noise in our cities. And so on, trade-off by trade-off, we should divert our productive capacities from the production of existing goods and services to the production of a cleaner, quieter, more pastoral nation up to—and no further than—the point at which we value more highly the next washing machine or hospital that we would have to do without than we value the next unit of environmental improvement that the diverted resources would create.

Now this proposition seems to me unassailable but so general and abstract as to be unhelpful—at least unadministerable in the form stated. It assumes we can measure in some way the incremental units of human satisfaction yielded by very different types of goods. The proposition must remain a pious abstraction until I can explain how this measurement process can occur. In subsequent chapters I will attempt to show that we can do this—in some contexts with great precision and in other contexts only by rough approximation. But I insist that the proposition stated describes the result for which we should be striving—and again, that it is always useful to know what your target is even if your weapons are too crude to score a bull's eye.

The Ethics of Respect for Nature

PAUL W. TAYLOR

I. HUMAN-CENTERED AND LIFE-CENTERED SYSTEMS OF ENVIRONMENTAL ETHICS

In this paper I show how the taking of a certain ultimate moral attitude toward nature, which I call "respect for nature," has a central place in the foundations of a life-centered system of environmental ethics. I hold that a set of moral norms (both standards of character and rules of conduct) governing human treatment of the natural world is a rationally grounded set if and only if, first, commitment to those norms is a practical entailment of adopting the attitude of respect for nature as an ultimate moral attitude, and second, the adopting of that attitude on the part of all rational agents can itself be justified. When the basic characteristics of the attitude of respect for nature are made clear, it will be seen that a life-centered system of environmental ethics need not be holistic or organicist in its conception of the kinds of entities that are deemed the appropriate objects of moral concern and consideration. Nor does such a system require that the concepts of ecological homeostasis, equilibrium, and integrity provide us with normative principles from which could be derived (with the addition of factual knowledge) our obligations with regard to natural ecosystems. The "balance of nature" is not itself a moral norm, however important may be the role it plays in our general outlook on the natural world that underlies the attitude of respect of nature. I argue that finally it is the good (well-being, welfare) of individual organisms, considered as entities having inherent worth, that determines our moral relations with the Earth's wild communities of life.

In designating the theory to be set forth as life-centered, I intend to contrast it with all anthropocentric views. According to the latter, human actions affecting the natural environment and its nonhuman

Paul W. Taylor, Excerpts from "The Ethics of Respect for Nature," *Environmental Ethics* Vol. 3, No. 3 (1981): 197–218. Reprinted by permission of Paul Taylor.

inhabitants are right (or wrong) by either of two criteria: they have consequences which are favorable (or unfavorable) to human well-being, or they are consistent (or inconsistent) with the system of norms that protect and implement human rights. From this human-centered standpoint it is to humans and only to humans that all duties are ultimately owed. We may have responsibilities *with regard to* the natural ecosystems and biotic communities of our planet, but these responsibilities are in every case based on the contingent fact that our treatment of those ecosystems and communities of life can further the realization of human values and/or human rights. We have no obligation to promote or protect the good of nonhuman living things, independently of this contingent fact.

A life-centered system of environmental ethics is opposed to human-centered ones precisely on this point. From the perspective of a life-centered theory, we have prima facie moral obligations that are owed to wild plants and animals themselves as members of the Earth's biotic community. We are morally bound (other things being equal) to protect or promote their good for *their* sake. Our duties to respect the integrity of natural ecosystems, to preserve endangered species, and to avoid environmental pollution stem from the fact that these are ways in which we can help make it possible for wild species populations to achieve and maintain a healthy existence in a natural state. Such obligations are due those living things out of recognition of their inherent worth. They are entirely additional to and independent of the obligations we owe to our fellow humans. Although many of the actions that fulfill one set of obligations will also fulfill the other, two different grounds of obligation are involved. Their well-being, as well as human well-being, is something to be realized *as an end in itself*.

If we were to accept a life-centered theory of environmental ethics, a profound reordering of our moral universe would take place. We would begin to look at the whole of the Earth's biosphere in a new light. Our duties with respect to the "world" of nature would be seen as making prima facie claims upon us to be balanced against our duties with respect to the "world" of human civilization. We could no longer simply take the human point of view and consider the effects of our actions exclusively from the perspective of our own good.

II. THE GOOD OF A BEING AND THE CONCEPT OF INHERENT WORTH

What would justify acceptance of a life-centered system of ethical principles? In order to answer this it is first necessary to make clear the fundamental moral attitude that underlies and makes intelligible the commitment to live by such a system. It is then necessary to examine the considerations that would justify any rational agent's adopting that moral attitude.

Two concepts are essential to the taking of a moral attitude of the sort in question. A being which does not "have" these concepts, that is, which is unable to grasp their meaning and conditions of applicability, cannot be said to have the attitude as part of its moral outlook. These concepts are, first, that of the good (well-being, welfare) of a living thing, and second, the idea of an entity possessing inherent worth. I examine each concept in turn.

(1) Every organism, species population, and community of life has a good of its own which moral agents can intentionally further or damage by their actions. To say that an entity has a good of its own is simply to say that, without reference to any *other* entity, it can be benefited or harmed. One can act in its overall interest or contrary to its overall interest, and environmental conditions can be good for it (advantageous to it) or bad for it (disadvantageous to it). What is good for an entity is what "does it good" in the sense of enhancing or preserving its life and well-being. What is bad for an entity is something that is detrimental to its life and well-being.

We can think of the good of an individual non-human organism as consisting in the full development of its biological powers. Its good is realized to the extent that it is strong and healthy. It possesses whatever capacities it needs for successfully coping with its environment and so preserving its existence throughout the various stages of the normal life cycle of its species. The good of a population or community of such individuals consists in the population or community maintaining itself from generation to generation as a coherent system of genetically and ecologically related organisms whose average good is at an optimum level for the given environment. (Here *average good* means that the degree of realization of the good of *individual organisms* in the population or community is, on average, greater than would be the case under any other ecologically functioning order of interrelations among those species populations in the given ecosystem.)

The idea of a being having a good of its own, as I understand it, does not entail that the being must have interests or take an interest in what affects its life for better or for worse. We can act in a being's interest or contrary to its interest without its being interested in what we are doing to it in the sense of wanting or not wanting us to do it. It may, indeed, be wholly unaware that favorable and unfavorable events are taking place in its life. I take it that trees, for example, have no knowledge or desires or feelings. Yet it is undoubtedly the case that trees can be harmed or benefited by our actions. We can crush their roots by running a bulldozer too close to them. We can see to it that they get adequate nourishment and moisture by fertilizing and watering the soil around them. Thus we can help or hinder them in the realization of their good. It is the good of trees themselves that is thereby affected. We can similarly act so as to further the good of an entire tree population of a certain species (say, all the redwood trees in a California valley) or the good of a whole community of plant life in a given wilderness area, just as we can do harm to such a population or community.

When constructed in this way, the concept of a being's good is not coextensive with sentience or the capacity for feeling pain. William Frankena has argued for a general theory of environmental ethics in which the ground of a creature's being worthy of moral consideration is its sentience. I have offered some criticisms of this view elsewhere, but the full refutation of such a position, it seems to me, finally depends on the positive reasons for accepting a life-centered theory of a kind I am defending in this essay.

It should be noted further that I am leaving open the question of whether machines—in particular, those which are not only goal-directed, but also self-regulating—can properly be said to have a good of their own. Since I am concerned only with human treatment of wild organisms, species populations, and communities of life as they occur in our planet's natural ecosystems, it is to those entities alone that the concept "having a good of its own" will here be applied. I am not denying that other living things, whose genetic origin and environmental conditions have been produced, controlled, and manipulated by humans for human ends, do have a good of their own in the same sense as do wild plants and animals. It is not my purpose in this essay, however, to set out or defend the principles that should guide our conduct with regard to their good. It is only insofar as their production and use by humans have good or ill effects upon natural ecosystems and their wild inhabitants that the ethics of respect for nature comes into play.

(2) The second concept essential to the moral attitude of respect for nature is the idea of inherent worth. We take that attitude toward wild living things (individuals, species populations, or whole biotic communities) when and only when we regard them as entities possessing inherent worth. Indeed, it is only because they are conceived in this way that moral agents can think of themselves as having validly blinding duties, obligations, and responsibilities that are *owed* to them as their *due*. I am not at this juncture arguing why they *should* be so regarded; I consider it at length below. But so regarding them is a presupposition of our taking the attitude of respect toward them and accordingly understanding ourselves as bearing certain moral relations to them. This can be shown as follows:

What does it mean to regard an entity that has a good of its own as possessing inherent worth? Two general principles are involved: the principle of moral consideration and the principle of intrinsic value.

According to the principle of moral consideration, wild living things are deserving of the concern and consideration of all moral agents simply in virtue of their being members of the Earth's community of life. From the moral point of view their good must be taken into account whenever it is affected for better or worse by the conduct of rational agents. This holds no matter what species the creature belongs to. The good of each is to be accorded some value and so acknowledged as having some weight in the deliberation of all rational agents. Of course, it may be necessary for such agents to act in ways contrary to the good of this or that particular organism or group of organisms in order to further the good of others, including the good of humans. But the principle of moral consideration prescribes that, with respect to each being an entity having its own good, every individual is deserving of consideration.

The principle of intrinsic value states that, regardless of what kind of entity it is in other respects, if it is a member of the Earth's community of life, the realization of its good is something *intrinsically* valuable. This means that its good is prima facie worthy of being preserved or promoted as an end in itself and for the sake of the entity whose good it is. Insofar as we regard any organism, species population, or life community as an entity having inherent worth, we believe that it must never be treated as if it were a mere object or thing whose entire value lies in being instrumental to the good of some other entity. The well-being of each is judged to have value in and of itself.

Combining these two principles, we can now define what it means for a living thing or group of living things to possess inherent worth. To say that it possesses inherent worth is to say that its good is deserving of the concern and consideration of all moral agents, and that the realization of its good has intrinsic value, to be pursued as an end in itself and for the sake of the entity whose good it is.

The duties owed to wild organisms, species populations, and communities of life in the Earth's natural ecosystems are grounded on their inherent worth. When rational, autonomous agents regard such entities as possessing inherent worth, they place intrinsic value on the realization of their good and so hold themselves responsible for performing actions that will have this effect and for refraining from actions having the contrary effect.

III. THE ATTITUDE OF RESPECT FOR NATURE

Why should moral agents regard wild living things in the natural world as possessing inherent worth? To answer this question we must first take into account the fact that, when rational, autonomous agents subscribe to the principles of moral consideration and intrinsic value and so conceive of wild living things as having that kind of worth, such agents are *adopting a certain ultimate moral attitude toward the natural world*. This is the attitude I call "respect for nature." It parallels the attitude of respect for persons in human ethics. When we adopt the attitude of respect for persons as the proper (fitting, appropriate) attitude to take toward all persons as persons, we consider the fulfillment of the basic interests of each individual to have intrinsic value. We thereby make a moral commitment to live a certain kind of life in relation to other persons. We place ourselves under the direction of a system of standards and rules that we consider validly binding on all moral agents as such.

Similarly, when we adopt the attitude of respect for nature as an ultimate moral attitude we make a commitment to live by certain normative principles. These principles constitute the rules of conduct and standards of character that are to govern our treatment of the natural world. This is, first, an *ultimate* commitment because it is not derived from any higher norm. The attitude of respect for nature is not grounded on some other, more general, or more fundamental attitude. It sets the total framework for our responsibilities toward the natural world. It can be justified, as I show below, but its justification cannot consist in referring to a more general attitude or a more basic normative principle.

Second, the commitment is a *moral* one because it is understood to be a disinterested matter of principle. It is this feature that distinguishes the attitude of respect for nature from the set of feelings and dispositions that comprise the love of nature. The latter stems from one's personal interest in a response to the natural world. Like the affectionate feelings we have toward certain individual human beings, one's love of nature is nothing more than the particular way one feels about the natural environment and its wild inhabitants. And just as our love for an individual person differs from our respect for all persons as such (whether we happen to love them or not), so love of nature differs from respect for nature. Respect for nature is an attitude we believe all moral agents ought to have simply as moral agents, regardless of whether or not they also love nature. Indeed, we have not truly taken the attitude of respect for nature ourselves unless we believe this. To put it in a Kantian way, to adopt the attitude of respect for nature is to take a stance that one wills it to be a universal law for all rational beings. It is to hold that stance categorically, as being validly applicable to every moral agent without exception, irrespective of whatever personal feelings toward nature such an agent might have or might lack.

Although the attitude of respect for nature is in this sense a disinterested and universalizable attitude, anyone who does adopt it has certain steady, more or less permanent dispositions. These dispositions, which are themselves to be considered disinterested and universalizable, comprise three interlocking sets: dispositions to seek certain ends, dispositions to carry on one's practical reasoning and deliberation in a certain way, and dispositions to have certain feelings. We may accordingly analyze the attitude of respect for nature into the following components. (a) The disposition to aim at, and to take steps to bring about, as final and disinterested ends, the promoting and protecting of the good of organisms, species populations, and life communities in natural ecosystems. (These ends are "final" in not being pursued as means to further ends. They are "disinterested" in being independent of the self-interest of the agent.) (b) The disposition to consider actions that tend to realize those ends to be prima facie obligatory *because* they have that tendency. (c) The disposition to experience positive and negative feelings toward states of affairs in the world *because* they are favorable or unfavorable to the good of organisms, species populations, and life communities in natural ecosystems.

The logical connection between the attitude of respect for nature and the duties of a life-centered system of environmental ethics can now be made clear. Insofar as one sincerely takes that attitude and so has the three sets of dispositions, one will at the same time be disposed to comply with certain rules of duty (such as nonmaleficence and noninterference) and with standards of character (such as fairness and benevolence) that determine the obligations and virtues of moral agents with regard to the Earth's wild living things. We can say that the actions one performs and the character traits one develops in fulfilling these moral requirements are the way one *expresses* or *embodies* the attitude in one's conduct and character. In his famous essay, "Justice as Fairness," John Rawls describes the rules of the duties of human morality (such as fidelity, gratitude, honesty, and justice) as "forms of conduct in which recognition of others as persons is manifested."[1] I hold that the rules of duty governing our treatment of the natural world and its inhabitants are forms of conduct in which the attitude of respect for nature is manifested.

IV. THE JUSTIFIABILITY OF THE ATTITUDE OF RESPECT FOR NATURE

I return to the question posed earlier, which has not yet been answered: why *should* moral agents regard wild living things as possessing inherent worth? I now argue that the only way we can answer this question is by showing how adopting the attitude of respect for nature is justified for all moral agents. Let us suppose that we were able to establish that there are good reasons for adopting the attitude, reasons which are intersubjectively valid for every rational agent. If there are such reasons, they would justify anyone's having the three sets of dispositions mentioned above as constituting what it means to have the attitude. Since these include the disposition to promote or protect the good of wild living things as a disinterested and ultimate end, as well as the disposition to perform actions for the reason that they tend to realize that end, we see that such dispositions commit a person to the principles of moral consideration and intrinsic value. To be disposed to further, as an end in itself, the

good of any entity in nature just because it is that kind of entity, is to be disposed to give consideration to *every* such entity and to place intrinsic value on the realization of its good. Insofar as we subscribe to these two principles we regard living things as possessing inherent worth. Subscribing to the principles is what it *means* to so regard them. To justify the attitude of respect for nature, then, is to justify commitment to these principles and thereby to justify regarding wild creatures as possessing inherent worth.

We must keep in mind that inherent worth is not some mysterious sort of objective property belonging to living things that can be discovered by empirical observation or scientific investigation. To ascribe inherent worth to an entity is not to describe it by citing some feature discernible by sense perception or inferable by inductive reasoning. Nor is there a logically necessary connection between the concept of a being having a good of its own and the concept of inherent worth. We do not contradict ourselves by asserting that an entity that has a good of its own lacks inherent worth. In order to show that such an entity "has" inherent worth we must give good reasons for ascribing that kind of value to it (placing that kind of value upon it, conceiving of it to be valuable in that way). Although it is humans (persons, valuers) who must do the valuing, for the ethics of respect for nature, the value so ascribed is not a human value. That is to say, it is not a value derived from considerations regarding human well-being or human rights. It is a value that is ascribed to nonhuman animals and plants themselves, independently of their relationship to what humans judge to be conducive to their own good.

Whatever reasons, then, justify our taking the attitude of respect for nature as defined above are also reasons that show why we *should* regard the living things of the natural world as possessing inherent worth. We saw earlier that, since the attitude is an ultimate one, it cannot be derived from a more fundamental attitude nor shown to be a special case of a more general one. On what sort of grounds, then, can it be established?

The attitude we take toward living things in the natural world depends on the way we look at them, on what kind of beings we conceive them to be, and on how we understand the relations we bear to them. Underlying and supporting your attitude is a certain *belief system* that constitutes a particular world view or outlook on nature and the place of human life in it. To give good reasons for adopting the attitude of respect for nature, then, we must first articulate the belief system which underlies and supports that attitude. If it appears that the belief system is internally coherent and well-ordered, and if, as far as we can now tell, it is consistent with all known scientific truths relevant to our knowledge of the object of the attitude (which in this case includes the whole set of the Earth's natural ecosystems and their communities of life), then there remains the task of indicating why scientifically informed and rational thinkers with a developed capacity of reality awareness can find it acceptable as a way of conceiving of the natural world and our place in it. To the extent we can do this we provide at least a reasonable argument for accepting the belief system and the ultimate moral attitude it supports.

I do not hold that such a belief system can be *proven* to be true, either inductively or deductively. As we shall see, not all of its components can be stated in the form of empirically verifiable propositions. Nor is its internal order governed by purely logical relationships. But the system as a whole, I contend, constitutes a coherent, unified, and rationally acceptable "picture" or "map" of a total world. By examining each of its main components and seeing how they fit together, we obtain a scientifically informed and well-ordered conception of nature and the place of humans in it.

This belief system underlying the attitude of respect for nature I call (for want of a better name) "the biocentric outlook on nature." Since it is not wholly analyzable into empirically confirmable assertions, it should not be thought of as simply a compendium of the biological sciences concerning our planet's ecosystems. It might best be described as a philosophical world view, to distinguish it from a scientific theory or explanatory system. However, one of its major tenets is the great lesson we have learned from the science of ecology: the interdependence of all living things in an organically unified order whose balance and stability are necessary conditions for the realization of the good of its constituent biotic communities.

Before turning to an account of the main components of the biocentric outlook, it is convenient here to set forth the overall structure of my theory of environmental ethics as it has now emerged. The ethics of respect for nature is made up of three basic elements: a belief system, an ultimate moral attitude, and a set of rules of duty and standards of character. These elements are connected with each other in the following manner. The belief system provides a certain outlook on nature which supports and makes intelligible an autonomous agent's adopting, as an ultimate moral attitude, the attitude of respect for nature. It supports and makes intelligible the attitude in the sense that, when an autonomous agent understands its moral relations to the natural world in terms of this outlook, it recognizes the attitude of respect to be the only *suitable* or *fitting* attitude to take toward all wild forms of life in the Earth's biosphere. Living things are now viewed as *the appropriate objects of the attitude of respect* and are accordingly regarded as entities possessing inherent worth. One then places intrinsic value on the promotion and protection of their good. As a consequence of this, one makes a moral commitment to abide by a set of rules of duty and to fulfill (as far as one can by one's own efforts) certain standards of good character. Given one's adoption of the attitude of respect, one makes that moral commitment because one considers those rules and standards to be validly binding on all moral agents. They are seen as embodying forms of conduct and character structures in which the attitude of respect for nature is manifested.

This three-part complex which internally orders the ethics of respect for nature is symmetrical with a theory of human ethics grounded on respect for persons. Such a theory includes, first, a conception of oneself and others as persons, that is, as centers of autonomous choice. Second, there is the attitude of respect for persons as persons. When this is adopted as an ultimate moral attitude it involves the disposition to treat every person as having inherent worth or "human dignity." Every human being, just in virtue of her or his humanity, is understood to be worthy of moral consideration, and intrinsic value is placed on the autonomy and well-being of each. This is what Kant meant by conceiving of persons as ends in themselves. Third, there is an ethical system of duties which are acknowledged to be owed by everyone to everyone. These duties are forms of conduct in which public recognition is given to each individual's inherent worth as a person.

This structural framework for a theory of human ethics is meant to leave open the issue of consequentialism (utilitarianism) versus nonconsequentialism (deontology). That issue concerns the particular kind of system of rules defining the duties of moral agents toward persons. Similarly, I am leaving open in this paper the question of what particular kind of system of rules defines our duties with respect to the natural world.

V. THE BIOCENTRIC OUTLOOK ON NATURE

The biocentric outlook on nature has four main components. (1) Humans are thought of as members of the Earth's community of life, holding that membership on the same terms as apply to all the nonhuman members. (2) The Earth's natural ecosystems as a totality are seen as a complex web of interconnected elements, with the sound biological functioning of each being dependent on the sound biological function of the others. (This is the component referred to above as the great lesson that the science of ecology has taught us). (3) Each individual organism is conceived of as a teleological center of life, pursuing its own good in its own way. (4) Whether we are concerned with standards of merit or with the concept of inherent worth, the claim that humans by their very nature are superior to other species is a groundless claim and, in the light of elements (1), (2), and (3) above, must be rejected as nothing more than an irrational bias in our own favor.

The conjunction of these four ideas constitutes the biocentric outlook on nature. In the remainder of this paper I give a brief account of the first three components, followed by a more detailed analysis of the fourth. I then conclude by indicating how this outlook provides a way of justifying the attitude of respect for nature.

VI. HUMANS AS MEMBERS OF THE EARTH'S COMMUNITY OF LIFE

We share with other species a common relationship to the Earth. In accepting the biocentric outlook we take the fact of our being an animal species to be a fundamental feature of our existence. We consider it an essential aspect of "the human condition." We do not deny the differences between ourselves and other species, but we keep in the forefront of our consciousness the fact that in relation to our planet's natural ecosystems we are but one species population among many. Thus we acknowledge our origin in the very same evolutionary process that gave rise to all other species and we recognize ourselves to be confronted with similar environmental challenges to those that confront them. The laws of genetics, of natural selection, and of adaptation apply equally to all of us as biological creatures. In this light we consider ourselves as one with them, not set apart from them. We, as well as they, must face certain basic conditions of existence that impose requirements on us for our survival and well-being. Each animal and plant is like us in having a good of its own. Although our human good (what is of true value in human life, including the exercise of individual autonomy in choosing our own particular value systems) is not like the good of a nonhuman animal or plant, it can no more be realized than their good can without the biological necessities for survival and physical health.

When we look at ourselves from the evolutionary point of view, we see that not only are we very recent arrivals on Earth, but that our emergence as a new species on the planet was originally an event of no particular importance to the entire scheme of things. The Earth was teeming with life long before we appeared. Putting the point metaphorically, we are relative newcomers, entering a home that has been the residence of others for hundreds of millions of years, a home that must now be shared by all of us together.

The comparative brevity of human life on Earth may be vividly depicted by imagining the geological time scale in spatial terms. Suppose we start with algae, which have been around for at least 600 million years. (The earliest protozoa actually predated this by several *billion* years.) If the time that algae have been here were represented by the length of a football field (300 feet), then the period during which sharks have been swimming in the world's oceans and spiders have been spinning their webs would occupy three quarters of the length of the field; reptiles would show up at about the center of the field; mammals would cover the last third of the field; hominids (mammals of the family *Hominidae*) the last two feet; and the species *Homo sapiens* the last six inches.

Whether this newcomer is able to survive as long as other species remains to be seen. But there is surely something presumptuous about the way humans look down on the "lower" animals, especially those that have become extinct. We consider the dinosaurs, for example, to be biological failures, though they existed on our planet for 65 million years. One writer has made the point with beautiful simplicity:

> We sometimes speak of the dinosaurs as failures; there will be time enough for that judgment when we have lasted even for one tenth as long. . . .[2]

The possibility of the extinction of the human species, a possibility which starkly confronts us in the contemporary world, makes us aware of another respect in which we should not consider ourselves privileged beings in relation to other species. This is the fact that the well-being of humans is dependent upon the ecological soundness and health of many plant and animal communities, while their soundness and health does not in the least depend upon human well-being. Indeed, from their standpoint the very existence of humans is quite unnecessary. Every last man, woman, and child could disappear from the face of the Earth without any significant detrimental consequence for the good of wild animals and plants. On the contrary, many of them would be greatly benefited. The destruction of their habitats by human "developments" would cease. The poisoning and pol-luting of their environment would come to an end. The Earth's land, air, and water would no longer be subject to the degradation they are now undergoing as the result of large-scale technology and uncontrolled population growth. Life communities in natural ecosystems would gradually return to their former healthy state. Tropical forests, for example, would again be able to make their full contribution to a life-sustaining atmosphere for the whole planet. The rivers, lakes, and oceans of the world would (perhaps) eventually become clean again. Spilled oil, plastic trash, and even radioactive waste might finally, after many centuries, cease doing their terrible work. Ecosystems would return to their proper balance, suffering only the disruptions of natural events such as volcanic eruptions and glaciation. From these the community of life could recover, as it has so often done in the past. But the ecological disasters now perpetrated on it by humans—disasters from which it might never recover—these it would no longer have to endure.

If, then, the total, final, absolute extermination of our species (by our own hands?) should take place and if we should not carry all the others with us into oblivion, not only would the Earth's community of life continue to exist, but in all probability its well-being would be enhanced. Our presence, in short, is not needed. If we were to take the standpoint of the community and give voice to its true interest, the ending of our six-inch epoch would most likely be greeted with a hearty "Good riddance!"

VII. THE NATURAL WORLD AS AN ORGANIC SYSTEM

To accept the biocentric outlook and regard ourselves and our place in the world from its perspective is to see the whole natural order of the Earth's biosphere as a complex but unified web of interconnected organisms, objects, and events. The ecological relationships between any community of living things and their environment form an organic whole of functionally interdependent parts. Each ecosystem is a small universe itself in which the interactions of its various species populations comprise an intricately woven network of cause-effect relations. Such dynamic but at the same time relatively stable structures as food chains, predator-prey relations, and plant succession in a forest are self-regulating, energy-recycling mechanisms that preserve the equilibrium of the whole.

As far as the well-being of wild animals and plants is concerned, this ecological equilibrium must not be destroyed. The same holds true of the well-being of humans. When one views the realm of nature from the perspective of the biocentric outlook, one never forgets that in the long run the integrity of the entire biosphere of our planet is essential to the realization of the good of its constituent communities of life, both human and nonhuman.

Although the importance of this idea cannot be overemphasized, it is by now so familiar and so widely acknowledged that I shall not further elaborate on it here. However, I do wish to point out that this "holistic" view of the Earth's ecological systems does not itself constitute a moral norm. It is a factual aspect of biological reality, to be understood as a set of causal connections in ordinary empirical terms. Its significance for humans is the same as its significance for nonhumans, namely, in setting basic conditions for the realization of the good of living things. Its ethical implications for our treatment of the natural environment lie entirely in the fact that our *knowledge* of these causal connections is an essential *means* to fulfilling the aims we set for ourselves in adopting the attitude of respect for nature. In addition, its theoretical implications for the ethics of respect for nature lie in the fact that it (along with the other elements of the biocentric outlook) makes the adopting of that attitude a rational and intelligible thing to do.

VIII. INDIVIDUAL ORGANISMS AS TELEOLOGICAL CENTERS OF LIFE

As our knowledge of living things increases, as we come to a deeper understanding of their life cycles, their interactions with other organisms, and the manifold ways in which they adjust to the environment, we become more fully aware of how each of them is carrying out its biological functions according to the laws of its species-specific nature. But besides this, our increasing knowledge and understanding also develop in us a sharpened awareness of the uniqueness of each individual organism. Scientists who have made careful studies of particular plants and animals, whether in the field or in laboratories, have often acquired a knowledge of their subjects as identifiable individuals. Close observation over extended periods of time has led them to an appreciation of the unique "personalities" of their subjects. Sometimes a scientist may come to take a special interest in a particular animal or plant, all the while remaining strictly objective in the gathering and recording of data. Nonscientists may likewise experience this development of interest when, as amateur naturalists, they make accurate observations over sustained periods of close acquaintance with an individual organism. As one becomes more and more familiar with the organism and its behavior, one becomes fully sensitive to the particular way it is living out its life cycle. One may become fascinated by it and even experience some involvement with its good and bad fortunes (that is, with the occurrence of environmental conditions favorable or unfavorable to the realization of its good). The organism comes to mean something to one as a unique, irreplaceable individual. The final culmination of this process is the achievement of a genuine understanding of its point of view and, with that understanding, an ability to "take" that point of view. *Conceiving of it as a center of life, one is able to look at the world from its perspective.*

This development from objective knowledge to the recognition of individuality to full awareness of an organism's standpoint, is a process of heightening our consciousness of what it means to be an individual living thing. We grasp the particularity of the organism as a teleological center of life, striving to preserve itself and to realize its own good in its own unique way.

It is to be noted that we need not be falsely anthropomorphizing when we conceive of individual plants and animals in this manner. Understanding them as teleological centers of life does not necessitate "reading into" them human characteristics. We need not, for example, consider them to have consciousness. Some of them may be aware of the world around them and others may not. Nor need we deny that different kinds and levels of awareness are exemplified when consciousness in some form is present. But conscious or not, all are equally teleological centers of life in the sense that each is a unified system of goal-oriented activities directed toward their preservation and well-being.

When considered from an ethical point of view, a teleological center of life is an entity whose "world" can be viewed from the perspective of *its* life. In looking at the world from that perspective we recognize objects and events occurring in its life as being beneficent, maleficent, or indifferent. The first are occurrences which increase its powers to preserve its existence and realize its good. The second decrease or destroy those powers. The third have neither of these effects on the entity. With regard to our human role as moral agents, we can conceive of a teleological center of life as a being whose standpoint we can take in making judgments about what events in the world are good or evil, desirable or undesirable. In making these judgments it is what promotes or protects the being's own good, not what benefits moral agents themselves, that sets the standard of evaluation. Such judgments can be made about anything that happens to the entity which is favorable or unfavorable in relation to its good. As was pointed out earlier, the entity itself need not have any (conscious) *interest* in what is happening to it for such judgments to be meaningful and true.

It is precisely judgments of this sort that we are disposed to make when we take the attitude of respect for nature. In adopting that attitude those judgments are given weight as reasons for action in our practical deliberation. They become morally relevant facts in the guidance of our conduct.

IX. THE DENIAL OF HUMAN SUPERIORITY

This fourth component of the biocentric outlook on nature is the single most important idea in establishing the justifiability of the attitude of respect for nature. Its central role is due to the special relationship it bears to the first three components of the outlook. This relationship will be brought out after the concept of human superiority is examined and analyzed.

In what sense are humans alleged to be superior to other animals? We are different from them in having certain capacities that they lack. But why should these capacities be a mark of superiority? From what point of view are they judged to be signs of superiority and what sense of superiority is meant? After all, various nonhuman species have capacities that humans lack. There is the speed of a cheetah, the vision of an eagle, the agility of a monkey. Why should not these be taken as signs of *their* superiority over humans.

One answer that comes immediately to mind is that these capacities are not as *valuable* as the human capacities that are claimed to make us superior. Such uniquely human characteristics as rational thought, aesthetic creativity, autonomy and self-determination, and moral freedom, it might be held, have a higher value than the capacities found in other species. Yet we must ask: valuable to whom, and on what grounds?

The human characteristics mentioned are all valuable to humans. They are essential to the preservation and enrichment of our civilization and culture. Clearly it is from the human standpoint that they are being judged to be desirable and good. It is not difficult here to recognize a begging of the question. Humans are claiming human superiority from a strictly human point of view, that is, from a point of view in which the good of humans is taken as the standard of judgment. All we need to do is to look at the capacities of nonhuman animals (or plants, for that matter) from the standpoint of *their* good to find a contrary judgment of superiority. The speed of the cheetah, for example, is a sign of its superiority to humans when considered from the standpoint of the good of its species. If it were as slow a runner as a human, it would not be able to survive. And so for all the other abilities of nonhumans which further their good but which are lacking in humans. In each case the claim to human superiority would be rejected from a nonhuman standpoint.

When superiority assertions are interpreted in this way, they are based on judgments of *merit*.

To judge the merits of a person or an organism one must apply grading or ranking standards to it. (As I show below, this distinguishes judgments of merit from judgments of inherent worth.) Empirical investigation then determines whether it has the "good-making properties" (merits) in virtue of which it fulfills the standards being applied. In the case of humans, merits may be either moral or nonmoral. We can judge one person to be better than (superior to) another from the moral point of view by applying certain standards to their character and conduct. Similarly, we can appeal to nonmoral criteria in judging someone to be an excellent piano player, a fair cook, a poor tennis player, and so on. Different social purposes and roles are implicit in the making of such judgments, providing the frame of reference for the choice of standards by which the nonmoral merits of people are determined. Ultimately such purposes and roles stem from a society's way of life as a whole. Now a society's way of life may be thought of as the cultural form given to the realization of human values. Whether moral or nonmoral standards are being applied, then, all judgments of people's merits finally depend on human values. All are made from an exclusively human standpoint.

The question that naturally arises at this juncture is: why should standards that are based on human values be assumed to be the only valid criteria of merit and hence the only true signs of superiority? This question is especially pressing when humans are being judged superior in merit to nonhumans. It is true that a human being may be a better mathematician than a monkey, but the monkey may be a better tree climber than a human being. If we humans value mathematics more than tree climbing, that is because our conception of civilized life makes the development of mathematical ability more desirable than the ability to climb trees. But is it not unreasonable to judge nonhumans by the values of human civilization, rather than by values connected with what it is for a member of *that* species to live a good life? If all living things have a good of their own, it at least makes sense to judge the merits of nonhumans by standards derived from *their* good. To use only standards based on human values is already to commit oneself to holding that humans are superior to nonhumans, which is the point in question.

A further logical flaw arises in connection with the widely held conviction that humans are *morally* superior beings because they possess, while others lack, the capacities of a moral agent (free will, accountability, deliberation, judgment, practical reason). This view rests on a conceptual confusion. As far as moral standards are concerned, only beings that have the capacities of a moral agent can properly be judged to be *either* moral (morally good) *or* immoral (morally deficient). Moral standards are simply not applicable to beings that lack such capacities. Animals and plants cannot therefore be said to be morally inferior in merit to humans. Since the only beings that can have moral merits *or be deficient in such merits* are moral agents, it is conceptually incoherent to judge humans as superior to nonhumans on the ground that humans have moral capacities while nonhumans don't.

Up to this point I have been interpreting the claim that humans are superior to other living things as a grading or ranking judgment regarding their comparative merits. There is, however, another way of understanding the idea of human superiority. According to this interpretation, humans are superior to nonhumans not as regards their merits but as regards their inherent worth. Thus the claim of human superiority is to be understood as asserting that all humans, simply in virtue of their humanity, have *a greater inherent worth* than other living things.

The inherent worth of an entity does not depend on its merits. To consider something as possessing inherent worth, we have seen, is to place intrinsic value on the realization of its good. This is done regardless of whatever particular merits it might have or might lack, as judged by a set of grading or ranking standards. In human affairs, we are all familiar with the principle that one's worth as a person does not vary with one's merits or lack of merits. The same can hold true of animals and plants. To regard such entities as possessing inherent worth entails disregarding their merits and deficiencies, whether they are being judged from a human standpoint or from the standpoint of their own species.

The idea of one entity having more merit than another, and so being superior to it in merit, makes perfectly good sense. Merit is a grading or ranking concept, and judgments of comparative merit are based on the different degrees to which things satisfy a given standard. But what can it mean to talk about one thing being superior to another in inherent worth? In order to get at what is being asserted in such a claim it is helpful first to look at the social origin of the concept of degrees of inherent worth.

The idea that humans can possess different degrees of inherent worth originated in societies having rigid class structures. Before the rise of modern democracies with their egalitarian outlook, one's membership in a hereditary class determined one's social status. People in the upper classes were looked up to, while those in the lower classes were looked down upon. In such a society one's social superiors and social inferiors were clearly defined and easily recognized.

Two aspects of these class-structured societies are especially relevant to the idea of degrees of inherent worth. First, those born into the upper classes were deemed more worthy of respect than those born into the lower orders. Second, the superior worth of upper class people had nothing to do with their merits nor did the inferior worth of those in the lower classes rest on their lack of merits. One's superiority or inferiority entirely derived from a social position one was born into. The modern concept of a meritocracy simply did not apply. One could not advance into a higher class by any sort of moral or nonmoral achievement. Similarly, an aristocrat held his title and all the privileges that went with it just because he was the eldest son of a titled nobleman. Unlike the bestowing of knighthood in contemporary Great Britain, one did not earn membership in the nobility by meritorious conduct.

We who live in modern democracies no longer believe in such hereditary social distinctions. Indeed, we would wholeheartedly condemn them on moral grounds as being fundamentally unjust. We have come to think of class systems as a paradigm of social injustice, it being a central principle of the democratic way of life that among humans there are no superiors and no inferiors. Thus we have rejected the whole conceptual framework in which people are judged to have different degrees of inherent worth. That idea is incompatible with our notion of human equality based on the doctrine that all humans, simply in virtue of their humanity, have the same inherent worth. (The belief in universal human rights is one form that this egalitarianism takes.)

The vast majority of people in modern democracies, however, do not maintain an egalitarian outlook when it comes to comparing human beings with other living things. Most people consider our own species to be superior to all other species and this superiority is understood to be a matter of inherent worth, not merit. There may exist thoroughly vicious and depraved humans who lack all merit. Yet because they are human they are thought to belong to a higher class of entities than any plant or animal. That one is born into the species *Homo sapiens* entitles one to have lordship over those who are one's inferiors, namely, those born into other species. The parallel with hereditary social classes is very close. Implicit in this view is a hierarchical conception of nature according to which an organism has a position of superiority or inferiority in the Earth's community of life simply on the basis of its genetic background. The "lower" orders of life are looked down upon and it is considered perfectly proper that they serve the interests of those belonging to the highest order, namely humans. The intrinsic value we place on the well-being of our fellow humans reflects our recognition of their rightful positions as our equals. No such intrinsic value is to be placed on the good of other animals, unless we choose to do so out of fondness or affection for them. But their well-being imposes no moral requirement on us. In this respect there is an absolute difference in moral status between ourselves and them.

This is the structure of concepts and beliefs that people are committed to insofar as they regard humans to be superior in inherent worth to all other species. I now wish to argue that this structure of concepts and beliefs is completely groundless. If we accept the first three components of the biocentric outlook and from that perspective look at the major philosophical traditions which have supported that structure, we find it to be at bottom nothing more than the expression of an irrational bias in our own favor. The philosophical traditions themselves rest on very questionable assumptions or else simply beg the question. I briefly consider three of the main traditions to substantiate the point. These are classical Greek humanism, Cartesian dualism, and the Judeo-Christian concept of the Great Chain of Being.

The inherent superiority of humans over other species was implicit in the Greek definition of man as a rational animal. Our animal nature was identified with "brute" desires that need the order and restraint of reason to rule them (just as reason is the special virtue of those who rule in the ideal state). Rationality was then seen to be the key to our superiority over animals. It enables us to live on a higher plane and endows us with a nobility and worth that other creatures lack. This familiar way of comparing humans with other species is deeply ingrained in our Western philosophical outlook. The point to consider here is that this view does not actually provide an argument *for* human superiority but rather makes explicit the framework of thought that is implicitly used by those who think of humans as inherently superior to nonhumans. The Greeks who held that humans, in virtue of their rational capacities, have a kind of worth greater than that of any nonrational being, never looked at rationality as but one capacity of living things among many others. But when we consider rationality from the standpoint of the first three elements of the ecological outlook, we see that its value lies in its importance for *human* life. Other creatures achieve their species-specific good without the need of rationality, although they often make use of capacities that humans lack. So the humanistic outlook of classical Greek thought does not give us a neutral (non-question-begging) ground on which to construct a scale of degrees of inherent worth possessed by different species of living things.

The second tradition, centering on the Cartesian dualism of soul and body, also fails to justify the claim to human superiority. That superiority is supposed to derive from the fact that we have souls while animals do not. Animals are mere automata and lack

the divine element that makes us spiritual beings. I won't go into the now familiar criticisms of this two-substance view. I only add the point that, even if humans are composed of an immaterial, unextended soul and a material, extended body, this in itself is not a reason to deem them of greater worth than entities that are only bodies. Why is a soul substance a thing that adds value to its possessor? Unless some theological reasoning is offered here (which many, including myself, would find unacceptable on epistemological grounds), no logical connection is evident. An immaterial something which thinks is better than a material something which does not think only if thinking itself has value, either intrinsically or instrumentally. Now it is intrinsically valuable to humans alone, who value it as an end in itself, and it is instrumentally valuable to those who benefit from it, namely humans.

For animals that neither enjoy thinking for its own sake nor need it for living the kind of life for which they are best adapted, it has no value. Even if "thinking" is broadened to include all forms of consciousness, there are still many living things that can do without it and yet live what is for their species a good life. The anthropocentricity underlying the claim to human superiority runs throughout Cartesian dualism.

A third major source of the idea of human superiority is the Judeo-Christian concept of the Great Chain of Being. Humans are superior to animals and plants because their Creator has given them a higher place on the chain. It begins with God at the top, and then moves to the angels, who are lower than God but higher than humans, then to humans, positioned between the angels and the beasts (partaking of the nature of both), and then on down to the lower levels occupied by nonhuman animals, plants, and finally inanimate objects. Humans, being "made in God's image," are inherently superior to animals and plants by virtue of their being closer (in their essential nature) to God.

The metaphysical and epistemological difficulties with this conception of a hierarchy of entities are, in my mind, insuperable. Without entering into this matter here, I only point out that if we are unwilling to accept the metaphysics of traditional Judaism and Christianity, we are again left without good reasons for holding to the claim of inherent human superiority.

The foregoing considerations (and others like them) leave us with but one ground for the assertion that a human being, regardless of merit, is a higher kind of entity than any other living thing. This is the mere fact of the genetic makeup of the species *Homo sapiens*. But this is surely irrational and arbitrary. Why should the arrangement of genes of a certain type be a mark of superior value, especially when this fact about an organism is taken by itself, unrelated to any other aspect of its life? We might just as well refer to any other genetic makeup as a ground of superior value. Clearly we are confronted here with a wholly arbitrary claim that can only be explained as an irrational bias in our own favor.

That the claim is nothing more than a deep-seated prejudice is brought home to us when we look at our relation to other species in the light of the first three elements of the biocentric outlook. Those elements taken conjointly give us a certain overall view of the natural world and of the place of humans in it. When we take this view we come to understand other living things, their environmental conditions, and their ecological relationships in such a way as to awake in us a deep sense of our kinship with them as fellow members of the Earth's community of life. Humans and nonhumans alike are viewed together as integral parts of one unified whole in which all living things are functionally interrelated. Finally, when our awareness focuses on the individual lives of plants and animals, each is seen to share with us the characteristic of being a teleological center of life striving to realize its own good in its own unique way.

As this entire belief system becomes part of the conceptual framework through which we understand and perceive the world, we come to see ourselves as bearing a certain moral relation to nonhuman forms of life. Our ethical role in nature takes on a new significance. We begin to look at other species as we look at ourselves, seeing them as beings which have a good they are striving to realize just as we have a good we are striving to realize. We accordingly develop the disposition to view the world from the standpoint of their good as well as from the standpoint of our own good. Now if the groundlessness of the claim that humans are inherently superior to other species were brought clearly before our minds, we would not remain intellectually neutral toward that claim but would reject it as being fundamentally at variance with our total world outlook. In the absence of any good reasons for holding it, the assertion of human superiority would then appear simply as the expression of an irrational and self-serving prejudice that favors one particular species over several million others.

Rejecting the notion of human superiority entails its positive counterpart: the doctrine of species impartiality. One who accepts that doctrine regards all living things as possessing inherent worth—the *same* inherent worth, since no one species has been shown to be either "higher" or "lower" than any other. Now we saw earlier that, insofar as one thinks of a living thing as possessing inherent worth, one considers it to be the appropriate object of the attitude of respect and believes that attitude to be the only fitting or suitable one for all moral agents to take toward it.

Here, then, is the key to understanding how the attitude of respect is rooted in the biocentric outlook on nature. The basic connection is made through the denial of human superiority. Once we reject the claim that humans are superior either in merit or in worth to other living things, we are ready to adopt the attitude of respect. The denial of human superiority is itself the result of taking the perspective on nature built into the first three elements of the biocentric outlook.

Now the first three elements of the biocentric outlook, it seems clear, would be found acceptable to any rational and scientifically informed thinker who is fully "open" to the reality of the lives of nonhuman organisms. Without denying our distinctively human characteristics, such a thinker can acknowledge the fundamental respects in which we are members of the Earth's community of life and in which the biological conditions necessary for the realization of our human values are inextricably linked with the whole system of nature. In addition, the conception of individual living things as teleological centers of life simply articulates how a scientifically informed thinker comes to understand them as the result of increasingly careful and detailed observations. Thus, the biocentric outlook recommends itself as an acceptable system of concepts and beliefs to anyone who is clear-minded, unbiased, and factually enlightened, and who has a developed capacity of reality awareness with regard to the lives of individual organisms. This, I submit, is as good a reason for making the moral commitment involved in adopting the attitude of respect for nature as any theory of environmental ethics could possibly have.

X. MORAL RIGHTS AND THE MATTER OF COMPETING CLAIMS

I have not asserted anywhere in the foregoing account that animals or plants have moral rights. This omission was deliberate. I do not think that the reference class of the concept, bearer of moral rights, should be extended to include nonhuman living things. My reasons for taking this position, however, go beyond the scope of this paper. I believe I have been able to accomplish many of the same ends which those who ascribe rights to animals or plants wish to accomplish. There is no reason, moreover, why plants and animals, including whole species populations and life communities, cannot be accorded *legal* rights under my theory. To grant them legal protection could be interpreted as giving them legal entitlement to be protected, and this, in fact, would be a means by which a society that subscribed to the ethics of respect for nature could give public recognition to their inherent worth.

There remains the problem of competing claims, even when wild plants and animals are not thought of as bearers of moral rights. If we accept the biocentric outlook and accordingly adopt the attitude of respect for nature as our ultimate moral attitude, how do we resolve conflicts that arise from our respect for persons in the domain of human ethics and our respect for nature in the domain of environmental ethics? This is a question that cannot adequately be dealt with here. My main purpose in this paper has been to try to establish a base point from which we can start working toward a solution to the problem. I have shown why we cannot just begin with an initial presumption in favor of the interests of our own species. It is after all within our power as moral beings to place limits on human population and technology with the deliberate intention of sharing the Earth's bounty with other species. That such sharing is an ideal difficult to realize even in an approximate way does not take away its claim to our deepest moral commitment.

NOTES

1. John Rawls, "Justice As Fairness," *Philosophical Review* 67 (1958): 183.

2. Stephen R. L. Clark, *The Moral Status of Animals* (Oxford: Clarendon Press, 1977), p. 112.

Are All Species Equal?

DAVID SCHMIDTZ

I. RESPECT FOR NATURE

Species egalitarianism is the view that all species have equal moral standing.[1] To have moral standing is, at a minimum, to command respect, to be something more than a mere thing. Is there any reason to believe that all species have moral standing in even this most minimal sense? If so—that is, if all species command respect—is there any reason to believe they all command *equal* respect?

The following sections summarise critical responses to the most famous philosophical argument for species egalitarianism. I then try to explain why other species command our respect but also why they do not command equal respect. The intuition that we should have respect for nature is part of what motivates people to embrace species egalitarianism, but one need not be a species egalitarian to have respect for nature. I close by questioning whether species egalitarianism is even compatible with respect for nature.

II. THE GROUNDING OF SPECIES EGALITARIANISM

According to Paul Taylor, anthropocentrism 'gives either exclusive or primary consideration to human interests above the good of other species.'[2] The alternative to anthropocentrism is biocentrism, and it is biocentrism that, in Taylor's view, grounds species egalitarianism:

The beliefs that form the core of the biocentric outlook are four in number:

(a) The belief that humans are members of the Earth's Community of life in the same sense and on the same terms in which other living things are members of that community.

(b) The belief that the human species, along with all other species, are integral elements in a system of interdependence.

(c) The belief that all organisms are teleological centres of life in the sense that each is a unique individual pursuing its own good in its own way.

(d) The belief that humans are not inherently superior to other living beings.

Taylor concludes, 'Rejecting the notion of human superiority entails its positive counterpart: the doctrine of species impartiality. One who accepts that doctrine regards all living things as possessing inherent worth—the *same* inherent worth, since no one species has been shown to be either higher or lower than any other.'[3]

Taylor does not claim that this is a valid argument, but he thinks that if we concede (a), (b), and (c), it would be unreasonable not to move to (d), and then to his egalitarian conclusion. Is he right? For those who accept Taylor's three premises (and who thus interpret those premises in terms innocuous enough to render them acceptable), there are two responses. First, we may go on to accept (d), following Taylor, but then still deny that there is any warrant for moving from there to Taylor's egalitarian conclusion. Having accepted that our form of life is not superior, we might choose instead to regard it as inferior. More plausibly, we might view our form of life as noncomparable. We simply do not have the same kind of value as nonhumans. The question of how we compare to nonhumans has a simple answer: we do not compare to them.

Alternatively, we may reject (d) and say humans are indeed inherently superior but our superiority is a moot point. Whether we are inherently superior (that is, superior as a form of life) does not matter much. Even if we are superior, the fact remains that within the web of ecological interdependence mentioned in premises (a) and (b), it would be a mistake to ignore the needs and the telos of the other species referred to in premise (c). Thus, there are two ways of rejecting Taylor's argument for species egalitarianism. Each, on its face, is compatible with the respect for nature that motivates Taylor's egalitarianism in the first place.

Taylor's critics, such as James Anderson and William French, have taken the second route. They reject (d). After discussing their arguments, and building on some while rejecting others, I explore some of our reasons to have respect for nature and ask whether they translate into reasons to be species egalitarians.

III. IS SPECIES EGALITARIANISM HYPOCRITICAL?

Paul Taylor and Arne Naess are among the most intransigent of species egalitarians, yet they allow that human needs override the needs of nonhumans.[4] William C. French argues that they cannot have it both ways.[5] French perceives a contradiction between the egalitarian principles that Taylor and Naess officially endorse and the unofficial principles they offer as the real principles by which we should live. Having proclaimed that we are all equal, French asks, what licenses Taylor and Naess to say that, in cases of conflict, nonhuman interests can legitimately be sacrificed to vital human interests?

French has a point. James C. Anderson makes a similar point.[6] Yet, somehow the inconsistency of Taylor and Naess is too obvious. Perhaps their position is not as blatantly inconsistent as it appears. Let me suggest how Taylor and Naess could respond to French. Suppose I find myself in a situation of mortal combat with an enemy soldier. If I kill my enemy to save my life, that does not entail that I regard my enemy as inherently inferior (i.e., as an inferior form of life). Likewise, if I kill a bear to save my life, that does not entail that I regard the bear as inherently inferior. Therefore, Taylor and Naess can, without hypocrisy, deny that species egalitarianism requires a radically self-effacing pacifism.

What, then, does species egalitarianism require? It requires us to avoid mortal combat whenever we can, not just with other humans but with living things in general. On this view, we ought to regret finding ourselves in kill-or-be-killed situations that we could have avoided. There is no point in regretting the fact that we must kill in order to eat, though, for there is no avoiding that. Species egalitarianism is compatible with our having a limited license to kill.

What seems far more problematic for species egalitarianism is that it seems to suggest that it makes no difference *what* we kill. Vegetarians typically think it is worse to kill a cow than to kill a potato. Are they wrong? Yes they are, according to species egalitarianism. In this respect, species egalitarianism cannot be right. I do believe we have reason to respect nature. But we fail to give nature due respect if we say we should have no more respect for a cow than for a potato.

IV. IS SPECIES EGALITARIANISM ARBITRARY?

Suppose interspecies comparisons are possible. Suppose the capacities of different species, and whatever else gives species moral standing, are commensurable. In that case, it could turn out that all species are equal, but that would be quite a fluke.

Taylor says a being has intrinsic worth if and only if it has a good of its own. Anderson does not disagree, but he points out that if we accept Taylor's idea of a thing having a good of its own, then that licenses us to notice differences among the various kinds of 'good of its own.' (We can notice differences without being committed to ranking them.) For example, we can distinguish, along Aristotelian lines, vegetative, animal, and cognitive goods of one's own. To have a vegetative nature is to be what Taylor, in premise (c), calls a teleological centre of life. A being with an animal nature is a teleological centre of life, and more. A being with a cognitive as well as animal nature is a teleological centre of life, and more still. Cognitive nature may be something we share with whales, dolphins, and higher primates. It is an empirical question. Anderson's view is that so long as we do not assume away this possibility, valuing cognitive capacity is not anthropocentric. The question is what would make *any* species superior to another (p. 348).

As mentioned earlier, Taylor defines anthropocentrism as giving exclusive or primary consideration to human interests above the good of other species. So, when we acknowledge that cognitive capacity is one valuable capacity among others, are we giving exclusive or primary considerations to human interests? Anderson thinks not, and surely he is right. Put it this way: if biocentrism involves resolving to ignore the fact that cognitive capacity is something we value—if biocentrism amounts to a resolution to value only those capacities that all living things share—then biocentrism is at least as arbitrary and question-begging as anthropocentrism.

It will not do to defend species egalitarianism by singling out a property that all species possess, arguing that this property is morally important, and then concluding that all species are therefore of equal moral importance. The problem with this sort of argument is that, where there is one property that provides a basis for moral standing, there might be others. Other properties might be possessed by some but not all species, and might provide bases for different kinds or degrees of moral standing.

V. THE MULTIPLE BASES OF MORAL STANDING

Taylor is aware of the Aristotelian classification scheme, but considers its hierarchy of capacities to be question-begging. Taylor himself assumes that human rationality is on a par with a cheetah's foot-speed. In this case, though, perhaps it is Taylor who begs the question. It hardly seems unreasonable to see the difference between the foot-speed of chimpanzees and cheetahs as a difference of degree, while seeing the difference between the sentience of a chimpanzee and the nonsentience of a tree as a difference in kind.

Anthropocentrists might argue that the good associated with cognitive capacity is superior to the good associated with vegetative capacity. Could they be wrong? Let us suppose they are wrong. For argument's sake, let us suppose *vegetative* capacity is the superior good. Even so, the exact nature of the good associated with an organism's vegetative capacity will depend upon the organism's other capacities. For example, Anderson (p. 358) points out that even if health in a human and health in a tree are instances of the same thing, they need not have the same moral standing. Why not? Because health in a human has an instrumental value that health in a tree lacks. John Stuart Mill's swine can take pleasure in its health but trees cannot. Animals have a plant's capacities plus more. In turn, humans (and possibly dolphins, apes, and so on) have an animal's capacities plus more. The comparison between Socrates and swine therefore is less a matter of comparing swine to non-swine and more a matter of comparing swine to 'swine-plus' (Anderson, p. 361). Crucially, Anderson's argument for the superiority of Socrates over swine does not presume that one capacity is higher than another. We do not need to make any assumptions about the respective merits of animal or vegetative versus cognitive capacities in order to conclude that the capacities of 'swine-plus' are superior to those of swine.

We may of course conclude that *one* of the grounds of our moral standing (i.e., our vegetative natures) is something we share with all living things. Beyond that, nothing about equality even suggests itself. In particular, it begs no questions to notice that there are grounds for moral standing that we do not share with all living things.

VI. IN PRAISE OF SPECIESISM

William French invites us to see species rankings not 'as an assessment of some inherent superiority, but rather as a considered moral recognition of the fact that greater ranges of vulnerability are generated by broader ranges of complexity and capacities' (p. 56). One species outranks another not because it is a superior form of life but rather because it is a more vulnerable form of life. French, if I understand correctly, interprets vulnerability as a matter of having *more* to lose. This interpretation is problematic. It implies that a millionaire, having more to lose than a pauper, is by that fact more vulnerable than the pauper. Perhaps this interpretation is forced upon French, though. If French had instead chosen a more natural interpretation—if he had chosen to interpret vulnerability as a matter of *probability* of loss—then a ranking by vulnerability would not be correlated to complex capacities in the way he wants. Ranking by probability of loss would change on a daily basis, and the top-ranked species often would be an amphibian.

If we set aside questions about how to interpret vulnerability, there remains a problem with French's proposal. If having complex capacities is not itself morally important, then being in danger of losing them is not morally important either. Vulnerability, on any interpretation, is essentially of derivative importance; any role it could play in ranking species must already be played by the capacities themselves.

Yet, although I reject French's argument, I do not reject his inegalitarian conclusion. The conclusion that mice are the moral equals of chimpanzees is about as insupportable as a conclusion can be. Suppose that, for some reason, we take an interest in how chimpanzees rank compared to mice. Perhaps we wonder what we would do in an emergency where we could save a drowning chimpanzee or a drowning mouse but not both. More realistically, we might wonder whether, other things equal, we have any reason to use mice in our medical experiments rather than chimpanzees. Species egalitarianism seems to say not.

Suppose we decide upon reflection that, from our human perspective, chimpanzees are superior to mice and humans are superior to chimpanzees. Would the perceived superiority of our form of life give us reason to think we have no obligations whatsoever to mice, or to chimpanzees? Those who believe we have fewer obligations to inferior species might be pressed to say whether they also would allow that we have fewer obligations to inferior human beings. Lawrence Johnson, for example, rhetorically asks whether it is worse to cause a person pain if the person is a Nobel Prize winner.[7] Well, why not? Echoing Peter Singer, Johnson argues that if medical researchers had to choose between harvesting the organs of a chimpanzee or a brain-damaged human baby, 'one thing we cannot justify is trying to have it both ways. If rationality is what makes the basic moral difference, then we cannot maintain that the brain-damaged infant ought to be exempt from utilisation just because it is human

while at the same time allowing that the animal can be used if utility warrants' (p. 52).

Does this seem obvious? It should not. Johnson presumes that rationality is relevant to justification at the *token* level when speciesists (i.e., those who believe some species, the human species in particular, are superior to others) presumably would invoke rationality as a justification at the *type* level. One can say rationality makes a moral difference at the type level without thereby taking any position on whether rationality makes a moral difference at the token level. A speciesist could say humanity's characteristic rationality mandates respect for humanity, not merely for particular humans who exemplify human rationality. Similarly, once we note that chimpanzees have characteristic cognitive capacities that mice lack, we do not need to compare individual chimpanzees and mice on a case by case basis in order to have a moral justification for planning to use a mouse rather than a chimpanzee in an experiment.

Of course, some chimpanzees lack the characteristic features in virtue of which chimpanzees command respect as a species, just as some humans lack the characteristic features in virtue of which humans command respect as a species. It is equally obvious that some chimpanzees have cognitive capacities (for example) that are superior to the cognitive capacities of some humans. But whether every human being is superior to every chimpanzee is beside the point. The point is that we can, we do, and we should make decisions on the basis of our recognition that mice, chimpanzees, and humans are relevantly different types. We can have it both ways after all. Or so a speciesist could argue.

VII. EQUALITY AND TRANSCENDENCE

Even if speciesists are right to see a nonarbitrary distinction between humans and other species, though, the fact remains that, as Anderson (p. 362) points out, claims of superiority do not easily translate into justifications of domination. We can have reasons to treat nonhuman species with respect, regardless of whether we consider them to be on a moral par with *homo [sic] sapiens*.

What kind of reasons do we have for treating other species with respect? We might have respect for chimpanzees or even mice on the grounds that they are sentient. Even mice have a rudimentary point of view and rudimentary hopes and dreams, and we might well respect them for that. But what about plants? Plants, unlike mice and chimpanzees, do not care what happens to them. It is literally true that they could not care less. So, why should we care? Is it even possible for us to have any good reason, other than a purely instrumental reason, to care what happens to plants?

When we are alone in a forest wondering whether it would be fine to chop down a tree for fun, our perspective on what happens to the tree is, so far as we know, the only perspective there is. The tree does not have its own. Thus, explaining why we have reason to care about trees requires us to explain caring from our point of view, since that (we are supposing) is all there is. In that case, we do not have to satisfy *trees* that we are treating them properly; rather, we have to satisfy *ourselves*. So, again, can we have noninstrumental reasons for caring about trees—for treating them with respect?

One reason to care (not the only one) is that gratuitous destruction is a failure of self-respect. It is a repudiation of the kind of self-awareness and self-respect that we can achieve by repudiating wantonness. So far as I know, no one finds anything puzzling in the idea that we have reason to treat our lawns or living rooms with respect. Lawns and living rooms have instrumental value, but there is more to it than that. Most of us have the sense that taking reasonable care of our lawns and living rooms is somehow a matter of self-respect, not merely a matter of preserving their instrumental value. Do we have similar reasons to treat forests with respect? I think we do. There is an aesthetic involved, the repudiation of which would be a failure of self-respect. (Obviously, not everyone feels the same way about forests. Not everyone feels the same way about lawns and living rooms, either. But the point here is to make sense of respect for nature, not to argue that respect for nature is in fact universal or that failing to respect nature is irrational.)[8] If and

when we identify with a Redwood, in the sense of being inspired by it, having respect for its size and age and so on, then as a psychological fact, we really do face moral questions about how we ought to treat it. If and when we come to see a Redwood in that light, subsequently turning our backs on it becomes a kind of self-effacement. The values that we thereby fail to take seriously are *our* values, not the tree's.

A related way of grounding respect for nature is suggested by Jim Cheney's remark that 'moral regard is appropriate wherever we are *able* to manage it—in light of our sensibilities, knowledge, and cultural/personal histories. . . . The limits of moral regard are set only by the limitations of one's own (or one's species' or one's community's) ability to respond in a caring manner.'[9] Should we believe Cheney's rather startling proposal that moral regard is appropriate whenever we can manage it? One reason to take it very seriously is that exercising our capacity for moral regard is a way of expressing respect for that capacity. Developing that capacity is a form of self-realization.

Put it this way. I am arguing that the attitude we take toward gazelles (for example) raises issues of self-respect insofar as we see ourselves as relevantly like gazelles. My reading of Cheney suggests a different and complementary way of looking at the issue. Consider that lions owe nothing to gazelles. Therefore, if we owe it to gazelles not to hunt them, it must be because we are *unlike* lions, not (or not only) because we are *like* gazelles.

Unlike lions, we have a choice about whether to hunt gazelles, and we are capable of deliberating about that choice in a reflective way. We are capable of caring about the gazelle's pain, the gazelle's beauty, the gazelle's hopes and dreams (such as they are), and so forth. And if we do care, then in a more or less literal way, something is wrong with us—we are less than fully human—if we cannot adjust our behaviour in the light of what we care about. If we do not care, then we are missing something. For a human being, to lack a broad respect for living things and beautiful things and well-functioning things is to be stunted in a way.

Our coming to see other species as commanding respect is itself a way of transcending our animal natures. It is ennobling. It is part of our animal natures unthinkingly to see ourselves as superior, and to try to dominate accordingly; our capacity to see ourselves as equal is one of the things that makes us different. Thus, our capacity to see ourselves as equal may be one of the things that makes us superior. Coming to see all species as equal may not be the best way of transcending our animal natures—it does not work for me—but it is one way. Another way of transcending our animal natures and expressing due respect for nature is simply to not worry so much about ranking species. This latter way is, I think, better. It is more respectful of our own reflective natures. It does not dwell on rankings. It does not insist on seeing equality where a more reflective being simply would see what is there to be seen and would not shy away from respecting the differences as well as the commonalities. The whole idea of ranking species, even as equals, sometimes seems like a child's game. It seems beneath us.

VIII. RESPECT FOR EVERYTHING

Thus, a broad respect for living or beautiful or well-functioning things need not translate into equal respect. It need not translate into universal respect, either. I can appreciate mosquitoes to a degree. My wife (a biochemist who studies mosquito immune systems) even finds them beautiful, or so she says. My own appreciation, by contrast, is thin and grudging and purely intellectual. In neither degree nor kind is it anything like the appreciation I have for my wife, or for human beings in general, or even for the rabbits I sometimes find eating my flowers in the morning. Part of our responsibility as moral agents is to be somewhat choosy about what we respect and how we respect it. I can see why people shy away from openly accepting that responsibility, but they still have it.

Johnson says speciesism is as arbitrary as racism unless we can show that the differences are morally relevant (p. 51). This is, to be sure, a popular sentiment among radical environmentalists and animal liberationists. But are we really like racists when we think it is worse to kill a dolphin than to kill a tuna?

The person who says there is a relevant similarity between speciesism and racism has the burden of proof: go ahead and identify the similarity. Is seeing moral significance in biological differences between chimpanzees and potatoes anything like seeing moral significance in biological differences between races? I think not.

Is it true that we need good reason to *exclude* plants and animals from the realm of things we regard as commanding respect? Or do we need reason to *include* them? Should we be trying to identify properties in virtue of which a thing forfeits presumptive moral standing? Or does it make more sense to be trying to identify properties in virtue of which a thing commands respect? The latter seems more natural to me, which suggests the burden of proof lies with those who claim we should have respect for other species.

I would not say, though, that this burden is unbearable. One reason to have regard for other species has to do with self-respect. (As I said earlier, when we mistreat a tree that we admire, the values we fail to respect are our values, not the tree's.) A second reason has to do with self-realisation. (As I said, exercising our capacity for moral regard is a form of self-realisation.) Finally, at least some species seem to share with human beings precisely those cognitive and affective characteristics that lead us to see human life as especially worthy of esteem. Johnson describes experiments in which rhesus monkeys show extreme reluctance to obtain food by means that would subject monkeys in neighbouring cages to electric shock (p. 64n). He describes the case of Washoe, a chimpanzee who learned sign language. Anyone who has tried to learn a foreign language ought to be able to appreciate how astonishing an intellectual feat it is that an essentially nonlinguistic creature could learn a language—a language that is not merely foreign but the language of another species.

Johnson believes Washoe has moral standing (pp. 27–31), but he does not believe that the moral standing of chimpanzees, and indeed of all living creatures, implies that we must resolve never to kill (p. 136). Thus, Johnson supports killing introduced animal species (feral dogs, rabbits, and so forth) to prevent the extermination of Australia's native species, including native plant species (p. 174).

Is Johnson guilty of advocating the speciesist equivalent of ethnic cleansing? Has he shown himself to be no better than a racist? I think not. Johnson is right to want to take drastic measures to protect Australia's native flora, and the idea of respecting trees is intelligible. Certainly one thing I feel in the presence of Redwoods is something like a feeling of respect. But I doubt that what underlies Johnson's willingness to kill feral dogs is mere respect for Australia's native plants. I suspect that his approval of such killings turns on the needs and aesthetic sensibilities of human beings, not just the interests of plants.[10] For example, if the endangered native species happened to be a malaria-carrying mosquito, I doubt that Johnson would advocate wiping out an exotic but minimally intrusive species of amphibian in order to save the mosquitoes.

Aldo Leopold urged us to see ourselves as plain citizens of, rather than conquerors of the biotic community, but there are some species with whom we can never be fellow citizens.[11] The rabbits eating my flowers in the back yard are neighbours, and I cherish their company, minor frictions notwithstanding. I feel no sense of community with mosquitoes, though, and not merely because they are not warm and furry. Some mosquito species are so adapted to making human beings miserable that moral combat is not accidental; rather, combat is a natural state. It is how such creatures live. Recall Cheney's remark that the limits of moral regard are set by the limits of our ability to respond in a caring manner. I think it is fair to say human beings are not able to respond to malaria-carrying mosquitoes in a caring manner. At very least, most of us would think less of a person who did respond to them in a caring manner. We would regard the person's caring as a parody of respect for nature.

The conclusion that *all* species have moral standing is unmotivated. For human beings, viewing apes as having moral standing is a form of self-respect. Viewing viruses as having moral standing is not. It is good to have a sense of how amazing living things

are, but being able to marvel at living things is not the same as thinking all species have moral standing. Life as such commands respect only in the limited but nonetheless important sense that for self-aware and reflective creatures who want to act in ways that make sense, deliberately killing something is an act that does not make sense unless we have good reason to do it. Destroying something for no good reason is (at best) the moral equivalent of vandalism.

IX. THE HISTORY OF THE DEBATE

There is an odd project in the history of philosophy that equates what seem to be three distinct projects:

1. determining our essence;
2. specifying how we are different from all other species;
3. specifying what makes us morally important.

Equating these three projects has important ramifications. Suppose for the sake of argument that what makes us morally important is that we are capable of suffering. If what makes us morally important is necessarily the same property that constitutes our essence, then our essence is that we are capable of suffering. And if our essence necessarily is what makes us different from all other species, then we can deduce that dogs are not capable of suffering.

Likewise with rationality. If rationality is our essence, then rationality is what makes us morally important and also what makes us unique. Therefore, we can deduce that chimpanzees are not rational. Alternatively, if some other animal becomes rational, does that mean our essence will change? Is that why some people find Washoe, the talking chimpanzee, threatening?

The three projects, needless to say, should not be conflated in the way philosophy seems historically to have conflated them, but we can reject species equality without conflating them. If we like, we can select a property with respect to which all species are the same, then argue that that property confers moral standing, then say all species have moral standing. To infer that all species have the same standing, though, would be to ignore the possibility that there are other morally important properties with respect to which not all species are equal.

There is room to wonder whether species egalitarianism is even compatible with respect for nature. Is it true that we should have no more regard for dolphins than for tuna? Is it true that the moral standing of chimpanzees is no higher than that of mosquitoes? I worry that these things are not only untrue, but also disrespectful. Dolphins and chimpanzees command more respect than species egalitarianism allows.

There is no denying that it demeans us to destroy species we find beautiful or otherwise beneficial. What about species in which we find neither beauty nor benefit? It is, upon reflection, obviously in our interest to enrich our lives by finding them beautiful or beneficial, if we can. By and large, we must agree with Leopold that it is too late for conquering the biotic community. Our most pressing task now is to find ways of fitting in. Species egalitarianism is one way of trying to understand how we fit in. In the end, it is not an acceptable way. Having respect for nature and being a species egalitarian are two different things.

NOTES

1. A species egalitarian may or may not believe that individual living things all have equal moral standing. A species egalitarian may think a given whooping crane matters more than a given bald eagle because the cranes are endangered, despite believing that the differences between the two species qua species are not morally important.

2. Paul W. Taylor (1983) In defense of biocentrism, *Environmental Ethics*, 5: 237–43, here p. 240.

3. Taylor (1994), [*Respect for Nature* (Princeton, NJ: Princeton University Press)], p. 35.

4. Arne Naess (1973) The shallow and the deep, long-range ecology movement: a summary, *Inquiry*, 16: 95–100.

5. William C. French (1995) Against biospherical egalitarianism, *Environmental Ethics*, 17: 39–57, here pp. 44ff.

6. James C. Anderson (1993) Species equality and the foundations of moral theory, *Environmental Values*, 2: 347–65, here p. 350.

7. Lawrence Johnson (1991) *A Morally Deep World* (New York, Cambridge University Press), p. 52.

8. Thus, the objective is to explain how a rational agent could have respect for trees, not to argue that a rational agent could not fail to have respect. In utilitarian terms, a person whose utility function leaves no room to derive pleasure from respecting trees is not irrational for failing to respect trees, but people whose utility functions include a potential for deriving pleasure from respecting trees have reason (other things equal) to enrich their lives by realising that potential.

9. Jim Cheney (1987) Eco-feminism and deep ecology, *Environmental Ethics* 9: 115–45, here p. 144.

10. Johnson believes ecosystems as such have moral standing and that, consequently, 'we should always stop short of entirely destroying or irreparably degrading any ecosystem' (p. 276). 'Chopping some trees is one thing, then, but destroying a forest is something else' (p. 276). But this is impossible to square with his remark that there 'is an ecosystem in a tiny puddle of water in a rotting stump' (p. 265). Thus, when Johnson says ecosystems should never be destroyed, he does not mean ecosystems per se. Rather he means forests, deserts, marshes, and so on—ecosystems that are recognisable as habitat either for humans or for species that humans care about.

11. Aldo Leopold (1966, first published in 1949) *Sand County Almanac* (New York, Oxford University Press) p. 240.

The Land Ethic

ALDO LEOPOLD

When god-like Odysseus returned from the wars in Troy, he hanged all on one rope a dozen slave-girls of his household whom he suspected of misbehavior during his absence.

This hanging involved no question of propriety. The girls were property. The disposal of property was then, as now, a matter of expediency, not of right and wrong.

Concepts of right and wrong were not lacking from Odysseus' Greece: witness the fidelity of his wife through the long years before at last his black-prowed galleys clove the wine-dark seas for home. The ethical structure of that day covered wives, but had not yet been extended to human chattels. During the three thousand years which have since elapsed, ethical criteria have been extended to many fields of conduct, with corresponding shrinkages in those judged by expediency only.

This extension of ethics, so far studied only by philosophers, is actually a process in ecological evolution. Its sequences may be described in ecological as well as in philosophical terms. An ethic, ecologically, is a limitation on freedom of action in the struggle for existence. An ethic, philosophically, is a differentiation of social from anti-social conduct. These are two definitions of one thing. The thing has its origin in the tendency of interdependent individuals or groups to evolve modes of co-operation. The ecologist calls these symbioses. Politics and economics are advanced symbioses in which the original free-for-all competition has been replaced, in part, by co-operative mechanisms with an ethical content.

The complexity of co-operative mechanisms has increased with population density, and with the efficiency of tools. It was simpler, for example, to define

the anti-social uses of sticks and stones in the days of the mastodons than of bullets and billboards in the age of motors.

The first ethics dealt with the relation between individuals; the Mosaic Decalogue is an example. Later accretions dealt with the relation between the individual and society. The Golden Rule tries to integrate the individual to society; democracy to integrate social organization to the individual.

There is as yet no ethic dealing with man's relation to land and to the animals and plants which grow upon it. Land, like Odysseus' slave-girls, is still property. The land-relation is still strictly economic, entailing privileges but not obligations.

The extension of ethics to this third element in human environment is, if I read the evidence correctly, an evolutionary possibility and an ecological necessity. It is the third step in a sequence. The first two have already been taken. Individual thinkers since the days of Ezekiel and Isaiah have asserted that the despoliation of land is not only inexpedient but wrong. Society, however, has not yet affirmed their belief. I regard the present conservation movement as the embryo of such an affirmation.

An ethic may be regarded as a mode of guidance for meeting ecological situations so new or intricate, or involving such deferred reactions, that the path of social expediency is not discernible to the average individual. Animal instincts are modes of guidance for the individual in meeting such situations. Ethics are possibly a kind of community instinct in-the-making.

THE COMMUNITY CONCEPT

All ethics so far evolved rest upon a single premise: that the individual is a member of a community of interdependent parts. His instincts prompt him to compete for his place in the community, but his ethics prompt him also to co-operate (perhaps in order that there may be a place to compete for).

The land ethic simply enlarges the boundaries of the community to include soils, waters, plants, and animals, or collectively: the land.

This sounds simple: do we not already sing our love for and obligation to the land of the free and the home of the brave? Yes, but just what and whom do we love? Certainly not the soil, which we are sending helter-skelter downriver. Certainly not the waters, which we assume have no function except to turn turbines, float barges, and carry off sewage. Certainly not the plants, of which we exterminate whole communities without batting an eye. Certainly not the animals, of which we have already extirpated many of the largest and most beautiful species. A land ethic of course cannot prevent the alteration, management, and use of these 'resources,' but it does affirm the right to continued existence, and, at least in spots, their continued existence in a natural state.

In short, a land ethic changes the role of *Homo sapiens* from conquerer of the land-community to plain member and citizen of it. It implies respect for his fellow-members, and also respect for the community as such.

In human history, we have learned (I hope) that the conquerer role is eventually self-defeating. Why? Because it is implicit in such a role that the conqueror knows, *ex cathedra*, just what makes the community clock tick, and just what and who is valuable, and what and who is worthless, in community life. It always turns out that he knows neither, and this is why his conquests eventually defeat themselves.

In the biotic community, a parallel situation exists. Abraham knew exactly what the land was for: it was to drop milk and honey into Abraham's mouth. At the present moment, the assurance with which we regard this assumption is inverse to the degree of our education.

The ordinary citizen today assumes that science knows what makes the community clock tick; the scientist is equally sure that he does not. He knows that the biotic mechanism is so complex that its workings may never be fully understood.

* * *

SUBSTITUTES FOR A LAND ETHIC

When the logic of history hungers for bread and we hand out a stone, we are at pains to explain how much the stone resembles bread. I now describe some of the stones which serve in lieu of a land ethic.

One basic weakness in a conservation system based wholly on economic motives is that most members of the land community have no economic value. Wildflowers and songbirds are examples. Of the 22,000 higher plants and animals native to Wisconsin, it is doubtful whether more than 5 per cent can be sold, fed, eaten, or otherwise put to economic use. Yet these creatures are members of the biotic community, and if (as I believe) its stability depends on its integrity, they are entitled to continuance.

When one of these non-economic categories is threatened, and if we happen to love it, we invent subterfuges to give it economic importance. At the beginning of the century songbirds were supposed to be disappearing. Ornithologists jumped to the rescue with some distinctly shaky evidence to the effect that insects would eat us up if birds failed to control them. The evidence had to be economic in order to be valid.

It is painful to read these circumlocutions today. We have no land ethic yet, but we have at least drawn nearer the point of admitting that birds should continue as a matter of biotic right, regardless of the presence or absence of economic advantage to us.

A parallel situation exists in respect of predatory mammals, raptorial birds, and fish-eating birds. Time was when biologists somewhat overworked the evidence that these creatures preserve the health of game by killing weaklings, or that they control rodents for the farmer, or that they prey only on 'worthless' species. Here again, the evidence had to be economic in order to be valid. It is only in recent years that we hear the more honest argument that predators are members of the community, and that no special interest has the right to exterminate them for the sake of a benefit, real or fancied, to itself. Unfortunately this enlightened view is still in the talk stage. In the field the determination of predators goes merrily on: witness the impending erasure of the timber wolf by fiat of Congress, the Conservation Bureaus, and many state legislatures.

Some species of trees have been 'read out of the party' by economics-minded foresters because they grow too slowly, or have too low a sale value to pay as timber crops: white cedar, tamarack, cypress, beech, and hemlock are examples. In Europe, where forestry is ecologically more advanced, the non-commercial tree species are recognized as members of the native forest community, to be preserved as such, within reason. Moreover some (like beech) have been found to have a valuable function in building up soil fertility. The interdependence of the forest and its constituent tree species, ground flora, and fauna is taken for granted.

Lack of economic value is sometimes a character not only of species or groups, but of entire biotic communities: marshes, bogs, dunes, and 'deserts' are examples. Our formula in such cases is to relegate their conservation to government as refuges, monuments, or parks. The difficulty is that these communities are usually interspersed with more valuable private lands; the government cannot possibly own or control such scattered parcels. The net effect is that we have relegated some of them to ultimate extinction over large areas. If the private owner were ecologically minded, he would be proud to be the custodian of a reasonable proportion of such areas, which add diversity and beauty to his farm and to his community.

* * *

To sum up: a system of conservation based solely on economic self-interest is hopelessly lopsided. It tends to ignore, and thus eventually to eliminate, many elements in the land community that lack commercial value, but that are (as far as we know) essential to its healthy functioning. It assumes, falsely, I think, that the economic parts of the biotic clock will function without the uneconomic parts. It tends to relegate to government many functions eventually too large, too complex, or too widely dispersed to be performed by government.

* * *

THE LAND PYRAMID

An ethic to supplement and guide the economic relation to land presupposes the existence of some mental image of land as a biotic mechanism. We can be ethical only in relation in something we can see, feel, understand, love, or otherwise have faith in.

The image commonly employed in conservation education is 'the balance of nature.' For reasons too lengthy to detail here, this figure of speech fails to describe accurately what little we know about the land mechanism. A much truer image is the one employed in ecology: the biotic pyramid.

* * *

Plants absorb energy from the sun. This energy flows through a circuit called the biota, which may be represented by a pyramid consisting of layers. The bottom layer is the soil. A plant layer rests on the soil, an insect layer on the plants, a bird and rodent layer on the insects, and so on up through various animal groups to the apex layer, which consists of the larger carnivores.

The species of a layer are alike not in where they came from, or in what they look like, but rather in what they eat. Each successive layer depends on those below it for food and often for other services, and each in turn furnishes food and services to those above. Proceeding upward, each successive layer decreases in numerical abundance. Thus, for every carnivore there are hundreds of his prey, thousands of their prey, millions of insects, uncountable plants. The pyramidal form of the system reflects this numerical progression from apex to base. Man shares an intermediate layer with the bears, raccoons, and squirrels which eat both meat and vegetables.

The lines of dependency for food and other services are called food chains. Thus soil-oak-deer-Indian is a chain that has now been largely converted to soil-corn-cow-farmer. Each species, including ourselves, is a link in many chains. The deer eats a hundred plants other than oak, and the cow a hundred plants other than corn. Both, then, are links in a hundred chains. The pyramid is a tangle of chains so complex as to seem disorderly, yet the stability of the system proves it to be a highly organized structure. Its functioning depends on the co-operation and competition of its diverse parts.

In the beginning, the pyramid of life was low and squat; the food chains short and simple. Evolution has added layer after layer, link after link. Man is one of thousands of accretions to the height and complexity of the pyramid. Science has given us many doubts, but it has given us at least one certainty: the trend of evolution is to elaborate and diversify the biota.

Land, then, is not merely soil; it is a fountain of energy flowing through a circuit of soils, plants, and animals. Food chains are the living channels which conduct energy upward; death and decay return it to the soil. The circuit is not closed; some energy is dissipated in decay, some is added by absorption from the air, some is stored in soils, peats, and long-lived forests; but it is a sustained circuit, like a slowly augmented revolving fund of life. There is always a net loss by downhill wash, but this is normally small and offset by the decay of rocks. It is deposited in the ocean and, in the course of geological time, raised to form new lands and new pyramids.

The velocity and character of the upward flow of energy depend on the complex structure of the plant and animal community, much as the upward flow of sap in a tree depends on its complex cellular organization. Without this complexity, normal circulation would presumably not occur. Structure means the characteristic numbers, as well as the characteristic kinds and functions, of the component species. This interdependence between the complex structure of the land and its smooth functioning as an energy unit is one of its basic attributes.

When a change occurs in one part of the circuit, many other parts must adjust themselves to it. Change does not necessarily obstruct or divert the flow of energy; evolution is a long series of self-induced changes, the net result of which has been to elaborate the flow mechanism and to length the circuit. Evolutionary changes, however, are usually slow and local. Men's invention of tools has enabled him to make changes of unprecedented violence, rapidity, and scope.

* * *

THE OUTLOOK

It is inconceivable to me that an ethical relation to land can exist without love, respect, and admiration for land, and a high regard for its value. By value, I of course mean something far broader than mere economic value; I mean value in the philosophical sense.

* * *

The 'key-log' which must be moved to release the evolutionary process for an ethic is simply this: quit thinking about decent land-use as solely an economic problem. Examine each question in terms of what is ethically and esthetically right, as well as what is economically expedient. A thing is right when it tends to preserve the integrity, stability, and beauty of the biotic community. It is wrong when it tends otherwise.

It of course goes without saying that economic feasibility limits the tether of what can or cannot be done for land. It always has and it always will. The fallacy the economic determinists have tied around our collective neck, and which we now need to cast off, is the belief that economics determines *all* land-use. This is simply not true. An innumerable host of actions and attitudes, comprising perhaps the bulk of all land relations, is determined by the land-users' tastes and predilections, rather than by his purse. The bulk of all land relations hinges on investments of time, forethought, skill, and faith rather than on investments of cash. As a land-user thinketh, so is he.

I have purposely presented the land ethic as a product of social evolution because nothing so important as an ethic is ever 'written.' Only the most superficial student of history supposes that Moses 'wrote' the Decalogue; it evolved in the minds of a thinking community, and Moses wrote a tentative summary of it for a 'seminar.' I say tentative because evolution never stops.

The evolution of a land ethic is an intellectual as well as emotional process. Conservation is paved with good intentions which prove to be futile, or even dangerous, because they are devoid of critical understanding either of the land, or of economic land-use. I think it is a truism that as the ethical frontier advances from the individual to the community, its intellectual content increases.

The mechanism of operation is the same for any ethic: social approbation for right actions: social disapproval for wrong actions.

By and large, our present problem is one of attitudes and implements. We are remodeling the Alhambra with a steam-shovel, and we are proud of our yardage. We shall hardly relinquish the shovel, which after all has many good points, but we are in need of gentler and more objective criteria for its successful use.

CASES FOR ANALYSIS

1. Tigers and Humans

Tigers are rapidly disappearing from India. A century ago, India may have been home to as many as 100,000 tigers; now there are less than 3,600—perhaps far less. Poachers kill the big cats and sell the fur and bones to be used mainly in traditional Chinese medicine. Poachers, however, are not the only menace. As one report says,

[T]he threats to the tiger are as varied and complex as the lands they roam: disappearing natural habitat shared with millions of people, a tiger tourism industry that has alienated villagers, a communist rebellion in a core swath of tiger lands and a conservation effort mired in bureaucracy. . . .

The Palamau Tiger Reserve is a case in point. Two hundred villages dot its landscape, peopled by 100,000 impoverished tribesmen. Each day they extract 30 tons of firewood from the forests, and large patches of woodlands are being cleared for grazing and mining.*

Give reasons for your answers to the following questions: To save the tigers, should local residents be forced to give up their lifestyle, which threatens tiger habitats? Should native peoples be forced to give up elements of their folk or religious healing practices that require tiger pelts and bones? If tigers and people cannot possibly coexist in the same area (so that either of them must be forcibly moved to another habitat), which should be forced to move? Is it morally permissible to kill a few tigers to save the entire species? Or do the rights of each individual count more than the species?

*Gavin Rabinowitz, "India Hunts for Ways to Save Its Tigers," NBCNEWS.com, 17 February 2006, http://www.nbcnews.com/id/11347534/ns/world_news-world_environment/t/india-hunts-way-save-its -tigers/#.VOj9DFPF9RY (21 February 2015).

2. Saving the Glaciers

The glaciers have been disappearing from Glacier National Park in Montana and adjoining Waterton National Park in Canada. In 1850, Glacier is said to have had 150 glaciers; in 2006 there were 27. In response to this trend, various organizations petitioned for the parks to be designated endangered by being placed on the danger list of the World Heritage Committee. As one report says,

> Endangered status would require the World Heritage Committee to find ways to mitigate how climate change affects the park, [the law professor who wrote the petition] said . . . Better fuel efficiency for automobiles and stronger energy efficiency standards for buildings and appliances are among the ways to reduce greenhouse pollution that contributes to warming, the petition [said].

But some denounced the petition as unnecessary and unsupported by scientific data, while one group of scientists estimated that if climate trends continue, Glacier Park's glaciers will disappear completely by 2030.†

Justify your answers: Suppose the glaciers' melting would have no appreciable effect on the environment except that they would no longer exist. Would conservationists still be justified in trying to save the glaciers? If so, how could they justify their efforts? If not, why not? Suppose the glaciers could be saved only if the government spends $10 billion on pollution controls—money that would have to be taken away from social programs. Would this cost be worth it? Why or why not?

†"Associated Press, Endangered Status for Glacier National Park?" NBCNEWS.com, 16 February 2006, http://www.nbcnews.com/id/11389665/ns/us_news-environment/t/endangered-status-glacier-national -park/#.VOj_I1PF9RY (21 February 2015).

---

3. Ivory-Billed Woodpecker v. Irrigation

While ornithologists continue to debate whether the ivory-billed woodpecker still lingers in the bayous of Arkansas, the rare bird, once presumed extinct, is now being used by conservationists in their fight against a federally funded and potentially devastating irrigation project.

This Monday, a Little Rock federal court will hear a case against the U.S. Army Corps of Engineers' Grand Prairie Area Demonstration Project. Plaintiffs ask that all work be halted on the project until appropriate environmental studies can be performed to evaluate its effect on the woodpecker.

Lisa Swann of the National Wildlife Federation states that the Grand Prairie project would be "a recipe for disaster" for the near extinct bird, though the U.S. Army Corps maintains that the $319 million project, which would replenish exhausted groundwater aquifers in a 242,000-acre agricultural region, is completely safe.

The corps biologist, Ed Lambert, argues that their "biological assessment" performed last spring has proven that the Grand Prairie project will bring no harm to the woodpecker.

Plans for Grand Prairie have been underway since the 1980s, when studies found that the ground water aquifers of east-central Arkansas were in danger of depletion by rice growers. The corps has been working with area farmers to build reservoirs that will eventually be filled with water pumped from the White River.

According to the corps, Grand Prairie will not only aid farmers, but will create new wetland habitat for waterfowl and shorebirds. The water piped in from the White River could also replenish the slowly shrinking hardwood forests of Arkansas and reintroduce thousands of acres of native grassland.

However, Swann's group and other environmentalists see the project differently. They argue that the project will waste huge amounts of tax dollars and only benefit farmers. The National Wildlife Federation stated in one publication that the "mammoth sucking machine" will damage wetlands and pollute the water, threatening ducks, mussels, and a variety of other species in the region who rely on clean and safe water.

The celebrity of these species is the ivory-billed woodpecker. Long believed extinct, any sighting since the 1940s was given little credit by experts, as the bird is commonly mistaken for the smaller pileated woodpecker, which has similar coloring.

One expert, however, began to investigate these sightings. Tim Gallagher of the Cornell Lab of Ornithology and editor of *Living Bird* magazine began to study the mysterious ivory-bill in the 1970s. Eventually, his research led him to Gene Sparling, who claimed to have seen a red-crested male while kayaking in the wetlands of eastern Arkansas.

During the winter of 2004, Gallagher set out to catch a glimpse of the elusive bird himself, accompanied by Sparling and a fellow birder, and on February 27, Gallagher succeeded in spotting a male ivory-bill. Further expeditions ensued, and on April 28, 2005, an article in *Science* was published proclaiming that the ivory-bill was no longer extinct.[*]

Assume that the woodpecker does exist and that the water project would wipe it out. Should the project proceed or be cancelled? Why? How might a species egalitarian (biocentrist) answer this? A species nonegalitarian? An ecological holist?

[*]Based on Mike Stuckey, "New Star of the Bird world Stars in Lawsuit, Too," MSNBC.com, 25 January 2006, www.nbcnews.com/id/10929337/ (20 January 2012).

CHAPTER 16

Animal Rights

One of philosophy's most important functions is to help us critically examine beliefs that we often simply accept without question. Philosophy seems to have played this role especially well in the issue of animal rights, for it was a philosopher who helped engender the current animal rights movement by arguing that something was very wrong with the traditional attitude toward animals (that is, nonhuman animals) and their treatment. The traditional notion is that an animal is merely a resource that humans may dispose of as they see fit: an animal is food, fuel, or fun—something with instrumental value only. Peter Singer was the philosopher who challenged the received wisdom, declaring in his 1975 book *Animal Liberation* that its subject was the "tyranny of human over nonhuman animals. This tyranny has caused and today is still causing an amount of pain and suffering that can only be compared with that which resulted from the centuries of tyranny by white humans over black humans."[1]

The traditional attitude toward animals has been influential in the West for centuries. It sprang from several sources, including Judeo-Christian thought and the arguments of several distinguished philosophers. The book of *Genesis* declares that God created humans in his own image, "saying to them, 'Be fruitful, multiply, fill the earth and conquer it. Be masters of the fish of the sea, the birds of heaven and all living animals on the earth'" (Genesis 1.28). Aristotle claims that all of nature exists "specifically

for the sake of man," that animals are merely instruments for humankind. Thomas Aquinas is remarkably explicit about humans' proper attitude toward animals:

> Hereby is refuted the error of those who said it is sinful for a man to kill dumb animals: for by divine providence they are intended for man's use in the natural order. Hence it is no wrong for man to make use of them, either by killing them or in any other way whatever.[2]

Aquinas also says that we should avoid being cruel to animals—but only because cruelty to animals might lead to cruelty to humans. Animal cruelty in itself, he explains, is no wrong. Likewise, René Descartes thinks animals are ours to use any way we want. After all, he asserts, animals are not sentient—they are machines, like mechanical clocks, devoid of feelings and incapable of experiencing pleasure or pain. Immanuel Kant, who thinks that people are not means to an end but ends in themselves, contends that animals are means to the end known as man. Today few would agree with Descartes that animals cannot experience pain, but the traditional idea that animals have no (or low) moral standing is widespread.

Those who reject the traditional attitude remind us that beliefs about the moral status of animals influence how animals are treated in the real

---

[1]Peter Singer, *Animal Liberation*, 2nd ed. (New York: New York Review of Books, 1990), i.

[2]Thomas Aquinas, *Summa Theologica*, from *Basic Writings of Saint Thomas Aquinas*, ed. and annotated Anton C. Pegis (New York: Random House, 1945), Second Part of the Second Part, Question 64, Article 1.

world—and that treatment, they say, is horrendous on a vast scale. In 2013 in the United States alone, more than 9 billion animals were slaughtered for food—cows, poultry, calves, pigs, sheep, and lambs.[3] Critics have charged that the animals are subjected to appalling suffering, including lifelong confinement in spaces so small the animals can hardly move, isolation of veal calves in small crates (and, some say, in almost total darkness), routine mutilation or surgery such as branding and cutting off pigs' tails and chicken's beaks, and the slaughter of chickens and livestock without first stunning them or using any other methods to minimize pain and suffering.[4]

In addition, each year millions of animals—from mice to dogs to primates—are used in laboratory experiments all over the world. Some of this research—no one knows how much—causes significant animal suffering. According to a U.S. government report, in 2004 about 8 percent of larger animals used in experiments (excluding mice and rats) endured "pain or distress" that could not be relieved with medication.

These concerns push us toward the key moral questions that we try to sort out in this chapter: Do animals have instrumental value only? Do they have rights? Do we owe them any moral respect or concern at all? Is it morally permissible to experiment on animals, to raise and kill them for food, to cause them unnecessary pain and suf-

[3]U.S. Department of Agriculture, National Agricultural Statistical Services, *Livestock Slaughter: 2013 Summary;* USDA, NASS, *Poultry Slaughter: 2013 Summary.*
[4]Geoffrey Becker, "Humane Treatment of Farm Animals: Overview and Issues," Congressional Research Service Report RS21978, 18 November 2005 (updated 13 September 2010), www.nationalaglawcenter.org/assets/crs/RS21978.pdf (20 January 2012); People for the Ethical Treatment of Animals, "Petition for Agency Action to Fully Comply with the Mandates of the Humane Methods of Livestock Slaughter Act," 11 December 2001, www.peta.org/feat/usda/petition.html (3 December 2006).

fering? Do animals have the same moral worth as an infant, a mentally incompetent man, a woman with severe senile dementia, or a man in a persistent vegetative state?

ISSUE FILE: BACKGROUND

Fortunately, on these issues there is at least a parcel of common ground. First, almost no one believes, as Descartes did, that animals are equivalent to windup clocks, mechanisms without feelings. Science and common sense suggest that many animals (mostly vertebrates) are *sentient*—that is, they can have experiences. They can experience bodily sensations such as pain and pleasure as well as emotions such as fear and frustration. Sentient beings are thought to have the capacity to suffer. Second, virtually everyone thinks that being cruel to animals—unnecessarily causing them pain or misery—is wrong. Even when we consider this judgment carefully and critically, it seems inescapable. Third, there is general agreement, among philosophers at least, that sentient animals are worthy of some degree of moral respect or concern. Most disputes turn on interpretations of this last point: Exactly how much moral concern do we owe animals? Do they deserve the same level of moral consideration that we give to humans? Do they deserve less? How should we treat them?

Such questions are essentially about the moral status, or moral considerability, of animals. As noted in the previous chapter, something has moral status if it is a suitable candidate for moral concern or respect in its own right, regardless of its relationships to humans. Ethically, we cannot treat a being that has moral status just any way we want, as if it were a mere thing. Whatever we do to such a being, we must take its moral status into account. Another way of expressing the notion of moral status is to say that any being with moral status is an object of **direct moral consideration** or concern. That is, such a being is worthy of moral concern for its own sake, not because of its relationship to others. A being that is the object of **indirect moral consideration** is granted respect or concern because of its relationship to other individuals. Human beings are objects of direct moral consideration; some say that animals such as dogs, pigs, and rabbits are too. A screwdriver is not the kind of thing that can be the object of direct moral concern, but it may be of indirect moral concern because of its value to a human being. Some people insist that all nonhuman animals are of indirect moral concern, deriving whatever value they have from their usefulness to humans. Many others reject this view, asserting that sentient animals have independent moral status.

Moral status is typically understood to be something that comes in degrees and that can be overridden or discounted in some circumstances. Philosophers speak of varying levels or weights of moral considerability. Some contend that animals have the same moral status as normal adult humans—that, for example, the interests of animals are as morally important as the comparable interests of humans. Some argue that humans deserve more moral respect or concern than animals, that the interests of humans always take precedence over those of animals. Many maintain that moral considerability varies depending on the species (human or nonhuman), with humans enjoying the greatest degree of moral considerability and other species being assigned lower degrees on a sliding scale. But philosophers disagree on the basis for assigning the different rankings. Whatever a being's moral status, it is usually not viewed as absolute; sometimes it may be overridden or canceled by factors thought to be more important. Some people think, for example, that a dog's moral status prohibits humans from beating it just for fun but may allow beatings under some circumstances—say, to prevent it from straying into traffic and causing an accident.

Frequently people use the term **animal rights** as a synonym for *moral status*. When they say that animals have rights, they mean only that animals deserve some degree of direct moral considerability. But often the term is used in a more restricted way to refer to a particularly strong type of moral status. In this stronger sense, for an animal to have rights is for it to be entitled to a kind of moral respect that cannot be overridden (or cannot be overridden easily) by other considerations. Those who accept this notion of animal rights may argue that animals should *never* be condemned to factory farms or used in medical experimentation, even if such treatment would make millions of humans happy. Such rights are analogous to rights that people are supposed to have. People are thought to have a right, for instance, not to be unjustly imprisoned—even if their imprisonment would increase the overall happiness of society as a whole. (We take a closer look at strong animal rights in the next section.)

Before examining arguments that animals have moral status or rights, we should cite a few arguments to the contrary. Some people claim that only human beings have moral status and that animals, if they matter at all, have only indirect value as resources or tools for people. If cruelty to animals is wrong, it is wrong only because it makes humans callous or upsets people or damages personal property. The usual tack of those who reject moral status for animals is to argue that only beings that possess a particular property have moral status—a property that animals do not possess while humans do. The proposed status-granting properties are numerous and include having a soul, nurturing strong family bonds, using language, being a member of the human species, and being a person or a moral agent.

The notion that animals lack souls and therefore have no moral status is, of course, a traditional religious view defended on traditional religious grounds. Generally philosophers do not take this path, because their focus is on reason and arguments rather than on faith and because philosophical analysis has rendered the concept of a soul problematic or controversial.

CRITICAL THOUGHT: Should We Abolish Dog Racing?

Consider this verbal snapshot of the greyhound-racing issue:

> Many greyhounds live in miserable conditions, and many of them are put to death after their racing careers are over. For those who object to animal suffering, the preferred step would be to ensure that greyhounds are allowed decent lives—and to hope that the racing industry is compatible with the goal. But if it is simply impractical for law to ensure that greyhounds live minimally decent lives, some people would argue that greyhound racing should be abolished.*

What position would you take on the moral permissibility of this practice? What argument would you make to support your position? (After reading this chapter, return to this box and reconsider your judgment.)

*Cass R. Sunstein, "Introduction: What Are Animal Rights?" in *Animal Rights: Current Debates and New Directions*, ed. Sunstein and Martha C. Nussbaum (Oxford: Oxford University Press, 2004), 9.

The claim that animals have no moral standing because they do not have the kind of strong family relationships exhibited by humans has been undermined not by philosophy but by science. The same goes for the parallel claim regarding animals' language skills. One philosopher sums up the relevant empirical findings:

> [M]any species of non-humans develop long-lasting kinship ties—orangutan mothers stay with their young for eight to ten years and while they eventually part company, they continue to maintain their relationships. Less solitary animals, such as chimpanzees, baboons, wolves, and elephants maintain extended family units built upon complex individual relationships, for long periods of time. Meerkats in the Kalahari desert are known to sacrifice their own safety by staying with sick or injured family members so that the fatally ill will not die alone. . . . While the lives of many, perhaps most, non-humans in the wild are consumed with struggle for survival, aggression and battle, there are some non-humans whose lives are characterized by expressions of joy, playfulness, and a great deal of sex. Recent studies in cognitive ethology have suggested that some non-humans engage in manipulative and deceptive activity, can construct "cognitive maps" for navigation,

and some non-humans appear to understand symbolic representation and are able to use language.[5]

A more common claim is that just *being human*—having the DNA of the human species, in other words—is the property that gives a being moral considerability. If so, then nonhumans do not and cannot have moral status. This view has seemed initially plausible to some, but critics have wondered why simply having human DNA would bestow moral status on a creature.

Perhaps the most telling objection against the human species argument is based on a simple thought experiment. Suppose we humans encounter extraterrestrial creatures who have all the same attributes and capabilities that we have—self-consciousness, intelligence, language skills, reasoning ability, emotions, and more. We would presumably have to admit that these beings have

---

[5]Lori Gruen, "The Moral Status of Animals," *The Stanford Encyclopedia of Philosophy* (Fall 2003 ed.), ed. Edward N. Zalta, http://plato.stanford.edu/entries/moral-animal/ (23 February 2015).

full moral status, just as we do. Yet they are not human. They may not even be carbon-based life forms. Physically they may be nothing like any member of the human species. This strange (but possible) state of affairs suggests that being human is not a necessary condition for having moral status.

Taking a cue from Kant, some philosophers contend that only persons or moral agents can be candidates for moral considerability—and animals do not make the cut. Persons are typically regarded as rational beings who are free to choose their own ends and determine their own actions and values. Moral agents are beings who can make moral judgments and act according to moral reasons or principles. So the basic claim is that since all or most animals are not persons or moral agents, they can have no moral standing. They simply lack the necessary property.

As many critics have pointed out, using personhood and moral agency as criteria for determining moral status has a troublesome drawback: it excludes not only animals from moral considerability but some humans as well. This difficulty is common to all lack-of-some-necessary-property arguments, which we will examine more closely in the next section.

In any case, many think that all these standards for moral status are in a sense beside the point. To them it is obvious that regardless of whether an animal possesses these "higher" capacities and characteristics, it can suffer. They reason that if it can suffer, then it can be wronged by deliberately causing it to suffer. If deliberately hurting it is wrong, it must have some level of moral considerability.

MORAL THEORIES

How might a utilitarian assess the treatment of non-human animals? What would he or she say about their moral status? The most famous answers to these questions come from the utilitarian philosopher Peter Singer, credited with kindling through his writings what is popularly known as the animal rights movement. His most celebrated book, *Animal Liberation*, helped spark serious debates about the treatment of animals, the meat industry, and vegetarianism—debates that continue to this day. Classic utilitarianism says that the right action is the one that produces the best balance of happiness over unhappiness (or pleasure over pain), *everyone considered*. Singer's approach is to include *both* animals and humans in this "everyone." The pain and pleasure of *all* sentient beings must be considered when we are deciding which action maximizes the good.

This inclusion of *all* animals (human and nonhuman) in utilitarian calculations is not new, however—it was, in fact, advocated by utilitarianism's founder, Jeremy Bentham (1748–1832):

> The day *may* come when the rest of the animal creation may acquire those rights which never could have been withholden from them but by the hand of tyranny. The French have already discovered that the blackness of the skin is no reason why a human being should be abandoned without redress to the caprice of a tormentor. It may one day come to be recognized that the number of the legs, the villosity of the skin, or the termination of the *os sacrum*, are reasons equally insufficient for abandoning a sensitive being to the same fate. What else is it that should trace the insuperable line? Is it the faculty of reason, or perhaps the faculty of discourse? But a full grown horse or dog is beyond comparison a more rational, as well as a more conversable animal, than an infant of a day, or a week, or even a month, old. But suppose they were otherwise, what would it avail? The question is not, Can they reason? nor Can they *talk?* but, *Can they suffer?*[6]

For both Bentham and Singer, what makes a being worthy of moral concern, what requires us to include it in the moral community, is its ability to experience pain and pleasure—its ability to

---

[6]Jeremy Bentham, *An Introduction to Principles of Morals and Legislation* (1789; reprint, New York: Hafner, 1948), 311.

suffer. Why do humans have moral status? Not, says the utilitarian, because of their capacity for reason, social relationships, and personhood—but because of their capacity for suffering. Likewise, because sentient animals can suffer, they too have moral status. Furthermore, Bentham and Singer argue that because both humans and animals can suffer, they both deserve *equal moral consideration*. As Singer says,

> [T]he interests of every being affected by an action are to be taken into account and given the same weight as the like interests of any other being. . . . If a being suffers, there can be no moral justification for refusing to take that suffering into consideration. No matter what the nature of the being, the principle of equality requires that its suffering be counted equally with the like suffering—in so far as rough comparisons can be made—of any other being. If a being is not capable of suffering, or of experiencing enjoyment or happiness, there is nothing to be taken into account.[7]

According to Singer, those who do not give equal moral consideration to both human and nonhuman animals are guilty of **speciesism**—discrimination against nonhuman animals just because of their species. Speciesism, he says, is wrong for the same reason that racism and sexism are wrong: it violates the principle of equal consideration—that is, equal consideration of comparable interests.

Equal consideration of comparable interests, however, does not mean equal treatment. Humans and animals have some interests in common (such as avoiding pain), and they differ dramatically in the possession of other interests (humans are capable of enjoying art and studying philosophy, but animals are not). Singer's utilitarianism demands that when comparable interests are involved, those of humans and those of animals must be given equal weight. A pig's suffering is just as

important as a man's or a woman's. If a pig and a man were both experiencing intense pain, we must not assume that the man's pain should be taken more seriously. We should regard the agony of both beings with equal concern. But when interests are not comparable, we need not pretend that they are. We may, for example, give weight to a woman's interest in enjoying a good book, but we would give no weight to this interest in a dog, because a dog has no such interest.

What are the implications of Singer's view for the treatment of animals? For one thing, it implies that our system of meat production is wrong and should be abolished. There is general agreement that currently the meat industry causes immense suffering to millions of sentient creatures. In standard utilitarian calculations if we weigh this extreme suffering against the moderate pleasures it produces (the gustatory enjoyment of humans), we see that the meat industry generates a net balance of evil over good. The alternative to having a meat industry—vegetarianism—would result in far more good than evil. As Singer puts it,

> Since, as I have said, none of these [meat industry] practices cater for anything more than our pleasures of taste, our practice of rearing and killing other animals in order to eat them is a clear instance of the sacrifice of the most important interests of other beings in order to satisfy trivial interests of our own. To avoid speciesism we must stop this practice, and each of us has a moral obligation to cease supporting this practice.[8]

Some see a problem in Singer's stance, however, because his call for eliminating meat production and embracing vegetarianism does not seem to be fully warranted by his arguments. By Singer's own lights, a humane form of meat production may be morally permissible. If animals could be raised and killed without suffering—if their lives could be pleasant and their deaths painless—then

---

[7]Peter Singer, "All Animals Are Equal," *Philosophical Exchange* 1 (1974): 106, 107–8.

[8]Singer, "All Animals Are Equal," 109.

CRITICAL THOUGHT: Should We Experiment on Orphaned Babies?

Consider this controversial argument against speciesism by Peter Singer:

> In the past, argument about vivisection has often missed the point, because it has been put in absolutist terms: Would the abolitionist be prepared to let thousands die if they could be saved by experimenting on a single animal? The way to reply to this purely hypothetical question is to pose another: would the experimenter be prepared to perform his experiment on an orphaned human infant, if that were the only way to save many lives? (I say "orphan" to avoid the complication of parental feelings, although in doing so I am being overfair to the experimenter, since the nonhuman subjects of experiments are not orphans.) If the experimenter is not prepared to use an orphaned human infant, then his readiness to use nonhumans is simple discrimination, since adult apes, cats, mice, and other mammals are more aware of what is happening to them, more self-directing and, so far as we can tell, at least as sensitive to pain, as any human infant.*

What is Singer's point here? Is he advocating the practice of experimenting on orphaned human infants? Suppose you disagree with Singer. What argument would you make against his position?

*Peter Singer, "All Animals Are Equal," *Philosophical Exchange* 1 (1974): 110.

---

there might be a net balance of good over evil in the process. Then both meat production and meat eating might be acceptable. It seems that Singer's arguments could be used to support reform of the meat production industry just as easily as its total elimination.

As for scientific experimentation on animals, Singer thinks that it might be permissible if the benefits gained from the research outweigh any suffering involved. "[I]f a single experiment could cure a major disease, that experiment would be justifiable," he says.[9] However, he believes that in practice, animal experimentation usually results in more evil than good because often the benefits to humans are negligible.

How would a nonconsequentialist view the treatment of animals? Probably the most influential example of the nonconsequentialist approach is that of Tom Regan, another philosopher who has helped define and inspire the animal rights movement. He argues for *animal rights* proper—that is, animal rights in the restricted sense of having moral considerability that cannot be easily overridden, not in the weaker, generic sense of simply possessing moral status. According to Regan,

> The genius and the retarded child, the prince and the pauper, the brain surgeon and the fruit vendor, Mother Theresa and the most unscrupulous used car salesman—all have inherent value, all possess it *equally*, and *all have an equal right to be treated with respect*, to be treated in ways that do not reduce them to the status of things, as if they exist as resources for others.[10]

Regan maintains that such equal inherent value and equal rights apply to animals just as much as they do to humans. More specifically, he says, they apply to all mature mammals, human and nonhuman. Creatures with inherent value

[9]Singer, *Animal Liberation*, 77–78.

[10]Tom Regan, "The Case for Animal Rights," in *In Defense of Animals*, ed. Peter Singer (Oxford: Blackwell, 1985), 21.

> **QUICK REVIEW**
>
> *direct moral consideration*—Moral consideration for a being's own sake, rather than because of its relationship to others.
>
> *indirect moral consideration*—Moral consideration on account of a being's relationship to others.
>
> *animal rights*—Possession by animals of (1) moral status; (2) strong moral consideration that cannot be easily overridden.
>
> *speciesism*—Discrimination against nonhuman animals just because of their species.

must be treated, in Kant's famous phrase, as ends in themselves, not merely as means to an end. Their value or their treatment does not depend on some utilitarian calculation of pain and pleasure. According to Regan, humans and animals have equal value and equal rights because they share particular mental capacities; they are sensitive, experiencing beings—or as Regan says, "experiencing subjects of a life":

> [W]e are each of us the experiencing subject of a life, a conscious creature having an individual welfare that has importance to us whatever our usefulness to others. We want and prefer things, believe and feel things, recall and expect things. And all these dimensions of our life, including our pleasure and pain, our enjoyment and suffering, our satisfaction and frustration, our continued existence or our untimely death—all make a difference to the quality of our life as lived, as experienced, by us as individuals. As the same is true of those animals who concern us (those who are eaten and trapped, for example), they too must be viewed as the experiencing subjects of a life, with inherent value of their own.[11]

How should we treat animals, then, if they have such rights and if these rights are equal to our

own? Regan's theory (what he calls the rights view) implies that if it would be wrong to dissect, hurt, torture, eat, cage, hunt, or trap a human, then it would also be wrong to do the same to an animal—and the amount of good that might be produced by such acts is irrelevant. Therefore, Regan concludes, all forms of animal experimentation should be abolished. "Because these animals are treated routinely, systematically as if their value were reducible to their usefulness to others," Regan says, "they are routinely, systematically treated with a lack of respect, and thus are their rights routinely, systematically violated."[12] On the same grounds, he thinks that commercial animal agriculture and commercial and sport hunting and trapping should also be abolished.

MORAL ARGUMENTS

Do animals really have equal rights in the strict sense just mentioned? That is, do nonhuman animals have the same right to respect and moral concern that humans have? Using Tom Regan's rights view as inspiration without sticking strictly to his line of reasoning, let us examine some simple (and simplified) arguments for and against this proposition.

For our purposes, we can state the argument for the rights view like this:

1. Nonhuman animals (normal, fully developed mammals) are experiencing subjects of a life (or "experiencing subjects," for short), just as humans are.

2. All experiencing subjects have equal inherent value.

3. All those with equal inherent value are entitled to equal moral rights (the equal right to be treated with respect).

4. Therefore, nonhuman animals have equal moral rights.

[11]Regan, "The Case for Animal Rights," 22.

[12]Regan, "The Case for Animal Rights," 24.

This is a valid argument; the conclusion does follow from the three premises. So we have good reason to accept the conclusion if the premises are true. Are they? Premise 1 is an empirical claim about the mental capacities of animals (again, normal, fully developed mammals). There is scientific evidence suggesting that animals do have at least most of the capacities in question. For simplicity's sake, then, let us assume that Premise 1 is true.

Premises 2 and 3 are much more difficult to sort out. We should not accept them unless there are good reasons for doing so. Good reasons would involve separate arguments that support each of them. Regan has provided such arguments, and several critics have responded to them. Some have said, for example, that the notion of inherent value is obscure and that the link between inherent value and moral rights is unclear. Many others have sidestepped these issues and attacked the conclusion directly, arguing that regardless of whether animals have some moral rights, they surely do not have the *same* moral rights that humans do—that is, the equal right to be treated with respect.

Those who take this latter approach begin with an advantage. Our moral common sense suggests that there must be some sort of difference between the moral status of most humans and that of most animals. We tend to think that accidentally running over a man with our car is morally worse than doing the same to a rabbit. Most of us believe that there is an important moral difference between imprisoning women in cages for later slaughter and doing the same to chickens or hogs—even if we also deem the latter cruel and immoral.

Our intuition about such things can be wrong, of course. So those who reject equal moral rights for animals have offered other considerations. The philosopher Mary Anne Warren, for example, argues that animals do indeed have some moral rights but that there are reasons for thinking that these rights are weaker or less demanding than the rights of humans. For one thing, she notes, the human right to freedom is stronger or more extensive than the animal right to freedom. This right prohibits the unlawful imprisonment of humans, even if the prison is comfortable and spacious. Human dignity and the satisfaction of human aspirations and desires demand a higher degree of freedom of movement than would be required for the satisfaction of the needs or interests of many nonhuman animals. Imprisonment of animals in areas that allow them to satisfy their needs and pursue their natural inclinations, Warren says, "need not frustrate the needs or interests of animals in any significant way, and thus do not clearly violate their rights." In a similar vein, Warren argues that both humans and animals have a prima facie right to life, but this right is generally weaker for animals than for humans. As she puts it, "Human lives, one might say, have greater intrinsic value, because they are worth more *to their possessors*."[13] Humans have hopes, plans, and purposes that make them value continued existence; animals, apparently, lack this forward-looking perspective. Warren adds that nonhuman animals nevertheless have a right to life because, among other things, their premature demise robs them of any future pleasures they might have had.

Regan has responded to such arguments for unequal rights for animals by offering a common counterargument. In general, the arguments contend that animals have less inherent value (and therefore weaker moral rights) because animals lack something that adult humans have—perhaps the ability to reason, intelligence, autonomy, intellect, or some other valuable property. But, Regan says, if this contention is true, then we must say that some humans who lack these characteristics (retarded children or people with serious mental

[13]Mary Anne Warren, "The Rights of the Nonhuman World," in *Environmental Philosophy: A Collection of Readings*, eds. Robert Elliot and Arran Gare (University Park: Pennsylvania State University Press, 1983), 116.

illness, for example) also have less inherent value than normal adult humans and therefore less robust moral rights. In other words, if these critics of equal rights are correct, we are fully justified in treating these "deficient humans" as we would nonhuman animals. "But it is not true," he says, "that such humans . . . have less inherent value than you or I. Neither, then, can we rationally sustain the view that animals like them in being experiencing subjects of a life have less inherent value. *All* who have inherent value have it *equally*, whether they be human animals or not."[14]

SUMMARY

The traditional attitude toward animals is that they are merely resources that humans can dispose of as they see fit; animals have instrumental value only. But many reject the traditional view and put forward reasons for supposing that animals have moral status. Something has moral status if it is a suitable candidate for moral concern or respect in its own right.

Some people claim that only humans have moral status and that animals have just indirect value to humans. The usual approach of those who reject moral status for animals is to argue that a being is entitled to moral status only if it possesses particular properties—and that animals do not possess them. These status-granting properties include having a soul, having strong family bonds, using language,

---

[14]Regan, "The Case for Animal Rights," 23.

---

being a member of the human species, and being a person or a moral agent.

One of the more common claims is that one must be human to have moral status. Critics, however, have asked what it is about being human that gives one moral status. A thought experiment used against this claim asks us to imagine meeting extraterrestrial creatures who are self-conscious, intelligent, rational, and like ourselves in many other ways. We would presumably have to admit that the aliens have moral status just as we do, even though they are not human. Being human, then, seems not to be necessary for having moral status.

The most famous utilitarian approach to the treatment of animals is that of the philosopher Peter Singer. He argues that the pain and pleasure of animals as well as that of humans must be included in utilitarian calculations. What makes a being worthy of moral concern, he says, is its capacity for suffering, and since both humans and animals can suffer, they both deserve equal moral consideration. Consequently, Singer maintains that our system of meat production is wrong and should be abolished.

The most notable nonconsequentialist approach to the treatment of animals is that of Tom Regan. He argues for strong animal rights on the grounds that all "experiencing subjects of a life" have equal inherent value and therefore an equal right to be treated with respect. Experiencing subjects of a life include healthy, mature mammals (humans and nonhumans). Regan maintains that because such animals have equal rights, all commercial animal agriculture and sport hunting and trapping should be abolished.

READINGS

All Animals Are Equal

PETER SINGER

In recent years a number of oppressed groups have campaigned vigorously for equality. The classic instance is the Black Liberation movement, which demands an end to the prejudice and discrimination that has made blacks second-class citizens. The immediate appeal of the black liberation movement and its initial, if limited success made it a model for other oppressed groups to follow. We became familiar with liberation movements for Spanish-Americans, gay people, and a variety of other minorities. When a majority group—women—began their campaign, some thought we had come to the end of the road. Discrimination on the basis of sex, it has been said, is the last universally accepted form of discrimination, practiced without secrecy or pretense even in those liberal circles that have long prided themselves on their freedom from prejudice against racial minorities.

One should always be wary of talking of "the last remaining form of discrimination." If we have learnt anything from the liberation movements, we should have learnt how difficult it is to be aware of latent prejudice in our attitudes to particular groups until this prejudice is forcefully pointed out.

A liberation movement demands an expansion of our moral horizons and an extension or reinterpretation of the basic moral principle of equality. Practices that were previously regarded as natural and inevitable come to be seen as the result of an unjustifiable prejudice. Who can say with confidence that all his or her attitudes and practices are beyond criticism? If we wish to avoid being numbered amongst the oppressors, we must be prepared to re-think even our most fundamental attitudes. We need to consider them from the point of view of those most disadvantaged by our attitudes, and the practices that follow from these attitudes. If we can make this unaccustomed mental switch we may discover a pattern in our attitudes and practices that consistently operates so as to benefit one group—usually the one to which we ourselves belong—at the expense of another. In this way we may come to see that there is a case for a new liberation movement. My aim is to advocate that we make this mental switch in respect of our attitudes and practices towards a very large group of beings: members of species other than our own—or, as we popularly though misleadingly call them, animals. In other words, I am urging that we extend to other species the basic principle of equality that most of us recognise should be extended to all members of our own species.

All this may sound a little far-fetched, more like a parody of other liberation movements than a serious objective. In fact, in the past the idea of "The Rights of Animals" really has been used to parody the case for women's rights. When Mary Wollstonecraft, a forerunner of later feminists, published her *Vindication of the Rights of Women* in 1792, her ideas were widely regarded as absurd, and they were satirized in an anonymous publication entitled *A Vindication of the Rights of Brutes*. The author of this satire (actually Thomas Taylor, a distinguished Cambridge philosopher) tried to refute Wollstonecraft's reasonings by showing that they could be carried one stage further. If sound when applied to women, why should the arguments not be applied to dogs, cats and horses? They seemed to hold equally well for these "brutes": yet to hold that brutes had rights was manifestly absurd; therefore the reasoning by which this conclusion had been reached must be unsound, and if unsound when applied to brutes, it must also be unsound when applied to women, since the very same arguments had been used in each case.

Peter Singer, "All Animals Are Equal," *Philosophical Exchange* Vol. 1 (1974). Copyright © Peter Singer 1974. Reprinted by permission of the author.

One way in which we might reply to this argument is by saying that the case for equality between men and women cannot validly be extended to non-human animals. Women have a right to vote, for instance, because they are just as capable of making rational decisions as men are; dogs, on the other hand, are incapable of understanding the significance of voting, so they cannot have the right to vote. There are many other obvious ways in which men and women resemble each other closely, while humans and other animals differ greatly. So, it might be said, men and women are similar beings, and should have equal rights, while humans and non-humans are different and should not have equal rights.

The thought behind this reply to Taylor's analogy is correct up to a point, but it does not go far enough. There *are* important differences between humans and other animals, and these differences must give rise to *some* differences in the rights that each have. Recognizing this obvious fact, however, is no barrier to the case for extending the basic principle of equality to non-human animals. The differences that exist between men and women are equally undeniable, and the supporters of Women's Liberation are aware that these differences may give rise to different rights. Many feminists hold that women have the right to an abortion on request. It does not follow that since these same people are campaigning for equality between men and women they must support the right of men to have abortions too. Since a man cannot have an abortion, it is meaningless to talk of his right to have one. Since a pig can't vote, it is meaningless to talk of its right to vote. There is no reason why either Women's Liberation or Animal Liberation should get involved in such nonsense. The extension of the basic principle of equality from one group to another does not imply that we must treat both groups in exactly the same way, or grant exactly the same rights to both groups. Whether we should do so will depend on the nature of the members of the two groups. The basic principle of equality, I shall argue, is equality of consideration; and equal consideration for different beings may lead to different treatment and different rights.

So there is a different way of replying to Taylor's attempt to parody Wollstonecraft's arguments, a way which does not deny the differences between humans and non-humans, but goes more deeply into the question of equality, and concludes by finding nothing absurd in the idea that the basic principle of equality applies to so-called "brutes." I believe that we reach this conclusion if we examine the basis on which our opposition to discrimination on grounds of race or sex ultimately rests. We will then see that we would be on shaky ground if we were to demand equality for blacks, women, and other groups of oppressed humans while denying equal consideration to non-humans.

When we say that all human beings, whatever their race, creed or sex, are equal, what is it that we are asserting? Those who wish to defend a hierarchical, inegalitarian society have often pointed out that by whatever test we choose, it simply is not true that all humans are equal. Like it or not, we must face the fact that humans come in different shapes and sizes; they come with differing moral capacities, differing intellectual abilities, differing amounts of benevolent feeling and sensitivity to the needs of others, differing abilities to communicate effectively, and differing capacities to experience pleasure and pain. In short, if the demand for equality were based on the actual equality of all human beings, we would have to stop demanding equality. It would be an unjustifiable demand.

Still, one might cling to the view that the demand for equality among human beings is based on the actual equality of the different races and sexes. Although humans differ as individuals in various ways, there are no differences between the races and sexes *as such*. From the mere fact that a person is black, or a woman, we cannot infer anything else about that person. This, it may be said, is what is wrong with racism and sexism. The white racist claims that whites are superior to blacks, but this is false—although there are differences between individuals, some blacks are superior to some whites in all of the capacities and abilities that could conceivably be relevant. The opponent of sexism would say the same: a person's sex is no guide to his or her abilities, and this is why it is unjustifiable to discriminate on the basis of sex.

This is a possible line of objection to racial and sexual discrimination. It is not, however, the way that someone really concerned about equality would choose, because taking this line could, in some circumstances, force one to accept a most inegalitarian society. The fact that humans differ as individuals, rather than as races or sexes, is a valid reply to someone who defends a hierarchical society like, say, South Africa, in which all whites are superior in status to all blacks. The existence of individual variations that cut across the lines of race or sex, however, provides us with no defence at all against a more sophisticated opponent of equality, one who proposes that, say, the interests of those with I.Q. ratings above 100 be preferred to the interests of those with I.Q.s below 100. Would a hierarchical society of this sort really be so much better than one based on race or sex? I think not. But if we tie the moral principle of equality to the factual equality of the different races or sexes, taken as a whole, our opposition to racism and sexism does not provide us with any basis for objecting to this kind of inegalitarianism.

There is a second important reason why we ought not to base our opposition to racism and sexism on any kind of factual equality, even the limited kind asserts that variations in capacities and abilities are spread evenly between the different races and sexes: we can have no absolute guarantee that these abilities and capacities really are distributed evenly, without regard to race or sex, among human beings. So far as actual abilities are concerned, there do seem to be certain measurable differences between both races and sexes. These differences do not, of course, appear in each case, but only when averages are taken. More important still, we do not yet know how much of these differences is really due to the different genetic endowments of the various races and sexes, and how much is due to environmental differences that are the result of past and continuing discrimination. Perhaps all of the important differences will eventually prove to be environmental rather than genetic. Anyone opposed to racism and sexism will certainly hope that this will be so, for it will make the task of ending discrimination a lot easier; nevertheless it would be dangerous to rest the case against racism and sexism on the belief that all significant differences are environmental in origin. The opponent of, say, racism

who takes this line will be unable to avoid conceding that if differences in ability did after all prove to have some genetic connection with race, racism would in some way be defensible.

It would be folly for the opponent of racism to stake his whole case on a dogmatic commitment to one particular outcome of a difficult scientific issue which is still a long way from being settled. While attempts to prove that differences in certain selected abilities between races and sexes are primarily genetic in origin have certainly not been conclusive, the same must be said of attempts to prove that these differences are largely the result of environment. At this stage of the investigation we cannot be certain which view is correct, however much we may hope it is the latter.

Fortunately, there is no need to pin the case for equality to one particular outcome of this scientific investigation. The appropriate response to those who claim to have found evidence of genetically-based differences in ability between the races or sexes is not to stick to the belief that the genetic explanation must be wrong, whatever evidence to the contrary may turn up: instead we should make it quite clear that the claim to equality does not depend on intelligence, moral capacity, physical strength, or similar matters of fact. Equality is a moral ideal, not a simple assertion of fact. There is no logically compelling reason for assuming that a factual difference in ability between two people justifies any difference in the amount of consideration we give to satisfying their needs and interests. The principle of the equality of human beings is not a description of an alleged actual equality among humans: it is a prescription of how we should treat humans.

Jeremy Bentham incorporated the essential basis of moral equality into his utilitarian system of ethics in the formula: "Each to count for one and none for more than one." In other words, the interests of every being affected by an action are to be taken into account and given the same weight as the like interests of any other being. A later utilitarian, Henry Sidgwick, put the point in this way: "The good of any one individual is of no more importance, from the point of view (if I may say so) of the Universe, than the good of any other."[1] More recently, the leading figures in contemporary moral philosophy have shown a great deal of agreement in specifying as a fundamental presupposition of their moral theories some similar requirement which operates so as to give everyone's interests equal consideration—although they cannot agree on how this requirement is best formulated.

It is an implication of this principle of equality that our concern for others ought not to depend on what they are like, or what abilities they possess—although precisely what this concern requires us to do may vary according to the characteristics of those affected by what we do. It is on this basis that the case against racism and the case against sexism must both ultimately rest; and it is in accordance with this principle that speciesism is also to be condemned. If possessing a higher degree of intelligence does not entitle one human to use another for his own ends, how can it entitle humans to exploit non-humans?

Many philosophers have proposed the principle of equal consideration of interests, in some form or other, as a basic moral principle; but, as we shall see in more detail shortly, not many of them have recognised that this principle applies to members of other species as well as to our own. Bentham was one of the few who did realize this. In a forward-looking passage, written at a time when black slaves in the British dominions were still being treated much as we now treat non-human animals, Bentham wrote:

> The day *may* come when the rest of the animal creation may acquire those rights which never could have been witholden from them but by the hand of tyranny. The French have already discovered that the blackness of the skin is no reason why a human being should be abandoned without redress to the caprice of a tormentor. It may one day come to be recognised that the number of the legs, the villosity of the skin, or the termination of the *os sacrum*, are reasons equally insufficient for abandoning a sensitive being to the same fate. What else is it that should trace the insuperable line? Is it the faculty of reason, or perhaps the faculty of discourse? But a full-grown horse or dog is beyond comparison a more rational, as well as a more conversable animal, than an infant of a day, or a week, or even a month, old. But suppose they were otherwise, what would it avail? The question is not, Can they reason? nor Can they *talk*? but, *Can they suffer?*[2]

In this passage Bentham points to the capacity for suffering as the vital characteristic that gives a being the right to equal consideration. The capacity for suffering—or more strictly, for suffering and/or enjoyment or happiness—is not just another characteristic like the capacity for language, or for higher mathematics. Bentham is not saying that those who try to mark "the insuperable line" that determines whether the interests of a being should be considered happen to have selected the wrong characteristic. The capacity for suffering and enjoying things is a pre-requisite for having interests at all, a condition that must be satisfied before we can speak of interests in any meaningful way. It would be nonsense to say that it was not in the interests of a stone to be kicked along the road by a schoolboy. A stone does not have interests because it cannot suffer. Nothing that we can do to it could possibly make any difference to its welfare. A mouse, on the other hand, does have an interest in not being tormented, because it will suffer if it is.

If a being suffers, there can be no moral justification for refusing to take that suffering into consideration. No matter what the nature of the being, the principle of equality requires that its suffering be counted equally with the like suffering—in so far as rough comparisons can be made—of any other being. If a being is not capable of suffering, or of experiencing enjoyment or happiness, there is nothing to be taken into account. This is why the limit of sentience (using the term as a convenient, if not strictly accurate, shorthand for the capacity to suffer or experience enjoyment or happiness) is the only defensible boundary of concern for the interests of others. To mark this boundary by some characteristic like intelligence or rationality would be to mark it in an arbitrary way. Why not choose some other characteristic, like skin color?

The racist violates the principle of equality by giving greater weight to the interests of members of his own race, when there is a clash between their interests and the interests of those of another race. Similarly the speciesist allows the interests of his own species to override the greater interests of members of other species. The pattern is the same in each case. Most human beings are speciesists. I shall now very briefly describe some of the practices that show this.

For the great majority of human beings, especially in urban, industrialized societies, the most direct form of contact with members of other species is at mealtimes: we eat them. In doing so we treat them purely as means to our ends. We regard their life and well-being as subordinate to our taste for a particular kind of dish. I say "taste" deliberately—this is purely a matter of pleasing our palate. There can be no defence of eating flesh in terms of satisfying nutritional needs, since it has been established beyond doubt that we could satisfy our need for protein and other essential nutrients far more efficiently with a diet that replaced animal flesh by soy beans, or products derived from soy beans, and other high-protein vegetable products.[3]

It is not merely the act of killing that indicates what we are ready to do to other species in order to gratify our tastes. The suffering we inflict on the animals while they are alive is perhaps an even clearer indication of our speciesism than the fact that we are prepared to kill them.[4] In order to have meat on the table at a price that people can afford, our society tolerates methods of meat production that confine sentient animals in cramped, unsuitable conditions for the entire durations of their lives. Animals are treated like machines that convert fodder into flesh, and any innovation that results in a higher "conversion ratio" is liable to be adopted. As one authority on the subject has said, "cruelty is acknowledged only when profitability ceases."[5] So hens are crowded four or five to a cage with a floor area of twenty inches by eighteen inches, or around the size of a single page of the *New York Times*. The cages have wire floors, since this reduces cleaning costs, though wire is unsuitable for the hens' feet; the floors slope, since this makes the eggs roll down for easy collection, although this makes it difficult for the hens to rest comfortably. In these conditions all the birds' natural instincts are thwarted: they cannot stretch their wings fully, walk freely, dust-bathe, scratch the ground, or build a nest. Although they have never known other conditions, observers have noticed that the birds vainly try to perform these actions. Frustrated at their inability to do so, they often develop what farmers call "vices," and peck each other to death. To prevent this, the beaks of young birds are often cut off.

This kind of treatment is not limited to poultry. Pigs are now also being reared in cages inside sheds. These animals are comparable to dogs in intelligence, and need a varied, stimulating environment if they are not to suffer from stress and boredom. Anyone who kept a dog in the way in which pigs are frequently kept would be liable to prosecution, in England at least, but because our interest in exploiting pigs is greater than our interest in exploiting dogs, we object to cruelty to dogs while consuming the produce of cruelty to pigs. Of the other animals, the condition of veal calves is perhaps worst of all, since these animals are so closely confined that they cannot even turn around or get up and lie down freely. In this way they do not develop unpalatable muscle. They are also made anaemic and kept short of roughage, to keep their flesh pale, since white veal fetches a higher price; as a result they develop a craving for iron and roughage, and have been observed to gnaw wood off the sides of their stalls, and lick greedily at any rusty hinge that is within reach.

Since, as I have said, none of these practices cater for anything more than our pleasures of taste, our practice of rearing and killing other animals in order to eat them is a clear instance of the sacrifice of the most important interests of other beings in order to satisfy trivial interests of our own. To avoid speciesism we must stop this practice, and each of us has a moral obligation to cease supporting the practice. Our custom is all the support that the meat-industry needs. The decision to cease giving it that support may be difficult, but it is no more difficult than it would have been for a white Southerner to go against the traditions of his society and free his slaves; if we do not change our dietary habits, how can we censure those slaveholders who would not change their own way of living?

The same form of discrimination may be observed in the widespread practice of experimenting on other species in order to see if certain substances are safe for human beings, or to test some psychological theory about the effect of severe punishment on learning, or to try out various new compounds just in case something turns up. People sometimes think that all this experimentation is for vital medical purposes, and so will reduce suffering overall. This comfortable belief is very wide of the mark. Drug companies test new shampoos and cosmetics that they are intending to put on the market by dropping them into the eyes of rabbits, held open by metal clips, in order to observe what damage results. Food additives, like artificial colorings and preservatives, are tested by what is known as the "LD_{50}"—a test designed to find the level of consumption at which 50% of a group of animals will die. In the process, nearly all of the animals are made very sick before some finally die, and others pull through. If the substance is relatively harmless, as it often is, huge doses have to be force-fed to the animals, until in some cases sheer volume or concentration of the substance causes death.

Much of this pointless cruelty goes on in the universities. In many areas of science, non-human animals are regarded as an item of laboratory equipment, to be used and expended as desired. In psychology laboratories experimenters devise endless variations and repetitions of experiments that were of little value in the first place. To quote just one example, from the experimenter's own account in a psychology journal: at the University of Pennsylvania, Perrin S. Cohen hung six dogs in hammocks with electrodes taped to their hind feet. Electric shock of varying intensity was then administered through the electrodes. If the dog learnt to press its head against a panel on the left, the shock was turned off, but otherwise it remained on indefinitely. Three of the dogs, however, were required to wait periods varying from 2 to 7 seconds while being shocked before making the response that turned off the current. If they failed to wait, they received further shocks. Each dog was given from 26 to 46 "sessions" in the hammock, each session consisting of 80 "trials" or shocks, administered at intervals of one minute. The experimenter reported that the dogs, who were unable to move in the hammock, barked or bobbed their heads when the current was applied. The reported findings of the experiment were that there was a delay in the dogs' responses that increased proportionately to the time the dogs were required to endure the shock, but a gradual increase in the intensity of the shock had no systematic effect in the timing of the response. The experiment was funded by the National Institutes of Health, and the United States Public Health Service.

In this example, and countless cases like it, the possible benefits to mankind are either nonexistent or fantastically remote; while the certain losses to members of other species are very real. This is, again, a clear indication of speciesism.

In the past, argument about vivesection has often missed this point, because it has been put in absolutist terms: would the abolitionist be prepared to let thousands die if they could be saved by experimenting on a single animal? The way to reply to this purely hypothetical question is to pose another: would the experimenter be prepared to perform his experiment on an orphaned human infant, if that were the only way to save many lives? (I say "orphan" to avoid the complication of parental feelings, although in doing so I am being overfair to the experimenter, since the nonhuman subjects of experiments are not orphans.) If the experimenter is not prepared to use an orphaned human infant, then his readiness to use nonhumans is simple discrimination, since adult apes, cats, mice and other mammals are more aware of what is happening to them, more self-directing and, so far as we can tell, at least as sensitive to pain, as any human infant. There seems to be no relevant characteristic that human infants possess that adult mammals do not have to the same or a higher degree. (Someone might try to argue that what makes it wrong to experiment on a human infant is that the infant will, in time and if left alone, develop into more than the nonhuman, but one would then, to be consistent, have to oppose abortion, since the fetus has the same potential as the infant—indeed, even contraception and abstinence might be wrong on this ground, since the egg and sperm, considered jointly, also have the same potential. In any case, this argument still gives us no reason for selecting a nonhuman, rather than a human with severe and irreversible brain damage, as the subject for our experiments.)

The experimenter, then, shows a bias in favor of his own species whenever he carries out an experiment on a nonhuman for a purpose that he would not think justified him in using a human being at an equal or lower level of sentience, awareness, ability to be self-directing, etc. No one familiar with the kind of results yielded by most experiments on animals can have the slightest doubt that if this bias were eliminated the number of experiments performed would be a minute fraction of the number performed today.

Experimenting on animals, and eating their flesh, are perhaps the two major forms of speciesism in our society. By comparison, the third and last form of speciesism is so minor as to be insignificant, but it is perhaps of some special interest to those for whom this paper was written. I am referring to speciesism in contemporary philosophy.

Philosophy ought to question the basic assumptions of the age. Thinking through, critically and carefully, what most people take for granted is, I believe, the chief task of philosophy, and it is this task that makes philosophy a worthwhile activity. Regrettably, philosophy does not always live up to its historic role. Philosophers are human beings and they are subject to all the preconceptions of the society to which they belong. Sometimes they succeed in breaking free of the prevailing ideology: more often they become its most sophisticated defenders. So, in this case, philosophy as practiced in the universities today does not challenge anyone's preconceptions about our relations with other species. By their writings, those philosophers who tackle problems that touch upon the issue reveal that they make the same unquestioned assumptions as most other humans, and what they say tends to confirm the reader in his or her comfortable speciesist habits.

I could illustrate this claim by referring to the writings of philosophers in various fields—for instance, the attempts that have been made by those interested in rights to draw the boundary of the sphere of rights so that it runs parallel to the biological boundaries of the species *homo sapiens*, including infants and even mental defectives, but excluding those other beings of equal or greater capacity who are so useful to us at mealtimes and in our laboratories. I think it would be a more appropriate conclusion to this paper, however, if I concentrated on the problem with which we have been centrally concerned, the problem of equality.

It is significant that the problem of equality, in moral and political philosophy, is invariably formulated in terms of human equality. The effect of this is that the question of the equality of other animals does not confront the philosopher, or student, as an issue in itself—and this is already an indication of the failure of philosophy to challenge accepted beliefs. Still, philosophers have found it difficult to discuss the issue of human equality without raising, in a paragraph or two, the question of the status of other animals. The reason for this, which should be apparent from what I have said already, is that if humans are to be regarded as equal to one another, we need some sense of "equal" that does not require any actual, descriptive equality of capacities, talents or other qualities. If equality is to be related to any actual characteristics of humans, these characteristics must be some lowest common denominator, pitched so low that no human lacks them—but then the philosopher comes up against the catch that any such set of characteristics which covers *all* humans will not be possessed *only by humans*. In other words, it turns out that in the only sense in which we can truly say, as an assertion of fact, that all humans are equal, at least some members of other species are also equal—equal, that is, to each other and to humans. If, on the other hand, we regard the statement "All humans are equal" in some non-factual way, perhaps as a prescription, then, as I have already argued, it is even more difficult to exclude non-humans from the sphere of equality.

This result is not what the egalitarian philosopher originally intended to assert. Instead of accepting the radical outcome to which their own reasonings naturally point, however, most philosophers try to reconcile their beliefs in human equality and animal inequality by arguments that can only be described as devious.

As a first example, I take William Frankena's well-known article "The Concept of Social Justice." Frankena opposes the idea of basing justice on merit, because he sees that this could lead to highly inegalitarian results. Instead he proposes the principle that:

> . . . all men are to be treated as equals, not because they are equal, in any respect but simply because they are human. They are human because they have emotions and desires, and are able to think, and hence are capable of enjoying a good life in a sense in which other animals are not.[6]

But what is this capacity to enjoy the good life which all humans have, but no other animals? Other animals have emotions and desires, and appear to be capable of enjoying a good life. We may doubt that they can think—although the behavior of some apes, dolphins and even dogs suggests that some of them can—but what is the relevance of thinking? Frankena goes on to admit that by "the good life" he means "not so much the morally good life as the happy or satisfactory life," so thought would appear to be unnecessary for enjoying the good life; in fact to emphasise the need for thought would make difficulties for the egalitarian since only some people are capable of leading intellectually satisfying lives—or morally good lives. This makes it difficult to see what Frankena's principle of equality has to do with simply being *human*. Surely every sentient being is capable of leading a life that is happier or less miserable than some alternative life, and hence has a claim to be taken into account. In this respect the distinction between humans and non-humans is not a sharp division, but rather a continuum along which we move gradually, and with overlaps between the species, from simple capacities for enjoyment and satisfaction, or pain and suffering, to more complex ones.

Faced with a situation in which they see a need for some basis for the moral gulf that is commonly thought to separate humans and animals, but can find no concrete difference that will do the job without undermining the equality of humans, philosophers tend to waffle. They resort to high-sounding phrases like "the intrinsic dignity of the human individual";[7] they talk of the "intrinsic worth of all men" as if men (humans?) had some worth that other beings did not,[8] or they say that humans, and only humans, are "ends in themselves," while "everything other than a person can only have value for a person."[9]

This idea of a distinctive human dignity and worth has a long history; it can be traced back directly to the Renaissance humanists, for instance to Pico della Mirandola's *Oration on the Dignity of Man*. Pico and other humanists based their estimate of human dignity on the idea that man possessed the central, pivotal position in the "Great Chain of Being" that led from the lowliest forms of matter to God himself; this view of the universe, in turn, goes back to both classical and Judeo-Christian doctrines. Contemporary philosophers have cast off these metaphysical and religious shackles and freely invoke the dignity of mankind without needing to justify the idea at all. Why should we not attribute "intrinsic dignity" or "intrinsic worth" to ourselves? Fellow-humans are unlikely to reject the accolades we so generously bestow on them, and those to whom we deny the honor are unable to object. Indeed, when one thinks only of humans, it can be very liberal, very progressive, to talk of the dignity of all human beings. In so doing, we implicitly condemn slavery, racism, and other violations of human rights. We admit that we ourselves are in some fundamental sense on a par with the poorest, most ignorant members of our own species. It is only when we think of humans as no more than a small sub-group of all the beings that inhabit our planet that we may realize that in elevating our own species we are at the same time lowering the relative status of all other species.

The truth is that the appeal to the intrinsic dignity of human beings appears to solve the egalitarian's problems only as long as it goes unchallenged. Once we ask *why* it should be that all humans—including infants, mental defectives, psychopaths, Hitler, Stalin and the rest—have some kind of dignity or worth that no elephant, pig or chimpanzee can ever achieve, we see that this question is as difficult to answer as our original request for some relevant fact that justifies the inequality of humans and other animals. In fact, these two questions are really one: talk of intrinsic dignity or moral worth only takes the problem back one step, because any satisfactory defence of the claim that all and only humans have intrinsic dignity would need to refer to some relevant capacities or characteristics that all and only humans possess. Philosophers frequently introduce ideas of dignity, respect and worth at the point at which other reasons appear to be lacking, but this is hardly good enough. Fine phrases are the last resource of those who have run out of arguments.

In case there are those who still think it may be possible to find some relevant characteristic that distinguishes all humans from all members of other species, I shall refer again, before I conclude, to the existence of some humans who quite clearly are below the level of awareness, self-consciousness, intelligence, and sentience, of many non-humans. I am thinking of humans with severe and irreparable brain damage, and also of infant humans. To avoid the complication of the relevance of a being's potential, however, I shall henceforth concentrate on permanently retarded humans.

Philosophers who set out to find a characteristic that will distinguish humans from other animals rarely take the course of abandoning these groups of humans by lumping them in with the other animals. It is easy to see why they do not. To take this line without re-thinking our attitudes to other animals would entail that we have the right to perform painful experiments on retarded humans for trivial reasons; similarly it would follow that we had the right to rear and kill these humans for food. To most philosophers these consequences are as unacceptable as the view that we should stop treating non-humans in this way.

Of course, when discussing the problem of equality it is possible to ignore the problem of mental defectives, or brush it aside as if somehow insignificant. This is the easiest way out. What else remains? My final example of speciesism in contemporary philosophy has been selected to show what happens when a writer is prepared to face the question of human equality and animal inequality without ignoring the existence of mental defectives, and without resorting to obscurantist mumbo-jumbo. Stanley Benn's clear and honest article "Egalitarianism and Equal Consideration of Interests"[10] fits this description.

Benn after noting the usual "evident human inequalities" argues, correctly I think, for equality of consideration as the only possible basis for egalitarianism. Yet Benn, like other writers, is thinking only of "equal consideration of human interests." Benn is quite open in his defence of this restriction of equal consideration:

> . . . not to possess human shape *is* a disqualifying condition. However faithful or intelligent a dog may be, it would be a monstrous sentimentality to attribute to him interests that could be weighed in an equal balance with those of human beings . . . if, for instance,

one had to decide between feeding a hungry baby or a hungry dog, anyone who chose the dog would generally be reckoned morally defective, unable to recognize a fundamental inequality of claims.

> This is what distinguishes our attitude to animals from our attitude to imbeciles. It would be odd to say that we ought to respect equally the dignity or personality of the imbecile and of the rational man . . . but there is nothing odd about saying that we should respect their interests equally, that is, that we should give to the interests of each the same serious consideration as claims to considerations necessary for some standard of well-being that we can recognize and endorse.

Benn's statement of the basis of the consideration we should have for imbeciles seems to me correct, but why should there be any fundamental inequality of claims between a dog and a human imbecile? Benn sees that if equal consideration depended on rationality, no reason could be given against using imbeciles for research purposes, as we now use dogs and guinea pigs. This will not do: "But of course we do distinguish imbeciles from animals in this regard," he says. That the common distinction is justifiable is something Benn does not question; his problem is how it is to be justified. The answer he gives is this:

> . . . we respect the interests of men and give them priority over dogs not *insofar* as they are rational, but because rationality is the human norm. We say it is *unfair* to exploit the deficiencies of the imbecile who falls short of the norm, just as it would be unfair, and not just ordinarily dishonest, to steal from a blind man. If we do not think in this way about dogs, it is because we do not see the irrationality of the dog as a deficiency or a handicap, but as normal for the species. The characteristics, therefore, that distinguish the normal man from the normal dog make it intelligible for us to talk of other men having interests and capacities, and therefore claims, of precisely the same kind as we make on our own behalf. But although these characteristics may provide the point of the distinction between men and other species, they are not in fact the qualifying conditions for membership, or the distinguishing criteria of the class of morally considerable persons; and this is precisely because a man does not become a member of a different species, with its own standards of normality, by reason of not possessing these characteristics.

The final sentence of this passage gives the argument away. An imbecile, Benn concedes, may have no characteristics superior to those of a dog; nevertheless this does not make the imbecile a member of "a different species" as the dog is. *Therefore* it would be "unfair" to use the imbecile for medical research as we use the dog. But why? That the imbecile is not rational is just the way things have worked out, and the same is true of the dog—neither is any more responsible for their mental level. If it is unfair to take advantage of an isolated defect, why is it fair to take advantage of a more general limitation? I find it hard to see anything in this argument except a defence of preferring the interests of members of our own species because they are members of our own species. To those who think there might be more to it, I suggest the following mental exercise. Assume that it has been proven that there is a difference in the average, or normal, intelligence quotient for two different races, say whites and blacks. Then substitute the term "white" for every occurrence of "men" and "black" for every occurrence of "dog" in the passage quoted; and substitute "high I.Q." for "rationality" and when Benn talks of "imbeciles" replace this term by "dumb whites"—that is, whites who fall well below the normal white I.Q. score. Finally, change "species" to "race." Now re-read the passage. It has become a defence of a rigid, no-exceptions division between whites and blacks, based on I.Q. scores, *not withstanding an admitted overlap* between whites and blacks in this respect. The revised passage is, of course, outrageous, and this not only because we have made fictitious assumptions in our substitutions. The point is that in the original passage Benn was defending a rigid division in the amount of consideration due to members of different species, despite admitted cases of overlap. If the original did not, at first reading strike us as being as outrageous as the revised version does, this is largely because although we are not racists ourselves, most of us are speciesists. Like the other articles, Benn's stands as a warning of the case with which the best minds can fall victim to a prevailing ideology.

NOTES

1. *The Methods of Ethics* (7th Ed.) p. 382.

2. *Introduction to the Principles of Morals and Legislation*, ch. XVII.

3. In order to produce 1 lb. of protein in the form of beef or veal, we must feed 21 lbs. of protein to the animal. Other forms of livestock are slightly less inefficient, but the average ratio in the U.S. is still 1:8. It has been estimated that the amount of protein lost to humans in this way is equivalent to 90% of the annual world protein deficit.

4. Although one might think that killing a being is obviously the ultimate wrong one can do to it, I think that the infliction of suffering is a clearer indication of speciesism because it might be argued that at least part of what is wrong with killing a human is that most humans are conscious of their existence over time, and have desires and purposes that extend into the future. Of course, if one took this view one would have to hold that killing a human infant or mental defective is not in itself wrong, and is less serious than killing certain higher mammals that probably do have a sense of their own existence over time.

5. Ruth Harrison, *Animal Machines* (Stuart, London, 1964).

6. In R. Brandt (ed.) *Social Justice* (Prentice Hall, Englewood Cliffs, 1962): the passage quoted appears on p. 19.

7. Frankena, *op. cit.*, p. 23.

8. H. A. Bedau, "Egalitarianism and the Idea of Equality" in *Nomos IX: Equality*, ed. J. R. Pennock and J. W. Chapman, New York, 1967.

9. G. Vlastos, "Justice and Equality" in Brandt. *Social Justice*, p. 48.

10. *Nomos IX: Equality:* the passages quoted are on p. 62ff.

The Case for Animal Rights

TOM REGAN

I regard myself as an advocate of animal rights—as a part of the animal rights movement. That movement, as I conceive it, is committed to a number of goals, including:

- the total abolition of the use of animals in science;
- the total dissolution of commercial animal agriculture;
- the total elimination of commercial and sport hunting and trapping.

There are, I know, people who profess to believe in animal rights but do not avow these goals. Factory farming, they say, is wrong—it violates animals' rights—but traditional animal agriculture is all right. Toxicity tests of cosmetics on animals violates their rights, but important medical research—cancer research, for example—does not. The clubbing of baby seals is abhorrent, but not the harvesting of adult seals. I used to think I understood this reasoning. Not any more. You don't change unjust institutions by tidying them up.

What's wrong—fundamentally wrong—with the way animals are treated isn't the details that vary from case to case. It's the whole system. The forlornness of the veal calf is pathetic, heart wrenching; the pulsing pain of the chimp with electrodes planted deep in her brain is repulsive; the slow, tortuous death of the raccoon caught in the leg-hold trap is agonizing. But what is wrong isn't the pain, isn't the suffering, isn't the deprivation. These compound what's wrong. Sometimes—often—they make it much, much worse. But they are not the fundamental wrong.

The fundamental wrong is the system that allows us to view animals as *our resources*, here for *us*—to be eaten, or surgically manipulated, or exploited for sport or money. Once we accept this view of animals—as our resources—the rest is as predictable as it is regrettable. Why worry about their loneliness, their pain, their death? Since animals exist for us, to benefit us in one way or another, what harms them really doesn't matter—or matters only if it starts to bother us, makes us feel a trifle uneasy when we eat our veal escalope, for example. So, yes, let us get veal calves out of solitary confinement, give them more space, a little straw, a few companions. But let us keep our veal escalope.

But a little straw, more space and a few companions won't eliminate—won't even touch—the basic wrong that attaches to our viewing and treating these animals as our resources. A veal calf killed to be eaten after living in close confinement is viewed and treated in this way: but so, too, is another who is raised (as they say) 'more humanely'. To right the wrong of our treatment of farm animals requires more than making rearing methods 'more humane'; it requires the total dissolution of commercial animal agriculture.

How we do this, whether we do it or, as in the case of animals in science, whether and how we abolish their use—these are to a large extent political questions. People must change their beliefs before they change their habits. Enough people, especially those elected to public office, must believe in change—must want it—before we will have laws that protect the rights of animals. This process of change is very complicated, very demanding, very exhausting, calling for the efforts of many hands in education, publicity, political organization and activity, down to the licking of envelopes and stamps. As a trained and practising philosopher, the sort of contribution I can make is limited but, I like to think, important. The currency of philosophy is ideas—their meaning and rational foundation—not the nuts and bolts of the legislative process, say, or the mechanics of community organization. That's what I have been exploring over the past ten years or so in my essays and talks and, most recently, in my book, *The Case for Animal Rights*. I believe the major conclusions I reach in the book are true because they are supported by the weight of the best arguments. I believe the idea of animal rights has reason, not just emotion, on its side.

In the space I have at my disposal here I can only sketch, in the barest outline, some of the main features of the book. It's main themes—and we should not be surprised by this—involve asking and answering deep, foundational moral questions about what morality is, how it should be understood and what is the best moral theory, all considered. I hope I can convey something of the shape I think this theory takes. The attempt to do this will be (to use a word a friendly critic once used to describe my work) cerebral, perhaps too cerebral. But this is misleading. My feelings about how animals are sometimes treated run just as deep and just as strong as those of my more volatile compatriots. Philosophers do—to use the jargon of the day—have a right side to their brains. If it's the left side we contribute (or mainly should), that's because what talents we have reside there.

How to proceed? We begin by asking how the moral status of animals has been understood by thinkers who deny that animals have rights. Then we test the mettle of their ideas by seeing how well they stand up under the heat of fair criticism. If we start our thinking in this way, we soon find that some people believe that we have no duties directly to animals, that we owe nothing to them, that we can do nothing that wrongs them. Rather, we can do wrong acts that involve animals, and so we have duties regarding them, though none to them. Such views may be called indirect duty views. By way of illustration: suppose your neighbour kicks your dog. Then your neighbour has done something wrong. But not to your dog. The wrong that has been done is a wrong to you. After all, it is wrong to upset people, and your neighbour's kicking your dog upsets you. So you are the one who is wronged, not your dog. Or again: by kicking your dog your neighbour damages your property. And since it is wrong to damage another person's property, your neighbour has done something wrong—to you, of course, not to your dog. Your neighbour no more wrongs your dog than your car would

be wronged if the windshield were smashed. Your neighbour's duties involving your dog are indirect duties to you. More generally, all of our duties regarding animals are indirect duties to one another—to humanity.

How could someone try to justify such a view? Someone might say that your dog doesn't feel anything and so isn't hurt by your neighbour's kick, doesn't care about the pain since none is felt, is as unaware of anything as is your windshield. Someone might say this, but no rational person will, since, among other considerations, such a view will commit anyone who holds it to the position that no human being feels pain either—that human beings also don't care about what happens to them. A second possibility is that though both humans and your dog are hurt when kicked, it is only human pain that matters. But, again, no rational person can believe this. Pain is pain wherever it occurs. If your neighbour's causing you pain is wrong because of the pain that is caused, we cannot rationally ignore or dismiss the moral relevance of the pain that your dog feels.

Philosophers who hold indirect duty views—and many still do—have come to understand that they must avoid the two defects just noted: that is, both the view that animals don't feel anything as well as the idea that only human pain can be morally relevant. Among such thinkers the sort of view now favoured is one or other form of what is called *contractarianism*.

Here, very crudely, is the root idea: morality consists of a set of rules that individuals voluntarily agree to abide by, as we do when we sign a contract (hence the name contractrarianism). Those who understand and accept the terms of the contract are covered directly; they have rights created and recognized by, and protected in, the contract. And these contractors can also have protection spelled out for others who, though they lack the ability to understand morality and so cannot sign the contract themselves, are loved or cherished by those who can. Thus young children, for example, are unable to sign contracts and lack rights. But they are protected by the contract none the less because of the sentimental interests of others, most notably their parents. So we have, then, duties involving these children, duties regarding them, but no duties to them. Our duties in their case are indirect duties to other human beings, usually their parents.

As for animals, since they cannot understand contracts, they obviously cannot sign; and since they cannot sign, they have no rights. Like children, however, some animals are the objects of the sentimental interest of others. You, for example, love your dog or cat. So those animals that enough people care about (companion animals, whales, baby seals, the American bald eagle), though they lack rights themselves, will be protected because of the sentimental interests of people. I have, then, according to contractarianism, no duty directly to your dog or any other animal, not even the duty not to cause them pain or suffering; my duty not to hurt them is a duty I have to those people who care about what happens to them. As for other animals, where no or little sentimental interest is present—in the case of farm animals, for example, or laboratory rats—what duties we have grow weaker and weaker, perhaps to vanishing point. The pain and death they endure, though real, are not wrong if no one cares about them.

When it comes to the moral status of animals' contractarianism could be a hard view to refute if it were an adequate theoretical approach to the moral status of human beings. It is not adequate in this latter respect, however, which makes the question of its adequacy in the former case, regarding animals, utterly moot. For consider: morality, according to the (crude) contractarian position before us, consists of rules that people agree to abide by. What people? Well, enough to make a difference—enough, that is, *collectively* to have the power to enforce the rules that are drawn up in the contract. That is very well and good for the signatories but not so good for anyone who is not asked to sign. And there is nothing in contractarianism of the sort we are discussing that guarantees or requires that everyone will have a chance to participate equally in framing the rules of morality. The result is that this approach to ethics could sanction the most blatant forms of social, economic, moral and political injustice, ranging from a repressive caste system to systematic racial or sexual discrimination. Might, according to this theory, does make right. Let those who are the victims of injustice suffer as they

will. It matters not so long as no one else—no contractor, or too few of them—cares about it. Such a theory takes one's moral breath away . . . as if, for example, there would be nothing wrong with apartheid in South Africa if few white South Africans were upset by it. A theory with so little to recommend it at the level of the ethics of our treatment of our fellow humans cannot have anything more to recommend it when it comes to the ethics of how we treat our fellow animals.

The version of contractarianism just examined is, as I have noted, a crude variety, and in fairness to those of a contractarian persuasion it must be noted that much more refined, subtle and ingenious varieties are possible. For example, John Rawls, in his *A Theory of Justice*, sets forth a version of contractarianism that forces contractors to ignore the accidental features of being a human being—for example, whether one is whiter or black, male or female, a genius or of modest intellect. Only by ignoring such features, Rawls believes, can we ensure that the principles of justice that contractors would agree upon are not based on bias or prejudice. Despite the improvement a view such as Rawls's represents over the cruder forms of contractarianism, it remains deficient: it systematically denies that we have direct duties to those human beings who do not have a sense of justice—young children, for instance, and many mentally retarded humans. And yet it seems reasonably certain that, were we to torture a young child or a retarded elder, we would be doing something that wronged him or her, not something that would be wrong if (and only if) other humans with a sense of justice were upset. And since this is true in the case of these humans, we cannot rationally deny the same in the case of animals.

Indirect duty views, then, including the best among them, fail to command our rational assent. Whatever ethical theory we should accept rationally, therefore, it must at least recognize that we have some duties directly to animals, just as we have some duties directly to each other. The next two theories I'll sketch attempt to meet this requirement.

The first I call the cruelty-kindness view. Simply stated, this says that we have a direct duty to be kind to animals and a direct duty not to be cruel to them.

Despite the familiar, reassuring ring of these ideas, I do not believe that this view offers an adequate theory. To make this clearer, consider kindness. A kind person acts from a certain kind of motive—compassion or concern, for example. And that is a virtue. But there is no guarantee that a kind act is a right act. If I am a generous racist, for example, I will be inclined to act kindly towards members of my own race, favouring their interests above those of others. My kindness would be real and, so far as it goes, good. But I trust it is too obvious to require argument that my kind acts may not be above moral reproach—may, in fact, be positively wrong because rooted in injustice. So kindness, notwithstanding its status as a virtue to be encouraged, simply will not carry the weight of a theory of right action.

Cruelty fares no better. People or their acts are cruel if they display either a lack of sympathy for or, worse, the presence of enjoyment in another's suffering. Cruelty in all its guises is a bad thing, a tragic human failing. But just as a person's being motivated by kindness does not guarantee that he or she does what is right, so the absence of cruelty does not ensure that he or she avoids doing what is wrong. Many people who perform abortions, for example, are not cruel, sadistic people. But that fact alone does not settle the terribly difficult question of the morality of abortion. The case is no different when we examine the ethics of our treatment of animals. So, yes, let us be for kindness and against cruelty. But let us not suppose that being for the one and against the other answers questions about moral right and wrong.

Some people think that the theory we are looking for is utilitarianism. A utilitarian accepts two moral principles. The first is that of equality: everyone's interests count, and similar interests must be counted as having similar weight or importance. White or black, American or Iranian, human or animal—everyone's pain or frustration matter, and matter just as much as the equivalent accepts is that of utility: do the act that will bring about the best balance between satisfaction and frustration for everyone affected by the outcome.

As a utilitarian, then, here is how I am to approach the task of deciding what I morally ought to do: I must ask who will be affected if I choose to do one thing rather than another, how much each individual will be affected, and where the best results are most likely to lie—which option, in other words, is most likely to bring about the best results, the best balance between satisfaction and frustration. That option, whatever it may be, is the one I ought to choose. That is where my moral duty lies.

The great appeal of utilitarianism rests with its uncompromising *egalitarianism:* everyone's interests count and count as much as the like interests of everyone else. The kind of odious discrimination that some forms of contractarianism can justify—discrimination based on race or sex, for example—seems disallowed in principle by utilitarianism, as is speciesism, systematic discrimination based on species membership.

The equality we find in utilitarianism, however, is not the sort an advocate of animal or human rights should have in mind. Utilitarianism has no room for the equal moral rights of different individuals because it has no room for their equal inherent value or worth. What has value for the utilitarian is the satisfaction of an individual's interests, not the individual whose interests they are. A universe in which you satisfy your desire for water, food and warmth is, other things being equal, better than a universe in which these desires are frustrated. And the same is true in the case of an animal with similar desires. But neither you nor the animal have any value in your own right. Only your feelings do.

Here is an analogy to help make the philosophical point clearer: a cup contains different liquids, sometimes sweet, sometimes bitter, sometimes a mix of the two. What has value are the liquids: the sweeter the better, the bitterer the worse. The cup, the container, has no value. It is what goes into it, not what they go into, that has value. For the utilitarian you and I are like the cup; we have no value as individuals and thus no equal value. What has value is what goes into us, what we serve as receptacles for; our feelings of satisfaction have positive value, our feelings of frustration negative value.

Serious problems arise for utilitarianism when we remind ourselves that it enjoins us to bring about the best consequences. What does this mean? It doesn't mean the best consequences for me alone, or for my family or friends, or any other person taken individually. No, what we must do is, roughly, as follows: we must add up (somehow!) the separate satisfactions and frustrations of everyone likely to be affected by our choice, the satisfactions in one column, the frustrations in the other. We must total each column for each of the options before us. That is what it means to say the theory is aggregative. And then we must choose that option which is most likely to bring about the best balance of totalled satisfactions over totalled frustrations. Whatever act would lead to this outcome is the one we ought morally to perform—it is where our moral duty lies. And that act quite clearly might not be the same one that would bring about the best results for me personally, or for my family or friends, or for a lab animal. The best aggregated consequences for everyone concerned are not necessarily the best for each individual.

That utilitarianism is an aggregative theory—different individuals' satisfactions or frustrations are added, or summed, or totalled—is the key objection to their theory. My Aunt Bea is old, inactive, a cranky, sour person, though not physically ill. She prefers to go on living. She is also rather rich. I could make a fortune if I could get my hands on her money, money she intends to give me in any event, after she dies, but which she refuses to give me now. In order to avoid a huge tax bite, I plan to donate a handsome sum of my profits to a local children's hospital. Many, many children will benefit from my generosity, and much joy will be brought to their parents, relatives and friends. If I don't get the money rather soon, all these ambitions will come to naught. The once-in-a-lifetime opportunity to make a real killing will be gone. Why, then, not kill my Aunt Bea? Oh, of course I *might* get caught. But I'm no fool and besides, her doctor can be counted on to co-operate (he has an eye for the same investment and I happen to know a good deal about his shady past). The deed can be done . . . professionally, shall we say. There is *very* little chance of getting caught. And as for my conscience being guilt-ridden, I am a resourceful sort of fellow and will take more than sufficient comfort—as I lie on the beach at Acapulco—in contemplating the joy and health I have brought to so many others.

Suppose Aunt Bea is killed and the rest of the story comes out as told. Would I have done anything wrong? Anything immoral? One would have thought that I had. Not according to utilitarianism. Since what I have done has brought about the best balance between totalled satisfaction and frustration for all those affected by the outcome, my action is not wrong. Indeed, in killing Aunt Bea the physician and I did what duty required.

This same kind of argument can be repeated in all sorts of cases, illustrating, time after time, how the utilitarian's position leads to results that impartial people find morally callous. It *is* wrong to kill my Aunt Bea in the name of bringing about the best results for others. A good end does not justify an evil means. Any adequate moral theory will have to explain why this is so. Utilitarianism fails in this respect and so cannot be the theory we seek.

What to do? Where to begin anew? The place to begin, I think, is with the utilitarian's view of the value of the individual—or, rather, lack of value. In its place, suppose we consider that you and I, for example, do have value as individuals—what we'll call *inherent value*. To say we have such value is to say that we are something more than, something different from, mere receptacles. Moreover, to ensure that we do not pave the way for such injustices as slavery or sexual discrimination, we must believe that all who have inherent value have it equally, regardless of their sex, race, religion, birthplace and so on. Similarly to be discarded as irrelevant are one's talents or skills, intelligence and wealth, personality or pathology, whether one is loved and admired or despised and loathed. The genius and the retarded child, the prince and the pauper, the brain surgeon and the fruit vendor, Mother Teresa and the most unscrupulous used-car salesman—all have inherent value, all possess it equally, and all have an equal right to be treated with respect, to be treated in ways that do not reduce them to the status of things, as if they existed as resources for others. My value as an individual is independent of my usefulness to you. Yours is not dependent on your usefulness to me. For either of us to treat the other in ways that fail to show respect for the other's independent value is to act immorally, to violate the individual's rights.

Some of the rational virtues of this view—what I call the rights view—should be evident. Unlike (crude) contractarianism, for example, the rights view *in principle* denies the moral tolerability of any and all forms of racial, sexual or social discrimination; and unlike utilitarianism, this view *in principle* denies that we can justify good results by using evil means that violate an individual's rights—denies, for example, that it could be moral to kill my Aunt Bea to harvest beneficial consequences for others. That would be to sanction the disrespectful treatment of the individual in the name of the social good, something the rights view will not—categorically will not—ever allow.

The rights view, I believe, is rationally the most satisfactory moral theory. It surpasses all other theories in the degree to which it illuminates and explains the foundation of our duties to one another—the domain of human morality. On this score it has the best reasons, the best arguments, on its side. Of course, if it were possible to show that only human beings are included within its scope, then a person like myself, who believes in animal rights, would be obliged to look elsewhere.

But attempts to limit its scope to humans only can be shown to be rationally defective. Animals, it is true, lack many of the abilities humans possess. They can't read, do higher mathematics, build a bookcase or make *baba ghanoush*. Neither can many human beings, however, and yet we don't (and shouldn't) say that they (these humans) therefore have less inherent value, less of a right to be treated with respect, than do others. It is the *similarities* between those human beings who most clearly, most non-controversially have such value (the people reading this, for example), not our differences, that matter most. And the really crucial, the basic similarity is simply this: we are each of us the experiencing subject of a life, a conscious creature having an individual welfare that has importance to us whatever our usefulness to others. We want and prefer things, believe and feel things, recall and expect things. And all these dimensions of our life, including our pleasure and pain, our enjoyment and suffering, our satisfaction and frustration, our continued existence or our untimely death—all make a difference to the quality of our life as lived, as

experienced, by us as individuals. As the same is true of those animals that concern us (the ones that are eaten and trapped, for example), they too must be viewed as the experiencing subjects of a life, with inherent value of their own.

Some there are who resist the idea that animals have inherent value. 'Only humans have such value,' they profess. How might this narrow view be defended? Shall we say that only humans have the requisite intelligence, or autonomy, or reason? But there are many, many humans who fail to meet these standards and yet are reasonably viewed as having value above and beyond their usefulness to others. Shall we claim that only humans belong to the right species, the species *Homo sapiens*? But this is blatant speciesism. Will it be said, then, that all—and only—humans have immortal souls? Then our opponents have their work cut out for them. I am myself not ill-disposed to the proposition that there are immortal souls. Personally, I profoundly hope I have one. But I would not want to rest my position on a controversial ethical issue on the even more controversial question about who or what has an immortal soul. That is to dig one's hole deeper, not to climb out. Rationally, it is better to resolve moral issues without making more controversial assumptions than are needed. The question of who has inherent value is such a question, one that is resolved more rationally without the introduction of the idea of immortal souls than by its use.

Well, perhaps some will say that animals have some inherent value, only less than we have. Once again, however, attempts to defend this view can be shown to lack rational justification. What could be the basis of our having more inherent value than animals? Their lack of reason, or autonomy, or intellect? Only if we are willing to make the same judgement in the case of humans who are similarly deficient. But it is not true that such humans—the retarded child, for example, or the mentally deranged—have less inherent value than you or I. Neither, then, can we rationally sustain the view that animals like them in being the experiencing subjects of a life have less inherent value. *All* who have inherent value have it *equally*, whether they be human animals or not.

Inherent value, then, belongs equally to those who are the experiencing subjects of a life. Whether it belongs to others—to rocks and rivers, trees and glaciers, for example—we do not know and may never know. But neither do we need to know, if we are to make the case for animal rights. We do not need to know, for example, how many people are eligible to vote in the next presidential election before we can know whether I am. Similarly, we do not need to know how many individuals have inherent value before we can know that some do. When it comes to the case for animal rights, then, what we need to know is whether the animals that, in our culture, are routinely eaten, hunted and used in our laboratories, for example, are like us in being subjects of a life. And we do know this. We do know that many—literally, billions and billions—of these animals are the subjects of a life in the sense explained and so have inherent value if we do. And since, in order to arrive at the best theory of our duties to one another, we must recognize our equal inherent value as individuals, reason—not sentiment, not emotion—reason compels us to recognize the equal inherent value of these animals and, with this, their equal right to be treated with respect.

That, *very* roughly, is the shape and feel of the case for animal rights. Most of the details of the supporting argument are missing. They are to be found in the book to which I alluded earlier. Here, the details go begging, and I must, in closing, limit myself to four final points.

The first is how the theory that underlies the case for animal rights shows that the animal rights movement is a part of, not antagonistic to, the human rights movement. The theory that rationally grounds the rights of animals also grounds the rights of humans. Thus those involved in the animal rights movement are partners in the struggle to secure respect for human rights—the rights of women, for example, or minorities, or workers. The animal rights movement is cut from the same moral cloth as these.

Second, having set out the broad outlines of the rights view, I can now say why its implications for farming and science, among other fields, are both clear and uncompromising. In the case of the use of animals in science, the rights view is categorically abolitionist. Lab animals are not our tasters; we are not their kings. Because these animals are treated routinely, systematically as if their value were reducible to their usefulness to others, they are routinely, systematically treated with a lack of respect, and thus are their rights routinely, systematically violated. This is just as true when they are used in trivial, duplicative, unnecessary or unwise research as it is when they are used in studies that hold out real promise of human benefits. We can't justify harming or killing a human being (my Aunt Bea, for example) just for these sorts of reason. Neither can we do so even in the case of so lowly a creature as a laboratory rat. It is not just refinement or reduction that is called for, not just larger, cleaner cages, not just more generous use of anaesthetic or the elimination of multiple surgery, not just tidying up the system. It is complete replacement. The best we can do when it comes to using animals in science is—not to use them. That is where our duty lies, according to the rights view.

As for commercial animal agriculture, the rights view takes a similar abolitionist position. The fundamental moral wrong here is not that animals are kept in stressful close confinement or in isolation, or that their pain and suffering, their needs and preferences are ignored or discounted. All these *are* wrong, of course, but they are not fundamentally wrong. They are symptoms and effects of the deeper, systematic wrong that allows these animals to be viewed and treated as lacking independent value, as resources for us—as, indeed, a renewable resource. Giving farm animals more space, more natural environments, more companions does not right the fundamental wrong, any more than giving lab animals more anaesthesia or bigger, cleaner cages would right the fundamental wrong in their case. Nothing less than the total dissolution of commercial animal agriculture will do this, just as, for similar reasons I won't develop at length here, morality requires nothing less than the total elimination of hunting and trapping for commercial and sporting ends. The rights view's implications, then, as I have said, are clear and uncompromising.

My last two points are about philosophy, my profession. It is, most obviously, no substitute for political action. The words I have written here and in other places by themselves don't change a thing. It is what we do with the thoughts that the words express—our acts, our deeds—that changes things. All that philosophy can do, and all I have attempted, is to offer a vision of what our deeds should aim at. And the why. But not the how.

Finally, I am reminded of my thoughtful critic, the one I mentioned earlier, who chastised me for being too cerebral. Well, cerebral I have been: indirect duty views, utilitarianism, contractarianism—hardly the stuff deep passions are made of. I am also reminded, however, of the image another friend once set before me—the image of the ballerina as expressive of disciplined passion. Long hours of sweat and toil, of loneliness and practice, of doubt and fatigue: those are the discipline of her craft. But the passion is there too, the fierce drive to excel, to speak through her body, to do it right, to pierce our minds. That is

the image of philosophy I would leave with you, not 'too cerebral' but *disciplined passion*. Of the discipline enough has been seen. As for the passion: there are times, and these not infrequent, when tears come to my eyes when I see, or read, or hear of the wretched plight of animals in the hands of humans. Their pain, their suffering, their loneliness, their innocence, their death. Anger. Rage. Pity. Sorrow. Disgust. The whole creation groans under the weight of the evil we humans visit upon these mute, powerless creatures. It *is* our hearts, not just our heads, that call for an end to it all, that demand of us that we overcome, for them, the habits and forces behind their systematic oppression. All great movements, it is written, go through three stages: ridicule, discussion, adoption. It is the realization of this third stage, adoption, that requires both our passion and our discipline, our hearts and our heads. The fate of animals is in our hands. God grant we are equal to the task.

Difficulties with the Strong Animal Rights Position

Mary Anne Warren

Tom Regan has produced what is perhaps the definitive defense of the view that the basic moral rights of at least some non-human animals are in no way inferior to our own. In *The Case for Animal Rights*, he argues that all normal mammals over a year of age have the same basic moral rights.[1] Non-human mammals have essentially the same right not to be harmed or killed as we do. I shall call this "the strong animal rights position," although it is weaker than the claims made by some animal liberationists in that it ascribes rights to only some sentient animals.

Mary Anne Warren, "A Critique of Regan's Animal Rights Theory," *Between the Species* Vol. 2, No. 4 (Fall 1987): 433–441. Reprinted with permission from Between the Species.

I will argue that Regan's case for the strong animal rights position is unpersuasive and that this position entails consequences which a reasonable person cannot accept. I do not deny that some non-human animals have moral rights; indeed, I would extend the scope of the rights claim to include all sentient animals, that is, all those capable of having experiences, including experiences of pleasure or satisfaction and pain, suffering, or frustration.[2] However, I do not think that the moral rights of most non-human animals are identical in strength to those of persons.[3] The rights of most non-human animals may be overridden in circumstances which would not justify overriding the rights of persons. There are, for instance, compelling realities which sometimes require that we kill animals for reasons which could not justify the killing of persons. I will call this view "the weak animal rights" position, even though it ascribes rights to a wider range of animals than does the strong animal rights position.

I will begin by summarizing Regan's case for the strong animal rights position and noting two problems with it. Next, I will explore some consequences of the strong animal rights position which I think are unacceptable. Finally, I will outline the case for the weak animal rights position.

REGAN'S CASE

Regan's argument moves through three stages. First, he argues that normal, mature mammals are not only sentient but have other mental capacities as well. These include the capacities for emotion, memory, belief, desire, the use of general concepts, intentional action, a sense of the future, and some degree of self-awareness. Creatures with such capacities are said to be subjects-of-a-life. They are not only alive in the biological sense but have a psychological identity over time and an existence which can go better or worse for them. Thus, they can be harmed or benefited. These are plausible claims, and well defended. One of the strongest parts of the book is the rebuttal of philosophers, such as R. G. Frey, who object to the application of such mentalistic terms to creatures that do not use a human-style language. The second and third stages of the argument are more problematic.

In the second stage, Regan argues that subjects-of-a-life have inherent value. His concept of inherent value grows out of his opposition to utilitarianism. Utilitarian moral theory, he says, treats individuals as "mere receptacles" for morally significant value, in that harm to one individual may be justified by the production of a greater net benefit to other individuals. In opposition to this, he holds that subjects-of-a-life have a value independent of both the value they may place upon their lives or experiences and the value others may place upon them.

Inherent value, Regan argues, does not come in degrees. To hold that some individuals have more inherent value than others is to adopt a "perfectionist" theory, i.e., one which assigns different moral worth

to individuals according to how well they are thought to exemplify some virtue(s), such as intelligence or moral autonomy. Perfectionist theories have been used, at least since the time of Aristotle, to rationalize such injustices as slavery and male domination, as well as the unrestrained exploitation of animals. Regan argues that if we reject these injustices, then we must also reject perfectionism and conclude that all subjects-of-a-life have equal inherent value. Moral agents have no more inherent value than moral patients, i.e., subjects-of-a-life who are not morally responsible for their actions.

In the third phase of the argument, Regan uses the thesis of equal inherent value to derive strong moral rights for all subjects-of-a-life. This thesis underlies the Respect Principle, which forbids us to treat beings who have inherent value as mere receptacles, i.e., mere means to the production of the greatest overall good. This principle, in turn, underlies the Harm Principle, which says that we have a direct *prima facie* duty not to harm beings who have inherent value. Together, these principles give rise to moral rights. Rights are defined as valid claims, claims to certain goods and against certain beings, i.e., moral agents. Moral rights generate duties not only to refrain from inflicting harm upon beings with inherent value but also to come to their aid when they are threatened by other moral agents. Rights are not absolute but may be overridden in certain circumstances. Just what these circumstances are we will consider later. But first, let's look at some difficulties in the theory as thus far presented.

THE MYSTERY OF INHERENT VALUE

Inherent value is a key concept in Regan's theory. It is the bridge between the plausible claim that all normal, mature mammals—human or otherwise—are subjects-of-a-life and the more debatable claim that they all have basic moral rights of the same strength. But it is a highly obscure concept, and its obscurity makes it ill-suited to play this crucial role.

Inherent value is defined almost entirely in negative terms. It is not dependent upon the value which either the inherently valuable individual or anyone else may place upon that individual's life or experiences. It is not (necessarily) a function of sentience or any other mental capacity, because, Regan says, some entities which are not sentient (e.g., trees, rivers, or rocks) may, nevertheless, have inherent value (p. 246). It cannot attach to anything other than an individual; species, eco-systems, and the like cannot have inherent value.

These are some of the things which inherent value is not. But what is it? Unfortunately, we are not told. Inherent value appears as a mysterious non-natural property which we must take on faith. Regan says that it is a *postulate* that subjects-of-a-life have inherent value, a postulate justified by the fact that it avoids certain absurdities which he thinks follow from a purely utilitarian theory (p. 247). But why is the postulate that *subjects-of-a-life* have inherent value? If the inherent value of a being is completely independent of the value that it or anyone else places upon its experiences, then why does the fact that it has certain sorts of experiences constitute evidence that it has inherent value? If the reason is that subjects-of-a-life have an existence which can go better or worse for them, then why isn't the appropriate conclusion that all sentient beings have inherent value, since they would all seem to meet that condition? Sentient but mentally unsophisticated beings may have a less extensive range of possible satisfactions and frustrations, but why should it follow that they have—or may have—no inherent value at all?

In the absence of a positive account of inherent value, it is also difficult to grasp the connection between being inherently valuable and having moral rights. Intuitively, it seems that value is one thing, and rights are another. It does not seem incoherent to say that some things (e.g., mountains, rivers, redwood trees) are inherently valuable and yet are not the sorts of things which can have moral rights. Nor does it seem incoherent to ascribe inherent value to some things which are not individuals, e.g., plant or animal species, though it may well be incoherent to ascribe moral rights to such things.

In short, the concept of inherent value seems to create at least as many problems as it solves. If inherent value is based on some natural property, then why

not try to identify that property and explain its moral significance, without appealing to inherent value? And if it is not based on any natural property, then why should we believe in it? That it may enable us to avoid some of the problems faced by the utilitarian is not a sufficient reason, if it creates other problems which are just as serious.

IS THERE A SHARP LINE?

Perhaps the most serious problems are those that arise when we try to apply the strong animal rights position to animals other than normal, mature mammals. Regan's theory requires us to divide all living things into two categories: those which have the same inherent value and the same basic moral rights that we do, and those which have no inherent value and presumably no moral rights. But wherever we try to draw the line, such a sharp division is implausible.

It would surely be arbitrary to draw such a sharp line between normal, mature mammals and all other living things. Some birds (e.g., crows, magpies, parrots, mynahs) appear to be just as mentally sophisticated as most mammals and thus are equally strong candidates for inclusion under the subject-of-a-life criterion. Regan is not in fact advocating that we draw the line here. His claim is only that normal mature mammals are clear cases, while other cases are less clear. Yet, on his theory, there must be such a sharp line *somewhere*, since there are no degrees of inherent value. But why should we believe that there is a sharp line between creatures that are subjects-of-a-life and creatures that are not? Isn't it more likely that "subjecthood" comes in degrees, that some creatures have only a little self-awareness, and only a little capacity to anticipate the future, while some have a little more, and some a good deal more?

Should we, for instance, regard fish, amphibians, and reptiles as subjects-of-a-life? A simple yes-or-no answer seems inadequate. On the one hand, some of their behavior is difficult to explain without the assumption that they have sensations, beliefs, desires, emotions, and memories; on the other hand, they do not seem to exhibit very much self-awareness or very much conscious anticipation of future events. Do they have enough mental sophistication to count as subjects-of-a-life? Exactly how much is enough?

It is still more unclear what we should say about insects, spiders, octopi, and other invertebrate animals which have brains and sensory organs but whose minds (if they have minds) are even more alien to us than those of fish or reptiles. Such creatures are probably sentient. Some people doubt that they can feel pain, since they lack certain neurological structures which are crucial to the processing of pain impulses in vertebrate animals. But this argument is inconclusive, since their nervous systems might process pain in ways different from ours. When injured, they sometimes act as if they are in pain. On evolutionary grounds, it seems unlikely that highly mobile creatures with complex sensory systems would not have developed a capacity for pain (and pleasure), since such a capacity has obvious survival value. It must, however, be admitted that we do not *know* whether spiders can feel pain (or something very like it), let alone whether they have emotions, memories, beliefs, desires, self-awareness, or a sense of the future.

Even more mysterious are the mental capacities (if any) of mobile microfauna. The brisk and efficient way that paramecia move about in their incessant search for food *might* indicate some kind of sentience, in spite of their lack of eyes, ears, brains, and other organs associated with sentience in more complex organisms. It is conceivable—though not very probable—that they, too, are subjects-of-a-life.

The existence of a few unclear cases need not pose a serious problem for a moral theory, but in this case, the unclear cases constitute most of those with which an adequate theory of animal rights would need to deal. The subject-of-a-life criterion can provide us with little or no moral guidance in our interactions with the vast majority of animals. That might be acceptable if it could be supplemented with additional principles which would provide such guidance. However, the radical dualism of the theory precludes supplementing it in this way. We are forced to say that either a spider has the same right to life as you and I do, or it has no right to life whatever—and that only the gods know which of these alternatives is true.

Regan's suggestion for dealing with such unclear cases is to apply the "benefit of the doubt" principle. That is, when dealing with beings that may or may not be subjects-of-a-life, we should act as if they are. But if we try to apply this principle to the entire range of doubtful cases, we will find ourselves with moral obligations which we cannot possibly fulfill. In many climates, it is virtually impossible to live without swatting mosquitoes and exterminating cockroaches, and not all of us can afford to hire someone to sweep the path before we walk, in order to make sure that we do not step on ants. Thus, we are still faced with the daunting task of drawing a sharp line somewhere on the continuum of life forms—this time, a line demarcating the limits of the benefit of the doubt principle.

The weak animal rights theory provides a more plausible way of dealing with this range of cases, in that it allows the rights of animals of different kinds to vary in strength. . . .

WHY ARE ANIMAL RIGHTS WEAKER THAN HUMAN RIGHTS?

How can we justify regarding the rights of persons as generally stronger than those of sentient beings which are not persons? There are a plethora of bad justifications, based on religious premises or false or unprovable claims about the differences between human and non-human nature. But there is one difference which has a clear moral relevance: people are at least sometimes capable of being moved to action or inaction by the force of reasoned argument. Rationality rests upon other mental capacities, notably those which Regan cites as criteria for being a subject-of-a-life. We share these capacities with many other animals. But it is not just because we are subjects-of-a-life that we are both able and morally compelled to recognize one another as beings with equal basic moral rights. It is also because we are able to "listen to reason" in order to settle our conflicts and cooperate in shared projects. This capacity, unlike the others, may require something like a human language.

Why is rationality morally relevant? It does not make us "better" than other animals or more "perfect."

It does not even automatically make us more intelligent. (Bad reasoning reduces our effective intelligence rather than increasing it.) But it is morally relevant insofar as it provides greater possibilities for cooperation and for the nonviolent resolution of problems. It also makes us more dangerous than non-rational beings can ever be. Because we are potentially more dangerous and less predictable than wolves, we need an articulated system of morality to regulate our conduct. Any human morality, to be workable in the long run, must recognize the equal moral status of all persons, whether through the postulate of equal basic moral rights or in some other way. The recognition of the moral equality of other persons is the price we must each pay for their recognition of our moral equality. Without this mutual recognition of moral equality, human society can exist only in a state of chronic and bitter conflict. The war between the sexes will persist so long as there is sexism and male domination; racial conflict will never be eliminated so long as there are racist laws and practices. But to the extent that we achieve a mutual recognition of equality, we can hope to live together, perhaps as peacefully as wolves, achieving (in part) through explicit moral principles what they do not seem to need explicit moral principles to achieve.

Why not extend this recognition of moral equality to other creatures, even though they cannot do the same for us? The answer is that we cannot. Because we cannot reason with most non-human animals, we cannot always solve the problems which they may cause without harming them—although we are always obligated to try. We cannot negotiate a treaty with the feral cats and foxes, requiring them to stop preying on endangered native species in return for suitable concessions on our part.

> if rats invade our houses . . . we cannot reason with them, hoping to persuade them of the injustice they do us. We can only attempt to get rid of them.[4]

Aristotle was not wrong in claiming that the capacity to alter one's behavior on the basis of reasoned argument is relevant to the full moral status which he accorded to free men. Of course, he was wrong in his other premise, that women and slaves by their nature cannot reason well enough to function as autonomous moral agents. Had that premise been true, so would his conclusion that women and slaves are not quite the moral equals of free men. In the case of most non-human animals, the corresponding premise is true. If, on the other hand, there are animals with whom we can (learn to) reason, then we are obligated to do this and to regard them as our moral equals.

Thus, to distinguish between the rights of persons and those of most other animals on the grounds that only people can alter their behavior on the basis of reasoned argument does not commit us to a perfectionist theory of the sort Aristotle endorsed. There is no excuse for refusing to recognize the moral equality of some people on the grounds that we don't regard them as quite as rational as we are, since it is perfectly clear that most people can reason well enough to determine how to act so as to respect the basic rights of others (if they choose to), and that is enough for moral equality.

But what about people who are clearly not rational? It is often argued that sophisticated mental capacities such as rationality cannot be essential for the possession of equal basic moral rights, since nearly everyone agrees that human infants and mentally incompetent persons have such rights, even though they may lack those sophisticated mental capacities. But this argument is inconclusive, because there are powerful practical and emotional reasons for protecting non-rational human beings, reasons which are absent in the case of most non-human animals. Infancy and mental incompetence are human conditions which all of us either have experienced or are likely to experience at some time. We also protect babies and mentally incompetent people because we care for them. We don't normally care for animals in the same way, and when we do—e.g., in the case of much-loved pets—we may regard them as having special rights by virtue of their relationship to us. We protect them not only for their sake but also for our own, lest we be hurt by harm done to them. Regan holds that such "side-effects" are irrelevant to moral rights, and perhaps they are. But in ordinary usage, there is no sharp line between moral rights and those moral protections which are not rights. The extension of strong moral protections to infants and the mentally impaired in no way proves that non-human animals have the same basic moral rights as people.

WHY SPEAK OF "ANIMAL RIGHTS" AT ALL?

If, as I have argued, reality precludes our treating all animals as our moral equals, then why should we still ascribe rights to them? Everyone agrees that animals are entitled to some protection against human abuse, but why speak of animal *rights* if we are not prepared to accept most animals as our moral equals? The weak animal rights position may seem an unstable compromise between the bold claim that animals have the same basic moral rights that we do and the more common view that animals have no rights at all.

It is probably impossible to either prove or disprove the thesis that animals have moral rights by producing an analysis of the concept of a moral right and checking to see if some or all animals satisfy the conditions for having rights. The concept of a moral right is complex, and it is not clear which of its strands are essential. Paradigm rights holders, i.e., mature and mentally competent persons, are *both* rational and morally autonomous beings and sentient subjects-of-a-life. Opponents of animal rights claim that rationality and moral autonomy are essential for the possession of rights, while defenders of animal rights claim that they are not. The ordinary concept of a moral right is probably not precise enough to enable us to determine who is right on purely definitional grounds.

If logical analysis will not answer the question of whether animals have moral rights, practical considerations may, nevertheless, incline us to say that they do. The most plausible alternative to the view that animals have moral rights is that, while they do not have *rights*, we are, nevertheless, obligated not to be cruel to them. Regan argues persuasively that the injunction to avoid being cruel to animals is inadequate to express our obligations towards animals, because it focuses on the mental states of those who cause animal suffering, rather than on the harm done to the animals themselves (p. 158). Cruelty is inflict-ing pain or suffering and either taking pleasure in that pain or suffering or being more or less indifferent to it. Thus, to express the demand for the decent treatment of animals in terms of the rejection of cruelty is to invite the too easy response that those who subject animals to suffering are not being cruel because they regret the suffering they cause but sincerely believe that what they do is justified. The injunction to avoid cruelty is also inadequate in that it does not preclude the killing of animals—for any reason, however trivial—so long as it is done relatively painlessly.

The inadequacy of the anti-cruelty view provides one practical reason for speaking of animal rights. Another practical reason is that this is an age in which nearly all significant moral claims tend to be expressed in terms of rights. Thus, the denial that animals have rights, however carefully qualified, is likely to be taken to mean that we may do whatever we like to them, provided that we do not violate any human rights. In such a context, speaking of the rights of animals may be the only way to persuade many people to take seriously protests against the abuse of animals.

Why not extend this line of argument and speak of the rights of trees, mountains, oceans, or anything else which we may wish to see protected from destruction? Some environmentalists have not hesitated to speak in this way, and, given the importance of protecting such elements of the natural world, they cannot be blamed for using this rhetorical device. But, I would argue that moral rights can meaningfully be ascribed only to entities which have some capacity for sentience. This is because moral rights are protections designed to protect rights holders from harms or to provide them with benefits which matter *to them*. Only beings capable of sentience can be harmed or benefited in ways which matter to them, for only such beings can like or dislike what happened to them or prefer some conditions to others. Thus, sentient animals, unlike mountains, rivers, or species, are at least logically possible candidates for moral rights. This fact, together with the need to end current abuses of animals—e.g., in scientific research . . . —provides a plausible case for speaking of animal rights.

CONCLUSION

I have argued that Regan's case for ascribing strong moral rights to all normal, mature mammals is unpersuasive because (1) it rests upon the obscure concept of inherent value, which is defined only in negative terms, and (2) it seems to preclude any plausible answer to questions about the moral status of the vast majority of sentient animals. . . .

The weak animal rights theory asserts that (1) any creature whose natural mode of life includes the pursuit of certain satisfactions has the right not to be forced to exist without the opportunity to pursue those satisfactions; (2) that any creature which is capable of pain, suffering, or frustration has the right that such experiences not be deliberately inflicted upon it without some compelling reason; and (3) that no sentient being should be killed without good reason. However, moral rights are not an all-or-nothing affair. The strength of the reasons required to override the rights of a non-human organism varies, depending upon—among other things—the probability that it is sentient and (if it is clearly sentient) its probable degree of mental sophistication.

NOTES

1. Tom Regan, *The Case for Animal Rights* (Berkeley: University of California Press, 1983). All page references are to this edition.

2. The capacity for sentience, like all of the mental capacities mentioned in what follows, is a disposition. Dispositions do not disappear whenever they are not currently manifested. Thus, sleeping or temporarily unconscious persons or non-human animals are still sentient in the relevant sense (i.e., still capable of sentience), so long as they still have the neurological mechanisms necessary for the occurrence of experiences.

3. It is possible, perhaps probable, that some non-human animals—such as cetaceans and anthropoid apes—should be regarded as persons. If so, then the weak animal rights position holds that these animals have the same basic moral rights as human persons.

4. Bonnie Steinbock, "Speciesism and the Idea of Equality," *Philosophy* 53 (1978): 253.

Speciesism and the Idea of Equality

Bonnie Steinbock

Most of us believe that we are entitled to treat members of other species in ways which would be considered wrong if inflicted on members of our own species. We kill them for food, keep them confined, use them in painful experiments. The moral philosopher has to ask what relevant difference justifies this difference in treatment. A look at this question will lead us to re-examine the distinctions which we have assumed make a moral difference.

Bonnie Steinbock, "Speciesism and the Idea of Eqality" in *Philosophy*, April 1978, vol. 53, no. 204, pp. 247–256. Reprinted with the permission of Cambridge University Press.

It has been suggested by Peter Singer[1] that our current attitudes are 'speciesist', a word intended to make one think of 'racist' or 'sexist'. The idea is that membership in a species is in itself not relevant to moral treatment, and that much of our behaviour and attitudes towards non-human animals is based simply on this irrelevant fact.

There is, however, an important difference between racism or sexism and 'speciesism'. We do not subject animals to different moral treatment simply because they have fur and feathers, but because they are in fact different from human beings in ways that could be morally relevant. It is false that women are incapable of being benefited by education, and therefore that claim cannot serve to justify preventing them from attending school. But this is not false of cows and dogs, even chimpanzees. Intelligence is thought to be a morally relevant capacity because of its relation to the capacity for moral responsibility.

What is Singer's response? He agrees that non-human animals lack certain capacities that human animals possess, and that this may justify different *treatment*. But it does not justify giving less consideration to their needs and interests. According to Singer, the moral mistake which the racist or sexist makes is not essentially the factual error of thinking that blacks or women are inferior to white men. For even if there were no factual error, even if it were true that blacks and women are less intelligent and responsible than whites and men, this would not justify giving less consideration to their needs and interests. It is important to note that the term 'speciesism' is in one way like, and in another way unlike, the terms 'racism' and 'sexism'. What the term 'speciesism' has in common with these terms is the reference to focusing on a characteristic which is, in itself, irrelevant to moral treatment. And it is worth reminding us of this. But Singer's real aim is to bring us to a new understanding of the idea of equality. The question is, on what do claims to equality rest? The demand for *human* equality is a demand that the interests of all human beings be considered equally, unless there is a moral justification for not doing so. But why should the interests of all human beings be considered equally? In order to answer this question, we have to give some sense to the phrase, 'All men (human beings) are created equal'. Human beings are manifestly *not* equal, differing greatly in intelligence, virtue and capacities. In virtue of what can the claim to equality be made?

It is Singer's contention that claims to equality do not rest on factual equality. Not only do human beings differ in their capacities, but it might even turn out that intelligence, the capacity for virtue, etc., are not distributed evenly among the races and sexes:

The appropriate response to those who claim to have found evidence of genetically based differences in ability between the races or sexes is not to stick to the belief that the genetic explanation must be wrong, whatever evidence to the contrary may turn up; instead we should make it quite clear that the claim to equality does not depend on intelligence, moral capacity, physical strength, or similar matters of fact. Equality is a moral ideal, not a simple assertion of fact. There is no logically compelling reason for assuming that a factual difference in ability between two people justifies any difference in the amount of consideration we give to satisfying their needs and interests. The principle of equality of human beings is not a description of an alleged actual equality among humans: it is a prescription of how we should treat humans.[2]

In so far as the subject is human equality, Singer's view is supported by other philosophers. Bernard Williams, for example, is concerned to show that demands for equality cannot rest on factual equality among people, for no such equality exists.[3] The only respect in which all men are equal, according to Williams, is that they are all equally men. This seems to be a platitude, but Williams denies that it is trivial. Membership in the species *homo sapiens* in itself has no special moral significance, but rather the fact that all men are human serves as a *reminder* that being human involves the possession of characteristics that are morally relevant. But on what characteristics does Williams focus? Aside from the desire for self-respect (which I will discuss later), Williams is not concerned with uniquely human capacities. Rather, he focuses on the capacity to feel pain and the capacity to feel affection. It is in virtue of these capacities, it seems, that the idea of equality is to be justified.

Apparently Richard Wasserstrom has the same idea as he sets out the racist's 'logical and moral mistakes' in 'Rights, Human Rights and Racial Discrimination'.[4] The racist fails to acknowledge that the black person is as capable of suffering as the white person. According to Wasserstrom, the reason why a person is said to have a right not to be made to suffer acute physical pain is that we all do in fact value freedom from such pain. Therefore, if anyone has a right to be free from suffering acute physical pain, *everyone* has this right, for there is no possible basis of discrimination. Wasserstrom says, 'For, if all persons do have equal capacities of these sorts and if the existence of these capacities is the reason for ascribing these rights to anyone, then all persons ought to have the right to claim equality of treatment in respect to the possession and exercise of these rights'.[5] The basis of equality, for Wasserstrom as for Williams, lies not in some uniquely human capacity, but rather in the fact that all human beings are alike in their capacity to suffer. Writers on equality have focused on this capacity, I think, because it functions as some sort of lowest common denominator, so that whatever the other capacities of a human being, he is entitled to equal consideration because, like everyone else, he is capable of suffering.

If the capacity to suffer is the reason for ascribing a right to freedom from acute pain, or a right to well being, then it certainly looks as though these rights must be extended to animals as well. This is the conclusion Singer arrives at. The demand for human equality rests on the equal capacity of all human beings to suffer and to enjoy well being. But if this is the basis of the demand for equality, then this demand must include all beings which have an equal capacity to suffer and enjoy well being. That is why Singer places at the basis of the demand for equality, not intelligence or reason, but sentience. And equality will mean, not equality of treatment, but 'equal consideration of interests'. The equal consideration of interests will often mean quite different treatment, depending on the nature of the entity being considered. (It would be as absurd to talk of a dog's right to vote, Singer says, as to talk of a man's right to have an abortion.)

It might be thought that the issue of equality depends on a discussion of rights. According to this line of thought, animals do not merit equal consideration of interests because, unlike human beings, they do not, or cannot, have rights. But I am not going to discuss rights, important as the issue is. The fact that an entity does not have rights does not necessarily imply that its interests are going to count for less than the interests of entities which are right-bearers. According to the view of rights held by H. L. A. Hart

and S. I. Benn, infants do not have rights, nor do the mentally defective, nor do the insane, in so far as they all lack certain minimal conceptual capabilities for having rights.[6] Yet it certainly does not seem that either Hart or Benn would agree that *therefore* their interests are to be counted for less, or that it is morally permissible to treat them in ways in which it would not be permissible to treat right-bearers. It seems to mean only that we must give different sorts of reasons for our obligations to take into consideration the interests of those who do not have rights.

We have reasons concerning the treatment of other people which are clearly independent of the notion of rights. We would say that it is wrong to punch someone because doing that infringes his rights. But we could also say that it is wrong because doing that hurts him, and that is, ordinarily, enough of a reason not to do it. Now this particular reason extends not only to human beings, but to all sentient creatures. One has a *prima facie* reason not to pull the cat's tail (whether or not the cat has rights) because it hurts the cat. And this is the only thing, normally, which is relevant in this case. The fact that the cat is not a 'rational being', that it is not capable of moral responsibility, that it cannot make free choices or shape its life—all of these differences from us having nothing to do with the justifiability of pulling its tail. Does this show that rationality and the rest of it are irrelevant to moral treatment?

I hope to show that this is not the case. But first I want to point out that the issue is not one of cruelty to animals. We all agree that cruelty is wrong, whether perpetrated on a moral or non-moral, rational or non-rational agent. Cruelty is defined as the infliction of unnecessary pain or suffering. What is to count as necessary or unnecessary is determined, in part, by the nature of the end pursued. Torturing an animal is cruel, because although the pain is logically necessary for the action to be torture, the end (deriving enjoyment from seeing the animal suffer) is monstrous. Allowing animals to suffer from neglect or for the sake of large profits may also be thought to be unnecessary and therefore cruel. But there may be some ends, which are very good (such as the advancement of medical knowledge), which can be accomplished by subjecting animals to pain in experiments. Although most people would agree that the pain inflicted on animals used in medical research ought to be kept to a minimum, they would consider pain that cannot be eliminated 'necessary' and therefore not cruel. It would probably not be so regarded if the subjects were non-voluntary human beings. Necessity, then, is defined in terms of human benefit, but this is just what is being called into question. The topic of cruelty to animals, while important from a practical viewpoint, because much of our present treatment of animals involves the infliction of suffering for no good reason, is not very interesting philosophically. What is philosophically interesting is whether we are justified in having different standards of necessity for human suffering and for animal suffering.

Singer says, quite rightly I think, 'If a being suffers, there can be no moral justification for refusing to take that suffering into consideration'.[7] But he thinks that the principle of equality requires that, no matter what the nature of the being, its suffering be counted equally with the like suffering of any other being. In other words sentience does not simply provide us with reasons for acting; it is the *only* relevant consideration for equal consideration of interests. It is this view that I wish to challenge.

I want to challenge it partly because it has such counter-intuitive results. It means, for example, that feeding starving children before feeding starving dogs is just like a Catholic charity's feeding hungry Catholics before feeding hungry non-Catholics. It is simply a matter of taking care of one's own, something which is usually morally permissible. But whereas we would admire the Catholic agency which did not discriminate, but fed all children, first come, first served, we would feel quite differently about someone who had this policy for dogs and children. Nor is this, it seems to me, simply a matter of a sentimental preference for our own species. I might feel much more love for my dog than for a strange child—and yet I might feel morally obliged to feed the child

before I fed my dog. If I gave in to the feelings of love and fed my dog and let the child go hungry, I would probably feel guilty. This is not to say that we can simply rely on such feelings. Huck Finn felt guilty at helping Jim escape, which he viewed as stealing from a woman who had never done any harm. But while the existence of such feelings does not settle the morality of an issue, it is not clear to me that they can be explained away. In any event, their existence can serve as a motivation for trying to find a rational justification for considering human interests above non-human ones.

However, it does seem to me that this *requires* a justification. Until now, common sense (and academic philosophy) have seen no such need. Benn says, 'No one claims equal consideration for all mammals—human beings count, mice do not, though it would not be easy to say *why* not. . . . Although we hesitate to inflict unnecessary pain on sentient creatures, such as mice or dogs, we are quite sure that we do not need to show good reasons for putting human interests before theirs.'[8]

I think we do have to justify counting our interests more heavily than those of animals. But how? Singer is right, I think, to point out that it will not do to refer vaguely to the greater value of human life, to human worth and dignity:

> Faced with a situation in which they see a need for some basis for the moral gulf that is commonly thought to separate humans and animals, but can find no concrete difference that will do this without undermining the equality of humans, philosophers tend to waffle. They resort to high-sounding phrases like 'the intrinsic dignity of the human individual'. They talk of 'the intrinsic worth of all men' as if men had some worth that other beings do not have or they say that human beings, and only human beings, are 'ends in themselves', while 'everything other than a person can only have value for a person'. . . . Why should we not attribute 'intrinsic dignity' or 'intrinsic worth' to ourselves? Why should we not say that we are the only things in the universe that have intrinsic value? Our fellow human beings are unlikely to reject the accolades we so generously bestow upon them, and

those to whom we deny the honour are unable to object.[9]

Singer is right to be sceptical of terms like 'intrinsic dignity' and 'intrinsic worth'. These phrases are no substitute for a moral argument. But they may point to one. In trying to understand what is meant by these phrases, we may find a difference or differences between human beings and non-human animals that will justify different treatment while not undermining claims for human equality. While we are not compelled to discriminate among people because of different capacities, if we can find a significant difference in capacities between human and non-human animals, this could serve to justify regarding human interests as primary. It is not arbitrary or smug, I think, to maintain that human beings have a different moral status from members of other species because of certain capacities which are characteristic of being human. We may not all be equal in these capacities, but all human beings possess them to some measure, and non-human animals do not. For example, human beings are normally held to be responsible for what they do. In recognizing that someone is responsible for his or her actions, you accord that person a respect which is reserved for those possessed of moral autonomy, or capable of achieving such autonomy. Secondly, human beings can be expected to reciprocate in a way that non-human animals cannot. Non-human animals cannot be motivated by altruistic or moral reasons; they cannot treat you fairly or unfairly. This does not rule out the possibility of an animal being motivated by sympathy or pity. It does rule out altruistic motivation in the sense of motivation due to the recognition that the needs and interests of others provide one with certain reasons for acting'.[10] Human beings are capable of altruistic motivation in this sense. We are sometimes motivated simply by the recognition that someone else is in pain, and that pain is a bad thing, no matter who suffers it. It is this sort of reason that I claim cannot motivate an animal or an entity not possessed of fairly abstract concepts. (If some non-human animals do possess the requisite concepts—perhaps chimpanzees who have learned a language—they might well be capable of altruistic motivation.) This means that our moral dealings with animals are necessarily much more limited than our dealings with other human beings. If rats invade our houses, carrying disease and biting our children, we cannot reason with them, hoping to persuade them of the injustice they do us. We can only attempt to get rid of them. And it is this that makes it reasonable for us to accord them a separate and not equal moral status, even though their capacity to suffer provides us with some reason to kill them painlessly, if this can be done without too much sacrifice of human interests. Thirdly, as Williams points out, there is the 'desire for self-respect': 'a certain human desire to be identified with what one is doing, to be able to realize purposes of one's own, and not to be the instrument of another's will unless one has willingly accepted such a role.[11] Some animals may have some form of this desire, and to the extent that they do, we ought to consider their interest in freedom and self-determination. (Such considerations might affect our attitudes toward zoos and circuses.) But the desire for self-respect *per se* requires the intellectual capacities of human beings, and this desire provides us with special reasons not to treat human beings in certain ways. It is an affront to the dignity of a human being to be a slave (even if a well-treated one); this cannot be true for a horse or a cow. To point this out is of course only to say that the justification for the treatment of an entity will depend on the sort of entity in question. In our treatment of other entities, we must consider the desire for autonomy, dignity and respect, but only where such a desire exists. Recognition of different desires and interests will often require different treatment, a point Singer himself makes.

But is the issue simply one of different desires and interests justifying and requiring different treatment? I would like to make a stronger claim, namely, that certain capacities, which seem to be unique to human beings, entitle their possessors to a privileged position in the moral community. Both rats and human beings dislike pain, and so we have a *prima facie* reason not to inflict pain on either. But if we can free human beings from crippling diseases, pain and death through experimentation which involves making animals suffer, and if this is the only way to achieve such results, then I think that such experimentation is justified because human lives are more valuable than animal lives. And this is because of certain capacities and abilities that normal human beings have which animals apparently do not, and which human beings cannot exercise if they are devastated by pain or disease.

My point is not that the lack of the sorts of capacities I have been discussing gives us a justification for treating animals just as we like, but rather that it is these differences between human beings and non-human animals which provide a rational basis for different moral treatment and consideration. Singer focuses on sentience alone as the basis of equality, but we can justify the belief that human beings have a moral worth that non-human animals do not, in virtue of specific capacities, and without resorting to 'high-sounding phrases'.

Singer thinks that intelligence, the capacity for moral responsibility, for virtue, etc., are irrelevant to equality, because we would not accept a hierarchy based on intelligence any more than one based on race. We do not think that those with greater capacities ought to have their interests weighed more heavily than those with lesser capacities, and this, he thinks, shows that differences in such capacities are irrelevant to equality. But it does not show this at all. Kevin Donaghy argues (rightly, I think) that what entitles us human beings to a privileged position in the moral community is a certain minimal level of intelligence, which is a prerequisite for morally relevant capacities.[12] The fact that we would reject a hierarchical society based on degree of intelligence does not show that a minimal level of intelligence cannot be used as a cut-off point, justifying giving greater consideration to the interests of those entities which meet this standard.

Interestingly enough, Singer concedes the rationality of valuing the lives of normal human beings over the lives of non-human animals.[13] We are not required to value equally the life of a normal human

being and the life of an animal, he thinks, but only their suffering. But I doubt that the value of an entity's life can be separated from the value of its suffering in this way. If we value the lives of human beings more than the lives of animals, this is because we value certain capacities that human beings have and animals do not. But freedom from suffering is, in general, a minimal condition for exercising these capacities, for living a fully human life. So, valuing human life more involves regarding human interests as counting for more. That is why we regard human suffering as more deplorable than comparable animal suffering.

But there is one point of Singer's which I have not yet met. Some human beings (if only a very few) are less intelligent than some non-human animals. Some have less capacity for moral choice and responsibility. What status in the moral community are these members of our species to occupy? Are their interests to be considered equally with ours? Is experimenting on them permissible where such experiments are painful or injurious, but somehow necessary for human well being? If it is certain of our capacities which entitle us to a privileged position, it looks as if those lacking those capacities are not entitled to a privileged position. To think it is justifiable to experiment on an adult chimpanzee but not on a severely mentally incapacitated human being seems to be focusing on membership in a species where that has no moral relevance. (It is being 'speciesist' in a perfectly reasonable use of the word.) How are we to meet this challenge?

Donaghy is untroubled by this objection. He says that it is fully in accord with his intuitions, that he regards the killing of a normally intelligent human being as far more serious than the killing of a person so severely limited that he lacked the intellectual capacities of an adult pig. But this parry really misses the point. The question is whether Donaghy thinks that the killing of a human being so severely limited that he lacked the intellectual capacities of an adult pig would be less serious than the killing of that pig. If superior intelligence is what justifies privileged status in the moral community, then the pig who is smarter than a human being ought to have superior moral status. And I doubt that this is fully in accord with Donaghy's intuitions.

I doubt that anyone will be able to come up with a concrete and morally relevant difference that would justify, say, using a chimpanzee in an experiment rather than a human being with less capacity of reasoning, moral responsibility, etc. Should we then experiment on the severely retarded? Utilitarian considerations aside (the difficulty of comparing intelligence between species, for example), we feel a special obligation to care for the handicapped members of our own species, who cannot survive in this world without such care. Non-human animals manage very well, despite their 'lower intelligence' and lesser capacities; most of them do not require special care from us. This does not, of course, justify experimenting on them. However, to subject to experimentation those people who depend on us seems even worse than subjecting members of other species to it. In addition, when we consider the severely retarded, we think, 'That could be me'. It makes sense to think that one might have been born retarded, but not to think that one might have been born a monkey. And so, although one can imagine oneself in the monkey's place, one feels a closer identification with the severely retarded human being. Here we are getting away from such things as 'morally relevant differences' and are talking about something much more difficult to articulate, namely, the role of feeling and sentiment in moral thinking. We would be *horrified* by the use of the retarded in medical research. But what are we to make of this horror? Has it moral significance or is it 'mere' sentiment, of no more import than the sentiment of whites against blacks? It is terribly difficult to know how to evaluate such feelings. I am not going to say more about this, because I think that the treatment of severely incapacitated human beings does not pose an insurmountable objection to the privileged status principle. I am willing to admit that my horror at the thought of experiments being performed on severely mentally incapacitated human beings in cases in which I would find it justifiable and preferable to perform the same experiments on non-

human animals (capable of similar suffering) may not be a moral emotion. But it is certainly not wrong of us to extend special care to members of our own species, motivated by feelings of sympathy, protectiveness, etc. If this is speciesism, it is stripped of its tone of moral condemnation. It is not racist to provide special care to members of your own race; it is racist to fall below your moral obligation to a person because of his or her race. I have been arguing that we are morally obliged to consider the interests of all sentient creatures, but not to consider those interests equally with human interests. Nevertheless, even this recognition will mean some radical changes in our attitude toward and treatment of other species.

NOTES

1. Peter Singer, *Animal Liberation* (A New York Review Book, 1975).

2. Singer, 5.

3. Bernard Williams, 'The Idea of Equality', *Philosophy, Politics and Society* (Second Series), Laslett and Runciman (eds.) (Blackwell, 1962), 110–131, reprinted in *Moral Concepts*, Feinberg (ed.) (Oxford, 1970), 153–171.

4. Richard Wasserstrom, 'Rights, Human Rights, and Racial Discrimination', *Journal of Philosophy* 61, No. 20 (1964), reprinted in *Human Rights*, A. I. Melden (ed.) (Wadsworth, 1970), 96–110.

5. Ibid., 106.

6. H. L. A. Hart, 'Are There Any Natural Rights?', *Philosophical Review* 64 (1955), and S. I. Benn, 'Abortion, Infanticide, and Respect for Persons', *The Problem of Abortion*, Feinberg (ed.) (Wadsworth, 1973), 92–104.

7. Singer, 9.

8. Benn, 'Equality, Moral and Social', *The Encyclopedia of Philosophy* 3, 40.

9. Singer, 266–267.

10. This conception of altruistic motivation comes from Thomas Nagel's *The Possibility of Altruism* (Oxford, 1970).

11. Williams, op. cit., 157.

12. Kevin Donaghy, 'Singer on Speciesism', *Philosophic Exchange* (Summer 1974).

13. Singer, 22.

CASES FOR ANALYSIS

1. Animal Testing

Protesters for and against animal testing have predicted an escalating conflict after the two sides clashed during weekend demonstrations in Oxford. Both groups pledged to step up campaigns which have already resulted in death threats aimed at advocates of animal testing and panic buttons installed at the home of a leading provivisection protester.

Pro-Test, the group which organised the Oxford rally of scientists, students and patients, plans a march in London which it hopes will draw 5,000 supporters. A spokesman for Speak, the animal rights group campaigning against a new animal research laboratory in Oxford, said the Pro-Test demonstration had left it "fired up" to take tougher action.

Spokesman Mel Broughton said: "They should be worried, not because they are in any danger of violence, but because they have fired us up even more against them and the university." . . .

Many researchers stayed away from the march, fearing reprisals against them and their families. Professor Tipu Aziz, a leading neurosurgeon, said: "This country has thousands of researchers paralysed by fear. That's a travesty of democracy." . . .

A spokesman for the Animal Liberation Front, Robin Webb, yesterday described the Pro-Test marchers as "irrelevant."

"The ALF supporters will completely ignore this protest group and will continue targeting institutions and companies which are directly involved in building the proposed facility," he said.

The Medical Research Council's chief executive, Colin Blakemore, described the Pro-Test demonstration as "immensely gratifying. For a long time, we have needed this kind of collective response. The people want this thuggery and nastiness off the streets of Oxford."*

Which side in this conflict do you sympathize with more? Why? Suppose you are a member of Pro-Test. How would you argue in favor of scientific animal testing? Say you are an ALF supporter. What arguments could you make for the banning of most (or all) animal testing? Is either side justified in using violence or the threat of violence to further its cause? Why or why not?

*Robert Booth, "Opposing Sides in Animal Testing Row Pledge to Step-Up Action," from *The Guardian*, February 27, 2006. Copyright © 2006 Guardian News and Media Ltd. Reprinted with permission.

2. Seal Hunting and the Fate of the Inuit

In the 1980s, postcards were distributed to 12 million United States and United Kingdom households depicting the infamous Canadian Atlantic fisher swinging a bat at a baby seal and eliciting an overwhelming emotional response. Major legislative bodies relented to public pressure with a staggering impact on wildlife management. The collapse of the sealskin market marked a victory for protesters who had waged the most effective, international mass media campaign ever undertaken.

The moral victory for animal rights activists not only hurt Newfoundlanders, it adversely affected thousands of Canadian Inuit living in tiny, remote, Arctic hamlets. Antifur protesters lump all seal-hunting methods together. It is tragic but not surprising that there has been virtually no media coverage of the devastating economic, social, and cultural impact of the collapse of the seal skin market on Inuit. If outsiders had known more about Inuit life, perhaps they would not have so easily dismissed all seal-hunting as unethical and cruel.

Canadian Inuit, who number about 46,000, are part of a circumpolar Inuit community numbering about 150,000 in Greenland, Alaska, and Russia. For Canadian Inuit, the seal is not just a source of cash through fur sales, but the keystone of their culture. Although Inuit harvest and hunt many species that inhabit the desert tundra and ice platforms, the seal is their mainstay. . . .

Inuit no longer use seal oil lamps or kudlik for heating, as did their grandparents. But seal meat, which is extremely high in protein, minerals, and vitamins and very low in fat, is still the most valued meat in many parts of the Arctic. Seal skin mittens and boots continue to provide the greatest protection against the harsh Arctic climate.

Like most people, Inuit respond to structural changes by adapting and innovating. They were already dependent on costly hunting supplies by the 1980s. When fur prices plummeted after the sealskin boycott, their credit and cash flow from furs dried up while the cost of supplies rose. Many families could no longer afford hunting equipment. Their fragile economy was imperiled and their vulnerability increased. Their social order was ruptured as they were deprived of the complex social aspect of sharing seal meat.

Their historical, legal, social, and economic situation already placed them at alarmingly higher risks of poverty and violence than other Canadians even when they live outside the North, as 10,000 Inuit have chosen to do. Life expectancy among the Inuit is 10 years lower than other Canadians. Rates of infant mortality, unemployment, illnesses such as diabetes, violence against women, and overcrowded housing are chillingly high.

One of the most brutal aspects of the lack of cultural continuity is the epidemic of youth suicide striking small communities in clusters where one death rapidly engenders another. But the Inuit, having endured myths and misinformation about their culture for decades, have carried on. . . .

The Inuit are resourceful people who deserve more respectful attention from outsiders.[†]

Provide reasons for your answers: Would a utilitarian like Peter Singer be likely to support a ban on all seal hunting even though it would devastate the Inuit? Would he be likely to approve of the Inuit's hunting if they could always kill the seals painlessly? Would a nonconsequentialist like Tom Regan disapprove of the hunting of the seals under all circumstances? If the fate of the Inuit and the seals was to be decided by either Singer or Regan, which philosopher do you think the Inuit would prefer?

[†]Kirt Ejesiak and Maureen Flynn-Burhoe, "Animal Rights vs. Inuit Rights," *The Boston Goble*, May 8, 2005. Reprinted by permission of the authors.

3. Snakes and Snake Charmers

Mumbai, India (*Daily News & Analysis*)—Every year around Nagpanchami, animal welfare activists play an interesting game of snakes and ladders with snake charmers in the city. The good news, say activists, is that the snakes finally seem to be winning. On Sunday, the Bombay Society for Prevention of Cruelty to Animals (BSPCA) rescued four snakes from Kurla and CST, said snake handler Sunil Ranade who works with the BSPCA.

Snake charmers use the reptiles to make money during the Hindu snake festival. "They earn up to Rs3,000 on Nagpanchami because people pay to watch cobras drink milk," Ranade said.

Thanks to the raids conducted by NGOs like the BSPCA and the Plant and Animal Welfare Society (PAWS), the cruel practice of feeding milk to the snakes has considerably reduced, activists say. "In 1996–97, 670 snakes were seized in the raids. But last year (2005), we rescued just 30. The number of snake charmers coming into the city is gradually going down," said Ranade.

Nilesh Bhanage, general secretary, PAWS-Thane said, "We have been conducting raids since 1998. Then, we seized around 40 snakes on Nagpanchami." But last year, Bhanage's team rescued one cobra. "On Sunday, we found no snakes in Bhandup, Mulund, Kanjur Marg and Vikhroli," said Sunish Subramaniam of PAWS-Mumbai. "This is a good sign as it means snake charmers are afraid of the law," explained Bhanage. The Black cobra, a species highly in demand on Nagpanchami, is usually caught from Rajasthan, Punjab and Haryana.

"The snake charmers keep the snakes hungry for a month so that they can drink the milk offered by the devotees; but, in fact, snakes can't digest milk. They also break their venomous fangs which make the snakes unable to protect themselves. These snakes can't be released back into the wild as they cannot hunt," explained Bhanage.

Wildlife activists say the snakes are bought for Rs400. "In the city they fetch between Rs1,000 and Rs3,000," said Ranade.

"After the festival, the snakes are killed and their skin sold. A skin in good condition can fetch as much as Rs3,000."[‡]

Give reasons for your answers: Do you think the activists were justified in rescuing the snakes from the charmers? Is snake charming itself animal abuse? Do snakes have moral rights? Should snake charming be banned—even if it is the only way some people can make a living? What do you think a utilitarian would say about this practice?

‡Deepa Suryanardyan, "Snake Goes Up the Ladder," *Daily News & Analysis*, July 30, 2006. Reprinted by permission of Diligent Media Corporation, Ltd.

CHAPTER 17

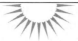

Political Violence: War, Terrorism, and Torture

When has *Homo sapiens* ever been nonviolent? Probably never. The evolution of humans parallels the evolution of their instruments for killing each other. Violence seems as much a part of human life as it ever was, except that the efficiency of our violent methods has improved. Spears can dispatch one person at a time, but smart bombs can kill by the dozens, and nuclear weapons can eliminate the human race altogether.

Fortunately while human beings have been inflicting violence, they have also been raising moral questions about its use. The central concern is this: when, if ever, are we morally justified in resorting to it? Is *every* use of violence wrong, as Buddhist and Christian doctrines have insisted? To just about everyone, violence is inherently bad, an evil in itself. If so, how can perpetrating it ever be morally permissible? If we condemn an aggressor for his assault on the innocent, what should we say when the innocent rise up and kill him in self-defense? Should we condemn them too? Is violence ever justified to protect something less valuable than your life—your property, your rights, your reputation, your income?

All these questions apply with double force to *political* violence, the resort to violence for political ends. War, terrorism, torture, revolution, assassination, civil war, and violent demonstrations—these are all paradigm cases of violence with political aims. Unlike personal violence (for example, muggings, shootings, and rapes), political violence is large in its scale and its effects. A war can involve millions; terrorism can terrify thousands.

In recent years, philosophers have paid a lot of attention to the morality of violence, especially to issues arising from political violence in the form of war, terrorism, and torture. They have clarified concepts, sharpened the focus of moral debate, and arrived at some well argued answers to the major questions. In this chapter, we examine some of this important philosophical work.

ISSUE FILE: BACKGROUND

We all know what violence is. Or do we? In fact, the term *violence* in common usage has multiple meanings and is difficult to pin down. Consider: we often refer to the violence of a storm, or to a violent mood, or to the violence of social injustice, or to the violence done by anything we disapprove of (as in "censorship is violence against the human spirit" or "your remarks are violent acts against minorities"). But if we are to make sense of moral arguments regarding violence, we must be clear about the meaning of the term. For the purposes of this discussion, we can define violence (against people) as some philosophers have: the physical or psychological attack on, or the vigorous abuse of, persons, causing their suffering, injury, or death. (Violence can also involve the destroying or damaging of property.) By this definition, striking, shoving, stabbing, raping, and shooting someone are clear instances of violence, and so are political acts such as wars, terrorism, torture, and the like. We would also count as violence the severe harming of a person psychologically through verbal abuse or humiliation. Denying people the right to vote, perpetuating social inequalities, and defaming a person may be immoral or illegal, but these actions are not examples of violence as just defined.

Most people hold that since violence is inherently bad, it should be used only if there is strong moral justification for it. In other words, violence is prima facie wrong—wrong unless there are good reasons for thinking it morally permissible. Thus people often speak of war and other modes of violence as things to be *resorted to*, actions to be taken only after other options are exhausted.

But why is violence wrong? One answer often given is that it constitutes a violation of people's rights—their right to life, self-determination, respect as a person, or immunity from harm. Another view is that violence is prima facie wrong because it runs afoul of the moral principles of justice, freedom, and utility (human welfare). Some argue that the wrongness of violence arises from its detrimental effects on society: it's wrong because it makes society worse off than if no violence were present. This is one way to articulate a consequentialist notion of violence, but there are others, all based on the premise that violence is (generally) wrong because its bad consequences (usually) outweigh the good.

The most destructive, horrifying violence known to humans is practiced in war. War is a form of political violence because its essence is violent conflict between political communities, usually for the purpose of deciding who gets to effect political changes. Ever since philosophers began examining the ethics of war over two millennia ago, the main moral questions have been (1) How—if at all—can war be justified? and (2) Assuming it can be justified, how should it be conducted? Most serious responses to these questions have fallen into three major categories, traditionally labeled *realism, pacifism*, and *just war theory*. **Realism** (as applied to warfare) is the view that moral standards are not applicable to war, which must be judged only on prudence, on how well war serves state interests.

War cannot be immoral, only more or less advantageous for the state. Eminent realists of the past include the philosophers Niccolò Machiavelli (1469–1527) and Thomas Hobbes (1588–1679); modern realists include Reinhold Niebuhr and Henry Kissinger, former U.S. secretary of state for the Nixon administration.

Realists may argue that morality has no part to play in warfare because all moral statements are meaningless or unknowable or because moral norms do not apply to states, just to persons. The former claim denies that there can be appeals to any moral standards at all and is therefore vulnerable to the usual arguments that philosophers make against such moral skepticism (see Chapter 2). To the latter view, some nonrealists may reply that there is no good reason to think that states are exempt from moral judgments. Nonrealists may also insist that despite the seemingly unrestrained brutality of war, common sense suggests that sometimes moral norms do apply to warfare. According to this position, even when people favor a war of extreme, indeed savage, measures, they tend to believe that there are at least some moral limits to what can be done. Most would probably balk at the use of nuclear weapons, or the deliberate killing of children, or the mass rape of all noncombatant women.

Pacifism is the view that war is never morally permissible. (The term is also often used to refer to the broader idea that all violence is wrong or that all killing is wrong.) Pacifists in this sense are opposed to all wars regardless of the reasons behind them. They may or may not, however, be against all uses of personal violence, or violence between individuals. They may believe, for example, that personal violence in self-defense or in law enforcement may be justified. To make their case, pacifists may argue in a consequentialist vein that war is never justified, because it always produces more bad than good. The catastrophic loss of life and the widespread destruction of war can never offset whatever political or material gains are achieved; riches, land, oil, or power cannot outweigh the carnage. Pacifists may also rely on a nonconsequentialist argument like this: War is always wrong because in the deliberate killing of human beings it violates a fundamental right—the right to life. This right—which may have either a religious or secular basis—is absolute, admitting no exceptions.

The usual objection to the consequentialist approach is that though war is horrific and often (perhaps usually) produces more bad than good, at least sometimes the results may be good overall. It is possible, this argument goes, that waging a war could save the lives of many more people than are killed in the conflict or that fighting one small war could prevent a much larger one. A common objection to the pacifist's nonconsequentialist line is that even though a person has a right to life, we may be morally justified in killing him or her in self-defense if there is no other way to save our own lives. Thus sometimes killing in war is regrettable but necessary—and therefore morally permissible.

Just war theory is the doctrine that war may be morally permissible under stipulated conditions. It is a centuries-old attempt to understand how war—an enduring form of systematic killing—can be reconciled with our moral presumptions *against* killing. It specifies when resorting to war may be morally justified and how armed conflict should be conducted to meet the minimal demands of morality. Thomas Aquinas produced the most influential discourse on the doctrine, which has been evolving ever since as both religious and secular thinkers have tried to improve it. Just war theory has become the most widely used lens through which the ethics of war is viewed these days. As one theorist points out,

> To be sure, this tradition has often found expression in church law and theological reflection; yet it also appears in codifications and theories of international law, in military manuals on how rightly to conduct war, and—as Michael Walzer has shown in

Just and Unjust Wars—in the judgments and reactions of common people.[1]

Just war theory is concerned with two main issues: (1) the justification for resorting to war (traditionally labeled **jus ad bellum,** or "the justice of war") and (2) the moral permissibility of acts in war (**jus in bello,** or "justice in war"). Theorists have addressed *jus ad bellum* by specifying that going to war can be morally permissible only if certain requirements are met. In the following list, Aquinas urged the first three requirements, and later thinkers embraced them and added several more. According to the theory, only if all the requirements are met can a war be considered just.

1. *The cause must be just.* War is such a horrifying business that only a just cause—a morally legitimate reason—can justify going to war. The most commonly cited just cause is self-defense against attack. The usual thinking is that precisely as individuals are entitled to use violence to defend themselves against violent personal attacks, so states have the right to defend against unjust attacks from another state. The implication here is that states have no right to *instigate* a war.

Many theorists define a just cause broadly: a just cause is resistance to substantial aggression, which has been defined as "the type of aggression that violates people's most fundamental rights."[2] This resistance includes self-defense against external threat, of course. But it also may encompass defending the innocent from deadly attack (as in genocide or "ethnic cleansing," for example), defending people whose basic human rights are being violated by a brutal regime, or defending other states from unjust external attack. Some early theorists thought

[1]James Turner Johnson, "Threats, Values, and Defense: Does the Defense of Values by Force Remain a Moral Possibility?" *Parameters* 15, no. 1 (Spring 1985).

[2]James P. Sterba, "Reconciling Pacifists and Just War Theorists," *Social Theory and Practice* 18, no. 1 (Spring 1992): 21.

that wars could be justifiably fought to convert or punish those of a different religion—a view now rejected by Western philosophers and theologians but still strongly supported in some parts of the world.

Some people argue that war in self-defense is justified only in response to an actual attack; others maintain that an attack need not be actual but only feared—that is, a "preventive war" may be justified. But many contend that to start a war on such grounds is to act on a mere fear of the unknown and to invite other states to launch attacks for no good reason (or for ulterior motives). In response to this worry, a number of theorists maintain that a war is justified only if the threat of attack from another state is "immediate and imminent," which means something like "clearly about to happen." Such a war is properly called preemptive. Much of the debate about the United States's launching

a preemptive strike against Iraq in 2003 has been about whether this "immediate and imminent" standard was met as well as about whether the standard is relevant when there might be a danger from weapons of mass destruction.

2. *The war must be sanctioned by proper authority.* The resort to war must be approved by a state's rightful government. As Aquinas says, a just war requires "the authority of the sovereign by whose command the war is to be waged. For it is not the business of a private individual to declare war."[3]

3. *The war should be fought with the right intentions.* Wars must be waged for the sake of the just

[3] Thomas Aquinas, *Summa Theologica,* in *Basic Writings of Saint Thomas Aquinas,* ed. and annotated Anton C. Pegis (New York: Random House, 1945), Second Part of the Second Part, Question 40, Article 1.

CRITICAL THOUGHT: Preemptive War on Iraq

According to most forms of just war theory, a preemptive attack against a state is justified only if that state presents a substantial danger that is "immediate and imminent." As some commentators on just war theory explain, "To establish this condition [of immediate and imminent threat], evidence of planning that is virtually completed needs to be shown."* Now consider this description of the run-up to the U.S. preemptive strike on Iraq in 2003.

> [President George W. Bush] claimed that he was justified [in going to war with Iraq] so as to prevent (really to preempt) Iraq from attacking the United States. But such talk of prevention is imprecise, for it may refer either to a necessary preemption of an impending attack or merely to an unjustified fear as a pretext for war based on other motivations. In his 2003 State of the Union speech, Bush said that "The British government has learned that Saddam Hussein recently sought significant quantities of uranium from Africa."

Such a claim was meant to show that Iraq posed an imminent, not merely a speculative threat to the United States. In addition, Bush said that he was not required to wait for the United States to be attacked, or even to wait for all of the evidence needed to show that Iraq might attack.[†]

Assume this passage is an accurate depiction of the pre-war situation and is the only relevant information available to you. Would you judge the threat from Iraq to be "immediate and imminent"? Why or why not? Based on what you have learned about just war theory in this chapter, do you think a fair-minded just war theorist would say the attack on Iraq was justified or unjustified? Why? Do *you* believe that starting the war was just? What are your reasons?

*Larry May, Eric Rovie, and Steven Viner, introduction to *The Morality of War: Classical and Contemporary Readings,* eds. May, Rovie, and Viner (Upper Saddle River, NJ: Pearson/Prentice Hall, 2006), xi.
†Ibid.

cause, not moved by some illegitimate motives such as bloodlust, greed, empire expansion, and ethnic hatred. Aquinas continues,

> [I]t is necessary that the belligerents should have a rightful intention, so that they intend the advancement of good, or the avoidance of evil. . . . For it may happen that the war is declared by the legitimate authority, and for a just cause, and yet be rendered unlawful through a wicked intention.

4. *Armed conflict should be a last resort.* For a war to be just, all peaceful means of sorting out differences between adversaries should be tried first. Diplomacy, economic pressure, world opinion—all these avenues and others should be exhausted before employing guns and bombs.

5. *The good resulting from war must be proportional to the bad.* The good expected to come from fighting for a just cause must be weighed against the tremendous evils that will inevitably accompany war—death, destruction, pain, and loss on a mass scale.

6. *There must be a reasonable chance of success.* Futile wars should not be waged. Mass killing with no likelihood of achieving anything is unjust. So only if success is reasonably probable should a state resort to war.

Just war theorists believe that it is possible for a resort to war to be morally permissible while the conduct of that war is morally abhorrent. They therefore are concerned not only with *jus ad bellum* but also with *jus in bello,* right action during the meting out of the violence. They explicitly reject the popular notion that once war commences, there are no moral restraints whatsoever on what can be done to anyone or anything during the conflict. Michael Walzer, the leading contemporary advocate for just war theory, asserts that the popular view is "profoundly wrong":

> War is indeed ugly, but there are degrees of ugliness and humane men must, as always, be concerned with degrees. . . . Surely there is a point at which the means employed for the sake of this or that political goal come into conflict with a more general human purpose: the maintenance of moral standards and the survival of some sort of international society. At that point, political arguments against the use of such means are overshadowed, or ought to be, by moral arguments. At that point, war is not merely ugly but criminal.[4]

Traditionally, requirements for *jus in bello*—the so-called rules of war—have included:

1. *Discrimination.* Those fighting a war must distinguish between combatants and noncombatants, never deliberately targeting the latter. People who should not be intentionally attacked are said to have **noncombatant immunity,** a status traditionally reserved for women, children, the elderly, and the sick and injured. Though some noncombatants are almost certain to be killed or harmed in any war, such tragedies are supposed to be unavoidable or unintended and therefore pardonable.

The distinction between combatant and noncombatant is often not very clear, especially when a conflict involves fighters wearing civilian clothes and operating among peaceful inhabitants. Michael Walzer offers a helpful distinction by saying that noncombatants are those who are not "engaged in harm." But some thinkers have tended to blur the line between people usually thought to have immunity and those who do not. They ask, Should people be given immunity if they cheer on their combatants, give them food, and shelter them? Are they really to be regarded as "innocent civilians"?

In any case, the prohibition against intentionally attacking noncombatants is enshrined in international law and widely regarded as the most fundamental "rule of war."

2. *Proportionality.* The use of force should be proportional to the rightful aims of the war—"overkill" is disallowed. Even in bitter conflict, combatants should not kill or destroy more than necessary to achieve the just ends for which the war is waged.

3. *No evil means.* Many just war theorists maintain that certain tactics and weapons in war are

[4]Michael Walzer, "Moral Judgment in Time of War," *Dissent* 14, no. 3 (May–June 1967): 284.

"evil in themselves" and thus should never be used regardless of a war's aims. Such evil means are said to include genocide, biological or chemical warfare (use of anthrax and nerve gas, for example), nuclear attack, and rape.

4. *Benevolent quarantine.* Soldiers who surrender to their enemies have rights and should be treated accordingly. They must be given "benevolent quarantine" as prisoners of war (POWs)—humane captivity in safe confines removed from the battlefield. In that environment they must not be subjected to execution, torture, starvation, or other forms of serious abuse.

Blood brother to war is the grisly phenomenon of terrorism, an old scourge that has persisted into the twenty-first century. The ethical questions it evokes are thornier than they might seem at first glance: What is terrorism? Is terrorism ever justified? Who commits terrorist acts? Can states commit terrorist acts? Is the United States or any other country guilty of terrorism? For example, was the Allied bombing of German cities in World War II (in which hundreds of thousands of civilians died) a case of state terrorism? How should we treat terrorists? How should we respond to terrorist violence? How much, if at all, should we curtail civil liberties to protect ourselves against terrorism? Can we evaluate the morality of terrorism in the same way we assess the morality of war (by using, for example, just war theory)?

Most people probably think they know what terrorism is, yet it is notoriously difficult to define. One of the main challenges is to differentiate terrorism from acts of war and violent crimes. In the definition adopted by the U.S. Department of State, terrorism is "premeditated, politically motivated violence perpetrated against noncombatant targets by subnational groups or clandestine agents, usually intended to influence an audience."[5] According to a 1974 British government definition, terrorism is

"the use of violence for political ends, and includes any use of violence for the purpose of putting the public, or any section of the public, in fear."[6] For our discussion we can use a definition that comprises key elements in common usage or philosophical writing: **terrorism** is violence against noncombatants for political, religious, or ideological ends.

Some think terrorism is a recent phenomenon. But scholars who define terrorism broadly maintain that its history is long and bloody. The term *terrorism* sprang from the French Revolution's Reign of Terror, in which the new state sanctioned the use of terror against its enemies, real or imagined, executing thousands of mostly ordinary citizens. In the nineteenth century, anarchists aimed to inspire the masses to revolution with terrifying deeds against established regimes. They achieved worldwide attention and spread public alarm—but no revolution—by assassinating several state leaders, including President William McKinley in the United States and Tsar Alexander II in Russia.

The twentieth century had a shockingly large share of terrorism, in both old and new forms driven by familiar and unfamiliar motives. Terrorism in the first half of the century was mostly nationalist (as were terrorist groups in Ireland, Palestine, Algeria, and the Balkans), state-sponsored (by, for example, the Serbian and Bulgarian governments), and state-administered (as in Nazi Germany, Stalinist Russia, and several South American dictatorships). Its preferred form was assassination and mass killing. The second half witnessed more state-sponsored terrorism and the predominance of terrorism that was ideological or religious. Terrorism in this period was distinguished by its heavy reliance on the horrors of airline hijackings, kid-

---

[5]U.S. Department of State, *Patterns of Global Terrorism 2003* (Washington, DC: U.S. Department of State 2004), xii.

[6]*International Encyclopedia of Terrorism,* 1997 ed., s.v. "The Official View"; quoted in *A Military Guide to Terrorism in the Twenty-first Century,* U.S. Army Training and Doctrine Command, 15 August 2005, version 3.0, available at www.fas.org/irp/threat/terrorism/index (4 December 2006), 1–3.

nappings, and suicide bombings. According to the Center for Defense Information,

> Through the 1960s and 1970s, the numbers of those groups that might be described as terrorist swelled to include not only nationalists, but those motivated by ethnic and ideological considerations. The former included groups such as the Palestinian Liberation Organization (and its many affiliates), the Basque ETA, and the Provisional Irish Republican Army, while the latter comprised organizations such as the Red Army Faction (in what was then West Germany) and the Italian Red Brigades. As with the emergence of modern terrorism almost a century earlier, the United States was not immune from this latest wave, although there the identity-crisis-driven motivations of the white middle-class Weathermen starkly contrasted with the ghetto-bred malcontent [sic] of the Black Panther movement.[7]

Since around the mid-1990s, the threat of religiously inspired terrorism has expanded dramatically. In 1998, there were 37 incidents of religious terrorism worldwide resulting in 758 deaths. In 2001, there were 99 incidents and 3,275 deaths, most of which occurred in the September 11 attacks on the United States. In 2005, religious terrorists killed 2,061 people throughout the world in 606 incidents.[8] In 2009, there were nearly 15,000 deaths from terrorist attacks of all kinds; 9,280 of these were caused by Sunni Islamic extremists, while 1,052 were committed by Christian extremists.[9] The Council on Foreign Affairs reports that

Religious terrorists seek to use violence to further what they see as divinely commanded purposes, often targeting broad categories of foes in an attempt to bring about sweeping changes. Religious terrorists come from many faiths, as well as from small cults. . . . Because religious terrorists are concerned not with rallying a constituency of fellow nationalists or ideologues but with pursuing their own vision of divine will, they lack one of the major constraints that historically has limited the scope of terror attacks, experts say. As [the terrorism expert Bruce] Hoffman puts it, the most extreme religious terrorists can sanction "almost limitless violence against a virtually open-ended category of targets: that is, anyone who is not a member of the terrorists' religion or religious sect."[10]

Among the more infamous terrorist incidents of the past forty-plus years are the following, as described by the U.S. Department of State:

Munich Olympic Massacre, September 5, 1972: Eight Palestinian "Black September" terrorists seized eleven Israeli athletes in the Olympic Village in Munich, West Germany. In a bungled rescue attempt by West German authorities, nine of the hostages and five terrorists were killed.

Iran Hostage Crisis, November 4, 1979: After President Carter agreed to admit the Shah of Iran into the United States, Iranian radicals seized the U.S. Embassy in Tehran and took 66 American diplomats hostage. Thirteen hostages were soon released, but the remaining 53 were held until their release on January 20, 1981.

Grand Mosque Seizure, November 20, 1979: 200 Islamic terrorists seized the Grand Mosque in Mecca, Saudi Arabia, taking hundreds of pilgrims hostage. Saudi and French security forces retook the shrine after an intense battle in which some 250 people were killed and 600 wounded.

Pan Am 103 Bombing, December 21, 1988: Pan American Airlines Flight 103 was blown up over Lockerbie, Scotland, by a bomb believed to have been placed on the aircraft by Libyan terrorists in Frankfurt, West Germany. All 259 people on board were killed.

---

[7]Mark Burgess, "A Brief History of Terrorism," Center for Defense Information, 2 July 2003, http://www.pogo.org/our-work/straus-military-reform-project/cdi-archive/a-brief-history-of-terrorism.html (24 February 2015).

[8]National Memorial Institute for the Prevention of Terrorism (MIPT), *Terrorism Knowledge Base*, www.tkb.org/Home.jsp (27 January 2006).

[9]National Counterterrorism Center, *2009 Report on Terrorism*, 30 April 2010, http://www.riskintel.com/wp-content/uploads/downloads/2011/10/2009_report_on_terrorism.pdf (24 February 2015).

[10]Council on Foreign Relations, "Types of Terrorism," *Council on Foreign Affairs*, http://cfrterrorism.org/terrorism/types.html (27 January 2006).

World Trade Center Bombing, February 26, 1993: The World Trade Center in New York City was badly damaged when a car bomb planted by Islamic terrorists exploded in an underground garage. The bomb left 6 people dead and 1,000 injured. The men carrying out the attack were followers of Umar Abd al-Rahman, an Egyptian cleric who preached in the New York City area.

Bombing of the Federal Building in Oklahoma City, April 19, 1995: Right-wing extremists Timothy McVeigh and Terry Nichols destroyed the Federal Building in Oklahoma City with a massive truck bomb that killed 166 and injured hundreds more in what was up to then the largest terrorist attack on American soil.

Terrorist Attacks on U.S. Homeland, September 11, 2001: Two hijacked airliners crashed into the twin towers of the World Trade Center. Soon thereafter, the Pentagon was struck by a third hijacked plane. A fourth hijacked plane, suspected to be bound for a high-profile target in Washington, crashed into a field in southern Pennsylvania. The attacks killed 3,025 U.S. citizens and other nationals. President Bush and Cabinet officials indicated that Osama bin Laden was the prime suspect and that they considered the United States in a state of war with international terrorism. . . .

Car Bomb Explosion in Bali, October 12, 2002: A car bomb exploded outside the Sari Club Discotheque in Denpasar, Bali, Indonesia, killing 202 persons and wounding 300 more. Most of the casualties, including 88 of the dead, were Australian tourists. Seven Americans were among the dead. Al-Qaeda claimed responsibility. Two suspects were later arrested and convicted. Iman Samudra, who had trained in Afghanistan with al-Qaeda and was suspected of belonging to Jemaah Islamiya, was sentenced to death on September 10, 2003.[11]

To this list we could add many more incidents, and probably most shocking among them would be these: The March 11, 2004, attacks in Madrid and the July 7, 2005, bombings in London. In Madrid a coordinated series of bombs exploded on four commuter trains, killing 191 people and injuring more than 1,500. Investigators blamed Islamic militants connected to cells in Europe. In London, almost simultaneously four jihadists set off bombs on a double-decker bus and three subway trains, killing themselves and fifty-two other people and injuring hundreds. In 2008 in Mumbai, India, Pakistan-based militants killed 174 people in a shooting rampage. And in 2011, a man described as a Christian right-wing extremist set off a large bomb in Oslo, Norway, killing eight people, then systematically murdered 69 others at an island youth camp.

The most recent events in global terrorism are also the most frightening. In 2014 large swaths of Iraqi and Syrian territory were taken over by a group known as the Islamic State of Iraq and Syria (ISIS). It is made up of thousands of Islamist militants drawn from the Syrian civil war, jihadist elements in Iraq, and volunteers from Europe, the United States, and elsewhere. ISIS aspires to be a caliphate, an Islamic nation, calling itself the Islamic State, but its methods are terrorist on a mass scale:

> The stories, the videos, the acts of unfathomable brutality have become a defining aspect of ISIS, which controls a nation-size tract of land and has now pushed Iraq to the precipice of dissolution. Its adherents kill with such abandon that even the leader of al-Qaeda has disavowed them. . . .
>
> [I]n terms of impact, the acts of terror have been wildly successful. From beheadings to summary executions to amputations to crucifixions, the terrorist group has become the most feared organization in the Middle East. That fear, evidenced in fleeing Iraqi soldiers and 500,000 Mosul residents, has played a vital role in the group's march toward Baghdad. In many cases, police and soldiers literally ran, shedding their uniforms as they went, abandoning large caches of weapons.[12]

---

[11]U.S. Department of State, Office of the Historian, Bureau of Public Affairs, "Significant Terrorist Incidents, 1961–2003: A Brief Chronology," March 2004, http://fas.org/irp/threat/terror_chron.html (24 February 2015).

[12]Terrence McCoy, "ISIS, Beheadings and the Success of Horrifying Violence," *Washington Post*, June 13, 2014, http://www.washingtonpost.com/news/morning-mix/wp/2014/06/13/isis-beheadings-and-the-success-of-horrifying-violence/ (31 October 2014).

ISIS is now a transnational movement with the wherewithal to inspire followers around the world. Its strength is increasing, and Western and Middle Eastern countries have failed to stop it. In the West, a major worry is that ISIS may spawn not just a few but thousands of hardened, battle-tested terrorists.

The question that all terrorism provokes is, What should be our moral response to it? Many argue that a violent response is the wrong response, that a "war on terror" is misguided and morally impermissible. The proper response, they say, is dialogue with aggressors, a criminal justice approach instead of military force, and the eradication of the true causes of terrorism—poverty, oppression, suffering, and injustice. As one observer has said,

> In my view, the most effective counterterrorism approach would arise from a foreign policy that took the sufferings of people in other countries seriously. A progressive orientation would stand in contrast to today's official counterterrorism, which views suffering as irrelevant, or even as a reason to inflate the terrorist danger.[13]

The opposing view is that violence may in fact be a morally justified reaction to terrorism—that is, morally justified by the lights of just war theory. As noted earlier, just war theory is the timeworn doctrine that war may be morally permissible if particular requirements are met. It lays out the conditions under which resorting to war would be morally justified and specifies the criteria for judging the morality of how it is fought. Some contend that all the criteria can sometimes be met, justifying a carefully measured military response to terrorist attacks. Thus one observer argues that

> according to just war theory, defending against this sort of terrorism is a just cause; that within significant constraints sovereign political authorities can have authority to undertake military actions for the sake of this just cause, notwithstanding the nature of organization of the terrorists; and that a political community

can pursue such a cause with right intention, even though in the world as it is military efforts to defend against terrorism may well not meet this condition.[14]

Others say that government antiterrorism activities and policies (what has been called the "war on terror") have gone too far by undermining civil liberties in the name of security. A prime concern is that some overreaching antiterrorism laws meant to be temporary can easily become permanent. Critics have also charged that repressive governments have used the war on terror as an excuse to violate the human rights and civil liberties of innocent people deemed undesirable by the state.

A more fundamental—and controversial—moral issue is whether terrorist actions can ever be morally justified. Many argue on various grounds that terrorism is never morally permissible, regardless of the merits of the terrorists' cause. The philosopher Haig Khatchadourian, for example, argues that acts of terrorism are always wrong because (1) they violate basic principles of just war theory and, (2) except in rare cases where other overriding moral principles apply, they violate their victims' right to be treated as moral persons. Regarding reason (1), Khatchadourian claims that terrorism in all forms violates the just war principles of discrimination and proportionality. Concerning reason (2), he says that

> Treating people as moral persons means treating them with consideration in two closely related ways. First, it means respecting their autonomy as individuals with their own desires and interests, plans and projects, commitments and goals. That autonomy is clearly violated if they are humiliated, coerced and terrorized, taken hostage or kidnapped, and above all, killed. Second, consideration . . . includes sensitivity to and consideration of their feelings and desires, aspirations, projects, and goals. That in turn is an integral part of treating their life as a whole—including their relationships and memories—as a thing of value. Finally, it includes respecting their

[13] Richard Falk, "Thinking about Terrorism," *The Nation*, 28 June 1986; note that this view was expressed long before the events of September 11, 2001.

[14]Joseph M. Boyle Jr., "Just War Doctrine and the Military Response to Terrorism," *Journal of Political Philosophy* 11, no. 2 (2003): 153–70.

"culture or ethnic, religious or racial identity or heritage." These things are the very antithesis of what terrorism does to its victims and the victimized.[15]

Similarly the just war theorist Michael Walzer asserts that terrorism is wrong because it is an indiscriminate attack on the innocent. He thinks that a terrorist attack is worse than rape or murder because these crimes are at least directed at specific persons for particular reasons, even if those reasons are perverse. But terrorist violence is aimed at no one in particular for no purpose that could be linked to a specific person. For the terrorist, any innocent person who happens to fit into a broad category is as good a target as any other. "Terrorists are like killers on a rampage," says Walzer, "except that their rampage is not just expressive of rage or madness; the rage is purposeful and programmatic. It aims at a general vulnerability: Kill these people in order to terrify those."[16]

Not everyone agrees, however. A few thinkers, while deploring terrorist violence, argue that in some cases terrorism may be morally permissible. In fact, some maintain that particular instances of terrorism can even meet the requirements of just war theory and therefore be justified in the same way that acts of war are justified. For example, one proponent of this view argues that when a stateless group has its right of self-determination thwarted, it may have a just cause—and an organization representing the group can be "a morally legitimate authority to carry out violence as a last resort to defend the group's rights."[17]

Disputes about the moral permissibility of terrorist actions can quickly bring us back to arguments about a plausible definition of terrorism.

[15]Haig Khatchadourian, *The Morality of Terrorism* (New York: Peter Lang, 1998), 31–32.
[16]Michael Walzer, "Terrorism: A Critique of Excuses," in *Problems of International Justice*, ed. Steven Luper-Foy (Boulder, CO: Westview Press, 1988), 238.
[17]Andrew Valls, "Can Terrorism Be Justified?" in *Ethics in International Affairs: Theories and Cases*, ed. Valls (Lanham, MD: Rowman and Littlefield, 2000), 65–79.

Suppose, for instance, that the preferred definition of terrorism is a variation on the one proposed earlier: deliberate use of violence against noncombatants for political or ideological purposes. This definition would apply to many acts that seem to be unambiguous examples of terrorism—the September 11 attacks, the Munich Olympics massacre, the Bali car bombing of October 2002, and many others. But what about the following cases in which noncombatants were also deliberately killed for political reasons: the Allied bombings of Dresden and other German cities in World War II and the atomic obliteration of Hiroshima and Nagasaki? According to our revised definition, aren't these also terrorist acts? And if so, could not the United States and Britain be classified as terrorist states?

Some are willing to accept such implications of our definition (or similar ones). They think that deliberately targeting noncombatants for political or ideological purposes is never morally acceptable—no matter who does the targeting. So for them, the World War II city bombings were indeed instances of terrorism, and the states doing the bombing were acting as terrorists. Others avoid these repugnant implications by working from a definition that confines terrorism to **nonstate actors**—that is, to individuals or groups that are not sovereign states. (Recall the definition of terrorism offered by the U.S. Department of State—"premeditated, politically motivated violence perpetrated against noncombatant targets by subnational groups or clandestine agents[.]") Terrorism then would be the killing of innocents by al Qaeda or the Red Brigades, but not by a sovereign polity like the United States. Walzer, however, takes the line that terrorism is never morally justified but that some of the city bombings in World War II *were* justified (and therefore were not terrorism) because they were done in a "supreme emergency"—circumstances in which civilization itself is threatened with eminent destruction.

Often where there is war or terrorism, there is also torture. As with other forms of political violence, the vexing question is whether torture is

CRITICAL THOUGHT: Terrorists or Freedom Fighters?

On January 5, 2006, BBC News reported on two of the many suicide bombings that have occurred throughout Iraq. One bomb was detonated in Karbala near an important Shia shrine. It killed 60 people and injured over 100. The other bomb exploded at a Ramadi police recruiting center, killing another 60. At the time, talks were going on among Shia, Sunni, and Kurdish groups to form a coalition government. Iraqi President Jalal Talabini appeared to think that the bombings were meant to cause tension between religious groups and wreck the political process. "These groups of dark terror," he said, "will not succeed through these cowardly acts in dissuading Iraqis in their bid to form a government of national unity."*

Assume that the attacks were terrorist acts carried out by Iraqis intent on ridding Iraq of its Western occupiers and their influence on the government of Iraq (an assumption that may or may not be correct). In that case, was the terrorism morally justified? Why or why not? Should the attackers be called "freedom fighters" instead of terrorists? Could the terrorist acts meet all the conditions of just war theory?

*"Iraq Suicide Bomb Blasts Kill 120," BBC News Online, 5 January 2006, http://news.bbc.co.uk/2/hi/middle_east/4583232 .stm (24 February 2015).

ever morally justified. And the most challenging version of this question is whether it is permissible to use torture to prevent terrorist carnage.

Torture is the intentional inflicting of severe pain or suffering on people to punish or intimidate them or to extract information from them. It has been used by both secular and religious authorities for centuries and continues to this day to be applied to hapless victims throughout the world. This, despite worldwide condemnation of the practice and its absolute prohibition in international law, including by United Nations treaties and the Geneva Conventions.

For generations the United States officially opposed torture and prosecuted both American soldiers and the nation's enemies for using harsh methods against captives. But the administration of George W. Bush was accused of authorizing and employing interrogation tactics that had long been regarded as torture. The subjects were suspected terrorists, and the purpose of the severe approach was to wrest from them some information that might help authorities crush terrorist groups or

prevent future terrorist attacks. Reports show that "waterboarding" (simulated drowning) and other extreme techniques were used against detainees in U.S.-run facilities overseas.

Three issues dominate the debates over the morality of torture: (1) Does torture work? (2) Is torture ever morally acceptable? and (3) What should be the state's policy regarding the use of torture?

As usually understood, question 1 is about whether torture is effective in getting reliable information from suspects. Science has yet to definitively answer the question, and the views of expert interrogators conflict. Many intelligence officers claim that torture rarely, if ever, yields useful information; other experts assert that torture occasionally produces valuable data. People in both camps worry about the indirect effect of using harsh methods—the damage to American prestige and influence, the increased likelihood of our enemies using torture against us, and the slide down the slippery slope toward the wider use of more brutal means.

For many nonconsequentialists, the answer to question 2 is an absolutist no—torture is the use of a person merely as a means, a clear instance of a lack of respect for a human being. Torture is therefore always wrong. But most people are probably not absolutists; they think that in rare cases there could be exceptions to a no-torture rule. (We consider a popular argument for this view in the "Moral Arguments" section.)

Question 3 is a separate issue entirely. Whether or not we believe that torture would be morally justified in a particular instance, we might take a very different view about legalizing or institutionalizing it. On this matter, there are three main positions: (1) torture should be illegal and never sanctioned in any circumstances; (2) torture should be illegal and officially condemned but unofficially (and secretly) used when necessary; and (3) torture should be a legal instrument of the state, although administered under strict guidelines and oversight.

Those taking the first approach insist that legalizing torture would have devastating consequences. It would corrupt democratic institutions, diminish our moral authority in the world, cause torture to become routine and widespread in society, and arouse worldwide resentment and anger toward us.

Those who prefer the second approach believe that torture may sometimes be necessary but that acknowledging its use could cause many of the problems that worry those in the first group. Their critics accuse them of hypocrisy, but they see no good alternative to this clandestine, "under the radar" strategy.

The third approach is preferred by many who deplore the hypocrisy of the second group but are convinced that the use of torture is inevitable. They hold that if torture is legalized, its use can be better controlled than in any unofficial arrangement, and its abuses and proliferation can be limited. Alan Dershowitz advocates this third way, recommending a system in which official interrogators may use torture only after they acquire permission—"torture warrants"—from a judge.

MORAL THEORIES

Both consequentialist and nonconsequentialist perspectives have been given major roles in the ethics of war and peace. On the consequentialist side, utilitarianism has been used both to support and to undermine pacifism. Some have argued, for example, that by utilitarian lights, antiwar pacifism must be true. The philosopher Thomas Nagel provides some examples of such pacifist arguments:

> It may even be argued that war involves violence on such a scale that it is never justified on utilitarian grounds—the consequences of refusing to go to war will never be as bad as the war itself would be, even if atrocities were not committed. Or in a more sophisticated vein it might be claimed that a uniform policy of never resorting to military force would do less harm in the long run, if followed consistently, than a policy of deciding each case on utilitarian grounds (even though on occasion particular applications of the pacifist policy might have worse results than a specific utilitarian decision).[18]

Whether good consequences produced by a pacifist stance would always in fact outweigh the bad of war making is, of course, a question of nonmoral fact—and some utilitarians assert that the facts do not help the pacifist's case. These critics say there is no evidence to support the notion that a policy of pacifism always results in less death and suffering. As one philosopher says,

> [I]t is worthwhile to point out that the general history of the human race certainly offers no support for the supposition that turning the other cheek always produces good effects on the aggressor. Some aggressors, such as the Nazis, were apparently "egged on" by the "pacifist" attitude of their victims.[19]

Utilitarians can push this kind of argument even further and say that resorting to war is sometimes justified because it results in a better balance

[18]Thomas Nagel, "War and Massacre," *Philosophy & Public Affairs* 1, no. 2 (Winter 1972): 123–43.
[19]Jan Narveson, "Pacifism: A Philosophical Analysis," *Ethics* 75, no. 4 (1965): 623–24.

of good over bad, everyone considered, than not going to war. (Obviously, they too would need to back up such an empirical claim.) To be consistent, they would also want to base the moral rightness of military actions in war (*jus in bello*) on utilitarian considerations.

As we saw earlier, utilitarian elements are built into just war theory, which is a coherent system of both consequentialist and nonconsequentialist requirements. In our previous list of *jus ad bellum* conditions, the last three requirements are usually taken as consequentialist: (4) last resort, (5) good proportional to the bad, and (6) reasonable chance of success. And the *jus in bello* conditions of discrimination and proportionality are often viewed as rules for maximizing the good for both combatants and noncombatants.

When justifying views on the resort to war, both pacifists and nonpacifists may take a nonconsequentialist approach, appealing to fundamental moral principles rather than to the results of actions. As we have seen, pacifists typically rest their case on the right to life; nonpacifists, on the right of self-defense or the defense of basic human rights generally. The former regard their moral principle as absolute—it allows no exceptions—but the latter may not.

As you would expect, there can be stark differences on many critical matters between the consequentialist and nonconsequentialist. One such issue is the treatment of noncombatants. Absolutist nonconsequentialists maintain that the intentional killing of noncombatants is always morally wrong regardless of the circumstances, but consequentialists insist that sometimes there are exceptions:

Regarding the absolute prohibition on intentional killing of noncombatants, absolutists have been termed "immunity theorists." Immunity theorists hold that it is always morally impermissible to intentionally kill noncombatants in war. Noncombatants are "innocent" and thus immune from attack. . . .

. . . Consequentialists believe that actions in war can be morally justified depending on the end or aim of the action. If it is morally sufficient, the end can justify the means. . . . From this perspective, consequentialists, unlike absolutists, can morally justify the intentional killing of noncombatants or "innocents" in war. A controversial example addressed in this debate is the bombing of Hiroshima and Nagasaki in World War II. Consequentialists can morally justify these bombings. Absolutists, however, contend that these bombings were immoral because these bombings targeted noncombatants.[20]

How would traditional moral theories have us view the moral justification of terrorism? It seems that act-utilitarianism would have to sanction at least some terrorist attacks. The act-utilitarian must admit that it is possible for a terrorist action to yield the best overall results in a situation—and "best overall results" is the overriding factor here. But a utilitarian could not consistently condone terrorist actions that served only the interests of a particular group, for the theory demands that right actions produce the greatest overall happiness, *everyone considered*. Many (or perhaps most) acts of terrorism are clearly meant to exclusively favor a specific segment of a population; everyone is deliberately *not* considered.

Some writers contend that even though consequentialist moral theories can justify terrorism, the theories can do so "only under conditions that terrorists in the flesh will find it difficult to satisfy."[21] Consider: Consequentialism would demand that the terrorist acts be effective and efficient and that there be no nonterrorist actions likely to yield better or equal results. Such theories would require that the aim to be achieved be worth the horrific damage that a terrorist act can produce.

---

[20]Larry May, Eric Rovie, and Steve Viner, in *The Morality of War: Classical and Contemporary Readings,* eds. May, Rovie, and Viner (Upper Saddle River, NJ: Pearson/Prentice Hall, 2006), 200.

[21]R. G. Frey and Christopher W. Morris, "Terrorism," in *Violence, Terrorism, and Justice,* eds. Frey and Morris (Cambridge: Cambridge University Press, 1991), 1–11.

Terrorists themselves sometimes justify their actions on consequentialist grounds: They assert that only terrorism can help them achieve their objectives. But many observers are skeptical of terrorism's power to attain *any* political ends, especially the goal of liberation from an oppressive regime. Walzer observes, "I doubt that terrorism has ever achieved national liberation—no nation that I know of owes its freedom to a campaign of random murder."[22] Certainly terrorism can frighten the public and increase the terrorists' notoriety, but winning a political struggle is a much rougher road. If terrorism is indeed an ineffective strategy, then this fact could form the backbone of a consequentialist argument *against* terrorist acts.

Nonconsequentialist moral theories (or nonconsequentialist moral principles) often yield condemnations of terrorism in all forms. A traditional natural law theorist would insist that terrorism is always wrong because it violates the prohibition against intentionally killing the innocent. Natural law's doctrine of double effect—which disallows intentional bad actions even if they achieve good results—would lead to this conclusion (assuming the definition of terrorism given earlier). Some people, of course, could try to counter this view by rejecting the doctrine of double effect or by questioning the concept of moral innocence. A Kantian theorist or other nonconsequentialist could argue that terrorism is not morally permissible because it violates innocent persons' human rights, their right to life, or their autonomy or because terrorism uses people merely as a means to an end.

Many philosophers view terrorism from the perspective of just war theory. Some of them argue that terrorism is wrong because it violates key conditions of just war theory—in particular, discrimination, proportionality (both *jus ad bellum* and *jus in bello*), last resort, and just cause. As we saw earlier, some reject this claim and maintain that just war theory, rightly interpreted, shows that in some

[22]Walzer, "Terrorism," 240.

instances terrorism may be justified because it meets all the conditions.

A nonconsequentialist is likely to consider torture wrong in all circumstances—wrong because it violates the rights of persons, primarily by severely diminishing their autonomy as individuals. A consequentialist could either accept or reject the use of torture, depending on her assessment of the likely effects. She could decide that torture is justified in rare cases in which it could prevent a massive terrorist attack or lead to the destruction of a terrorist cell involved in the killing of hundreds or thousands of people. She could also argue that when all the consequences of torturing someone are carefully weighed, torture is never the best option. Its negative ramifications always outweigh the positive.

MORAL ARGUMENTS

Perhaps the simplest argument against political violence is based on the commonsense presumption that violence of any kind is inherently (prima facie) wrong and therefore requires very strong reasons for believing that in a particular case it is justified. One form this argument could take is this: Violence is inherently wrong; there are no good reasons to suppose that it is ever justified; therefore, violence (including political violence) is always wrong. This argument puts the burden of proof on those who allege that sometimes violence is permissible.

But the problem for anyone who relies on this line is that many people have been happy to take up this burden, arguing in the case of war, terrorism, or torture that there are indeed strong reasons why violence is occasionally justified. Likewise, many who insist on nonviolence have not been content to rest their case on this burden-of-proof argument. They have tried to show that strong arguments can independently support their position.

As we have seen, it's possible to argue for and against the resort to war using either a consequentialist or nonconsequentialist tact. Just war theory is a mix of both these approaches, and it has probably been the focus of most of the philosophical disputes concerning war and peace.

One set of arguments about war that continues to provoke intense debate is **humanitarian intervention.** The conventional model of a justified resort to war is: one sovereign state defending itself against another's aggression. A state's self-defense is thought to be just cause for unleashing the dogs of war. But humanitarian intervention is a different sort of scenario, for it involves a state (or states) going to war to defend people of another state against the murderous aggression of their own regime. The aggression may appear in the form of genocide, ethnic cleansing, forced starvation, and mass imprisonment or slavery—the kinds of atrocities that occurred forty years ago in Cambodia and Uganda, and more recently in Somalia, East Timor, Kosovo, Rwanda, and Libya. The situations that are said to cry out for humanitarian intervention are both compelling and alien to early just war theory:

> The standard cases have a standard form: a government, an army, a police force, tyrannically controlled, attacks its own people or some subset of its own people, a vulnerable minority, say, territorially based or dispersed throughout the country. . . . The attack takes place within the country's borders; it doesn't require any boundary crossings; it is an exercise of sovereign power. There is no aggression, no invading army to resist and beat back. Instead, the rescuing forces are the invaders; they are the ones who, in the strict sense of international law, begin the war. But they come into a situation where the moral stakes are clear: the oppressors or, better, the state agents of oppression are readily identifiable; their victims are plain to see.[23]

To get to the heart of these matters, we want to ask, Is humanitarian intervention ever morally permissible? Those who say yes—the interventionists—might offer an argument like this:

[23]Michael Walzer, "The Argument about Humanitarian Intervention," *Dissent* 49, no. 1 (Winter 2002), http://www.dissentmagazine.org/article/the-argument-about-humanitarian-intervention (26 February 2015).

1. An individual has a duty to try to stop an unjust and potentially fatal attack against someone (to intervene), even if defending the victim requires using violence against the attacker (assuming that the defender is capable of acting without too much personal risk, and there is no other way to stop the attack).

2. Humanitarian intervention by a state (or states) is exactly analogous to this type of personal intervention on behalf of seriously threatened victims.

3. Therefore, states have a duty of humanitarian intervention (under the right circumstances).

This argument is, of course, inductive—an argument by analogy. Probably few people would balk at Premise 1: it is a simple moral principle drawn from commonsense morality. Some might insist that a principle declaring that we have a *duty* to intervene is too strong—better to say that in the right circumstances, intervening is *morally permissible*, not obligatory. Though this complaint may have merit, let us stay with the original wording for simplicity's sake.

Premise 2 is the weak link here. For an argument by analogy to be strong, the two things being compared must be sufficiently similar in relevant ways. In this case, the intervention of an individual to halt an attack on another person must be relevantly similar to an intervention by sovereign states to stop aggression by another state against people within the state's borders. But noninterventionists might claim that the argument is weak because the personal and national circumstances are different in important respects. One difference is the well-established doctrine of international conduct that one sovereign state may not meddle in the internal affairs of another. This noninterference principle, says the noninterventionist, seems much stronger than any analogous rule on the personal level. Even interfering in a family conflict in which one family member is being brutally assaulted by the others may seem morally permissible sometimes, while analogous interference in a state's internal conflicts seems less morally clear cut.

There is much more that can be said both for and against Premise 2, but let us turn to another interventionist argument:

1. All persons have certain supremely important, basic rights—for example, rights to life, to self-determination, and to freedom from harm—rights that must not be violated by either people or states.

2. People who have these basic rights violated are entitled to use force to defend them, and it is morally permissible for other people or states to use force to help in that defense (humanitarian intervention).

3. People or states that violate others' basic rights forfeit their own right not to have force used against them.

4. Therefore, humanitarian intervention is morally permissible in defense of basic rights.

Interventionists are likely to get very little disagreement about either Premise 1 or Premise 3. For a majority of moral philosophers, the concepts of moral rights and their forfeiture are plausible elements in most of the major moral traditions. But Premise 2 is controversial. The idea of people using force in self-defense (to protect their lives or property, for example) is part of commonsense morality, but noninterventionists have questioned the defense of others' rights that involves crossing borders and violating state sovereignty. A critical problem, they would argue, is that the principle embodied in Premise 2 would have us ignore the rights of sovereign states to defend human rights—yet state sovereignty is itself a well-established principle of international relations. So we have a conflict of moral principles. In a utilitarian vein, noninterventionists may also argue that a policy of humanitarian intervention that ignores state sovereignty and attends to the countless violations of rights by a state could lead to perpetual wars everywhere. Some noninterventionists allow that intervention

may indeed be necessary in certain extraordinary cases involving genocide, massacres, and other extreme horrors. But they think that intervention should be reserved for these horrors, otherwise, perpetual war will in fact be the norm.

In this era of the "war on terror" and the worldwide threat of terrorist acts, moral arguments on terrorism are both extremely important and often controversial. Probably the liveliest—and, to some, the most disturbing—disputes have to do with the moral permissibility of terrorist acts. Consider the tragic events of September 11, 2001. Many people the world over assume without question that those who caused that horrific loss of life committed acts of terrorism that were morally wrong and monstrously evil. And many careful thinkers have come to the same conclusions, albeit by a more reflective, reasoned route. Plenty of people in both groups believe that terrorism is always morally wrong. But some equally reflective observers who are just as horrified by September 11 argue that terrorism may sometimes be permissible (and that many who disagree are being inconsistent, perhaps even hypocritical). We may even hear arguments for the permissibility of terrorism from people sympathetic to certain terrorist causes. Let us look more closely at some of these disputes. First, consider this argument:

1. If the killing of innocents is sometimes morally permissible in war, then it is morally permissible in terrorism (defined here as the intentional killing of innocents for political purposes).

2. The killing of innocents is sometimes morally permissible in war.

3. Therefore, the killing of innocents is sometimes morally permissible in terrorism.

This conclusion asserts that we cannot condemn all acts of terrorism out of hand, for some may be morally justified. The argument is that, as most people believe, killing innocents in wartime is sometimes permissible. Noncombatants are usually killed and maimed in war because combat so often happens near or among them. Still, most people are willing to accept this "collateral damage" as the inevitable—but regrettable—consequence of waging war. Some civilian deaths are unavoidable but morally permissible. Yet if they are morally acceptable in war, they must be morally acceptable aspects of terrorism. After all, both kinds of violence involve the death of innocents during hostilities directed at political ends.

Many critics of this argument would accept Premise 2 but reject Premise 1, insisting that there is a morally significant difference between the killing of innocents in war and in terrorist attacks. They would say that the killing of noncombatants in war is morally permissible because it is unintended; noncombatant deaths happen inadvertently as combatants are targeted. Terrorist killings, however, are wrong because they are intentional. The deliberate slaughter of innocents is never morally acceptable. Obviously, this response is an appeal to the doctrine of double effect.

But some would not accept this appeal, reasoning along the following lines:

> While the principle of double effect is plausible in some cases, it is severely defective. To see this, suppose that the September 11 attackers had only intended to destroy the Pentagon and the World Trade Center and had no desire to kill anyone. Suppose that they knew, however, that thousands would die in the attack on the buildings. And suppose, following the attack, they said "We are not murderers. We did not mean to kill these people."
>
> What would be our reaction? I very much doubt that we would think them less culpable. They could not successfully justify or excuse their actions by saying that although they foresaw the deaths of many people, these deaths were not part of their aim. We would certainly reject this defense. But if we would reject the appeal to double effect in this case, then we should do so in others.[24]

Not everyone would agree with this reasoning, but let us move on to a related argument:

1. Deliberately killing innocents for political or ideological reasons is morally wrong.
2. Deliberately killing noninnocents for such reasons may be morally permissible (as in war or revolution, for example).
3. Some people commonly thought to be innocents are actually noninnocents (they are pseudo-innocents).
4. Therefore, deliberately killing pseudo-innocents for political or ideological reasons may in some cases be morally permissible.

This argument states formally what is often alleged more casually: some actions usually condemned as instances of terrorism (involving the deliberate killing of innocents) are *not* terrorist acts at all because the "innocents" are not really innocent. This claim (common in some cultures and often uttered by terrorists themselves) is that some people should be judged noninnocents if they, for example, indirectly aid or sympathize with a hated regime, or happen to belong to the same race or religion as those presumed guilty of committing some acts of injustice or oppression, or are simply part of a system or enterprise that adversely affects a favored group. Such an attitude has been held by many, most infamously by Osama bin Laden:

> The ruling to kill the Americans and their allies—civilian and military—is an individual duty for every Muslim who can do it in any country in which it is possible to do, in order to liberate the Al Aksa Mosque and the holy mosque from their grip, and in order for their families to move out of all the lands of Islam, defeated and unable to threaten any Muslim.[25]

---

[24]Stephen Nathanson, "Can Terrorism Be Morally Justified?" in *Morality in Practice*, ed. James P. Sterba, 7th ed. (Belmont, CA: Wadsworth/Thomson, 2004), 607.

[25]From Jeffrey Goldberg, "Inside Jihad U.: The Education of a Holy Warrior," *New York Times Magazine,* June 2000; quoted in Louis P. Pojman, "The Moral Response to Terrorism and the Cosmopolitan Imperative," in *Terrorism and International Justice,* ed. James P. Sterba (New York: Oxford University Press, 2003).

The precise distinction between innocents and noninnocents (or combatants and noncombatants) in war is controversial among philosophers. But most of these thinkers do acknowledge a clear difference between the two concepts, and many reject the sort of blurring of the distinctions common among those who wish to justify terrorism. A typical argument against such justifications is that if the distinctions are discarded, then anyone and everyone could be deemed guilty and therefore a legitimate target of terrorism. For example, if ordinary individuals who buy bananas and thereby contribute to an economy run by a bloodthirsty dictatorship somehow share the blame for the regime's crimes, then any man, woman, or child could share the guilt—and deserve the terrorist's justice.

Attributing guilt to people because of such remote connections to wrongdoing, critics say, seems to reduce the notions of guilt and innocence to absurdity.

Probably the strongest—and most controversial—argument for the political use of torture is based on the so-called ticking-bomb scenario. Suppose a bomb will soon detonate in a major American city, killing a hundred thousand innocent people. The only way to prevent this massive loss of life is to torture the terrorist who planted the bomb until he reveals its location. Would it be morally permissible to waterboard or electrocute him until he talks? (Note that this is a separate question from torture's legality.) Many think the obvious answer is yes and that there is strong moral justification for using torture in this case. What considerations could lead to this conclusion? Here is one philosopher's answer (referring to a similar version of the ticking-bomb situation):

> Consider the following points: (1) The police reasonably believe that torturing the terrorist will probably save thousands of lives; (2) the police know that there is no other way to save those lives; (3) the threat to

QUICK REVIEW

realism (as applied to warfare)—The view that moral standards are not applicable to war, and that war instead must be judged on how well it serves state interests.

pacifism—The view that war is never morally permissible.

just war theory—The doctrine that war may be morally permissible under stipulated conditions.

jus ad bellum—The justification for resorting to war; the justice of war.

jus in bello—The moral permissibility of acts in war; justice in war.

noncombatant immunity—The status of a person who should not be intentionally attacked in war.

terrorism (as defined in this chapter)—Violence against noncombatants for political, religious, or ideological ends.

terrorism (the definition preferred by the U.S. State Department)—Premeditated, politically motivated violence perpetrated against noncombatant targets by subnational groups or clandestine agents, usually intended to influence an audience.

nonstate actors—Individuals or groups that are not sovereign states.

torture—The intentional inflicting of severe pain or suffering on people to punish or intimidate them or extract information from them.

humanitarian intervention—The act of a state (or states) going to war to defend people of another state against the murderous aggression of their own regime.

life is more or less imminent; (4) the thousands about to be murdered are innocent—the terrorist has no good, let alone decisive, justificatory moral reason for murdering them; (5) the terrorist is known to be (jointly with other terrorists) morally responsible for planning, transporting, and arming the nuclear device and, if it explodes, he will be (jointly with other terrorists) morally responsible for the murder of thousands.[26]

Some take a deontological approach to this issue and declare that torture is always wrong in all circumstances (a common absolutist position). Critics of this view say that it is suspect because torturing people usually seems to be morally not as bad as killing them. If so, it would be implausible to assert that torturing the terrorist is absolutely forbidden but that not torturing him and letting thousands die would be morally permissible.

Others who are opposed to torture believe that ticking-bomb scenarios are too contrived to be taken seriously; such states of affairs simply don't happen in the real world. The usual response to this is that in light of what we know about terrorist tactics and aims (and about police cases that resemble ticking-bomb scenarios), we have good reasons to believe the opposite—ticking-bomb situations are indeed possible.

SUMMARY

Political violence is the resort to violence for political ends. War, terrorism, torture, revolution, assassination, civil war, and violent demonstrations are examples. Violence is the physical or psychological attack on, or the vigorous abuse of, persons, causing their suffering, injury, or death. (Violence can also involve the destroying or damaging of property.) Violence is considered prima facie wrong—wrong unless there are good rea-

sons for thinking it morally permissible. Thus people often speak of war and other modes of violence as things to be *resorted to*, actions to be taken only after other options are exhausted.

Violence is thought to be wrong for several reasons. Some argue that violence constitutes a violation of people's rights—their right to life, self-determination, respect as a person, or immunity from harm. Another view is that violence is wrong because it runs afoul of the moral principles of justice, freedom, and utility (human welfare). The consequentialist position is that violence is (generally) wrong because its bad consequences (usually) outweigh the good.

The main ethical questions regarding war and peace are (1) how—if at all—can the resort to war be justified? and (2) assuming it can be justified, how should it be conducted? Most serious answers to such questions come from three distinct perspectives. Realism is the view that moral standards are not applicable to war, though considerations of prudence are. Pacifism is the view that war is never morally permissible. Just war theory is the doctrine that war may be morally permissible under stipulated conditions.

Depending on how they judge the empirical evidence, utilitarians may with logical consistency take either a pacifist or nonpacifist stand on war. Nonconsequentialists may also consistently support or reject pacifism. Pacifists typically rest their case on the nonconsequentialist principle of the right to life. Nonpacifists may back their case with the nonconsequentialist principles of the right to self-defense or of human rights generally.

Terrorism is violence against noncombatants for political, religious, or ideological ends. The key question that terrorism provokes is, What should be our moral response to it? Should it always and everywhere be condemned? Or is terrorism sometimes justified? One way to grapple with terrorism is to try to apply the requirements of just war theory to terrorist acts. Many philosophers argue that by the lights of just war theory, terrorism is never morally permissible. Others contend that it is possible for terrorism to meet just war criteria and thereby prove itself justified. Even without reference to just war theory, some argue that terrorism is always wrong because

[26]Seumas Miller, "Torture," *Stanford Encyclopedia of Philosophy*, 29 April 2011, http://plato.stanford.edu/entries/torture/ (26 February 2015).

it violates the victims' right to be treated as moral persons, or because it is an indiscriminate attack on the innocent.

A consequentialist moral theory would likely condone terrorism if it maximized happiness or welfare for all concerned, but in actual cases this requirement may make terrorism very difficult to justify.

Torture is the intentional inflicting of severe pain or suffering on people to punish or intimidate them or to extract information from them. Three issues dominate the debates over the morality of torture: (1) Does torture work? (2) Is torture ever morally acceptable? and (3) What should be the state's policy regarding the use of torture?

READINGS

Reconciling Pacifists and Just War Theorists

James P. Sterba

Traditionally pacifism and just war theory have represented radically opposed responses to aggression. Pacifism has been interpreted to rule out any use of violence in response to aggression. Just war theory has been interpreted to permit a measured use of violence in response to aggression. It has been thought that the two views might sometimes agree in particular cases—for example, that pacifists and just war theorists might unconditionally oppose nuclear war, but beyond that it has been generally held that the two views lead to radically opposed recommendations. In this paper, I hope to show that this is not the case. I will argue that pacifism and just war theory, in their most morally defensible interpretations, can be substantially reconciled both in theory and practice.

In traditional just war theory there are two basic elements: an account of just cause and an account of just means. Just cause is usually specified as follows:

1) There must be substantial aggression;
2) Nonbelligerent correctives must be either hopeless or too costly; and
3) Belligerent correctives must be neither hopeless nor too costly.

Needless to say, the notion of substantial aggression is a bit fuzzy, but it is generally understood to be the

James P. Sterba, Excerpts from "Reconciling Pacifists and Just War Theorists," *Social Theory and Practice* Vol.18, No. 1 (Spring 1992): 21–38. Reprinted with permission of Social Theory and Practice.

type of aggression that violates people's most fundamental rights. To suggest some specific examples of what is and is not substantial aggression, usually the taking of hostages is regarded as substantial aggression while the nationalization of particular firms owned by foreigners is not so regarded. But even when substantial aggression occurs, frequently nonbelligerent correctives are neither hopeless nor too costly. And even when nonbelligerent correctives are either hopeless or too costly, in order for there to be a just cause, belligerent correctives must be neither hopeless nor too costly.

Traditional just war theory assumes, however, that there are just causes and goes on to specify just means as imposing two requirements:

1) Harm to innocents should not be directly intended as an end or a means.
2) The harm resulting from the belligerent means should not be disproportionate to the particular defensive objective to be attained.

While the just means conditions apply to each defensive action, the just cause conditions must be met by the conflict as a whole.

It is important to note that these requirements of just cause and just means are not essentially about war at all. Essentially, they constitute a theory of just defense that can apply to war but can also apply to a wide range of defensive actions short of war. Of course, what needs to be determined is whether these requirements can be justified. Since just war theory is usually opposed to pacifism, to secure a non-question-begging justification for the theory and its requirements we need to proceed as much as possible from premises that are common to pacifists and just war theorists alike. The difficulty here is that there is not just one form of pacifism but many. So we need to determine which form of pacifism is most morally defensible.

Now when most people think of pacifism they tend to identify it with a theory of nonviolence. We can call this view "nonviolent pacifism." It maintains that:

> Any use of violence against other human beings is morally prohibited.

It has been plausibly argued, however, that this form of pacifism is incoherent. In a well-known article, Jan Narveson rejects nonviolent pacifism as incoherent because it recognizes a right to life yet rules out any use of force in defense of that right.[1] The view is incoherent, Narveson claims, because having a right entails the legitimacy of using force in defense of that right at least on some occasions.

Given the cogency of objections of this sort, some have opted for a form of pacifism that does not rule out all violence but only lethal violence. We can call this view "nonlethal pacifism." It maintains that

> Any lethal use of force against other human beings is morally prohibited.

In defense of nonlethal pacifism, Cheyney Ryan has argued that there is a substantial issue between the pacifist and the nonpacifist concerning whether we can or should create the necessary distance between ourselves and other human beings in order to make the act of killing possible.[2] To illustrate, Ryan cites George Orwell's reluctance to shoot at an enemy soldier who jumped out of a trench and ran along the top of a parapet half-dressed and holding up his trousers with both hands. Ryan contends that what kept Orwell from shooting was that he couldn't think of the soldier as a thing rather than a fellow human being.

However, it is not clear that Orwell's encounter supports nonlethal pacifism. For it may be that what kept Orwell from shooting the enemy soldier was not his inability to think of the soldier as a thing rather

than a fellow human being but rather his inability to think of the soldier who was holding up his trousers with both hands as a threat or a combatant. Under this interpretation, Orwell's decision not to shoot would accord well with the requirements of just war theory.

Let us suppose, however, that someone is attempting to take your life. Why does that permit you, the defender of nonlethal pacifism might ask, to kill the person making the attempt? The most cogent response, it seems to me, is that killing in such a case is not evil, or at least not morally evil, because anyone who is wrongfully engaged in an attempt upon your life has already forfeited his or her right to life by engaging in such aggression.[3] So, provided that you are reasonably certain that the aggressor is wrongfully engaged in an attempt upon your life, you would be morally justified in killing, assuming that it is the only way of saving your own life.

There is, however, a form of pacifism that remains untouched by the criticisms I have raised against both nonviolent pacifism and nonlethal pacifism. This form of pacifism neither prohibits all violence nor even all uses of lethal force. We can call the view "anti-war pacifism" because it holds that

> Any participation in the massive use of lethal force in warfare is morally prohibited.

In defense of anti-war pacifism, it is undeniable that wars have brought enormous amounts of death and destruction in their wake and that many of those who have perished in them are noncombatants or innocents. In fact, the tendency of modern wars has been to produce higher and higher proportions of noncombatant casualties, making it more and more difficult to justify participation in such wars. At the same time, strategies for nonbelligerent conflict resolution are rarely intensively developed and explored before nations choose to go to war, making it all but impossible to justify participation in such wars.

To determine whether the requirements of just war theory can be reconciled with those of anti-war pacifism, however, we need to consider whether we should distinguish between harm intentionally inflicted upon innocents and harm whose infliction of innocents is merely foreseen. On the one hand, we could favor a uniform restriction against the infliction of harm upon innocents that ignores the intended/foreseen distinction. On the other hand, we could favor a differential restriction which is more severe against the intentional infliction of harm upon innocents but is less severe against the infliction of harm that is merely foreseen. What needs to be determined, therefore, is whether there is any rationale for favoring this differential restriction on harm over a uniform restriction. But this presupposes that we can, in practice, distinguish between what is foreseen and what is intended, and some have challenged whether this can be done. So first we need to address this challenge.

Now the practical test that is frequently appealed to in order to distinguish between foreseen and intended elements of an action is the Counterfactual Test. According to this test, two questions are relevant:

1) Would you have performed the action if only the good consequences would have resulted and not the evil consequences?
2) Would you have performed the action if only the evil consequences resulted and not the good consequences?

If an agent answers "Yes" to the first question and "No" to the second, some would conclude that (1) the action is an intended means to the good consequences; (2) the good consequences are an intended end; and (3) the evil consequences are merely foreseen.

But how well does this Counterfactual Test work? Douglas Lackey has argued that the test gives the wrong result in any case where the "act that produces an evil effect produces a larger good effect."[4] Lackey cites the bombing of Hiroshima as an example. That bombing is generally thought to have had two effects: the killing of Japanese civilians and the shortening of the war. Now suppose we were to ask:

1) Would Truman have dropped the bomb if only the shortening of the war would have resulted but not the killing of the Japanese civilians?
2) Would Truman have dropped the bomb if only the Japanese civilians would have been killed and the war not shortened?

And suppose that the answer to the first question is that Truman would have dropped the bomb if only the shortening of the war would have resulted but not the killing of the Japanese civilians, and the answer to the second question is that Truman would not have dropped the bomb if only the Japanese civilians would have been killed and the war not shortened. Lackey concludes from this that the killing of civilians at Hiroshima, self-evidently a means for shortening the war, is by the Counterfactual Test classified not as a means but as a mere foreseen consequence. On these grounds, Lackey rejects the Counterfactual Test as an effective device for distinguishing between the foreseen and the intended consequences of an action.

Unfortunately, this is to reject the Counterfactual Test only because one expects too much from it. It is to expect the test to determine all of the following:

1) Whether the action is an intended means to the good consequences;
2) Whether the good consequences are an intended end of the action; and
3) Whether the evil consequences are simply foreseen consequences.

In fact, this test is only capable of meeting the first two of these expectations. And the test clearly succeeds in doing this for Lackey's own example, where the test shows the bombing of Hiroshima to be an intended means to shortening the war, and shortening the war an intended consequence of the action.

To determine whether the evil consequences are simply foreseen consequences, however, an additional test is needed, which I shall call the Nonexplanation Test. According to this test, the relevant question is:

> Does the bringing about of the evil consequences help explain why the agent undertook the action as a means to the good consequences?

If the answer is "No," that is, if the bringing about of the evil consequences does not help explain why the agent undertook the action as a means to the good consequences, the evil consequences are merely foreseen. But if the answer is "Yes," the evil consequences are an intended means to the good consequences.

Of course, there is no guaranteed procedure for arriving at an answer to the Nonexplanation Test. Nevertheless, when we are in doubt concerning whether the evil consequences of an act are simply foreseen, seeking an answer to the Nonexplanation Test will tend to be the best way of reasonably resolving that doubt. For example, applied to Lackey's example, the Nonexplanation Test comes up with a "Yes," since the evil consequences in this example do help explain why the bombing was undertaken to shorten the war. For according to the usual account, Truman ordered the bombing to bring about the civilian deaths which by their impact upon Japanese morale were expected to shorten the war. So, by the Nonexplanation Test, the civilian deaths were an intended means to the good consequences of shortening the war.

Assuming then that we can distinguish in practice between harm intentionally inflicted upon innocents and harm whose infliction on innocents is merely foreseen, we need to determine whether there is any rationale for favoring a differential restriction that is more severe against the intentional infliction of harm upon innocents but is less severe against the infliction of harm that is merely foreseen over a uniform restriction against the infliction of harm upon innocents that ignores the intended/foreseen distinction.

Let us first examine the question from the perspective of those suffering the harm. Initially, it might appear to matter little whether the harm would be intended or just foreseen by those who cause it. From the perspective of those suffering harm, it might appear that what matters is simply that the overall amount of harm be restricted irrespective of whether it is foreseen or intended. But consider—don't those who suffer harm have more reason to protest when the harm is done to them by agents who are directly engaged in causing harm to them than when the harm is done incidentally by agents whose ends and means are good? Don't we have more reason to protest when we are being used by others than when we are affected by them only incidentally?

Moreover, if we examine the question from the perspective of those causing harm, additional support for this line of reasoning can be found. For it would seem that we have more reason to protest a restriction against foreseen harm than we have reason to protest a comparable restriction against intended harm. This is because a restriction against foreseen harm limits our actions when our ends and means are good whereas a restriction against intended harm only limits our actions when our ends or means are evil or harmful, and it would seem that we have greater grounds for acting when both our ends and means are good than when they are not. Consequently, because we have more reason to protest when we are being used by others than when we are being affected by them only incidentally, and because we have more reason to act when both our ends and means are good than when they are not, we should favor the foreseen/intended distinction that is incorporated into just means.

It might be objected, however, that at least sometimes we could produce greater good overall by violating the foreseen/intended distinction of just means and acting with the evil means of intentionally harming innocents. On this account, it might be argued that it should be permissible at least sometimes to intentionally harm innocents in order to achieve greater good overall.

Now it seems to me that this objection is well-taken in so far as it is directed against an absolute restriction upon intentional harm to innocents. It seems clear that there are expectations to such a restriction when intentional harm to innocents is:

1) trivial (for example, as in the case of stepping on someone's foot to get out of a crowded subway);
2) easily repairable (for example, as in the case of lying to a temporarily depressed friend to keep him from committing suicide); or
3) greatly outweighed by the consequences of the action, especially to innocent people (for example, as in the case of shooting one of two hundred civilian hostages to prevent in the only way possible the execution of all two hundred).

Yet while we need to recognize these executions to an absolute restriction upon intentional harm to innocents, there is good reason not to permit simply maximizing good consequences overall because that would place unacceptable burdens upon particular individuals. More specifically, it would be an unacceptable burden on innocents to allow them to be intentionally harmed in cases other than the exceptions we have just enumerated. And, allowing for these exceptions, we would still have reason to favor a differential restriction against harming innocents that is more severe against the intentional infliction of harm upon innocents but is less severe against the infliction of harm upon innocents that is merely foreseen. Again, the main grounds for this preference is that we would have more reason to protest when we are being used by others than when we are being affected by them only incidentally, and more reason to act when both our ends and means are good than when they are not.

So far, I have argued that there are grounds for favoring a differential restriction on harm to innocents that is more severe against intended harm and less severe against foreseen harm. I have further argued that this restriction is not absolute so that when the evil intended is trivial, easily repairable or greatly outweighed by the consequences, intentional harm to innocents can be justified. Moreover, there is no reason to think that anti-war pacifists would reject either of these conclusions. Anti-war pacifists are opposed to any participation in the massive use of lethal force in warfare, yet this need not conflict with the commitment of just war theorists to a differential but nonabsolute restriction on harm to innocents as a requirement of just means.[5] Where just war theory goes wrong, according to anti-war pacifists, is not in its restriction on harming innocents but rather in its failure to adequately determine when belligerent correctives are too costly to constitute a just cause or lacking in the proportionality required by just means. According to anti-war pacifists, just war theory provides insufficient restraint in both of these areas. Now to evaluate this criticism, we need to consider a wide range of cases where killing or inflicting serious harm on others in defense of oneself or others might be thought to be justified, beginning with the easiest cases to assess from the perspectives of anti-war pacifism and the just war theory and then moving on to cases that are more difficult to assess from those perspectives.

Case 1 where only the intentional or foreseen killing of an unjust aggressor would prevent one's own death.[6] This case clearly presents no problems. In the first place, anti-war pacifists adopted their view because they were convinced that there were instances of justified killing. And, in this case, the only person killed is an unjust aggressor. So surely anti-war pacifists would have to agree with just war theorists that one justifiably kill an unjust aggressor if it is the only way to save one's life.

Case 2 where only the intentional or foreseen killing of an unjust aggressor and the foreseen killing of one innocent bystander would prevent one's own death and that of five other innocent people.[7] In this case, we have the foreseen killing of an innocent person as well as the killing of the unjust aggressor, but since it is the only way to save one's own life and the lives of five other innocent people, anti-war pacifists and just war theorists alike would have reason to judge it morally permissible. In this case, the intended life-saving benefits to six innocent people is judged to outweigh the foreseen death of one innocent person and the intended or foreseen death of the unjust aggressor.

Case 3 where only the intentional or foreseen killing of an unjust aggressor and the foreseen killing of one innocent bystander would prevent the death of five other innocent people. In this case, despite the fact that we lack the justification of self-defense, saving the lives of five innocent people in the only way possible should still provide anti-war pacifists and just war theorists with sufficient grounds for granting the moral permissibility of killing an unjust aggressor, even when the killing of an innocent bystander is a foreseen consequence. In this case, the intended lifesaving benefits to five innocent people would still outweigh the foreseen death of one innocent person and the intended or foreseen death of the unjust aggressor.

Case 4 where only the intentional or foreseen killing of an unjust aggressor and the foreseen killing of five innocent people would prevent the death of two innocent people. In this case, neither anti-war pacifists nor just war theorists would find the cost and proportionality requirements of just war theory to be met. Too many innocent people would have to be killed to save too few. Here the fact that the deaths of the innocents would be merely foreseen does not outweigh the fact that we would have to accept the deaths of five innocents and the death of the unjust aggressor in order to be able to save two innocents.

Notice that up to this point in interpreting these cases, we have simply been counting the number of innocent deaths involved in each case and opting for whichever solution minimized the loss of innocent lives that would result. Suppose, however, that an unjust aggressor is not threatening the lives of innocents but only their welfare or property. Would the taking of the unjust aggressor's life in defense of the welfare and property of innocents be judged proportionate? Consider the following case.

Case 5 where only the intentional or foreseen killing of an unjust aggressor would prevent serious injury to oneself and five other innocent people. Since in this case the intentional or foreseen killing of the unjust aggressor is the only way of preventing serious injury to oneself and five other innocent people, then, by analogy with Cases 1–3, both anti-war pacifists and just war theorists alike would have reason to affirm its moral permissibility. Of course, if there were any other way of stopping unjust aggressors in such cases short of killing them, that course of action would clearly be required. Yet if there is no alternative, the intentional or foreseen killing of the unjust aggressor to prevent serious injury to oneself and/or five other innocent people would be justified.

In such cases, the serious injury could be bodily injury, as when an aggressor threatens to break one's limbs, or it could be serious psychological injury, as when an aggressor threatens to inject mind-altering drugs, or it could be a serious threat to property. Of course, in most cases where serious injury is threatened, there will be ways of stopping aggressors short of killing them. Unfortunately, this is not always possible.

In still other kinds of cases, stopping an unjust aggressor would require indirectly inflicting serious harm, but not death, upon innocent bystanders. Consider the following cases.

Case 6 where only the intentional or foreseen infliction of serious harm upon an unjust aggressor and the foreseen infliction of serious harm upon one innocent bystander would prevent serious harm to oneself and five other innocent people.

Case 7 where only the intentional or foreseen infliction of serious harm upon an unjust aggressor and the foreseen infliction of serious harm upon one innocent bystander would prevent serious harm to five other innocent people.

In both of these cases, serious harm is indirectly inflicted upon one innocent bystander in order to pre-vent greater harm from being inflicted by an unjust aggressor upon other innocent people. In Case 6, we also have the justification of self-defense, which is lacking in Case 7. Nevertheless, with regard to both cases, anti-war pacifists and just war theorists should agree that preventing serious injury to five or six innocent people in the only way possible renders it morally permissible to inflict serious injury upon an unjust aggressor, even when the serious injury of one innocent person is a foreseen consequence. In these cases, by analogy with Cases 2 and 3, the foreseen serious injury of one innocent person and the intended or foreseen injury of the unjust aggressor should be judged proportionate given the intended injury-preventing benefits to five or six other innocent people.

Up to this point there has been the basis for general agreement among anti-war pacifists and just war theorists as to how to interpret the proportionality requirement of just means, but in the following case this no longer obtains.

Case 8 where only the intentional or foreseen killing of an unjust aggressor and the foreseen killing of one innocent bystander would prevent serious injuries to the members of a much larger group of people.

The interpretation of this case is crucial. In this case, we are asked to sanction the loss of an innocent life in order to prevent serious injuries to the members of a much larger group of people. Unfortunately, neither anti-war pacifists nor just war theorists have explicitly considered this case. Both anti-war pacifists and just war theorists agree that we can inflict serious injury upon an unjust aggressor and an innocent bystander to prevent greater injury to other innocent people, as in Cases 6 and 7, and that one can even intentionally or indirectly kill an unjust aggressor to prevent serious injury to oneself or other innocent people as in Case 5. Yet neither anti-war pacifists nor just war theorists have explicitly addressed the question of whether we can indirectly kill an innocent bystander in order to prevent serious injuries to the members of a much larger group of innocent people. Rather they have tended to confuse Case 8 with Case 5 where it is agreed that one can justifiably kill an unjust aggressor in order to prevent serious injury to oneself or five other innocent people. In Case 8, however, one is doing something quite different: one is killing an innocent bystander in order to prevent serious injury to oneself and five other innocent people.

Now this kind of trade-off is not accepted in standard police practice. Police officers are regularly instructed not to risk innocent lives simply to prevent serious injury to other innocents. Nor is there any reason to think that a trade-off that is unacceptable in standard police practice would be acceptable in larger scale conflicts. Thus, for example, even if the Baltic republics could have effectively freed themselves from the Soviet Union by infiltrating into Moscow several bands of saboteurs who would then attack several military and government installations in Moscow, causing an enormous loss of innocent lives, such trade-offs would not have been justified. Accordingly, it follows that if the proportionality requirement of just war theory is to be met, we must save more innocent lives than we cause to be lost, we must prevent more injuries than we bring about, and we must not kill innocents, even indirectly, simply to prevent serious injuries to ourselves and others.

Of course, sometimes our lives and well-being are threatened together. Or better, if we are unwilling to sacrifice our well-being then our lives are threatened as well. Nevertheless, if we are justified in our use of lethal force to defend ourselves in cases where we will indirectly kill innocents, it is because our lives are also threatened, not simply our well-being. And the same holds for when we are defending others.

What this shows is that the constraints imposed by just war theory on the use of belligerent correctives are actually much more severe than anti-war pacifists have tended to recognize. In determining when belligerent correctives are too costly to constitute a just cause or lacking in the proportionality required by just means, just war theory under its most morally defensible interpretation:

1) allows the use of belligerent means against unjust aggressors only when such means minimize the loss and injury to innocent lives overall;
2) allows the use of belligerent means against unjust aggressors to indirectly threaten innocent lives only

to prevent the loss of innocent lives, not simply to prevent injury to innocents; and

3) allows the use of belligerent means to directly or indirectly threaten or even take the lives of unjust aggressors when it is the only way to prevent serious injury to innocents.

Now it might be objected that all that I have shown through the analysis of the above eight cases is that killing in defense of oneself or others is morally permissible, not that it is morally required or morally obligatory. That is true. I have not established any obligation to respond to aggression with lethal force in these cases, but only that it is morally permissible to do so. For one thing, it is difficult to ground an obligation to use lethal force on self-defense alone, as would be required in Case 1 or in one version of Case 5. Obligations to oneself appear to have an optional quality that is absent from obligations to others. In Cases 2–3 and 5–7, however, the use of force would prevent serious harm or death to innocents, and here I contend it would be morally obligatory if either the proposed use of force required only a relatively small personal sacrifice from us or if we were fairly bound by convention or a mutual defense agreement to come to the aid of others. In such cases, I think we can justifiably speak of a moral obligation to kill or seriously harm in defense of others.

Another aspect of Cases 1–3 and 5–7 to which someone might object is that it is the wrongful actions of others that put us into situations where I am claiming that we are morally justified in seriously harming or killing others. But for the actions of unjust aggressors, we would not be in situations where I am claiming that we are morally permitted or required to seriously harm or kill.

Yet doesn't something like this happen in a wide range of cases when wrongful actions are performed? Suppose I am on the way to the bank to deposit money from a fund-raiser, and someone accosts me and threatens to shoot me if I don't hand over the money. If I do hand over the money, I would be forced to do something I don't want to do, something that involves a loss to myself and others. But surely it is morally permissible for me to hand over the money in this case. And it may even be morally required for me to do so if resistance would lead to the shooting of others in addition to myself. So it does seem that bad people, by altering the consequences of our actions, can alter our obligations as well. What our obligations are under nonideal conditions are different from what they would be under ideal conditions. If a group of thugs comes into this room and make it very clear that they intend to shoot me if each of you doesn't give them one dollar, I think, and I would hope that you would also think, that each of you now has an obligation to give the thugs one dollar when before you had no such obligation. Likewise, I think that the actions of unjust aggressors can put us into situations where it is morally permissible or even morally required for us to seriously harm or kill when before it was not.

Now it might be contended that anti-war pacifists would concede the moral permissibility of Cases 1–3 and 5–7 but still maintain that any participation in the massive use of lethal force in warfare is morally prohibited. The scale of the conflict, anti-war pacifists might contend, makes all the difference. Of course, if this simply means that many large-scale conflicts will have effects that bear no resemblance to Cases 1–3 or 5–7, this can hardly be denied. Still, it is possible for some large-scale conflicts to bear a proportionate resemblance to the above cases. For example, it can be argued plausibly that India's military action against Pakistan in Bangladesh and the Tanzanian incursion into Uganda during the rule of Idi Amin resemble Cases 3, 5, or 7 in their effects upon innocents.[8] What this shows is that anti-war pacifists are not justified in regarding every participation in the massive use of lethal force in warfare as morally prohibited. Instead, anti-war pacifists must allow that at least in some real-life cases, wars and other large-scale military operations both have been and will be morally permissible.

This concession from anti-war pacifists, however, needs to be matched by a comparable concession from just war theorists themselves, because too frequently they have interpreted their theory in morally indefensible ways. When just war theory is given a morally defensible interpretation, I have argued that the theory favors a strong just means prohibition against intentionally harming innocents. I have also argued that the theory favors the use of belligerent means only when such means 1) minimize the loss and injury to innocent lives overall; 2) threaten innocent lives only to prevent the loss of innocent lives, not simply to prevent injury to innocents; and 3) threaten or even take the lives of unjust aggressors when it is the only way to prevent serious injury to innocents.

Obviously, just war theory, so understood, is going to place severe restrictions on the use of belligerent means in warfare. In fact, most of the actual uses of belligerent means in warfare that have occurred turn out to be unjustified. For example, the U.S. involvement in Nicaragua, El Salvador, and Panama, Soviet involvement in Afghanistan, Israeli involvement in the West Bank and the Gaza Strip all violate the just cause and just means provisions of just war theory as I have defended them. Even the recent U.S.-led war against Iraq violated both the just cause and just means provisions of just war theory.[9] In fact, one strains to find examples of justified applications of just war theory in recent history. Two examples I have already referred to are India's military action against Pakistan in Bangladesh and the Tanzanian incursion into Uganda during the rule of Idi Amin. But after mentioning these two examples it is difficult to go on. What this shows is that when just war theory and anti-war pacifism are given their most morally defensible interpretations, both views can be reconciled. In this reconciliation, the few wars and large-scale conflicts that meet the stringent requirements of just war theory are the only wars and large-scale conflicts to which anti-war pacifists cannot justifiably object.[10] We can call the view that emerges from this reconciliation "just war pacifism." It is the view which claims that due to the stringent requirements of just war theory, only very rarely will participation in a massive use of lethal force in warfare be morally justified. It is the view on which I rest my case for the reconciliation of pacifism and just war theory.[11]

NOTES

1. Jan Narveson, "Pacifism: A Philosophical Analysis," *Ethics* 75 (1965): 259–71.

2. Cheyney Ryan, "Self-Defense, Pacifism and the Possibility of Killing," *Ethics* 93 (1983): 514–24.

3. Alternatively, one might concede that even in this case killing is morally evil, but still contend that it is morally justified because it is the lesser of two evils.

4. Douglas P. Lackey, "The Moral Irrelevance of the Counterforce/Countervalue Distinction," *The Monist* 70 (1987): 255–76.

5. This is because the just means restrictions protect innocents quite well against the infliction of intentional harm.

6. By an "unjust aggressor" I mean someone who the defender is reasonably certain is wrongfully engaged in an attempt upon her life or the lives of other innocent people.

7. What is relevant in this case is that the foreseen deaths are a relatively small number (one in this case) compared to the number of innocents whose lives are saved (six in this case). The primary reason for using particular numbers in this case and those that follow is to make it clear that at this stage of the argument no attempt is being made to justify the large-scale killing that occurs in warfare.

8. Although there is a strong case for India's military action against Pakistan in Bangladesh and the Tanzanian incursion into Uganda during the rule of Idi Amin, there are questions that can be raised about the behavior of Indian troops in Bangladesh following the defeat of the Pakistanian forces and about the regime Tanzania put in power in Uganda.

9. The just cause provision was violated because the extremely effective economic sanctions were not given enough time to work. It was estimated that when compared to past economic blockades, the blockade against Iraq had a near 100% chance of success if given about a year to work. (See *The New York Times*, January 14, 1991.) The just means provision was violated because the number of combatant and noncombatant deaths was disproportionate. As many as 120,000 Iraqi soldiers were killed, according to U.S. intelligence sources.

10. Of course, anti-war pacifists are right to point out that virtually all wars that have been fought have led to unforeseen harms and have been fought with less and less discrimination as the wars progressed. Obviously, these are considerations that in just war theory must weigh heavily against going to war.

11. Of course, more needs to be done to specify the requirements of just war pacifism. One fruitful way to further specify these requirements is to appeal to a hypothetical social contract decision procedure as has been done with respect to other practical problems. Here I have simply tried to establish the defensibility of just war pacifism without appealing to any such procedure. Yet once the defensibility of just war pacifism has been established, such a decision procedure will prove quite useful in working out its particular requirements.

Against "Realism"

MICHAEL WALZER

For as long as men and women have talked about war, they have talked about it in terms of right and wrong. And for almost as long, some among them have derided such talk, called it a charade, insisted that war lies beyond (or beneath) moral judgment. War is a world apart, where life itself is at stake, where human nature is reduced to its elemental forms, where self-

interest and necessity prevail. Here men and women do what they must to save themselves and their communities, and morality and law have no place. *Inter arma dilent leges*: in time of war the law is silent.

Sometimes this silence is extended to other forms of competitive activity, as in the popular proverb, "All's fair in love and war." That means that anything goes—any kind of deceit in love, any kind of violence in war. We can neither praise nor blame; there is nothing to say. And yet we are rarely silent. The language we use to talk about love and war is so rich with moral meaning that it could hardly have been developed except through centuries of argument. Faithfulness, devotion, chastity, shame, adultery, seduction, betrayal; aggressive, self-defense, appeasement, cruelty, ruthlessness, atrocity, massacre—all these words are judgments, and judging is as common a human activity as loving or fighting.

It is true, however, that we often lack the courage of our judgments, and especially so in the case of military conflict. The moral posture of mankind is not well represented by that popular proverb about love and war. We would do better to mark a contrast rather than a similarity: before Venus, censorious; before Mars, timid. Not that we don't justify or condemn particular attacks, but we do so hesitantly and uncertainly (or loudly and recklessly), as if we were not sure that our judgments reach to the reality of war.

THE REALIST ARGUMENT

Realism is the issue. The defenders of *silent leges* claim to have discovered an awful truth: what we conventionally call inhumanity is simply humanity under pressure. War strips away our civilized adornments and reveals our nakedness. They describe that nakedness for us, not without a certain relish: fearful, self-concerned, driven, murderous. They aren't wrong in any simple sense. The words are sometimes descriptive. Paradoxically, the description is often a kind of apology: yes, our soldiers committed atrocities in the course of the battle, but that's what war does to people, that's what war is like. The proverb, all's fair, is invoked in defense of conduct that appears to be unfair. And one urges silence on the law when one is engaged in activities that would otherwise be called unlawful. So there are arguments here that will enter into my own argument: justifications and excuses, references to necessity and duress, that we can recognize as forms of moral discourse and that have or don't have force in particular cases. But there is also a general account of war as a realm of necessity and duress, the purpose of which is to make discourse about particular cases appear to be ideal chatter, a mask of noise with which we conceal, even from ourselves, the awful truth. It is that general account that I have to challenge before I can begin my own work, and I want to challenge it at its source and in its most compelling

form, as it is put forward by the historian Thucydides and the philosopher Thomas Hobbes. These two men, separated by 2,000 years, are collaborators of a kind, for Hobbes translated Thucydides' *History of the Peloponnesian Wars* and then generalized its argument in his own *Leviathan*. It is not my purpose here to write a full philosophical response to Thucydides and Hobbes. I wish only to suggest, first by argument and then by example, that the judgment of war and of wartime conduct is a serious enterprise.

The Melian Dialogue

The dialogue between the Athenian generals Cleomedes and Tisias and the magistrates of the island state of Melos is one of the high points of Thucydides' *History* and the climax of his realism. Melos was a Spartan colony, and its people had "therefore refused to be subject, as the rest of the islands were, unto the Athenians; but rested at first neutral; and afterwards, when the Athenians put them to it by wasting of their lands, they entered into open war."[1] This is a classic account of aggression, for to commit aggression is simply to "put people to it" as Thucydides describes. But such a description, he seems to say, is merely external; he wants to show us the inner meaning of war. His spokesmen are the two Athenian generals, who demand a parley and then speak as generals have rarely done in military history. Let us have no fine words about justice, they say. We for our part will not pretend that, having defeated the Persians, our empire is deserved; you must not claim that having done no injury to the Athenian people, you have a right to be let alone. We will talk instead of what is feasible and what is necessary. For this is what war is really like: "they that have odds of power exact as much as they can, and the weak yield to such conditions as they can get."

It is not only the Melians here who bear the burdens of necessity. The Athenians are driven, too; they must expand their empire, Cleomedes and Tisias believe, or lose what they already have. The neutrality of Melos "will be an argument of our weakness, and your hatred of our power, among those we have rule over." It will inspire rebellion throughout the islands, wherever men and women are "offended with the necessity of subjection"—and what subject is not offended, eager for freedom, resentful of his con-querors? When the Athenian generals say that men "will everywhere reign over such as they be too strong for," they are not only describing the desire for glory and command, but also the more narrow necessity of inter-state politics: reign or be subject. If they do not conquer when they can, they only reveal weakness and invite attack; and so, "by a necessity of nature" (a phrase Hobbes later made his own), they conquer when they can.

The Melians, on the other hand, are too weak to conquer. They face a harsher necessity: yield or be destroyed. "For you have not in hand a match of valor upon equal terms . . . but rather a consultation upon your safety . . ." The rulers of Melos, however, value freedom above safety: "If you then to retain your command, and your vassals to get loose from you, will undergo the utmost danger: would it not in us, that be already free, be great baseness and cow-ardice, if we should not encounter anything what-soever rather than suffer ourselves to be brought into bondage?" Though they know that it will be a "hard matter" to stand against the power and fortune of Athens, "nevertheless we believe that, for fortune, we shall be nothing inferior, as having the gods on our side, because we stand innocent against men unjust." And as for power, they hope for assistance from the Spartans, "who are of necessity obliged, if for no other cause, yet for consanguinity's sake and for their own honor to defend us." But the gods, too, reign where they can, reply the Athenian generals, and consan-guinity and honor have nothing to do with necessity. The Spartans will (necessarily) think only of them-selves: "most apparently of all men, they hold for honorable that which pleaseth and for just that which profiteth."

So the argument ended. The magistrates refused to surrender; the Athenians laid seige to their city; the Spartans sent no help. Finally, after some months of fighting, in the winter of 416 B.C., Melos was betrayed by several of its citizens. When further resistance seemed impossible, the Melians "yielded themselves to the discretion of the Athenians: who slew all the men of military age, made slaves of the women and chil-dren; and inhabited the place with a colony sent thither afterwards of 500 men of their own."

The dialogue between the generals and the mag-istrates is a literary and philosophical construction of Thucydides. The magistrates speak as they well might have done, but their conventional piety and heroism is only a foil to what the classical critic Dionysius calls the "depraved shrewdness" of the Athenian generals.[2] It is the generals who have often seemed unbelievable. Their words, writes Dionysius, were appropriate to oriental monarchs . . . but unfit to be spoken by Athenians . . ."[3] Perhaps Thucydides means us to notice the unfitness, not so much of the words but of the policies they were used to defend, and thinks we might have missed it had he permitted the generals to speak as they probably in fact spoke, weaving "fair pretenses" over their vile actions. We are to under-stand that Athens is no longer itself. Cleomedes and Tisias do not represent that noble people who fought the Persians in the name of freedom and whose poli-tics and culture, as Dionysius says, "exercised such a humanizing influence on everyday life." They repre-sent instead the imperial decadence of the city state. It is not that they are war criminals in the modern sense; that idea is alien to Thucydides. But they embody a certain loss of ethical balance, of restraint and moderation. Their statesmanship is flawed, and their "realistic" speeches provide an ironic contrast to the blindness and arrogance with which the Atheni-ans only a few months later launched the disastrous expedition to Sicily. The *History,* on this view, is a tragedy and Athens itself the tragic hero.[4] Thucydides has given us a morality play in the Greek style. We can glimpse his meaning in Euripides' *The Trojan Women,* written in the immediate aftermath of the conquest of Melos and undoubtedly intended to sug-gest the human significance of slaughter and slavery—and to predict a divine retribution:[5]

How ye are blind
Ye treaders down of cities, ye that cast
Temples to desolation, and lay waste
Tombs, the untrodden sanctuaries where lie
The ancient dead; yourselves so soon to die!

But Thucydides seems in fact to be making a rather different, and a more secular, statement than this quotation suggests, and not about Athens so much as about war itself. He probably did not mean the harshness of the Athenian generals to be taken as a sign of depravity, but rather as a sign of impatience, toughmindedness, honesty—qualities of mind not inappropriate in military commanders. He is arguing, as Werner Jaeger has said, that "the principle of force forms a realm of its own, with laws of its own," distinct and separate from the laws of moral life.[6] This is certainly the way Hobbes read Thucydides, and it is the reading with which we must come to grips. For if the realm of force is indeed distinct and if this is an accurate account of its laws, then one could no more criticize the Athenians for their wartime policies than one could criticize a stone for falling downwards. The slaughter of the Melians is explained by reference to the circumstances of war and the necessities of nature; and again, there is nothing to say. Or rather, one can *say* anything, call necessity cruel and war hellish; but while these statements may be true in their own terms, they do not touch the political realities of the case or help us understand the Athenian decision.

It is important to stress, however, that Thucydides has told us nothing at all about the Athenian decision. And if we place ourselves, not in the council room at Melos where a cruel policy was being expounded, but in the assembly at Athens where that policy was first adopted, the argument of the generals has a very different ring. In the Greek as in the English language, the word *necessity* "doubles the parts of indispensable and inevitable."[7] At Melos, Cleomedes and Tisias mixed the two of these, stressing the last. In the assembly they could have argued only about the first, claiming, I suppose, that the destruction of Melos was necessary (indispensable) for the preservation of the empire. But this claim is rhetorical in two senses. First, it evades the moral question of whether the preservation of the empire was itself necessary. There were some Athenians, at least, who had doubts about that, and more who doubted that the empire had to be a uniform system of domination and subjection (as the policy adopted for Melos suggested). Secondly, it

exaggerates the knowledge and foresight of the generals. They are not saying with certainty that Athens will fall unless Melos is destroyed; their argument has to do with probabilities and risks. And such arguments are always arguable. Would the destruction of Melos really reduce Athenian risks? Are there alternative policies? What are the likely costs of this one? Would it be right? What would other people think of Athens if it were carried out?

Once the debate begins, all sorts of moral and strategic questions are likely to come up. And for the participants in the debate, the outcome is not going to be determined "by a necessity of nature," but by the opinions they hold or come to hold as a result of the arguments they hear and then by the decisions they freely make, individually and collectively. Afterwards, the generals claim that a certain decision was inevitable; and that, presumably, is what Thucydides wants us to believe. But the claim can only be made afterwards, for inevitability here is mediated by a process of political deliberation, and Thucydides could not know what was inevitable until that process had been completed. Judgments of necessity in this sense are always retrospective in character—the work of historians, not historical actors.

Now, the moral point of view derives its legitimacy from the perspective of the actor. When we make moral judgments, we try to recapture that perspective. We reiterate the decision-making process, or we rehearse our own future decisions, asking what we would have done (or what we would do) in similar circumstances. The Athenian generals recognize the importance of such questions, for they defend their policy certain "that you likewise, and others that should have the same power which we have, would do the same." But that is a dubious knowledge, especially so once we realize that the "Melian decree" was sharply opposed in the Athenian assembly. Our standpoint is that of citizens debating the decree. What *should* we do?

We have no account of the Athenian decision to attack Melos or of the decision (which may have been taken at the same time) to kill and enslave its people. Plutarch claims that it was Alcibiades, chief architect of the Sicilian expedition, who was "the principal cause of the slaughter . . . having spoken in favor of the decree."[8] He played the part of Cleon in the debate that Thucydides does record, that occurred some years earlier, over the fate of Mytilene. It is worth glancing back at that earlier argument. Mytilene had been an ally of Athens from the time of the Persian War; it was never a subject city in any formal way, but bound by treaty to the Athenian cause. In 428, it rebelled and formed an alliance with the Spartans. After considerable fighting, the city was captured by Athenian forces, and the assembly determined "to put to death . . . all the men of Mytilene that were of age, and to make slaves of the women and children: laying to their charge the revolt itself in that they revolted not being in subjection as others were . . ."[9] But the following day the citizens "felt a kind of repentance . . . and began to consider what a great and cruel decree it was, that not the authors only, but that the whole city should be destroyed." It is this second debate that Thucydides has recorded, or some part of it, giving us two speeches, that of Cleon upholding the original decree and that of Diodotus urging its revocation. Cleon argues largely in terms of collective guilt and retributive justice; Diodotus offers a critique of the deterrent effects of capital punishment. The assembly accepts Diodotus' position, convinced apparently that the destruction of Mytilene would not uphold the force of treaties or ensure the stability of the empire. It is the appeal to interest that triumphs—as has often been pointed out—though, it should be remembered that the occasion for the appeal was the repentance of the citizens. Moral anxiety, not political calculation, leads them to worry about the effectiveness of their decree.

In the debate over Melos, the positions must have been reversed. Now there was no retributivist argument to make, for the Melians had done Athens no injury. Alcibiades probably talked like Thucydides' generals, though with the all-important difference I have already noted. When he told his fellow citizens that the decree was necessary, he didn't mean that it was ordained by the laws that govern the realm of force; he meant merely that it was needed (in his view) to reduce the risks of rebellion among the subject cities of the Athenian empire. And his opponents

probably argued, like the Melians, that the decree was dishonorable and unjust and would more likely excite resentment than fear throughout the islands, that Melos did not threaten Athens in any way, and that other policies would serve Athenian interests and Athenian self-esteem. Perhaps they also reminded the citizens of their repentance in the case of Mytilene and urged them once again to avoid the cruelty of massacre and enslavement. How Alcibiades won out, and how close the vote was, we don't know. But there is no reason to think that the decision was predetermined and debate of no avail: no more with Melos than with Mytilene. Stand in imagination in the Athenian assembly, and one can still feel a sense of freedom.

But the realism of the Athenian generals has a further thrust. It is not only a denial of the freedom that makes moral decision possible; it is a denial also of the meaningfulness of moral argument. The second claim is closely related to the first. If we must act in accordance with our interests, driven by our fears of one another, then talk about justice cannot possibly be anything more than talk. It refers to no purposes that we can make our own and to no goals that we can share with others. That is why the Athenian generals could have woven "fair pretenses" as easily as the Melian magistrates; in discourse of this sort anything can be said. The words have no clear references, no certain definitions, no logical entailments. They are, as Hobbes writes in *Leviathan,* "ever used with relation to the person that useth them," and they express that person's appetites and fears and nothing else. It is only "most apparent" in the Spartans, but true for everyone, that "they hold for honorable that which pleaseth them and for just that which profiteth." Or, as Hobbes later explained, the names of the virtues and vices are of "uncertain signification."[10]

> For one calleth wisdom, what another calleth fear; and one cruelty what another justice; one prodigality, what another magnanimity . . . etc. And therefore such names can never be true grounds of any ratiocination.

"Never"—until the sovereign, who is also the supreme linguistic authority, fixes the meaning of the moral vocabulary; but in the state of war, *"never"* without qualification, because in that state, by definition, no

sovereign rules. In fact, even in civil society, the sovereign does not entirely succeed in bringing certainty into the world of virtue and vice. Hence moral discourse is always suspect, and war is only an extreme case of the anarchy of moral meanings. It is generally true, but especially so in time of violent conflict that we can understand what other people are saying only if we see through their "fair pretenses" and translate moral talk into the harder currency of interest talk. When the Melians insist that their cause is just, they are saying only that they don't want to be subject; and had the generals claimed that Athens deserved its empire, they would simply have been expressing the lust for conquest or the fear of overthrow.

This is a powerful argument because it plays upon the common experience of moral disagreement—painful, sustained, exasperating, and endless. For all its realism, however, it fails to get at the realities of that experience or to explain its character. We can see this clearly, I think, if we look again at the argument over the Mytilene decree. Hobbes may well have had this debate in mind when he wrote, "and one [calleth] cruelty what another justice . . ." The Athenians repented of their cruelty, writes Thucydides, while Cleon told them that they had not been cruel at all but justly severe. Yet this was in no sense a disagreement over the meaning of words. Had there been no common meanings, there could have been no debate at all. The cruelty of the Athenians consisted in seeking to punish not only the authors of the rebellion but others as well, and Cleon agreed that that would indeed be cruel. He then went on to argue, as he had to do given his position, that in Mytilene there were no "others." "Let not the fault be laid upon a few, and the people absolved. For they have all alike taken arms against us . . ."

I cannot pursue the argument further, since Thucydides doesn't, but there is an obvious rejoinder to Cleon, having to do with the status of the women and children of Mytilene. This might involve the deployment of additional moral terms (innocence, for example); but it would not hang—any more than the argument about cruelty and justice hangs—on idiosyncratic definitions. In fact, definitions are not at issue here, but descriptions and interpretations. The Atheni-

ans shared a moral vocabulary, shared it with the people of Mytilene and Melos; and allowing for cultural differences, they share it with us too. They had no difficulty, and we have none, in understanding the claim of the Melian magistrates that the invasion of their island was unjust. It is in applying the agreed-upon words to actual cases that we come to disagree. These disagreements are in part generated and always compounded by antagonistic interests and mutual fears. But they have other causes, too, which help to explain the complex and disparate ways in which men and women (even when they have similar interests and no reason to fear one another) position themselves in the moral world. There are, first of all, serious difficulties of perception and information (in war and politics generally), and so controversies arise over "the facts of the case." There are sharp disparities in the weight we attach even to values we share, as there are in the actions we are ready to condone when these values are threatened. There are conflicting commitments and obligations that force us into violent antagonism even when we see the point of one another's positions. All this is real enough, and common enough: it makes morality into a world of good-faith quarrels as well as a world of ideology and verbal manipulation.

In any case, the possibilities for manipulation are limited. Whether or not people speak in good faith, they cannot say just anything they please. Moral talk is coercive; one thing leads to another. Perhaps that's why the Athenian generals did not want to begin. A war called unjust is not, to paraphrase Hobbes, a war misliked; it is a war misliked for particular reasons, and anyone making the charge is required to provide particular sorts of evidence. Similarly, if I claim that I am fighting justly, I must also claim that I was attacked ("put to it," as the Melians were), or threatened with attack, or that I am coming to the aid of a victim of someone else's attack. And each of these claims has its own entailments, leading me deeper and deeper into a world of discourse where, though I can go on talking indefinitely, I am severely constrained in what I can say. I must say this or that, and at many points in a long argument this or that will be true or false. We don't have to translate moral talk into interest talk in order to understand it; morality refers in its own way to the real world.

Let us consider a Hobbist example. In Chapter XXI of *Leviathan,* Hobbes urges that we make allowance for the "natural timorousness" of mankind. "When armies fight, there is on one side, or both a running away; yet when they do it not out of treachery, but fear, they are not esteemed to do it unjustly, but dishonorably." Now, judgments are called for here: we are to distinguish cowards from traitors. If these are words of "inconstant signification," the task is impossible and absurd. Every traitor would please natural timorousness, and we would accept the plea or not depending on whether the soldier was a friend or an enemy, an obstacle to our advancement or an ally and supporter. I suppose we sometimes do behave that way, but it is not the case (nor does Hobbes, when it comes to cases, suppose that it is) that the judgments we make can only be understood in these terms. When we charge a man with treason, we have to tell a very special kind of story about him, and we have to provide concrete evidence that the story is true. If we call him a traitor when we cannot tell that story, we are not using words inconstantly, we are simply lying.

STRATEGY AND MORALITY

Morality and justice are talked about in much the same way as military strategy. Strategy is the other language of war, and while it is commonly said to be free from the difficulties of moral discourse, its use is equally problematic. Though generals agree on the meaning of strategic terms—entrapment, retreat, flanking maneuver, concentration of forces, and so on—they nevertheless disagree about strategically appropriate courses of action. They argue about what ought to be done. After the battle, they disagree about what happened, and if they were defeated, they argue about who was to blame. Strategy, like morality, is a language of justification.[11] Every confused and cowardly commander describes his hesitations and panics as part of an elaborate plan; the strategic vocabulary is as available to him as it is to a competent commander. But that is not to say that its terms are meaningless. It would be a great triumph for the incompetent if they were, for

we would then have no way to talk about incompetence. No doubt, "one calleth retreat what another calleth strategic redeployment . . ." But we do know the difference between these two, and though the facts of the case may be difficult to collect and interpret, we are nevertheless able to make critical judgments.

Similarly, we can make moral judgments: moral concepts and strategic concepts reflect the real world in the same way. They are not merely normative terms, telling soldiers (who often don't listen) what to do. They are descriptive terms, and without them we would have no coherent way of talking about war. Here are soldiers moving away from the scene of a battle, marching over the same ground they marched over yesterday, but fewer now, less eager, many without weapons, many wounded: we call this a retreat. Here are soldiers lining up the inhabitants of a pleasant village, men, women, and children, and shooting them down: we call this a massacre.

It is only when their substantive content is fairly clear that moral and strategic terms can be used imperatively, and the wisdom they embody expressed in the form of rules. Never refuse quarter to a soldier trying to surrender. Never advance with your flanks unprotected. One might construct out of such commands a moral or a strategic war plan, and then it would be important to notice whether or not the actual conduct of the war conformed to the plan. We can assume that it would not. War is recalcitrant to this sort of theoretical control—a quality it shares with every other human activity, but which it seems to possess to an especially intense degree. In *The Charterhouse of Parma,* Stendhal provides a description of the battle of Waterloo that is intended to mock the very idea of a strategic plan. It is an account of combat as chaos, therefore not an account at all but a denial, so to speak, that combat is accountable. It should be read alongside some strategic analysis of Waterloo like that of Major General Fuller, who views the battle as an organized series of maneuvers and counter-maneuvers.[12] The strategist is not unaware of confusion and disorder in the field; nor is he entirely unwilling to see these as aspects of war itself, the natural effects of the stress of battle. But he sees them also as matters of command responsibility, failures of discipline or control. He suggests that strategic imperatives have been ignored; he looks for lessons to be learned.

The moral theorist is in the same position. He too must come to grips with the fact that his rules are often violated or ignored—and with the deeper realization that, to men at war, the rules often don't seem relevant to the extremity of their situation. But however he does this, he does not surrender his sense of war as a human action, purposive and premeditated, for whose effects someone is responsible. Confronted with the many crimes committed in the course of a war, or with the crime of aggressive war itself, he searches for human agents. Nor is he alone in this search. It is one of the most important features of war, distinguishing it from the other scourges of mankind, that the men and women caught up in it are not only victims, they are also participants. All of us are inclined to hold them responsible for what they do (though we may recognize the plea of duress in particular cases). Reiterated over time, our arguments and judgments shape what I want to call *the moral reality of war*—that is, all those experiences of which moral language is descriptive or within which it is necessarily employed.

It is important to stress that the moral reality of war is not fixed by the actual activities of soldiers but by the opinions of mankind. That means, in part, that it is fixed by the activity of philosophers, lawyers, publicists of all sorts. But these people don't work in isolation from the experience of combat, and their views have value only insofar as they give shape and structure to that experience in ways that are plausible to the rest of us. We often say, for example, that in time of war soldiers and statesmen must make agonizing decisions. The pain is real enough, but it is not one of the natural effects of combat. Agony is not like Hobbist fear: it is entirely the product of our moral views, and it is common in war only insofar as those views are common. It was not some unusual Athenian who "repented" of the decision to kill the men of Mytilene, but the citizens generally. They repented, and they were able to understand one another's repentance, because they shared a sense of what cruelty meant. It is by the assignment of such meanings that we make war what it is—which is to say that it could be (and it probably has been) something different.

What of a soldier or statesman who does not feel the agony? We say of him that he is morally ignorant or morally insensitive, much as we might say of a general who experienced no difficulty making a (really) difficult decision that he did not understand the strategic realities of his own position or that he was reckless and insensible of danger. And we might go on to argue, in the case of the general, that such a man has no business fighting or leading others in battle, that he ought to know that his army's right flank, say, is vulnerable, and ought to worry about the danger and take steps to avoid it. Once again, the case is the same with moral decisions: soldiers and statesmen ought to know the dangers of cruelty and injustice and worry about them and take steps to avoid them.

HISTORICAL RELATIVISM

Against this view, however, Hobbist relativism is often given a social or historical form: moral and strategic knowledge, it is said, changes over time or varies among political communities, and so what appears to me as ignorance may look like understanding to someone else. Now, change and variation are certainly real enough, and they make for a tale that is complex in the telling. But the importance of that tale for ordinary moral life and, above all, for the judgment of moral conduct is easily exaggerated. Between radically separate and dissimilar cultures, one can expect to find radical dichotomies in perception and understanding. No doubt the moral reality of war is not the same for us as it was for Genghis Khan; nor is the strategic reality. But even fundamental social and political transformations within a particular culture may well leave the moral world intact or at least sufficiently whole so that we can still be said to share it with our ancestors. It is rare indeed that we do not share it with our contemporaries, and by and large we learn how to act among our contemporaries by studying the actions of those who have preceded us. The assumption of that study is that they saw the world much as we do. That is not always true, but it is true enough of the time to give stability and coherence to our moral lives (and to our military lives). Even when world views and high ideals have been abandoned—as the glorification of aristocratic chivalry was abandoned in early modern times—notions about right conduct are remarkably persistent: the military code survives the death of warrior idealism. I shall say more about this survival later on, but I can demonstrate it now in a general way by looking at an example from feudal Europe, an age in some ways more distant from us than Greece of the city states, but with which we nevertheless share moral and strategic perceptions.

Three Accounts of Agincourt

Actually, the sharing of strategic perceptions is in this case the more dubious of the two. Those French knights so many of whom died at Agincourt had notions about combat very different from our own. Modern critics have still felt able to criticize their "fanatical adherence to the old method of fighting" (King Henry, after all, fought differently) and even to offer practical suggestions: the French attack, writes Oman, "should have been accompanied by a turning movement around the woods . . ."[13] Had he not been "overconfident," the French commander would have seen the advantages of the move. We can talk in a similar way about the crucial moral decision that Henry made toward the end of the battle, when the English thought their victory secure. They had taken many prisoners, who were loosely assembled behind the lines. Suddenly, a French attack aimed at the supply tents far in the rear seemed to threaten a renewal of the fighting. Here is Holinshed's sixteenth century account of the incident (virtually copied from an earlier chronicle):[14]

> . . . certain Frenchmen on horseback . . . to the number of six hundred horsemen, which were the first that fled, hearing that the English tents and pavilions were a good way distant from the army, without any sufficient guard to defend the same . . . entered upon the king's camp and there . . . robbed the tents, broke up chests, and carried away caskets and slew such servants as they found to make any resistance. . . . But when the outcry of the lackeys and boys which ran away for fear of the Frenchmen . . . came to the king's ears, he doubting lest his enemies should gather together again, and begin a new field; and mistrusting further that the prisoners would be an aid to his enemies . . . contrary

to his accustomed gentleness, commanded by sound of trumpet that every man . . . should incontinently slay his prisoner.

The moral character of the command is suggested by the words "accustomed gentleness" and "incontinently." It involved a shattering of personal and conventional restraints (the latter well-established by 1415), and Holinshed goes to some lengths to explain and excuse it, stressing the king's fear that the prisoners his forces held were about to rejoin the fighting. Shakespeare, whose *Henry V* closely follows Holinshed, goes further, emphasizing the slaying of the English servants by the French and omitting the chronicler's assertion that only those who resisted were killed:[15]

> *Fluellen.* Kill the [b]oys and the baggage! 'Tis expressly against the law of arms. 'Tis as arrant a piece of knavery, mark you now, as can be offert.

At the same time, however, he cannot resist an ironical comment:

> *Gower.* . . . they have burned and carried away all that was in the king's tent, wherefore the king most worthily hath caused every soldier to cut his prisoner's throat. O, 'tis a gallant king!

A century and a half later, David Hume gives a similar account, without the irony, stressing instead the king's eventual cancellation of his order:[16]

> . . . some gentlemen of Picardy . . . had fallen upon the English baggage, and were doing execution on the unarmed followers of the camp, who fled before them. Henry, seeing the enemy on all sides of him, began to entertain apprehensions from his prisoners; and he thought it necessary to issue a general order for putting them to death; but on discovering the truth, he stopped the slaughter, and was still able to save a great number.

Here the moral meaning is caught in the tension between "necessary" and "slaughter." Since slaughter is the killing of men as if they were animals—it "makes a massacre," wrote the poet Dryden, "what was a war"—it cannot often be called necessary. If the prisoners were so easy to kill, they were probably not dangerous enough to warrant the killing. When he grasped the actual situation, Henry, who was (so Hume wants us to believe) a moral man, called off the executions.

French chroniclers and historians write of the event in much the same way. It is from them that we learn that many of the English knights refused to kill their prisoners—not, chiefly, out of humanity, rather for the sake of the ransom they expected; but also "thinking of the dishonor that the horrible executions would reflect on themselves."[17] English writers have focused more, and more worriedly, on the command of the king; he was, after all, their king. In the later nineteenth century, at about the same time as the rules of war with respect to prisoners were being codified, their criticism grew increasingly sharp: "a brutal butchery," "cold-blooded wholesale murder."[18] Hume would not have said that, but the difference between that and what he did say is marginal, not a matter of moral or linguistic transformation.

To judge Henry ourselves we would need a more circumstantial account of the battle than I can provide here.[19] Even given that account, our opinions might differ, depending on the allowance we were willing to make for the stress and excitement of battle. But that is a clear example of a situation common in both strategy and morality, where our sharpest disagreements are structured and organized by our underlying agreements, by the meanings we share. For Holinshed, Shakespeare, and Hume—traditional chronicler, Renaissance playwright, and Enlightenment historian— and for us too, Henry's command belongs to a category of military acts that requires scrutiny and judgment. It is *as a matter of fact* morally problematic, because it accepts the risks of cruelty and injustice. In exactly the same way, we might regard the battle plan of the French commander as strategically problematic, because it accepted the risks of a frontal assault on a prepared position. And, again, a general who did not recognize these risks is properly said to be ignorant of morality or strategy.

In moral life, ignorance isn't all that common; dishonesty is far more so. Even those soldiers and statesmen who don't feel the agony of a problematic decision generally know that they should feel it. Harry Truman's flat statement that he never lost a night's sleep over his decision to drop the atomic bomb on Hiroshima is not the sort of thing political leaders often say. They usually find it preferable to stress the painfulness of decision-making; it is one of the burdens of office, and it is best if the burdens appear to be borne. I suspect that many officeholders even experience pain simply because they are expected to. If they don't, they lie about it. The clearest evidence for the stability of our values over time is the unchanging character of the lies soldiers and statesmen tell. They lie in order to justify themselves, and so they describe for us the lineaments of justice. Wherever we find hypocrisy, we also find moral knowledge. The hypocrite is like that Russian general in Solzhenitsyn's *August 1914*, whose elaborate battle reports barely concealed his total inability to control or direct the battle. He knew at least that there was a story to tell, a set of names to attach to things and happenings, so he tried to tell the story and attach the names. His effort was not mere mimicry; it was, so to speak, the tribute that incompetence pays to understanding. The case is the same in moral life: there really is a story to tell, a way of talking about wars and battles that the rest of us recognize as morally appropriate. I don't mean that particular decisions are necessarily right or wrong, or simply right or wrong, only that there is a way of seeing the world so that moral decision-making makes sense. The hypocrite knows that this is true, though he may actually see the world differently.

Hypocrisy is rife in wartime discourse, because it is especially important at such a time to appear to be in the right. It is not only that the moral stakes are high; the hypocrite may not understand that; more crucially, his actions will be judged by other people, who are not hypocrites, and whose judgments will affect their policies toward him. There would be no point to hypocrisy if this were not so, just as there would be no point to lying in a world where no one told the truth. The hypocrite presumes on the moral understanding of the rest of us, and we have no choice, I think, except to take his assertions seriously and put them to the test of moral realism. He pretends to think and act as the rest of us expect him to do. He tells us that he is fighting according to the moral war plan: he does not aim at civilians, he grants quarter to soldiers trying to surrender, he never tortures prisoners, and so on. These claims are true or false, and though it is not easy to judge them (nor is the war plan really so simple), it is important to make the effort. Indeed, if we call ourselves moral men and women, we must make the effort, and the evidence is that we regularly do so. If we had all become realists like the Athenian generals or like Hobbists in a state of war, there would be an end alike to both morality and hypocrisy. We would simply tell one another, brutally and directly, what we wanted to do or have done. But the truth is that one of the things most of us want, even in war, is to act or to seem to act morally. And we want that, most simply, because we know what morality means (at least, we know what it is generally thought to mean).

* * *

NOTES

1. This and subsequent quotations are from *Hobbes' Thucydides,* ed. Richard Schlatter (New Brunswick, N.J., 1975), pp. 377–85 (*The History of The Peloponesian War,* 5:84–116).

2. Dionysius of Halicarnassus, *On Thucydides,* trans. W. Kendrick Pritchett (Berkeley, 1975), pp. 31–33.

3. Even oriental monarchs are not quite so toughminded as the Athenian generals. According to Herodotus, when Xerxes first disclosed his plans for an invasion of Greece, he spoke in more conventional terms: "I will bridge the Hellespont and march an army through Europe into Greece, and punish the Athenians for the outrage they committed upon my father and upon us." (*The Histories,* Book 7, trans. Aubrey de Selincourt) The reference is to the burning of Sardis, which we may take as the pretext for the Persian invasion. The example bears out Francis Bacon's assertion that "there is that justice imprinted in the nature of men that they enter not upon wars (whereof so many calamities do ensue) but upon some, at least specious, grounds and quarrels." (Essay 29, "Of the True Greatness of Kingdoms and Estates")

4. See F. M. Cornford, *Thucydides Mythistoricus* (London, 1907), esp. ch. XIII.

5. *The Trojan Women,* trans. Gilbert Murray (London, 1905), p. 16.

6. Werner Jaeger, *Paideia: the Ideals of Greek Culture,* trans. Gilbert Highet (New York, 1939), I, 402.

7. H. W. Fowler, *A Dictionary of Modern English Usage,* second ed., rev. Sir Ernest Gowers (New York, 1965), p. 168; cf. Jaeger, I, 397.

8. *Plutarch's Lives,* trans. John Dryden, rev. Arthur Hugh Clough (London, 1910), I, 303. Alcibiades also "selected for himself one of the captive Melian women . . ."

9. *Hobbes' Thucydides,* pp. 194–204 (*The History of the Peloponnesian War,* 3:36–49).

10. Thomas Hobbes, *Leviathan,* ch. IV.

11. Hence we can "unmask" strategic discourse just as Thucydides did with moral discourse. Imagine that the two Athenian generals, after their dialogue with the Melians, return to their camp to plan the coming battle. The senior in command speaks first: "Don't give me any fine talk about the need to concentrate our forces or the importance of strategic surprise. We'll simply call for a frontal assault; the men will organize themselves as best they can; things are going to be confused anyway. I need a quick victory here, so that I can return to Athens covered with glory before the debate on the Sicilian campaign begins. We'll have to accept some risks; but that doesn't matter since the risks will be yours, not mine. If we are beaten, I'll contrive to blame you. That's what war is like." Why is strategy the language of hard-headed men? One sees through it so easily . . .

12. *The Charterhouse of Parma,* I, chs. 3 and 4; J. F. C. Fuller, *A Military History of the Western World* (n.p., 1955), II, ch. 15.

13. C. W. C. Oman, *The Art of War in the Middle Ages* (Ithaca, N.Y., 1968), p. 137.

14. Raphael Holinshed, *Chronicles of England, Scotland, and Ireland,* excerpted in William Shakespeare, *The Life of Henry V* (Signet Classics, New York, 1965), p. 197.

15. *Henry V,* 4:7, ll. 1–11.

16. David Hume, *The History of England* (Boston, 1854), II, 358.

17. René de Belleval, *Azincourt* (Paris, 1865), pp. 105–6.

18. See the summary of opinions in J. H. Wylie, *The Reign of Henry the Fifth* (Cambridge, England, 1919), II, 171ff.

19. For an excellent and detailed account, which suggests that Henry's action cannot be defended, see John Keegan, *The Face of Battle* (New York, 1976), pp. 107–12.

Can Terrorism Be Morally Justified?

Stephen Nathanson

Can terrorism be morally justified?

Even asking this question can seem like an insult—both to victims of terrorist actions and to moral common sense. One wants to say: if the murder of innocent people by terrorists is not clearly wrong, what is?

But the question is more complicated than it looks. We can see this by broadening our focus and considering some of the other beliefs held by people who condemn terrorism. Very few of us accept the pacifist view that all violence is wrong. Most of us believe that some acts of killing and injuring people are morally justified. Indeed, most of us think that war is sometimes justified, even though it involves organized, large-scale killing, injuring, and destruction and even though innocent civilians are usually among the victims of war. So, most of us believe that even the killing of innocent people is sometimes morally justified. It is this fact that makes the condemnation of terrorism morally problematic. We pick out terrorism for special condemnation because its victims are civilian, noncombatants rather than military or governmental officials, but we also believe that such killings are sometimes morally permissible.

Seen in a broader context, moral judgments of terrorism often seem hypocritical. They often presuppose self-serving definitions of "terrorism" that allow people to avoid labeling actions that they approve as instances of terrorism, even though these actions are indistinguishable from other acts that are branded with this negative label. On other occasions, moral judgments of terrorism rest on biased, uneven applications of moral principles to the actions of friends and foes. Principles that are cited to condemn the actions of foes are ignored when similar actions are committed by friends.

We need to ask then: Can people who believe that war is sometimes morally permissible consistently condemn terrorist violence? Or are such condemnations necessarily hypocritical and self-serving?

If we are to avoid hypocrisy, then we need both (a) a definition of terrorism that is neutral with respect to who commits the actions, and (b) moral judgments of terrorism that derive from the consistent, even-handed applications of moral criteria.

This paper aims to achieve both of these things. First, I begin with a definition of terrorism and then discuss why terrorism is always wrong. In addition, I want to show that the condemnation of terrorism does not come without other costs. A consistent approach to terrorism requires us to revise some common judgments about historical events and forces us to reconsider actions in which civilians are killed as "collateral damage" (i.e., side effects) of military attacks.

My aim, then, is to criticize both terrorist actions and a cluster of widespread moral views about violence and war. This cluster includes the following beliefs:

1. Terrorism is always immoral.
2. The allied bombing of cities in World War II was morally justified because of the importance of defeating Nazi Germany and Japan.
3. It is morally permissible to kill civilians in war if these killings are not intended.

The trouble with this cluster is that the first belief expresses an absolute prohibition of acts that kill innocent people while the last two are rather permissive. If we are to avoid inconsistency and hypocrisy, we must revise our views either (a) by accepting that terrorism is sometimes morally permissible, or (b) by judging that city bombings and many collateral damage killings are morally wrong. I will defend the second of these options.

Stephen Nathanson, From "Can Terrorism be Morally Justified?" in *Morality in Practice*, ed. James P. Sterba, 7th ed. (Belmont, CA: Wadsworth/Thomson, 2004), 602–10. Reprinted with permission from Stephen Nathanson.

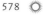

DEFINING TERRORISM

I offer the following definition of terrorism to launch my discussion of the moral issues. Terrorist acts have the following features:

1. They are acts of serious, deliberate violence or destruction.
2. They are generally committed by groups as part of a campaign to promote a political or social agenda.
3. They generally target limited numbers of people but aim to influence a larger group and/or the leaders who make decisions for the group.
4. They either kill or injure innocent people or pose a serious threat of such harms to them.

This definition helps in a number of ways. First, it helps us to distinguish acts of terrorism from other acts of violence. Nonviolent acts are not terrorist acts; nor are violent actions that are unrelated to a political or social agenda. Ironically, some terrible kinds of actions are not terrorist because they are too destructive. As condition 3 tells us, terrorism generally targets limited numbers of people in order to influence a larger group. Acts of genocide that aim to destroy a whole group are not acts of terrorism, but the reason why makes them only worse, not better.

Second, the definition helps us to identify the moral crux of the problem with terrorism. Condition 1 is not the problem because most of us believe that some acts of violence are morally justified. Condition 2 can't be the problem because anyone who believes in just causes of war must accept that some causes are so important that violence may be a legitimate way to promote them. Condition 3 is frequently met by permissible actions, as when we punish some criminals to deter other people from committing crimes. Condition 4 seems closer to what is essentially wrong with terrorism. If terrorism is always immoral, it is because it kills and injures innocent people.

As I have already noted, however, morally conscientious people sometimes want to justify acts that kill innocent people. If a blanket condemnation of terrorism is to be sustained, then we must either condemn all killings of innocent people, or we must find morally relevant differences between the killing of innocents by terrorists and the killing of innocents by others whose actions we find morally acceptable.

TERRORISM AND CITY BOMBING: THE SAME OR DIFFERENT?

Many people who condemn terrorism believe that city bombing in the war against Nazism was justified, even though the World War II bombing campaigns intentionally targeted cities and their inhabitants. This view is defended by some philosophical theorists, including Michael Walzer, in his book *Just and Unjust Wars,* and G. Wallace in "Terrorism and the Argument from Analogy."[1] By considering these theorists, we can see if there are relevant differences that allow us to say that terrorism is always wrong but that the World War II bombings were morally justified.

One of the central aims of Michael Walzer's *Just and Unjust Wars* is to defend what he calls the "war convention," the principles that prohibit attacks on civilians in wartime. Walzer strongly affirms the principle of noncombatant immunity, calling it a "fundamental principle [that] underlies and shapes the judgments we make of wartime conduct." He writes:

> A legitimate act of war is one that does not violate the rights of the people against whom it is directed. . . . [N]o one can be threatened with war or warred against, unless through some act of his own he has surrendered or lost his rights.[2]

Unlike members of the military, civilians have not surrendered their rights in any way, and therefore, Walzer says, they may not be attacked.

Given Walzer's strong support for noncombatant immunity and his definition of terrorism as the "method of random murder of innocent people," it is no surprise that he condemns terrorism. At one point, after describing a terrorist attack on an Algerian milk bar frequented by teenagers, he writes:

> Certainly, there are historical moments when armed struggle is necessary for the sake of human freedom. But if dignity and self-respect are to be the outcomes of that struggle, it cannot consist of terrorist attacks against children.[3]

Here and elsewhere, Walzer denounces terrorism because it targets innocent people.

Nonetheless, he claims that the aerial attacks on civilians by the British early in World War II were justified. In order to show why, he develops the concept of a "supreme emergency." Nazi Germany, he tells us, was no ordinary enemy; it was an "ultimate threat to everything decent in our lives."[4] Moreover, in 1940, the Nazi threat to Britain was imminent. German armies dominated Europe and sought to control the seas. Britain feared an imminent invasion by a country that threatened the basic values of civilization.

According to Walzer, the combination of the enormity and the imminence of the threat posed by Nazi Germany produced a supreme emergency, a situation in which the rules prohibiting attacks on civilians no longer held. If killing innocents was the only way to ward off this dreadful threat, then it was permissible. Since air attacks on German cities were the only means Britain had for inflicting harm on Germany, it was morally permissible for them to launch these attacks.

Walzer does not approve all of the city bombing that occurred in World War II. The emergency lasted, he thinks, only through 1942. After that, the threat diminished, and the constraints of the war convention should once again have been honored. In fact, the bombing of cities continued throughout the war, climaxing in massive attacks that killed hundreds of thousands of civilians: the bombing of Dresden, the fire bombings of Japanese cities by the United States, and the atomic bombings of Hiroshima and Nagasaki. According to Walzer, none of these later attacks were justified because the supreme emergency had passed.

While Walzer's discussion begins with the special threat posed by Nazism, he believes that supreme emergencies can exist in more ordinary situations. In the end, he supports the view that if a single nation is faced by "a threat of enslavement or extermination[,]" then its "soldiers and statesmen [may] override the rights of innocent people for the sake of their own political community. . . ."[5] While he expresses this view with "hesitation and worry," he nevertheless broadens the reach of the concept of "supreme emergency" to include circumstances that arise in many wars.

The problem for Walzer is that his acceptance of the broad "supreme emergency" exception threatens to completely undermine the principle of noncombatant immunity that lies at the heart of his own view of the ethics of warfare. How can the principle of noncombatant immunity be fundamental if it can be overridden in some cases? Moreover, his condemnation of terrorism is weakened because it seems to be possible that people might resort to terrorism in cases that qualify as supreme emergencies, as when their own people are threatened by extermination or enslavement. Walzer's defense of the bombing of cities, then, seems to be inconsistent with his sweeping denunciation of terrorism.

WALLACE'S ARGUMENT FROM ANALOGY

While Walzer does not directly address the tension between the two parts of his view, G. Wallace explicitly tries to defend the view that terrorism is wrong and that the bombing of cities was justified. According to Wallace, the bombing campaign was justified because it satisfied all four of the following criteria:

1. It was a measure of last resort.
2. It was an act of collective self-defense.
3. It was a reply in kind against a genocidal, racist aggressor.
4. It had some chances of success.

He then asks whether acts of terrorism might be justified by appeal to these very same criteria.

Wallace's answer is that the [acts of] terrorism cannot meet these criteria. Or, more specifically, he says that while any one of the criteria might be met by a terrorist act, all four of them cannot be satisfied. Why not? The problem is not with criteria 2 and 3; a community might well be oppressed by a brutal regime and might well be acting in its own defense. In these respects, its situation would be like that of Britain in 1940.

But, Wallace claims, conditions 1 and 4 cannot both be satisfied in this case. If the community has a good chance of success through the use of terrorism (thus satisfying condition 4), then other means of opposition might work as well, and terrorism will fail to be a last resort. Hence it will not meet condition 1. At the same time, if terrorist tactics are a last resort because all other means of opposition will fail, then the terrorist tactics are also likely to fail, in which case condition 4 is not met.

What Wallace has tried to show is that there are morally relevant differences between terrorism and the city bombings by Britain. Even if some of the criteria for justified attacks on civilians can be met by would-be terrorists, all of them cannot be. He concludes that "[E]ven if we allow that conditions (1) and (4) can be met separately, their joint satisfaction is impossible."[6]

Unfortunately, this comforting conclusion—that the British city bombing was justified but that terrorism cannot be—is extremely implausible. Both terrorism and city bombing involve the intentional killing of innocent human beings in order to promote an important political goal. Wallace acknowledges this but claims that the set of circumstances that justified city bombing could not possibly occur again so as to justify terrorism.

There is no basis for this claim, however. Wallace accepts that the right circumstances occurred in the past, and so he should acknowledge that it is at least possible for them to occur in the future. His conclusion ought to be that if city bombing was justifiable, then terrorism is in principle justifiable as well. For these reasons, I believe that Wallace, like Walzer, is logically committed to acknowledging the possibility of morally justified terrorism.

This is not a problem simply for these two authors. Since the historical memory of city bombing in the United States and Britain sees [such tactics] as justifiable means of war, the dilemma facing these authors faces our own society. We condemn terrorists for intentionally killing innocent people while we think it was right to use tactics in our own wars that did the same. Either we must accept the view that terrorism can sometimes be justified, or we must come to see our own bombings of cities as violations of the prohibitions on killing civilians in wartime.

TERRORISM, COLLATERAL DAMAGE, AND THE PRINCIPLE OF DOUBLE EFFECT

Many of us believe that wars are sometimes justified, but we also know that even if civilians are not intentionally killed, the deaths of civilians is a common feature of warfare. Indeed, during the twentieth century, civilian deaths became a larger and larger proportion of the total deaths caused by war. A person who believes that wars may be justified but that terrorism cannot be must explain how this can be.

One common approach focuses on the difference between intentionally killing civilians, as terrorists do, and unintentionally killing civilians, as sometimes happens in what we regard as legitimate acts of war. According to this approach, terrorism is wrong because it is intentional while so-called "collateral damage" killings and injuries are morally permissible because they are not intended.

This type of view is developed by Igor Primoratz in "The Morality of Terrorism."[7] Primoratz attempts to show why terrorism is morally wrong and how it differs from other acts of wartime killing that are morally permissible.

First, he makes it clear that, by definition, terrorism always involves the intentional killing of innocent people. He then offers a number of arguments to show why such killings are wrong. The first two have to do with the idea that persons are moral agents who are due a high level of respect and concern. He writes:

> [E]very human being is an individual, a person separate from other persons, with a unique, irreproducible thread of life and a value that is not commensurate with anything else.[8]

Given the incommensurable value of individual persons, it is wrong to try to calculate the worth of some hoped-for-goal by comparison with the lives and deaths of individual people. This kind of calculation violates the ideal of giving individual lives our utmost respect and concern. Terrorists ignore this central moral ideal. They treat innocent people as political pawns, ignoring their individual worth and seeing their deaths simply as means toward achieving their goals.

In addition, Primoratz argues, terrorists ignore the moral relevance of guilt and innocence in their treatment of individuals. They attack people who have no responsibility for the alleged evils that the terrorists oppose and thus violate the principle that people should be treated in accord with what they deserve.

Terrorists, Pirmoratz tells us, also forsake the ideal of moral dialogue amongst equals. They not only decide who will live and who will die, but they feel no burden to justify their actions in ways that the victims might understand and accept. People who take moral ideas seriously engage in open discussion in order to justify their actions. They engage others in moral debate. Ideally, according to Primoratz, a moral person who harms others should try to act on reasons that are so compelling that they could be acknowledged by their victims. Terrorist acts cannot be justified to their victims, and terrorists are not even interested in trying to do so.

Though these ideas are sketched out rather than fully developed, Primoratz successfully expresses some important moral values. Drawing on these values, he concludes that terrorism is incompatible with "some of the most basic moral beliefs many of us hold."[9]

Primoratz vs. Trotsky

Having tried to show why terrorism is wrong, Primoratz considers an objection put forward by Leon Trotsky, who defended terrorism as a revolutionary tactic. Trotsky claims that people who approve traditional war but condemn revolutionary violence are in a weak position because the differences between these are morally arbitrary. If wars that kill innocent people can be justified, Trotsky claims, then so can revolutions that kill innocent people.

Primoratz replies by arguing that there is an important moral difference between terrorism and some acts of war that kill innocent people. While he acknowledges that the "suffering of civilians . . . is surely inevitable not only in modern, but in almost all wars," Primoratz stresses that the moral evaluation of acts of killing requires that we "attend not only to the suffering inflicted, but also to the way it is inflicted."[10] By this, he means that we need, among other things, to see what the person who did the act intended.

To illustrate his point, he contrasts two cases of artillery attacks on a village. In the first case, the artillery attack is launched with the explicit goal of killing the civilian inhabitants of the village. The civilians are the target of the attack. This attack is the equivalent of terrorism since both intentionally target innocent people, and just like terrorism, it is immoral.

In a second case, the artillery attack is aimed at "soldiers stationed in the village." While the soldiers know that innocent people will be killed, that is not their aim.

> Had it been possible to attack the enemy unit without endangering the civilians in any way, they would certainly have done so. This was not possible, so they attacked although they knew that the attack would cause civilian casualties too; but they did their best to reduce those inevitable, but undesired consequences as much as possible.[11]

In this second case, the civilian deaths and injuries are collateral damage produced by an attack on a legitimate military target. That is the key difference between terrorism and legitimate acts of war. Terrorism is intentionally directed at civilians, while legitimate acts of war do not aim to kill or injure civilians, even when this is their effect.

Primoratz concludes that Trotsky and other defenders of terrorism are wrong when they equate war and terrorism. No doubt, the intentional killing of civilians does occur in war, and when it does Primoratz would condemn it for the same reason he condemns terrorism. But if soldiers avoid the intentional killing of civilians, then their actions can be morally justified, even when civilians die as a result of what they do. As long as soldiers and revolutionaries avoid the intentional killing of innocent people, they will not be guilty of terrorist acts.

Problems with Primoratz's View

Primoratz's view has several attractive features. Nonetheless, it has serious weaknesses.

In stressing the role of intentions, Primoratz appeals to the same ideas expressed by what is called the "principle of double effect." According to this principle, we should evaluate actions by their intended goals rather than their actual consequences. An act that produces collateral damage deaths is an unintentional killing and hence is not wrong in the way that the same act would be if the civilians' deaths were intended.

While the principle of double effects is plausible in some cases, it is actually severely defective. To see this, suppose that the September 11 attackers had only intended to destroy the Pentagon and the World

Trade Center and had no desire to kill anyone. Suppose that they knew, however, that thousands would die in the attack on the buildings. And suppose, following the attack, they said "We are not murderers. We did not mean to kill these people."

What would be our reaction? I very much doubt that we would think them less culpable. They could not successfully justify or excuse their actions by saying that although they foresaw the deaths of many people, these deaths were not part of their aim. We would certainly reject this defense. But if we would reject the appeal to double effect in this case, then we should do so in others.

In Primoratz's example, the artillery gunners attack the village with full knowledge of the high probability of civilian deaths. The artillery gunners know they will kill innocent people, perhaps even in large numbers, and they go ahead with the attack anyway. If it would not be enough for my imagined September 11 attackers to say that they did not intend to kill people, then it is not enough for Primoratz's imagined soldiers to say that they did not mean to kill the villagers when they knew full well that this would result from their actions.

If we accept Primoratz's defense of collateral damage killings, his argument against terrorism is in danger of collapsing because terrorists can use Primoratz's language to show that their actions, too, may be justifiable. If Primoratz succeeds in justifying the collateral damage killings and if the distinction between these killings and terrorism cannot rest solely on whether the killings are intentional, then the criteria that he uses may justify at least some terrorist acts. Like the soldiers in his example, the terrorists may believe that the need for a particular attack is "so strong and urgent that it prevailed over the prohibition of killing or maiming a comparatively small number of civilians." Consistency would require Primoratz to agree that the terrorist act was justified in this case.

Recall, too, Primoratz's claim that actions need to be capable of being justified to the victims themselves. Would the victims of the artillery attack accept the claim that the military urgency justified the "killing or maiming a comparatively small number of civilians?"[12] Why should they accept the sacrifice of their own lives on the basis of this reasoning?

In the end, then, Primoratz does not succeed in showing why terrorism is immoral while collateral damage killing can be morally justified. Like Wallace and Walzer, he has trouble squaring the principles that he uses to condemn terrorism with his own approval of attacks that produce foreseeable collateral damage deaths.

The problem revealed here is not merely a problem for a particular author. The view that collateral damage killings are permissible because they are unintended is a very widespread view. It is the view that United States officials appealed to when our bombings in Afghanistan produced thousands of civilian casualties. Our government asserted that we did not intend these deaths to occur, that we were aiming at legitimate targets, and that the civilian deaths were merely collateral damage. Similar excuses are offered when civilians are killed by cluster bombs and land mines, weapons whose delayed detonations injure and kill people indiscriminately, often long after a particular attack is over.

There are many cases in which people are morally responsible for harms that they do not intend to bring about, but if these harms can be foreseen, their claims that they "did not mean to do it" are not taken seriously. We use labels like "reckless disregard" for human life or "gross negligence" to signify that wrongs have been done, even though they were not deliberate. When such actions lead to serious injury and death, we condemn such actions from a moral point of view, just as we condemn terrorism. The principle of double effect does not show that these condemnations are mistaken. If we want to differentiate collateral damage killings from terrorism so as to be consistent in our moral judgments, we will need something better than the principle of double effect and the distinction between intended and unintended effects.

A SKETCH OF A DEFENSE

I want to conclude by sketching a better rationale for the view that terrorist attacks on civilians are always wrong but that some attacks that cause civilian deaths and injuries as unintended consequences are morally justified.

I have argued that a central problem with standard defenses of collateral damage killings is that they lean too heavily on the distinction between what is intended and what is foreseen. This distinction, when used with the doctrine of double effect, is too slippery and too permissive. As I noted above, it might provide an excuse for the September 11 attacks if (contrary to fact) the attacks were only targeting the World Trade Center *building* and the Pentagon *building* and did not actually aim to kill innocent civilians.

Michael Walzer makes a similar criticism of the double effect principle. "Simply not to intend the death of civilians is too easy," he writes. "What we look for in such cases is some sign of a positive commitment to save civilian lives."[13] Walzer calls his revised version the principle of "double intention." It requires military planners and soldiers to take positive steps to avoid or minimize these evils, even if these precautions increase the danger to military forces.

Walzer's rule is a step in the right direction, but we need to emphasize that the positive steps must be significant. They cannot be *pro forma* or minimal efforts. In order to show a proper respect for the victims of these attacks, serious efforts must be made to avoid death and injury to them. I suggest the following set of requirements for just, discriminate fighting, offering them as a sketch rather than a full account. The specifics might have to be amended, but the key point is that serious efforts must be made to avoid harm to civilians. Not intending harm is not enough. In addition, military planners must really exert themselves. They must, as we say, *bend over backwards* to avoid harm to civilians. For example, they must:

1. Target attacks as narrowly as possible on military resources;
2. Avoid targets where civilian deaths are extremely likely;
3. Avoid the use of inherently indiscriminate weapons (such as land mines and cluster bombs) and inherently indiscriminate strategies (such as high-altitude bombing of areas containing both civilian enclaves and military targets); and
4. Accept that when there are choices between damage to civilian lives and damage to military personnel, priority should be given to saving civilian lives.

If a group has a just cause for being at war and adheres to principles like these, then it could be said to be acknowledging the humanity and value of those who are harmed by its actions. While its attacks might expose innocent people to danger, its adherence to these principles would show that it was not indifferent to their well-being. In this way, it would show that its actions lack the features that make terrorism morally objectionable.

Why is this? Because the group is combining its legitimate effort to defend itself or others with serious efforts to avoid civilian casualties. The spirit of their effort is captured in the phrase I have already used: "bending over backwards." The "bend over backwards" ideal is superior to the principle of double effect in many ways. First, it goes beyond the weak rule of merely requiring that one not intend to kill civilians. Second, while the double effect rule's distinction between intended and unintended results permits all sorts of fudges and verbal tricks, the "bend over backwards" rule can be applied in a more objective and realistic way. It would be less likely to approve sham compliance than is the doctrine of double effect.

The "bend over backwards" rule might even satisfy Primoratz's requirement that acts of violence be justifiable to their victims. Of course, no actual victim is likely to look favorably on attacks by others that will result in the victim's death or serious injury. But suppose we could present the following situation to people who might be victims of an attack (a condition that most of us inhabit) and have them consider it from something like Rawls's veil of ignorance. We would ask them to consider the following situation:

- Group A is facing an attack by group B; if successful, the attack will lead to death or the severest oppression of group A.

- The only way that group A can defend itself is by using means that will cause death and injury to innocent members of group B.
- You are a member of one of the groups, but you do not know which one.

Would you approve of means of self-defense that will kill and injure innocent members of B in order to defend group A?

In this situation, people would not know whether they would be victims or beneficiaries of whatever policy is adopted. In this circumstance, I believe that they would reject a rule permitting either intentional or indiscriminate attacks on civilians. Thus, they would reject terrorism as a legitimate tactic, just as they would reject indiscriminate attacks that kill and injure civilians.

At the same time, I believe that they would approve a rule that combined a right of countries to defend themselves against aggression with the restrictions on means of fighting contained in the "bend over backwards" rule. This would have the following benefits. If one were a member of a group that had been attacked, one's group would have a right of self-defense. At the same time, if one were an innocent citizen in the aggressor country, the defenders would be required to take serious steps to avoid injury or death to you and other civilians.

If people generally could accept such a rule, then actions that adhere to that rule would be justifiable to potential victims as well as potential attackers. This would include actions that cause civilian casualties but that adhere to the "bend over backwards" principle.

I believe that this sort of approach achieves what nonpacifist critics of terrorism want to achieve. I provide a principled basis for condemning terrorism, no matter who it is carried out by, and a principled justification of warfare that is genuinely defensive. Moreover, the perspective is unified in a desirable way. Terrorist actions cannot be morally justified because the *intentional* targeting of civilians is the most obvious kind of violation of the "bend over backwards" rule.

At the same time that these principles allow for the condemnation of terrorism, they are immune to charges of hypocrisy because they provide a basis for criticizing not only terrorist acts but also the acts of any group that violates the "bend over backwards" rule, either by attacking civilians directly or by failing to take steps to avoid civilian deaths.

CONCLUSION

Can terrorism be morally justified? Of course not. But if condemnations of terrorism are to have moral credibility, they must rest on principles that constrain our own actions and determine our judgments of what we ourselves do and have done. To have moral credibility, opponents of terrorism must stand by the principles underlying their condemnations, apply their principles in an evenhanded way, and bend over backwards to avoid unintended harms to civilians. Only in this way can we begin inching back to a world in which those at war honor the moral rules that prohibit the taking of innocent human lives. As long as condemnations of terrorism are tainted by hypocrisy, moral judgments will only serve to inflame people's hostilities rather than reminding them to limit and avoid serious harms to one another.

NOTES

1. Michael Walzer, *Just and Unjust Wars* (New York: Basic Books, 1977); Gerry Wallace, "Terrorism and the Argument from Analogy," *Journal of Moral and Social Studies*, vol. 6 (1991), 149–160.

2. Walzer, 135.

3. Walzer, 205.

4. Walzer, 253.

5. Walzer, 254.

6. Wallace, 155–156.

7. Igor Primoratz, "The Morality of Terrorism?" *Journal of Applied Philosophy*, vol. 14 (1997), 222.

8. Primoratz, 224.

9. Primoratz, 225.

10. Primoratz, 227.

11. Primoratz, 227.

12. Primoratz, 228.

13. Walzer, 155–156.

The Case for Torturing the Ticking Bomb Terrorist

ALAN M. DERSHOWITZ

The arguments in favor of using torture as a last resort to prevent a ticking bomb from exploding and killing many people are both simple and simple-minded. Bentham constructed a compelling hypothetical case to support his utilitarian argument against an absolute prohibition on torture:

> Suppose an occasion were to arise, in which a suspicion is entertained, as strong as that which would be received as a sufficient ground for arrest and commitment as for felony—a suspicion that at this very time a considerable number of individuals are actually suffering, by illegal violence inflictions equal in intensity to those which if inflicted by the hand of justice, would universally be spoken of under the name of torture. For the purpose of rescuing from torture these hundred innocents, should any scruple be made of applying equal or superior torture, to extract the requisite information from the mouth of one criminal, who having it in his power to make known the place where at this time the enormity was practising or about to be practised, should refuse to do so? To say nothing of wisdom, could any pretence be made so much as to the praise of blind and vulgar humanity, by the man who to save one criminal, should determine to abandon 100 innocent persons to the same fate?

If the torture of one guilty person would be justified to prevent the torture of a hundred innocent persons, it would seem to follow—certainly to Bentham—that it would also be justified to prevent the murder of thousands of civilians in the ticking bomb case. Consider two hypothetical situations that are not, unfortunately, beyond the realm of possibility. In fact, they are both extrapolations on actual situations we have faced.

Several weeks before September 11, 2001, the Immigration and Naturalization Service detained Zacarias Moussaoui after flight instructors reported suspicious statements he had made while taking flying lessons and paying for them with large amounts of cash. The government decided not to seek a warrant to search his computer. Now imagine that they had, and that they discovered he was part of a plan to destroy large occupied buildings, but without any further details. They interrogated him, gave him immunity from prosecution, and offered him large cash rewards and a new identity. He refused to talk. They then threatened him, tried to trick him, and employed every lawful technique available. He still refused. They even injected him with sodium [pentothal] and other truth serums, but to no avail. The attack now appeared to be imminent, but the FBI still had no idea what the target was or what means would be used to attack it. We could not simply evacuate all buildings indefinitely. An FBI agent proposes the use of nonlethal torture—say, a sterilized needle inserted under the fingernails to produce unbearable pain without any threat to health or life, or the method used in the film *Marathon Man*, a dental drill through an unanesthetized tooth.

The simple cost-benefit analysis for employing such nonlethal torture seems overwhelming: it is surely better to inflict nonlethal pain on one guilty terrorist who is illegally withholding information needed to prevent an act of terrorism than to permit a large number of innocent victims to die. Pain is a lesser and more remediable harm than death; and the lives of a thousand innocent people should be valued more than the bodily integrity of one guilty person. If the variation on the Moussaoui case is not sufficiently compelling to make this point, we can always raise the stakes. Several weeks after September 11, our government received reports that a ten-kiloton nuclear weapon may have been stolen from Russia and was on its way to New York City, where it would be detonated and kill hundreds of thousands of people. The reliability of the source, code named Dragonfire, was uncertain, but assume for purposes of this hypothetical extension of the actual case that the source was a captured terrorist—like the one tortured by the Philippine authorities—who knew precisely how and where the weapon was being brought into New York and was to be detonated. Again, everything short of torture is tried, but to no avail. It is not absolutely certain torture will work, but it is our last, best hope for preventing a cataclysmic nuclear devastation in a city too large to evacuate in time. Should nonlethal torture be tried? Bentham would certainly have said yes.

The strongest argument against any resort to torture, even in the ticking bomb case, also derives from Bentham's utilitarian calculus. Experience has shown that if torture, which has been deemed illegitimate by the civilized world for more than a century, were now to be legitimated—even for limited use in one extraordinary type of situation—such legitimation would constitute an important symbolic setback in the worldwide campaign against human rights abuses. Inevitably, the legitimation of torture by the world's leading democracy would provide a welcome justification for its more widespread use in other parts of the world. Two Bentham scholars, W. L. Twining and P. E. Twining, have argued that torture is unacceptable even if it is restricted to an extremely limited category of cases:

> There is at least one good practical reason for drawing a distinction between justifying an isolated act of torture in an extreme emergency of the kind postulated above and justifying the *institutionalisation* of torture as a regular practice. The circumstances are so extreme in which most of us would be prepared to justify resort to torture, if at all, the conditions we would impose would be so stringent, the practical problems of devising and enforcing adequate safeguards so difficult and the risks of abuse so great that it would be unwise and dangerous to entrust any government, however enlightened, with such a power. Even an out-and-out utilitarian can support an absolute prohibition against institutionalised torture on the ground that no government in the world can be trusted not to abuse the power and to satisfy in practice the conditions he would impose.

Bentham's own justification was based on *case* or *act* utilitarianism—a demonstration that in a *particu-*

lar case, the benefits that would flow from the limited use of torture would outweigh its costs. The argument against any use of torture would derive from *rule* utilitarianism—which considers the implications of establishing a precedent that would inevitably be extended beyond its limited case utilitarian justification to other possible evils of lesser magnitude. Even terrorism itself could be justified by a case utilitarian approach. Surely one could come up with a singular situation in which the targeting of a small number of civilians—blowing up a German kindergarten by the relatives of inmates in a Nazi death camp, for example, and threatening to repeat the targeting of German children unless the death camps were shut down.

The reason this kind of single-case utilitarian justification is simple-minded is that it has no inherent limiting principle. If nonlethal torture of one person is justified to prevent the killing of many important people, then what if it were necessary to use lethal torture—or at least torture that posed a substantial risk of death? What if it were necessary to torture the suspect's mother or children to get him to divulge the information? What if it took threatening to kill his family, his friends, his entire village? Under a simple-minded quantitative case utilitarianism, anything goes as long as the number of people tortured or killed does not exceed the number that would be saved. This is morality by numbers, unless there are other constraints on what we can properly do. These other constraints can come from rule utilitarianisms or other principles of morality, such as the prohibition against deliberately punishing the innocent. Unless we are prepared to impose some limits on the use of torture or other barbaric tactics that might be of some use in preventing terrorism, we risk hurtling down a slippery slope into the abyss of amorality and ultimately tyranny. Dostoevsky captured the complexity of this dilemma in *The Brothers Karamazov* when he had Ivan pose the following question to Alyosha: "Imagine that you are creating a fabric of human destiny with the object of making men happy in the end, giving them peace at least, but that it was essential and inevitable to torture to death only one tiny creature—that baby beating its breast with its fist, for instance—and to found that edifice on its unavenged tears, would you consent to be the architect on those conditions? Tell me the truth."

A willingness to kill an innocent child suggests a willingness to do anything to achieve a necessary result. Hence the slippery slope.

It does not necessarily follow from this understandable fear of the slippery slope that we can never consider the use of nonlethal infliction of pain, if its use were to be limited by acceptable principles of morality. After all, imprisoning a witness who refuses to testify after being given immunity is designed to be punitive—that is painful. Such imprisonment can, on occasion, produce more pain and greater risk of death than nonlethal torture. Yet we continue to threaten and use the pain of imprisonment to loosen the tongues of reluctant witnesses.

It is commonplace for police and prosecutors to threaten recalcitrant suspects with prison rape. As one prosecutor put it: "You're going to be the boyfriend of a very bad man." The slippery slope is an argument of caution, not a debate stopper, since virtually every compromise with an absolutist approach to rights carries the risk of slipping further. An appropriate response to the slippery slope is to build in a principled break. For example, if nonlethal torture were legally limited to convicted terrorists who had knowledge of future massive terrorist acts, were given immunity, and still refused to provide the information, there might still be objections to the use of torture, but they would have to go beyond the slippery slope argument.

The case utilitarian argument for torturing a ticking bomb terrorist is bolstered by an argument from analogy—an *a fortiori* argument. What moral principle could justify the death penalty for past individual murders and at the same time condemn nonlethal torture to prevent future mass murders? Bentham posed this rhetorical question as support for his argument. The death penalty is, of course, reserved for convicted murderers. But again, what if torture was limited to convicted terrorists who refused to divulge information about future terrorism? Consider as well the analogy to the use of deadly force against suspects fleeing from arrest for dangerous felonies of which they have not yet been convicted. Or military retaliations that produce the predictable and inevitable collateral killing of some innocent civilians. The case against torture, if made by a Quaker who opposes the death penalty, war, self-defense, and the use of lethal force against fleeing felons, is understandable. But for anyone who justifies killing on the basis of a cost-benefit analysis, the case against the use of nonlethal torture to save multiple lives is more difficult to make. In the end, absolute opposition to torture—even nonlethal torture in the ticking bomb case—may rest more on historical and aesthetic considerations than on moral or logical ones.

In debating the issue of torture, the first question I am often asked is, "Do you want to take us back to the Middle Ages?" The association between any form of torture and gruesome death is powerful in the minds of most people knowledgeable of the history of its abuses. This understandable association makes it difficult for many people to think about nonlethal torture as a technique for *saving* lives.

The second question I am asked is, "What kind of torture do you have in mind?" When I respond by describing the sterilized needle being shoved under the fingernails, the reaction is visceral and often visible— a shudder coupled with a facial gesture of disgust. Discussions of the death penalty on the other hand can be conducted without these kinds of reactions, especially now that we literally put the condemned prisoner "to sleep" by laying him out on a gurney and injecting a lethal substance into his body. There is no breaking of the neck, burning of the brain, bursting of internal organs, or gasping for breath that used to accompany hanging, electrocution, shooting, and gassing. The executioner has been replaced by a paramedical technician, as the aesthetics of death have become more acceptable. All this tends to cover up the reality that death is forever while nonlethal pain is temporary. In our modern age death is underrated, while pain is overrated.

I observed a similar phenomenon several years ago during the debate over corporal punishment that was generated by the decision of a court in Singapore to sentence a young American to medically supervised lashing with a cane. Americans who support the death penalty and who express little concern about inner-city prison conditions were outraged by the specter of a few welts on the buttocks of an American. It was an utterly irrational display of hypocrisy and double standards. Given a choice between a medically administered whipping and one month in a typical state lockup or prison, any rational and knowledgeable person would choose the lash. No one dies of welts or pain, but many inmates are raped, beaten, knifed, and otherwise mutilated and tortured in American prisons. The difference is that we don't see—and we don't want to see—what goes on behind their high walls. Nor do we want to think about it. Raising the issue of torture makes Americans think about a brutalizing and unaesthetic phenomenon that has been out of our consciousness for many years.

THE THREE—OR FOUR—WAYS

The debate over the use of torture goes back many years, with Bentham supporting it in a limited category of cases, Kant opposing it as part of his categorical imperative against improperly using people as means for achieving noble ends, and Voltaire's views on the matter being "hopelessly confused." The modern resort to terrorism has renewed the debate over how a rights-based society should respond to the prospect of using nonlethal torture in the ticking bomb situation. In the late 1980s the Israeli government appointed a commission headed by a retired Supreme Court justice to look into precisely that situation. The commission concluded that there are "three ways for solving this grave dilemma between the vital need to preserve the very existence of the state and its citizens, and maintain its character as a law-abiding state." The first is to allow the security service to continue to fight terrorism in "a twilight zone which is outside the realm of law." The second is "the way of the hypocrites: they declare that they abide by the rule of law, but turn a blind eye to what goes on beneath the surface." And the third, "the truthful road of the rule of law," is that the "law itself must insure a proper framework for the activity" of the security services in seeking to prevent terrorist acts.

There is of course a fourth road: namely to forgo any use of torture and simply allow the preventable terrorist act to occur. After the Supreme Court of Israel

outlawed the use of physical pressure, the Israeli security services claimed that, as a result of the Supreme Court's decision, at least one preventable act of terrorism had been allowed to take place, one that killed several people when a bus was bombed. Whether this claim is true, false, or somewhere in between is difficult to assess. But it is clear that if the preventable act of terrorism was of the magnitude of the attacks of September 11, there would be a great outcry in any democracy that had deliberately refused to take available preventive action, even if it required the use of torture. During numerous public appearances since September 11, 2001, I have asked audiences for a show of hands as to how many would support the use of nonlethal torture in a ticking bomb case. Virtually every hand is raised. The few that remain down go up when I ask how many believe that torture would actually be used in such a case.

Law enforcement personnel give similar responses. This can be seen in reports of physical abuse directed against some suspects that have been detained following September 11, reports that have been taken quite seriously by at least one federal judge. It is confirmed by the willingness of U.S. law enforcement officials to facilitate the torture of terrorist suspects by repressive regimes allied with our intelligence agencies. As one former CIA operative with thirty years of experience reported: "A lot of people are saying we need someone at the agency who can pull fingernails out. Others are saying, 'Let others use interrogation methods that we don't use.' The only question then is, do you want to have CIA people in the room?" The real issue, therefore, is not whether some torture would or would not be used in the ticking bomb case— it would. The question is whether it would be done openly, pursuant to a previously established legal procedure, or whether it would be done secretly, in violation of existing law.

Several important values are pitted against each other in this conflict. The first is the safety and security of a nation's citizens. Under the ticking bomb scenario this value may require the use of torture, if that is the only way to prevent the bomb from exploding and killing large numbers of civilians. The second value is the preservation of civil liberties and human rights.

This value requires that we not accept torture as a legitimate part of our legal system. In my debates with two prominent civil libertarians, Floyd Abrams and Harvey Silverglate, both have acknowledged that they would want nonlethal torture to be used if it could prevent thousands of deaths, but they did not want torture to be officially recognized by our legal system. As Abrams put it: "In a democracy sometimes it is necessary to do things off the books and below the radar screen." Former presidential candidate Alan Keyes took the position that although torture might be *necessary* in a given situation it could never be *right*. He suggested that a president *should* authorize the torturing of a ticking bomb terrorist, but that this act should not be legitimated by the courts or incorporated into our legal system. He argued that wrongful and indeed unlawful acts might sometimes be necessary to preserve the nation, but that no aura of legitimacy should be placed on these actions by judicial imprimatur.

This understandable approach is in conflict with the third important value: namely, open accountability and visibility in a democracy. "Off-the-book actions below the radar screen" are antithetical to the theory and practice of democracy. Citizens cannot approve or disapprove of governmental actions of which they are unaware. We have learned the lesson of history that off-the-book actions can produce terrible consequences. Richard Nixon's creation of a group of "plumbers" led to Watergate, and Ronald Reagan's authorization of an off-the-books foreign policy in Central America led to the Iran-Contra scandal. And these are only the ones we know about!

Perhaps the most extreme example of such a hypocritical approach to torture comes—not surprisingly—from the French experience in Algeria. The French army used torture extensively in seeking to prevent terrorism during a brutal colonial war from 1955 to 1957. An officer who supervised this torture, General Paul Aussaresses, wrote a book recounting what he had done and seen, including the torture of dozens of Algerians. "The best way to make a terrorist talk when he refused to say what he knew was to torture him," he boasted. Although the book was published decades after the war was over, the general was prosecuted—

but not for what he had done to the Algerians. Instead, he was prosecuted for *revealing* what he had done, and seeking to justify it.

In a democracy governed by the rule of law, we should never want our soldiers or our president to take any action that we deem wrong or illegal. A good test of whether an action should or should not be done is whether we are prepared to have it disclosed—perhaps not immediately, but certainly after some time has passed. No legal system operating under the rule of law should ever tolerate an "off-the-books" approach to necessity. Even the defense of necessity must be justified lawfully. The road to tyranny has always been paved with claims of necessity made by those responsible for the security of a nation. Our system of checks and balances requires that all presidential actions, like all legislative or military actions, be consistent with governing law. If it is necessary to torture in the ticking bomb case, then our governing laws must accommodate this practice. If we refuse to change our law to accommodate any particular action, then our government should not take that action.

Only in a democracy committed to civil liberties would a triangular conflict of this kind exist. Totalitarian and authoritarian regimes experience no such conflict, because they subscribe to neither the civil libertarian nor the democratic values that come in conflict with the value of security. The hard question is: which value is to be preferred when an inevitable clash occurs? One or more of these values must inevitably be compromised in making the tragic choice presented by the ticking bomb case. If we do not torture, we compromise the security and safety of our citizens. If we tolerate torture, but keep it off the books and below the radar screen, we compromise principles of democratic accountability. If we create a legal structure for limiting and controlling torture, we compromise our principled opposition to torture in all circumstances and create a potentially dangerous and expandable situation.

In 1678, the French writer François de La Rochefoucauld said that "hypocrisy is the homage that vice renders to virtue." In this case we have two vices: terrorism and torture. We also have two virtues: civil liberties and democratic accountability. Most civil libertarians I know prefer hypocrisy, precisely because it appears to avoid the conflict between security and civil liberties, but by choosing the way of the hypocrite these civil libertarians compromise the value of democratic accountability. Such is the nature of tragic choices in a complex world. As Bentham put it more than two centuries ago: "Government throughout is but a choice of evils." In a democracy, such choices must be made, whenever possible, with openness and democratic accountability, and subject to the rule of law.

Consider another terrible choice of evils that could easily have been presented on September 11, 2001—and may well be presented in the future: a hijacked passenger jet is on a collision course with a densely occupied office building; the only way to prevent the destruction of the building and the killing of its occupants is to shoot down the jet, thereby killing its innocent passengers. This choice now seems easy, because the passengers are certain to die anyway and their somewhat earlier deaths will save numerous lives. The passenger jet must be shot down. But what if it were only *probable*, not certain, that the jet would crash into the building? Say, for example, we know from cell phone transmissions that passengers are struggling to regain control of the hijacked jet, but it is unlikely they will succeed in time. Or say we have no communication with the jet and all we know is that it is off course and heading toward Washington, D.C., or some other densely populated city. Under these more questionable circumstances, the question becomes *who* should make this life and death choice between evils—a decision that may turn out tragically wrong?

No reasonable person would allocate this decision to a fighter jet pilot who happened to be in the area or to a local airbase commander—unless of course there was no time for the matter to be passed up the chain of command to the president or the secretary of defense. A decision of this kind should be made at the highest level possible, with visibility and accountability.

Why is this not also true of the decision to torture a ticking bomb terrorist? Why should that choice of evils be relegated to a local policeman, FBI agent, or CIA operative, rather than to a judge, the attorney general, or the president?

There are, of course, important differences between the decision to shoot down the plane and the decision to torture the ticking bomb terrorist. Having to shoot down an airplane, though tragic, is not likely to be a recurring issue. There is no slope down which to slip. Moreover, the jet to be shot down is filled with our fellow citizens—people with whom we can identify. The suspected terrorist we may choose to torture is a "they"—an enemy with whom we do not identify but with whose potential victims we do identify. The risk of making the wrong decision, or of overdoing the torture, is far greater, since we do not care as much what happens to "them" as to "us." Finally, there is something different about torture—even nonlethal torture—that sets it apart from a quick death. In addition to the horrible history associated with torture, there is also the aesthetic of torture. The very idea of deliberately subjecting a captive human being to excruciating pain violates our sense of what is acceptable. On a purely rational basis, it is far worse to shoot a fleeing felon in the back and kill him, yet every civilized society authorizes shooting such a suspect who poses dangers of committing violent crimes against the police or others. In the United States we execute convicted murderers, despite compelling evidence of the unfairness and ineffectiveness of capital punishment. Yet many of us recoil at the prospect of shoving a sterilized needle under the finger of a suspect who is refusing to divulge information that might prevent multiple deaths. Despite the irrationality of these distinctions, they are understandable, especially in light of the sordid history of torture.

We associate torture with the Inquisition, the Gestapo, the Stalinist purges, and the Argentine colonels responsible for the "dirty war." We recall it as a prelude to death, an integral part of a regime of gratuitous pain leading to a painful demise. We find it difficult to imagine a benign use of nonlethal torture to save lives.

Yet there was a time in the history of Anglo-Saxon law when torture was used to save life, rather than to take it, and when the limited administration of nonlethal torture was supervised by judges, including some who are well remembered in history. This fascinating story has been recounted by Professor John Langbein of Yale Law School, and it is worth summarizing here because it helps inform the debate over whether, if torture would in fact be used in a ticking bomb case, it would be worse to make it part of the legal system, or worse to have it done off the books and below the radar screen.

In his book on legalized torture during the sixteenth and seventeenth centuries, *Torture and the Law of Proof,* Langbein demonstrates the trade-off between torture and other important values. Torture was employed for several purposes. First, it was used to secure the evidence necessary to obtain a guilty verdict under the rigorous criteria for conviction required at the time—either the testimony of two eyewitnesses or the confession of the accused himself. Circumstantial evidence, no matter how compelling, would not do. As Langbein concludes, "no society will long tolerate a legal system in which there is no prospect in convicting unrepentant persons who commit clandestine crimes. Something had to be done to extend the system to those cases. The two-eyewitness rule was hard to compromise or evade, but the confession invited 'subterfuge.'" The subterfuge that was adopted permitted the use of torture to obtain confessions from suspects against whom there was compelling circumstantial evidence of guilt. The circumstantial evidence, alone, could not be used to convict, but it was used to obtain a torture warrant. That torture warrant was in turn used to obtain a confession, which then had to be independently corroborated—at least in most cases (witchcraft and other such cases were exempted from the requirement of corroboration).

Torture was also used against persons already convicted of capital crimes, such as high treason, who were thought to have information necessary to prevent attacks on the state.

Langbein studied eighty-one torture warrants, issued between 1540 and 1640, and found that in many of them, especially in "the higher cases of treasons, torture is used for discovery, and not for evidence." Torture was "used to protect the state": and

"mostly that meant preventive torture to identify and forestall plots and plotters." It was only when the legal system loosened its requirement of proof (or introduced the "black box" of the jury system) and when perceived threats against the state diminished that torture was no longer deemed necessary to convict guilty defendants against whom there had previously been insufficient evidence, or to secure preventive information.

The ancient Jewish system of jurisprudence came up with yet another solution to the conundrum of convicting the guilty and preventing harms to the community in the face of difficult evidentiary barriers. Jewish law required two witnesses and a specific advance warning before a guilty person could be convicted. Because confessions were disfavored, torture was not an available option. Instead, the defendant who had been seen killing by one reliable witness, or whose guilt was obvious from the circumstantial evidence, was formally acquitted, but he was then taken to a secure location and fed a concoction of barley and water until his stomach burst and he died. Moreover, Jewish law permitted more flexible forms of self-help against those who were believed to endanger the community.

Every society has insisted on the incapacitation of dangerous criminals regardless of strictures in the formal legal rules. Some use torture, others use informal sanctions, while yet others create the black box of a jury, which need not explain its commonsense verdicts. Similarly, every society insists that, if there are steps that can be taken to prevent effective acts of terrorism, these steps should be taken, even if they require some compromise with other important principles.

In deciding whether the ticking bomb terrorist should be tortured, one important question is whether there would be less torture if it were done as part of the legal system, as it was in sixteenth- and seventeenth-century England, or off the books, as it is in many countries today. The Langbein study does not definitively answer this question, but it does provide some suggestive insights. The English system of torture was more visible and thus more subject to public accountability, and it is likely that torture was employed less frequently in England than in France. "During these years when it appears that torture might have become routinized in English criminal procedure, the Privy Council kept the torture power under careful control and never allowed it to fall into the hands of the regular law enforcement officers," as it had in France. In England "no law enforcement officer . . . acquired the power to use torture without special warrant." Moreover, when torture warrants were abolished, "the English experiment with torture left no traces." Because it was under centralized control, it was easier to abolish than it was in France, where it persisted for many years.

It is always difficult to extrapolate from history, but it seems logical that a formal, visible, accountable, and centralized system is somewhat easier to control than an ad hoc, off-the-books, and under-the-radar-screen nonsystem. I believe, though I certainly cannot prove, that a formal requirement of a judicial warrant as a prerequisite to nonlethal torture would decrease the amount of physical violence directed against suspects. At the most obvious level, a double check is always more protective than a single check. In every instance in which a warrant is requested, a field officer has already decided that torture is justified and, in the absence of a warrant requirement, would simply proceed with the torture. Requiring that decision to be approved by a judicial officer will result in fewer instances of torture even if the judge rarely turns down a request. Moreover, I believe that most judges would require compelling evidence before they would authorize so extraordinary a departure from our constitutional norms, and law enforcement officials would be reluctant to seek a warrant unless they had compelling evidence that the suspect had information needed to prevent an imminent terrorist attack. A record would be kept of every warrant granted, and although it is certainly possible that some individual agents might torture without a warrant, they would have no excuse, since a warrant procedure would be available. They could not claim "necessity," because the decision as to whether the torture is indeed necessary has been taken out of their hands and placed in the hands of a judge. In addition, even if torture were deemed totally illegal without any exception, it would still occur, though the public would be less aware of its existence.

I also believe that the rights of the suspect would be better protected with a warrant requirement. He would be granted immunity, told that he was now compelled to testify, threatened with imprisonment if he refused to do so, and given the option of providing the requested information. Only if he refused to do what he was legally compelled to do—provide necessary information, which could not incriminate him because of the immunity—would he be threatened with torture. Knowing that such a threat was authorized by the law, he might well provide the information. If he still refused to, he would be subjected to judicially monitored physical measures designed to cause excruciating pain without leaving any lasting damage.

Let me cite two examples to demonstrate why I think there would be less torture with a warrant requirement than without one. Recall the case of the alleged national security wiretap placed on the phones of Martin Luther King by the Kennedy administration in the early 1960s. This was in the days when the attorney general could authorize a national security wiretap without a warrant. Today no judge would issue a warrant in a case as flimsy as that one. When Zacarias Moussaoui was detained after raising suspicions while trying to learn how to fly an airplane, the government did not seek a national security wiretap because its lawyers believed that a judge would not have granted one. If Moussaoui's computer could have been searched without a warrant, it almost certainly would have been.

It should be recalled that in the context of searches, our Supreme Court opted for a judicial check on the discretion of the police, by requiring a search warrant in most cases. The Court has explained the reason for the warrant requirement as follows: "The informed and deliberate determinations of magistrates . . . are to be preferred over the hurried action of officers." Justice Robert Jackson elaborated:

The point of the Fourth Amendment, which often is not grasped by zealous officers, is not that it denies law enforcement the support of the usual inferences which reasonable men draw from evidence. Its protection consists in requiring that those inferences be drawn by a neutral and detached magistrate instead of being judged by the officer engaged in the often competitive enterprise of ferreting out crime. Any assumption that evidence sufficient to support a magistrate's disinterested determination to issue a search warrant will justify the officers in making a search without a warrant would reduce the Amendment to nullity and leave the people's homes secure only in the discretion of police officers.

Although torture is very different from a search, the policies underlying the warrant requirement are relevant to the question whether there is likely to be more torture or less if the decision is left entirely to field officers, or if a judicial officer has to approve a request for a torture warrant. As Abraham Maslow once observed, to a man with a hammer, everything looks like a nail. If the man with the hammer must get judicial approval before he can use it, he will probably use it less often and more carefully.

There are other, somewhat more subtle, considerations that should be factored into any decision regarding torture. There are some who see silence as a virtue when it comes to the choice among such horrible evils as torture and terrorism. It is far better, they argue, not to discuss or write about issues of this sort, lest they become legitimated. And legitimation is an appropriate concern. Justice Jackson, in his opinion in one of the cases concerning the detention of Japanese-Americans during World War II, made the following relevant observation:

Much is said of the danger to liberty from the Army program for deporting and detaining these citizens of Japanese extraction. But a judicial construction of the due process clause that will sustain this order is a far more subtle blow to liberty than the promulgation of the order itself. A military order, however unconstitutional, is not apt to last longer than the military emergency. Even during that period a succeeding commander may revoke it all. But once a judicial opinion rationalizes such an order to show that it conforms to the Constitution, or rather rationalizes the Constitution to show that the Constitution sanctions such an order, the Court for all time has validated the principle of racial discrimination in criminal procedure and of transplanting American citizens. The principle then lies about like a loaded weapon ready for the hand of any authority that can bring forward a plausible claim of an urgent need. Every repetition imbeds that principle more deeply in our law and thinking and expands it to new purposes. All who observe the work of courts are familiar with what Judge Cardozo described as "the tendency of a principle to expand itself to the limit of its logic." A military commander may overstep the bounds of constitutionality, and it is an incident. But if we review and approve, that passing incident becomes the doctrine of the Constitution. There it has a generative power of its own, and all that it creates will be in its own image.

A similar argument can be made regarding torture: if an agent tortures, that is "an incident," but if the courts authorize it, it becomes a precedent. There is, however, an important difference between the detention of Japanese-American citizens and torture. The detentions were done openly and with presidential accountability; torture would be done secretly, with official deniability. Tolerating an off-the-book system of secret torture can also establish a dangerous precedent.

A variation on this "legitimation" argument would postpone consideration of the choice between authorizing torture and forgoing a possible tactic necessary to prevent an imminent act of terrorism until after the choice—presumably the choice to torture—has been made. In that way, the discussion would not, in itself, encourage the use of torture. If it were employed, then we could decide whether it was justified, excusable, condemnable, or something in between. The problem with that argument is that no FBI agent who tortured a suspect into disclosing information that prevented an act of mass terrorism would be prosecuted—as the policemen who tortured the kidnapper into disclosing the whereabouts of his victim were not prosecuted. In the absence of a prosecution, there would be no occasion to judge the appropriateness of the torture.

I disagree with these more passive approaches and believe that in a democracy it is always preferable to decide controversial issues in advance, rather than in the heat of battle. I would apply this rule to other tragic choices as well, including the possible use of a nuclear first strike, or retaliatory strikes—so long as the discussion was sufficiently general to avoid giving our potential enemies a strategic advantage by their knowledge of our policy.

Even if government officials decline to discuss such issues, academics have a duty to raise them and submit them to the marketplace of ideas. There may be danger in open discussion, but there is far greater danger in actions based on secret discussion, or no discussion at all.

Whatever option our nation eventually adopts—no torture even to prevent massive terrorism, no torture except with a warrant authorizing nonlethal torture, or no "officially" approved torture but its selective use beneath the radar screen—the choice is ours to make in a democracy. We do have a choice, and we should make it—before local FBI agents make it for us on the basis of a false assumption that we do not really "have a choice."

* * *

CASES FOR ANALYSIS

1. Intervention to Stop ISIS

In 2014 President Obama authorized airstrikes against a group of militant Islamists known as the Islamic State of Iraq and Syria (ISIS) to prevent them from possibly committing genocide against members of the Yezidi sect, a religious minority trapped on a mountaintop in northwest Iraq. In a speech, the president sought to justify the intervention:

> [A]t the request of the Iraqi government—we've begun operations to help save Iraqi civilians stranded on the mountain. As ISIL [ISIS] has marched across Iraq, it has waged a ruthless campaign against innocent Iraqis. And these terrorists have been especially barbaric towards religious minorities, including Christian and Yezidis, a small and ancient religious sect. Countless Iraqis have been displaced. And chilling reports describe ISIL militants rounding up families, conducting mass executions, and enslaving Yezidi women.
>
> In recent days, Yezidi women, men and children from the area of Sinjar have fled for their lives. And thousands—perhaps tens of thousands—are now hiding high up on the mountain, with little but the clothes on their backs. They're without food, they're without water. People are starving. And children are dying of thirst. Meanwhile, ISIL forces below have called for the systematic destruction of the entire Yezidi people, which would constitute genocide. So these innocent families are faced with a horrible choice: descend the mountain and be slaughtered, or stay and slowly die of thirst and hunger.
>
> I've said before, the United States cannot and should not intervene every time there's a crisis in the world. So let me be clear about why we must act, and act now. When we face a situation like we do on that mountain—with innocent people facing the prospect of violence on a horrific scale, when we have a mandate to help—in this case, a request from the Iraqi government—and when we have

the unique capabilities to help avert a massacre, then I believe the United States of America cannot turn a blind eye. We can act, carefully and responsibly, to prevent a potential act of genocide. That's what we're doing on that mountain.*

Was President Obama justified in ordering the armed intervention? What if the Iraqi government had not requested military action from the United States? Would the intervention be justified then? Why or why not? How would just war theory apply? How might a utilitarian evaluate the permissibility of the United States's military action? What might a nonconsequentialist say about it?

*Barack Obama, "Statement by the President," 7 August 2014, http://www.whitehouse.gov/the-press-office/2014/08/07/statement-president (27 February 2015).

2. War in Afghanistan

Consider this time line detailing the run-up to the U.S. invasion of Afghanistan in 2001.

September 11—Hijacked airliners are flown into the twin towers of the World Trade Center in New York and the Pentagon, outside Washington DC. A fourth plane crashes in Pennsylvania. In an address to the nation, President Bush describes the attacks as "deliberate and deadly terrorist acts." He says he has directed the U.S. intelligence and law enforcement communities "to find those responsible and bring them to justice," adding that the U.S. "will make no distinction between the terrorists who committed these acts and those who harbor them."

September 12—President Bush declares that the attacks were "acts of war." The United Nations Security Council passes Resolution 1368, recognizing "the inherent right of individual and collective self-defense" and calling on all states to work together to bring the perpetrators of the attacks to justice. The North Atlantic Council for the first time invokes Article 5 of NATO's founding treaty, stating that an armed attack against any member state shall be considered as an attack against all.

September 18—Congress passes a resolution giving the President authorization for the use of force "against those nations, organizations, or persons he determines planned, authorized, committed, or aided the terrorist attacks that occurred on September 11, 2001, or harbored such organizations or persons."

September 20—In an address to a joint session of Congress, President Bush says all the evidence suggests al-Qaeda was responsible for the attacks, and warns the Taliban regime that they must "hand over the terrorists, or they will share in their fate." The Department of Justice issues an Interim Rule stating that non-citizens can be detained for 48 hours without charge, or in the event of an "emergency or other extraordinary circumstance" for "an additional reasonable period of time." . . .

October 4—The British government issues a statement saying it is confident that Osama bin Laden and the al-Qaeda network "planned and carried out the atrocities of 11 September," and setting out the evidence for their conclusion.

October 7—U.S. military forces launch 'Operation Enduring Freedom' against Taliban and al-Qaeda facilities in Afghanistan. In a televised address, President Bush says U.S. actions "are designed to disrupt the use of Afghanistan as a terrorist base of operations, and to attack the military capability of the Taliban regime."[†]

Was the U.S. response to the September 11 attacks a legitimate act of self-defense? Why or why not? According to just war theory, was the U.S. invasion of Afghanistan justified? If so, how does the resort to warfare regarding each of the just war conditions? If not, why not? How does the decision to go to war fail any just war requirements?

[†]Anthony Dworkin and Ariel Meyerstein, "A Defining Moment—International Law Since September 11: A Timeline," Crimes of War Project, February 18, 2006. Reprinted with permission of the Crimes of War Project and the authors.

---

3. Terrorism and Torture

WASHINGTON—Most Americans and a majority of people in Britain, France and South Korea say torturing terrorism suspects is justified at least in rare instances, according to AP-Ipsos polling.

The United States has drawn criticism from human rights groups and many governments, especially in Europe, for its treatment of terror suspects. President Bush and other top officials have said the U.S. does not torture, but some suspects in American custody have alleged they were victims of severe mistreatment.

The polling, in the United States and eight of its closest allies, found that in Canada, Mexico and Germany people are divided on whether torture is ever justified. Most people opposed torture under any circumstances in Spain and Italy.

"I don't think we should go out and string everybody up by their thumbs until somebody talks. But if there is definitely a good reason to get an answer, we should do whatever it takes," said Billy Adams, a retiree from Tomball, Texas.

In America, 61 percent of those surveyed agreed torture is justified at least on rare occasions. Almost nine in 10 in South Korea and just over half in France and Britain felt that way.[‡]

Do you agree with most Americans that the use of torture is sometimes morally permissible in fighting terrorism? If so, what circumstances do you think would justify torture? If not, why not? How might a utilitarian justify (or oppose) torture? How might a Kantian theorist argue against torturing suspected terrorists?

[‡]Associated Press, "Poll Finds Broad Approval of Terrorist Torture," published on MSNBC.com, December 9, 2005. © The Associated Press. Reprinted by permission.

CHAPTER 18

Equality and Affirmative Action

A white man named Alan Bakke applies for admission to the Medical School of the University of California at Davis. Only one hundred slots are available, and there are many other applicants. His grades and admissions test scores, however, are good. The medical school denies him admission anyway—and grants admission to several others whose grades and scores are lower than his. As it turns out, the school has reserved sixteen of the available slots for minority students, many of whom had lower grades and test scores than Bakke. He sues, claiming that he has been denied admission solely because of his race. His case goes all the way to the Supreme Court, which is strongly divided but eventually decides in his favor. The majority opinion says that preferring members of a group solely on account of their race or ethnic origin is a clear-cut instance of discrimination. The Court finds that quota systems like the one used at the Davis Medical School are unconstitutional but that in some situations the use of race or minority status in admissions decisions may be permissible.

This famous Supreme Court case—*Regents of the University of California v. Bakke* (1978)—is one of many to grapple with the divisive and volatile issue of affirmative action, a social policy that is still being ferociously debated almost thirty years after the *Bakke* decision was handed down. It illustrates why this issue is so explosive, so complicated, and so important: disputes over affirmative action invariably involve complex collisions of beliefs and values about racism, sexism, discrimination, civil rights, justice, equality, desert, opportunity, and

social utility. Little wonder then that disagreements flare where agreement would be expected, and people often presumed to have different perspectives on the issue—liberals and conservatives, blacks and whites, men and women—may be just as likely to take the same side.

Affirmative action is notorious for touching off strong feelings that evoke simplistic, knee-jerk answers—precisely the kind of answers we want to avoid here. Only reflective, well-reasoned responses will do for moral questions like these: Are quota systems such as the one cited in the Bakke case morally permissible? Should people be given preference in college admissions or employment because they are members of a particular minority group? Should members of a minority group that was discriminated against in the past be given preferential treatment as compensation for that earlier discrimination? Is preferential treatment for minorities and women permissible even though it deprives white males of equal opportunities? Can affirmative action help create a more just and diverse society—or does it lead to a less just one, divided by race and culture?

ISSUE FILE: BACKGROUND

Affirmative action is a way of making amends for, or eradicating, discrimination based on race, ethnicity, and gender. It takes the form of policies and programs (usually mandated by government) designed to bring about the necessary changes in businesses, colleges, and other organizations. **Discrimination** in the sense used here is unfavorable treatment of people on irrelevant grounds. It refers to actions against people based on factors that cannot and should not be used to justify those actions. It includes, for example, failing to hire a qualified person just because she is a woman; refusing to give a good worker a raise in pay just because he is black or Hispanic; and denying an applicant admission to law school just because he is Asian.

The ideal that spawned affirmative action is this: all persons deserve equal respect and equal opportunity in employment and education. It is essentially an expression of the fundamental moral principle that *equals should be treated equally.* Two people should not be treated differently unless there are relevant differences between them—differences that would justify the dissimilar treatment.

Affirmative action in the United States evolved over the past half century from several groundbreaking laws, executive orders, and court cases. Most notable among these is the Civil Rights Act of 1964, enacted at a time when racial discrimination in the United States was a deeply implanted infection—painful, injurious, and widespread. Discrimination against minorities and women was rampant in the workplace, in college admissions offices, in government contracting, and in countless places of business, from barbershops to factories. Amounting to a direct assault on unequal treatment, the act outlawed discrimination in public accommodations (such as restaurants and hotels), public schools and universities, and business organizations of all kinds. Regarding the latter, the act declares

It shall be an unlawful employment practice for an employer—

(1) to fail or refuse to hire or discharge any individual or otherwise to discriminate against any individual with respect to his compensation, terms, conditions, or privileges of employment, because of such individuals' race, color, religion, sex, or national origin; or

(2) to limit, segregate, or classify his employees or applicants for employment in any way which would deprive or tend to deprive any individual of employment opportunities or otherwise adversely affect his status as an employee, because of such individual's race, color, religion, sex, or national origin.[1]

Later as the executive branch and the courts tried to interpret or implement antidiscrimination policies, affirmative action took on a broader meaning. Many companies and universities have gone beyond simply banning discriminatory practices. With prompting from the federal government, they have tried to institute equal opportunity ("to level the playing field") by ensuring that minority groups and women are represented in fair numbers (that is, numbers reflecting the proportion of such individuals in the whole community or the total workforce). But achieving fair or proportional representation has often required preferential treatment for the designated groups. Thus through the use of quotas or other means, members of the preferred groups have been favored over nonmembers, who typically are white males.

Thus we can say that there are actually two kinds of affirmative action—weak and strong.[2] **Weak affirmative action** is the use of policies and procedures to end discriminatory practices and ensure equal opportunity. It hews close to the spirit and the letter of the Civil Rights Act of 1964, which decrees in Title VI that "[No] person in the United States shall, on the ground of race, color or national origin, be excluded from participation in, denied the benefits of, or be subjected to discrimination under any program or activity receiv-

---

[1]Civil Rights Act of 1964, Section 601 of Title VI.
[2]Terms used by Louis P. Pojman in "The Case against Affirmative Action," *International Journal of Applied Philosophy* 12 (1998): 97–115 (reprinted in *Philosophy: The Quest for Truth,* ed. Louis P. Pojman [New York: Oxford University Press, 2006], 632–45). I attach very roughly the same meanings to them that Pojman does.

CRITICAL THOUGHT: Are Legacies Racist?

Take a look at this excerpt from a report on college "legacies" published in the *Christian Science
Monitor*:

WASHINGTON, D.C.—At Penn, they "take it very
seriously." At Michigan it "gets you extra points."
At Harvard, it "is not ignored," and at Notre Dame,
they are "very open" to it. "It" is "legacy": an admissions designation used by most private and some
public universities for applicants whose relatives
attended the school, and who, as such, get some
degree of preferential treatment. It's a practice as
old as colleges themselves, and is intended to boost
alumni support and donations and foster a sense of
community.

It's also racist, argue its critics.

Following fast on the footsteps of last year's
Supreme Court entry into the delicate area of

affirmative-action admissions, lawmakers are taking
a hard look at this so-called reverse affirmative
action, which gives an edge to those whose parents
and grandparents went to selective colleges at a
time when most minorities there were few and far
between[.]*

Are legacies indeed racist? If you think so, what
are your reasons? If you think not, what argument
would you put forth to support your belief? If you
were the president of a state college, what policy
toward legacies would you try to establish? Do
legacies violate the Civil Rights Act of 1964? Why
or why not?

*Danna Harman, "Family Ties: An Unfair Advantage?"
Christian Science Monitor, 6 February 2004.

---

ing Federal financial assistance." Weak affirmative
action can involve many strategies for expanding
equal opportunity, but it stops short of preferential treatment. As the philosopher Louis P. Pojman
explains it,

[Weak affirmative action] includes such things as dismantling of segregated institutions, widespread
advertisement to groups not previously represented
in certain privileged positions, special scholarships
for the disadvantaged classes (e.g., the poor, regardless of race or gender), and even using diversity or
under-representation of groups with a history of past
discrimination as a tie breaker when candidates for
these goods and offices are relatively equal. The goal
of *Weak Affirmative Action* is equal opportunity to
compete, not equal results. We seek to provide each
citizen regardless of race or gender a fair chance to
the most favored positions in society. There is no
more moral requirement to guarantee that 12% of
professors are Black than to guarantee that 85% of

the players in the National Basketball Association are
White.[3]

Weak affirmative action, then, is hardly controversial. Probably few people nowadays would
object to efforts to end discrimination against
minorities and women and to give people an equal
chance to get ahead. But strong affirmative action
is a different matter.

Strong affirmative action is the use of
policies and procedures to favor particular individuals because of their race, gender, or ethnic
background. It is a kind of preferential treatment
that is usually implemented through favoring
plans, quota systems, or other approaches. The
point of a quota system is to ensure that an organization has a predetermined number or percentage of minority members or women. Typically,
a proportion of available positions or slots are

[3]Pojman, "The Case against Affirmative Action," 98.

reserved for the preferred people, as was the arrangement at the Medical School of UC Davis in the Bakke case. Sometimes the result of using a quota system is that less qualified people are hired or accepted while equally or more qualified people are not—with the difference being only that the preferred ones are women or members of a minority.

Defenders of strong affirmative action have offered several justifications for it. A leading argument is that because in generations past minorities were treated cruelly and unjustly, they now deserve compensation for those terrible wrongs. Giving minorities preferential treatment in employment and education is the best way to make amends. As one philosopher puts it, "Racism was directed against Blacks whether they were talented, average, or mediocre, and attenuating the effects of racism requires distributing remedies similarly. Affirmative action policies compensate for the harms of racism (overt and institutional) through antidiscrimination laws and preferential policies."[4]

Another argument is that strong affirmative action is necessary to foster *diversity* in a population—diversity of race, ethnicity, gender, culture, and outlook. Diversity is rightly thought to be an extremely valuable commodity for any free society. It promotes understanding of cultures and viewpoints different from one's own, which in turn encourages tolerance and cooperation in an increasingly heterogeneous world. Some think it valuable enough to use strong affirmative action to achieve it.

As you would expect, diversity is thought to be critical to education—especially in universities, where the issue of promoting diversity through preferences has been vigorously debated. Many universities have tested the use of preferences for

diversity's sake, encouraged by the majority opinion in the Bakke case, which states that "The atmosphere of 'speculation, experiment and creation'—so essential to the quality of higher education—is widely believed to be promoted by a diverse student body."[5]

But strong affirmative action is strongly opposed by many who see it as *reverse discrimination*—unequal, preferential treatment against some people (mostly white males) to advance the interests of others (minorities and women). The main charge is that preferential treatment on the basis of race, gender, or minority status is *always* wrong. It is just as immoral when used against white males as it is when used against blacks or women. Speaking specifically of racial preferences, the philosopher Carl Cohen provides a succinct statement of this claim:

It uses categories that *must not* be used to distinguish among persons with respect to their entitlements in the community. Blacks and whites are equals, as blondes and brunettes are equals, as Catholics and Jews are equals, as Americans of every ancestry are equal. No matter who the beneficiaries may be or who the victims, preference on the basis of race is morally wrong. It was wrong in the distant past and in the recent past; it is wrong now; and it will always be wrong. Race preference violates the principle of human equality.[6]

MORAL THEORIES

In the debates over strong affirmative action, those who oppose it as well as those who endorse it appeal to conventional moral theories—both consequentialist and nonconsequentialist. Many who support strong affirmative action make the utili-

[4]Albert Mosley, "The Case for Affirmative Action," in *Philosophy: The Quest for Truth*, ed. Louis P. Pojman, 6th ed. (New York: Oxford University Press, 2006), 630.

[5]*Regents of the University of California v. Bakke*, 438 U.S. 265, 312 (1978).
[6]Carl Cohen, in *Affirmative Action and Racial Preference: A Debate*, by Carl Cohen and James P. Sterba (Oxford: Oxford University Press, 2003), 25.

CRITICAL THOUGHT: Are Whites-Only Scholarships Unjust?

After reading about weak and strong affirmative action in this chapter, consider the following news item:

> (CNN)—A whites-only scholarship to be awarded Wednesday by a student Republican organization at Roger Williams University in Bristol, Rhode Island, has drawn both controversy and support.
>
> "It all began two weeks ago as a way for the college Republican groups to express their opposition and tell people they are against race-based scholarships and affirmative action," June Speakman, faculty adviser for the College Republicans told CNN.
>
> "We never expected such an overwhelming response of e-mails and media attention."
>
> The scholarship is for $250, but College Republicans president Jason Mattera said he has received donations and pledges totaling $4,000 for future whites-only scholarships.
>
> Mattera is of Puerto Rican descent and was awarded a $5,000 scholarship from the Hispanic College Fund. He said he believes being eligible for such scholarships gives him "an inherent advantage over my white peers." He wants the university to award scholarships based on merit and not ethnicity.
>
> Applicants for the College Republicans' scholarship must be of Caucasian descent, have high hon-
> ors, write an essay, and show an impressive list of accomplishments, Mattera said. Sixteen people applied.
>
> Roger Williams University does not sponsor or endorse the scholarship, university spokesman Rick Goff told CNN.
>
> "The scholarship is entirely initiated by the College Republicans at the university," he said. . . .
>
> The state Republican Party has criticized the scholarship as having racist overtones.*

Is this whites-only scholarship an example of *weak* or *strong* affirmative action—or neither? Is it racist or discriminatory? If so, are blacks-only scholarships in the same category? If not, what distinguishes the one type of scholarship from the other? That is, what are your reasons for thinking that one is unjust while the other is not? Is there an implicit argument in the student organization's offering a whites-only scholarship? If so, what is it?

*Jennifer Styles, "Whites-Only Scholarship Generates Controversy," *CNN.com*, 20 February 2004, www.cnn.com /2004/EDUCATION/02/18/whites.only.scholars (27 February 2015). © 2004 Cable News Network. Reprinted courtesy of CNN.

---

tarian argument that these policies can have enormous benefits for minorities and women as well as for society as a whole. They contend, as suggested earlier, that preferential programs can increase racial and cultural diversity, which helps promote tolerance, mutual understanding, better use of people's talents, and—in higher education— enhanced learning. They also argue that preferential policies can have great social utility by creating role models for minorities and women whose self-esteem and hopes for success have been dimmed by generations of discrimination. They assert that role models are essential for demonstrating to young people that significant achievement is pos-

sible. Finally, some think the best argument is that strong affirmative action may be able to eradicate racism and transform our race-conscious society. A proponent of this view outlines the argument as follows:

[Affirmative action programs] rest on two judgments. The first is a judgment of social theory: that the United States will continue to be pervaded by racial divisions as long as the most lucrative, satisfying, and important careers remain mainly the prerogative of members of the white race, while others feel themselves systematically excluded from a professional and social elite. The second is a calculation of strategy: that increasing the number of blacks who are at work in the professions will, in the long run, reduce the sense of frustration and injustice and racial self-consciousness in the black community to the point at which blacks may begin to think of themselves as individuals who can succeed like others through talent and initiative. At that future point the consequences of nonracial admissions programs, whatever these consequences might be, could be accepted with no sense of racial barriers or injustice.[7]

Many opponents of strong affirmative action also make utilitarian appeals. Their most straightforward counterargument is that those who favor race or gender preferences are simply wrong about the consequences of the policies: the consequences are either not as beneficial as supposed or are actually injurious. Opponents try to undermine the diversity argument by insisting that racial and ethnic diversity does not necessarily result in diversity of ideas or outlooks, that no scientific evidence supports the notion that diversity policies yield benefits in education or learning, and that giving priority to racial or gender diversity in the workplace would severely undermine competence and efficiency, which are highly valued by society. They reject the role model argument on the grounds that role models selected by race or gender are not necessarily the role models we need. The best role models in education, they say, are people who are the best—the most competent, knowledgeable, inspiring, and decent—*whatever the color of their skin, their background, or their gender*. Many opposed to racial preferences doubt that such treatment can help eliminate racism and promote a color-blind society. In fact, they argue that racial preferences can often have the opposite effect:

Preference puts distinguished minority achievement under a cloud. It imposes upon every member of the

QUICK REVIEW

affirmative action—A way of making amends for, or eradicating, discrimination based on race, ethnicity, and gender.

discrimination—Unfavorable treatment of people on irrelevant grounds.

weak affirmative action—The use of policies and procedures to end discriminatory practices and ensure equal opportunity.

strong affirmative action—The use of policies and procedures to favor particular individuals because of their race, gender, or ethnic background.

preferred minority the demeaning burden of presumed inferiority. Preference *creates* that burden; it *makes* a stigma of the race of those who are preferred by race. An ethnic group given special favor by the community is *marked* as needing special favor—and the mark is borne prominently by every one of its members. Nasty racial stereotypes are reinforced, and the malicious imputation of inferiority is inescapable because it is tied to the color of the skin.[8]

As noted earlier, a common nonconsequentialist argument for strong affirmative action is based on the notion of compensatory justice: historically, minorities (blacks, Native Americans, Hispanics, and others) were the victims of racism by the white majority; justice requires that members of those minorities now be compensated for that past mistreatment; racial preferences in employment and education are appropriate compensation; therefore, racial preferences are morally permissible. As you might guess, many who wish to counter this argument also appeal to justice. They argue that compensation is just only (1) if it is given in proper

[7]Ronald Dworkin, "Bakke's Case: Are Quotas Unfair?" in *A Matter of Principle* (Cambridge, MA: Harvard University Press, 1985), 294.

[8]Cohen, *Affirmative Action,* 110.

measure to specific persons who have been harmed, and (2) if the specific persons who caused the harm do the compensating. But with racial preferences, this direct connection that morality seems to require is missing. The result, they contend, is that often the nonminority person who suffers because of compensatory justice (because he is well qualified but denied admission, for example) has had nothing to do with past racism, and the person who benefits from compensatory justice has suffered very little from racism (because he or she is well educated with above-average income, say). They conclude that racial preferences are unjust.

MORAL ARGUMENTS

Let us look a little closer at the argument from compensatory justice, giving particular attention to how a supporter of strong affirmative action might articulate and defend it. Consider this version of the argument, narrowly focused on compensatory claims that blacks might have against whites for historical discrimination:

1. In the past, blacks have been cruelly and systematically discriminated against by whites.

2. Blacks thus are owed just compensation for this ill treatment.

3. Strong affirmative action in the form of racial preferences is the most morally appropriate form of such compensation.

4. Therefore, racial preferences (in employment and education) should be used to compensate blacks for past discrimination.

First note that this argument is valid and that Premise 1 is true. Both those for and those against racial preferences would be likely to accept this premise, a statement of historical fact that few thoughtful people would dispute. Premises 2 and 3, on the other hand, are very contentious claims.

The most common way to support Premise 2 is to appeal to our moral intuitions about the jus-tice of compensating people who have been wronged. We tend to think that people who have been wronged do in fact deserve reparations, that valid grievances warrant redress. Many argue that blacks have been mistreated and discriminated against for so many generations that today they still suffer the lingering effects—they are disadvantaged before they even begin to compete for jobs, school admissions, and grades. Racial preferences help give them the edge that they need—and that they justly deserve as repayment for cruelties suffered in the past.

Those who reject Premise 2 counter that the principle of just compensation is certainly legitimate, but compensation in the form of racial preferences is not just. Compensation, they argue, should go to the particular persons who have been wronged, and the compensation should be paid by the specific persons who wronged them. But with racial preferences, they contend, the blacks who benefit are not all equally deserving of redress. The ancestors of contemporary blacks were almost certainly not equally wronged, not all wronged in the same fashion, and not all wronged more than some poor white males were wronged. As Carl Cohen says,

[M]any of Hispanic ancestry now enjoy here, and have long enjoyed, circumstances as decent and as well protected as those enjoyed by Americans of all other ethnicities. The same is true of African Americans, some of whom are impoverished and some of whom are rich and powerful. Rewards distributed on the basis of ethnic membership assume that the damage suffered by some were suffered by all—an assumption that we know to be false.[9]

Advocates of race preferences can counter this criticism with an analogy. In the United States, veterans receive preferential treatment when they apply for civil service jobs. Their applications are automatically given extra weight, which means

[9]Cohen, *Affirmative Action,* 27–28.

604 ☀ PART 4: ETHICAL ISSUES

that sometimes veterans may land jobs even when nonveteran applicants are equally qualified. The notion behind this policy is that a grateful nation owes veterans something for their service. The policy assumes that all veterans are owed preferential treatment even though some of them have served longer and more courageously than other of their comrades. So, the advocate of preferences asks, why should not blacks be treated according to a similar policy? Why should not all blacks be owed preferential treatment because of past discrimination—and owed it in equal measure even though some blacks have been wronged more than others?

Another kind of attack on Premise 2 focuses not on the people compensated but on those penalized so the debt can be paid. The claim is that racial preferences are unjust because they punish people who have done nothing to merit punishment. When blacks get preferential treatment in employment, the argument goes, some white males end up losing out—even though these whites had no part in past racism and may have never discriminated against anyone. Clearly, penalizing people for wrongdoing that they did not—and could not—commit is unjust; therefore, racial preferences are unjust.

A frequent reply to this argument is that the white males thought to be innocent victims of reverse discrimination are not as innocent as we might think. According to this response, white males are the recipients of advantages and privileges that have been unjustly extracted from blacks for generations—therefore, strong affirmative action does not take from white males anything that is rightfully theirs. The philosopher Judith Jarvis Thomson, an advocate of preferential hiring, makes the point in the following way:

No doubt few, if any, [young white male applicants] have themselves, individually, done any wrongs to blacks and women. But they have profited from the wrongs the community did. Many may actually have been direct beneficiaries of policies which excluded or downgraded blacks and women—perhaps in school admissions, perhaps in access to financial aid, perhaps elsewhere; and even those who did not directly benefit in this way had, at any rate, the advantage in the competition which comes of confidence in one's full membership, and of one's rights being recognized as a matter of course.[10]

Critics have tried to rebut this argument by questioning its underlying assumption—the notion that, as one philosopher puts it, "if someone gains from an unjust practice for which he is not responsible and even opposes, the gain is not really his and can be taken from him without injustice."[11] This rebuttal relies on the common-sense moral principle that a person who wrongs others is morally obligated to compensate them for that wrong but the wrongdoer's descendants are not. The sins of the parents cannot be transferred to the children.

Premise 3—that racial preferences are just and appropriate moral compensation for past discrimination—is defended by many, but probably most ably by Thomson:

[In] fact the nature of the wrongs done is such as to make jobs the best and most suitable form of compensation. What blacks and women were denied was full membership in the community; and nothing can more appropriately make amends for that wrong than precisely what will make them feel they now finally have it. And that means jobs. Financial compensation (the cost of which could be shared equally) slips through the fingers; having a job, and discovering you do it well, yield—perhaps better than anything else—that very self-respect which blacks and women have had to do without.[12]

[10]Judith Jarvis Thomson, "Preferential Hiring," *Philosophy & Public Affairs* 2, no. 4 (Summer 1973): 383–84.
[11]Robert Simon, "Preferential Hiring: A Reply to Judith Jarvis Thomson," *Philosophy & Public Affairs* 3, no. 3 (Spring 1974): 318.
[12]Thomson, "Preferential Hiring," 382–83.

Though several arguments can be tried against Premise 3, one in particular goes to the heart of the debate on racial preferences. It says that preferential treatment is not fitting compensation, because it ignores the true standard by which jobs and positions should be awarded—competence:

[T]he normal criterion of competence is a strong prima facie consideration when the most important positions are at stake. There are three reasons for this: (1) treating people according to their merits respects them as persons, as ends in themselves, rather than as means to social ends (if we believe that individuals possess a dignity that deserves to be respected, then we ought to treat that individual on the basis of his or her merits, not as a mere instrument for social policy); (2) society has given people expectations that if they attain certain levels of excellence they will be awarded appropriately; and (3) filling the most important positions with the best qualified is the best way to ensure efficiency in job-related areas and in society in general.[13]

SUMMARY

Affirmative action is meant to make up for or eliminate minority and gender discrimination, which is a form of unwarranted mistreatment. Affirmative action seeks to realize the ideal of equal respect and opportunity for all in employment and education.

[13]Pojman, "The Case against Affirmative Action," 101.

Weak affirmative action is generally not controversial, because it uses policies and procedures to ensure equal opportunity without demanding that one group be preferred over another. Strong affirmative action, on the other hand, is controversial, because it makes use of minority and gender preferences.

Those who defend strong affirmative action argue that it is needed to compensate certain groups for mistreatment and discrimination of the past. It is also thought to level the playing field—to give minorities and women an edge in the competition for jobs and educational admissions. Some also contend that such preferences are justified because they help promote cultural, ethnic, and intellectual diversity, a beneficial force for free societies. Strong affirmative action is opposed by many who think it is reverse discrimination, unequal treatment that penalizes white males to give advantages to blacks and women. These critics generally reject all forms of preferential treatment whether they favor white males or not.

Arguments for and against strong affirmative action can appeal to both consequentialist and nonconsequentialist theories. Some argue that preferential treatment is justified because it has positive consequences for minorities and for society as a whole. Others argue that such policies do not work as advertised and actually harm the people they are meant to help. Nonconsequentialist arguments appeal to justice, asserting either that affirmative action programs are just (doing compensatory justice, for example) or unjust (distorting compensatory justice).

READINGS

Reverse Discrimination as Unjustified

LISA H. NEWTON

I have heard it argued that "simple justice" requires that we favor women and blacks in employment and educational opportunities, since women and blacks were "unjustly" excluded from such opportunities for so many years in the not so distant past. It is a strange argument, an example of a possible implication of a true proposition advanced to dispute the proposition itself, like an octopus absent-mindedly slicing off his head with a stray tentacle. A fatal confusion underlies this argument, a confusion fundamentally relevant to our understanding of the notion of the rule of law.

Two senses of justice and equality are involved in this confusion. The root notion of justice, progenitor of the other, is the one that Aristotle (*Nichomachean Ethics* 5. 6; *Politics* 1. 2; 3. 1) assumes to be the foundation and proper virtue of the political association. It is the condition which free men establish among themselves when they "share a common life in order that their association bring them self-sufficiency"—the regulation of their relationship by law, and the establishment, by law, of equality before the law. Rule of law is the name and pattern of this justice; its equality stands against the inequalities—of wealth, talent, etc.—otherwise obtaining among its participants, who by virtue of that equality are called "citizens." It is an achievement—complete, or, more frequently, partial—of certain people in certain concrete situations. It is fragile and easily disrupted by powerful individuals who discover that the blind equality of rule of law is inconvenient for their interests. Despite its obvious instability, Aristotle assumed that the establishment of justice in this sense, the creation of citizenship, was a permanent possibility for

men and that the resultant association of citizens was the natural home of the species. At levels below the political association, this rule-governed equality is easily found; it is exemplified by any group of children agreeing together to play a game. At the level of the political association, the attainment of this justice is more difficult, simply because the stakes are so much higher for each participant. The equality of citizenship is not something that happens of its own accord, and without the expenditure of a fair amount of effort it will collapse into the rule of a powerful few over an apathetic many. But at least it has been achieved, at some times in some places; it is always worth trying to achieve, and eminently worth trying to maintain, wherever and to whatever degree it has been brought into being.

Aristotle's parochialism is notorious; he really did not imagine that persons other than Greeks could associate freely in justice, and the only form of association he had in mind was the Greek *polis*. With the decline of the *polis* and the shift in the center of political thought, his notion of justice underwent a sea change. To be exact, it ceased to represent a political type and became a moral ideal: the ideal of equality as we know it. This ideal demands that all men be included in citizenship—that one Law govern all equally, that all men regard all other men as fellow citizens, with the same guarantees, rights, and protections. Briefly, it demands that the circle of citizenship achieved by any group be extended to include the entire human race. Properly understood, its effect on our associations can be excellent: it congratulates us on our achievement of rule of law as a process of government but refuses to let us remain complacent until we have expanded the associations to include others within the ambit of the rules, as often and as far as possible. While one man is a slave, none of us may feel truly free. We are constantly prodded by this ideal to look for possible justifiable discrimination, for inequalities not absolutely required for the functioning of the society and advantageous to all. And after twenty centuries of pressure, not at all constant, from this ideal, it might be said that some progress has been made. To take the cases in point for this problem, we are now prepared to assert, as Aristotle would never have been, the equality of sexes and of persons of different colors. The ambit of American citizenship, once restricted to white males of property, has been extended to include all adult free men, then all adult males including ex-slaves, then all women. The process of acquisition of full citizenship was for these groups a sporadic trail of half-measures, even now not complete; the steps on the road to full equality are marked by legislation and judicial decisions which are only recently concluded and still often not enforced. But the fact that we can now discuss the possibility of favoring such groups in hiring shows that over the area that concerns us, at least, full equality is presupposed as a basis for discussion. To that extent, they are full citizens, fully protected by the law of the land.

It is important for my argument that the moral idea of equality be recognized as logically distinct from the condition (or virtue) of justice in the political sense. Justice in this sense exists *among* a citizenry, irrespective of the number of the populace included in that citizenry. Further, the moral idea is parasitic upon the political virtue, for "equality" is unspecified—it means nothing until we are told in what respect that equality is to be realized. In a political context, "equality" is specified as "equal rights"—equal access to the public realm, public goods and offices, equal treatment under the law—in brief, the equality of citizenship. If citizenship is not a possibility, political equality is unintelligible. The ideal emerges as a generalization of the real condition and refers back to that condition for its content.

Now, if justice (Aristotle's justice in the political sense) is equal treatment under law for all citizens, what is injustice? Clearly, injustice is the violation of that equality, discriminating for or against a group of citizens, favoring them with special immunities and privileges or depriving them of those guaranteed to the others. When the southern employer refuses to hire blacks in white-collar jobs, when Wall Street will only hire women as secretaries with new titles, when Mississippi high schools routinely flunk all black boys above ninth grade, we have examples of injustice, and we work to restore the equality of the public realm by ensuring that equal opportunity will be provided in such cases in the future. But of course, when the employers and the schools *favor* women and blacks, the same injustice is done. Just as the previous discrimination did, this reverse discrimination violates the public equality which defines citizenship and destroys the rule of law for the areas in which these favors are granted. To the extent that we adopt a program of discrimination, reverse or otherwise, justice in the political sense is destroyed, and none of us, specifically affected or not, is a citizen, a bearer of rights—we are all petitioners for favors. And to the same extent, the ideal of equality is undermined, for it has content only where justice obtains, and by destroying justice we render the ideal meaningless. It is, then, an ironic paradox, if not a contradiction in terms, to assert that the ideal of equality justifies the violation of justice; it is as if one should argue, with William Buckley, that an ideal of humanity can justify the destruction of the human race.

Logically, the conclusion is simple enough: all discrimination is wrong prima facie because it violates justice, and that goes for reverse discrimination too. No violation of justice among the citizens may be justified (may overcome the prima facie objection) by appeal to the ideal of equality, for that ideal is logically dependent upon the notion of justice. Reverse discrimination, then, which attempts no other justification than an appeal to equality, is wrong. But let us try to make the conclusion more plausible by suggesting some of the implications of the suggested practice of reverse discrimination in employment and education. My argument will be that the problems raised there are insoluble, not only in practice, but in principle.

We may argue, if we like, about what "discrimination" consists of. Do I discriminate against blacks if I admit none to my school when none of the black applicants are qualified by the tests I always give?

How far must I go to root out cultural bias from my application forms and tests before I can say that I have not discriminated against those of different cultures? Can I assume that women are not strong enough to be roughnecks on my oil rigs, or must I test them individually? But this controversy, the most popular and well-argued aspect of the issue, is not as fatal as two others which cannot be avoided: if we are regarding the blacks as a "minority" victimized by discrimination, what is a "minority"? And for any group—blacks, women, whatever—that has been discriminated against, what amount of reverse discrimination wipes out the initial discrimination? Let us grant as true that women and blacks were discriminated against, even where laws forbade such discrimination, and grant for the sake of argument that a history of discrimination must be wiped out by reverse discrimination. What follows?

First, are there other groups which have been discriminated against? For they should have the same right of restitution. What about American Indians, Chicanos, Appalachian Mountain whites, Puerto Ricans, Jews, Cajuns, and Orientals? And if these are to be included, the principle according to which we specify a "minority" is simply the criterion of "ethnic (sub) group," and we're stuck with every hyphenated American in the lower-middle class clamoring for special privileges for *his* group—and with equal justification. For be it noted, when we run down the Harvard roster, we find not only a scarcity of blacks (in comparison with the proportion in the population) but an even more striking scarcity of those second-, third-, and fourth-generation ethnics who make up the loudest voice of Middle America. Shouldn't they demand *their* share? And eventually, the WASPs will have to form their own lobby, for they too are a minority. The point is simply this: there is no "majority" in America who will not mind giving up just a bit of their rights to make room for a favored minority. There are only other minorities, each of which is discriminated against by the favoring. The initial injustice is then repeated dozens of times, and if each minority is granted the same right of restitution as the others, an entire area of rule governance is dissolved into a pushing and shoving match between self-interested groups. Each works to catch the public eye and political popularity by whatever means of advertising and power politics lend themselves to the effort, to capitalize as much as possible on temporary popularity until the restless mob picks another group to feel sorry for. Hardly an edifying spectacle, and in the long run no one can benefit: the pie is no larger—it's just that instead of setting up and enforcing rules for getting a piece, we've turned the contest into a free-for-all, requiring much more effort for no larger a reward. It would be in the interests of all the participants to reestablish an objective rule to govern the process, carefully enforced and the same for all.

Second, supposing that we do manage to agree in general that women and blacks (and all the others) have some right of restitution, some right to a privileged place in the structure of opportunities for a while, how will we know when that while is up? How much privilege is enough? When will the guilt be gone, the price paid, the balance restored? What recompense is right for centuries of exclusion? What criterion tells us when we are done? Our experience with the Civil Rights movement shows us that agreement on these terms cannot be presupposed: a process that appears to some to be going at a mad gallop into a black takeover appears to the rest of us to be at a standstill. Should a practice of reverse discrimination be adopted, we may safely predict that just as some of us begin to see "a satisfactory start toward righting the balance," others of us will see that we "have already gone too far in the other direction" and will suggest that the discrimination ought to be reversed again. And such disagreement is inevitable, for the point is that we could not *possibly* have any criteria for evaluating the kind of recompense we have in mind. The context presumed by any discussion of restitution is the context of rule of law: law sets the rights of men and simultaneously sets the method for remedying the violation of those rights. You may exact suffering from others and/or damage payments for yourself if and only if the others have violated your rights; the suffering you have endured is not sufficient reason for them to suffer. And remedial rights exist only where there is law: primary human rights are useful guides to legislation but cannot stand as reasons for awarding remedies for injuries sustained. But then, the context presupposed by any discussion of restitution is the context of pre-existent full citizenship. No remedial rights could exist for the excluded; neither in law nor in logic does there exist a right to *sue* for a standing to sue.

From these two considerations, then, the difficulties with reverse discrimination become evident. Restitution for a disadvantaged group whose rights under the law have been violated is possible by legal means, but restitution for a disadvantaged group whose grievance is that there was no law to protect them simply is not. First, outside of the area of jus-tice defined by the law, no sense can be made of "the group's rights," for no law recognizes that group or the individuals in it, qua members, as bearers of rights (hence *any* group can constitute itself as a disadvantaged minority in some sense and demand similar restitution). Second, outside of the area of protection of law, no sense can be made of the violation of rights (hence the amount of the recompense cannot be decided by any objective criterion). For both reasons, the practice of reverse discrimination undermines the foundation of the very ideal in whose name it is advocated; it destroys justice, law, equality, and citizenship itself, and replaces them with power struggles and popularity contests.

The Case against Affirmative Action

LOUIS P. POJMAN

Hardly a week goes by but that the subject of Affirmative Action does not come up. Whether in the form of preferential hiring, nontraditional casting, quotas, "goals and time tables," minority scholarships, race-norming, reverse discrimination, or employment of members of underutilized groups, the issue confronts us as a terribly perplexing problem. Affirmative action was one of the issues that divided the Democratic and Republican parties during the 1996 election, the Democrats supporting it ("Mend it don't end it") and the Republicans opposing it ("affirmative action is reverse racism"). During the last general election (November 7, 1996) California voters by a 55% to 45% vote approved Proposition 209 (called the "California Civil Rights Initiative") which made it illegal to discriminate on the basis of race or gender, hence ending Affirmative Action in public institutions in California. The Supreme Court

Louis Pojman, "The Case Against Affirmative Action" from *International Journal of Applied Philosophy*, 1998, Vol. 12, No.1, pp. 97–115. Reprinted by permission of Philosophy Documentation Center.

recently refused to rule on the appeal, thus leaving it to the individual states to decide how they will deal with this issue. Both sides have reorganized for a renewed battle. Meanwhile, on Nov. 11, 1977, the European Union's High Court of Justice in Luxembourg approved Affirmative Action programs giving women preferential treatment in the 15 European Union countries.

Let us agree that despite the evidences of a booming economy, the poor are suffering grievously, with children being born into desperate material and psychological poverty; for them the ideal of "equal opportunity for all" is a cruel joke. Many feel that the federal government has abandoned its guarantee to provide the minimum necessities for each American, so that the pace of this tragedy seems to be worsening daily. In addition to this, African-Americans have a legacy of slavery and unjust discrimination to contend with, and other minorities have also suffered from injustice. Women have their own peculiar history of being treated unequally in relevant ways. What is the answer to this national problem? Is it increased welfare? More job training? More support for education? Required licensing of parents to have children? Negative income tax? More support for families or for mothers with small children? All of these have merit and should be part of the national debate. But, my thesis is, however tragic the situation may be (and we may disagree on just how tragic it is), one policy is *not* a legitimate part of the solution and that is *reverse, unjust discrimination* against young white males. Strong Affirmative Action, which implicitly advocates reverse discrimination, while no doubt well intentioned, is morally heinous, asserting, by implication, that *two wrongs make a right.*

The *Two Wrongs Make a Right* Thesis goes like this: Because *some* Whites once enslaved some Blacks, the descendants of those slaves (some of whom may now enjoy high incomes and social status) have a right to opportunities and offices over better qualified Whites and who had nothing to do with either slavery or the oppression of Blacks (and who may even have suffered hardship comparable to that of poor Blacks). In addition, Strong Affirmative Action creates a new Hierarchy of the Oppressed: Blacks get primary preferential treatment, women second, Native Americans third, Hispanics fourth, Handicapped fifth, and Asians sixth and so on until White males, no matter how needy or well qualified, must accept the leftovers. Naturally, combinations of oppressed classes (e.g., a one-eyed, Black Hispanic female) trump all single classifications. The equal protection clause of the Fourteenth Amendment becomes reinterpreted as "Equal protection for all equals, but some equals are more equal than others."

Before analyzing arguments concerning Affirmative Action, I must define my terms.

By *Weak Affirmative Action* I mean policies that will increase the opportunities of disadvantaged people to attain social goods and offices. It includes such things as dismantling of segregated institutions, widespread advertisement to groups not previously represented in certain privileged positions, special scholarships for the disadvantaged classes (e.g., the poor, regardless of race or gender), and even using diversity or under-representation of groups with a history of past discrimination as a tie breaker when candidates for these goods and offices are relatively equal. The goal of *Weak Affirmative Action* is equal opportunity to compete, not equal results. We seek to provide each citizen regardless of race or gender a fair chance to the most favored positions in society. There is no more moral requirement to guarantee that 12% of professors are Black than to guarantee that 85% of the players in the National Basketball Association are White.

By *Strong Affirmative Action* I mean preferential treatment on the basis of race, ethnicity or gender (or some other morally irrelevant criterion), discriminating in favor of underrepresented groups against overrepresented groups, aiming at roughly equal results. *Strong Affirmative Action* is *reverse discrimination*. It says it is right to do wrong to correct a wrong. This is the policy currently being promoted under the name of *Affirmative Action,* so I will use that term or "AA" for short throughout this essay to stand for this version of affirmative action. I will not argue for or against the principle of *Weak Affirmative Action.* Indeed, I think it has some moral weight. *Strong Affirmative Action* has none, or so I will argue.

This essay concentrates on AA policies with regard to race, but the arguments can be extended to cover ethnicity and gender. I think that if a case for Affirmative Action can be made it will be as a corrective to racial oppression. I will examine [nine] arguments regarding AA. The first six will be *negative,* attempting to show that the best arguments for Affirmative Action fail. The last three will be *positive* arguments for policies opposing Affirmative Action.

I. A CRITIQUE OF ARGUMENTS FOR AFFIRMATIVE ACTION

A. The Need for Role Models

This argument is straightforward. We all have need of role models, and it helps to know that others like us can be successful. We learn and are encouraged to strive for excellence by emulating our heroes and "our kind of people" who have succeeded.

In the first place it's not clear that role models of one's own racial or sexual type are necessary (let alone sufficient) for success. One of my heroes was Gandhi, an Indian Hindu, another was my grade school science teacher, Miss DeVoe, and another Martin Luther King, behind whom I marched in Civil Rights demonstrations. More important than having role models of one's "own type" is having genuinely good people, of whatever race or gender, to emulate. Our common humanity should be a sufficient basis for us to see the possibility of success in people of virtue and merit. To yield to the demand, however tempting it may be, for "role-models-just-like-us" is to treat people like means not ends. It is to elevate morally irrelevant particularity over relevant traits, such as ability and integrity. We don't need people exactly like us to find inspiration. As Steve Allen once quipped, "If I had to follow a role model exactly, I would have become a nun."

Furthermore, even if it is of some help to people with low self-esteem to gain encouragement from seeing others of their particular kind in successful positions, it is doubtful whether this is a sufficient reason to justify preferential hiring or reverse discrimination. What good is a role model who is inferior to other professors or physicians or business personnel? The best way to create role models is to promote people because they are the best qualified for the job. It is the violation of this fact that is largely responsible for the widespread whisper in the medical field (at least in New York), "Never go to a Black physician under 40" (referring to the fact that AA has affected the medical system during the past twenty years). Fight the feeling how I will, I cannot help wondering on seeing a Black or woman in a position of honor, "Is she in this position because she merits it or because of Affirmative Action?" Where Affirmative Action is the policy, the "figment of pigment" creates a stigma of undeservedness, whether or not it is deserved.[1]

Finally, entertain this thought experiment. Suppose we discovered that tall handsome white males somehow made the best role models for the most people, especially poor people. Suppose even large numbers of minority people somehow found inspiration in their sight. Would we be justified in hiring tall handsome white males over better qualified short Hispanic women, who were deemed less role-model worthy?

B. The Compensation Argument

The argument goes like this: blacks have been wronged and severely harmed by whites. Therefore white society should compensate blacks for the injury caused them. Reverse discrimination in terms of preferential hiring, contracts, and scholarships is a fitting way to compensate for the past wrongs.

This argument actually involves a distorted notion of compensation. Normally, we think of compensation as owed by a specific person A to another person B whom A has wronged in a specific way C. For example, if I have stolen your car and used it for a period of time to make business profits that would have gone to you, it is not enough that I return your car. I must pay you an amount reflecting your loss and my ability to pay. If I have made $5,000 and only have $10,000 in assets, it would not be possible for you to collect $20,000 in damages—even though that is the amount of loss you have incurred.

Sometimes compensation is extended to groups of people who have been unjustly harmed by the greater society. For example, the United States government has compensated the Japanese-Americans who were interred during the Second World War, and the West German government has paid reparations to the survivors of Nazi concentration camps. But here a specific people have been identified who were wronged in an identifiable way by the government of the nation in question.

On the face of it, demands by blacks for compensation do not fit the usual pattern. Southern States with Jim Crow laws could be accused of unjustly harming blacks, but it is hard to see that the United States government was involved in doing so. Much of the harm done to blacks was the result of private discrimination, not state action. So the Germany/US analogy doesn't hold. Furthermore, it is not clear that all blacks were harmed in the same way or whether some were *unjustly* harmed or harmed more than poor whites and others (e.g., short people). Finally, even if identifiable blacks were harmed by identifiable social practices, it is not clear that most forms of Affirmative Action are appropriate to restore the situation. The usual practice of a financial payment seems more appropriate than giving a high level job to someone unqualified or only minimally qualified, who, speculatively, might have been better qualified had he not been subject to racial discrimination. If John is the star tailback of our college team with a promising professional future, and I accidentally (but culpably) drive my pickup truck over his legs, and so cripple him, John may be due compensation, but he is not due the tailback spot on the football team.

Still, there may be something intuitively compelling about compensating members of an oppressed group who are minimally qualified. Suppose that the Hatfields and the McCoys are enemy clans and some youths from the Hatfields go over and steal diamonds and gold from the McCoys, distributing it within the Hatfield economy. Even though we do not know which Hatfield youths did the stealing, we would want to restore the wealth, as far as possible, to the McCoys. One way might be to tax the Hatfields, but another might be to give preferential treatment in terms of scholarships and training programs and hiring to the McCoys.

This is perhaps the strongest argument for Affirmative Action, and it may well justify some weaker versions of AA, but it is doubtful whether it is sufficient to justify strong versions with quotas and goals and time tables in skilled positions. There are at least two reasons for this. First, we have no way of knowing how many people of any given group would have achieved some given level of competence had the world been different. This is especially relevant if my objections to the Equal Results Argument (below) are correct. Secondly, the normal criterion of competence is a strong prima facie consideration when the most important positions are at stake. There are three reasons for this: (1) treating people according to their merits respects them as persons, as ends in themselves, rather than as means to social ends (if we believe that individuals possess a dignity which deserves to be respected, then we ought to treat that individual on the basis of his or her merits, not as a mere instrument for social policy); (2) society has given people expectations that if they attain certain levels of excellence they will be awarded appropri-

ately; and (3) filling the most important positions with the best qualified is the best way to ensure efficiency in job-related areas and in society in general. These reasons are not absolutes. They can be overridden.[2] But there is a strong presumption in their favor, so that a burden of proof rests with those who would override them.

At this point we get into the problem of whether innocent non-blacks should have to pay a penalty in terms of preferential hiring of blacks. We turn to that argument.

C. The Argument for Compensation from Those Who Innocently Benefitted from Past Injustice

Young White males as innocent beneficiaries of unjust discrimination against blacks and women have no grounds for complaint when society seeks to level the tilted field. They may be innocent of oppressing blacks, other minorities, and women, but they have unjustly benefitted from that oppression or discrimination. So it is perfectly proper that less qualified women and blacks be hired before them.

The operative principle is: He who knowingly and willingly benefits from a wrong must help pay for the wrong. Judith Jarvis Thomson puts it this way. "Many [white males] have been direct beneficiaries of policies which have downgraded blacks and women . . . and even those who did not directly benefit . . . had, at any rate, the advantage in the competition which comes of the confidence in one's full membership [in the community], and of one's right being recognized as a matter of course."[3] That is, white males obtain advantages in self-respect and self-confidence deriving from a racist/sexist system which denies these to blacks and women.

Here is my response to this argument: As I noted in the previous section, compensation is normally individual and specific. If A harms B regarding x, B has a right to compensation from A in regards to x. If A steals B's car and wrecks it, A has an obligation to compensate B for the stolen car, but A's son has no obligation to compensate B. Furthermore, if A dies or disappears, B has no moral right to claim that society compensate him for the stolen car—though if he has insurance, he can make such a claim to the insurance company. Sometimes a wrong cannot be compensated, and we just have to make the best of an imperfect world.

Suppose my parents, divining that I would grow up to have an unsurpassable desire to be a basketball player, bought an expensive growth hormone for me. Unfortunately, a neighbor stole it and gave it to little Michael, who gained the extra 13 inches—my 13 inches—and shot up to an enviable 6 feet 6 inches. Michael, better known as Michael Jordan, would have been a runt like me but for his luck. As it is he profited from the injustice, and excelled in basketball, as I would have done had I had my proper dose.

Do I have a right to the millions of dollars that Jordan made as a professional basketball player—the unjustly innocent beneficiary of my growth hormone? I have a right to something from the neighbor who stole the hormone and it might be kind of Jordan to give me free tickets to the [Bulls'] basketball games, and remember me in his will. As far as I can see, however, he does not *owe* me anything, either legally or morally.

Suppose further that Michael Jordan and I are in high school together and we are both qualified to play basketball, only he is far better than I. Do I deserve to start in his position because I would have been as good as he is had someone not cheated me as a child? Again, I think not. But if being the lucky beneficiary of wrongdoing does not entail that Jordan (or the coach) owes me anything in regards to basketball, why should it be a reason to engage in preferential hiring in academic positions or highly coveted jobs? If minimal qualifications are not adequate to override excellence in basketball, even when the minimality is a consequence of wrongdoing, why should they be adequate in other areas?

D. The Diversity Argument

It is important that we learn to live in a pluralistic world, learning to get along with those of other races, conditions, and cultures, so we should have schools and employment situations as fully integrated as pos-

sible. In a shrinking world we need to appreciate each other's culture and specific way of looking at life. Diversity is an important symbol and educative device. Thus, proponents of AA argue, preferential treatment is warranted to perform this role in society.

Once again, there is some truth in these concerns. Diversity of ideas challenges us to scrutinize our own values and beliefs, and diverse customs have aesthetic and moral value, helping us to appreciate the novelty and beauty in life. Diversity may expand our moral horizons. But, again, while we can admit the value of diversity, it hardly seems adequate to override the moral requirement to treat each person with equal respect. *Diversity for diversity's sake is moral promiscuity,* since it obfuscates rational distinctions, undermines treating individuals as ends, treating them, instead as mere means (to the goals of social engineering), and, furthermore, unless those hired are highly qualified, the diversity factor threatens to become a fetish. At least at the higher levels of business and the professions, *competence* far outweighs considerations of diversity. I do not care whether the group of surgeons operating on me reflect racial or gender balance, but I do care that they are highly qualified. Neither do most football or basketball fans care whether their team reflects ethnic and gender diversity, but demand the best combination of players available. And likewise with airplane pilots, military leaders, business executives, and, may I say it, teachers and university professors. One need not be a white male to teach, let alone, appreciate Shakespeare, nor need one be Black to teach, let alone appreciate, Alice Walker's *Color Purple.*

There may be times when diversity may seem to be "crucial" to the well-being of a diverse community, such as for a police force. Suppose that White policemen tend to overreact to young Black males and the latter group distrust White policemen. Hiring more less qualified Black policemen, who would relate better to these youth, may have overall utilitarian value. But such a move, while we might take it as a lesser evil, could have serious consequences in allowing the demographic prejudices to dictate social policy. A better strategy would be to hire the best police, that is, those who can perform in disciplined, intelligent manner, regardless of their race. A White policeman must be able to arrest a Black burglar, even as a Black policeman must be able to arrest a White rapist. The quality of the police man or woman, not their race or gender is what counts.

On the other hand, if a Black policeman, though lacking some of the formal skills of the White policeman, really is able to do a better job in the Black community, this might constitute a case of merit, not Affirmative Action. As Stephen Kershnar points out, this is similar to the legitimacy of hiring Chinese men to act as undercover agents in Chinatown.[4]

E. The Equal Results Argument

Some philosophers and social scientists hold that human nature is roughly identical, so that on a fair playing field the same proportion from every race and ethnic group and both genders would attain to the highest positions in every area of endeavor. It would follow that any inequality of results itself is evidence for inequality of opportunity.

History is important when considering governmental rules like Test 21 because low scores by blacks can be traced in large measure to the legacy of slavery and racism: segregation, poor schooling, exclusion from trade unions, malnutrition, and poverty have all played their roles. Unless one assumes that blacks are naturally less able to pass the test, the conclusion must be that the results are themselves socially and legally constructed, not a mere given for which law and society can claim no responsibility.

The conclusion seems to be that genuine equality eventually requires equal results. Obviously blacks have been treated unequally throughout US history, and just as obviously the economic and psychological effects of that inequality linger to this day, showing up in lower income and poorer performance in school and on tests than whites achieve. Since we have no reason to believe that differences in performance can be explained by factors other than history, equal results are a good benchmark by which to measure progress made toward genuine equality. (John Arthur, *The Unfinished Constitution* [Belmont, CA: Wadsworth Publishing Co, 1990], p. 238)

Sterling Harwood seems to support a similar theory when he writes, "When will [AA] end? When will affirmative action stop compensating blacks? As soon as the unfair advantage is gone, affirmative action will stop. The elimination of the unfair advantage can be determined by showing that the percentage of blacks hired and admitted at least roughly equaled the percentage of blacks in the population."[5]

Albert G. Mosley develops a similar argument. "Establishing Blacks' presence at a level commensurate with their proportion in the relevant labor market need not be seen as an attempt to actualize some valid prediction. Rather, given the impossibility of determining what level of representation Blacks would have achieved were it not for racial discrimination, the assumption of proportional representation is the only *fair* assumption to make. This is not to argue that Blacks should be maintained in such positions, but their contrived exclusion merits equally contrived rectification."[6] The result of a just society should be equal numbers in proportion to each group in the work force.

However, Arthur, Mosley, and Harwood fail even to consider studies that suggest that there are innate differences between races, sexes, and groups. If there are genetic differences in intelligence, temperament, and other qualities within families, why should we not expect such differences between racial groups and the two genders? Why should the evidence for this be completely discounted?

Mosley's reasoning is as follows: Since we don't know for certain whether groups proportionately differ in talent, we should presume that they are equal in every respect. So we should presume that if we were living in a just society, there would be roughly proportionate representation in every field (e.g., equal representation of doctors, lawyers, professors, carpenters, airplane pilots, basketball players, and criminals). Hence, it is only fair—productive of justice—to aim at proportionate representation in these fields.

But the logic is flawed. Under a situation of ignorance we should not presume equality or inequality of representation—but conclude that we *don't know* what the results would be in a just society. Ignorance doesn't favor equal group representation any more than it favors unequal group representation. It is neutral between them.

Consider this analogy. Suppose that you were the owner of a National Basketball Association team. Suppose that I and other frustrated White basketball players bring a class-action suit against you and all the other team owners, claiming that you have subtly and systematically discriminated against White and Asian basketball players who make up less than 20% of the NBA players. You reply that you and the other owners are just responding to individual merit, we respond that the discrimination is a function of deep prejudice against White athletes, especially basketball players, who are discouraged in every way from competing on fair terms with Blacks who dominate the NBA. You would probably wish that the matter of unequal results was not brought up in the first place, but once it has been, would you not be in your rights to defend yourself by producing evidence, showing that *average* physiological differences exist between Blacks and Whites and Asians, so that we should not presume unjust discrimination?

Similarly, the proponents of the Doctrine of Equal Results open the door to a debate over average ability in ethnic, racial and gender groups. The proponent of equal or fair opportunity would just as soon downplay this feature in favor of judging people as individuals by their merit (hard though that may be). But if the proponent of AA insists on the Equal Results Thesis, we are obliged to examine the Equal Abilities Thesis, on which it is based—the thesis that various ethnic and gender groups all have the same distribution of talent on the relevant characteristic. With regard to cognitive skills we must consult the best evidence we have on average group differences. We need to compare average IQ scores, SAT scores, standard personality testing, success in academic and professional areas and the like. If the evidence shows that group differences are nonexistent, the AA proponent may win, but if the evidence turns out to be against the Equal Abilities Thesis, the AA proponent loses. Consider for a start that the average white and Asian scores 195 points higher on the SAT tests and that on virtually all IQ tests for the past seven or eight decades the average Black IQ is 85 as opposed to the average White and Asian IQ at over 100, or that males and females differ significantly on cognitive ability tests. Females outperform males in reading comprehension, perceptual speed, and associative memory (ratios of 1.4 to 2.2), but males typically outnumber females among high scoring individuals in mathematics, science and social science (by a ratio of 7.0 in the top 1% of overall mathematics distribution).[7] The results of average GRE, LSAT, MCAT scores show similar patterns or significant average racial difference. The Black scholar Glenn Loury notes, "In 1990 black high school seniors from families with annual incomes of $70,000 or more scored an average of 855 on the SAT, compared with average scores of 855 and 879 respectively for Asian-American and white seniors whose families had incomes between $10,000 and 20,000 per year."[8] Note, we are speaking about statistical averages. There are brilliant and retarded people in each group.

When such statistics are discussed many people feel uncomfortable and want to drop the subject. Perhaps these statistics are misleading, but then we need to look carefully at the total evidence. The proponent of equal opportunity urges us to get beyond racial and gender criteria in assignment of offices and opportunities and treat each person, not as an *average* White or Black or female or male, but as a *person* judged on his or her own merits.

Furthermore, on the logic of Mosley and company, we should take aggressive AA against Asians and Jews since they are overrepresented in science, technology, and medicine, and we should presume that Asians and Jews are no more talented than average. So that each group receives its fair share, we should ensure that 12% of the philosophers in the United States are Black, reduce the percentage of Jews from an estimated 15% to 2%—thus firing about 1,300 Jewish philosophers. The fact that Asians are producing 50% of Ph.D.s in science and math in this country and blacks less than 1% clearly shows, on this reasoning, that we are providing special secret advantages to Asians. By this logic, we should reduce the quota of Blacks in the NBA to 12%.

But why does society have to enter into this results game in the first place? Why do we have to decide whether all difference is environmental or genetic? Perhaps we should simply admit that we lack sufficient evidence to pronounce on these issues with any certainty—but if so, should we not be more modest in insisting on equal results? Here's a thought experiment. Take two families of different racial groups, Green and Blue. The Greens decide to have only two children, to spend all their resources on them, and to give them the best possible education. The two Green kids respond well and end up with achievement test scores in the 99th percentile. The Blues fail to practice family planning and have 15 children. They can only afford 2 children, but lack of ability or whatever prevents them from keeping their family size down. Now they need help for their large family. Why does society have to step in and help them? Society did not force them to have 15 children. Suppose that the achievement test scores of the 15 children fall below the 25th percentile. They cannot compete with the Greens. But now enters AA. It says that it is society's fault that the Blue children are not as able as the Greens and that the Greens must pay extra taxes to enable the Blues to compete. No restraints are put on the Blues regarding family size. This seems unfair to the Greens. Should the Green children be made to bear responsibility for the consequences of the Blues' voluntary behavior?

My point is simply that philosophers like Arthur, Harwood, and Mosley need to cast their net wider and recognize that demographics and childbearing and -rearing practices are crucial factors in achievement. People have to take some responsibility for their actions. The equal results argument (or axiom) misses a greater part of the picture.

F. The "No One Deserves His Talents" Argument Against Meritocracy

According to this argument, the competent do not deserve their intelligence, their superior character, their industriousness, or their discipline; therefore they have no right to the best positions in society; therefore it is not unjust to give these positions to less (but still minimally) qualified blacks and women. In one form this argument holds that since no one deserves anything, society may use any criteria it pleases to distribute goods. The criterion most often designated is social utility. Versions of this argument are found in the writings of John Arthur, John Rawls, Bernard Boxill, Michael Kinsley, Ronald Dworkin, and Richard Wasserstrom. Rawls writes, "No one deserves his place in the distribution of native endowments, any more than one deserves one's initial starting place in society. The assertion that a man deserves the superior character that enables him to make the effort to cultivate his abilities is equally problematic; for his character depends in large part upon fortunate family and social circumstances for which he can claim no credit. The notion of desert seems not to apply to these cases."[9] Michael Kinsley is even more adamant.

Opponents of affirmative action are hung up on a distinction that seems more profoundly irrelevant: treating individuals versus treating groups. What is the moral difference between dispensing favors to people on their "merits" as individuals and passing out society's benefits on the basis of group identification?

Group identifications like race and sex are, of course, immutable. They have nothing to do with a person's moral worth. But the same is true of most of what comes under the label "merit." The tools you need for getting ahead in a meritocratic society—not all of them but most: talent, education, instilled cultural values such as ambition—are distributed just as arbitrarily as skin color. They are fate. The notion that people somehow "deserve" the advantages of these characteristics in a way they don't "deserve" the advantage of their race is powerful, but illogical.[10]

It will help to put the argument in outline form.

1. Society may award jobs and positions as it sees fit as long as individuals have no claim to these positions.

2. To have a claim to something means that one has earned it or deserves it.

3. But no one has earned or deserves his intelligence, talent, education or cultural values which produce superior qualifications.

4. If a person does not deserve what produces something, he does not deserve its products.

5. Therefore better qualified people do not deserve their qualifications.

6. Therefore, society may override their qualifications in awarding jobs and positions as it sees fit (for social utility or to compensate for previous wrongs).

So it is permissible if a minimally qualified black or woman is admitted to law or medical school ahead of a white male with excellent credentials or if a less qualified person from an "underutilized" group gets a professorship ahead of an eminently better qualified white male. Sufficiency and underutilization together outweigh excellence.

My response: Premise 4 is false. To see this, reflect that just because I do not deserve the money that I have been given as a gift (for instance) does not mean that I am not entitled to what I get with that money. If you and I both get a gift of $100 and I bury mine in the sand for 5 years while you invest yours wisely and double its value at the end of five years, I cannot complain that you should split the increase 50/50 since neither of us deserved the original gift. If we accept the notion of responsibility at all, we must hold that persons deserve the fruits of their labor and conscious choices. Of course, we might want to distinguish moral from legal desert and argue that, morally speaking, effort is more important than outcome, whereas, legally speaking, outcome may be more important. Nevertheless, there are good reasons in terms of efficiency, motivation, and rough justice for holding a strong prima facie principle of giving scarce high positions to those most competent.

The attack on moral desert is perhaps the most radical move that egalitarians like Rawls and company have made against meritocracy, and the ramifications of their attack are far reaching. Here are some implications: Since I do not deserve my two good eyes or two good kidneys, the social engineers may take one of each from me to give to those needing an eye or a kidney—even if they have damaged their organs by their own voluntary actions. Since no one deserves anything, we do not deserve pay for our labors or praise for a job well done or first prize in the race we win. The notion of moral responsibility vanishes in a system of levelling.

But there is no good reason to accept the argument against desert. We do act freely and, as such, we are responsible for our actions. We deserve the fruits of our labor, reward for our noble feats and punishment for our misbehavior.

We have considered six arguments for Affirmative Action and have found no compelling case for Strong AA and only one plausible argument (a version of the compensation argument) for Weak AA. We must now turn to the arguments against Affirmative Action to see whether they fare any better.

II. ARGUMENTS AGAINST AFFIRMATIVE ACTION

A. Affirmative Action Requires Discrimination Against a Different Group

Weak AA weakly discriminates against new minorities, mostly innocent young white males, and Strong Affirmative Action strongly discriminates against these new minorities. As I argued in I. C, this discrimination is unwarranted, since, even if some compensation to blacks were indicated, it would be unfair to make innocent white males bear the whole brunt of the payments. Recently I had this experience. I knew a brilliant philosopher, with outstanding publications in first level journals, who was having difficulty getting a tenure-track position. For the first time in my life I offered to make a phone call on his behalf to a university to which he had applied. When I got the Chair of the Search Committee, he offered that the committee was under instructions from the Administration to hire a woman or a Black. They had one of each on their short-list, so they weren't even considering the applications of White males. At my urging he retrieved my friend's file, and said, "This fellow looks far superior to the two candidates we're interviewing, but there's nothing I can do about it." Cases like this come to my attention regularly. In fact, it is poor white youth who become the new pariahs on the job market. The children of the wealthy have little trouble getting into the best private grammar schools and, on the basis of superior early education, into the best universities, graduate schools, managerial and professional positions. Affirmative Action simply shifts injustice, setting Blacks, Hispanics, Native Americans, Asians and women against young white males, especially ethnic and poor white males. It makes no more sense to discriminate in favor of a rich Black or female who had the opportunity of the best family and education available against a poor White, than it does to discriminate in favor of White males against Blacks or women. It does little to rectify the goal of providing equal opportunity to all.

At the end of his essay supporting Affirmative Action, Albert Mosley points out that other groups besides Blacks have been benefitted by AA, "women, the disabled, the elderly."[11] He's correct in including the elderly, for through powerful lobbies, such as the AARP, they do get special benefits, including medicare, and may sue on the grounds of being discriminated against due to *Agism*, prejudice against older people. Might this not be a reason to reconsider Affirmative Action? Consider the sheer rough percentages of those who qualify for AA programs.

GROUP	PERCENTAGE in Population
1. Women	52%
2. Blacks	12%
3. Hispanics	9%
4. Native Americans	2%
5. Asians	4%
6. Physically & Mentally Disabled	10%
7. Welfare recipients	6%
8. The Elderly	25% (est. Adults over 60)
9. Italians (in New York City)	3%
Totals	123%

The elderly can sue on the grounds of Agism, receive entitlements in terms of Social Security and Medicare, and have the AARP lobbying on their behalf. Recently, it has been proposed that homosexuals be included in oppressed groups deserving Affirmative Action. At Northeastern University in 1996 the faculty governing body voted to grant homosexuals Affirmative Action status at this university. How many more percentage points would this add? Several authors have advocated putting all poor people on the list. And if we took handicaps seriously would we not add ugly people, obese people, and, especially, short people, for which there is ample evidence of discrimination? How about left-handed people (about 9% of the population)—they can't play shortstop or third base and have to put up with a right-handedly biased world. The only group not on the list is that of White males. Are they, especially healthy, middle class young White males, becoming the new "oppressed class"? Should we add them to our list?

Respect for persons entails that we treat each person as an end in him or herself, not simply as a means to be used for social purposes. What is wrong about discrimination against Blacks is that it fails to treat Black people as individuals, judging them instead by their skin color not their merit. What is wrong about discrimination against women is that it fails to treat them as individuals, judging them by their gender, not their merit. What is equally wrong about *Affirmative Action* is that it fails to treat White males with dignity as individuals, judging them by *both their race and gender,* instead of their merit. *Current Strong Affirmative Action is both racist and sexist.*

B. Affirmative Action Encourages Mediocrity and Incompetence

A few years ago Rev. Jesse Jackson joined protesters at Harvard Law School in demanding that the Law School faculty hire black women. Jackson dismissed Dean of the Law School, Robert C. Clark's standard of choosing the best qualified person for the job as "Cultural anemia." "We cannot just define who is qualified in the most narrow vertical academic terms," he said. "Most people in the world are yellow, brown, black, poor, non-Christian and don't speak English, and they can't wait for some white males with archaic rules to appraise them."[12] It might be noted that if Jackson is correct about the depth of cultural decadence at Harvard, blacks might be well advised to form and support their own more vital law schools and leave places like Harvard to their archaism.

At several universities, the administration has forced departments to hire members of minorities even when far superior candidates were available. Shortly after obtaining my PhD in the late 70s I was mistakenly identified as a black philosopher (I had a civil rights record and was once a black studies major) and was flown to a major university, only to be rejected for a more qualified candidate when it discovered that I was white.

Stories of the bad effects of Affirmative Action abound. The philosopher Sidney Hook writes that "At one Ivy League university, representatives of the Regional HEW[13] demanded an explanation of why there were no women or minority students in the Graduate Department of Religious Studies. They were told that a reading knowledge of Hebrew and Greek was presupposed. Whereupon the representatives of HEW advised orally: 'Then end those old fashioned programs that require irrelevant languages. And start up programs on relevant things which minority group students can study without learning languages.' "[14]

Nicholas Capaldi notes that the staff of HEW itself was one-half women, three-fifths members of minorities, and one-half black—a clear case of racial overrepresentation.

In 1972 officials at Stanford University discovered a proposal for the government to monitor curriculum in higher education: the "Summary Statement . . . Sex Discrimination Proposed HEW Regulation to Effectuate Title IX of the Education Amendment of 1972" to "establish and use internal procedure for reviewing curricula, designed both to ensure that they do not reflect discrimination on the basis of sex and to resolve complaints concerning allegations of such discrimination, pursuant to procedural standards to be prescribed by the Director of the office of Civil Rights." Fortunately, Secretary of HEW Caspar Weinberger discovered the intrusion and assured Stanford University that he would never approve of it.

Government programs of enforced preferential treatment tend to appeal to the lowest possible common denominator. Witness the 1974 HEW Revised Order No. 14 on Affirmative Action expectations for preferential hiring: "Neither minorities nor female employees should be required to possess higher qualifications than those of the lowest qualified incumbents."

Furthermore, no test may be given to candidates unless it is *proved* to be relevant to the job.

No standard or criteria which have, by intent or effect, worked to exclude women or minorities as a class can be utilized, unless the institution can demonstrate the necessity of such standard to the performance of the job in question.

Whenever a validity study is called for . . . the user should include . . . an investigation of suitable alternative selection procedures and suitable alternative methods of using the selection procedure which have as little adverse impact as possible. . . . Whenever the user is shown an alternative selection procedure with evidence of less adverse impact and substantial evidence of validity for the same job in similar circumstances, the user should investigate it to determine the appropriateness of using or validating it in accord with these guidelines.[15]

At the same time Americans are wondering why standards in our country are falling and the Japanese and Koreans are getting ahead. Affirmative Action with its twin idols, Sufficiency of Qualification and Diversity, is the enemy of excellence. I will develop this thought in the next section.

C. An Argument from the Principle of Merit

Traditionally, we have believed that the highest positions in society should be awarded to those who are best qualified. The Koran states that "A ruler who appoints any man to an office, when there is in his dominion another man better qualified for it, sins against God and against the State." Rewarding excellence both seems just to the individuals in the competition and makes for efficiency. Note that one of the most successful acts of racial integration, the Brooklyn Dodger's recruitment of Jackie Robinson in the late 40s, was done in just this way, according to merit. If Robinson had been brought into the major league as a mediocre player or had batted .200 he would have been scorned and sent back to the minors where he belonged.

As mentioned earlier, merit is not an absolute value, but there are strong *prima facie* reasons for awarding positions on that basis, and it should enjoy a weighty presumption in our social practices.

In a celebrated article Ronald Dworkin says that "Bakke had no case" because society did not owe Bakke anything. That may be, but then why does it owe anyone anything? Dworkin puts the matter in Utility terms, but if that is the case, society may owe Bakke a place at the University of California/Davis, for it seems a reasonable rule-utilitarian principle that achievement should be awarded in society. We generally want the best to have the best positions, the best qualified candidate to win the political office, the most brilliant and competent scientist to be chosen for the most challenging research project, the best qualified pilots to become commercial pilots, only the best soldiers to become generals. Only when little is at stake do we weaken the standards and content ourselves with sufficiency (rather than excellence)—there are plenty of jobs where "sufficiency" rather than excellence is required. Perhaps we have even come to feel that medicine or law or university professorships are so routine that they can be performed by minimally qualified people—in which case AA has a place.

Note! no one is calling for quotas or proportional representation of *underutilized* groups in the National Basketball Association where blacks make up 80% of the players. But, surely, if merit and merit alone reigns in sports, should it not be valued at least as much in education and industry?

The case for meritocracy has two pillars. One pillar is a deontological argument which holds that we ought to treat people as ends and not merely means. By giving people what they deserve as *individuals,* rather than as members of *groups* we show respect for their inherent worth. If you and I take a test, and you get 95% of the answers correct, and I only get 50% correct, it would be unfair to you for both of us to receive the same grade, say an A, and even more unfair to give me a higher grade A+ than your B+. Although I have heard cases where teachers have been instructed to "race norm" in grading (giving Blacks and Hispanics higher grades for the same numerical scores), most proponents of AA stop short of advocating such a practice. But, I would ask them, what's really the difference between taking the overall average of a White and a Black and "race norming" it? If teachers shouldn't do it, why should administrators?

The second pillar for meritocracy is utilitarian. In the end, we will be better off by honoring excellence. We want the best leaders, teachers, policemen, physicians, generals, lawyers, and airplane pilots that we can possibly produce in society. So our program should be to promote equal opportunity, as much as is feasible in a free market economy, and reward people according to their individual merit.

CONCLUSION

Let me sum up my discussion. The goal of the Civil Rights movement and of moral people everywhere has been justice for all, including equal opportunity. The question is: how best to get there. Civil Rights legislation removed the unjust legal barriers, opening the way towards equal opportunity, but it did not tackle the deeper causes that produce differential results. Weak Affirmative Action aims at encouraging minorities to strive for excellence in all areas of life, without unduly jeopardizing the rights of majorities. The problem of Weak Affirmative Action is that it easily slides into Strong Affirmative Action where quotas, goals and timetables," "equal results"—in a word—*reverse discrimination*—prevail and are forced onto groups, thus promoting mediocrity, inefficiency, and resentment. Furthermore, AA aims at the higher levels of society—universities and skilled jobs, but if we want to improve our society, the best way to do it is to concentrate on families, children, early education, and the like, so all are prepared to avail themselves of opportunity. Affirmative Action, on the one hand, is too much, too soon and on the other hand, too little, too late.

In addition to the arguments I have offered, Affirmative Action, rather than unite people of good will in the common cause of justice, tends to balkanize us into segregation-thinking. Professor Derrick Bell of Harvard Law School recently said that the African American Supreme Court Judge Clarence Thomas, in his opposition to Affirmative Action "doesn't think black." Does Bell really claim that there is a standard and proper "Black" (and presumably a White) way of thinking? Ideologues like Bell, whether radical Blacks like himself, or Nazis who advocate "think Aryan," both represent the same thing: cynicism about rational debate, the very antithesis of the quest for impartial truth and justice. People who believe in reason to resolve our differences will oppose this kind of balkanization of the races.

Martin Luther said that humanity is like a man mounting a horse who always tends to fall off on the other side of the horse. This seems to be the case with Affirmative Action. Attempting to redress the discriminatory iniquities of our history, our well-intentioned social engineers now engage in new forms of discriminatory iniquity and thereby think that they have successfully mounted the horse of racial harmony. They have only fallen off on the other side of the issue.

NOTES

1. This argument is related to *The Need of Breaking Stereotypes Argument*. Society may simply need to know that there are talented Blacks and women, so that it does not automatically assign them lesser respect or status. The right response is that hiring less qualified people is neither fair to those better qualified who are passed over nor an effective way to remove inaccurate stereotypes. If high competence is accepted as the criterion for hiring, then it is unjust to override it for purposes of social engineering. Furthermore, if Blacks and women are known to hold high positions simply because of reverse discrimination, they will still lack the respect due to those of their rank.

2. Merit sometimes may be justifiably overridden by need, as when parents choose to spend extra earnings on special education for their disabled child rather than for their gifted child. Sometimes we may override merit for utilitarian purposes. E.g., suppose you are the best short stop on a baseball team but are also the best catcher. You'd rather play short stop, but the manager decides to put you at catcher because, while your friend can do an adequate job at short, no one else is adequate at catcher. It's permissible for you to be assigned the job of catcher. Probably, some expression of appreciation would be due you.

3. Judith Jarvis Thomson, "Preferential Hiring," in Marshall Cohen, Thomas Nagel and Thomas Scanlon, eds., *Equality and Preferential Treatment* (Princeton: Princeton University Press, 1977).

4. Stephen Kershnar pointed this out in written comments (December 22, 1997).

5. Sterling Harwood, "The Justice of Affirmative Action," in Yearger Hudson and C. Peden, eds., *The Bill of Rights: Bicentennial Reflections* (Lewiston, NY: Edwin Mellen).

6. Albert G. Mosley in his and Nicholas Capaldi's *Affirmative Action: Social Justice or Unfair Preference?* (Rowman and Littlefield, 1996), p. 28.

7. Larry Hedges and Amy Nowell, "Sex Differences in Mental Test Scores, Variability, and Numbers of High-Scoring Individuals," *Science* 269 (July 1995), pp. 41–45.

8. Glen Loury, " 'Getting Involved': An Appeal for Greater Community Participation in the Public Schools," *Washington Post Education Review* (August 6, 1995).

9. John Rawls, *A Theory of Justice* (Harvard University Press, 1971), p. 104.

10. Michael Kinsley, "Equal Lack of Opportunity," *Harper's* (June 1983).

11. Albert Mosley, op. cit., p. 53.

12. *New York Times*, May 10, 1990.

13. HEW stands for the Federal Department of "Health, Education & Welfare."

14. Quoted by Nicholas Capaldi, *Out of Order: Affirmative Action and the Crisis of Doctrinaire Liberalism* (Buffalo, NY: Prometheus, 1985).

15. Capaldi, op. cit., p. 95

Affirmative Action and Quotas

RICHARD A. WASSERSTROM

* * *

Someone might say something like this [about affirmative action]: it is just wrong in principle ever to take an individual's race or sex into account. Persons just have a right never to have race or sex considered. No reasons need be given; we just know they have that right. This is a common way of talking today in moral philosophy, but I find nothing persuasive or attractive about it. I do not know that persons have such a right. I do not "see" it. Instead, I think I can give and have given reasons in my discussion of the social realities as well as my discussion of ideals for why they might be said to have rights not to be treated in certain ways. That is to say, I have tried to show something of what was wrong about the way blacks and women were and are treated in our culture. I have not simply proclaimed the existence of a right.

Another form of this objection is more convincing. The opponent of quotas and affirmative action programs might argue that any proponent of them is guilty of intellectual inconsistency, if not racism or sexism. At times past, employers, universities, and many social institutions did have racial or sexual quotas, when they did not practice overt racial or sexual exclusion, and it was clear that these quotas were pernicious. What is more, many of those who were most concerned to bring about the eradication of those racial quotes are now untroubled by the new programs which reinstitute them. And this is just a terrible sort of intellectual inconsistency which at worst panders to the fashion of the present moment and at best replaces intellectual honesty and integrity with understandable but misguided sympathy. The assimilationist ideal requires ignoring race and sex as distinguishing features of people.

Such an argument is a useful means by which to bring out the way in which the analysis I am proposing can respond. The racial quotas and practices of racial exclusion that were an integral part of the fabric of our culture, and which are still to some degree a part of it, were pernicious. They were a grievous wrong and it was and is important that all morally concerned individuals work for their eradication from our social universe. The racial quotas that are a part of contemporary affirmative action programs are, I think, commendable and right. But even if I am mistaken about the latter, the point is that there is no inconsistency involved in holding both views. For even if contemporary schemes of racial quotas are wrong, they are wrong for reasons very different from those that made quotas against blacks wrong.

As I have argued, the fundamental evil of programs that discriminated against blacks or women was that these programs were a part of a larger social universe which systematically maintained an unwarranted and unjust scheme which concentrated power, authority, and goods in the hands of white males. Programs which excluded or limited the access of blacks and women into these institutions were wrong both because of the direct consequences of these programs on the individuals most affected and because the system of racial and sexual superiority of which they were constituents was an immoral one in that it severely and without any adequate justification restricted the capacities, autonomy, and happiness of those who were members of the less favored categories.

Whatever may be wrong with today's affirmative action programs and quota systems, it should be clear that the evil, if any, is not the same. Racial and sexual minorities do not constitute the dominant social group. Nor is the conception of who is a fully developed member of the moral and social community one of an individual who is either female or black. Quotas which prefer women or blacks do not add to the already relatively overabundant supply of resources and opportunities at the disposal of white males. If

Richard A. Wasserstrom, excerpted from "Racism, Sexism, and Preferential Treatment: An Approach to the Topics" by Richard A. Wasserstrom, 24 UCLA Law Review 581 (1977). Reprinted by permission of the author.

racial quotas are to be condemned or if affirmative action programs are to be abandoned, it should be because they will not work well to achieve the desired result. It is not because they seek either to perpetuate an unjust society or to realize a corrupt ideal.

Still a third version of this objection might be that when used in affirmative action programs, race and sex are categories that are too broad in scope. They include some persons who do not have the appropriate characteristics and exclude some persons who do. If affirmative action programs made race and sex the sole criteria of selection, this would certainly be a plausible objection, although even here it is very important to see that the objection is no different in kind from that which applies to all legislation and rules. For example, in restricting the franchise to those who are eighteen and older, we exclude some who have all the relevant qualifications for voting and we include some who lack them. The fit can never be precise. Affirmative action programs almost always make race or sex a *relevant* condition, not a conclusive one. As such, they function the way all other classificatory schemes do. The defect, if there is one, is generic, and not peculiar to programs such as these.

There is finally the third objection: that affirmative action programs are wrong because they take race and sex into account rather than the only thing that matters—an individual's qualifications. Someone might argue that what is wrong with these programs is that they deprive persons who are more qualified by bestowing benefits on those who are less qualified in virtue of their being either black or female.

There are many things wrong with the objection based on qualifications. Not the least of them is that we do not live in a society in which there is even the serious pretense of a qualification requirement for many jobs of substantial power and authority. Would anyone claim that the persons who comprise the judiciary are there because they are the most qualified lawyers or the most qualified persons to be judges? Would anyone claim that Henry Ford II is the head of the Ford Motor Company because he is the most qualified person for the job? Or that the one hundred men who are Senators are the most qualified persons to be Senators? Part of what is wrong with

even talking about qualifications and merit is that the argument derives some of its force from the erroneous notion that we would have a meritocracy were it not for affirmative action.

But there is a theoretical difficulty as well, which cuts much more deeply into the argument about qualifications. The argument cannot be that the most qualified ought to be selected because the most qualified will perform most efficiently, for this instrumental approach was what the opponent of affirmative action thought was wrong with taking the instrumental perspective in the first place. To be at all persuasive, the argument must be that those who are the most qualified *deserve* to receive the benefits (the job, the place in law school, etc.) because they are the most qualified. And there is just no reason to think that this is a correct premise. There is a logical gap in the inference that the person who is most qualified to perform a task, *e.g.*, be a good student, deserves to be admitted as a student. Of course, those who deserve to be admitted should be admitted. But why do the most qualified deserve anything? There is just no necessary connection between academic merit (in the sense of qualification) and deserving to be a member of a student body. Suppose, for instance, that there is only one tennis court in the community. Is it clear that the two best tennis players ought to be the ones permitted to use it? Why not those who were there first? Or those who will enjoy playing the most? Or those who are the worst and therefore need the greatest opportunity to practice? Or those who have the chance to play least frequently?

We might, of course, have a rule that says that the best tennis players get to use the court before the others. Under such a rule, the best players would deserve the court more than the poorer ones. But that is just to push the inquiry back one stage. Is there any reason to think that good tennis players are entitled to such a rule? Indeed, the arguments that might be given for or against such a rule are many and varied. And few if any of the arguments that might support the rule would depend upon a connection between ability and desert.

Someone might reply that the most able students deserve to be admitted to the university because all of their earlier schooling was a kind of competition, with university admission being the prize awarded to the winners. They deserve to be admitted because that is what the rule of the competition provides. In addition, it would be unfair now to exclude them in favor of others, given the reasonable expectations they developed about the way in which their industry and performance would be rewarded. Minority admission programs, which inevitably prefer some who are less qualified over some who are more qualified, all possess this flaw.

There are several problems with this argument. The most substantial of them is that it is an empirically implausible picture of our social world. Most of what are regarded as the decisive characteristics for higher education have a great deal to do with things over which the individual has neither control nor responsibility: such things as home environment, socioeconomic class of parents, and, of course, the quality of the primary and secondary schools attended. Since individuals do not deserve having had any of these things vis-à-vis other individuals, they do not, for the most part, deserve their qualifications. And since they do not deserve their abilities they do not in any strong sense deserve to be admitted because of their abilities.

To be sure, if there is a rule which connects, say, performance at high school with admission to college, then there is a weak sense in which those who do well at high school deserve, for that reason alone, to be admitted to college. But then, as I have said, the merits of this rule need to be explored and defended. In addition, if persons have built up or relied upon their reasonable expectations concerning performance and admission, they have a claim to be admitted on this ground as well. But it is certainly not obvious that these claims of desert are any stronger or more compelling than competing claims based upon the needs of or advantages to women or blacks.

Qualifications are also potentially relevant in at least three other respects. In the first place, there is some minimal set of qualifications without which the benefits of participation in higher education cannot be obtained by the individuals involved. In the second place, the qualifications of the students within the university will affect to some degree or other the benefits obtainable to anyone within it. And finally, the qualifications of students within the university may also affect the way the university functions vis-à-vis the rest of the world. The university will do some things better and some things worse depending upon the qualifications of those who make it up. If the students are "less qualified," teachers may have to spend more time with them and less time on research. Some teachers may find teaching now more interesting. Others may find it less so. But all these considerations only establish that qualifications, in this sense, are relevant, not that they are decisive. This is wholly consistent with the claim that minority group membership is also a relevant but not a decisive consideration when it comes to matters of admission. And that is all that virtually any preferential treatment program—even one with quotas—has ever tried to claim.

I do not think I have shown programs of preferential treatment to be right and desirable, because I have not sought to answer all of the empirical questions that may be relevant. But I have, I hope, shown that it is wrong to think that contemporary affirmative action programs are racist or sexist in the centrally important sense in which many past and present features of our society have been and are racist and sexist. The social realities do make a fundamental difference. It is also wrong to think that these programs are in any strong sense either unjust or unprincipled. The case for programs of preferential treatment can plausibly rest on the view that the programs are not unfair (except in the weak sense described above) to white males, and on the view that it is unfair to continue the present set of unjust—often racist and sexist—institutions that comprise the social reality. The case for these programs also rests on the thesis that it is fair, given the distribution of power and influence in the United States, to redistribute in this way, and that such programs may reasonably be viewed as useful means by which to achieve very significant social ideals.

In Defense of Affirmative Action

Tom L. Beauchamp

Affirmative action policies have had their strongest appeal when discrimination that barred groups from desirable institutions persisted although forbidden by law. Policies that establish target goals, timetables, and quotas were initiated to ensure more equitable opportunities by counterbalancing apparently intractable prejudice and systemic favoritism. The policies that were initiated with such lofty ambitions are now commonly criticized on grounds that they establish quotas that unjustifiably elevate the opportunities of members of targeted groups, discriminate against equally qualified or even more qualified members of majorities, and perpetuate racial and sexual paternalism.

Affirmative action policies favoring *groups* have been controversial since former United States President Lyndon Johnson's 1965 executive order that required federal contractors to develop affirmative action policies.[1] Everyone now agrees that *individuals* who have been injured by past discrimination should be made whole for the inquiry, but it remains controversial whether and how past discrimination against groups justifies preferential treatment for the group's *current* members. Critics of group preferential policies hold that compensating individuals for unfair discrimination can alone be justified, but it is controversial whether individuals can be harmed merely by virtue of a group membership.[2]

Most who support affirmative action and those who oppose it both seek the best means to the same end: a color-blind, sex-blind society. Their goals do not differ. Nor do they entirely disagree over the means. If a color-blind, sex-blind society can be achieved and maintained by legal guarantees of equal opportunities to all, both parties agree that social

Tom L. Beauchamp, Reprinted with kind permission from Springer Science + Business Media: *Journal of Ethics*, excerpts from "In Defense of Affirmative Action," Vol. 2, No. 2 (1998), pp. 143–158, Tom L. Beauchamp, Copyright © 1998, Kluwer Academic Publishers.

policies should be restricted to this means. Here agreement ends. Those who support affirmative action do not believe such guarantees can be fairly and efficiently achieved other than by affirmative action policies. Those who seek an end to affirmative action believe that the goals can be achieved in other ways and that affirmative action policies themselves unjustifiably discriminate. I will be supporting affirmative action policies against this counterposition.

TWO PIVOTAL CONCEPTS

Like virtually all problems in practical ethics, the meaning of a few central terms can powerfully affect one's moral viewpoint. The terms "affirmative action" and "quotas" have proved particularly troublesome, because they have been defined in both minimal and maximal ways. The original meaning of "affirmative action" was minimalist. It referred to plans to safeguard equal opportunity, to protect against discrimination, to advertise positions openly, and to create scholarship programs to ensure recruitment from specific groups.[3] Few now oppose open advertisement and the like, and if this were all that were meant by "affirmative action," few would oppose it. However, "affirmative action" has assumed new and expanded meanings. Today it is typically associated with quotas and preferential policies that target specific groups, especially women or minority members.

I will not favor either the minimalist or the maximalist sense of "affirmative action." I will use the term to refer to positive steps taken to hire persons from groups previously and presently discriminated against, leaving open what will count as a "positive step" to remove discrimination. I thus adopt a broad meaning.

A number of controversies have also centered on the language of *quotas*.[4] A "quota," as I use the term, does not mean that fixed numbers of a group must be admitted, hired, or promoted—even to the point of including less qualified persons if they are the only available members of a targeted groups. Quotas are target numbers or percentages that an employer, admissions office, recruitment committee, and the like sincerely attempt to meet. Less qualified persons are occasionally hired or promoted under a policy that incorporates quotas; but it is no part of affirmative action or the meaning of "quotas" to hire persons who lack basic qualifications. Quotas are numerically expressible goals pursued in good faith and with due diligence.

The language of "quotas" can be toned down by speaking of hopes, objectives, and guidelines; but cosmetic changes of wording only thinly obscure a policy established to recruit from groups in which the goals are made explicitly by numbers. Thus, when John Sununu—presumably a strong opponent of quotas—told Secretary of Defense Richard Cheney that he "wanted 30 percent of the remaining 42 top jobs in the Defense Department to be filled by women and minorities,"[5] he was using a quota. Likewise, universities sometimes use quotas when the subtleties of faculty and staff hiring and promotion and student admission make no mention of them. For example, if the chair of a department says the department should hire 2 to 3 women in the next 5 available positions, the formula constitutes a quota, or at least a numerical target.

Reasons typically offered in defense of targeted affirmative action, with or without quotas, are the following: "We have many women students who need and do not have an ample number of role models and mentors." "The provost has offered a group of special fellowships to bring more minorities to the university." "More diversity is much needed in this department." "The goals and mission of this university strongly suggest a need for increased representation of women and minorities." In pursuing these objectives, members of departments and committees commonly act in ways that suggest they willingly endorse what either is or has a strong family resemblance to a specific target.

THE PREVALENCE OF DISCRIMINATION AS THE RATIONALE FOR AFFIRMATIVE ACTION

The moral problem of affirmative action is primarily whether specific targets, including quotas in the broad sense, can legitimately be used. To support affirmative action as a weapon against discrimination is not necessarily to endorse it in all institutions. Racial, sexual, and religious forms of discrimination affecting admission, hiring, and promotion have been substantially reduced in various sectors of US society, and perhaps even completely eliminated in some. The problem is that in other social sectors it is common to encounter discrimination in favor of a favored group or discrimination against disliked, distrusted, unattractive, or neglected groups. The pervasive attitudes underlying these phenomena are the most important background conditions of the debate over affirmative action, and we need to understand these pockets of discrimination in order to appreciate the attractions of affirmative action.

Statistics. Statistics constituting at least *prima facie* evidence of discrimination in society are readily available. These data indicate that in sizable parts of US society white males continue to receive the highest entry-level salaries when compared to all other social groups; that women with similar credentials and experience to those of men are commonly hired at lower positions or earn lower starting salaries than men and are promoted at one-half the rate of their male counterparts, with the consequence that the gap between salaries and promotion rates is still growing at an increasing rate; that 70% or more of white-collar positions are held by women, although they hold only about 10% of management positions; that three out of seven US employees occupy white-collar positions, whereas the ratio is but one of seven of African-Americans; and, finally, that a significant racial gap in unemployment statistics is a consistent pattern in the US, with the gap now greatest for college-educated, African-American males.[6] Whether these statistics demonstrate invidious discrimination is controversial, but additional data drawn from empirical studies reinforce the judgment that racial and sexual discrimination are reasons for and perhaps the best explanation of these statistics.

Housing. For example, studies of real estate rentals, housing sales, and home mortgage lending show a disparity in rejection rates—for example, loan rejection rates between white applicants and minority applicants. Wide disparities exist even after statistics are adjusted for economic differences; minority applicants are over 50% more likely to be denied a loan than white applicants of equivalent economic status. Other studies indicate that discrimination in sales of houses is prevalent in the US. Race appears to be as important as socioeconomic status in failing to secure both houses and loans, and studies also show that the approval rate for African-Americans increases in lending institutions with an increase in the proportion of minority employees in that institution.[7]

Jobs. A similar pattern is found in employment. In 1985 the Grier Partnership and the Urban League produced independent studies that reveal striking disparities in the employment levels of college-trained African-Americans and whites in Washington, DC, one of the best markets for African-Americans. Both studies found that college-trained African-Americans have much more difficulty than their white counterparts in securing employment. Both cite discrimination as the major underlying factor.[8]

In a 1991 study by the Urban Institute, employment practices in Washington, DC and Chicago were examined. Equally qualified, identically dressed white and African-American applicants for jobs were used to test for bias in the job market, as presented by newspaper-advertised positions. Whites and African-Americans were matched identically for speech patterns, age, work experience, personal characteristics, and physical build. Investigators found repeated discrimination against African-American male applicants. The higher the position, the higher the level of discrimination. The white men received job offers three times more often than the equally qualified African-Americans who interviewed for the same position. The authors of the study concluded that discrimination against African-American men is "widespread and entrenched."[9]

These statistics and empirical studies help frame racial discrimination in the US. Anyone who believes that only a narrow slice of surface discrimination exists will be unlikely to agree with what I have been and will be arguing, at least if my proposals entail strong affirmative action measures. By contrast, one who believes that discrimination is securely and almost invisibly entrenched in many sectors of society will be more likely to endorse or at least tolerate resolute affirmative action policies.

Although racism and sexism are commonly envisioned as intentional forms of favoritism and exclusion, intent to discriminate is not a necessary condition of discrimination. Institutional networks can unintentionally hold back or exclude persons. Hiring by personal friendships and word of mouth are common instances, as are seniority systems. Numerical targets are important remedies for these camouflaged areas, where it is particularly difficult to shatter patterns of discrimination and reconfigure the environment.[10]

The US Supreme Court has rightly upheld affirmative action programs with numerically expressed hiring formulas when intended to quash the effects of both intentional and unintentional discrimination.[11] The Court has also maintained that such formulas have sometimes been structured so that they unjustifiably exceed proper limits.[12] The particulars of the cases will determine how we are to balance different interests and considerations.

THE JUSTIFICATION OF AFFIRMATIVE ACTION

This balancing strategy is warranted. Numerical goals or quotas are justified if and only if they are necessary to overcome the discriminatory effects that could not otherwise be eliminated with reasonable efficiency. It is the intractable and often deeply hurtful character of racism and sexism that justified aggressive policies to remove their damaging effects. The history of affirmative action in the US, though short, is an impressive history of fulfilling once-failed promises, displacing disillusion, and protecting the most vulnerable members of US society against demeaning abuse. It has delivered the US from what was little more than a caste system and a companion of apartheid.

We have learned in the process that numerical formulas are sometimes essential tools, sometimes excessive tools, and sometimes permissible but optional tools—depending on the subtleties of the case. We can expect each case to be different, and for this reason we should be cautious about general pronouncements regarding the justifiability of numerical formulas—as well as the merit of merit-based systems and blinded systems. The better perspective is that until the facts of particular cases have been carefully assessed, we are not positioned to support or oppose any particular affirmative action policy or its abandonment.

The US Supreme Court has allowed these numerical formulas in plans that are intended to combat a manifest imbalance in traditionally segregated job categories (even if the particular workers drawn from minorities were not victims of past discrimination). In *Local 28 v. Equal Employment Opportunity Commission,* a minority hiring goal of 29.23 percent had been established. The Court held that such specific numbers are justified when dealing with persistent or egregious discrimination. The Court found that the history of Local 28 was one of complete "foot-dragging resistance" to the idea of hiring without discrimination in their apprenticeship training programs from minority groups. The Court argued that "affirmative race-conscious relief" may be the only reasonable means to the end of assuring equality of employment opportunities and to eliminate deeply ingrained discriminatory practices.[13]

In a 1989 opinion, by contrast, the US Supreme Court held in *City of Richmond v. J. A. Croson* that Richmond, Virginia, officials could not require contractors to set aside 30 percent of their budget for subcontractors who owned "minority business enterprises." This particular plan was not written to remedy the effects of prior or present discrimination. The Court found that *this way* of fixing a percentage based on race, in the absence of evidence of identified discrimination, denied citizens an equal opportunity to compete for subcontracts. Parts of the reasoning in this case were reaffirmed in the 1995 case of *Adarand Constructors Inc. v. Pena.*

Some writers have interpreted *Croson, Adarand,* and the 1997 decision of a three-judge panel of the 9th US Circuit Court of Appeals to the effect that California's voter-approved ban on affirmative action (Proposition 209) is constitutional as the dismantling of affirmative action plans that use numerical goals. Perhaps this prediction will turn out to be correct, but the US Supreme Court has consistently adhered to a balancing strategy that I believe captures the fitting way to frame issues of affirmative action.[14] It allows us to use race and sex as relevant bases of policies if and only if it is essential to do so in order to achieve a larger and justified social purpose.

These reasons for using race and sex in policies are far distant from the role of these properties in invidious discrimination. Racial discrimination and sexual discrimination typically spring from feelings of superiority and a sense that other groups deserve lower social status. Affirmative action entails no such attitude or intent. Its purpose is to restore to persons a status they have been unjustifiably denied, to help them escape stigmatization, and to foster relationships of interconnectedness in society.[15]

Affirmative action in pockets of the most vicious and visceral racism will likely be needed for another generation in the US, after which the US should have reached its goals of fair opportunity and equal consideration. Once these goals are achieved, affirmative action will no longer be justified and should be abandoned in the US. The goal to be reached at that point is not proportional representation, which has occasionally been used as a basis for fixing target numbers in affirmative action policies, but as such is merely a means to the end of discrimination, not an end to be pursued for its own sake. The goal is simply fair opportunity and equal consideration.

* * *

TOLERATING REVERSE DISCRIMINATION

It has often been said that reverse discrimination is caused by affirmative action policies and that this discrimination is no better than the racial or sexual discrimination that affirmative actions allegedly frustrates.[16] Some instances of such discriminatory exclusion do occur, of course, and compensation or rectification for an injured party is sometimes the appropriate response. However, some of these setbacks to the interests of those excluded by a policy may be no more objectionable than various burdens produced by social policies that advantage some members of society and disadvantage others. Inheritance laws, for example, favor certain members of society over others, whereas policies of eminent domain disadvantage persons who wish to retain what is legitimately their property in order to advance the public good. Such laws and outcomes are warranted by a larger public benefit and by justice-based considerations that conflict with the interests of the disadvantaged parties. The point is that disadvantages to majorities produced by affirmative action may be warranted by the promotion of social ideals of equal treatment for groups that were severely mistreated in the past.

In assessing the disadvantages that might be caused to members of majorities (primarily white males), we should remember that there are disadvantages to other parties that operate in the current system, many of which will not be affected by affirmative action or by its absence. For example, just as young white males may now be paying a penalty for wrongs committed by older white males (who will likely never be penalized), so the older members of minority groups and older women who have been most disadvantaged in the past are the least likely to gain an advantage from affirmative action policies. Paradoxically, the younger minority members and women who have suffered least from discrimination now stand to gain the most from affirmative action. Despite these unfairnesses, there is no clear way to remedy them.

Policies of affirmative action may have many other shortcomings as well. For example, they confer economic advantages upon some who do not deserve them and generate court battles, jockeying for favored position by a multiple array of minorities, a lowering of admission and work standards in some

institutions, heightened racial hostility, and continued suspicion that well-placed women and minority group members received their positions purely on the basis of quotas, thereby damaging their self-respect and the respect of their colleagues. Affirmative action is not a perfect social tool, but it is the best tool yet created as a way of preventing a recurrence of the far worse imperfections of our past policies of segregation and exclusion.

JUDGING THE PAST AND THE PRESENT

Looking back at this deplorable history and at the unprecedented development of affirmative action policies over the past thirty years in the US, what moral judgments can we reach about persons who either initiated these policies or those who failed to initiate such programs? Can we say that anyone has engaged in moral wrongdoing in implementing these policies, or exhibited moral failure in not implementing them? Addressing these questions should help us better judge the present in light of the past.

I will examine these questions through the classic AT&T affirmative action agreement in the 1970s. The salient facts of this case are as follows: The US Equal Employment Opportunity Commission (EEOC) had investigated AT&T in the 1960s on grounds of alleged discriminatory practices in hiring and promotion. In 1970 the EEOC stated that the firm engaged in "pervasive, system-wide, and blatantly unlawful discrimination in employment against women, African-Americans, Spanish-surnamed Americans, and other minorities."[17] The EEOC argued that the employment practices of AT&T violated several civil rights laws and had excluded women from all job classifications except low paying clerical and operator positions.

AT&T denied all charges and produced a massive array of statistics about women and minorities in the workforce. However, these statistics tended to undermine the corporation's own case. They showed that half the company's 700,000 employees were female, but that the women were all either secretaries or operators. It became apparent that the company categorized virtually all of its jobs in terms of men's work and women's work. The federal government was determined to obliterate this aspect of corporate culture in the belief that no other strategy would break the grip of this form of sexism. Eventually AT&T threw in the towel and entered a Consent Decree, which was accepted by a Philadelphia court in 1973. This agreement resulted in payments of $15 million in back wages to 13,000 women and 2,000 minority-group men and $23 million in raises to 36,000 employees who had been harmed by previous policies.

Out of this settlement came a companywide "model affirmative action plan" that radically changed the character of AT&T hiring and its promotion practices. The company agreed to create an "employee profile" in its job classifications to be achieved faster than would normally occur. It established racial and gender goals and intermediate targets in 15 job categories to be met in quarterly increments. The goals were determined by statistics regarding representative numbers of workers in the relevant labor market. The decree required that under conditions of a target failure, a less qualified (but qualified) person could take precedence over a more qualified person with greater seniority. This condition applied only to promotions, not to layoffs and rehiring, where seniority continued to prevail.

As was inevitable under this arrangement, reverse discrimination cases emerged. The well known McAleer case came before Judge Gerhard A. Gesell, who held in 1976 that McAleer was a faultless employee who became an innocent victim through an unfortunate but justifiable use of the affirmative action process.[18] Judge Gesell ruled that McAleer was entitled to monetary compensation (as damages), but not entitled to the promotion to which he thought he was entitled because the discrimination the Consent Decree had been designed to eliminate might be perpetuated if a qualified woman were not given the promotion.[19]

This AT&T case history, like many affirmative action cases, is a story of changed expectations and changing moral viewpoints. At the core of any framework for the evaluation of such cases is a distinction between *wrongdoing* and *culpability*, which derives from the need to evaluate the moral quality of actions by contrast to agents. For example, we might want to say that AT&T's hiring practices were wrong and that many employees were wronged by them, without judging anyone culpable for the wrongs done.

Virtually everyone is now agreed, including AT&T officials, that AT&T's hiring and promotion practices did involve unjustified discrimination and serious wrongdoing. Even basic moral principles were violated—for example, that one ought to treat persons with equal consideration and respect, that racial and sexual discrimination are impermissible, and the like. Less clear is whether the agents involved should be blamed. Several factors place limits on our ability to make judgments about the blameworthiness of agents—or at least the fairness of doing so. These factors include culturally induced moral ignorance, a changing circumstance in the specification of moral principles, and indeterminacy in an organization's division of labor and designation of responsibility. All were present to some degree in the AT&T case.

Judgments of exculpation depend, at least to some extent, on whether proper moral standards were acknowledged in the culture in which the events transpired—for example, in the professional ethics of the period. If we had possessed clear standards regarding the justice of hiring and promotion in the 1950s and 1960s, it would be easier to find AT&T officials culpable. The absence of such standards is a factor in our reflections about culpability and exculpation, but need not be part of our reflection on the wronging that occurred.

The fact of culturally induced moral ignorance does not by itself entail exculpation or a lack of accountability for states of ignorance. The issue is the degree to which persons are accountable for holding and even perpetuating or disseminating the beliefs that they hold when an opportunity to remedy or modify the beliefs exists. If such opportunities are unavailable, a person may have a valid excuse; but the greater the opportunity to eliminate ignorance the less is exculpation appropriate. Persons who permit their culturally induced moral ignorance to persist through a series of opportunities to correct the beliefs thereby increase their culpability.

The more persons are obstinate in not facing issues, and the more they fail to perceive the plight of other persons who may be negatively affected by their failure to act, the more likely are we to find their actions or inactions inexcusable. No doubt culturally induced moral ignorance was a mitigating factor in the 1960s and early 1970s, but I believe US history also shows that it was mixed with a resolute failure to face moral problems when it was widely appreciated that they were serious problems and were being faced by other institutions.

The central issue for my purposes is not whether discriminatory attitudes should be judged harshly in the pre-affirmative action situation at AT&T, but whether the affirmative action policy that was adopted itself involved wrongdoing or constituted, then or now, an activity for which we would blame persons who establish such policies. I do not see how agents could be blamed for maintaining and enforcing this program, despite its toughness. Given AT&T's history as well as the desperate situation of discrimination in US society, under what conditions could agents be culpable even if McAleer-type cases of reverse discrimination occasionally resulted? Even if we assume that McAleer and others were wronged in the implementation of the policy, it does not follow that the agents were culpable for their support of the policy.

Today, many corporate programs similar to the AT&T policy are in place. We can and should ask both whether persons are wronged by these policies and whether those who use the policies are culpable. The answer seems to me the same in the 1990s as it was in the 1970s: As long as there is persistent, intractable discrimination in society, the policies will be justified and the agents nonculpable, even if some persons are harmed and even wronged by the policies. To say that we should right wrongs done by the policies is not to say that we should abandon the policies themselves.

Indeed, I defend a stronger view: Affirmative action was a noble struggle against a crippling social ill in the 1960s and 1970s, and those who took part in the struggle deserve acknowledgement for their courage and foresight. Those who failed to seize the opportunity to enact affirmative action policies or some functional equivalent such as company-wide enforcement of equal opportunity are culpable for what, in many cases, were truly serious moral failures.

There is no reason to believe that, in this respect, the situation is changed today from the 1970s. Today persons in corporations, universities, and government agencies who are aware or should be aware that a high level of racism or sexism exists are culpable if they fail to move to counteract its invidious effects by affirmative policies or similarly serious interventions such as meaningful enforcement of fair opportunity. To say that we should judge the officers of these institutions culpable for their moral failures is not to say that there are no mitigating conditions for their failures, such as the mixed messages they have received over the past fifteen years from federal officials and the general cultural climate of moral indifference to the problem. At the same time, the mitigating conditions are weaker today than in the 1970s because the excuse of culturally induced moral ignorance is weaker. In general, there are now fewer excuses available for not taking an aggressive posture to combat discrimination than ever before.

All of this is not to say that we are never culpable for the way we formulate or implement affirmative action policies. One aspect of these policies for which we likely will be harshly judged in the future is a failure of truthfulness in publicly disclosing and advertising the commitments of the policies—for example, in advertising for new positions.[20] Once it has been determined that a woman or a minority group member will most likely be hired, institutions now typically place advertisements that include lines such as the following:

Women and minority-group candidates are especially encouraged to apply. The University of X is an equal opportunity, affirmative action employer.

Advertisements and public statements rarely contain more information about an institution's affirmative action objectives, although often more information might be disclosed that would be of material relevance to applicants. The following are examples of facts or objectives that might be disclosed: A department may have reserved its position for a woman or minority; the chances may be overwhelming that only a minority group member will be hired; the interview team may have decided in advance that only women will be interviewed; the advertised position may be the result of a university policy that offers an explicit incentive (perhaps a new position) to a department if a minority representative is appointed, etc. Incompleteness in disclosure and advertising sometimes stems from fear of legal liability, but more often from fear of departmental embarrassment and harm either to reputation or to future recruiting efforts.

The greater moral embarrassment, however, is our ambivalence and weak conceptions of what we are doing. Many, including academics, fear making public what they believe to be morally commendable in their recruiting efforts. There is something deeply unsatisfactory about a reluctance to disclose one's real position. This situation is striking, because the justification for the position is presumably that it is a morally praiseworthy endeavor. Here we have a circumstance in which the actions taken may not be wrong, but the agents are culpable for a failure to clearly articulate the basis of their actions and to allow those bases to be openly debated so that their true merits can be assessed by all affected parties.

CONCLUSION

During the course of the last thirty years, the widespread acceptance of racial segregation and sexual dominance in the US has surrendered to a more polite culture that accepts racial integration and sexual equality. This discernible change of attitude and institutional policy has led to an imposing public opposition to preferential treatment on the basis of race and sex in general. In this climate what should happen to affirmative action?

As long as our choices are formulated in terms of the false dilemma of either special preference for groups or individual merit, affirmative action is virtually certain to be overthrown. US citizens are now wary and weary of all forms of group preference, other than the liberty to choose one's preferred groups. I would be pleased to witness the defeat of affirmative action were the choice the simple one of group preference or individual merit. But it is not. Despite the vast changes of attitudes in thirty years of US culture, the underlying realities are naggingly familiar. Perhaps in another thirty years we can rid ourselves of the perils of affirmative action. But at present the public good and our sense of ourselves as a nation will be well served by retaining what would in other circumstances be odious policies. They merit preservation as long as we can say that, on balance, they serve us better than they disserve us.

NOTES

1. Executive Order 11246. C.F.R. 339 (1964–65).

2. See J. Angelo Corlett, "Racism and Affirmative Action," *Journal of Social Philosophy* 24 (1993), pp. 163–175; and Cass R. Sunstein, "The Limits of Compensatory Justice," in John Chapman (ed.), *Nomos XXXIII: Compensatory Justice* (New York: New York University Press, 1991), pp. 281–310.

3. See Thomas Nagel, "A Defense of Affirmative Action," Testimony before the Subcommittee on the Constitution of the Senate Judiciary Committee, June 18, 1981; and Louis Pojman, "The Moral Status of Affirmative Action," *Public Affairs Quarterly* 6 (1992), pp. 181–206.

4. See the analyses in Gertrude Ezorsky, *Racism and Justice* (Ithaca, NY: Cornell University Press, 1991); and Robert Fullinwider, *The Reverse Discrimination Controversy* (Totowa, NJ: Rowman and Allanheld, 1980).

5. Bob Woodward, *The Commanders* (New York: Simon and Schuster, 1991), p. 72.

6. Bron Taylor, *Affirmative Action at Work: Law, Politics, and Ethics* (Pittsburgh: University of Pittsburgh Press, 1991); Morley Gunderson, "Male–Female Wage Differentials and Policy Responses," *Journal of Economic Literature* 27 (1989), and Morley Gunderson, "Pay and Employment Equity in the United States and Canada," *International Journal of Manpower* 15 (1994), pp. 26–43; Patricia Gaynor and Garey Durden, "Measuring the Extent of Earnings Discrimination: An Update," *Applied Economics* 27 (1995), pp. 669–767; Marjorie L. Baldwin and William G. Johnson, "The Employment Effects of Wage Discrimination Against Black Men," *Industrial & Labor Relations Review* 49 (1996), pp. 302–316; Franklin D. Wilson, Marta Tienda, and Lawrence Wu, "Race and Unemployment:

Labor Market Experiences of Black and White Men, 1968–1988," *Work & Occupations* 22 (1995), pp. 245–270; National Center for Education Statistics, *Faculty in Higher Education Institutions, 1988, Contractor Survey Report,* compiled Susan H. Russell et al. (Washington: US Dept. of Education, 1990), pp. 5–13; Betty M. Vetter, ed., *Professional Women and Minorities: A Manpower Data Resource Service,* 8th ed. (Washington: Commission on Science and Technology, 1989); (anonymous) "Less Discrimination for Women but Poorer Prospect at Work than Men," *Management Services* 40 (1996), p. 6; Cynthia D. Anderson and Donald Tomaskovic-Devey, "Patriarchal Pressures: An Exploration of Organizational Processes that Exacerbate and Erode Gender Earnings Inequality," *Work & Occupations* 22 (1995), pp. 328–356; Thomas J. Bergman and G. E. Martin, "Tests for Compliance with Phases Plans to Equalize Discriminate Wages," *Journal of Applied Business Research* 11 (1994/1995), pp. 136–143.

7. Brent W. Ambrose, William T. Hughes, Jr., and Patrick Simmons, "Policy Issues concerning Racial and Ethnic Differences in Home Loan Rejection Rates," *Journal of Housing Research* 6 (1995), pp. 115–135; *A Common Destiny: Blacks and American Society,* ed. Gerald D. Jaynes and Robin M. Williams, Jr., Committee on the Status of Black Americans, Commission on Behavioral and Social Sciences and Education, National Research Council (Washington: NAS Press, 1989), pp. 12–13, 138–148; Sunwoong Kim, Gregory D. Squire, "Lender Characteristics and Racial Disparities in Mortgage Lending," *Journal of Housing Research* 6 (1995), pp. 99–113; Glenn B. Canner and Wayne Passmore, "Home Purchase Lending in Low-Income Neighborhoods and to Low-Income Borrowers," *Federal Reserve Bulletin* 81 (1995), pp. 71–103; Constance L. Hays, "Study Says Prejudice in Suburbs Is Aimed Mostly at Blacks," *The New York Times* (November 23, 1988), p. A16; John R. Walter, "The Fair Lending Laws and their Enforcement," *Economic Quarterly* 81 (1995), pp. 61–77; Stanley D. Longhofer, "Discrimination in Mortgage Lending: What Have We Learned?" *Economic Commentary* [Federal Reserve Bank of Cleveland] (August 15, 1996), pp. 1–4.

8. As reported by Rudolf A. Pyatt, Jr., "Significant Job Studies," *The Washington Post* (April 30, 1985), pp. D1–D2. See also Paul Burstein, *Discrimination, Jobs, and Politics* (Chicago: University of Chicago Press, 1985); Bureau of Labor Statistics, *Employment and Earnings* (Washington: US Dept. of Labor, Jan. 1989); *A Common Destiny,* op. cit., pp. 16–18, 84–88.

9. See Margery Austin Turner, Michael Fix, and Raymond Struyk, *Opportunities Denied, Opportunities Diminished: Discrimination in Hiring* (Washington, DC: The Urban Institute, 1991).

10. See Laura Purdy, "Why Do We Need Affirmative Action?" *Journal of Social Philosophy* 25 (1994), pp. 133–143; Farrell Bloch, *Antidiscrimination Law and Minority Employment: Recruitment Practices and Regulatory Constraints* (Chicago: University of Chicago Press, 1994); Joseph Sartorelli, "Gay Rights and Affirmative Action" in *Gay Ethics,* ed. Timothy F. Murphy (New York: Haworth Press, 1994); Taylor, *Affirmative Action at Work.*

11. *Fullilove v. Klutznick,* 448 U.S. 448 (1980); *United Steelworkers v. Weber,* 443 U.S. 193 (1979); *United States v. Paradise,* 480 U.S. 149 (1987); *Johnson v. Transportation Agency,* 480 U.S. 616 (1987); *Alexander v. Choate,* 469 U.S. 287, at 295.

12. *Firefighters v. Stotts,* 467 U.S. 561 (1984); *City of Richmond v. J. A. Croson Co.,* 109 S.Ct. 706 (1989); *Adarand Constructors Inc. v. Federico Pena,* 63 LW 4523 (1995); *Wygant v. Jackson Bd. of Education,* 476 U.S. 267 (1986); *Wards Cove Packing v. Atonio,* 490 U.S. 642.

13. In 1964 the New York Commission for Human Rights investigated the union and concluded that it excluded nonwhites through an impenetrable barrier of hiring by discriminatory selection. The state Supreme Court concurred and issued a "cease and desist" order. The union ignored it. Eventually, in a 1975 trial, the US District Court found a record "replete with instances of bad faith" and ordered a "remedial racial goal of 29% nonwhite membership" (based on the percentage of nonwhites in the local labor pool). Another court then found that the union had "consistently and egregiously violated" the law of the land (Title 7, in particular). In 1982 and 1983 court fines and civil contempt proceedings were issued. In the early 1980s virtually nothing had been done to modify the discriminatory hiring practices after 22 years of struggle.

14. For a very different view, stressing inconsistency, see Yong S. Lee, "Affirmative Action and Judicial Standards of Review: A Search for the Elusive Consensus," *Review of Public Personnel Administration* 12 (1991), pp. 47–69.

15. See Robert Ladenson, "Ethics in the American Workplace," *Business and Professional Ethics Journal* 14 (1995), pp. 17–31; Ezorsky, *Racism and Justice: The Case for Affirmative Action,* op. cit.; Thomas E. Hill, Jr., "The Message of Affirmative Action," *Social Philosophy and Policy* 8 (1991), pp. 108–129; Jorge L. Garcia, "The Heart of Racism," *Journal of Social Philosophy* 27 (1996), pp. 5–46.

16. See Robert Fullinwider, *The Reverse Discrimination Controversy,* op. cit.; Nicholas Capaldi, *Out of Order* (Buffalo, NY, 1985); F. R. Lynch, *Invisible Victims: White Males and the Crisis of Affirmative Action* (Westport, CT: Greenwood Press, 1989); Barry R. Gross, eds., *Reverse Discrimination* (Buffalo: Prometheus Books, 1977).

17. US Equal Employment Opportunity Commission, "Petition to Intervene," Federal Communications Commission Hearings on AT&T Revised Tariff Schedule (December 10, 1970), p. 1.

18. *McAleer v. American Telephone and Telegraph Company*, 416 F. Supp. 435 (1976); "AT&T Denies Job Discrimination Charges, Claims Firm Is Equal Employment Leader," *The Wall Street Journal* (December 14, 1970), p.6; Richard M. Hodgetts, "AT&T versus the Equal Employment Opportunity Commission," in *The Business Enterprise: Social Challenge, Social Response* (Philadelphia, W. B. Saunders Company, 1977), pp. 176–182.

19. According to a representative of the legal staff in AT&T's Washington Office (phone conversation on March 10, 1982).

20. See Steven M. Cahn, "Colleges Should be Explicit about Who Will be Considered for Jobs," *The Chronicle of Higher Education* (April 5, 1989), p. B3.

CASES FOR ANALYSIS

1. Racial Preferences for Whites?

Affirmative action is most often thought of as a racial preference for marginalized peoples—a way to ensure that those who are often discriminated against have places in schools and workplaces. But some insist that the roots of affirmative action are firmly grounded in a racial preference for whites.

One commentator argues that the abolition of white indentured servants perfectly encapsulates white racial preference, for though white slavery was no longer legal in the United States as of the nineteenth century, black and indigenous workers remained in bondage. Racial preference for whites was the guiding principle behind the 1790 Naturalization Act, which granted U.S. citizenship to almost any immigrant of European ancestry, but excluded blacks, Asians, and American Indians. Asian exclusion laws, segregation, and Manifest Destiny, which led to the annexation of half of Mexico, are also products of affirmative action for whites.

He points out that as recently as the 1960s, the Federal Housing Administration provided loans almost exclusively to white families. From the 1930s to the 1960s, approximately 15 million whites were able to obtain homes with FHA loans, while people of color received no such aid.

He concludes that the group that has benefited most through affirmative action programs is white America. The laws and public policies of the United States have been shaped and molded by white racial preference, and many of the social and economic inequalities we face today are the result of years of affirmative action for whites.*

Do you agree with this commentator that racial preferences for whites have always been a major part of U.S. history? If so, do you think that the U.S. government should make amends for such past inequalities? Why or why not? If racial preferences for whites have indeed always been widespread, were they always unjust as well? Suppose they were unjust. Would racial preferences in favor of *nonwhites* now be just? Why or why not?

*Based on Tim Wise, "The Mother of All Racial Preferences," Znet, 24 May 2003, https://zcomm.org /zcommentary/the-mother-of-all-racial-preferences-by-tim-wise/. Originally appeared as a ZNet Commentary at www.zmag.org.

2. Are Racial Preferences Harmful?

Over the past few years, researchers have begun to produce large datasets that make it possible to compare the fortunes of minority students who attend universities that use varying levels of admissions preferences. In many contexts, scholars find that students perform better, both in the short-term and the long-term, when students' credentials are closer to those of their classmates. When students are surrounded by peers who have much higher credentials, they often have more trouble persisting in a difficult major, graduating from college or getting a good job.

This phenomenon is known as the "mismatch effect," and last month I published a study in the *Stanford Law Review,* trying to determine whether the mismatch effect operates in law schools. . . . My study focused on black law students and compared black and white outcomes.

I found that law schools almost universally use very large preferences for blacks to achieve something very close to racial proportionality. The credentials gap between white and black students is about 30 times larger than it would be in a race-blind regime.

Starting a highly competitive curriculum with a large academic disadvantage, blacks wind up clustered in the bottom tenth of the class at nearly all law schools. I estimate the mismatch effect increases the number of black dropouts from law school by 40%, and increases the number of blacks failing their first bar exam by 80%.

The mismatch effect appears to operate in the job market as well. Law firms—once thought to be single-minded in their determination to recruit lawyers from the most elite schools possible—turn out to weigh law school grades more heavily than school prestige. The typical black law graduate, I estimate, loses about $10,000 in annual earnings because large preferences induce her to make a bad trade-off between law school prestige and law school grades.[†]

This study is controversial, but suppose it shows what the researcher says it does. Would you then favor *dismantling* preferences for black law students? Would you favor *maintaining* law school preference systems if they helped black students rather than harmed them? Why or why not? Some people advocate using preferences in higher education to redress the wrongs of past discrimination. To be logically consistent, should they disregard evidence suggesting that preferences hurt blacks?

[†]Richard Sander, "Preferences Hurt Black Law Students," UCLA Today, Vol. 25, No. 10 (February 2005). Used by permission of the author.

3. Diversity in Undergraduate Admissions

In 1998, California's ban on affirmative action went into effect in undergraduate admissions, and the effect at Berkeley was considerable. In its first year without race-based preferences, the school accepted its least diverse freshman class in 17 years, admitting 56 percent fewer blacks and 49 percent fewer Latinos than in 1997. Six months later, in February 1999, several civil rights groups filed a class-action suit against the university on behalf of 750 minority students denied admission in the fall. The suit focused on the school's policy of weighting grade point averages with credit for Advanced Placement (AP) classes, and pointed to the fact that many minority students attend high schools without AP classes. The school countered that it had no other way to differentiate between all of its applicants with 4.0 averages. In 1998, more than 14,000 students with 4.0 averages applied for just 8,400 spots in the freshman class.[‡]

Provide reasons for your answers to the following questions. Is diversity in student population an important value in higher education? Is achieving it important enough to justify race-based preferences in admissions? Was Berkeley's system of weighting grade point averages with credit for AP classes fair to minority students who did not have access to such classes? Should admissions schemes take into account students' disadvantaged backgrounds?

[‡]*Frontline*, "Secrets of the SAT: Challenging Race Sensitive Admissions Policies—A Summary of Important Rulings," *PBS Online*, first aired 5 October 1999, http://www.pbs.org/wgbh/pages/frontline/shows/sats/ (28 February 2015). From WGBH Educational Foundation Copyright © 2007 WGBH/Boston.

CHAPTER 19

Global Economic Justice

A plain fact of the moral life is that in ethical matters small and large, personal and abstract, we wrestle with issues of justice. Whatever our moral outlook, we must sometimes ask, What is just? **Justice** is about persons getting what is fair or what is their due. In the name of justice, we condemn racial discrimination, unequal pay for equal work, and judicial punishment based on a judge's prejudice. For justice's sake, we strive to treat people the same unless there is a morally relevant reason for treating them differently—that is, we try to treat equals equally. For reasons of justice, we act—or feel obliged to act—to change the way things are, to try to make the world or ourselves more just.

Among the more vexing questions of justice are those that emerge when we become aware of people in dire need of something we have, something we could easily supply. Then the questions are, Do we have a duty to give to the needy in order to somehow ease their misery? Do they have a right to some of what we have? If so, how much should we relinquish to them? Would we be justified in refusing to give? Such queries trouble us on two levels—*locally* (pertaining to needy people nearby: in our neighborhood, community, or country) and *globally* (regarding the poor and hungry in other countries). The former has always been a concern. The latter presses us harder than ever because, thanks to our technology and wealth, we now know a great deal about the suffering of people in distant lands and we have the wherewithal to do something about it. In this chapter,

we explore the global question, What are our obligations to the impoverished, hungry, dying strangers who are half a world away and whom we will never meet?

ISSUE FILE: BACKGROUND

For many people, this moral issue is compelling because the wretchedness of the world's poor is profound and the economic gap between rich and poor is wide. According to the latest estimates, 1.2 billion people are living in extreme poverty, and about one in five persons in the developing world lives on less than $1.25 a day. About 99 million children under the age of five are underweight for their age—a sign of severe malnutrition. The mortality rate for children under five is 48 deaths per 1,000 live births. Eighteen thousand children die each day, mostly from preventable causes.[1]

Economic inequality across the globe has always been with us, but now its scale is larger than most people realize. The eighty-five richest people on the

---

[1]World Bank, "Poverty Overview," Oct. 8, 2014, http://www.worldbank.org/en/topic/poverty/overview (28 February 2015); United Nations, Departrment of Economic and Social Affairs, "The Millennium Development Goals Report, 2014," July 30, 2014, http://www.un.org/millenniumgoals/2014%20MDG%20report/MDG%202014%20English%20web.pdf (28 February 2015); UNICEF, "The State of the World's Children 2014 in Numbers," January 2014, http://www.unicef.org/sowc2014/numbers/ (28 February 2015).

planet now own as much as the entire poorest half of the world's population. People in the poorest half of the world possess only about 0.7 percent of the world's wealth. The richest 1 percent of people own almost half of all wealth—which amounts to $110 trillion. Perhaps it is not surprising that in 2005 the wealthiest 20 percent of the world consumed over 75 percent of its goods, whereas the poorest consumed only 1.5 percent.[2]

Most careful thinkers agree on such facts and react with dismay and sympathy, but they disagree on the proper moral response to the massive suffering. The disagreements hinge on which moral theory is accepted and on how certain elements of morality are interpreted.

One factor is our distance from those who need help. Suppose you come upon a child drowning in a stream. With very little inconvenience to yourself you could easily save her, and you are the only person in a position to do so. If you walk away, no one will be the wiser. Would you save her? Most people probably would, and many would think they had a *duty* to save her. That is, not to save her would be wrong.

But imagine that the child is not 20 feet away from you but 1 mile or 100 miles or 5,000 miles away. If you somehow had the power to rescue her despite the distance involved, would you be obligated to do so? Most of us assume that we have duties to help those close to us—our family, friends, neighbors, or fellow citizens. After all, we have relationships with these people, and we are often in a good position to aid them. But many believe we have no duty at all to help distant peoples, strangers with whom we have no social or emotional connection. Distance changes our moral obligations; charity begins at home. Others argue that distance is irrelevant. As one philosopher says, "It makes no moral difference whether the person I can help is a neighbor's child ten yards from me or a Bengali whose name I shall never know, ten thousand miles away."[3]

Another important element in debates over aid to the needy is the notion of rights. A **right** is a person's claim or entitlement to something, a moral demand that obligates others to act accordingly. Someone's **negative right** obligates others *not to interfere* with that person's obtaining something. Someone's **positive right** obligates others *to help that person* obtain something.

Many insist that people possess only negative rights—that is, persons are entitled to be free of coercion or harm or improper restraint. Those who take this line maintain that they have no duty to help the needy, whether near or far. Their obligation is to refrain from interfering in others' lives. They may, out of a sense of charity, give to the destitute, but they are not *morally required* to give anything. Others argue that people have both negative and positive rights and that we thus are obligated to aid the less fortunate, including the poor and hungry of the world. They may contend that everyone has a right to the necessities of life and that the affluent are, therefore, duty bound to provide them. The have-nots possess a right to the resources of the haves. Exactly how much the have-nots are entitled to, however, is a matter of debate.

Some argue that we must aid the needy of other lands because we have a **duty of beneficence,** a moral obligation to benefit others. The impoverished may not have a right to our resources, but we nevertheless should give what we can to them. If we can help the poor without sacrificing too much

---

[2]Oxfam International, "Working for the Few," 2014, http://www.oxfam.org/en/research/working-few (28 February 2015); United Nations Development Programme (UNDP), "Human Development Report 1998: Consumption for Human Development" (New York, 1998), http://hdr.undp.org/sites/default/files/reports/259/hdr_1998_en_complete_nostats.pdf (28 February 2015).

[3]Peter Singer, "Famine, Affluence, and Morality," *Philosophy and Public Affairs* 1, no. 1 (Spring 1972), 23–32.

of what we have, the argument goes, we should do so.

For a few conscientious people, beneficence seems to require extraordinary sacrifice—they feel obliged to give until their own standard of living is jeopardized. Others accept a duty of beneficence toward the distant needy but try to balance it against other duties, including those to their families and to themselves.

People in this latter group often appeal to a common distinction in morality—that between obligatory and supererogatory actions. Obligatory actions are what duty requires; **supererogatory actions** are above and beyond the demands of duty. Supererogatory conduct is not required, but it is praiseworthy. Some think their duty of beneficence is limited and that giving more than required is supererogatory—commendable but optional. Others (many utilitarians, for example) do not recognize supererogatory actions. To them, duty demands that we benefit others as much as possible all the time. If maximum moral effort is required of all our actions, then no actions are supererogatory. On this view, we should give until it hurts, perhaps to the point of greatly reducing our own wealth.

MORAL THEORIES

Concerns about justice emerge in different regions of the moral life. As we saw in earlier chapters, they appear in deliberations about fair punishment for wrongdoing, an issue known as **retributive justice.** Questions regarding the fair distribution of society's goods (income, rights, welfare aid, etc.) are topics of **distributive justice.** The latter applies not only to justice within a society but also to justice among societies—for example, to the global distribution of wealth and resources among rich and poor countries and among rich and poor individuals.

Theories of distributive justice try to explain what makes a particular allocation of economic goods fair or just. They may be part of a broader moral theory such as Kantian ethics or utilitarianism, or they may stand alone as distinctive conceptions of justice. Either way, they often have something interesting to say about the morality of helping or not helping impoverished people of distant lands.

Libertarian theories emphasize individual liberties and negative rights. Exemplified in the writings of Robert Nozick, John Hospers, and others, these perspectives reject positive rights as a violation of personal freedom because such rights force people to contribute to the welfare of others.

VITAL STATS:
The Planet's Poor and Hungry

- In 2010, 1.2 billion people lived in extreme poverty.
- Every day, 18,000 children under age five die from preventable causes.
- From 2011 to 2013, 842 million people suffered from chronic hunger.
- About 805 million people continue to go hungry.
- The richest 1 percent of people own almost half of all wealth—which amounts to $110 trillion.
- In 2012, 748 million people relied on unsafe drinking water.
- An estimated 801,000 children under five years of age die each year from diarrhea, mostly from unsafe drinking water and unsanitary conditions.

Data from United Nations, "Millennium Development Report 2014," http://www.un.org/millenniumgoals /reports.shtml (1 March 2015); International Food Policy Research Institute, *2014 Global Hunger Index*, http ://www.ifpri.org/publication/2014-global-hunger-index (1 March 2015); Oxfam International, "Working for the Few," 2014, http://www.oxfam.org/en/research/working -few (1 March 2015); Centers for Disease Control and Prevention, "Global Water, Sanitation, and Hygiene," 2012, http://www.cdc.gov/healthywater/global/assessing .html (1 March 2015).

The central point is that people have a right not to be interfered with and to do whatever they want with their own property as long as they do not violate the liberty rights of others. John Hospers expresses the view like this:

> The political philosophy that is called libertarianism . . . is the doctrine that every person is the owner of his own life, and that no one is the owner of anyone else's life; and that consequently every human being has the right to act in accordance with his own choices, unless those actions infringe on the equal liberty of other human beings to act in accordance with *their* choices.[4]

The libertarian asserts that we have no duty to help the poor and hungry of the world; we are not obligated to share our resources with those less fortunate. If we aid the needy, we do so as an act of charity, not because duty commands.

Critics of the libertarian doctrine say that it conflicts with commonsense morality. In strictly libertarian terms, we have no duty to save a drowning child even though we could do so with minimal trouble. But surely when saving her life costs us so little, the critics say, we have a strong duty of beneficence to pull her from the water. The notion that saving her is not morally obligatory but merely optional seems implausible.

Consequentialist or utilitarian theories have been marshaled both to commend the aiding of distant peoples and to deplore it. Taking a utilitarian tack, Peter Singer argues that we can increase the overall good, or utility, in the world if the affluent give large portions of their wealth to the needy in other countries. He thinks his approach would dramatically lower the standard of living for the rich and drastically reduce the suffering of the poor, resulting in a general decrease in misery, starvation, and death. He tries to show that

transferring our surplus of goods to those who have little or nothing is not a supererogatory gesture but an inescapable moral obligation.

Others who argue in a consequentialist vein have ended up opposing aid to the world's starving millions. In their view, uncontrolled population growth is the cause of global poverty and starvation. They contend that in developing countries, population growth is usually unrestrained, so population increases over time, inevitably outstripping available food supplies. Famine soon follows, and many die; but then the balance between population and available food is restored. Giving the starving people food to avert famine would temporarily prevent mass starvation and allow the population to increase again—but that would only postpone the inevitable famine. When this catastrophe does come, many more people will suffer and die than if food were never donated. Thus, on consequentialist grounds, these critics of food aid argue that feeding the hungry in countries where population is unchecked will just lead to greater tragedy. Our moral duty, they say, is not to feed the hungry.

Critics question nearly every assumption behind this argument. They dispute the notions that population growth is the primary cause of famine, that giving food aid is the only option for preventing starvation, and that rich nations bear no responsibility for the plight of the poor in developing countries.

Egalitarian theories hold that justice requires equal distributions of goods among all persons. Some egalitarians insist that everyone be allotted a certain minimum amount of vital goods such as food and medical care. Others claim that only a truly equal share of everything is just. Since all persons have equal value and deserve equal respect, they have equal rights to the world's resources. The world's food, for example, should be shared equally by everyone on the planet. This global equality is the supreme value, even though it requires taking goods from the better-off to give to the needy,

---

[4]John Hospers, "What Libertarianism Is," in *The Libertarian Alternative*, ed. Tibor R. Machan (Chicago: Nelson-Hall, 1974), 3.

thus curtailing the personal liberties of some for the betterment of others.

This latter point provokes considerable criticism from those who believe that individual liberties should take precedence over economic equality—libertarians, for example. They think ensuring that people can use their own legitimately acquired resources as they see fit is more important than guaranteeing that everyone's needs are met.

MORAL ARGUMENTS

Among the more influential arguments on obligations to the world's needy is Peter Singer's utilitarian case for making major personal sacrifices to aid impoverished, starving people. His argument is straightforward:

1. "[S]uffering and death from lack of food, shelter, and medical care are bad."[5]

2. "[I]f it is in our power to prevent something bad from happening, without thereby sacrificing anything of comparable moral importance, we ought, morally, to do it."[6]

3. Therefore, we are morally obligated to prevent suffering caused by the lack of these necessities.

Singer asserts that our moral duty applies to needy people regardless of their distance from us. "If we accept any principle of impartiality, universalizability, equality, or whatever," he says, "we cannot discriminate against someone merely because he is far away from us (or we are far away from him)."[7]

The argument shows, Singer says, that giving money to famine relief is not an act of charity, a supererogatory gesture—but a moral duty:

> Because giving money is regarded as an act of charity, it is not thought that there is anything wrong with not giving. . . . On the contrary, we ought to give the money away, and it is wrong not to do so.[8]

But how much should we give? The second premise requires a drastic change in conventional moral attitudes toward the extent of our obligations:

> [W]e ought to give until we reach the level of marginal utility—that is, the level at which, by giving more, I would cause as much suffering to myself or my dependents as I would relieve by my gift. This would mean, of course, that one would reduce oneself to very near the material circumstances of a Bengali refugee.[9]

Singer offers a weaker version of the second premise, even though he thinks the stronger one is closer to the truth: we are duty bound to prevent something bad from happening as long as we can prevent it without "sacrificing anything morally significant."[10] This principle would require us to contribute to famine relief when doing so would not cost us anything of real importance. If by aiding the poor we would have to forgo buying new clothes or a fancier car, so be it.

Even if we all adopted only the weaker principle, Singer says, society would likely be transformed:

> Even if we accepted the principle only in its moderate form, however, it should be clear that we would have to give away enough to ensure that the consumer society, dependent as it is on people spending on trivia rather than giving to famine relief, would slow down and perhaps disappear entirely.[11]

Critics of Singer's strong premise charge that it disregards essential features of the moral life. We may have a duty to help those in need, but we also have obligations involving rights. John Arthur contends, for example, that each person has rights that should not be relinquished even to help

---

[5]Singer, "Famine, Affluence, and Morality," 231.
[6]Singer, 231.
[7]Singer, 232.

[8]Singer, 235.
[9]Singer, 241.
[10]Singer, 231.
[11]Singer, 241.

others in dire need. Each of us could help others by giving away a kidney or an eye—we could save a life or restore sight to a blind person, and our loss would not be comparable to the terrible loss experienced by someone who will die or be blind for lack of our help. But this much sacrifice is not obligatory:

> If anything is clear, however, it is that our [moral] code does not *require* such heroism; you are entitled to keep your second eye and kidney. . . . The reason for this is often expressed in terms of rights; it's your body, you have a right to it, and that weighs against whatever duty you have to help. To sacrifice a kidney to a stranger is to do more than is required, it's heroic.[12]

Singer's critics hold that desert is another factor we must weigh when deciding whether to give food to the hungry. As Arthur says,

> Suppose, for example, an industrious farmer manages through hard work to produce a surplus of food for the winter while a lazy neighbor spends his summer fishing. Must our industrious farmer ignore his hard work and give the surplus away because his neighbor or his family will suffer? What again seems clear is that we have more than one factor to weigh. Not only should we compare the consequences of his keeping it with his giving it away; we also should weigh the fact that one farmer deserves the food, he earned it through his hard work.[13]

Others who question Singer's view concede that we have an obligation to aid distant people but maintain that we also have a duty to help those with whom we have a special relationship. As one philosopher explains,

> I may have a duty to give of my surplus to help save drowning children in a distant land, but I have a stronger duty to help those with whom I have intimate or contractual ties.[14]

Like Singer, Garrett Hardin also takes a consequentialist approach to the morality of aiding the needy, but he arrives at a very different conclusion. He argues that the rich should *not* aid the poor and hungry because doing so will only invite catastrophe for rich and poor alike.

His argument proceeds by way of metaphors, the most well known being the lifeboat. Rich countries are lifeboats carrying the affluent people of the world in an ocean swarming with the drowning poor, who are desperately trying to scramble into the boats or grasp some of the food on board. Like a country, each lifeboat is limited in the number of people it can sustain, and to maintain a margin of safety it should carry fewer passengers than its maximum capacity. If a boat takes on any more passengers or throws vital supplies to the unfortunates swimming nearby, everyone—rich and poor—will perish. Either the boat will capsize, or those on board will slowly starve. Thus, the only reasonable option is to refuse to help the drowning people. Sadly, millions will be lost, but those already on board will be saved. The conclusion to be drawn, Hardin says, is that the moral duty of affluent countries is not to give aid to the starving, overpopulated ones.

Many take issue with Hardin's argument (and metaphors). A chief complaint is that the lifeboat argument is simplistic, that it ignores some hard facts about rich and poor nations. For instance, Hardin implies that the lifeboats of the rich have no interaction with the poor. But many deny this, asserting that for years rich countries have been taking advantage of poor ones and, therefore, bear some responsibility for the wretched plight of the impoverished:

> Haven't colonization and commercial arrangements worked to increase the disparity between the rich and the poor nations of the earth? We extract cheap raw materials from poor nations and sell those nations expensive manufactured goods (for example, radios, cars, computers, and weapons) instead of appropriate agricultural goods and training. The structure of tariffs and internal subsidies discriminates selectively against

---

[12]John Arthur, "Equality, Entitlements, and the Distribution of Income," *Philosophy for the 21st Century*, ed. Steven M. Cohn (New York: Oxford University Press, 2003), 677.

[13]Arthur, 678.

[14]Louis P. Pojman, ed., *Life and Death: A Reader in Moral Problems*, 2nd ed. (Belmont, CA: Wadsworth, 2000), 180.

QUICK REVIEW

justice—The morality of persons getting what is fair or what is their due.

right—A claim or entitlement to something; a moral demand that obligates others to honor it.

negative right—A person's right that obligates others not to interfere with that person's obtaining something.

positive right—A person's right that obligates others to help that person obtain something.

duty of beneficence—A moral obligation to benefit others.

supererogatory actions—Conduct that is above and beyond duty; not required, but praiseworthy.

retributive justice—Justice concerning fair punishment for wrongdoing.

distributive justice—Justice concerning the fair distribution of society's goods.

libertarian theory of justice—A doctrine emphasizing individual liberties and negative rights, and rejecting positive rights as a violation of personal freedom.

egalitarian theory of justice—A doctrine holding that justice requires equal distribution of goods and social benefits among all persons.

---

underdeveloped nations. Multinational corporations place strong inducements on poor countries to produce cash crops such as coffee and cocoa instead of food crops needed to feed their own people. . . . Hardin's lifeboat metaphor grimly obscures the fact that we have profited and are profiting from the economic conditions in the third world.[15]

The lifeboat metaphor suggests that supplies are fixed, but critics protest that the reality is far different:

[15]Pojman, 175.

In the real world, the quantity has strict limits, but these are far from having been reached. . . . Nor are we forced to devote fixed proportions of our efforts and energy to automobile travel, pet food, packaging, advertising, corn-fed beef, "defense," and other diversions, many of which cost far more than foreign aid does. The fact is that enough food is now produced to feed the world's population adequately. That people are malnourished is due to distribution and to economics, not to agricultural limits.[16]

The gist of these counterarguments is that the survival of rich countries is not really at stake and that feeding the hungry will not necessarily capsize any boats. The critics conclude that Hardin offers no good reason for our not aiding the needy.

SUMMARY

Justice is about persons getting what is fair or what is their due. Distributive justice pertains to the fair distribution of society's goods and applies to both national and international issues. A central justice issue in global economics is, What is the moral duty of the affluent to the needy of the world?

In answering this question, libertarian theories—which emphasize negative rights—say that we have no duties to the poor. The poor have only negative rights of noninterference; they have no positive rights to be aided by others. Consequentialist theories have been used both to advocate helping the poor and to refrain from helping them, their proponents arguing that the overall benefits and harms of aid are the deciding factor. Egalitarian theories maintain that justice requires equal distributions of goods among all persons.

Peter Singer argues that we should make huge sacrifices to aid the impoverished of the world: if it is in our power to prevent something bad from happening without sacrificing anything of comparable moral importance, we should do it. Garrett Hardin contends that we have an opposite duty—not to help the needy. Both Singer and Hardin argue that their preferred course of action results in the overall best consequences.

[16]William W. Murdoch and Allan Oaten, "Population and Food: Metaphors and the Reality," *BioScience* 25, no. 9 (September 1975): 561.

R E A D I N G S

On Justice

JOHN RAWLS

THE ROLE OF JUSTICE

Justice is the first virtue of social institutions, as truth is of systems of thought. A theory however elegant and economical must be rejected or revised if it is untrue; likewise laws and institutions no matter how efficient and well-arranged must be reformed or abolished if they are unjust. Each person possesses an inviolability founded on justice that even the welfare of society as a whole cannot override. For this reason justice denies that the loss of freedom for some is made right by a greater good shared by others. It does not allow that the sacrifices imposed on a few are outweighed by the larger sum of advantages enjoyed by many. Therefore in a just society the liberties of equal citizenship are taken as settled; the rights secured by justice are not subject to political bargaining or to the calculus of social interests. The only thing that permits us to acquiesce in an erroneous theory is the lack of a better one; analogously, an injustice is tolerable only when it is necessary to avoid an even greater injustice. Being first virtues of human activities, truth and justice are uncompromising.

These propositions seem to express our intuitive conviction of the primacy of justice. No doubt they are expressed too strongly. In any event I wish to inquire whether these contentions or others similar to them are sound, and if so how they can be accounted for. To this end it is necessary to work out a theory of justice in the light of which these assertions can be interpreted and assessed. I shall begin by considering the role of the principles of justice. Let us assume, to fix ideas, that a society is a more or less self-sufficient association of persons who in their

John Rawls, Reprinted by permission of the publisher from *A Theory of Justice: Revised Edition* by John Rawls, pp. 3–5, 10–19, 52–54, Cambridge, Mass.: The Belknap Press of Harvard University Press, Copyright © 1971, 1999 by the President and Fellows of Harvard College.

relations to one another recognize certain rules of conduct as binding and who for the most part act in accordance with them. Suppose further that these rules specify a system of cooperation designed to advance the good of those taking part in it. Then, although a society is a cooperative venture for mutual advantage, it is typically marked by a conflict as well as by an identity of interests. There is an identity of interests since social cooperation makes possible a better life for all than any would have if each were to live solely by his own efforts. There is a conflict of interests since persons are not indifferent as to how the greater benefits produced by their collaboration are distributed, for in order to pursue their ends they each prefer a larger to a lesser share. A set of principles is required for choosing among the various social arrangements which determine this division of advantages and for underwriting an agreement on the proper distributive shares. These principles are the principles of social justice: they provide a way of assigning rights and duties in the basic institutions of society and they define the appropriate distribution of the benefits and burdens of social cooperation.

Now let us say that a society is well-ordered when it is not only designed to advance the good of its members but when it is also effectively regulated by a public conception of justice. That is, it is a society in which (1) everyone accepts and knows that the others accept the same principles of justice, and (2) the basic social institutions generally satisfy and are generally known to satisfy these principles. In this case while men may put forth excessive demands on one another, they nevertheless acknowledge a common point of view from which their claims may be adjudicated. If men's inclination to self-interest makes their vigilance against one another necessary, their public sense of justice makes their secure association together possible. Among individuals with disparate aims and purposes a shared conception of justice establishes the bonds of civic friendship; the general desire for justice limits the pursuit of other ends. One may think of a public conception of justice as constituting the fundamental charter or a well-ordered human association.

* * *

THE MAIN IDEA OF THE THEORY OF JUSTICE

My aim is to present a conception of justice which generalizes and carries to a higher level of abstraction the familiar theory of the social contract as found, say, in Locke, Rousseau, and Kant. In order to do this we are not to think of the original contract as one to enter a particular society or to set up a particular form of government. Rather, the guiding idea is that the principles of justice for the basic structure of society are the object of the original agreement. They are the principles that free and rational persons concerned to further their own interests would accept in an initial position of equality as defining the fundamental terms of their association. These principles are to regulate all further agreements; they specify the kinds of social cooperation that can be entered into and the forms of government that can be established. This way of regarding the principles of justice I shall call justice as fairness.

Thus we are to imagine that those who engage in social cooperation choose together, in one joint act, the principles which are to assign basic rights and duties and to determine the division of social benefits. Men are to decide in advance how they are to regulate their claims against one another and what is to be the foundation charter of their society. Just as each person must decide by rational reflection what constitutes his good, that is, the system of ends which it is rational for him to pursue, so a group of persons must decide once and for all what is to count among them as just and unjust. The choice which rational men would make in this hypothetical situation of equal liberty, assuming for the present that this choice problem has a solution, determines the principles of justice.

In justice as fairness the original position of equality corresponds to the state of nature in the traditional theory of the social contract. This original position is not, of course, thought of as an actual historical state of affairs, much less as a primitive condition of culture. It is understood as a purely hypothetical situation characterized so as to lead to a certain conception of justice. Among the essential features of this situation is that no one knows his place in society, his class position or social status, nor does any one know his fortune in the distribution of natural assets and abilities, his intelligence, strength, and the like. I shall even assume that the parties do not know their conceptions of the good or their special psychological propensities. The principles of justice are chosen behind a veil of ignorance. This ensures that no one is advantaged or disadvantaged in the choice of principles by the outcome of natural chance or the contingency of social circumstances. Since all are similarly situated and no one is able to design principles to favor his particular condition, the principles of justice are the result of a fair agreement or bargain. For given the circumstances of the original position, the symmetry of everyone's relations to each other, this initial situation is fair between individuals as moral persons, that is, as rational beings with their own ends and capable, I shall assume, of a sense of justice. The original position is, one might say, the appropriate initial status quo, and thus the fundamental agreements reached in it are fair. This explains the propriety of the name "justice as fairness": it conveys the idea that the principles of justice are agreed to in an initial situation that is fair. The name does not mean that the concepts of justice and fairness are the same, any more than the phrase "poetry as metaphor" means that the concepts of poetry and metaphor are the same.

Justice as fairness begins, as I have said, with one of the most general of all choices which persons might make together, namely, with the choice of the first principles of a conception of justice which is to regulate all subsequent criticism and reform of institutions. Then, having chosen a conception of justice, we can suppose that they are to choose a constitution and a legislature to enact laws, and so on, all in accordance with the principles of justice initially agreed upon. Our social situation is just if it is such that by this sequence of hypothetical agreements we would have contracted into the general system of rules which defines it. Moreover, assuming that the original position does determine a set of principles (that is, that a particular conception of justice would be chosen), it will then be true that whenever social institutions satisfy these principles those engaged in them can say to one another that they are cooperating on terms to which they would agree if they were free and equal persons whose relations with respect to one another were fair. They could all view their arrangements as meeting the stipulations which they would acknowledge in an initial situation that embodies widely accepted and reasonable constraints on the choice of principles. The general recognition of this fact would provide the basis for a public acceptance of the corresponding principles of justice. No society can, of course, be a scheme of cooperation which men enter voluntarily in a literal sense; each person finds himself placed at birth in some particular position in some particular society, and the nature of this position materially affects his life prospects. Yet a society satisfying the principles of justice as fairness comes as close as a society can to being a voluntary scheme, for it meets the principles which free and equal persons would assent to under circumstances that are fair. In this sense its members are autonomous and the obligations they recognize self-imposed.

One feature of justice as fairness is to think of the parties in the initial situation as rational and mutually disinterested. This does not mean that the parties are egoists, that is, individuals with only certain kinds of interests, say in wealth, prestige, and domination. But they are conceived as not taking an interest in one another's interests. They are to presume that even their spiritual aims may be opposed, in the way that the aims of those of different religions may be opposed. Moreover, the concept of rationality must be interpreted as far as possible in the narrow sense, standard in economic theory, of taking the most effective means to given ends.

* * *

In working out the conception of justice as fairness one main task clearly is to determine which principles of justice would be chosen in the original position. To do this we must describe this situation in some detail and formulate with care the problem of choice which it presents. These matters I shall take up in the immediately succeeding chapters. It may be observed, however, that once the principles of justice are thought of as arising from an original agreement in a situation of equality, it is an open question whether the principle of utility would be acknowledged. Offhand it hardly seems likely that persons who view themselves as equals, entitled to press their claims upon one another, would agree to a principle which may require lesser life prospects for some simply for the sake of a greater sum of advantages enjoyed by others. Since each desires to protect his interests, his capacity to advance his conception of the good, no one has a reason to acquiesce in an enduring loss for himself in order to bring about a greater net balance of satisfaction. In the absence of strong and lasting benevolent impulses, a rational man would not accept a basic structure merely because it maximized the algebraic sum of advantages irrespective of its permanent effects on his own basic rights and interests. Thus it seems that the principle of utility is incompatible with the conception of social cooperation among equals for mutual advantage. It appears to be inconsistent with the idea of reciprocity implicit in the notion of a well-ordered society. Or, at any rate, so I shall argue.

I shall maintain instead that the persons in the initial situation would choose two rather different principles: the first requires equality in the assignment of basic rights and duties, while the second holds that social and economic inequalities, for example inequalities of wealth and authority, are just only if they result in compensating benefits for everyone, and in particular for the least advantaged members of society. These principles rule out justifying institutions on the grounds that the hardships of some are offset by a greater good in the aggregate. It may be expedient but it is not just that some should have less in order that others may prosper. But there is no injustice in the greater benefits earned by a few provided that the situation of persons not so fortunate is thereby improved. The intuitive idea is that since everyone's well-being depends upon a scheme of cooperation without which no one could have a satisfactory life, the division of advantages should be such as to draw forth the willing cooperation of everyone taking part in it, including those less well situated. The two principles mentioned seem to be a fair basis on which those better endowed, or more fortunate in their social position, neither of which we can be said to deserve, could expect the willing cooperation of others when some workable scheme is a necessary condition of the welfare of all. Once we decide to look for a conception of justice that prevents the use of the accidents of natural endowment and the contingencies of social circumstance as counters in a quest for political and economic advantage, we are led to these principles. They express the result of leaving aside those aspects of the social world that seem arbitrary from a moral point of view.

* * *

THE ORIGINAL POSITION AND JUSTIFICATION

I have said that the original position is the appropriate initial status quo which insures that the fundamental agreements reached in it are fair. This fact yields the name "justice as fairness." It is clear, then, that I want to say that one conception of justice is more reasonable than another, or justifiable with respect to it, if rational persons in the initial situation would choose its principles over those of the other for the role of justice. Conceptions of justice are to be ranked by their acceptability to persons so circumstanced. Understood in this way the question of justification is settled by working out a problem of deliberation: we have to ascertain which principles it would be rational to adopt given the contractual situation. This connects the theory of justice with the theory of rational choice.

If this view of the problem of justification is to succeed, we must, of course, describe in some detail the nature of this choice problem. A problem of rational decision has a definite answer only if we

know the beliefs and interests of the parties, their relations with respect to one another, the alternatives between which they are to choose, the procedure whereby they make up their minds, and so on. As the circumstances are presented in different ways, correspondingly different principles are accepted. The concept of the original position, as I shall refer to it, is that of the most philosophically favored interpretation of this initial choice situation for the purposes of a theory of justice.

But how are we to decide what is the most favored interpretation? I assume, for one thing, that there is a broad measure of agreement that principles of justice should be chosen under certain conditions. To justify a particular description of the initial situation one shows that it incorporates these commonly shared presumptions. One argues from widely accepted but weak premises to more specific conclusions. Each of the presumptions should by itself be natural and plausible; some of them may seem innocuous or even trivial. The aim of the contract approach is to establish that taken together they impose significant bounds on acceptable principles of justice. The ideal outcome would be that these conditions determine a unique set of principles; but I shall be satisfied if they suffice to rank the main traditional conceptions of social justice.

One should not be misled, then, by the somewhat unusual conditions which characterize the original position. The idea here is simply to make vivid to ourselves the restrictions that it seems reasonable to impose on arguments for principles of justice, and therefore on these principles themselves. Thus it seems reasonable and generally acceptable that no one should be advantaged or disadvantaged by natural fortune or social circumstances in the choice of principles. It also seems widely agreed that it should be impossible to tailor principles to the circumstances of one's own case. We should insure further that particular inclinations and aspirations, and persons' conceptions of their good do not affect the principles adopted. The aim is to rule out those principles that it would be rational to propose for acceptance, however little the chance of success, only if one knew certain things that are irrelevant from the standpoint of justice. For example, if a man knew that he was wealthy, he might find it rational to advance the principle that various taxes for welfare measures be counted unjust; if he knew that he was poor, he would most likely propose the contrary principle. To represent the desired restrictions one imagines a situation in which everyone is deprived of this sort of information. One excludes the knowledge of those contingencies which sets men at odds and allows them to be guided by their prejudices. In this manner the veil of ignorance is arrived at in a natural way. This concept should cause no difficulty if we keep in mind the constraints on arguments that it is meant to express. At any time we can enter the original position, so to speak, simply by following a certain procedure, namely, by arguing for principles of justice in accordance with these restrictions.

It seems reasonable to suppose that the parties in the original position are equal. That is, all have the same rights in the procedure for choosing principles; each can make proposals, submit reasons for their acceptance, and so on. Obviously the purpose of these conditions is to represent equality between human beings as moral persons, as creatures having a conception of their good and capable of a sense of justice. The basis of equality is taken to be similarity in these two respects. Systems of ends are not ranked in value; and each man is presumed to have the requisite ability to understand and to act upon whatever principles are adopted. Together with the veil of ignorance, these conditions define the principles of justice as those which rational persons concerned to advance their interests would consent to as equals when none are known to be advantaged or disadvantaged by social and natural contingencies.

There is, however, another side to justifying a particular description of the original position. This is to see if the principles which would be chosen match our considered convictions of justice or extend them in an acceptable way. We can note whether applying these principles would lead us to make the same judgments about the basic structure of society which we now make intuitively and in which we have the greatest confidence; or whether, in cases where our present judgments are in doubt and given with hesi-

tation, these principles offer a resolution which we can affirm on reflection. There are questions which we feel sure must be answered in a certain way. For example, we are confident that religious intolerance and racial discrimination are unjust. We think that we have examined these things with care and have reached what we believe is an impartial judgment not likely to be distorted by an excessive attention to our own interests. These convictions are provisional fixed points which we presume any conception of justice must fit. But we have much less assurance as to what is the correct distribution of wealth and authority. Here we may be looking for a way to remove our doubts. We can check an interpretation of the initial situation, then, by the capacity of its principles to accommodate our firmest convictions and to provide guidance where guidance is needed.

In searching for the most favored description of this situation we work from both ends. We begin by describing it so that it represents generally shared and preferably weak conditions. We then see if these conditions are strong enough to yield a significant set of principles. If not, we look for further premises equally reasonable. But if so, and these principles match our considered convictions of justice, then so far well and good. But presumably there will be discrepancies. In this case we have a choice. We can either modify the account of the initial situation or we can revise our existing judgments, for even the judgments we take provisionally as fixed points are liable to revision. By going back and forth, sometimes altering the conditions of the contractual circumstances, at others withdrawing our judgments and conforming them to principle, I assume that eventually we shall find a description of the initial situation that both expresses reasonable conditions and yields principles which match our considered judgments duly pruned and adjusted. This state of affairs I refer to as reflective equilibrium. It is an equilibrium because at last our principles and judgments coincide; and it is reflective since we know to what principles our judgments conform and the premises of their derivation. At the moment everything is in order. But this equilibrium is not necessarily stable. It is liable to be upset by further examination of the conditions which should be imposed on the contractual situation and by particular cases which may lead us to revise our judgments. Yet for the time being we have done what we can to render coherent and to justify our convictions of social justice. We have reached a conception of the original position.

I shall not, of course, actually work through this process. Still, we may think of the interpretation of the original position that I shall present as the result of such a hypothetical course of reflection. It represents the attempt to accommodate within one scheme both reasonable philosophical conditions on principles as well as our considered judgments of justice. In arriving at the favored interpretation of the initial situation there is no point at which an appeal is made to self-evidence in the traditional sense either of general conceptions or particular convictions. I do not claim for the principles of justice proposed that they are necessary truths or derivable from such truths. A conception of justice cannot be deduced from self-evident premises or conditions on principles; instead, its justification is a matter of the mutual support of many considerations, of everything fitting together into one coherent view.

A final comment. We shall want to say that certain principles of justice are justified because they would be agreed to in an initial situation of equality. I have emphasized that this original position is purely hypothetical. It is natural to ask why, if this agreement is never actually entered into, we should take any interest in these principles, moral or otherwise. The answer is that the conditions embodied in the description of the original position are ones that we do not in fact accept. Or if we do not, then perhaps we can be persuaded to do so by philosophical reflection. Each aspect of the contractual situation can be given supporting grounds. Thus what we shall do is to collect together into one conception a number of conditions on principles that we are ready upon due consideration to recognize as reasonable. These constraints express what we are prepared to regard as limits on fair terms of social cooperation. One way to look at the idea of the original position, therefore, is to see it as an expository device which sums up the meaning of these conditions and helps us to extract

their consequences. On the other hand, this conception is also an intuitive notion that suggests its own elaboration, so that led on by it we are drawn to define more clearly the standpoint from which we can best interpret moral relationships. We need a conception that enables us to envision our objective from afar: the intuitive notion of the original position is to do this for us.

* * *

TWO PRINCIPLES OF JUSTICE

I shall now state in a provisional form the two principles of justice that I believe would be agreed to in the original position. The first formulation of these principles is tentative. As we go on I shall consider several formulations and approximate step by step the final statement to be given much later. I believe that doing this allows the exposition to proceed in a natural way.

The first statement of the two principles reads as follows.

> First: each person is to have an equal right to the most extensive scheme of equal basic liberties compatible with a similar scheme of liberties for others.
>
> Second: social and economic inequalities are to be arranged so that they are both (a) reasonably expected to be to everyone's advantage, and (b) attached to positions and offices open to all.

* * *

These principles primarily apply as I have said, to the basic structure of society and govern the assignment of rights and duties and regulate the distribution of social and economic advantages. Their formulation presupposes that, for the purposes of a theory of justice, the social structure may be viewed as having two more or less distinct parts, the first principle applying to the one, the second principle to the other. Thus we distinguish between the aspects of the social system that define and secure the equal basic liberties and the aspects that specify and establish social and economic inequalities. Now it is essential to observe that the basic liberties are given by a list of such liberties. Important among these are political liberty (the right to vote and to hold public office) and freedom of speech and assembly: liberty of conscience and freedom of thought: freedom of the person, which includes freedom from psychological oppression and physical assault and dismemberment (integrity of the person); the right to hold personal property and freedom from arbitrary arrest and seizure as defined by the concept of the rule of law. These liberties are to be equal by the first principle.

The second principle applies, in the first approximation, to the distribution of income and wealth and to the design of organizations that make use of differences in authority and responsibility. While the distribution of wealth and income need not be equal, it must be to everyone's advantage, and at the same time, positions of authority and responsibility must be accessible to all. One applies the second principle by holding positions open, and then, subject to this constraint, arranges social and economic inequalities so that everyone benefits.

These principles are to be arranged in a serial order with the first principle prior to the second. This ordering means that infringements of the basic equal liberties protected by the first principle cannot be justified, or compensated for, by greater social and economic advantages. These liberties have a central range of application within which they can be limited and compromised only when they conflict with other basic liberties. Since they may be limited when they clash with one another, none of these liberties is absolute; but however they are adjusted to form one system, this system is to be the same for all. It is diffi-

cult, and perhaps impossible, to give a complete specification of these liberties independently from the particular circumstances—social, economic, and technological—of a given society. The hypothesis is that the general form of such a list could be devised with sufficient exactness to sustain this conception of justice. Of course, liberties not on the list, for example, the right to own certain kinds of property (e.g., means of production) and freedom of contract as understood by the doctrine of laissez-faire are not basic; and so they are not protected by the priority of the first principle. Finally, in regard to the second principle, the distribution of wealth and income, and positions of authority and responsibility, are to be consistent with both the basic liberties and equality of opportunity.

The two principles are rather specific in their content, and their acceptance rests on certain assumptions that I must eventually try to explain and justify. For the present, it should be observed that these principles are a special case of a more general conception of justice that can be expressed as follows.

All social values—liberty and opportunity, income and wealth, and the social bases of self-respect—are to be distributed equally unless an unequal distribution of any, or all, of these values is to everyone's advantage.

Injustice, then, is simply inequalities that are not to the benefit of all.

* * *

The Entitlement Theory of Justice

ROBERT NOZICK

* * *

The term "distributive justice" is not a neutral one. Hearing the term "distribution," most people presume that some thing or mechanism uses some principle or criterion to give out a supply of things. Into this process of distributing shares some error may have crept. So it is an open question, at least, whether redistribution should take place; whether we should do again what has already been done once, though poorly. However, we are not in the position of children who have been given portions of pie by someone who now makes last minute adjustments to rectify careless cutting. There is no *central* distribution, no person or group entitled to control all the resources, jointly deciding how they are to be doled out. What each person gets, he gets from others who give to him in exchange for something, or as a gift. In a free society, diverse persons control different resources, and new holdings arise out of the voluntary exchanges and actions of persons. There is no more a distributing or distribution of shares than there is a distributing of mates in a society in which persons choose whom they shall marry. The total result is the product of many individual decisions which the different individuals involved are entitled to make. Some uses of the term "distribution," it is true, do not imply a previous distributing appropriately judged by some criterion (for example, "probability distribution"); nevertheless, * * * it would be best to use a terminology that clearly is neutral. We shall speak of people's holdings; a principle of justice in holdings describes (part of) what justice tells us (requires) about holdings. I shall state first what I take to be the correct view about justice in holdings, and then turn to the discussion of alternate views.

THE ENTITLEMENT THEORY

The subject of justice in holdings consists of three major topics. The first is the *original acquisition of holdings*, the appropriation of unheld things. This includes the issues of how unheld things may come to be held, the process, or processes, by which unheld things may come to be held, the things that may come to be held by these processes, the extent of what comes to be held by a particular process, and so on. We shall refer to the complicated truth about this topic, which we shall not formulate here, as the principle of justice in acquisition. The second topic concerns the *transfer of holdings* from one person to another. By what processes may a person transfer holdings to another? How may a person acquire a holding from another who holds it? Under this topic come general descriptions of voluntary exchange, and gift and (on the other hand) fraud, as well as reference to particular conventional details fixed upon in a given society. The complicated truth about this subject (with placeholders for conventional details) we shall call the principle of justice in transfer. (And we shall suppose it also includes principles governing how a person may divest himself of a holding, passing it into an unheld state.)

If the world were wholly just, the following inductive definition would exhaustively cover the subject of justice in holdings.

1. A person who acquires a holding in accordance with the principle of justice in acquisition is entitled to that holding.
2. A person who acquires a holding in accordance with the principle of justice in transfer, from someone else entitled to the holding, is entitled to the holding.
3. No one is entitled to a holding except by (repeated) applications of 1 and 2.

The complete principle of distributive justice would say simply that a distribution is just if everyone is entitled to the holdings they possess under the distribution.

A distribution is just if it arises from another just distribution by legitimate means. The legitimate means of moving from one distribution to another are specified by the principle of justice in transfer. The legitimate first "moves" are specified by the principle of justice in acquisition.[1] Whatever arises from a just situation by just steps is itself just. The means of change specified by the principle of justice in transfer preserve justice.

* * *

Not all actual situations are generated in accordance with the two principles of justice in holdings: the principle of justice in acquisition and the principle of justice in transfer. Some people steal from others, or defraud them, or enslave them, seizing their product and preventing them from living as they choose, or forcibly exclude others from competing in exchanges. None of these are permissible modes of transition from one situation to another. And some persons acquire holdings by means not sanctioned by the principle of justice in acquisition. The existence of past injustice (previous violations of the first two principles of justice in holdings) raises the third major topic under justice in holdings: the rectification of injustice in holdings. If past injustice has shaped present holdings in various ways, some identifiable and some not, what now, if anything, ought to be done to rectify these injustices? What obligations do the performers of injustice have toward those whose position is worse than it would have been had the injustice not been done? Or, than it would have been had compensation been paid promptly? How, if at all, do things change if the beneficiaries and those made worse off are not the direct parties in the act of injustice, but, for example, their descendants? Is an injustice done to someone whose holding was itself based upon an unrectified injustice? How far back must one go in wiping clean the historical slate of injustices? What may victims of injustice permissibly do in order to rectify the injustices being done to them, including the many injustices done by persons acting through their government? I do not know of a

thorough or theoretically sophisticated treatment of such issues. Idealizing greatly, let us suppose theoretical investigation will produce a principle of rectification. This principle uses historical information about previous situations and injustices done in them (as defined by the first two principles of justice and rights against interference), and information about the actual course of events that flowed from these injustices, until the present, and it yields a description (or descriptions) of holdings in the society. The principle of rectification presumably will make use of its best estimate of subjunctive information about what would have occurred (or a probability distribution over what might have occurred, using the expected value) if the injustice had not taken place. If the actual description of holdings turns out not to be one of the descriptions yielded by the principle, then one of the descriptions yielded must be realized.[2]

The general outlines of the theory of justice in holdings are that the holdings of a person are just if he is entitled to them by the principles of justice in acquisition and transfer, or by the principle of rectification of injustice (as specified by the first two principles). If each person's holdings are just, then the total set (distribution) of holdings is just.

* * *

HISTORICAL PRINCIPLES AND END-RESULT PRINCIPLES

The general outlines of the entitlement theory illuminate the nature and defects of other conceptions of distributive justice. The entitlement theory of justice in distribution is *historical*; whether a distribution is just depends upon how it came about. In contrast, *current time-slice principles* of justice hold that the justice of a distribution is determined by how things are distributed (who has what) as judged by some *structural* principle(s) of just distribution. A utilitarian who judges between any two distributions by seeing which has the greater sum of utility and, if the sums tie, applies some fixed equality criterion to choose the more equal distribution, would hold a current time-slice principle of justice. As would someone who had a fixed schedule of trade-offs between the sum of happiness and equality. According to a current time-slice principle, all that needs to be looked at, in judging the justice of a distribution, is who ends up with what; in comparing any two distributions one need look only at the matrix presenting the distributions. No further information need be fed into a principle of justice. It is a consequence of such principles of justice that any two structurally identical distributions are equally just. (Two distributions are structurally identical if they present the same profile, but perhaps have different persons occupying the particular slots. My having ten and your having five, and my having five and your having ten are structurally identical distributions.) Welfare economics is the theory of current time-slice principles of justice. The subject is conceived as operating on matrices representing only current information about distribution. This, as well as some of the usual conditions (for example, the choice of distribution is invariant under relabeling of columns), guarantees that welfare economics will be a current time-slice theory, with all of its inadequacies.

Most persons do not accept current time-slice principles as constituting the whole story about distributive shares. They think it relevant in assessing the justice of a situation to consider not only the distribution it embodies, but also how that distribution came about. If some persons are in prison for murder or war crimes, we do not say that to assess the justice of the distribution in the society we must look only at what this person has, and that person has, and that person has, . . . at the current time. We think it relevant to ask whether someone did something so that he *deserved* to be punished, deserved to have a lower share. Most will agree to the relevance of further information with regard to punishments and penalties. Consider also desired things. One traditional socialist view is that workers are entitled to the product and full fruits of their labor; they have earned it; a distribution is unjust if it does not give the workers what they are entitled to. Such entitlements are based upon some past history. No socialist holding this view would find it comforting to be told that because the actual distribution A happens to coincide structurally with the one he desires D, A therefore is no

less just than D; it differs only in that the "parasitic" owners of capital receive under A what the workers are entitled to under D, and the workers receive under A what the owners are entitled to under D, namely very little. This socialist rightly, in my view, holds onto the notions of earning, producing, entitlement, desert, and so forth, and he rejects current time-slice principles that look only to the structure of the resulting set of holdings. (The set of holdings resulting from what? Isn't it implausible that how holdings are produced and come to exist has no effect at all on who should hold what?) His mistake lies in his view of what entitlements arise out of what sorts of productive processes.

We construe the position we discuss too narrowly by speaking of *current* time-slice principles. Nothing is changed if structural principles operate upon a time sequence of current time-slice profiles and, for example, give someone more now to counterbalance the less he has had earlier. A utilitarian or an egalitarian or any mixture of the two over time will inherit the difficulties of his more myopic comrades. He is not helped by the fact that *some* of the information others consider relevant in assessing a distribution is reflected, unrecoverably, in past matrices. Henceforth, we shall refer to such unhistorical principles of distributive justice, including the current time-slice principles, as *end-result principles* or *end-state principles*.

In contrast to end-result principles of justice, *historical principles* of justice hold that past circumstances or actions of people can create differential entitlements or differential deserts to things. An injustice can be worked by moving from one distribution to another structurally identical one, for the second, in profile the same, may violate people's entitlements or deserts; it may not fit the actual history.

PATTERNING

The entitlement principles of justice in holdings that we have sketched are historical principles of justice. To better understand their precise character, we shall distinguish them from another subclass of the historical principles. Consider, as an example, the principle of distribution according to moral merit. This principle requires that total distributive shares vary directly with moral merit; no person should have a greater share than anyone whose moral merit is greater. (If moral merit could be not merely ordered but measured on an interval or ratio scale, stronger principles could be formulated.) Or consider the principle that results by substituting "usefulness to society" for "moral merit" in the previous principle. Or instead of "distribute according to moral merit," or "distribute according to usefulness to society," we might consider "distribute according to the weighted sum of moral merit, usefulness to society, and need," with the weights of the different dimensions equal. Let us call a principle of distribution *patterned* if it specifies that a distribution is to vary along with some natural dimension, weighted sum of natural dimensions, or lexicographic ordering of natural dimensions. And let us say a distribution is patterned if it accords with some patterned principle. (I speak of natural dimensions, admittedly without a general criterion for them, because for any set of holdings some artificial dimensions can be gimmicked up to vary along with the distribution of the set.) The principle of distribution in accordance with moral merit is a patterned historical principle, which specifies a patterned distribution. "Distribute according to I.Q." is a patterned principle that looks to information not contained in distributional matrices. It is not historical, however, in that it does not look to any past actions creating differential entitlements to evaluate a distribution; it requires only distributional matrices whose columns are labeled by I.Q. scores. The distribution in a society, however, may be composed of such simple patterned distributions, without itself being simply patterned. Different sectors may operate different patterns, or some combination of patterns may operate in different proportions across a society. A distribution composed in this manner, from a small number of patterned distributions, we also shall term "patterned." And we extend the use of "pattern" to include the overall designs put forth by combinations of end-state principles.

Almost every suggested principle of distributive justice is patterned: to each according to his moral merit, or needs, or marginal product, or how hard he tries, or the weighted sum of the foregoing, and so on. The principle of entitlement we have sketched is *not* patterned.[3] There is no one natural dimension or weighted sum or combination of a small number of natural dimensions that yields the distributions generated in accordance with the principle of entitlement. The set of holdings that results when some persons receive their marginal products, others win at gambling, others receive a share of their mate's income, others receive gifts from foundations, others receive interest on loans, others receive gifts from admirers, others receive returns on investment, others make for themselves much of what they have, others find things, and so on, will not be patterned.

* * *

HOW LIBERTY UPSETS PATTERNS

It is not clear how those holding alternative conceptions of distributive justice can reject the entitlement conception of justice in holdings. For suppose a distribution favored by one of these nonentitlement conceptions is realized. Let us suppose it is your favorite one and let us call this distribution D_1; perhaps everyone has an equal share, perhaps shares vary in accordance with some dimension you treasure. Now suppose that Wilt Chamberlain is greatly in demand by basketball teams, being a great gate attraction. (Also suppose contracts run only for a year, with players being free agents.) He signs the following sort of contract with a team: In each home game, twenty-five cents from the price of each ticket of admission goes to him. (We ignore the question of whether he is "gouging" the owners, letting them look out for themselves.) The season starts, and people cheerfully attend his team's games; they buy their tickets, each time dropping a separate twenty-five cents of their admission price into a special box with Chamberlain's name on it. They are excited about seeing him play; it is worth the total admission price to them. Let us suppose that in one season one million persons attend his home games, and Wilt Chamberlain winds up with $250,000, a much larger sum than the average income and larger even than anyone else has. Is he entitled to this income? Is this new distribution D_2, unjust? If so, why? There is *no* question about whether each of the people was entitled to the control over the resources they held in D_1; because that was the distribution (your favorite) that (for the purposes of argument) we assumed was acceptable. Each of these persons *chose* to give twenty-five cents of their money to Chamberlain. They could have spent it on going to the movies, or on candy bars, or on copies of *Dissent* magazine, or of *Monthly Review*. But they all, at least one million of them, converged on giving it to Wilt Chamberlain in exchange for watching him play basketball. If D_1 was a just distribution, and people voluntarily moved from it to D_2, transferring parts of their shares they were given under D_1 (what was it for if not to do something with?), isn't D_2 also just? If the people were entitled to dispose of the resources to which they were entitled (under D_1), didn't this include their being entitled to give it to, or exchange it with, Wilt Chamberlain? Can anyone else complain on grounds of justice? Each other person already has his legitimate share under D_1. Under D_1, there is nothing that anyone has that anyone else has a claim of justice against. After someone transfers something to Wilt Chamberlain, third parties *still* have their legitimate shares; *their* shares are not changed. By what process could such a transfer among two persons give rise to a legitimate claim of distributive justice on a portion of what was transferred, by a third party who had no claim of justice on any holding of the others *before* the transfer?[4] To cut off objections irrelevant here, we might imagine the exchanges occurring in a socialist society, after hours. After playing whatever basketball he does in his daily work, or doing whatever other daily work he does, Wilt Chamberlain decides to put in *overtime* to earn additional money. (First his work quota is set; he works time over that.) Or imagine it is a skilled juggler people like to see, who puts on shows after hours.

Why might someone work overtime in a society in which it is assumed their needs are satisfied? Perhaps because they care about things other than needs. I like to write in books that I read, and to have easy access to books for browsing at odd hours. It would be very pleasant and convenient to have the resources of Widener Library in my back yard. No society, I assume, will provide such resources close to each person who would like them as part of his regular allotment (under D_1). Thus, persons either must do without some extra things that they want, or be allowed to do something extra to get some of these things. On what basis could the inequalities that would eventuate be forbidden? Notice also that small factories would spring up in a socialist society, unless forbidden. I melt down some of my personal possessions (under D_1) and build a machine out of the material. I offer you, and others, a philosophy lecture once a week in exchange for your cranking the handle on my machine, whose products I exchange for yet other things, and so on. (The raw materials used by the machine are given to me by others who possess them under D_1, in exchange for hearing lectures.) Each person might participate to gain things over and above their allotment under D_1. Some persons even might want to leave their job in socialist industry and work full time in this private sector. I shall say something more about these issues in the next chapter. Here I wish merely to note how private property even in means of production would occur in a socialist society that did not forbid people to use as they wished some of the resources they are given under the socialist distribution D_1. The socialist society would have to forbid capitalist acts between consenting adults.

The general point illustrated by the Wilt Chamberlain example and the example of the entrepreneur in a socialist society is that no end-state principle or distributional patterned principle of justice can be continuously realized without continuous interference with people's lives. Any favored pattern would be transformed into one unfavored by the principle, by people choosing to act in various ways; for example, by people exchanging goods and services with other people, or giving things to other people, things the transferrers are entitled to under the favored distributional pattern. To maintain a pattern one must either continually interfere to stop people from transferring resources as they wish to, or continually (or periodically) interfere to take from some persons resources that others for some reason chose to transfer to them.

* * *

REDISTRIBUTION AND PROPERTY RIGHTS

Apparently, patterned principles allow people to choose to expend upon themselves, but not upon others, those resources they are entitled to (or rather, receive) under some favored distributional pattern D_1. For if each of several persons chooses to expend some of his D_1 resources upon one other person, then that other person will receive more than is D_1 share, disturbing the favored distributional pattern. Maintaining a distributional pattern is individualism with a vengeance! Patterned distributional principles do not give people what entitlement principles do, only better distributed. For they do not give the right to choose what to do with what one has; they do not give the right to choose to pursue an end involving (intrinsically, or as a means) the enhancement of another's position. To such views, families are disturbing; for within a family occur transfers that upset the favored distributional pattern. Either families themselves become units to which distribution takes place, the column occupiers (on what rationale?), or loving behavior is forbidden. We should note in passing the ambivalent position of radicals toward the family. Its loving relationships are seen as a model to be emulated and extended across the whole society, at the same time that it is denounced as a suffocating institution to be broken and condemned as a focus of parochial concerns that interfere with achieving radical goals. Need we say that it is not appropriate to enforce across the wider society the relationships of love and care appropriate within a family, relationships which are voluntarily undertaken?[5] Incidentally, love is an interesting instance of another relationship that is historical, in that (like justice) it depends upon what actually occurred. An adult may come to love another because of the other's characteristics; but it is the other person, and not the characteristics, that is loved. The love is not transferrable to someone else with the same characteristics, even to one who "scores" higher for these characteristics. And the love endures through changes of the characteristics that gave rise to it. One loves the particular person one actually encountered. Why love is historical, attaching to persons in this way and not to characteristics, is an interesting and puzzling question.

Proponents of patterned principles of distributive justice focus upon criteria for determining who is to receive holdings; they consider the reasons for which someone should have something, and also the total picture of holdings. Whether or not it is better to give than to receive, proponents of patterned principles ignore giving altogether. In considering the distribution of goods, income, and so forth, their theories are theories of recipient justice; they completely ignore any right a person might have to give something to someone. Even in exchanges where each party is simultaneously giver and recipient, patterned principles of justice focus only upon the recipient role and its supposed rights. Thus discussions tend to focus on whether people (should) have a right to inherit, rather than on whether people (should) have a right to bequeath or on whether persons who have a right to hold also have a right to choose that others hold in their place. I lack a good explanation of why the usual theories of distributive justice are so recipient oriented; ignoring givers and transferrers and their rights is of a piece with ignoring producers and their entitlements. But why is it *all* ignored?

Patterned principles of distributive justice necessitate *re*distributive activities. The likelihood is small that any actual freely-arrived-at set of holdings fits a given pattern; and the likelihood is nil that it will continue to fit the pattern as people exchange and give. From the point of view of an entitlement theory, redistribution is a serious matter indeed, involving, as it does, the violation of people's rights. (An exception is those takings that fall under the principle of the rectification of injustices.) From other points of view, also, it is serious.

Taxation of earnings from labor is on a par with forced labor.[6] Some persons find this claim obviously true: taking the earnings of n hours labor is like taking n hours from the person; it is like forcing the person to work n hours for another's purpose. Others find the claim absurd. But even these, *if* they object to forced labor, would oppose forcing unemployed hippies to work for the benefit of the needy.[7] And they would also object to forcing each person to work five extra hours each week for the benefit of the needy. But a system that takes five hours' wages in taxes does not seem to them like one that forces someone to work five hour, since it offers the person forced a wider range of choice in activities than does taxation in kind with the particular labor specified. (But we can imagine a gradation of systems of forced labor, from one that specifies a particular activity, to one that gives a choice among two activities, to . . . ; and so on up.) Furthermore, people envisage a system with something like a proportional tax on everything above the amount necessary for basic needs. Some think this does not force someone to work extra hours, since there is no fixed number of extra hours he is forced to work, and since he can avoid the tax entirely by earning only enough to cover his basic needs. This is a very uncharacteristic view of forcing for those who *also* think people are forced to do something *whenever* the alternatives they face are considerably worse. However, *neither* view is correct. The fact that others intentionally intervene, in violation of a side constraint against aggression, to threaten force to limit the alternatives, in this case to paying taxes or (presumably the worse alternative) bare subsistence, makes the taxation system one of forced labor and distinguishes it from other cases of limited choices which are not forcings.

The man who chooses to work longer to gain an income more than sufficient for his basic needs prefers some extra goods or services to the leisure and activities he could perform during the possible nonworking hours; whereas the man who chooses not to work the extra time prefers the leisure activities to the extra goods or services he could acquire by working more. Given this, if it would be illegitimate for a tax system to seize some of a man's leisure (forced labor) for the purpose of serving the needy, how can it be legitimate for a tax system to seize some of a man's goods for that purpose? Why should we treat the man whose happiness requires certain material goods or services differently from the man whose preferences and desires make such goods unnecessary for his happiness? Why should the man who prefers seeing a movie (and who has to earn money for a ticket) be open to the required call to aid the needy, while the person who prefers looking at a sunset (and hence need earn no extra money) is not? Indeed, isn't it surprising that redistributionists choose to ignore the man whose pleasures are so easily attainable without extra labor, while adding yet another burden to the poor unfortunate who must work for his pleasures? If anything, one would have expected the reverse. Why is the person with the nonmaterial or nonconsumption desire allowed to proceed unimpeded to his most favored feasible alternative, whereas the man whose pleasures or desires involve material things and who must work for extra money (thereby serving whomever considers his activities valuable enough to pay him) is constrained in what he can realize? Perhaps there is no difference in principle. And perhaps some think the answer concerns merely administrative convenience. (These questions and issues will not disturb those who think that forced labor to serve the needy or to realize some favored end-state pattern is acceptable.) In a fuller discussion we would have (and want) to extend our argument to include interest, entrepreneurial profits, and so on. Those who doubt that this extension can be carried through, and who draw the line here at taxation of income from labor, will have to state rather complicated patterned *historical* principles of distributive justice, since end-state principles would not distinguish *sources* of income in any way. It is enough for now to get away from end-state principles and to make clear how various patterned principles are dependent upon particular views about the sources or the illegitimacy or the lesser legitimacy of profits, interest, and so on; which particular views may well be mistaken.

What sort of right over others does a legally institutionalized end-state pattern give one? The central core of the notion of a property right in X, relative to which other parts of the notion are to be explained, is the right to determine what shall be done with X; the right to choose which of the constrained set of options concerning X shall be realized or attempted. The constraints are set by other principles or laws operating in the society; in our theory, by the

Lockean rights people possess (under the minimal state). My property rights in my knife allow me to leave it where I will, but not in your chest. I may choose which of the acceptable options involving the knife is to be realized. This notion of property helps us to understand why earlier theorists spoke of people as having property in themselves and their labor. They viewed each person as having a right to decide what would become of himself and what he would do, and as having a right to reap the benefits of what he did.

* * *

When end-result principles of distributive justice are built into the legal structure of a society, they (as do most patterned principles) give each citizen an enforceable claim to some portion of the total social product; that is, to some portion of the sum total of the individually and jointly made products. This total product is produced by individuals laboring, using means of production others have saved to bring into existence, by people organizing production or creating means to produce new things or things in a new way. It is on this batch of individual activities that patterned distributional principles give each individual an enforceable claim. Each person has a claim to the activities and the products of other persons, independently of whether the other persons enter into particular relationships that give rise to these claims, and independently of whether they voluntarily take these claims upon themselves, in charity or in exchange for something.

Whether it is done through taxation on wages or on wages over a certain amount, or through seizure of profits, or through there being a big *social pot* so that it's not clear what's coming from where and what's going where, patterned principles of distributive justice involve appropriating the actions of other persons. Seizing the results of someone's labor is equivalent to seizing hours from him and directing him to carry on various activities. If people force you to do certain work, or unrewarded work, for a certain period of time, they decide what you are to do and what purposes your work is to serve apart from your decisions. This process whereby they take this decision from you makes them a *part-owner* of you; it gives them a property right in you. Just as having

such partial control and power of decision, by right, over an animal or inanimate object would be to have a property right in it.

End-state and most patterned principles of distributive justice institute (partial) ownership by others of people and their actions and labor. These principles involve a shift from the classical liberals' notion of self-ownership to a notion of (partial) property rights in *other* people.

* * *

May a person emigrate from a nation that has institutionalized some end-state or patterned distributional principle? For some principles (for example, Hayek's) emigration presents no theoretical problem. But for others it is a tricky matter. Consider a nation having a compulsory scheme of minimal social provision to aid the neediest (or one organized so as to maximize the position of the worst-off group); no one may opt out of participating in it. (None may say, "Don't compel me to contribute to others and don't provide for me via this compulsory mechanism if I am in need.") Everyone above a certain level is forced to contribute to aid the needy. But if emigration from the country were allowed, anyone could choose to move to another country that did not have compulsory social provision but otherwise was (as much as possible) identical. In such a case, the person's *only* motive for leaving would be to avoid participating in the compulsory scheme of social provision. And if he does leave, the needy in his initial country will receive no (compelled) help from him. What rationale yields the result that the person be permitted to emigrate, yet forbidden to stay and opt out of the compulsory scheme of social provision? If providing for the needy is of overriding importance, this does militate against allowing internal opting out; but it also speaks against allowing external emigration. (Would it also support, to some extent, the kidnapping of persons living in a place without compulsory social provision, who could be forced to make a contribution to the needy in your community?) Perhaps the crucial component of the position that allows emigration solely to avoid certain arrangements, while not allowing anyone internally to opt out of them, is a concern for fraternal feelings within the country. "We don't want anyone here who doesn't contribute, who doesn't care enough about the others to contribute." That concern, in this case, would have to be tied to the view that forced aiding tends to produce fraternal feelings between the aided and the aider (or perhaps merely to the view that the knowledge that someone or other voluntarily is not aiding produces unfraternal feelings).

NOTES

1. Applications of the principle of justice in acquisition may also occur as part of the move from one distribution to another. You may find an unheld thing now and appropriate it. Acquisitions also are to be understood as included when, to simplify, I speak only of transitions by transfers.

2. If the principle of rectification of violations of the first two principles yields more than one description of holdings, then some choice must be made as to which of these is to be realized. Perhaps the sort of considerations about distributive justice and equality that I argue against play a legitimate role in *this* subsidiary choice. Similarly, there may be room for such considerations in deciding which otherwise arbitrary features a statute will embody, when such features are unavoidable because other considerations do not specify a precise line; yet a line must be drawn.

3. One might try to squeeze a patterned conception of distributive justice into the framework of the entitlement conception, by formulating a gimmicky obligatory "principle of transfer" that would lead to the pattern. For example, the principle that if one has more than the mean income one must transfer everything one holds above the mean to persons below the mean so as to bring them up to (but not over) the mean. We can formulate a criterion for a "principle of transfer" to rule out such obligatory transfers, or we can say that no correct principle of transfer, no principle of transfer in a free society will be like this. The former is probably the better course, though the latter also is true.

Alternatively, one might think to make the entitlement conception instantiate a pattern, by using matrix entries that express the relative strength of a person's entitlements as measured by some real-valued function. But even if the limitation to natural dimensions failed to exclude this function, the resulting edifice would *not* capture our system of entitlements to *particular* things.

4. Might not a transfer have instrumental effects on a third party, changing his feasible options? (But what if the two parties to the transfer independently had used their holdings in this fashion?) I discuss this question below, but note here that this question concedes the point for distributions of ultimate intrinsic noninstrumental goods (pure utility experiences, so to speak) that are transferable. It also might be objected that the transfer might make a third party more envious because it worsens his position relative to someone else. I find it incomprehensible how this can be thought to involve a claim of justice. * * *

Here and elsewhere in this chapter, a theory which incorporates elements of pure procedural justice might find what I say acceptable, *if* kept in its proper place; that is, if background institutions exist to ensure the satisfaction of certain conditions on distributive shares. But if these institutions are not themselves the sum or invisible-hand result of people's voluntary (nonaggressive) actions, the constraints they impose require justification. At no point does *our* argument assume any background institutions more extensive than those of the minimal night-watchman state, a state limited to protecting persons against murder, assault, theft, fraud, and so forth.

5. One indication of the stringency of Rawls' difference principle, which we attend to in the second part of this chapter, is its inappropriateness as a governing principle even within a family of individuals who love one another. Should a family devote its resources to maximizing the position of its least well off and least talented child, holding back the other children or using resources for their education and development only if they will follow a policy through their lifetimes of maximizing the position of their least fortunate sibling? Surely not. How then can this even be considered as the appropriate policy for enforcement in the wider society? (I discuss below what I think would be Rawls' reply: that some principles apply at the macro level which do not apply to micro-situations.)

6. I am unsure as to whether the arguments I present below show that such taxation merely *is* forced labor; so that "is on a par with" means "is one kind of." Or alternatively, whether the arguments emphasize the great similarities between such taxation and forced labor, to show it is plausible and illuminating to view such taxation in the light of forced labor. This latter approach would remind one of how John Wisdom conceives of the claims of metaphysicians.

7. Nothing hangs on the fact that here and elsewhere I speak loosely of *needs*, since I go on, each time, to reject the criterion of justice which includes it. If, however, something did depend upon the notion, one would want to examine it more carefully. For a skeptical view, see Kenneth Minogue, *The Liberal Mind* (New York: Random House, 1963), pp. 103–112.

Famine, Affluence, and Morality

PETER SINGER

As I write this, in November 1971, people are dying in East Bengal from lack of food, shelter, and medical care. The suffering and death that are occurring there now are not inevitable, not unavoidable in any fatalistic sense of the term. Constant poverty, a cyclone, and a civil war have turned at least nine million people into destitute refugees; nevertheless, it is not beyond the capacity of the richer nations to give enough assistance to reduce any further suffering to very small proportions. The decisions and actions of human beings can prevent this kind of suffering. Unfortunately, human beings have not made the necessary decisions. At the individual level, people have, with very few exceptions, not responded to the situation in any significant way. Generally speaking, people have not given large sums to relief funds; they have not written to their parliamentary representatives demanding increased government assistance; they have not demonstrated in the streets, held symbolic fasts, or done anything else directed toward providing the refugees with the means to satisfy their essential needs. At the government level, no government has given the sort of massive aid that would enable the refugees to survive for more than a few days. Britain, for instance, has given rather more than most countries. It has, to date, given £14,750,000. For comparative purposes, Britain's share of the nonrecoverable development costs of the Anglo-French Concorde project is already in excess of £275,000,000, and on present estimates will reach £440,000,000. The implication is that the British government values a supersonic transport more than thirty times as highly as it values the lives of the nine million refugees. Australia is another country which, on a per capita basis, is well up in the "aid to Bengal" table. Australia's aid, however, amounts to less than one-twelfth of the cost of Sydney's new opera house. The total amount given, from all sources, now stands are about £65,000,000. The estimated cost of keeping the refugees alive for one year is £464,000,000. Most of the refugees have now been in the camps for more than six months. The World Bank has said that India needs a minimum of £300,000,000 in assistance from other countries before the end of the year. It seems obvious that assistance on this scale will not be forthcoming. India will be forced to choose between letting the refugees starve or diverting funds from her own development program, which will mean that more of her own people will starve in the future.[1]

These are the essential facts about the present situation in Bengal. So far as it concerns us here, there is nothing unique about this situation except its magnitude. The Bengal emergency is just the latest and most acute of a series of major emergencies in various parts of the world, arising both from natural and from man-made causes. There are also many parts of the world in which people die from malnutrition and lack of food independent of any special emergency. I take Bengal as my example only because it is the present concern, and because the size of the problem has ensured that it has been given adequate publicity. Neither individuals nor governments can claim to be unaware of what is happening there.

What are the moral implications of a situation like this? In what follows, I shall argue that the way people in relatively affluent countries react to a situation like that in Bengal cannot be justified; indeed, the whole way we look at moral issues—our moral conceptual scheme—needs to be altered, and with it, the way of life that has come to be taken for granted in our society.

In arguing for this conclusion I will not, of course, claim to be morally neutral. I shall, however, try to argue for the moral position that I take, so that anyone who accepts certain assumptions, to be made explicit, will, I hope, accept my conclusion.

I begin with the assumption that suffering and death from lack of food, shelter, and medical care are bad. I think most people will agree about this, although one may reach the same view by different routes. I shall not argue for this view. People can hold all sorts of eccentric positions, and perhaps from some of them it would not follow that death by starvation is in itself bad. It is difficult, perhaps impossible, to refute such positions, and so for brevity I will henceforth take this assumption as accepted. Those who disagree need read no further.

My next point is this: if it is in our power to prevent something bad from happening, without thereby sacrificing anything of comparable moral importance, we ought, morally, to do it. By "without sacrificing anything of comparable moral importance" I mean without causing anything else comparably bad to happen, or doing something that is wrong in itself, or failing to promote some moral good, comparable in significance to the bad thing that we can prevent. This principle seems almost as uncontroversial as the last one. It requires us only to prevent what is bad, and not to promote what is good, and it requires this of us only when we can do it without sacrificing anything that is, from the moral point of view, comparably important. I could even, as far as the application of my argument to the Bengal emergency is concerned, qualify the point so as to make it: if it is in our power to prevent something very bad from happening, without thereby sacrificing anything morally significant, we ought, morally, to do it. An application of this principle would be as follows: if I am walking past a shallow pond and see a child drowning in it, I ought to wade in and pull the child out. This will mean getting my clothes muddy, but this is insignificant, while the death of the child would presumably be a very bad thing.

The uncontroversial appearance of the principle just stated is deceptive. If it were acted upon, even in its qualified form, our lives, our society, and our world would be fundamentally changed. For the principle takes, firstly, no account of proximity or distance. It makes no moral difference whether the person I can help is a neighbor's child ten yards from me or a Bengali whose name I shall never know, ten thousand miles away. Secondly, the principle makes no distinction between cases in which I am the only person who could possibly do anything and cases in which I am just one among millions in the same position.

I do not think I need to say much in defense of the refusal to take proximity and distance into account. The fact that a person is physically near to us, so that we have personal contact with him, may make it more likely that we *shall* assist him, but this does not show that we *ought* to help him rather than another who happens to be further away. If we accept any principle of impartiality, universalizability, equality, or whatever, we cannot discriminate against someone merely because he is far away from us (or we are far away from him). Admittedly, it is possible that we are in a better position to judge what needs to be done to help a person near to us than one far away, and perhaps also to provide the assistance we judge to be necessary. If this were the case, it would be a reason for helping those near to us first. This may once have been a justification for being more concerned with the poor in one's own town than with famine victims in India. Unfortunately for those who like to keep their moral responsibilities limited, instant communication and swift transportation have changed the situation. From the moral point of view, the development of the world into a "global village" has made an important, though still unrecognized, difference to our moral situation. Expert observers and supervisors, sent out by famine relief organizations or permanently stationed in famine-prone areas, can direct our aid to a refugee in Bengal almost as effectively as we could get it to someone in our own block. There would seem, therefore, to be no possible justification for discriminating on geographical grounds.

There may be a greater need to defend the second implication of my principle—that the fact that there are millions of other people in the same position, in respect to the Bengali refugees, as I am, does not make the situation significantly different from a situation in which I am the only person who can prevent something very bad from occurring. Again, of course, I admit that there is a psychological difference between the cases; one feels less guilty about doing nothing if one can point to others, similarly placed, who have also done nothing. Yet this can make no real difference to our moral obligations.[2] Should I consider that I am less obliged to pull the drowning child out of the pond if on looking around I see other people, no further away than I am, who have also noticed the child but are doing nothing? One has only to ask this question to see the absurdity of the view that numbers lessen obligation. It is a view that is an ideal excuse for inactivity; unfortunately most of the major evils—poverty, overpopulation, pollution—are problems in which everyone is almost equally involved.

The view that numbers do make a difference can be made plausible if stated in this way: if everyone in circumstances like mine gave £5 to the Bengal Relief Fund, there would be enough to provide food, shelter, and medical care for the refugees; there is no reason why I should give more than anyone else in the same circumstances as I am; therefore I have no obligation to give more than £5. Each premise in this argument is true, and the argument looks sound. It may convince us, unless we notice that it is based on a hypothetical premise, although the conclusion is not stated hypothetically. The argument would be sound if the conclusion were: if everyone in circumstances like mine were to give £5, I would have no obligation to give more than £5. If the conclusion were so stated, however, it would be obvious that the argument has no bearing on a situation in which it is not the case that everyone else gives £5. This, of course, is the actual situation. It is more or less certain that not everyone in circumstances like mine will give £5. So there will not be enough to provide the needed food, shelter, and medical care. Therefore by giving more than £5 I will prevent more suffering than I would if I gave just £5.

It might be thought that this argument has an absurd consequence. Since the situation appears to be that very few people are likely to give substantial amounts, it follows that I and everyone else in similar circumstances ought to give as much as possible, that is, at least up to the point at which by giving more one would begin to cause serious suffering for oneself and one's dependents—perhaps even beyond this point to the point of marginal utility, at which by giving more one would cause oneself and one's dependents as much suffering as one would prevent in Bengal. If everyone does this, however, there will be more than can be used for the benefit of the refugees, and some of the sacrifice will have been unnecessary. Thus, if everyone does what he ought to do, the result will not be as good as it would be if everyone did a little less than he ought to do, or if only some do all that they ought to do.

The paradox here arises only if we assume that the actions in question—sending money to the relief funds—are performed more or less simultaneously, and are also unexpected. For if it is to be expected that everyone is going to contribute something, then clearly each is not obliged to give as much as he would have been obliged to had others not been giving too. And if everyone is not acting more or less simultaneously, then those giving later will know how much more is needed, and will have no obligation to give more than is necessary to reach this amount. To say this is not to deny the principle that people in the same circumstances have the same obligations, but to point out that the fact that others have given, or may be expected to give, is a relevant circumstance: those giving after it has become known that many others are giving and those giving before are not in the same circumstances. So the seemingly absurd consequence of the principle I have put forward can occur only if people are in error about the actual circumstances—that is, if they think they are giving when others are not, but in fact they are giving when others are. The result of everyone doing what he really ought to do cannot be worse than the result of everyone doing less than he ought to do, although the result of everyone doing what he reasonably believes he ought to do could be.

If my argument so far has been sound, neither our distance from a preventable evil nor the number of other people who, in respect to that evil, are in the same situation as we are, lessens our obligation to mitigate or prevent that evil. I shall therefore take as established the principle I asserted earlier. As I have already said, I need to assert it only in its qualified form: if it is in our power to prevent something very bad from happening, without thereby sacrificing anything else morally significant, we ought, morally, to do it.

The outcome of this argument is that our traditional moral categories are upset. The traditional distinction between duty and charity cannot be drawn, or at least, not in the place we normally draw it. Giving money to the Bengal Relief Fund is regarded as an act of charity in our society. The bodies which collect money are known as "charities." These organizations see themselves in this way—if you send them a check, you will be thanked for your "generosity." Because giving money is regarded as an act of charity, it is not thought that there is anything wrong with not giving. The charitable man may be praised, but the man who is not charitable is not condemned. People do not feel in any way ashamed or guilty about spending money on new clothes or a new car instead of giving it to famine relief. (Indeed, the alternative does not occur to them.) This way of looking at the matter cannot be justified. When we buy new clothes not to keep ourselves warm but to look "well-dressed" we are not providing for any important need. We would not be sacrificing anything significant if we were to continue to wear our old clothes, and give the money to famine relief. By doing so, we would be preventing another person from starving. It follows from what I have said earlier that we ought to give money away, rather than spend it on clothes which we do not need to keep us warm. To do so is not charitable, or generous. Nor is it the kind of act which philosophers and theologians have called "supererogatory"—an act which it would be good to do, but not wrong not to do. On the contrary, we ought to give the money away, and it is wrong not to do so.

I am not maintaining that there are no acts which are charitable, or that there are no acts which it would be good to do but not wrong not to do. It may be possible to redraw the distinction between duty and charity in some other place. All I am arguing here is that the present way of drawing the distinction, which makes it an act of charity for a man living at the level of affluence which most people in the "developed nations" enjoy to give money to save someone else from starvation, cannot be supported. It is beyond the scope of my argument to consider whether the distinction should be redrawn or abolished altogether. There would be many other possible ways of drawing the distinction—for instance, one might decide that it is good to make other people as happy as possible, but not wrong not to do so.

Despite the limited nature of the revision in our moral conceptual scheme which I am proposing, the revision would, given the extent of both affluence and famine in the world today, have radical implications. These implications may lead to further objections, distinct from those I have already considered. I shall discuss two of these.

One objection to the position I have taken might be simply that it is too drastic a revision of our moral scheme. People do not ordinarily judge in the way I have suggested they should. Most people reserve their moral condemnation for those who violate some moral norm, such as the norm against taking another person's property. They do not condemn those who indulge in luxury instead of giving to famine relief. But given that I did not set out to present a morally neutral description of the way people make moral judgments, the way people do in fact judge has nothing to do with the validity of my conclusion. My conclusion follows from the principle which I advanced earlier, and unless that principle is rejected, or the arguments shown to be unsound, I think the conclusion must stand, however strange it appears.

* * *

The second objection to my attack on the present distinction between duty and charity is one which has from time to time been made against utilitarianism. It follows from some forms of utilitarian theory that we all ought, morally, to be working full time to increase the balance of happiness over misery. The position I have taken here would not lead to this conclusion in all circumstances, for if there were no bad occurrences that we could prevent without sacrificing something of comparable moral importance, my argument would have no application. Given the present conditions in many parts of the world, however, it does follow from my argument that we ought, morally, to be working full time to relieve great suffering of the sort that occurs as a result of famine or other disasters. Of course, mitigating circumstances can be adduced—for instance, that if we wear ourselves out through overwork, we shall be less effective than we would otherwise have been. Nevertheless, when all considerations of this sort have been taken into account, the conclusion remains: we ought to be preventing as much suffering as we can without sacrificing something else of comparable moral importance. This conclusion is one which we may be reluctant to face. I cannot see, though, why it should be regarded as a criticism of the position for which I have argued, rather than a criticism of our ordinary standards of behavior. Since most people are self-interested to some degree, very few of us are likely to do everything that we ought to do. It would, however, hardly be honest to take this as evidence that it is not the case that we ought to do it.

* * *

[Another] point raised by the conclusion reached earlier relates to the question of just how much we all ought to be giving away. One possibility, which has already been mentioned, is that we ought to give until we reach the level of marginal utility—that is, the level at which, by giving more, I would cause as much suffering to myself or my dependents as I would relieve by my gift. This would mean, of course, that one would reduce oneself to very near the material circumstances of a Bengali refugee. It will be recalled that earlier I put forward both a strong and a moderate version of the principle of preventing bad occurrences. The strong version, which required us to prevent bad things from happening unless in doing so we would be sacrificing something of comparable moral significance, does seem to require reducing ourselves to the level of marginal utility. I should also say that the strong version seems to me to be the correct one. I proposed the more moderate version—that we should prevent bad occurrences unless, to do so, we had to sacrifice something morally significant—only in order to show that even on this surely undeniable principle a great change in our way of life is required. On the more moderate principle, it may not follow that we ought to reduce ourselves to the level of marginal utility, for one might hold that to reduce

oneself and one's family to this level is to cause something significantly bad to happen. Whether this is so I shall not discuss, since, as I have said, I can see no good reason for holding the moderate version of the principle rather than the strong version. Even if we accepted the principle only in its moderate form, however, it should be clear that we would have to give away enough to ensure that the consumer society, dependent as it is on people spending on trivia rather than giving to famine relief, would slow down and perhaps disappear entirely. There are several reasons why this would be desirable in itself. The value and necessity of economic growth are now being questioned not only by conservationists, but by economists as well. There is no doubt, too, that the consumer society has had a distorting effect on the goals and purposes of its members. Yet looking at the matter purely from the point of view of overseas aid, there must be a limit to the extent to which we should deliberately slow down our economy; for it might be the case that if we gave away, say, forty percent of our Gross National Product, we would slow down the economy so much that in absolute terms we would be giving less than if we gave twenty-five percent of the much larger GNP that we would have if we limited our contribution to this smaller percentage.

I mention this only as an indication of the sort of factor that one would have to take into account in working out an ideal. Since Western societies generally consider one percent of the GNP an acceptable level for overseas aid, the matter is entirely academic. Nor does it effect the question of how much an individual should give in a society in which very few are giving substantial amounts.

It is sometimes said, though less often now than it used to be, that philosophers have no special role to play in public affairs, since most public issues depend primarily on an assessment of facts. On questions of fact, it is said, philosophers as such have no special expertise, and so it has been possible to engage in philosophy without committing oneself to any position on major public issues. No doubt there are some issues of social policy and foreign policy about which it can truly be said that a really expert assessment of the facts is required before taking sides or acting, but the issue of famine is surely not one of these. The facts about the existence of suffering are beyond dispute. Nor, I think, is it disputed that we can do something about it, either through orthodox methods of famine relief or through population control or both. This is therefore an issue on which philosophers are competent to take a position. The issue is one which faces everyone who has more money than he needs to support himself and his dependents, or who is in a position to take some sort of political action. These categories must include practically every teacher and student of philosophy in the universities of the Western world. If philosophy is to deal with matters that are relevant to both teachers and students, this is an issue that philosophers should discuss.

Discussion, though, is not enough. What is the point of relating philosophy to public (and personal) affairs if we do not take our conclusions seriously? In this instance, taking our conclusion seriously means acting upon it. The philosopher will not find it any easier than anyone else to alter his attitudes and way of life to the extent that, if I am right, is involved in doing everything that we ought to be doing. At the very least, though, one can make a start. The philosopher who does so will have to sacrifice some of the benefits of the consumer society, but he can find compensation in the satisfaction of a way of life in which theory and practice, if not yet in harmony, are at least coming together.

NOTES

1. There was also a third possibility: that India would go to war to enable the refugees to return to their lands. Since I wrote this paper, India has taken this way out. The situation is no longer that described above, but this does not affect my argument, as the next paragraph indicates.

2. In view of the special sense philosophers often give to the term, I should say that I use "obligation" simply as the abstract noun derived from "ought," so that "I have an obligation to" means no more, and no less, than "I ought to." This usage is in accordance with the definition of "ought" given up by the *Shorter Oxford English Dictionary*: "the general verb to express duty or obligation." I do not think any issue of substance hangs on the way the term is used; sentences in which I use "obligation" could all be rewritten, although somewhat clumsily, as sentences in which a clause containing "ought" replaces the term "obligation."

Lifeboat Ethics

GARRETT HARDIN

* * *

Before taking up certain substantive issues let us look at an alternative metaphor, that of a lifeboat. In developing some relevant examples the following numerical values are assumed. Approximately two-thirds of the world is desperately poor, and only one-third is comparatively rich. The people in poor countries have an average per capita GNP (Gross National Prod-

uct) of about $200 per year; the rich, of about $3,000. (For the United States it is nearly $5,000 per year.) Metaphorically, each rich nation amounts to a lifeboat full of comparatively rich people. The poor of the world are in other, much more crowded lifeboats. Continuously, so to speak, the poor fall out of their lifeboats and swim for a while in the water outside, hoping to be admitted to a rich lifeboat, or in some other way to benefit from the "goodies" on board. What should the passengers on a rich lifeboat do? This is the central problem of "the ethics of a lifeboat."

First we must acknowledge that each lifeboat is effectively limited in capacity. The land of every nation has a limited carrying capacity. The exact limit is a matter for argument, but the energy crunch is convincing more people every day that we have already exceeded the carrying capacity of the land. We have been living on "capital"—stored petroleum and coal—and soon we must live on income alone.

Let us look at only one lifeboat—ours. The ethical problem is the same for all, and is as follows. Here we sit, say 50 people in a lifeboat. To be generous, let us assume our boat has a capacity of 10 more, making 60. (This, however, is to violate the engineering principle of the "safety factor." A new plant disease or a bad change in the weather may decimate our population if we don't preserve some excess capacity as a safety factor.)

The 50 of us in the lifeboat see 100 others swimming in the water outside, asking for admission to the boat, or for handouts. How shall we respond to their calls? There are several possibilities.

One. We may be tempted to try to live by the Christian ideal of being "our brother's keeper," or by the Marxian ideal (Marx 1875) of "from each according to his abilities, to each according to his needs." Since the needs of all are the same, we take all the needy into our boat, making a total of 150 in a boat with a capacity of 60. The boat is swamped, and everyone drowns. Complete justice, complete catastrophe.

Two. Since the boat has an unused excess capacity of 10, we admit just 10 more to it. This has the disadvantage of getting rid of the safety factor, for which action we will sooner or later pay dearly. Moreover, *which* 10 do we let in? "First come, first served?" The best 10? The neediest 10? How do we *discriminate?* And what do we say to the 90 who are excluded?

Three. Admit no more to the boat and preserve the small safety factor. Survival of the people in the lifeboat is then possible (though we shall have to be on our guard against boarding parties).

The last solution is abhorrent to many people. It is unjust, they say. Let us grant that it is.

"I feel guilty about my good luck," say some. The reply to this is simple: *Get out and yield your place to others.* Such a selfless action might satisfy the conscience of those who are addicted to guilt but it would not change the ethics of the lifeboat. The needy person to whom a guilt-addict yields his place will not himself feel guilty about his sudden good luck. (If he did he would not climb aboard.) The net result of conscience-stricken people relinquishing their unjustly held positions is the elimination of their kind of conscience from the lifeboat. The lifeboat, as it were, purifies itself of guilt. The ethics of the lifeboat persist, unchanged by such momentary aberrations.

This then is the basic metaphor within which we must work out our solutions. Let us enrich the image step by step with substantive additions from the real world.

REPRODUCTION

The harsh characteristics of lifeboat ethics are heightened by reproduction, particularly by reproductive differences. The people inside the lifeboats of the wealthy nations are doubling in numbers every 87 years; those outside are doubling every 35 years, on the average. And the relative difference in prosperity is becoming greater.

Let us, for a while, think primarily of the U.S. lifeboat. As of 1973 the United States had a population of 210 million people, who were increasing by 0.8% per year, that is, doubling in number every 87 years.

Although the citizens of rich nations are outnumbered two to one by the poor, let us imagine an equal number of poor people outside our lifeboat—a mere 210 million poor people reproducing at a quite different rate. If we imagine these to be the combined populations of Colombia, Venezuela, Ecuador, Morocco, Thailand, Pakistan, and the Philippines, the average rate of increase of the people "outside" is 3.3% per year. The doubling time of this population is 21 years.

Suppose that all these countries, and the United States, agreed to live by the Marxian ideal, "to each according to his needs," the ideal of most Christians as well. Needs, of course, are determined by population size, which is affected by reproduction. Every nation regards its rate of reproduction as a sovereign right. If our lifeboat were big enough in the beginning it might be possible to live *for a while* by Christian-Marxian ideals. *Might.*

Initially, in the model given, the ratio of non-Americans to Americans would be one to one. But consider what the ratio would be 87 years later. By this time Americans would have doubled to a population of 420 million. The other group (doubling every 21 years) would now have swollen to 3,540 million. Each American would have more than eight people to share with. How could the lifeboat possibly keep afloat?

All this involves extrapolation of current trends into the future, and is consequently suspect. Trends may change. Granted: but the change will not necessarily be favorable. If—as seems likely—the rate of population increase falls faster in the ethnic group presently inside the lifeboat than it does among those now outside, the future will turn out to be even worse than mathematics predicts, and sharing will be even more suicidal.

RUIN IN THE COMMONS

The fundamental error of the sharing ethics is that it leads to the tragedy of the commons. Under a system of private property the man (or group of men) who own property recognize their responsibility to care for it, for if they don't they will eventually suffer. A farmer, for instance, if he is intelligent, will allow no more cattle in a pasture than its carrying capacity justifies. If he overloads the pasture, weeds take over, erosion sets in, and the owner loses in the long run.

But if a pasture is run as a commons open to all, the right of each to use it is not matched by an operational responsibility to take care of it. It is no use asking independent herdsmen in a commons to act responsibly, for they dare not. The considerate herdsman who refrains from overloading the commons suffers more than a selfish one who says his needs are greater. (As Leo Durocher says, "Nice guys finish last.") Christian-Marxian idealism is counterproductive. That it *sounds* nice is no excuse. With distribution systems, as with individual morality, good intentions are no substitute for good performance.

A social system is stable only if it is insensitive to errors. To the Christian-Marxian idealist a selfish person is a sort of "error." Prosperity in the system of the commons cannot survive errors. If *everyone* would

only restrain himself, all would be well; but it takes *only one less than everyone* to ruin a system of voluntary restraint. In a crowded world of less than perfect human beings—and we will never know any other—mutual ruin is inevitable in the commons. This is the core of the tragedy of the commons.

One of the major tasks of education today is to create such an awareness of the dangers of the commons that people will be able to recognize its many varieties, however disguised. There is pollution of the air and water because these media are treated as commons. Further growth of population and growth in the per capita conversion of natural resources into pollutants require that the system of the commons be modified or abandoned in the disposal of "externalities."

The fish populations of the oceans are exploited as commons, and ruin lies ahead. No technological invention can prevent this fate: in fact, all improvements in the art of fishing merely hasten the day of complete ruin. Only the replacement of the system of the commons with a responsible system can save oceanic fisheries.

The management of western range lands, though nominally rational, is in fact (under the steady pressure of cattle ranchers) often merely a government-sanctioned system of the commons, drifting toward ultimate ruin for both the rangelands and the residual enterprisers.

WORLD FOOD BANKS

In the international arena we have recently heard a proposal to create a new commons, namely an international depository of food reserves to which nations will contribute according to their abilities, and from which nations may draw according to their needs. Nobel laureate Norman Borlaug has lent the prestige of his name to this proposal.

A world food bank appeals powerfully to our humanitarian impulses. We remember John Donne's celebrated line, "Any man's death diminishes me." But before we rush out to see for whom the bell tolls let us recognize where the greatest political push for international granaries comes from, lest we be disillusioned later. Our experience with Public Law 480 clearly reveals the answer. This was the law that moved billions of dollars worth of U.S. grain to food-short, population-long countries during the past two decades. When P.L. 480 first came into being, a headline in the business magazine *Forbes* (Paddock and Paddock 1970) revealed the power behind it: "Feeding the World's Hungry Millions: How it will mean billions for U.S. business."

And indeed it did. In the years 1960 to 1970 a total of $7.9 billion was spent on the "Food for Peace" program, as P.L. 480 was called. During the years 1948 to 1970 an additional $49.9 billion were extracted from American taxpayers to pay for other economic aid programs, some of which went for food and food-producing machinery. (This figure does *not* include military aid.) That P.L. 480 was a give-away program was concealed. Recipient countries went through the motions of paying for P.L. 480 foods—with IOU's. In December 1973 the charade was brought to an end as far as India was concerned when the United States "forgave" India's $3.2 billion debt (Anonymous 1974). Public announcement of the cancellation of the debt was delayed for two months: one wonders why.

"Famine—[1975]!" (Paddock and Paddock 1970) is one of the few publications that points out the commercial roots of this humanitarian attempt. Though all U.S. taxpayers lost by P.L. 480, special interest groups gained handsomely. Farmers benefited because they were not asked to contribute the grain— it was bought from them by the taxpayers. Besides the direct benefit there was the indirect effect of increasing demand and thus raising prices of farm products generally. The manufacturers of farm machinery, fertilizers, and pesticides benefited by the farmers' extra efforts to grow more food. Grain elevators profited from storing the grain for varying lengths of time. Railroads made money hauling it to port, and shipping lines by carrying it overseas. Moreover, once the machinery for P.L. 480 was established an immense bureaucracy had a vested interest in its continuance regardless of its merits.

Very little was ever heard of these selfish interests when P.L. 480 was defended in public. The emphasis was always on its humanitarian effects. The combination of multiple and relatively silent selfish interests

with highly vocal humanitarian apologists constitutes a powerful lobby for extracting money from taxpayers. Foreign aid has become a habit that can apparently survive in the absence of any known justification. A news commentator in a weekly magazine (Lansner 1974), after exhaustively going over all the conventional arguments for foreign aid—self-interest, social justice, political advantage, and charity—and concluding that none of the known arguments really held water, concluded: "So the search continues for some logically compelling reasons for giving aid . . ." In other words. *Act now, Justify later*—if ever. (Apparently a quarter of a century is too short a time to find the justification for expending several billion dollars yearly.)

The search for a rational justification can be short-circuited by interjecting the word "emergency." Borlaug uses this word. We need to look sharply at it. What is an "emergency"? It is surely something like an accident, which is correctly defined as *an event that is certain to happen, though with a low frequency* (Hardin 1972a). A well-run organization prepares for everything that is certain, including accidents and emergencies. It budgets for them. It saves for them. It expects them—and mature decision-makers do not waste time complaining about accidents when they occur.

What happens if some organizations budget for emergencies and others do not? If each organization is solely responsible for its own well-being, poorly managed ones will suffer. But they should be able to learn from experience. They have a chance to mend their ways and learn to budget for infrequent but certain emergencies. The weather, for instance, always varies and periodic crop failures are certain. A wise and competent government saves out of the production of the good years in anticipation of bad years that are sure to come. This is not a new idea. The Bible tells us that Joseph taught this policy to Pharaoh in Egypt more than 2,000 years ago. Yet it is literally true that the vast majority of the governments of the world today have no such policy. They lack either the wisdom or the competence, or both. Far more difficult than the transfer of wealth from one country to another is the transfer of wisdom between sovereign powers or between generations.

"But it isn't their fault! How can we blame the poor people who are caught in an emergency? Why must we punish them?" The concepts of blame and punishment are irrelevant. The question is, what are the operational consequences of establishing a world food bank? If it is open to every country every time a need develops, slovenly rule will not be motivated to take Joseph's advice. Why should they? Others will bail them out whenever they are in trouble.

Some countries will make deposits in the world food bank and others will withdraw from it: there will be almost no overlap. Calling such a depository-transfer unit a "bank" is stretching the metaphor of *bank* beyond its elastic limits. The proposers, of course, never call attention to the metaphorical nature of the word they use.

THE RATCHET EFFECT

An "international food bank" is really, then, not a true bank but a disguised one-way transfer device for moving wealth from rich countries to poor. In the absence of such a bank, in a world inhabited by individually responsible sovereign nations, the population of each nation would repeatedly go through a cycle of the sort shown in Figure 1. P_2 is greater than P_1, either in absolute numbers or because a deterioration of the food supply has removed the safety factor and produced a dangerously low ratio of resources to population. P_2 may be said to represent a state of overpopulation, which becomes obvious upon the appearance of an "accident," e.g., a crop failure. If the

"emergency" is not met by outside help, the population drops back to the "normal" level—the "carrying capacity" of the environment—or even below. In the absence of population control by a sovereign, sooner or later the population grows to P_2 again and the cycle repeats. The long-term population curve (Hardin 1966) is an irregularly fluctuating one, equilibrating more or less about the carrying capacity.

A demographic cycle of this sort obviously involves great suffering in the restrictive phase, but such a cycle is normal to any independent country with inadequate population control. The third-century theologian Tertullian (Hardin 1969a) expressed what must have been the recognition of many wise men when he wrote: "The scourges of pestilence, famine, wars, and earthquakes have come to be regarded as a blessing to overcrowded nations, since they serve to prune away the luxuriant growth of the human race."

Only under a strong and farsighted sovereign—which theoretically could be the people themselves, democratically organized—can a population equilibrate at some set point below the carrying capacity, thus avoiding the pains normally caused by periodic and unavoidable disasters. For this happy state to be achieved it is necessary that those in power be able to contemplate with equanimity the "waste" of surplus food in times of bountiful harvests. It is essential that those in power resist the temptation to convert extra food into extra babies. On the public relations level it is necessary that the phrase "surplus food" be replaced by "safety factor."

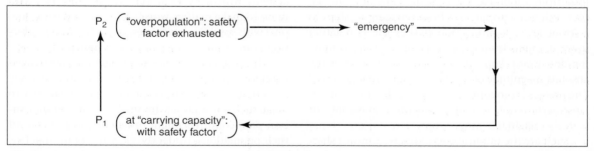

Fig. 1. The population cycle of a nation that has no effective, conscious population control, and which receives no aid from the outside. P_2 is greater than P_1.

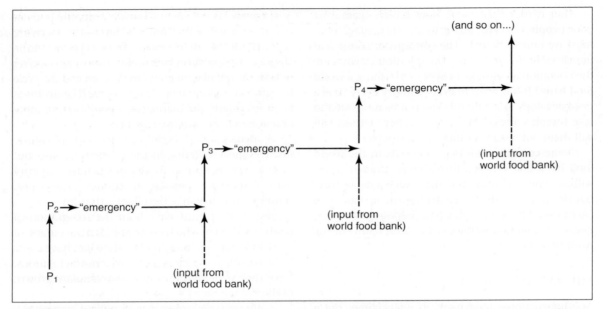

Fig. 2. The population escalator. Note that input from a world food bank acts like the pawl of a ratchet, preventing the normal population cycle shown in Figure 1 from being completed. $P_{II} + I$ is greater than P_{II}, and the absolute magnitude of the "emergencies" escalates. Ultimately the entire system crashes. The crash is not shown, and few can imagine it.

But wise sovereigns seem not to exist in the poor world today. The most anguishing problems are created by poor countries that are governed by rulers insufficiently wise and powerful. If such countries can draw on a world food bank in times of "emergency," the population *cycle* of Figure 1 will be replaced by the population *escalator* of Figure 2. The input of food from a food bank acts as the pawl of a ratchet, preventing the population from retracing its steps to a lower level. Reproduction pushes the population upward, inputs from the world bank prevent its moving downward. Population size escalates, as does the absolute magnitude of "accidents" and "emergencies." The process is brought to an end only by the total collapse of the whole system, producing a catastrophe of scarcely imaginable proportions.

Such are the implications of the well-meant sharing of food in a world of irresponsible reproduction.

I think we need a new word for systems like this. The adjective "melioristic" is applied to systems that produce continual improvement; the English word is derived from the Latin *meliorare*, to become or make better. Parallel with this it would be useful to bring in the word *pejoristic* (from the Latin *pejorare*, to become or make worse). This word can be applied to those systems which, by their very nature, can be relied upon to make matters worse. A world food bank coupled with sovereign state irresponsibility in reproduction is an example of a pejoristic system.

This pejoristic system creates an unacknowledged commons. People have more motivation to draw from than to add to the common store. The license to make such withdrawals diminishes whatever motivation poor countries might otherwise have to control their populations. Under the guidance of this ratchet, wealth can be steadily moved in one direction only, from the slowly-breeding rich to the rapidly-breeding poor, the process finally coming to a halt only when all countries are equally and miserably poor.

All this is terribly obvious once we are acutely aware of the pervasiveness and danger of the commons. But many people still lack this awareness and the euphoria of the "benign demographic transition" (Hardin 1973) interferes with the realistic appraisal of pejoristic mechanisms. As concerns public policy, the deductions drawn from the benign demographic transition are these:

1) If the per capita GNP rises the birth rate will fall; hence, the rate of population increase will fall, ultimately producing ZPG (Zero Population Growth).

2) The long-term trend all over the world (including the poor countries) is of a rising per capita GNP (for which no limit is seen).

3) Therefore, all political interference in population matters is unnecessary; all we need to do is foster economic "development"—*note the metaphor*—and population problems will solve themselves.

Those who believe in the benign demographic transition dismiss the pejoristic mechanism of Figure 2 in the belief that each input of food from the world outside fosters development within a poor country thus resulting in a drop in the rate of population increase. Foreign aid has proceeded on this assumption for more than two decades. Unfortunately it has produced no indubitable instance of the asserted effect. It has, however, produced a library of excuses. The air is filled with plaintive calls for more massive foreign aid appropriations so that the hypothetical melioristic process can get started.

* * *

REFERENCES

Anonymous. 1974. *Wall Street Journal* 19 Feb.

Borlaug, N. 1973. Civilization's future: a call for international granaries. *Bull. At. Sci.* 29: 7–15.

Boulding, K. 1966. The economics of the coming Spaceship earth. *In* H. Jarrett, ed. Environmental Quality in a Growing Economy. Johns Hopkins Press, Baltimore.

Buchanan, W. 1973. Immigration statistics. *Equilibrium* 1(3): 16–19.

Davis, K. 1963. Population. *Sci. Amer.* 209(3): 62–71.

Farvar, M. T., and J. P. Milton. 1972. The Careless Technology. Natural History Press, Garden City, N.Y.

Gregg, A. 1955. A medical aspect of the population problem. *Science* 121: 681–682.

Hardin, G. 1966. Chap. 9 *in* Biology: Its Principles and Implications, 2nd ed. Freeman, San Francisco.

———. 1968. The tragedy of the commons. *Science* 162: 1243–1248.

———. 1969a. Page 18 *in* Population, Evolution, and Birth Control, 2nd ed. Freeman, San Francisco.

———. 1969b. The economics of wilderness. *Nat. Hist.* 78(6): 20–27.

———. 1972a. Pages 81–82 *in* Exploring New Ethics for Survival: The Voyage of the Spaceship *Beagle*. Viking, N.Y.

———. 1972b. Preserving quality on Spaceship Earth. *In* J. B. Trefethen, ed. Transactions of the Thirty-Seventh North American Wildlife and Natural Resources Conference. Wildlife Management Institute, Washington, D.C.

———. 1973. Chap. 23 *in* Stalking the Wild Taboo. Kaufmann, Los Altos, Cal.

Harris, M. 1972. How green the revolution. *Nat. Hist.* 81(3): 28–30.

Langer, S. K. 1942. Philosophy in a New Key. Harvard University Press, Cambridge.

Lansner, K. 1974. Should foreign aid begin at home? *Newsweek*, 11 Feb. p. 32.

Marx, K. 1875. Critique of the Gotha program. Page 388 *in* R. C. Tucker, ed. The Marx-Engels Reader. Norton, N.Y., 1972.

Ophuls, W. 1974. The scarcity society. *Harpers* 248(1487): 47–52.

Paddock, W. C. 1970. How green is the green revolution? *BioScience* 20: 897–902.

Paddock, W., and E. Paddock. 1973. We Don't Know How. Iowa State University Press, Ames, Iowa.

Paddock, W., and P. Paddock. 1967. Famine—1975! Little, Brown, Boston.

Wilkes, H. G. 1972. The green revolution. *Environment* 14(8): 32–39.

CASES FOR ANALYSIS

1. Averting Famine

For years the small nation of Malawi in southern Africa remained on the verge of famine with high rates of acute child hunger, begging for emergency food aid from richer countries. But now the tables have turned, and Malawi is growing enough food to feed its people *and* sell much of the surplus to other nations. Rates of child hunger have dropped dramatically.

Why the change? With the soil in Malawi overfarmed and depleted, it was impossible for the country to feed itself. The situation improved only when Malawi began to ignore the advice of the World Bank and rich countries, which advised Malawi to get rid of fertilizer subsidies and to rely on the workings of free markets. After the disastrous harvest of 2005, Malawi reversed the trend and subsidized farmers' use of fertilizer—just as many Western countries do for their own farmers.

Malawi's success has prompted reappraisals of the capacity of agriculture to eliminate poverty and of a government's ability to spur self-sufficiency and growth through investments in agricultural production and know-how.*

If, as this story suggests, the World Bank and rich nations offered bad advice to Malawi, do they bear some responsibility for the subsequent food shortages? Does this story seem to support or undermine Garrett Hardin's views on helping the needy?

*Based on Celia W. Dugger, "Ending Famine, Simply by Ignoring the Experts," *New York Times*, 2 December 2007, http://www.nytimes.com/2007/12/02/world/africa/02malawi.html?scp=1&sq=ending+famine+simply+by+ignoring+the+experts&st=nyt&_r=0 (1 March 2015).

2. Developed Countries Failing the Poor

UNITED NATIONS—In criticism aimed primarily at the United States, Japan and the European Union, a U.N. report said rich donor nations have failed to deliver on promises to help the world's poorest countries and must increase aid by $18 billion a year.

The report released Thursday also criticized the failure of rich and poor nations to reach a trade pact in seven years of negotiations that would expand global trade opportunities for developing countries to reduce poverty. It called for redoubled efforts to conclude negotiations.

The report was issued ahead of a Sept. 25 meeting of world leaders at U.N. headquarters to step up efforts to achieve the Millennium Development Goals, adopted by world leaders at a summit in 2000. The goals include cutting extreme poverty by half, ensuring universal primary school education and starting to reverse the HIV/AIDS pandemic, all by 2015. . . .

U.N. Secretary-General Ban Ki-moon told a press conference that the report "sounds a strong alarm."

"The main message is that while there has been progress on several counts, delivery on commitments made by member states has been deficient, and has fallen behind schedule," he said. "We are already in the second half of our contest against poverty. We are running out of time." . . .

Ban noted that total aid from the world's major donor nations amounts to only 0.25% of their combined national income, far below the U.N. target of 0.7%. The only countries to reach or exceed that target were Denmark, Luxembourg, the Netherlands, Norway and Sweden.[†]

Is the failure of rich nations to aid the world's poorest countries morally wrong? Is the giving of aid a moral obligation for rich nations—or just a supererogatory act? What conclusion do you draw from the United States' failure to contribute its promised share of aid?

[†]Associated Press, "U.N. Report: Developed Countries Failing Poor," published on USAToday.com, September 4, 2008. © The Associated Press. Reprinted by permission.

---

3. Singer or Hardin?

CBC News—The Church World Service aid agency is warning that "immediate, massive intervention and assistance" are needed to prevent mass starvation in Kenya.

A team from the humanitarian agency reported recently that many fields are barren and cracked, dried out by the drought that is threatening a third of the east African country's population, or about 10 million people.

What was once among the most fertile land in Africa can now only support a few struggling plants suitable only for grazing cattle.

"We don't have any food," farmer Lizy Bimba, a Kwale resident, said in Swahili.

In one area, a local official reported that 85 per cent of 5,600 people are facing starvation, the Church World Service team said.

Other farmers have left the land to find what work they can.

"We have been forced to do this so that we get money to buy food," Musa Charo said in Swahili as he broke rocks to earn money to feed his 10 children.

The government declared the food shortage a national disaster on Jan. 16, the UN is appealing for international help and aid agencies warn that the problem will only get worse.[‡]

What would be the proper moral response of rich nations to this impending tragedy? Do you favor Garrett Hardin's approach in which rich countries would not send food aid? Or Peter Singer's path in which affluent individuals would be obligated to give much of their wealth to feed the hungry? Or a middle way in which the rich would have a duty to give some aid but would also have obligations to themselves and to their family and friends? Explain.

[‡]CBC News Staff, "Kenya Facing Mass Starvation: Aid Group." *CBC News*, January 31, 2009. Reprinted by permission of CBC Licensing.

GLOSSARY

abolitionists—Those who wish to abolish capital punishment.

abortion—The deliberate termination of a pregnancy by surgical or medical (with drugs) means.

act-egoism—The theory that to determine right action, you must apply the egoistic principle to individual acts.

active euthanasia—Euthanasia performed by taking a direct action to cause someone's death; "mercy killing."

act-utilitarianism—The theory that right actions are those that directly produce the greatest overall good, everyone considered.

advance directive—A legal document allowing physicians to withhold or withdraw treatments if a patient becomes terminally ill and unable to express his or her wishes.

affirmative action—A way of making amends for, or eradicating, discrimination based on race, ethnicity, and gender.

animal rights—Possession by animals of (1) moral status; (2) strong moral consideration that cannot be easily overridden.

anthropocentrism—The notion that only humans have moral status.

appeal to authority—The fallacy of relying on the opinion of someone thought to be an expert who is not.

appeal to ignorance—The fallacy of arguing that the absence of evidence entitles us to believe a claim.

appeal to the person—The fallacy (also known as *ad hominem*) of arguing that a claim should be rejected solely because of the characteristics of the person who makes it.

applied ethics—The application of moral norms to specific moral issues or cases, particularly those in a profession such as medicine or law.

argument—A group of statements, one of which is supposed to be supported by the rest.

begging the question—The fallacy of arguing in a circle—that is, trying to use a statement as both a premise in an argument and the conclusion of that argument. Such an argument says, in effect, *p* is true because *p* is true.

biocentrism—The view that all living entities have moral status, whether sentient or not.

capital punishment—Punishment by execution of someone officially judged to have committed a serious, or capital, crime.

categorical imperative—An imperative that we should follow regardless of our particular wants and needs; also, the principle that defines Kant's ethical system.

chromosome—One of forty-six molecules containing genes and residing in the cell's nucleus.

cloning—The production of a genetically identical copy of an existing biological entity through an asexual process.

cogent argument—A strong argument with true premises.

conception—The merging of a sperm cell and an ovum into a single cell; also called *fertilization*.

conclusion—The statement supported in an argument.

consequentialist theory—A theory asserting that what makes an action right is its consequences.

conventional view (of sexuality)—The idea that sex is morally acceptable only between a man and woman who are legally married to each other.

criminalization—Making the use (and possession) of drugs a criminal offense.

cultural relativism—The view that an action is morally right if one's culture approves of it.

decriminalization—Allowing people to use drugs without being liable to criminal prosecution and punishment.

deductive argument—An argument that is supposed to give logically conclusive support to its conclusion.

Defense of Marriage Act—A law passed by Congress in 1996 forbidding the federal government to recognize same-sex marriages, effectively denying federal benefits to gay and lesbian marriages.

descriptive ethics—The scientific study of moral beliefs and practices.

direct moral consideration—Moral consideration for a being's own sake, rather than because of its relationship to others.

discrimination—Unfavorable treatment of people on irrelevant grounds.

distributive justice—Justice concerning the fair distribution of society's goods.

divine command theory—A theory asserting that the morally right action is the one that God commands.

doctrine of double effect—The principle that performing a good action may be permissible even if it has bad effects, but performing a bad action for the purpose of achieving good effects is never permissible; any bad effects must be unintended.

drug—A non-food chemical substance that can affect the functions or makeup of the body.

drug addiction—An intense craving for a drug and compulsive, uncontrolled use of the drug despite harm done to the user or other people.

drug dependence—A condition in which discontinuing the use of a drug is extremely difficult, involving psychological or physical symptoms.

duty of beneficence—A moral obligation to benefit others.

ecological holist—One who believes that the fundamental unit of moral consideration in environmental ethics is the biosphere and its ecosystems.

ecological individualist—One who believes that the fundamental unit of moral consideration in environmental ethics is the individual.

egalitarian theory of justice—A doctrine holding that justice requires equal distributions of goods and social benefits among all persons.

emotivism—The view that moral utterances are neither true nor false but are expressions of emotions or attitudes.

equivocation—The fallacy of assigning two different meanings to the same term in an argument.

ethical egoism—The theory that the right action is the one that advances one's own best interests.

ethics (or moral philosophy)—The philosophical study of morality.

ethics of care—A perspective on moral issues that emphasizes close personal relationships and moral virtues such as compassion, love, and sympathy.

eudaimonia—Happiness, or flourishing.

euthanasia—Directly or indirectly bringing about the death of another person for that person's sake.

faulty analogy—The use of a flawed analogy to argue for a conclusion.

gene—A discrete section of genetic code.

gene therapy—An experimental technique for directly changing a person's genes to prevent or treat disease.

genetic engineering—Direct genetic intervention in an organism's genome to enhance traits and capabilities.

genetic enhancement—Genetic intervention to make people better than normal, to maximize human traits and capabilities.

genome—An organism's complete set of DNA.

Golden Mean—Aristotle's notion of a virtue as a balance between two behavioral extremes.

greatest happiness principle—According to Mill, the principle that "holds that actions are right in proportion as they tend to promote happiness, wrong as they tend to produce the reverse of happiness."

harm principle—The view that authorities are justified in restricting some people's freedom to prevent harm to others.

harm reduction—A policy of focusing not on decreasing the number of users of drugs or the quantity of available drugs in society but on reducing the harm that arises from drugs or drug laws.

hasty generalization—The fallacy of drawing a conclusion about an entire group of people or things based on an undersized sample of the group.

homosexuality—Sexual relations between people of the same sex.

humanitarian intervention—The act of a state (or states) going to war to defend people of another state against the aggression of their own regime.

hypothetical imperative—An imperative that tells us what we should do if we have certain desires.

imperfect duty—A duty that has exceptions.

indicator words—Terms that often appear in arguments to signal the presence of a premise or conclusion, or to indicate that an argument is deductive or inductive.

indirect moral consideration—Moral consideration on account of a being's relationship to others.

inductive argument—An argument that is supposed to offer probable support to its conclusion.

instrumentally (or extrinsically) valuable—Valuable as a means to something else.

intrinsically valuable—Valuable in itself, for its own sake.

invalid argument—A deductive argument that does not offer logically conclusive support for the conclusion.

involuntary euthanasia—Euthanasia performed on a person against his or her wishes.

jus ad bellum—The justification for resorting to war; the justice of war.

jus in bello—The moral permissibility of acts in war; justice in war.

justice—The morality of persons getting what is fair or what is their due.

just war theory—The doctrine that war may be morally permissible under stipulated conditions.

Kant's theory—A theory asserting that the morally right action is the one done in accordance with the categorical imperative.

legal moralism—The doctrine that the government is justified in curbing people's freedom to force them to obey moral rules.

legalization—Making the production and sale of drugs legal—that is, making their sale and production no longer a punishable crime.

liberal view (of sexuality)—The idea that as long as basic moral standards are respected, any sexual activity engaged in by informed, consenting adults is permissible.

libertarian theory of justice—A doctrine emphasizing individual liberties and negative rights, and rejecting positive rights as a violation of personal freedom.

means-ends principle—The rule that we must always treat people (including ourselves) as ends in themselves, never merely as a means.

metaethics—The study of the meaning and logical structure of moral beliefs.

moderate view (of sexuality)—The idea that sex is permissible, whether in marriage or not, if the consenting partners have a serious emotional connection.

morality—Beliefs concerning right and wrong, good and bad; they can include judgments, rules, principles, and theories.

moral statement—A statement affirming that an action is right or wrong or that a person (or one's motive or character) is good or bad.

moral status (or moral considerability)—The property of being a suitable candidate for direct moral concern or respect.

moral theory—An explanation of what makes an action right or what makes a person or thing good.

natural law theory—A theory asserting that the morally right action is the one that follows the dictates of nature.

negative right—A person's right that obligates others not to interfere with that person's obtaining something.

noncombatant immunity—The status of a person who should not be intentionally attacked in war.

nonconsequentialist theory—A theory asserting that the rightness of an action does not depend on its consequences.

nonmoral statement—A statement that does not affirm that an action is right or wrong or that a person (or one's motive or character) is good or bad.

nonstate actors—Individuals or groups that are not sovereign states.

nonvoluntary euthanasia—Euthanasia performed on a person who is not competent to decide the issue and has left no instructions regarding end-of-life preferences. In such cases, family or physicians usually make the decision.

normative ethics—The study of the principles, rules, or theories that guide our actions and judgments.

objectivism—The view that some moral principles are valid for everyone.

pacifism—The view that war is never morally permissible.

passive euthanasia—Euthanasia performed by withholding or withdrawing measures necessary for sustaining life.

paternalism principle—The view that authorities are sometimes justified in limiting people's freedom to prevent them from harming themselves.

perfect duty—A duty that has no exceptions.

person—A being thought to have full moral rights.

physician-assisted suicide—The killing of a person by the person's own hand with the help of a physician.

pornography—Sexually explicit images or text meant to cause sexual excitement or arousal.

positive right—A person's right that obligates others to help that person obtain something.

premise—A supporting statement in an argument.

principle of utility—Bentham's "principle which approves or disapproves of every action whatsoever, according to the tendency which it appears to have to augment or diminish the happiness of the party whose interest is in question."

psychological egoism—The view that the motive for all our actions is self-interest.

punishment—The deliberate and authorized causing of pain or harm to someone thought to have broken a law.

quickening—The point in fetal development when the mother can feel the fetus moving. (It occurs at about sixteen to twenty weeks.)

realism (as applied to warfare)—The view that moral standards are not applicable to war, and that it instead must be judged on how well it serves state interests.

reproductive cloning—The genetic duplication of a fully developed adult animal or human.

retentionists—Those who wish to retain the death penalty.

retributive justice—Justice concerning fair punishment for wrongdoing.

retributivism—The view that offenders deserve to be punished, or "paid back," for their crimes and to be punished in proportion to the severity of their offenses.

right—A claim or entitlement to something; a moral demand that obligates others to honor it.

rule-egoism—The theory that to determine right action, you must see if an act falls under a rule that if consistently followed would maximize your self-interest.

rule-utilitarianism—The theory that the morally right action is the one covered by a rule that if generally followed would produce the most favorable balance of good over evil, everyone considered.

same-sex marriage—Marriage, in the full legal sense, of gay and lesbian couples.

slippery slope—The fallacy of using dubious premises to argue that doing a particular action will inevitably lead to other actions that will result in disaster, so you should not do that first action.

sound argument—A valid argument with true premises.

species egalitarian—One who believes that all living things have equal moral status.

speciesism—Discrimination against nonhuman animals just because of their species.

species nonegalitarian—One who believes that some living things have greater moral status than others.

statement—An assertion that something is or is not the case.

straw man—The fallacy of misrepresenting someone's claim or argument so it can be more easily refuted.

strong affirmative action—The use of policies and procedures to favor particular individuals because of their race, gender, or ethnic background.

strong argument—An inductive argument that does in fact provide probable support for its conclusion.

subjective relativism—The view that an action is morally right if one approves of it.

supererogatory actions—Conduct that is "above and beyond" duty; not required, but praiseworthy.

terrorism (*as defined in the chapter*)—Violence against noncombatants for political, religious, or ideological ends.

terrorism (*the definition preferred by the U.S. State Department*)—Premeditated, politically motivated violence perpetrated against noncombatant targets by subnational groups or clandestine agents, usually intended to influence an audience.

therapeutic abortion—An abortion performed to protect the life or health of the mother.

torture—The intentional inflicting of severe pain or suffering on people to punish or intimidate them or extract information from them.

utilitarianism—A theory asserting that the morally right action is the one that produces the most favorable balance of good over evil, everyone considered.

valid argument—A deductive argument that does in fact provide logically conclusive support for its conclusion.

viability—The stage of fetal development at which the fetus is able to survive outside the uterus.

virtue—A stable disposition to act and feel according to some ideal or model of excellence.

virtue ethics—A theory of morality that makes virtue the central concern.

voluntary euthanasia—Euthanasia performed on a person with his or her permission.

weak affirmative action—The use of policies and procedures to end discriminatory practices and ensure equal opportunity.

weak argument—An inductive argument that does not give probable support to the conclusion.

zoocentrism—The notion that both human and nonhuman animals have moral status.

FURTHER READING

Chapter 1. Ethics and the Examined Life

Anita L. Allen, *New Ethics: A Guided Tour of the Twenty-First-Century Moral Landscape* (New York: Miramax, 2004).

Aristotle, *Nicomachean Ethics,* Book 2, Parts 1 and 4.

Simon Blackburn, *Being Good: A Short Introduction to Ethics* (Oxford: Oxford University Press, 2002).

Donald M. Borchert and David Stewart, *Exploring Ethics* (New York: Macmillan, 1986).

Steven M. Cahn and Joram G. Haber, eds., *Twentieth Century Ethical Theory* (Englewood Cliffs, NJ: Prentice Hall, 1995).

William K. Frankena, *Ethics,* 2nd ed. (Englewood Cliffs, NJ: Prentice-Hall, 1973).

Bernard Gert, *Morality: Its Nature and Justification* (New York: Oxford University Press, 1998).

Brooke Noel Moore and Robert Michael Stewart, *Moral Philosophy: A Comprehensive Introduction* (Belmont, CA: Mayfield, 1994).

Dave Robinson and Chris Garrett, *Introducing Ethics,* ed. Richard Appignanesi (New York: Totem Books, 2005).

Peter Singer, ed., *A Companion to Ethics,* corr. ed. (Oxford: Blackwell, 1993).

Paul Taylor, *Principles of Ethics: An Introduction* (Encino, CA: Dickenson, 1975).

Jacques P. Thiroux, *Ethics: Theory and Practice,* 3rd ed. (New York: Macmillan, 1986).

Thomas F. Wall, *Thinking Critically about Moral Problems* (Belmont, CA: Wadsworth, 2003).

G. J. Warnock, *The Object of Morality* (London: Methuen, 1971).

Chapter 2. Subjectivism, Relativism, and Emotivism

A. J. Ayer, *Language, Truth and Logic* (1936; reprint, New York: Dover, 1952).

Brand Blanshard, "Emotivism," in *Reason and Goodness* (1961; reprint, New York: G. Allen and Unwin, 1978).

Donald M. Borchert and David Stewart, "Ethical Emotivism," in *Exploring Ethics* (New York: Macmillan, 1986).

Richard B. Brandt, chapter 11 of *Ethical Theory: The Problems of Normative and Critical Ethics* (Englewood Cliffs, NJ: Prentice-Hall, 1959).

Jean Bethke Elshtain, "Judge Not?" *First Things,* no. 46 (October 1994): 36–40.

Fred Feldman, chapter 11 of *Introductory Ethics* (Englewood Cliffs, NJ: Prentice-Hall, 1978).

Chris Gowans, "Moral Relativism," *The Stanford Encyclopedia of Philosophy* (Spring 2004 ed.), ed. Edward N. Zalta, http://plato.stanford.edu/archives/spr2004/entries/moral-relativism (1 March 2015).

Melville Herskovits, *Cultural Relativism: Perspectives in Cultural Pluralism,* ed. Frances Herskovits (New York: Random House, 1972).

J. L. Mackie, *Ethics: Inventing Right and Wrong* (Harmondsworth: Penguin, 1977).

Theodore Schick Jr. and Lewis Vaughn, chapter 5 of *Doing Philosophy: An Introduction through Thought Experiments,* 2nd ed. (Boston: McGraw-Hill, 2003).

Peter Singer, ed., chapters 38 and 39 of *A Companion to Ethics,* corr. ed. (Oxford: Blackwell, 1993).

Walter T. Stace, "Ethical Relativism," in *The Concept of Morals* (1937; reprint, New York: Macmillan, 1965).

Paul Taylor, chapter 2 of *Principles of Ethics: An Introduction* (Encino, CA: Dickenson, 1975).

Chapter 3. Evaluating Moral Arguments

Richard Feldman, *Reason and Argument,* 2nd ed. (Upper Saddle River, NJ: Prentice Hall, 1999).

Richard M. Fox and Joseph P. DeMarco, *Moral Reasoning: A Philosophic Approach to Applied Ethics,* 2nd ed. (Fort Worth: Harcourt College Publishers, 2001).

Brooke Noel Moore and Richard Parker, *Critical Thinking,* 7th ed. (Boston: McGraw-Hill, 2004).

Lewis Vaughn, *The Power of Critical Thinking: Effective Reasoning about Ordinary and Extraordinary Claims* (New York: Oxford University Press, 2005).

Chapter 4. The Power of Moral Theories

John D. Arras and Nancy K. Rhoden, "The Need for Ethical Theory," in *Ethical Issues in Modern Medicine,* 3rd ed. (Mountain View, CA: Mayfield, 1989).

Richard B. Brandt, *Ethical Theory: The Problems of Normative and Critical Ethics* (Englewood Cliffs, NJ: Prentice-Hall, 1959).

C. D. Broad, *Five Types of Ethical Theory* (1930; reprint, London: Routledge & Kegan Paul, 1956).

John Hospers, *Human Conduct: Problems of Ethics,* shorter ed. (New York: Harcourt Brace Jovanovich, 1972).

John Rawls, "Some Remarks about Moral Theory," in *A Theory of Justice,* rev. ed. (Cambridge, MA: Harvard University Press, Belknap Press, 1999).

Chapter 5. Consequentialist Theories: Maximize the Good

Jeremy Bentham, "Of the Principle of Utility," in *An Introduction to the Principles of Morals and Legislation* (1789).

C. D. Broad, "Egoism as a Theory of Human Motives," in *Twentieth Century Ethical Theory,* ed. Steven M. Cahn and Joram G. Haber (Englewood Cliffs, NJ: Prentice-Hall, 1995).

Steven M. Cahn and Joram G. Haber, eds., *Twentieth Century Ethical Theory* (Englewood Cliffs, NJ: Prentice-Hall, 1995).

Fred Feldman, "Act Utilitarianism: Pro and Con," in *Introductory Ethics* (Englewood Cliffs, NJ: Prentice-Hall, 1978).

William Frankena, "Utilitarianism, Justice, and Love," in *Ethics,* 2nd ed. (Englewood Cliffs, NJ: Prentice-Hall, 1973).

C. E. Harris, "The Ethics of Utilitarianism," in *Applying Moral Theories,* 3rd ed. (Belmont, CA: Wadsworth, 1997).

Kai Nielsen, "A Defense of Utilitarianism," *Ethics* 82 (1972): 113–24.

Robert Nozick, "The Experience Machine," in *Anarchy, State and Utopia* (New York: Basic Books, 1974).

Louis P. Pojman, ed., *The Moral Life: An Introductory Reader in Ethics and Literature,* 2nd ed. (New York: Oxford University Press, 2004).

J. J. C. Smart, "Extreme and Restricted Utilitarianism," in *Essays Metaphysical and Moral: Selected Philosophical Papers* (Oxford: Blackwell, 1987).

Paul W. Taylor, "Ethical Egoism," in *Principles of Ethics: An Introduction* (Encino, CA: Dickenson, 1975).

Bernard Williams, "A Critique of Utilitarianism," in *Utilitarianism: For and Against,* ed. J. J. C. Smart and Williams (Cambridge: Cambridge University Press, 1973).

Chapter 6. Nonconsequentialist Theories: Do Your Duty

Stephen Buckle, "Natural Law," in *A Companion to Ethics,* ed. Peter Singer, corr. ed. (Oxford: Blackwell, 1993).

John Finnis, *Natural Law and Natural Rights* (Oxford: Clarendon Press; New York: Oxford University Press, 1980).

C. E. Harris, chapters 6 and 8 of *Applying Moral Theories,* 3rd ed. (Belmont, CA: Wadsworth, 1997).

Mark Murphy, "The Natural Law Tradition in Ethics," *The Stanford Encyclopedia of Philosophy* (Winter 2002 ed.), ed. Edward N. Zalta, http://plato.stanford.edu/archives /win2002/entries/natural-law-ethics (1 March 2015).

Kai Nielsen, *Ethics without God* (London: Pemberton; Buffalo, NY: Prometheus, 1973).

Robert Nozick, *Anarchy, State and Utopia* (New York: Basic Books, 1974).

Onora O'Neill, "Kantian Ethics," in *A Companion to Ethics,* ed. Peter Singer, corr. ed. (Oxford: Blackwell, 1993).

Louis P. Pojman, "Natural Law," in *Ethics: Discovering Right and Wrong,* 4th ed. (Belmont, CA: Wadsworth, 2002).

James Rachels, chapter 9 of *The Elements of Moral Philosophy,* 4th ed. (Boston: McGraw-Hill, 2003).

Paul Taylor, chapter 5 of *Principles of Ethics: An Introduction* (Encino, CA: Dickenson, 1975).

Thomas Aquinas, *Summa Theologica,* in *Basic Writings of Saint Thomas Aquinas,* ed. and annotated Anton C. Pegis (New York: Random House, 1945).

Robert N. Van Wyk, chapters 4 and 6 of *Introduction to Ethics* (New York: St. Martin's, 1990).

Chapter 7. Virtue Ethics: Be a Good Person

G. E. M. Anscombe, "Modern Moral Philosophy," *Philosophy* 33, no. 124 (January 1958): 1–19.

Philippa Foot, "Virtues and Vices," in *Virtues and Vices and Other Essays in Moral Philosophy* (Berkeley: University of California Press, 1978).

William K. Frankena, "Ethics of Virtue," in *Ethics,* 2nd ed. (Englewood Cliffs, NJ: Prentice-Hall, 1973).

Rosalind Hursthouse, "Virtue Ethics," *The Stanford Encyclopedia of Philosophy* (Fall 2003 ed.), ed. Edward N. Zalta, http://plato.stanford/archives/fall2003/entries/ ethics-virtue (1 March 2015).

Alasdair MacIntyre, "The Nature of the Virtues," in *After Virtue: A Study in Moral Theory* (Notre Dame, IN: University of Notre Dame Press, 1984).

Greg Pence, "Virtue Theory," in *A Companion to Ethics,* ed. Peter Singer, corr. ed. (Oxford: Blackwell, 1993).

Chapter 8. Abortion

Daniel Callahan, "Abortion Decisions: Personal Morality," in *Abortion: Law, Choice and Morality* (New York: Macmillan, 1970).

Sidney Callahan, "A Case for Pro-Life Feminism," *Commonweal* 25 (April 1986): 232–38.

Jane English, "Abortion and the Concept of a Person," *Canadian Journal of Philosophy* 5, no. 2 (October 1975): 233–43.

Joel Feinberg, "Abortion," in *Matters of Life and Death,* ed. Tom Regan, 3rd ed. (New York: McGraw-Hill, 1993).

Ronald Munson, "Abortion," in *Intervention and Reflection: Basic Issues in Medical Ethics,* ed. Munson, 7th ed. (Belmont, CA: Wadsworth, 2004).

John T. Noonan Jr., "An Almost Absolute Value in History," in *The Morality of Abortion: Legal and Historical Perspectives,* ed. Noonan (Cambridge, MA: Harvard University Press, 1970).

Louis P. Pojman and Francis J. Beckwith, eds., *The Abortion Controversy: 25 Years After Roe v. Wade: A Reader,* 2nd ed. (Belmont, CA: Wadsworth, 1998).

Roe v. Wade, 410 U.S. 113, 113–67 (1973). Justice Harry Blackmun, Majority Opinion of the Court.

Michael Tooley, *Abortion and Infanticide* (Oxford: Clarendon Press; New York: Oxford University Press, 1983).

Chapter 9. Altering Genes and Cloning Humans

Dan W. Brock, "Genetic Engineering," in *A Companion to Applied Ethics,* ed. R. G. Frey and Christopher Heath Wellman (Oxford: Blackwell Publishing, 2003), 356–57, 361–67.

Justine Burley, ed., *The Genetic Revolution and Human Rights* (Oxford: Oxford University Press, 1999).

Ruth Chadwick, "Gene Therapy," in *A Companion to Bioethics,* ed. Helga Kuhse and Peter Singer (Oxford: Blackwell Publishing, 2001), 189–97.

Cold Spring Harbor Laboratory, *DNA from the Beginning: An Animated Primer of 75 Experiments That Made Modern Genetics,* 2002, http://www.dnaftb.org/ (1 March 2015).

Walter Glannon, *Genes and Future People: Philosophical Issues in Human Genetics* (Boulder, CO: Westview Press, 2001).

Jonathan Glover, *Choosing Children: The Ethical Dilemmas of Genetic Intervention* (Oxford: Oxford University Press, 2006).

National Bioethics Advisory Commission, *Cloning Human Beings,* June 1997, https://bioethicsarchive.georgetown.edu/nbac/pubs/cloning1/cloning.pdf (1 March 2015).

President's Council on Bioethics, *Human Cloning and Human Dignity: An Ethical Inquiry,* 2002, https://repository.library.georgetown.edu/bitstream/handle/10822/559368/pcbe_cloning_report.pdf?sequence=1&isAllowed=y (1 March 2015).

Laura Purdy, "Genetics and Reproductive Risk: Can Having Children Be Immoral?" in *Genetics Now,* ed. John L. Buckley (Washington, D.C.: University Press of America, 1978).

Chapter 10. Euthanasia and Physician-Assisted Suicide

Tom L. Beauchamp, ed., *Intending Death: The Ethics of Assisted Suicide and Euthanasia* (Englewood Cliffs, NJ: Prentice Hall, 1995).

R. B. Brandt, "The Morality and Rationality of Suicide," in *A Handbook for the Study of Suicide,* ed. Seymour Perlin (New York: Oxford University Press, 1975).

Lonnie R. Bristow, President of the American Medical Association, statement on physician-assisted suicide to the U.S. House of Representatives Committee on the Judiciary, Subcommittee on the Constitution, 104th Cong., 2nd sess., *Congressional Record* 142 (29 April 1996).

Dan W. Brock, "Medical Decisions at the End of Life," in *A Companion to Bioethics,* ed. Helga Kuhse and Peter Singer (1998; reprint, Malden, MA: Blackwell, 2001).

Daniel Callahan, "When Self-Determination Runs Amok," *Hastings Center Report* 22, no. 2 (March/April 1992): 52–55.

Philippa Foot, "Euthanasia," *Philosophy & Public Affairs* 6, no. 2 (1977): 85–112.

Walter Glannon, "Medical Decisions at the End of Life," in *Biomedical Ethics* (New York: Oxford University Press, 2005).

John Lachs, "When Abstract Moralizing Runs Amok," *Journal of Clinical Ethics* 5, no. 1 (1994): 10–13.

Ronald Munson, "Euthanasia and Physician-Assisted Suicide," in *Intervention and Reflection: Basic Issues in Medical Ethics,* ed. Munson, 7th ed. (Belmont, CA: Wadsworth, 2004).

Jeffrey Olen and Vincent Barry, "Euthanasia," in *Applying Ethics: A Text with Readings,* 6th ed. (Belmont, CA: Wadsworth, 1999).

The President's Commission for the Study of Ethical Problems in Medicine and Biomedical and Behavioral Research (Washington, DC: Government Printing Office, 1983).

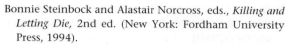

Bonnie Steinbock and Alastair Norcross, eds., *Killing and Letting Die,* 2nd ed. (New York: Fordham University Press, 1994).

Thomas D. Sullivan, "Active and Passive Euthanasia: An Impertinent Distinction?" *Human Life Review* 3, no. 3 (1977): 40–46.

Robert Young, "Voluntary Euthanasia," *The Stanford Encyclopedia of Philosophy* (Summer 2005 ed.), ed. Edward N. Zalta, http://plato.stanford.edu/archives /sum2005/entries/euthanasia-voluntary/ (1 March 2015).

Chapter 11. Capital Punishment

Hugo Adam Bedau, "Capital Punishment and Social Defense," in *Matters of Life and Death: New Introductory Essays in Moral Philosophy,* ed. Tom Regan, 2nd ed. (New York: Random House, 1986).

Hugo Adam Bedau and Paul Cassell, eds., *Debating the Death Penalty: Should America Have Capital Punishment? The Experts on Both Sides Make Their Best Case* (Oxford: Oxford University Press, 2004).

Gregg v. Georgia, 428 U.S. 153, 153–207 (1976). Justice Potter Stewart et al., Opinion of the Court.

Gregg v. Georgia, 428 U.S. 153, 231–41 (1976). Justice Thurgood Marshall, Dissenting Opinion.

Sidney Hook, "The Death Sentence," *New Leader,* 3 April 1961.

Alex Kozinski, "Tinkering with Death," *New Yorker,* 10 February 1997, 48–52.

Burton Leiser, "The Death Penalty Is Permissible," in *Liberty, Justice and Morals: Contemporary Value Conflicts,* 3rd ed. (New York: Macmillan, 1986).

John Stuart Mill, "Speech in Favor of Capital Punishment," 1868, http://ethics.sandiego.edu/books/Mill /Punishment/ (1 March 2015).

Stephen Nathanson, "An Eye for an Eye?" in *An Eye for an Eye? The Morality of Punishing by Death* (Totowa, NJ: Rowman and Littlefield, 1987).

Louis P. Pojman, "Why the Death Penalty Is Morally Permissible," in *Debating the Death Penalty: Should America Have Capital Punishment? The Experts on Both Sides Make Their Best Case,* eds. Hugo Bedau and Paul Cassell (Oxford: Oxford University Press, 2004).

William H. Shaw, "Punishment and the Criminal Justice System," in *Contemporary Ethics: Taking Account of Utilitarianism* (Malden, MA: Blackwell, 1999).

Ernest van den Haag, "On Deterrence and the Death Penalty," *Journal of Criminal Law, Criminology, and Police Science* 60, no. 2 (1969): 141–47.

Chapter 12. Drug Use, Harm, and Personal Liberty

Jonathan P. Caulkins, Angela Hawken, Beau Kilmer, and Mark Kleiman, *Marijuana Legalization: What Everyone Needs to Know* (New York: Oxford University Press, 2012).

Douglas Husak and Peter de Marneffe, *The Legalization of Drugs: For and Against,* (Cambridge: Cambridge University Press, 2005).

National Institute of Drug Abuse, "Medical Consequences of Drug Abuse," December 2012, http://www .drugabuse.gov/related-topics/medical-consequences -drug-abuse/mortality.

Pew Research Center, "America's New Drug Policy Landscape," April 2, 2014, http://www.people-press.org /2014/04/02/.

Substance Abuse and Mental Health Services Administration, Center for Behavioral Health Statistics and Quality, September 4, 2014, "The NSDUH Report: Substance Use and Mental Health Estimates from the 2013 National Survey on Drug Use and Health: Overview of Findings," Rockville, MD.

James Q. Wilson, "Against the Legalization of Drugs," *Commentary,* February 1990.

Chapter 13. Sexual Morality

Raymond A. Belliotti, "Sex," in *A Companion to Ethics,* ed. Peter Singer (Cambridge, MA: Blackwell, 1993).

Michael Levin, "Why Homosexuality Is Abnormal," *The Monist* 67 (April 1984): 251–83.

Roger Scruton, *Sexual Desire: A Moral Philosophy of the Erotic* (New York: Free Press, 1986).

Alan Soble, "Philosophy of Sexuality," in *The Internet Encyclopedia of Philosophy* (2006), http://www.iep.utm .edu/sexualit/ (1 March 2015).

Nancy Tuana and Laurie Shrage, "Sexuality," in *The Oxford Handbook of Practical Ethics,* ed. Hugh LaFollette (New York: Oxford University Press, 2003), 15–41.

Chapter 14. Same-Sex Marriage

Bruce Bawer, ed., *Beyond Queer: Challenging Gay Left Orthodoxy* (New York: Free Press, 1996).

John Corvino, ed., *Same Sex: Debating the Ethics, Science, and Culture of Homosexuality* (Lanham, MD: Rowman & Littlefield, 1997).

Richard D. Mohr, *The Little Book of Gay Rights* (Boston: Beacon Press, 1994).

Timothy F. Murphy, "Homosexuality and Nature: Happiness and the Law at Stake," *Journal of Applied Philosophy* 4, no. 2 (1987): 195–204.

Jonathan Rauch, "For Better or Worse? The Case for Gay (and Straight) Marriage," *The New Republic* (6 May 1996): 18–23.

Michael Ruse, *Homosexuality: A Philosophical Inquiry* (New York: Blackwell, 1988).

Congregation for the Doctrine of the Faith, "Considerations Regarding Proposals to Give Legal Recognition to Unions Between Homosexual Persons," June 2003.

Chapter 15. Environmental Ethics

Andrew Brennan and Yeuk-Sze Lo, "Environmental Ethics," *The Stanford Encyclopedia of Philosophy* (Summer 2002 ed.), ed. Edward N. Zalta, http://plato.stanford.edu/archives/sum2002/entries/ethics-environmental/ (1 March 2015).

J. Baird Callicott, "The Search for an Environmental Ethic," in *Matters of Life and Death: New Introductory Essays in Moral Philosophy,* ed. Tom Regan, 2nd ed. (New York: Random House, 1986).

Robert Elliot, "Environmental Ethics," in *A Companion to Ethics,* ed. Peter Singer, corr. ed. (Oxford: Blackwell, 1993).

Garrett Hardin, "The Tragedy of the Commons," *Science* 162 (13 December 1968): 1243–48.

Robert Heilbroner, "What Has Posterity Ever Done for Me?" *New York Times Magazine,* 19 January 1975, 14–15.

Aldo Leopold, "The Land Ethic," in *A Sand County Almanac: And Sketches Here and There* (1949; reprint, New York: Oxford University Press, 1981).

Arne Naess, "The Shallow and the Deep, Long-Range Ecological Movement," *Inquiry* 16 (Spring 1973): 95–100.

Holmes Rolston III, "Values in and Duties to the Natural World," in *Ecology, Economics, Ethics: The Broken Circle,* ed. F. Herbert Bormann and Stephen R. Kellert (New Haven: Yale University Press, 1991).

Albert Schweitzer, "Reverence for Life," in *Civilization and Ethics,* trans. John Naish (London: Black, 1923).

Christopher D. Stone, "Should Trees Have Standing? Toward Legal Rights for Natural Objects" in *Should Trees Have Standing? Toward Legal Rights for Natural Objects* (Los Altos, CA: William Kaufman, 1974).

Lynn White Jr., "The Historical Roots of Our Ecological Crisis," *Science* 155 (March 1967): 1203–7.

Chapter 16. Animal Rights

Carl Cohen, "The Case for the Use of Animals in Biomedical Research," *New England Journal of Medicine* 315 (October 1986): 865–70.

David DeGrazia, *Animal Rights: A Very Short Introduction* (Oxford: Oxford University Press, 2002).

R. G. Frey, "Animals," in *The Oxford Handbook of Practical Ethics,* ed. Hugh LaFollette (New York: Oxford University Press, 2003).

———, *Interests and Rights: The Case against Animals* (Oxford: Clarendon; New York: Oxford University Press, 1980).

Lori Gruen, "Animals," in *A Companion to Ethics,* ed. Peter Singer, corr. ed. (Oxford: Blackwell, 1993).

Mary Midgley, *Animals and Why They Matter* (Harmondsworth: Penguin, 1983).

James Rachels, *Created from Animals: The Moral Implications of Darwinism* (Oxford: Oxford University Press, 1990).

Tom Regan, *The Case for Animal Rights* (Berkeley: University of California Press, 1983).

Tom Regan and Peter Singer, eds. *Animal Rights and Human Obligations,* 2nd ed. (Englewood Cliffs, NJ: Prentice Hall, 1989).

Peter Singer, *Animal Liberation,* 2nd ed. (New York: New York Review of Books, 1990).

———, "Ethics beyond Species and beyond Instincts," in *Animal Rights: Current Debates and New Directions,* ed. Cass R. Sunstein and Martha C. Nussbaum (Oxford: Oxford University Press, 2004).

Bonnie Steinbock, "Speciesism and the Idea of Equality," *Philosophy* 53, no. 204 (April 1978): 247–56.

Cass R. Sunstein and Martha C. Nussbaum, eds., *Animal Rights: Current Debates and New Directions* (Oxford: Oxford University Press, 2004).

Mary Anne Warren, "The Rights of the Nonhuman World," in *Environmental Philosophy: A Collection of Readings,* eds. Robert Elliot and Arran Gare (University Park: Pennsylvania State University Press, 1983).

Chapter 17. Political Violence: War, Terrorism, and Torture

G. E. M. Anscombe, "War and Murder," in *Nuclear Weapons: A Catholic Response,* ed. Walter Stein (New York: Sheed and Ward, 1961).

Thomas Aquinas, *Summa Theologica,* Second Part of the Second Part, Questions 40, 64, and 69.

Joseph M. Boyle Jr., "Just War Doctrine and the Military Response to Terrorism," *Journal of Political Philosophy* 11, no. 2 (2003): 153–70.

R. G. Frey and Christopher W. Morris, eds., *Violence, Terrorism, and Justice* (Cambridge: Cambridge University Press, 1991).

Robert Fullinwider, "Terrorism, Innocence, and War," in *War After September 11,* ed. Verna V. Gehring (Lanham, MD: Rowman and Littlefield, 2003).

David Luban, "The War on Terrorism and the End of Human Rights," *Philosophy & Public Policy Quarterly* 22, no. 3 (Summer 2002): 9–14.

Larry May, Eric Rovie, and Steve Viner, eds., *The Morality of War: Classical and Contemporary Readings* (Upper Saddle River, NJ: Pearson/Prentice Hall, 2006).

Thomas Nagel, "War and Massacre," *Philosophy & Public Affairs* 1, no. 2 (Winter 1972): 123–43.

Jan Narveson, "Pacifism: A Philosophical Analysis," *Ethics* 75, no. 4 (1965): 259–71.

Brian Orend, "War," *The Stanford Encyclopedia of Philosophy* (Winter 2005 ed.), ed. Edward N. Zalta, http://plato.stanford.edu/archives/win2005/entries /war/ (1 March 2015).

Louis P. Pojman, "The Moral Response to Terrorism and the Cosmopolitan Imperative," in *Terrorism and International Justice*, ed. James P. Sterba (New York: Oxford University Press, 2003).

Henry Shue, "War," in *The Oxford Handbook of Practical Ethics*, ed. Hugh LaFollette (Oxford: Oxford University Press, 2003).

Charles Townshend, *Terrorism: A Very Short Introduction* (Oxford: Oxford University Press, 2002).

Andrew Valls, "Can Terrorism Be Justified?" in *Ethics in International Affairs*, ed. Valls (Lanham, MD: Rowman and Littlefield, 2000).

Michael Walzer, *Just and Unjust Wars: A Moral Argument with Historical Illustrations*, 2nd ed. (New York: Basic Books, 1992).

John Howard Yoder, *When War Is Unjust: Being Honest in Just-War Thinking*, 2nd ed. (Maryknoll, NY: Orbis Books, 1996).

Chapter 18. Equality and Affirmative Action

Bernard R. Boxill, "Equality, Discrimination and Preferential Treatment," in *A Companion to Ethics*, ed. Peter Singer (Oxford: Basil Blackwell, 1993), 333–342.

Steven M. Cahn, "Two Concepts of Affirmative Action," *Academe*, 83 (1997).

Carl Cohen and James P. Sterba, *Affirmative Action and Racial Preference* (New York: Oxford University Press, 2003).

Stephen Carter, *Reflections of an Affirmative Action Baby* (New York: Basic Books, 1993).

Ronald Dworkin, "Bakke's Case: Are Quotas Unfair?" in *A Matter of Principle* (Cambridge: Harvard University Press, 1985).

Walter Feinberg, "Affirmative Action," in *The Oxford Handbook of Practical Ethics*, ed. Hugh LaFollette (Oxford: Oxford University Press, 2003), 272–299.

Robert Fullinwider, "Affirmative Action," *The Stanford Encyclopedia of Philosophy* (Spring 2005 ed.), Edward N. Zalta, ed., http://plato.stanford.edu/archives/spr2005 /entries/affirmative-action/

Ira Katznelson, *When Affirmative Action Was White* (New York: Norton, 2005).

Albert Mosley, "The Case for Affirmative Action," in *Affirmative Action: Social Justice or Unfair Preference?* (New York: Rowman & Littlefield, 1997).

Justice Lewis Powell, Majority opinion in *Regents of the University of California v. Bakke* (1978).

Antonin Scalia, "The Disease as a Cure," *Washington University Law Quarterly*, no. 1, 1979.

Richard Wasserstrom, "A Defense of Programs of Preferential Treatment," *Phi Kappa Phi Journal*, LVIII (Winter 1978).

Chapter 19. Global Economic Justice

William Aiken and Hugh LaFollette, eds. *World Hunger and Morality,* 2nd ed. (Englewood Cliffs, NJ: Prentice-Hall, 1996).

Lester R. Brown, *Tough Choices: Facing the Challenge of Food Scarcity* (New York: Norton, 1996).

Joel E. Cohen, *How Many People Can the Earth Support?* (New York: Norton, 1995).

Nigel Dower, "World Poverty," in *A Companion to Ethics*, ed. Peter Singer (Cambridge, MA: Blackwell, 1993).

Steven Luper-Foy, ed., *Problems of International Justice* (Boulder, CO: Westview Press, 1988).

William W. Murdoch and Allan Oaten, "Population and Food: Metaphors and the Reality," *BioScience* 25 (1975): 561–67.

Onora O'Neill, *Faces of Hunger: An Essay on Poverty, Justice, and Development* (London: Allen & Unwin, 1986).

Thomas Pogge, *World Poverty and Human Rights: Cosmopolitan Responsibilities and Reforms,* 2nd ed. (Cambridge: Polity Press, 2008).

Louis P. Pojman, "World Hunger and Population," in *Life and Death: Grappling with the Moral Dilemmas of Our Time*, rev. 2nd ed. (Belmont, CA: Wadsworth, 2000).

Michael J. Sandel, ed., *Justice: A Reader* (New York: Oxford University Press, 2007).

Robert N. Van Wyk, "Perspectives on World Hunger and the Extent of Our Positive Duties," *Public Affairs Quarterly* 2, no. 2 (April 1988): 75–90.

ANSWERS TO ARGUMENT EXERCISES
(CHAPTER 3)

1. If John works out at the gym daily, he will be healthier. He is working out at the gym daily. So he will be healthier.

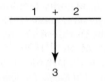

3. Ghosts do not exist. There is no reliable evidence showing that any disembodied persons exist anywhere.

5. The mayor is soft on crime. He cut back on misdemeanor enforcement and told the police department to be more lenient on traffic violators.

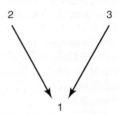

7. The president is either dishonest or incompetent. He's not incompetent, though, because he's an expert at getting self-serving legislation through Congress. I guess he's just dishonest.

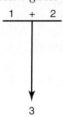

9. Can people without strong religious beliefs be moral? Countless people have been nonbelievers or nontheists and still behaved according to lofty moral principles. For example: the Buddhists of Asia and the Confucianists of China. Consider also the great secular philosophers from the ancient Greeks to the likes of David Hume and Bertrand Russell. So it's not true that those without strong religious beliefs cannot be moral.

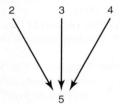

11. We shouldn't pay the lawnmower guy so much money because he never completes the work, and he will probably just gamble the money away because he has no self-control.

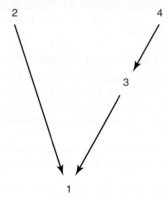

INDEX